# Clinical Drug Therapy

**FOURTH EDITION**

## Therapy

*Rationales for*
*Nursing Practice*

# Clinical Drug

**FOURTH EDITION**

# Therapy

## *Rationales for Nursing Practice*

**Anne Collins Abrams, R.N., M.S.N.**

*Associate Professor*
*Department of Baccalaureate Nursing*
*College of Allied Health and Nursing*
*Eastern Kentucky University*
*Richmond, Kentucky*


**CONSULTANT**

**Tracey L. Goldsmith, Pharm. D.**

*Clinical Manager*
*Department of Pharmacy Services*
*Hermann Hospital*
*Houston, Texas*

**J. B. Lippincott Company**
*Philadelphia*

**Sponsoring Editor:** *Margaret Belcher*
**Coordinating Editorial Assistant:** *Kimberly Oaks*
**Project Editor:** *Susan Deitch/Tom Gibbons*
**Indexer:** *Helene Taylor*
**Design Coordinator:** *Doug Smock*
**Interior Designer:** *Holly Reid McLaughlin*
**Cover Designer:** *Anne Bullen*
**Production Manager:** *Helen Ewan*
**Production Coordinator:** *Robert Randall*
**Compositor:** *Circle Graphics*
**Printer/Binder:** *Courier Book Company/Kendallville*
**Cover Printer:** *New England Book Components, Inc.*

Fourth Edition

6  5  4  3  2  1

**Library of Congress Cataloging-in-Publication Data**

Abrams, Anne Collins.
    Clinical drug therapy : rationales for nursing practice / Anne
Collins Abrams ; consultant, Tracey L. Goldsmith. — 4th ed.
        p.    cm.
    Includes bibliographical references and index.
    ISBN 0-397-55106-1
    1. Chemotherapy.    2. Nursing.    I. Goldsmith, Tracey L.
II. Title.
    [DNLM: 1. Drugs—nurses' instruction.    2. Drug Therapy—nurses'
instruction.    3. Nursing Process.    QV 55 A161c 1995]
    RM262.A27   1995
    615.5'8—dc20
DNLM/DLC
for Library of Congress                                          94-15844
                                                                     CIP

Any procedure or practice described in this book should be applied by the health-
care practitioner under appropriate supervision in accordance with professional
standards of care used with regard to the unique circumstances that apply in each
practice situation. Care has been taken to confirm the accuracy of information
presented and to describe generally accepted practices. However, the author, editors,
and publisher cannot accept any responsibility for errors or omissions or for any
consequences from application of the information in this book and make
no warranty express or implied, with respect to the contents of the book.

Every effort has been made to ensure drug selections and dosages are in
accordance with current recommendations and practice. Because of ongoing
research, changes in government regulations and the constant flow of information
on drug therapy, reactions and interactions, the reader is cautioned to check the
package insert for each drug for indications, dosages, warnings and precautions,
particularly if the drug is new or infrequently used.

## Dedication

To nursing students and practitioners, who invest time and effort in learning, thinking about, and applying drug knowledge in clinical practice.

To nursing faculty, who promote, encourage, and facilitate students' learning, thinking about, and applying drug knowledge in clinical practice.

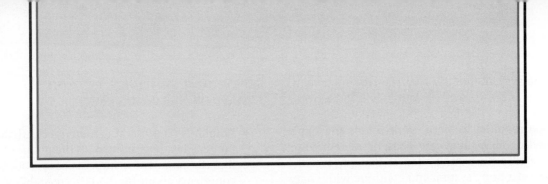

# Preface

## PURPOSE

The overall purpose of *Clinical Drug Therapy* is to promote rational, safe, and effective drug therapy. There are few areas of nursing with so much potential for help or harm to clients as the area of drug therapy, and a sound knowledge base is required to fulfill the nursing role. Thus, content and format are designed to present essential information clearly, facilitate attainment of an adequate knowledge base, and promote continued learning about drug therapy.

## BELIEFS AND ASSUMPTIONS

The author strongly believes that safe and effective drug therapy requires knowledge about the drug and the person receiving it. Such knowledge allows the nurse to anticipate therapeutic and adverse effects of drug administration and plan nursing care accordingly. Other beliefs and assumptions, which are considered infrequently in other nursing pharmacology texts, include the following:

- Nurses should prevent the need for drug therapy, when possible, through efforts to promote health and prevent symptoms and disorders that often are treated with drug therapy. These interventions are especially important now, with the increased emphasis on personal responsibility for health maintenance and health-care reform. Moreover, nurses are well qualified to counsel clients about healthful behaviors.
- When drug therapy is required, therapeutic effects can be enhanced by nursing interventions. For example, the simple intervention of ensuring adequate fluid intake promotes dissolution and absorption of oral tablets and capsules.
- Adverse drug effects may be prevented or minimized by nursing interventions. With an adequate knowledge base about the adverse effects associated with particular drugs and client characteristics that may increase risks of experiencing adverse effects, nurses may prevent adverse reactions or recognize them early enough to minimize their severity.
- Effective, non–drug-related interventions are generally safer than drug therapy. Thus, such interventions should be used instead of or in conjunction with drug therapy. When used with drug therapy, such interventions may promote lower drug dosage, less frequent administration, and fewer adverse effects.
- All drugs may cause adverse effects, including signs and symptoms of essentially any disease process. Consequently, nurses and other health-care providers need to actively assess clients for possible adverse effects and maintain a high index of suspicion that symptoms, especially new ones, may be drug induced.
- Nursing responsibility includes accurate administration of drugs, observation of client responses, and teaching clients about drug therapy.

## ORGANIZATIONAL FRAMEWORK

Content is organized into 11 sections, primarily by therapeutic drug groups and their effects on particular body systems. The main advantages of this approach are to reduce a massive amount of information to a more manageable size and to provide a foundation for learning about new drugs. The first section provides the basic information required to learn, understand, and apply drug knowledge in patient care. Most of the remaining sections begin with a brief chapter that reviews the physiology of a body system and continue with chapters that discuss drug groups used to treat disorders of that body system. In addition, separate sections discuss nutritional products, drugs used to treat infections, and drugs used to treat neoplastic, ophthalmic, and dermatologic disorders.

Within the text there are 10 chapters that are designed to provide background information and to facilitate understanding of content contained in the other chapters. These consist of the three introductory chapters and the seven physiology review chapters. The introductory chapters include a variety of topics such as drug names and sources, drug laws and standards, the receptor theory of drug action, and drug effects on body tissues (Chap. 1); dosage forms and routes and methods of accurate drug administration (Chap. 2); and guidelines for using the nursing process in relation to drug therapy (Chap. 3). The physiology chapters review characteristics basic to understanding drug effects on the central nervous (CNS), autonomic nervous, endocrine, immune, respiratory, cardiovascular, and digestive systems.

The heart of the text is the chapters that emphasize therapeutic classes of drugs and the prototypical or commonly used individual drugs within those classes. This chapter content includes a description of a condition for which a drug group is used; a general description of a drug group, including mechanism(s) of action, indications for use, and contraindications; and monographs or tables of individual drugs with recommended dosages and routes of administration.

Additional, clinically relevant information is then presented under three headings: Nursing Process, Principles of Therapy, and Nursing Actions. Nursing Process content emphasizes the importance of the nursing process in drug therapy, including assessment of the client's condition in relation to the drug group, nursing diagnoses, expected outcomes in terms of client characteristics, interventions and teaching indicated, and evaluation of the client's progress toward expected outcomes. Client teaching is differentiated from other interventions to emphasize its importance. Principles of Therapy include client-related and drug-related factors that influence choices of drugs, dosages, and routes of administration. Once a drug has been ordered, Nursing Actions state specific nursing responsibilities within the following categories: 1) administer accurately; 2) observe for therapeutic effects; 3) observe for adverse effects; 4) observe for drug interactions; and 5) teach clients.

## IMPORTANT FEATURES RETAINED FROM THE PREVIOUS EDITIONS

- Emphasis on presenting material clearly and comprehensibly. Beginning with the publication of the first edition in 1983, students have made favorable comments about the book's ''readability.''
- An organizational framework that allows the book to be used effectively as a textbook and as a reference. As a textbook, students can read chapters in their entirety to learn the characteristics of major drug classes, their prototypical drugs or commonly used representatives, their uses and effects in prevention or treatment of disease processes, and their implications for nursing practice. As a reference book, students can readily review selected topics for clinical laboratory practice or clinical nursing courses. Specific features that facilitate such uses include a consistent format and frequent headings that allow the reader to identify topics at a glance. In addition, *Clinical Drug Therapy* is indexed extensively by generic and trade names of drugs, nursing process, and other topics to provide rapid access to desired information.
- Emphasis on FDA-approved therapeutic drugs used to treat common disorders that are likely to be encountered in clinical nursing practice.
- Principles of therapy and guidelines for individualizing drug therapy in specific populations, particularly children and elderly adults. General principles about drug use in children and older adults are included in Chapter 3, whereas specific principles are included in most chapters throughout the book.
- Emphasis on nursing process before, during, and after drug therapy. A unique feature remains the inclusion of rationales for nursing actions, the purpose of which is to provide a strong knowledge base and scientific foundation.
- Emphasis on client teaching, the purpose of which is to promote active and knowledgeable client participation in drug therapy regimens.

## IMPORTANT FEATURES OF THE FOURTH EDITION

- **Updated drug information**. Most drug-related chapters have been revised extensively to reflect newer drugs and current use of older drugs. For example, approximately 100 new drugs have been added, and indications for use of several older drugs have been expanded (*e.g.*, angiotensin-converting enzyme inhibitors, beta-blockers, and calcium channel-blockers). In addition, several discontinued (by manufacturers), obsolete, or rarely used drugs have been deleted.

- **A new section and three new chapters related to drugs affecting the immune system.** These chapters include physiology of the immune system with a detailed description of immune cells and intercellular communication via cytokines and other chemical mediators. The chapter on immunostimulants provides an overview of one of the most exciting frontiers in treatment of human disease. The chapter on immunosuppressants describes drugs commonly used in organ and tissue transplants.
- **Expanded physiology content.** Cellular physiology is added in Chapter 1 because all body functions and disease processes and most drug actions occur at the cellular level. Neurophysiology is discussed more extensively in Chapter 4 to reflect increased knowledge of neurotransmitters and their roles in CNS functions and disorders. The actions of hormones at the cellular level are described in Chapter 22. The hormones are thought to act as "first messengers," whereas calcium, cyclic adenosine monophosphate, and possibly other intracellular substances act as "second messengers" to regulate cellular functions.
- **New illustrations**, including cellular structures and the receptor theory of drug action (Chap. 1) and neurotransmission (Chap. 4).
- **New tables**, including chemical mediators (Chap. 1), neurotransmitters (Chap. 4), cytokines (Chap. 45), immunostimulants (Chap. 47), and immunosuppressants (Chap. 48).
- **Appendices** related to Canadian drug names, Canadian drug laws and standards, the International System of Units (SI units), and selected miscellaneous drugs.
- **Additional new features** include
  - biotechnology (recombinant DNA or gene-splicing techniques) as an increasingly important source of drugs (Chap. 1)
  - gender and ethnic differences in responses to drug therapy (Chap. 1)
  - FDA drug approval processes (Chap. 1)
  - review questions at the end of each chapter.

## ANCILLARY TEACHING–LEARNING AIDS

Nursing students, like others, are expected to develop skills in critical thinking, information processing, decision making, collaboration, and problem solving. How can a teacher assist the student to develop these skills in relation to pharmacology? The goal of the ancillary package is to assist both student and teacher in this development. The following beliefs, concepts, and principles guided preparation of the materials.

- **Learning** is an active process of becoming informed or gaining knowledge through study and/or experience. Learning requires thinking about the material to be learned and manipulating it in ways to make the material meaningful to oneself. Thinking is a cognitive skill characterized by formulating ideas and considering them in relation to previous knowledge and experience. Just like psychomotor skills, cognitive skills can be enhanced by practice. Specific techniques include silent review and thinking about information; writing notes about text or lecture material; paraphrasing, summarizing, or self-questioning (mentally, verbally, or in writing); completing written worksheets, learning exercises and projects; and verbally questioning others or discussing the material with other students or faculty.
- **Teaching** is promoting learning. Specific techniques include providing information or knowledge; providing or assisting the student with finding sources of information; giving instructions; varying teaching strategies to accommodate different learning styles; providing opportunities to work independently and with others; providing examples that relate the material being studied to actual or anticipated "real-life" experiences; providing experience and practice in solving problems; and providing experience and practice in developing critical thinking skills.
- **Critical thinking** is careful, thoughtful, reasoned judgment. It is differentiated from personal opinion and superficial memorization of facts by the ability to obtain and use an appropriate quantity and quality of data for a given situation. Critical thinkers question assumptions, routines, and rituals, reconsider "known facts" when new information becomes available, and develop new "rules" when old ones fail or are unavailable.

**The Student Study Guide** aims to engage the student's interest and active participation by providing a variety of learning exercises and opportunities to practice cognitive skills as described above. Worksheets related to each chapter of the text (*e.g.*, matching and completion exercises; crossword puzzles) promote initial learning and review of terms, concepts, principles, and characteristics and uses of major drug groups. The worksheets can be completed independently or assigned and removed for review by the instructor. Clinical scenarios or case studies promote appropriate data gathering, critical analysis of both drug-related and client-related data, and application of the data in patient care. Review questions help students check their level of comprehension on chapter content.

**The Instructor's Manual** and test bank has two main

purposes: One is to facilitate use of the text in designing and implementing courses of study, whether in separate pharmacology courses or in nursing courses with integrated pharmacology. The second is to assist the instructor in evaluating students' knowledge of drug information and their ability to apply that information in client-care situations. To fulfill these purposes, learning objectives, major chapter elements, classroom and clinical teaching strategies, and test questions are stated for each chapter of the text. The multiple choice test items follow the format of NCLEX, and several transparency masters are provided. From these materials, each instructor can choose those relevant to his or her circumstances.

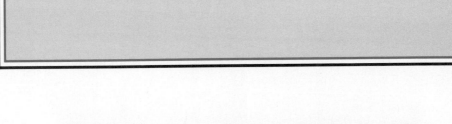

# Acknowledgments

Sincere appreciation is expressed to the following people who assisted in the preparation of this book and its ancillaries:

Tracey Goldsmith, Pharm. D., who reviewed all chapters and made helpful suggestions. This is the third edition for which Tracey has served as consultant, and her continuing efforts are acknowledged with gratitude.

Gail Ropelewski-Ryan, R.N., M.S.N., who coauthored the Student Study Guide and Instructor's Manual with Test Bank for the text.

Margaret Belcher, Senior Nursing Editor, and Susan Deitch, Project Editor, at J. B. Lippincott Company.

The following text reviewers, whose skillful directives strengthened the new chapters and appendices:

**Leonard V. Crowley,** M.D.

    Clinical Assistant Professor
    Department of Laboratory Medicine and Pathology
    Department of Family Practice and Community Health
    University of Minnesota
    College of Medicine
    Minneapolis, MN

**Tracey L. Goldsmith,** Pharm.D.

    Clinical Manager
    Department of Pharmacy Services
    Hermann Hospital
    Houston, TX

**Patricia F. Jassak,** M.S., R.N., O.C.N.

    Oncology Clinical Nurse Specialist
    Loyola University Medical Center
    Maywood, IL

**Barbara D. Kinsman,** R.N., M.S.N.

    Assistant Professor Nurse Education
    Corning Community College
    Corning, NY

**Judith Miller Klinefelter,** D.Ed., R.N., C.S.

    Assistant Professor of Nursing
    School of Nursing
    The Pennsylvania State University
    Hershey Medical Center
    Hershey, PA

**Kathryn A. Meier,** R.N.C., M.S.

    Nursing Instructor—High Risk Perinatal Nursing
    Lower Columbia College
    Longview, WA

**Harry E. Peery,** M.S., R.N.

    Lecturer, Departments of Physiology and Pharmacology
    University of Toronto, Faculty of Medicine
    Toronto, Ontario, Canada

# Contents

## SECTION I
## Introduction to Drug Therapy

### CHAPTER 1
### Introduction to Pharmacology                     3

Sources of Drugs   3
Drug Nomenclature   3
Sources of Drug Information   4
Federal Drug Laws and Standards   4
Cellular Physiology   6
Cellular Injury and Response to Injury   8
Mechanisms of Drug Movement   10
Pharmacokinetics   10
Pharmacodynamics   12
Variables That Affect Drug Actions   13
Adverse Effects of Drugs   17
Tolerance and Cross-tolerance   18

### CHAPTER 2
### Administering Medications                        20

Medication Systems   21
Medication Orders   21
Drug Preparations and Dosage Forms   22
Calculating Drug Dosages   22
Routes of Administration   24

### CHAPTER 3
### Nursing Process in Drug Therapy                  33

Using the Prototype Approach to Study Pharmacology   33
Legal Responsibilities of the Nurse   34
General Principles of Drug Therapy   37

## SECTION II
## Drugs Affecting the
## Central Nervous System

### CHAPTER 4
### Physiology of the Central Nervous System   47

Characteristics and Functions of the CNS   47
Classification of CNS Drugs   51

### CHAPTER 5
### Narcotic Analgesics
### and Narcotic Antagonists                         53

Pain   53
Description of Narcotic Analgesics   53
Classifications and Individual Drugs   54
Agonists-Antagonists   57
Principles of Therapy   59

### CHAPTER 6
### Analgesic–Antipyretic–Anti-inflammatory
### and Related Drugs                                66

Description   66
Prostaglandins   66
Mechanism of Action   67
Indications for Use   68
Contraindications for Use   68
Individual Drugs   68
Principles of Therapy   74

## CHAPTER 7

### Sedative-Hypnotics   81

Description  81
Sleep  81
Sedative-Hypnotic Drugs  81
Mechanism of Action  84
Indications for Use  84
Contraindications for Use  84
Principles of Therapy  85

## CHAPTER 8

### Antianxiety Drugs   89

Anxiety  89
Benzodiazepines  89
Individual Antianxiety Drugs  90
Principles of Therapy  93

## CHAPTER 9

### Antipsychotic Drugs   99

Psychosis  99
Antipsychotic Drugs  100
Individual Antipsychotic Drugs  100
Principles of Therapy  105

## CHAPTER 10

### Antidepressants   113

Depression  113
Antidepressant Drugs  116
Individual Antidepressants  116
Principles of Therapy  118

## CHAPTER 11

### Anticonvulsants   125

Seizure Disorders  125
Anticonvulsant Drugs  126
Individual Anticonvulsant Drugs  126
Principles of Therapy  130

## CHAPTER 12

### Antiparkinson Drugs   136

Parkinson's Disease  136
Antiparkinson Drugs  136
Individual Antiparkinson Drugs  137
Principles of Therapy  140

## CHAPTER 13

### Skeletal Muscle Relaxants   145

Skeletal Muscle Relaxants  145
Principles of Therapy  147

## CHAPTER 14

### Anesthetics   150

General Anesthesia  150
Regional Anesthesia  150
Adjuncts to Anesthesia  151

Individual Anesthetic Agents  152
Principles of Therapy  155

## CHAPTER 15

### Alcohol and Other Drug Abuse   163

Abuse and Dependence  163
Types of Drug Dependence  164
Selected Individual Drugs of Abuse  166
Principles of Therapy  171

## CHAPTER 16

### Central Nervous System Stimulants   176

Uses  176
Types of Stimulants  176
Central Nervous System Stimulants  177
Individual CNS Stimulants  177
Principles of Therapy  178

# SECTION III
# Drugs Affecting the Autonomic Nervous System

## CHAPTER 17

### Physiology of the Autonomic Nervous System   183

The Autonomic Nervous System  183
Characteristics of Autonomic Drugs  185

## CHAPTER 18

### Adrenergic Drugs   186

Description and Uses  186
Individual Adrenergic Drugs  187
Principles of Therapy  190

## CHAPTER 19

### Antiadrenergic Drugs   196

Description  196
Individual Antiadrenergic Drugs  198
Principles of Therapy  201

## CHAPTER 20

### Cholinergic Drugs   207

Description  207
Individual Cholinergic Drugs  208
Principles of Therapy  209

## CHAPTER 21

### Anticholinergic Drugs   213

Description  213
Individual Anticholinergic Drugs  215
Principles of Therapy  217

# SECTION IV
## Drugs Affecting the Endocrine System

### CHAPTER 22
**Physiology of the Endocrine System** 225

The Endocrine System 225
Endocrine System–Nervous System Interactions 225
General Characteristics of Hormones 226
General Characteristics of Hormonal Drugs 227

### CHAPTER 23
**Hypothalamic and Pituitary Hormones** 228

Description 228
Therapeutic Limitations 229
Individual Hormonal Agents 230
Principles of Therapy 232

### CHAPTER 24
**Corticosteroids** 236

Endogenous Corticosteroids 236
Exogenous Corticosteroids (Glucocorticoids) 239
Principles of Therapy 245

### CHAPTER 25
**Thyroid and Antithyroid Drugs** 253

Description and Uses 253
Thyroid Disorders 254
Individual Drugs 256
Principles of Therapy 259

### CHAPTER 26
**Hormones that Regulate Calcium and Phosphorus Metabolism** 265

Description 265
Hypocalcemia 268
Principles of Therapy: Drugs Used in Hypocalcemia 269
Hypercalcemia 272
Principles of Therapy: Drugs Used in Hypercalcemia 274

### CHAPTER 27
**Antidiabetic Drugs** 278

Endogenous Insulin 278
Diabetes Mellitus 279
Hypoglycemic Drugs 282
Principles of Therapy 287

### CHAPTER 28
**Estrogens, Progestins, and Oral Contraceptives** 297

Estrogens 297
Progesterone 298
Estrogens and Progestins Used as Drugs 298

Individual Estrogens, Progestins, and Oral Contraceptives 300
Principles of Therapy 302

### CHAPTER 29
**Androgens and Anabolic Steroids** 309

Androgens 309
Anabolic Steroids 309
Testosterone 309
Abuse of Androgenic and Anabolic Steroid Drugs 310
Characteristics of Androgenic and Anabolic Steroid Drugs 311
Principles of Therapy 313

# SECTION V
## Nutrients, Fluids, and Electrolytes

### CHAPTER 30
**Nutritional Products, Anorexiants, and Digestants** 319

Nutritional Products 319
Anorexiants and Digestants 319
Individual Nutritional Products for Oral or Tube Feeding 322
Intravenous Fluids 324
Pancreatic Enzymes 325
Principles of Therapy 326

### CHAPTER 31
**Vitamins** 333

Description and Uses 333
Principles of Therapy 341

### CHAPTER 32
**Minerals and Electrolytes** 346

Description and Uses 346
Individual Agents Used in Mineral-Electrolyte and Acid-Base Imbalances 348
Principles of Therapy 357

# SECTION VI
## Drugs Used to Treat Infections

### CHAPTER 33
**General Characteristics of Antimicrobial Drugs** 369

Host Defense Mechanisms 369
Microorganisms and Infections 369
Characteristics of Anti-infective Drugs 371
Principles of Therapy 374

**CHAPTER 34**

Penicillins                                                            380

Subgroups and Individual Penicillins   381
Principles of Therapy   384

**CHAPTER 35**

Cephalosporins                                                   388

Individual Cephalosporins   389
Principles of Therapy   389

**CHAPTER 36**

Aminoglycosides                                               396

Individual Aminoglycosides   397
Principles of Therapy   399

**CHAPTER 37**

Tetracyclines                                                     402

Principles of Therapy   404

**CHAPTER 38**

Macrolides                                                         407

Individual Macrolides   408
Principles of Therapy   408

**CHAPTER 39**

Miscellaneous Anti-infectives                           411

Beta-lactams   411
Quinolones   411
Polymyxins   412
Principles of Therapy   414

**CHAPTER 40**

Sulfonamides and Urinary Antiseptics             418

Sulfonamides   418
Urinary Antiseptics   418
Individual Drugs   421
Principles of Therapy   422

**CHAPTER 41**

Antitubercular Drugs                                        427

Tuberculosis   427
Treatment Regimens for Tuberculosis   427
Characteristics of Antitubercular Drugs   428
Individual Antitubercular Drugs   428
Principles of Therapy   430

**CHAPTER 42**

Antiviral Drugs                                                 434

General Characteristics of Viruses and Viral Infections   434
Antiviral Drugs   435
Individual Antiviral Drugs   435
Principles of Therapy   438

**CHAPTER 43**

Antifungal Drugs                                              442

Fungi and Fungal Infections   442
Antifungal Drugs   443
Individual Antifungal Drugs   443
Principles of Therapy   443

**CHAPTER 44**

Antiparasitics                                                   448

Protozoal Infections   448
Helminthiasis   449
Scabies and Pediculosis   450
Individual Antiparasitic Drugs   450
Principles of Therapy   456

**SECTION VII**
**Drugs Affecting the Immune System**

**CHAPTER 45**

Physiology of the Immune System                    463

Overview of Body Defense Mechanisms   463
Immunity   463
Immune Cells   465
Patient-Related Factors That Influence Immune Function
   469
Immune Disorders   470
Immunotherapy   471

**CHAPTER 46**

Immunizing Agents                                          472

Immunization   472
Agents for Active Immunity   472
Agents for Passive Immunity   478
Individual Immunizing Agents   478
Principles of Therapy   481

**CHAPTER 47**

Immunostimulants                                           486

Description   486
Individual Immunostimulants   488
Principles of Therapy   490

**CHAPTER 48**

Immunosuppressants                                        496

Description   496
Autoimmune Disorders   496
Tissue and Organ Transplants   497
Bone Marrow and Graft-Versus-Host Disease   498
Corticosteroids   498
Cytotoxic Agents   498
Principles of Therapy   501

# SECTION VIII
## Drugs Affecting the Respiratory System

### CHAPTER 49
**Physiology of the Respiratory System**    511

The Respiratory System   511
Disorders of the Respiratory System   512
Drug Therapy   513

### CHAPTER 50
**Bronchodilating and Antiasthmatic Drugs**   514

Respiratory Disorders   514
Drug Therapy   514
Individual Bronchodilating and Antiasthmatic Drugs   515
Principles of Therapy   520

### CHAPTER 51
**Antihistamines**   525

Individual Antihistamines   526
Principles of Therapy   529

### CHAPTER 52
**Nasal Decongestants, Antitussives, Mucolytics, and Cold Remedies**   533

Description   533
Nasal Decongestants   534
Antitussives   534
Expectorants   534
Mucolytics   534
Cold Remedies   534
Individual Drugs   534
Principles of Therapy   538

# SECTION IX
## Drugs Affecting the Cardiovascular System

### CHAPTER 53
**Physiology of the Cardiovascular System**   545

Heart   545
Blood Vessels   546
Blood   546
Drug Therapy in Cardiovascular Disorders   547

### CHAPTER 54
**Cardiotonic-Inotropic Agents Used in Congestive Heart Failure**   548

Congestive Heart Failure   548
Digitalis Glycosides   549
Indications for Use   550

Contraindications for Use   550
Individual Cardiotonic-Inotropic Agents   550
Principles of Therapy   553

### CHAPTER 55
**Antiarrhythmic Drugs**   560

Description   560
Cardiac Electrophysiology   560
Cardiac Arrhythmias   561
Antiarrhythmic Drugs   562
Classifications and Individual Drugs   562
Principles of Therapy   567

### CHAPTER 56
**Antianginal Drugs**   572

Angina Pectoris   572
Antianginal Drugs   572
Individual Antianginal Drugs   574
Principles of Therapy   577

### CHAPTER 57
**Drugs Used in Hypotension and Shock**   581

Hypotension and Shock   581
Antishock Drugs   581
Individual Drugs Used in Hypotension and Shock   582
Principles of Therapy   584

### CHAPTER 58
**Antihypertensive Drugs**   588

Regulation of Arterial Blood Pressure   588
Hypertension   589
Antihypertensive Drugs   589
Individual Drugs   590
Principles of Therapy   595

### CHAPTER 59
**Diuretics**   601

Description   601
Renal Physiology   601
Alterations in Renal Function   604
Diuretic Drugs   604
Principles of Therapy   607

### CHAPTER 60
**Anticoagulant, Antiplatelet, and Thrombolytic Agents**   613

Description   613
Blood Coagulation   613
Thrombotic and Thromboembolic Disorders   614
Individual Drugs   615
Principles of Therapy   619

CHAPTER 61
Antilipemics and Peripheral Vasodilators   626
Antilipemic Drugs and Peripheral Vasodilators   626
Atherosclerosis   626
Individual Drugs   627
Principles of Therapy   629


SECTION X
Drugs Affecting the Digestive System

CHAPTER 62
Physiology of the Digestive System   635
The Digestive System   635
Organs of the Digestive System   635
Secretions of the Digestive System   636
Effects of Drugs on the Digestive System   637

CHAPTER 63
Drugs Used in Peptic Ulcer Disease   638
Peptic Ulcer Disease   638
Types of Antiulcer Drugs   639
Individual Drugs   640
Principles of Therapy   644

CHAPTER 64
Laxatives and Cathartics   651
Description   651
Defecation   651
Laxatives and Cathartics   651
Principles of Therapy   655

CHAPTER 65
Antidiarrheals   659
Description   659
Antidiarrheal Drugs   660
Principles of Therapy   664

CHAPTER 66
Antiemetics   668
Nausea and Vomiting   668
Antiemetic Drugs   668
Principles of Therapy   672


SECTION XI
Drugs Used in Special Conditions

CHAPTER 67
Antineoplastic Drugs   679
Characteristics of Normal Cells   679
Characteristics of Malignant Neoplasms   679

Characteristics of Antineoplastic Drugs   683
Individual Drugs   685
Principles of Therapy   692

CHAPTER 68
Drugs Used in Ophthalmic Conditions   699
Structures of the Eye   699
Disorders of the Eye   700
Ophthalmic Drugs   700
Individual Drugs   701
Principles of Therapy   706

CHAPTER 69
Drugs Used in Dermatologic Conditions   712
Functions of the Skin   712
Disorders of the Skin   713
Types of Dermatologic Drugs   714
Individual Drugs   715
Principles of Therapy   721

CHAPTER 70
Drug Use During Pregnancy
and Lactation   726
Pregnancy and Lactation   726
Maternal-Placental-Fetal Circulation   726
Drug Effects on the Fetus   727
Fetal Therapeutics   728
Maternal Therapeutics   728
Abortifacients   734
Tocolytics   734
Drugs Used During Labor and Delivery at Term   734
Neonatal Therapeutics   736
Principles of Therapy   739


APPENDIX A
Miscellaneous Drugs   743
APPENDIX B
The International System of Units   745
APPENDIX C
Therapeutic Serum Drug Concentrations
for Selected Drugs   746
APPENDIX D
Canadian Drug Laws and Standards   747
APPENDIX E
Canadian Drug Names   748


INDEX   755

# Clinical Drug Therapy

**FOURTH**
**EDITION**

# Therapy

*Rationales for*
*Nursing Practice*

# Introduction to Drug Therapy

### CHAPTER 1

# Introduction to Pharmacology

Pharmacology is the study of drugs (chemicals) that alter functions of living organisms. Drug therapy involves the use of drugs to prevent, diagnose, or cure disease processes or to relieve signs and symptoms without curing the underlying disease. When prevention or cure is not a reasonable goal, relief of symptoms can greatly improve quality of life and ability to function in activities of daily living. Drugs may be given for local or systemic effects. Drugs that have local effects, such as dermatologic preparations and local anesthetics, act mainly at the site of application. Those that have systemic effects are absorbed into the bloodstream and circulated to various parts of the body. Most drugs are given for their systemic effects.

## Sources of drugs

Historically, drugs were mainly derived from plants (*e.g.*, morphine), animals (*e.g.*, insulin), and minerals (*e.g.*, iron). Now most drugs are synthetic chemical compounds manufactured in laboratories. Technologic advances have enabled production of synthetic versions of many drugs originally derived from plants and animals, as well as new drugs. Synthetic drugs are more standardized in chemical characteristics, more consistent in their effects, and less likely to produce allergic reactions. Semisynthetic drugs (*e.g.*, many antibiotics) are naturally occurring substances that have been chemically altered.

Biotechnology (also called recombinant deoxyribonucleic acid [DNA] technology and genetic engineering) is increasing in importance as a source of drugs. This technology includes methods for manipulating DNA and ribonucleic acid (RNA) and recombining genes into hybrid molecules that can be inserted into living organisms (*Escherichia coli* bacteria are often used) and repeatedly reproduced. Each hybrid molecule produces a genetically identical molecule, called a clone. Cloning makes it possible to identify the DNA sequence in a gene and produce the protein product encoded by a gene, including insulin and several other body proteins. Cloning also allows production of the relatively large amounts needed for therapeutic or research purposes.

## Drug nomenclature

Drugs are classified according to their effects on particular body systems, their therapeutic uses, and their chemical characteristics. For example, morphine can be classified as a central nervous system (CNS) depressant, a narcotic analgesic, and an opiate. Individual drugs that represent groups of drugs are called *prototypes*. Morphine is the prototype of narcotic analgesics and is the standard with which other narcotic analgesics are compared. Drug classifications and prototypes are extremely stable, and most new drugs can be assigned to a group and compared with an established prototype.

Individual drugs may have several different names,

but the two most commonly used are the generic name and the trade name. The *generic name* (*e.g.*, amoxicillin) is related to the chemical or official name and is independent of the manufacturer. The *trade* or *brand name* is designated and patented by the manufacturer. For example, amoxicillin is manufactured by several pharmaceutical companies, each of which assigns a specific trade name such as Amoxil or Polymox. (Trade names are capitalized; generic names are lower case.) Drugs may be prescribed and dispensed by generic or trade name.

## Sources of drug information

There are many sources of drug data. Among the most useful are pharmacology textbooks, drug reference books, and journal articles. For the beginning student of pharmacology, a textbook is usually the best source of information because it describes groups of drugs in relation to therapeutic uses. Thus, the student can get an overview of the major drug classifications and their effects. Nursing students usually need textbooks and other references to gain necessary drug knowledge and apply that knowledge to the nursing care of clients.

Drug reference books are most helpful in relation to individual drugs. Two authoritative sources are the *American Hospital Formulary Service* and *Drug Facts and Comparisons*. The former is published by the American Society of Hospital Pharmacists and updated periodically. The latter is published by the Facts and Comparisons division of the J.B. Lippincott Company and updated monthly (looseleaf edition) or annually (hardbound edition). A widely available but less authoritative source is the *Physicians' Desk Reference* (PDR). The PDR, published yearly, is a compilation of manufacturers' package inserts for selected drugs. In addition, several major publishers of nursing textbooks publish drug reference handbooks and many pharmacologic, medical, and nursing journals contain information on drugs. Journal articles often present detailed information about drug therapy for specific disease processes.

## Federal drug laws and standards

Current drug laws and standards have evolved over many years, often as an effort to protect consumers. Although state laws regulate some aspects of drug use and distribution, federal laws regulate most major aspects. The first federal law, the *Pure Food and Drug Act* of 1906, established official standards and requirements for accurate labeling of drug products. This law was amended in 1912 (Sherley Amendment) to prohibit fraudulent claims of efficacy and in 1914 (Harrison Narcotic Act) to restrict and regulate the importation, manufacture, sale, and use of opium, cocaine, marijuana, and other drugs that the act defined as narcotics.

The next major legal development was passage of the *Food, Drug, and Cosmetic Act* in 1938. This law was the first to require proof of safety before a new drug could be marketed. One amendment in 1945 required governmental certification of biologic products, such as insulin and antibiotics. A second amendment in 1952 (Durham-Humphrey Amendment) designated drugs that must be prescribed by a physician and dispensed by a pharmacist (prescription drugs). A third amendment in 1962 (Kefauver-Harris Amendment) required proof of effectiveness for drugs to remain commercially available and gave the federal government the authority to standardize drug names. Overall, this law and its amendments regulate the manufacture, distribution, advertising, and labeling of drugs in an attempt to ensure safety and effectiveness. It also confers official status on drugs listed in *The United States Pharmacopeia*. The names of these drugs may be followed by the letters *USP*. Official drugs must meet standards of purity and strength as determined by chemical analysis or animal response to specified doses (bioassay). The Food and Drug Administration (FDA) is charged with enforcing the law. In addition, the Public Health Service regulates vaccines and other biologic products, and the Federal Trade Commission can suppress misleading advertisements of nonprescription drugs.

In 1970, the *Comprehensive Drug Abuse Prevention and Control Act* was passed. Title II of this law, called the *Controlled Substances Act*, regulates distribution of narcotics and other drugs of abuse and categorizes these drugs according to therapeutic usefulness and potential for abuse. These categories are discussed in Box 1-1. In addition to federal laws, state laws also regulate the sale and distribution of controlled drugs.

Additional developments include the *Drug Regulation Reform Act* of 1978, which shortened the time required for developing and marketing new drugs, and the *Orphan Drug Act* of 1983, which provided incentives to manufacturers (decreased taxes and competition) for producing drugs to treat certain serious, uncommon disorders affecting relatively few people.

### DRUG APPROVAL PROCESSES

The FDA is responsible for approving new drugs and certain other aspects of drug use. The FDA reviews research studies (usually conducted or sponsored by a pharmaceutical company) about proposed new drugs; the organization does not test the drugs.

Prior to passage of the Food, Drug, and Cosmetic Act and its amendments, many drugs were marketed without confirmation of safety or efficacy. Since 1962, however, newly developed drugs have been extensively

# BOX 1-1. CATEGORIES OF CONTROLLED SUBSTANCES

## Schedule I

Drugs that are not approved for medical use and that have high abuse potentials are included in this category (heroin, lysergic acid diethylamide [LSD], peyote, mescaline, tetrahydrocannabinol, marijuana).

## Schedule II

These drugs are used medically and have high abuse potentials; abuse may lead to psychological or physical dependence. Included in this group are narcotic analgesics (*e.g.*, codeine, hydromorphone, methadone, meperidine, morphine, oxycodone, oxymorphone), central nervous system (CNS) stimulants (*e.g.*, cocaine, dextroamphetamine, methamphetamine, phenmetrazine, methylphenidate), and barbiturate sedative-hypnotics (amobarbital, pentobarbital, secobarbital).

## Schedule III

These drugs have less potential for abuse than those in Schedules I and II. Abuse may lead to psychological or physical dependence. Included are mixtures containing small amounts of controlled substances, such as codeine, barbiturates not listed in other schedules, an antidiarrheal (paregoric), and some CNS stimulants (benzphetamine, phendimetrazine). In addition, male sex hormones (androgens and anabolic steroids) became Schedule III controlled substances in 1991 because of their widespread overuse to enhance athletic prowess and bodybuilding.

## Schedule IV

Drugs in this category have some potential for abuse. Included are benzodiazepine antianxiety agents (*e.g.*, chlordiazepoxide, diazepam, lorazepam), benzodiazepine hypnotics (*e.g.*, flurazepam, temazepam); other sedative-hypnotics (phenobarbital, chloral hydrate, ethchlorvynol), and some prescription appetite suppressants (diethylpropion, fenfluramine, mazindol, phentermine).

## Schedule V

These products contain moderate amounts of controlled substances. They may be dispensed by the pharmacist without a physician's prescription but with some restrictions regarding amount, recordkeeping, and other safeguards. Included are antidiarrheal drugs, such as diphenoxylate and atropine (Lomotil).

withdrawn, usually because of adverse effects that become evident only when the drug is used in a large, diverse population.

### Testing and clinical trials

The testing process begins with animal studies to determine potential uses and effects. The next step involves FDA review of the data obtained in the animal studies. The drug then undergoes clinical trials in human subjects. Most clinical trials use a randomized, controlled experimental design that involves selection of subjects according to established criteria, random assignment of subjects to experimental groups, and administration of the test drug to one group and a control substance to another group.

In Phase I, a few doses are given to a few healthy volunteers to determine safe dosages, routes of administration, absorption, metabolism, excretion, and toxicity. In Phase II, a few doses are given to a few subjects with the disease or symptom for which the drug is being studied, and responses are compared with those of healthy subjects. In Phase III, the drug is given to a larger and more representative group of subjects with studies designed to reduce bias. In double blind, placebo-controlled designs, half of the patients receive the new drug and half receive a placebo, with neither patients nor researchers knowing who receives which formulation. In crossover studies, subjects serve as their own controls; each subject receives the experimental drug during half of the study and a placebo during the other half. Other research methods include control studies, in which some patients receive a known drug rather than a placebo, and subject matching, in which patients are paired with others of similar characteristics. Phase III studies help to determine whether the potential benefits of the drug outweigh the risks.

In Phase IV, the FDA evaluates the data from the first three phases for drug safety and effectiveness, allows the drug to be marketed for general use, and requires manufacturers to continue monitoring the drug's effects. Some adverse drug effects may become evident during the postmarketing phase as the drug is more widely used, especially in women of childbearing age, children, and the elderly because these groups are often excluded from earlier clinical trials.

### FDA approval

The FDA approves approximately 20 to 25 new drugs annually. Some policies and procedures were changed in 1985 and 1992 to accelerate the approval process for drugs, especially those for serious or life-threatening illnesses (*e.g.*, acquired immunodeficiency syndrome [AIDS], cancer, and Alzheimer's disease) for which

tested before being marketed for general use. The drugs are carefully evaluated at each step. Testing usually proceeds if there is evidence of safety and effectiveness but may be stopped at any time for inadequate effectiveness or excessive toxicity. Many potential drugs are discarded and never marketed; a few drugs are marketed but later

there is no cure. New drugs are categorized according to the following rating scale:

*1*—A new chemical compound, never before marketed as a pharmaceutical product in the United States

*1AA*—Drugs intended for treatment of AIDS, which are considered high priority and reviewed more rapidly than most other drugs

*1A*—Drugs with important therapeutic gains over other products already marketed for the same diseases or conditions

*1B*—Drugs with modest therapeutic gains over similar products already being marketed. Advantages of these drugs may include fewer or less serious adverse reactions or greater convenience in administration.

*1C*—Drugs with little or no advantage over existing products (often called "me too" drugs). Many new drugs fit into this category.

In recent years, the FDA assigned the National Academy of Sciences to review drugs introduced between 1938 and 1962 for efficacy. As a result, many drugs were rated as effective (evidence of effectiveness exists), probably effective (additional evidence needed to establish efficacy), possibly effective (little evidence available), and ineffective (no substantial evidence). Drugs rated as ineffective have been withdrawn; drugs rated as probably or possibly effective must be withdrawn within set time limits unless efficacy is substantiated.

The FDA also approves transfer of drugs from prescription to nonprescription (over-the-counter or OTC) status. Several drugs have received such approval, including clotrimazole (Gyne-Lotrimin), diphenhydramine (Benadryl), ibuprofen (Advil and others), and miconazole (Monistat 7). For drugs taken orally, recommended doses are usually lower for nonprescription products. Several other drugs are being considered for OTC availability.

## Cellular physiology

Because all body functions and disease processes and most drug actions take place at the cellular level, cellular physiology is reviewed. Each body cell has the capacity to function and respond to injury. Although cells differ in various tissues according to location and function, they have common characteristics as well. For example, all cells are normally able to exchange materials with their immediate environment to obtain energy from nutrients, synthesize complex molecules, and duplicate themselves. They also are able to communicate with each other through various body chemicals, such as neurotransmitters, hormones, and other substances.

Cells (see Fig. 1-1) are composed of *protoplasm*, which, in turn, is composed of water, proteins, lipids,

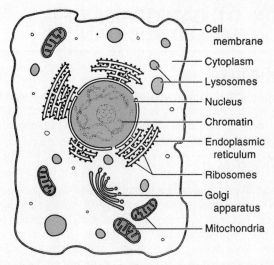

**FIGURE 1-1.** Schematic diagram of cell highlighting cytoplasmic organelles.

carbohydrates, and electrolytes (potassium, magnesium, phosphate, sulfate, and bicarbonate). Within the protoplasm are several structures. The *nucleus* directs cellular activities by determining the type and amount of proteins, enzymes, and other substances to be produced. The *cytoplasm* surrounds the nucleus and contains the working units of the cell. The *endoplasmic reticulum* (ER) contains ribosomes, which synthesize enzymes and other proteins. These include enzymes that synthesize glycogen, triglycerides, and steroids and those that detoxify drugs and other chemicals. Overall, the ER is important in the production of hormones by glandular cells and production of plasma proteins and drug-metabolizing enzymes by liver cells.

The *Golgi complex* stores hormones and other substances produced by the ER. It also packages these substances into secretory granules, which then move out of the Golgi complex into cytoplasm and, following an appropriate stimulus, are released from the cell through the process of exocytosis (see below).

*Mitochondria* generate energy for cellular activities and require oxygen. *Lysosomes* are membrane-enclosed vesicles that contain enzymes capable of breaking down nutrients (proteins, carbohydrates, fats), foreign substances, and the cell itself. During phagocytosis or when a cell becomes worn out or damaged, the membrane around the lysosome breaks, and the enzymes are released. Thus, lysosomal enzymes are important in the digestion of cellular debris and phagocytized antigens. However, lysosomal contents also are released into extracellular spaces, destroying surrounding cells. They may cause the tissue destruction that sometimes accompanies inflammatory reactions, including rheumatoid arthritis. In addition, the enzymes act on complement to produce component C5a and on kinins to produce bradykinin, both of which are inflammatory mediators (Box 1-2). Normally, the enzymes (proteases) are inacti-

# BOX 1-2. CHEMICAL MEDIATORS OF INFLAMMATION AND IMMUNITY

*Bradykinin* is one of the inactive polypeptide kinins present in body fluids. Kinins become physiologically active in the presence of tissue injury. When tissue cells are damaged, white blood cells (WBCs) increase in the area and ingest damaged cells to remove them from the area. When the WBCs die, they release enzymes that activate kinins. The activated kinins increase and prolong the vasodilation and increased vascular permeability caused by histamine. They also cause pain by stimulating nerve endings for pain in the area. Thus, bradykinin may aggravate and prolong the erythema, heat, and pain of local inflammatory reactions. It also increases mucous gland secretion.

*Complement* is a group of plasma proteins essential to normal inflammatory and immunologic processes. More specifically, complement destroys cell membranes of body cells (*e.g.*, red blood cells, lymphocytes, platelets) and pathogenic microorganisms (*e.g.*, bacteria, viruses). The system is initiated by an antigen-antibody reaction or by tissue injury. Components of the system (called C1 through C9) are activated in a cascade type of reaction in which each component becomes a proteolytic enzyme that splits the next component in the series. Activation yields products with profound inflammatory effects. C3a and C5a, also called anaphylatoxins, act mainly by liberating histamine from mast cells and platelets, and their effects are therefore similar to those of histamine. C3a is the most abundant cleavage product, and it causes or increases smooth muscle contraction, vasodilation, vascular permeability, degranulation of mast cells and basophils, and secretion of lysosomal enzymes by leukocytes. C5a performs the same functions as C3a and also promotes movement of neutrophils and macrophages into the injured area (chemotaxis). In addition, it activates the lipoxygenase pathway of arachidonic acid metabolism (see leukotrienes, below) in neutrophils and macrophages, thereby inducing formation of even more substances that increase vascular permeability and chemotaxis. Thus, C5a is a powerful inflammatory agent.

In the immune response, the complement system breaks down antigen-antibody complexes, especially those in which the antigen is a microbial agent. It enables the body to produce inflammation and localize an infective agent. More specific reactions include increased vascular permeability, chemotaxis, and opsonization (altering a microbe or other antigen so it can be more readily phagocytized).

*Cytokines* are mediators released by lymphocytes and other body cells in response to antigens. Unlike antibodies, their characteristics are not determined by the antigen that stimulates their production. Cytokines may act on the same cells that produce them, on surrounding cells, or on distant cells (like hormones) if sufficient amounts reach the bloodstream. Thus, these mediators act locally and systemically to produce inflammatory and immune responses, including increased vascular permeability and chemotaxis of macrophages, neutrophils, and basophils. Two major types of cytokines have been identified, interleukins (produced by leukocytes) and interferons (produced by T-lymphocytes or fibroblasts). Interleukin-1 mediates several inflammatory responses, in-

cluding fever, and interleukin-2 (also called T-cell growth factor) is required for the growth and function of T-lymphocytes. Interferons are a group of cytokines that protect nearby cells from invasion by intracellular microorganisms, such as viruses and rickettsiae. They also limit the growth of some cancer cells.

*Histamine* is stored in most body tissues, mainly in mast cells and basophils. Mast cells are especially abundant in skin and connective tissue. Histamine is discharged from mast cells into the vascular system in response to certain stimuli (*e.g.*, antigen-antibody reaction, tissue injury, extreme cold, and some drugs). Once released, histamine is highly vasoactive, causing vasodilation (increasing blood flow to the area and producing hypotension) and increasing permeability of capillaries and venules (producing edema). Other effects include contracting smooth muscles in the bronchi (producing bronchoconstriction and respiratory distress), gastrointestinal (GI) tract, and uterus; stimulating salivary, gastric, bronchial, and intestinal secretions; stimulating sensory nerve endings to cause pain and itching; and stimulating movement of eosinophils into injured tissue. Histamine is the first chemical mediator released in the inflammatory response and immediate hypersensitivity reactions (anaphylaxis)

When histamine is released from mast cells and basophils, it diffuses rapidly from its area of release into other tissues. It then acts on target tissues through both histamine-1 ($H_1$) and histamine-2 ($H_2$) receptors. $H_1$ receptors are located mainly on smooth muscle cells in blood vessels and the respiratory and GI tracts. When histamine binds with these receptors, resulting events include contraction of smooth muscle, increased venular permeability, production of nasal mucus, stimulation of sensory nerves, pruritus, and vasodilation of capillaries in the skin. $H_2$ receptors are also located in the airways, GI tract, and other tissues. When histamine binds to these receptors, there is increased secretion of gastric acid by parietal cells in the stomach mucosal lining, increased mucus secretion and bronchodilation in the airways, contraction of esophageal muscles, tachycardia, inhibition of lymphocyte function, and degranulation of basophils (with additional release of histamine and other mediators) in the bloodstream. In allergic reactions, both types of receptors mediate hypotension (in anaphylaxis), skin flushing, and headache. The peak effects of histamine occur within 1 to 2 minutes of its release and may last as long as 10 minutes, after which it is inactivated by histaminase (produced by eosinophils), or *N*-methyltransferase.

*Leukotrienes* are a group of chemical mediators formed by the lipoxygenase pathway of arachidonic acid metabolism. Arachidonic acid is a fatty acid released from the phospholipids of cell membranes in response to tissue injury. Leukotrienes help to regulate cellular responses to injury, including inflammation. Leukotrienes LTC4, LTD4, and LTE4 (formerly called slow-releasing substance of anaphylaxis or SRS-A because it is released slowly compared with histamine) cause sustained constriction of the bronchioles and are important mediators in bronchial asthma and immediate hypersensitivity reactions (anaphylaxis). The leukotrienes also may increase vascular

*(continued)*

## BOX 1-2. *(Continued)*

permeability, extravasation of WBCs, and chemotaxis of neu-trophils, basophils, eosinophils, and monocytes.

*Prostaglandins* are a group of chemical mediators formed by the cyclooxygenase pathway of arachidonic acid metabolism. Arachidonic acid is a fatty acid released from the phospho-lipids of cell membranes in response to tissue injury. Pros-taglandins are found in virtually all body tissues and act locally in the area where they are produced to regulate many cellular functions before being rapidly inactivated. The specific type of prostaglandin produced and its effects depend on the tissue involved, the stimulus, the hormonal environment, and other factors. In the inflammatory process, prostaglandins cause or potentiate the vasodilation, vascular permeability, pain, and edema caused by other mediators (*e.g.*, bradykinin, hista-mine) in areas of tissue damage. They also regulate smooth muscle in blood vessels and the GI, respiratory, and reproduc-tive systems; they protect GI mucosa from the erosive ef-fects of gastric acid; they regulate the amount and distribution

of renal blood flow; they control platelet function; and they maintain a patent ductus arteriosus in the fetus. More spe-cifically, prostaglandin $D_2$ causes bronchoconstriction; $E_2$ causes vasodilation, bronchodilation, increased activity of GI smooth muscle, increased sensitivity to pain, and fever; $F_2$ causes bronchoconstriction, increased uterine contraction, and increased activity of GI smooth muscle; $I_2$ (prostacyclin) causes vasodilation and decreased platelet aggregation; and thromboxane $A_2$ causes vasoconstriction and increased plate-let aggregation. Thus, prostaglandins may exert various and opposing effects in different body tissues.

*Serotonin* (5-hydroxytryptamine or 5-HT) is derived from the essential amino acid tryptophan and found in the brain (where it is an excitatory neurotransmitter), GI tract, and platelets. It is released by platelets activated by blood vessel injury. Its role in inflammatory and immune responses is not well understood. It reportedly causes vasoconstriction.

vated by enzyme inhibitors (antiproteases) in serum and synovial fluids, and excessive tissue destruction is pre-vented. The *cell membrane* separates intracellular con-tents from the extracellular environment, provides re-ceptors for hormones and other biologically active substances, participates in electrical events that occur in nerve and muscle cells, and helps to regulate growth and proliferation

Substances enter and leave the cell by several trans-port mechanisms. In addition to the basic mechanisms (*i.e.*, diffusion, osmosis, facilitated diffusion, and active transport), pinocytosis, phagocytosis, and exocytosis are important in inflammatory and immune processes. *Pi-nocytosis* involves ingestion of small amounts of extra-cellular fluid and dissolved particles and is an important mechanism for transport of proteins and electrolytes into cells. In this process, the cell membrane engulfs particles and forms a vesicle; the contents are eventually freed by lysosomal or other cytoplasmic enzymes. *Phagocytosis* resembles pinocytosis except that larger indentations occur in the cell membrane, which allow the cell to ingest large particles, such as bacteria and cell debris. Microorganisms and particles become attached to pha-gocytic cells where they are engulfed and killed or di-gested. *Exocytosis* is a mechanism for secreting intracellu-lar substances into extracellular spaces. In this process, a fluid-filled sac fuses to the inner side of the cell mem-brane and opens to the external cell surface where the contents are released into the extracellular fluid. Exo-cytosis allows removal of cellular debris and release of hormones and other substances synthesized inside the cell.

## Cellular injury and response to injury

Cellular injury may be caused by hypoxia, ischemia, microorganisms, chemicals, excessive heat or cold, radi-ation, and nutritional deficiencies or excesses. Chemi-cals, including therapeutic drugs, may injure the cell membrane and other cell structures, block enzymatic pathways, coagulate cell proteins (tissues), and disrupt the osmotic and ionic balance of the cell. Such injuries may result from the parent chemical or its metabolites. When cells are injured, the cell accumulates water, fats, and other normal components and excessive amounts or abnormal types of products synthesized within the cell. These reversible changes lead to edema and impaired cellular function. If the damage continues long enough or is not repaired, the changes become irreversible and result in cell death, tissue necrosis, and gangrene.

### INFLAMMATORY AND IMMUNE RESPONSES

Cellular response to injury involves inflammation, a generalized reaction to any tissue damage, which is an attempt to remove the damaging agent and repair the damaged tissue. The hemodynamic aspect of inflamma-tion includes vasodilation, which increases blood supply to the injured area, and increased capillary permeability, which allows fluid to leak into tissue spaces. The cellular aspect involves movement of leukocytes (white blood cells [WBCs]) into the area of injury. WBCs are attracted to the injured area by bacteria, tissue debris, plasma protein fractions (complement), and other substances in a process called chemotaxis. Once they reach the area, they phagocytize causative agents and tissue debris.

Specific WBCs are granulocytes (neutrophils, eosinophils, and basophils) and nongranulocytes (monocytes and lymphocytes). Granulocytes often contain inflammatory mediators or digestive enzymes in their cytoplasm. *Neutrophils*, the body's main defense against pathogenic bacteria, are the major group of leukocytes within the bloodstream. They respond to substances (*e.g.*, complement) released from infected or inflamed tissue that cause them to migrate to the affected tissue. There they localize the area of injury and phagocytize organisms or particles by releasing digestive enzymes and oxidative metabolites that kill engulfed pathogens or destroy other types of foreign particles. Neutrophils usually arrive within 90 minutes of injury, and their numbers increase greatly during the inflammatory process. They have a life span of approximately 10 hours and must be replaced frequently.

*Eosinophils* increase during allergic reactions and parasitic infections. In parasitic infections, they bind to and kill the parasites. In hypersensitivity reactions, they produce enzymes that inactivate histamine and leukotrienes (see Box 1-2) and may produce other enzymes that destroy antigen–antibody complexes. Despite these generally beneficial effects, eosinophils also may aggravate tissue damage by releasing cytotoxic substances. *Basophils* release histamine, a major chemical mediator in inflammatory and immediate hypersensitivity reactions.

Nongranulocytes arrive several hours after an injury, and monocytes usually replace neutrophils as the predominant WBC within 48 hours. Monocytes are the largest WBCs, and their life span is much longer than that of the granulocytes. Monocytes are able to phagocytize larger sizes and amounts of foreign material than neutrophils. In addition to their activity in the bloodstream, monocytes can leave blood vessels and enter tissue spaces (then called fixed tissue macrophages, although they can again become mobile and re-enter the bloodstream in some circumstances). Tissue macrophages are widely distributed in connective tissue and other areas (*e.g.*, Kupffer's cells in the liver, alveolar macrophages in the lungs, others in the lymph nodes and spleen) and form the mononuclear macrophage system (formerly called the reticuloendothelial system).

Both mobile and fixed monocytes are important in inflammatory and immune processes as the phagocytic cells digest or encapsulate foreign material and cellular debris. *Lymphocytes* include B cells, which are involved in antibody formation (humoral immunity), and T cells, which are involved in both cell-mediated and humoral immunity. Both types of lymphocytes play major roles in the immune response.

Inflammatory (and immune) responses produce their effects indirectly, through complex and overlapping interactions among cytokines and other chemical mediators. Cytokines are substances produced by human WBCs that induce WBC replication, phagocytosis, antibody production, fever, inflammation, and tissue repair (see Chap. 45). Chemical mediators are synthesized or released by mast cells, basophils, and other body cells. Once activated, mediators may exert their effects on tissues locally or at distant target sites. They also may induce or enhance other mediators. Histamine and other important mediators are described in Box 1-2.

## Characteristics of the inflammatory response

Local manifestations of inflammation include erythema, heat, edema, and pain. The erythema and heat result from vasodilation and increased blood supply, and edema results from leakage of blood plasma into the area. Pain is produced by the pressure of edema and secretions on nerve endings and by the chemical irritation of bradykinin, histamine, and other substances released by the damaged cells. Prostaglandins increase the pain and edema caused by other mediators. Systemic manifestations include leukocytosis, increased erythrocyte sedimentation rate, fever, headache, loss of appetite, lethargy, and weakness. Both local and systemic manifestations vary according to the cause and extent of tissue damage. Skeletal muscle may be broken down to provide the amino acids required for the synthesis of substances used to repair injured tissue, such as lymphokines, immunoglobulins, fibroblasts, and collagen.

Inflammation may be acute or chronic. Acute inflammation involves the hemodynamic and cellular responses to injury described previously. It is often precipitated by a self-limited stimulus, such as infection, which is rapidly controlled by host defenses. The inflamed area may heal completely with the injured tissue returning to normal or near-normal appearance and function; it may progress and develop a purulent exudate composed of WBCs, proteins, and tissue debris; or it may become chronic.

Chronic inflammation may result from recurrent or progressive episodes of acute inflammation or from a low-grade, smoldering type of tissue response to persistent irritants that are unable to penetrate deeply or spread rapidly (*e.g.*, foreign bodies; some viruses and bacteria, such as tuberculosis bacilli; and injured or altered tissue around a tumor or healing fracture). It follows a less consistent pattern and lasts longer, often months or years, and involves fewer neutrophils and more monocytes and lymphocytes in the affected area. It also produces more scar tissue, deformities, and impaired function. Little information is available about the chemical mediators of chronic inflammation, but immunologic mechanisms are thought to play an important role.

## Mechanisms of drug movement

To produce desired effects, drugs must reach adequate concentrations in blood and other tissue fluids surrounding responsive cells. Specific mechanisms of drug movement are passive diffusion, facilitated diffusion, and active transport.

*Passive diffusion* is the most common of these mechanisms. It involves movement of a drug from an area of higher concentration to one of lower concentration. For example, when an orally administered drug reaches the upper small intestine, its relatively high concentration promotes movement of its molecules into the bloodstream. The blood carries the molecules to other parts of the body; thus, drug concentration in the blood is low compared with that in the intestinal tract. When the drug molecules reach responsive cells, their greater concentration in the blood promotes movement of the drug into the fluids surrounding the cells or into the cells themselves. Passive diffusion continues until a state of equilibrium is reached between the amount of drug in the tissues and the amount in the blood.

*Facilitated diffusion* is a similar process, except that drug molecules combine with a carrier substance, such as an enzyme or other protein.

In *active transport*, drug molecules are moved from an area of lower concentration to one of higher concentration. This process requires a carrier substance and the release of cellular energy.

Drug movement and therefore drug action are affected by a drug's ability to cross cell membranes. For example, a drug given orally must pass through the cell membranes that line the intestinal tract, lymphatic vessels, and capillary walls to reach the bloodstream and circulate through the body. Cell membranes are complex structures composed of lipid and protein. Lipid-soluble drugs cross cell membranes by dissolving in the lipid layer; water-soluble drugs cross cell membranes through pores or channel openings. Lipid-soluble drugs can cross cell membranes more easily than water-soluble ones. Thus, most drugs are lipid-soluble.

## Pharmacokinetics

Pharmacokinetics involves drug movement through the body (*i.e.*, "what the body does to the drug"). Specific processes are absorption, distribution, metabolism (biotransformation), and excretion.

## ABSORPTION

*Absorption* is the process that occurs between the time a drug enters the body and the time it enters the bloodstream to be circulated. The rate and extent of absorption are affected by the dosage form of the drug, its route of administration, gastrointestinal function, and other variables. Dosage form is a major determinant of a drug's bioavailability (the amount of drug absorbed into the bloodstream).

Most oral drugs must be swallowed, dissolved in gastric fluid, and reach the small intestine before they are absorbed. Liquid medications are usually absorbed faster than tablets or capsules because they need not be dissolved. Increases in gastric emptying time and intestinal motility usually lead to increased drug absorption by promoting contact with absorptive mucous membrane. However, they also may decrease absorption because some drugs are degraded in gastric fluids, and others may move through the intestinal tract too rapidly to be absorbed. For most drugs, the presence of food in the stomach slows the rate of absorption and may decrease the amount of drug absorbed.

Drugs injected into subcutaneous or intramuscular tissues are usually absorbed more rapidly than oral drugs because they move directly from the injection site to the bloodstream. Absorption is especially rapid from intramuscular sites because muscle tissue has an abundant blood supply. Because they are placed directly in the bloodstream, drugs injected intravenously bypass the barriers to absorption encountered by other drugs.

Other absorptive sites include the skin, mucous membranes, and lungs. Most drugs applied to the skin are given for local effects (*e.g.*, sunscreens). Systemic absorption from intact skin is minimal but may be considerable when the skin is inflamed or damaged. Also, a number of drugs have been specifically formulated for transdermal systemic absorption (*e.g.*, estrogen, nitroglycerin, scopolamine, clonidine). Many drugs applied to mucous membranes also are given for local effects. However, systemic absorption occurs from the mucosa of the oral cavity, nose, eye, vagina, and rectum. Drugs absorbed through mucous membranes pass directly into the bloodstream. The lungs have a large surface area for absorption of anesthetic gases and a few other drugs.

## DISTRIBUTION

The term *distribution* refers to the transport of drug molecules within the body. Once a drug is injected or absorbed into the bloodstream, it is carried by the blood and tissue fluids to its sites of pharmacologic action, metabolism, and excretion. Distribution depends largely on the adequacy of the blood circulation. Drugs are distributed rapidly to organs receiving a large blood supply, such as the heart, liver, and kidneys. Distribution to other internal organs, muscle, fat, and skin is usually slower.

An important factor in drug distribution is *protein binding*. Most drugs form a complex with plasma proteins, mainly albumin, which act as carriers. Drug molecules bound to plasma proteins are pharmacologically inactive because the large size of the complex keeps them in the bloodstream and prevents them from reaching sites of action, metabolism, and excretion. *Only the free or unbound portion of a drug acts on body cells.* As the free drug acts on cells, the decrease in plasma drug levels causes some of the bound drug to be released. Protein binding allows some of a drug dose to be stored and released as needed. This, in turn, maintains more even blood levels and reduces the risk of drug toxicity.

Protein binding also is the basis for some important drug-drug interactions. A drug with a strong attraction to protein binding sites may displace a less tightly bound drug. The displaced drug then becomes pharmacologically active, and the overall effect is the same as taking a larger dose of the displaced drug.

Plasma protein binding can be seen as a method by which the body stores drugs. Some drugs also are stored in muscle, fat, or other body tissues and released gradually when plasma drug levels fall. Drugs that are highly bound to plasma proteins or stored extensively in other tissues tend to have a long duration of action.

Drug distribution in the CNS is unique. Many drugs do not enter the brain and cerebrospinal fluid, at least in therapeutic concentrations, because they cannot pass the blood-brain barrier, a group of cells that acts as a selectively permeable membrane to protect the CNS. However, the blood-brain barrier also can make drug therapy of CNS disorders more difficult.

Drug distribution during pregnancy and lactation also is unique (see Chap. 70). During pregnancy, most drugs cross the placenta and may affect the fetus. During lactation, many drugs enter breast milk and may affect the nursing infant.

## METABOLISM

The term *metabolism* refers to the way in which drugs are inactivated or biotransformed by the body. Most often, an active drug is changed into one or more inactive metabolites, which are then excreted. Some active drugs yield metabolites that are also active and that continue to exert their effects on body cells until they are metabolized further or excreted. Other drugs are initially inactive and exert no pharmacologic effects until they are metabolized.

Most drugs are lipid-soluble, a characteristic that aids their movement across cell membranes. However, the kidneys, which are the primary excretory organs, can excrete only water-soluble substances. Therefore, one function of metabolism is to convert fat-soluble drugs into water-soluble metabolites.

Most drugs are metabolized by enzymes in the liver (called the microsomal, mixed-function oxidase or the cytochrome P-450 enzyme system); the plasma, kidneys, lungs, and gastrointestinal mucosa also contain drug-metabolizing enzymes. These enzymes, which are complex proteins in structure, catalyze the chemical reactions of oxidation, reduction, hydrolysis, and conjugation with endogenous substances, such as glucuronic acid, sulfate, and others. With chronic administration, some drugs activate the hepatic enzymes, thereby accelerating drug metabolism. In a process called *enzyme induction*, the drugs stimulate liver cells to produce larger amounts of drug-metabolizing enzymes. Larger amounts of the enzymes then allow larger amounts of a drug to be metabolized during a given time. As a result, larger doses of the rapidly metabolized drug may be required to produce therapeutic effects.

Drugs that induce enzyme activity also may increase the rate of metabolism for endogenous steroidal hormones (*e.g.*, cortisol, estrogens, testosterone, and vitamin D). High protein diets may aid production of drug-metabolizing enzymes. Metabolism also can be decreased or delayed in a process called *enzyme inhibition*, which most often occurs with concurrent administration of two or more drugs that compete for the same metabolizing enzymes. In this instance, smaller doses of the slowly metabolized drug may be needed to avoid adverse reactions and toxicity from drug accumulation. The rate of drug metabolism also is reduced in infants, owing to the immaturity of their hepatic enzyme system; in people with impaired blood flow to the liver or severe hepatic or cardiovascular disease; and in people on low-protein diets.

When drugs are given orally, they are absorbed from the gastrointestinal tract and carried to the liver through the portal circulation. Some drugs are extensively metabolized in the liver, with only a portion of a drug dose reaching the systemic circulation for distribution to sites of action. This phenomenon is called the *first-pass effect*.

## EXCRETION

The term *excretion* refers to elimination of a drug from the body. Effective excretion requires adequate functioning of the circulatory system and of the organs of excretion (kidneys, bowel, lungs, and skin). Most drugs are excreted by the kidneys and eliminated unchanged or as metabolites in the urine. Some drugs or metabolites are excreted in bile, then eliminated in feces; others are excreted in bile, reabsorbed, returned to the liver (called *enterohepatic recirculation*), metabolized, and eventually excreted in urine. Some oral drugs are not absorbed and are excreted in the feces. The lungs mainly remove volatile substances, such as anesthetic gases. The skin has minimal excretory function. Factors impairing excretion, especially severe renal disease, lead to drug accumulation and potentially severe adverse reactions.

### SERUM HALF-LIFE

*Serum half-life*, also called *elimination half-time*, is the time required for the serum concentration of a drug to decrease by 50%. It is determined primarily by the drug's rates of metabolism and excretion. A drug with a short half-life requires more frequent administration than one with a long half-life.

When a drug is given at a stable dose, approximately four or five half-lives are required to achieve steady-state concentrations and develop equilibrium between tissue and serum concentrations. Because maximal therapeutic effects do not occur until equilibrium is established, some drugs are not fully effective for days or weeks. To maintain steady-state conditions, the amount of drug given daily must equal the amount eliminated from the body.

## Pharmacodynamics

Pharmacodynamics involves drug actions on target cells and the resulting alterations in cellular biochemical reactions and functions (*i.e.*, "what the drug does to the body").

### RECEPTOR THEORY OF DRUG ACTION

Like the physiologic substances (*e.g.*, hormones and neurotransmitters) that normally regulate cell functions, most drugs exert their effects by chemically binding with receptors at the cellular level (Fig. 1-2). Receptors are mainly proteins located on the surfaces of cell membranes or within cells. Specific receptors include *enzymes* involved in essential metabolic or regulatory processes (*e.g.*, dihydrofolate reductase, acetylcholinesterase), *proteins* involved in transport (*e.g.*, sodium, potassium adenosine triphosphatase) or structural processes (*e.g.*, tubulin), and *nucleic acids* (*e.g.*, DNA) involved in cellular protein synthesis, reproduction, and other metabolic activities.

When drug molecules bind with receptor molecules, the resulting drug-receptor complex initiates physiochemical reactions that stimulate or inhibit normal cellular functions. One type of reaction involves activation, inactivation, or other alterations of intracellular enzymes. Because almost all cellular functions are catalyzed by enzymes, drug-induced changes can markedly increase or decrease the rate of cellular metabolism. For

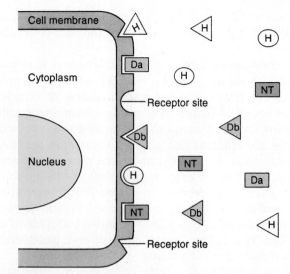

*FIGURE 1-2.* Cell membrane contains receptors for physiologic substances such as hormones (H) and neurotransmitters (NT). These substances stimulate or inhibit cellular function. Drug molecules (Da and Db) also interact with receptors to stimulate or inhibit cellular function.

example, an epinephrine-receptor complex increases the activity of the intracellular enzyme adenyl cyclase, which then causes the formation of cyclic adenosine monophosphate (cAMP). The cAMP, in turn, can initiate any one of many different intracellular actions, the exact effect depending on the type of cell.

A second type of reaction involves changes in the permeability of cell membranes to one or more ions. The receptor protein is a structural component of the cell membrane, and its binding to a drug molecule may open or close ion channels. In nerve cells, for example, sodium or calcium ion channels may open and allow movement of the ion(s) into the cell. This usually causes the cell membrane to depolarize and excite the cell. At other times, potassium channels may open and allow movement of potassium ions out of the cell. This action inhibits neuronal excitability and function. In muscle cells, movement of the ions into the cells may alter intracellular functions, such as the direct effect of calcium ions in stimulating muscle contraction.

A third reaction may modify the synthesis, release, or inactivation of the neurohormones (*e.g.*, acetylcholine, norepinephrine, serotonin) that regulate many physiologic processes.

Additional elements and characteristics of the receptor theory include:

1.  The site and extent of drug action on body cells are determined primarily by specific characteristics of receptors and drugs. Receptors vary in type, location, number, and functional capacity. For example, many different types of receptors have been identified. Most

types occur in most body tissues, such as receptors for epinephrine and norepinephrine (whether from stimulation of the sympathetic nervous system or administration of drug formulations) and receptors for hormones, including growth hormone, thyroid hormone, and insulin. Some occur in fewer body tissues, such as receptors for opiates and benzodiazepines in the brain and subgroups of receptors for epinephrine in the heart (called beta$_1$-adrenergic receptors) and lungs (beta$_2$-adrenergic receptors). Receptor type and location influence drug action. The receptor is often described as a lock into which the drug molecule fits as a key, and only those drugs able to chemically bond to the receptors in a particular body tissue can exert pharmacologic effects on that tissue. Thus, all body cells do not respond to all drugs, even though virtually all cell receptors are exposed to any drug molecules circulating in the bloodstream.

The number of receptor sites available to interact with drug molecules also affects the extent of drug action. It is likely that a minimal number of receptors must be occupied by drug molecules to produce pharmacologic effects. Thus, if many receptors are available but only a few are occupied by drug molecules, few drug effects occur. In this instance, increasing drug dosage increases pharmacologic effects. Conversely, if only a few receptors are available for many drug molecules, receptors may be saturated. In this instance, if most or all receptor sites are occupied, increasing drug dosage produces no additional pharmacologic effect.

Drugs vary even more widely than receptors. Because all drugs are chemical substances, chemical characteristics determine drug actions and pharmacologic effects. For example, a drug's chemical structure affects its ability to reach tissue fluids around a cell and bind with its cell receptors. Minor changes in drug structure may produce major changes in pharmacologic effects. Another major factor is the concentration of drug molecules that reach receptor sites in body tissues. Drug- and patient-related variables that affect drug actions are further described below.

2. When drug molecules chemically bind with cell receptors, pharmacologic effects are agonism or antagonism. *Agonists* are drugs that stimulate cell function or produce effects similar to those produced by naturally occurring hormones, neurotransmitters, and other substances. *Antagonists* are drugs that inhibit cell function by occupying receptor sites. This prevents natural body substances or other drugs from occupying the receptor sites and activating cell functions. Presumably, once drug action occurs, whether agonism or antagonism, drug molecules detach from receptor molecules (*i.e.*, the chemical binding is reversible).

3. Receptors are dynamic cellular components that can

be synthesized by body cells and altered by endogenous substances and exogenous drugs. For example, prolonged stimulation of body cells with an agonist usually reduces the number or sensitivity of receptors. As a result, the cell becomes less responsive to the agonist (a process called receptor desensitization, refractoriness, or down regulation). Prolonged inhibition of normal cellular functions with an antagonist may increase receptor number or sensitivity. If the antagonist is suddenly reduced or stopped, the cell becomes excessively responsive to an agonist (a process called hyperreactivity, supersensitivity, or up regulation). These changes in receptors may explain why some drugs need to be tapered in dosage and discontinued gradually if withdrawal symptoms are to be avoided.

## NONRECEPTOR DRUG ACTIONS

A relatively small number of drugs act by mechanisms other than combining with receptor sites on cells. These include:

1. Antacids, which act chemically to neutralize the hydrochloric acid produced by gastric parietal cells.
2. Osmotic diuretics (*e.g.*, mannitol), which increase the osmolarity of plasma and pull water out of tissues into the bloodstream.
3. Drugs that are structurally similar to nutrients required by body cells (*e.g.*, purines and pyrimidines) and that can be incorporated into cellular constituents, such as nucleic acids. This interferes with normal cell functioning. Several anticancer drugs act by this mechanism.
4. Metal chelating agents, which combine with toxic metals (*e.g.*, lead) to form a complex that can be more readily excreted.

# Variables that affect drug actions

Expected responses to drugs are largely based on those occurring when a particular drug is given to healthy adult males (18–65 years old) of average weight (150 lb, or 70 kg). However, increasing awareness that consumers of therapeutic drugs vary widely in their responses is leading to increased emphasis on controlled studies in more representative patient populations for which a drug is intended (including women, children, the elderly, and patients with particular diseases or symptoms). In any client, though, responses may be altered by both drug- and client-related variables, some of which are described below.

## DRUG-RELATED VARIABLES

### Dosage

Although the terms *dose* and *dosage* are often used interchangeably, dose usually indicates the amount to be given at one time, while dosage refers to the frequency, size, and number of doses. Dosage is a major determinant of drug actions and responses, both therapeutic and adverse. If the amount is too small or administered infrequently, no pharmacologic action occurs because the drug does not reach an adequate concentration at cellular receptor sites. If the amount is too large or administered too often, toxicity (poisoning) may occur. Because dosage includes the amount of the drug and the frequency of administration, overdosage may occur with a single large dose or with chronic ingestion of smaller amounts. Doses that produce signs and symptoms of toxicity are called *toxic doses*. Doses that cause death are called *lethal doses*.

Dosages recommended in drug literature are usually those that produce particular responses in 50% of the people tested. These dosages generally produce a mixture of therapeutic and adverse effects. The dosage of a particular drug depends on many characteristics of the drug (purpose for use, potency, pharmacokinetics, route of administration, dosage form, and others) and of the recipient (age, weight, state of health, and function of cardiovascular, renal, and hepatic systems). Thus, the recommended dosages are intended as guidelines for individualizing dosages.

### Route of administration

Routes of administration affect drug actions and responses largely by influencing absorption and distribution. For rapid drug action and response, the intravenous route is most effective because the drug is injected directly into the bloodstream. For many drugs, the intramuscular route also produces drug action within a few minutes because muscles have an abundant blood supply. The oral route generally produces slower drug action than parenteral routes. Absorption and action of topical drugs vary according to the drug formulation, whether the drug is applied to skin or mucous membranes, and other factors.

### Drug-diet interactions

Food may alter absorption of oral drugs. In many instances, food slows absorption of oral drugs by slowing gastric emptying time and altering gastrointestinal secretions and motility. When tablets or capsules are taken with or soon after food, they dissolve more slowly; therefore, drug molecules are delivered to absorptive sites in the intestine more slowly. Food also may decrease absorption by combining with a drug to form an insoluble drug-food complex. In other instances, however, certain drugs or dosage forms demonstrate enhanced absorption with certain types of meals. For example, a fatty meal increases absorption of some sustained-release forms of theophylline.

In addition, some foods contain substances that react with certain drugs. One such interaction occurs between tyramine-containing foods and monoamine oxidase (MAO) inhibitor drugs. Tyramine causes the release of norepinephrine, a potent vasoconstrictive agent, from the adrenal medulla and sympathetic neurons. Normally, norepinephrine is active for only a few milliseconds before it is inactivated by MAO; however, because MAO inhibitors prevent inactivation of norepinephrine, ingesting tyramine-containing foods with an MAO inhibitor may produce severe hypertension or intracranial hemorrhage. MAO inhibitors include the antidepressants isocarboxazid (Marplan) and phenelzine (Nardil) and the antineoplastic procarbazine (Matulane). Tyramine-rich foods to be avoided by clients taking MAO inhibitors include beer, wine, aged cheeses, yeast products, chicken livers, and pickled herring.

An interaction may occur between oral anticoagulants, such as warfarin (Coumadin), and foods containing vitamin K. Because vitamin K antagonizes the action of oral anticoagulants, large amounts of green leafy vegetables, such as spinach and other greens, may offset anticoagulant effects and predispose the person to thromboembolic disorders.

A third interaction occurs between tetracycline, an antibiotic, and dairy products, such as milk and cheese. The drug combines with the calcium in milk products to form an insoluble, unabsorbable compound that is excreted in the feces.

### Drug-drug interactions

The action of a particular drug may be increased or decreased by its interaction with another drug in the body. Most interactions occur whenever the interacting drugs are present in the body; some, especially those affecting absorption of oral drugs, occur when the interacting drugs are given at or near the same time.

Interactions that can increase the therapeutic or adverse effects of drugs are as follows:

1. *Additive effects* occur when two drugs with similar pharmacologic actions are taken.
     ***Example***: alcohol + sedative drug → increased sedation
2. *Synergism or potentiation* occurs when two drugs with different sites or mechanisms of action produce greater effects when taken together than either does when taken alone.

*Example*: acetaminophen (non-narcotic analgesic) + codeine (narcotic analgesic) → increased analgesia

3. *Interference* by one drug with the metabolism or elimination of a second drug may result in intensified effects of the second drug.

*Examples*: isoniazid (an antituberculosis drug) + phenytoin (an anticonvulsant) → potentiation of the effects of phenytoin on the CNS. In this instance, isoniazid inhibits enzymatic breakdown of phenytoin. Probenecid (a uricosuric drug) + penicillin (an antibiotic) → increased antibacterial effect of penicillin. Probenecid inhibits excretion of penicillin by kidney tubules. Cimetidine (an antiulcer drug) inhibits drug metabolizing enzymes in the liver and therefore interferes with the metabolism of many drugs (*e.g.*, benzodiazepine antianxiety and hypnotic drugs, calcium channel blockers, tricyclic antidepressants, some antiarrhythmics, beta-blockers and anticonvulsants, theophylline, and warfarin). When these drugs are given concurrently with cimetidine, they are more likely to cause adverse reactions and toxic effects.

4. *Displacement* of one drug from plasma protein binding sites by a second drug increases the effects of the displaced drug. This increase occurs because the molecules of the displaced drug, freed from their bound form, become pharmacologically active.

*Example*: aspirin (an anti-inflammatory–analgesic–antipyretic agent) + warfarin (an anticoagulant) → increased anticoagulant effect

Interactions in which drug effects are decreased are grouped under the term *antagonism*. Examples of such interactions are as follows:

1. In some situations, a drug that is a specific antidote is given to antagonize the toxic effects of another drug.

*Example*: naloxone (a narcotic antagonist) + morphine (a narcotic analgesic) → relief of narcotic-induced respiratory depression. Naloxone molecules displace morphine molecules from their receptor sites on nerve cells so that the morphine molecules cannot continue to exert their depressant effects.

2. Decreased intestinal absorption of oral drugs occurs when drugs combine to produce nonabsorbable compounds.

*Example*: aluminum or magnesium hydroxide (antacids) + tetracycline (an antibiotic) → binding of tetracycline to aluminum or magnesium, causing decreased absorption and decreased antibiotic effect of tetracycline

3. Activation of drug-metabolizing enzymes in the liver increases the metabolism rate of any drug metabolized primarily in the liver. Some anticonvulsants, antitubercular drugs, barbiturates, and antihistamines are known "enzyme inducers."

*Example*: phenobarbital (a barbiturate) + warfarin (an anticoagulant) → decreased effects of warfarin

4. Increased excretion occurs when urinary pH is changed and renal reabsorption is blocked.

*Example*: sodium bicarbonate + phenobarbital → increased excretion of phenobarbital. The sodium bicarbonate alkalinizes the urine, raising the number of barbiturate ions in the renal filtrate. The ionized particles cannot pass easily through renal tubular membranes. Therefore, less drug is reabsorbed into the blood, and more is excreted by the kidneys.

## CLIENT-RELATED VARIABLES

### Age

The effects of age on drug action are most pronounced in neonates, infants, and older adults. In children, drug action depends largely on age and developmental stage. During pregnancy, drugs cross the placenta and may harm the fetus. Fetuses have no effective mechanisms for metabolizing or eliminating drugs because their liver and kidney functions are immature. Newborn infants (birth to 1 month) also handle drugs inefficiently. Drug distribution, metabolism, and excretion differ markedly in neonates, especially premature babies, because their organ systems are not fully developed. Older infants (1 month to 1 year) reach approximately adult levels of protein binding and kidney function, but liver function and the blood-brain barrier are still immature.

Children (1–12 years) experience a period of increased activity of drug-metabolizing enzymes so that some drugs are rapidly metabolized and eliminated. Although the onset and duration of this period have not been established, a few studies have been done with particular drugs. Theophylline, for example, is cleared much faster in a 7-year-old child than in a neonate or adult (18–65 years). After about 12 years of age, healthy children handle drugs similarly to healthy adults.

In older adults (65 years and older), physiologic changes may alter all pharmacokinetic processes. Changes in the gastrointestinal tract include decreased gastric acidity, decreased blood flow, and decreased motility. Despite these changes, however, there is relatively little difference in absorption. Changes in the cardiovascular system include decreased cardiac output and therefore slower distribution of drug molecules to their sites of action, metabolism, and excretion. In the liver, there is decreased blood flow and probably a decreased number of metabolizing enzymes. Thus, many drugs are metabolized more slowly, have a longer action, and are more likely to accumulate with chronic administration. In the kidneys, there is decreased blood flow, decreased glomerular filtration rate, and decreased tubular secretion of drugs. All these changes tend to slow excretion and promote accumulation of drugs in the body. Impaired kidney and liver function greatly increase the risks of adverse drug effects. In addition, older adults are more likely to have acute and chronic illnesses that require multiple drugs or long-term drug therapy. Thus, possibilities for interactions among drugs and between drugs and diseased organs are greatly multiplied.

## Body weight

Body weight affects drug action mainly in relation to dose. The ratio between the amount of drug given and body weight influences drug distribution and concentration at sites of action. Generally, people heavier than average need larger doses, provided that renal, hepatic, and cardiovascular functions are adequate. Recommended doses for many drugs are listed in terms of grams or milligrams per kilogram of body weight.

## Genetic and ethnic characteristics

Drugs are given to elicit certain responses that are relatively predictable for the majority of drug recipients. However, some individuals experience inadequate therapeutic effects, and some experience unusual or exaggerated effects, including increased toxicity. These interindividual variations in drug response are often attributed to genetic or ethnic differences in drug pharmacokinetics or pharmacodynamics. As a result, there is increased awareness that genetic and ethnic characteristics are important factors and that diverse groups need to be included in clinical trials.

### Pharmacogenetics

*Pharmacogenetics* is a relatively new area of study that is concerned with genetically related variability in responses to drugs. A person's genetic characteristics may influence drug action in several ways. For example, genes determine the types and amounts of proteins produced in the body. When most drugs enter the body, they interact with proteins (*e.g.*, in plasma, tissues, cell membranes, and drug-receptor sites) to reach their sites of action and with other proteins (*e.g.*, drug-metabolizing enzymes in the liver and other organs) to be biotransformed and eliminated from the body. Presumably, genetic characteristics that alter any of these proteins could alter drug pharmacokinetics or pharmacodynamics.

One of the earliest pharmacokinetic genetic variations to be identified was the observation that some people taking usual doses of isoniazid (an antitubercular drug),

hydralazine (an antihypertensive agent), or procainamide (an antiarrhythmic) lacked therapeutic effects, while other people developed toxicity. Research established that these drugs are normally metabolized by acetylation, a chemical conjugation process in which the drug molecule combines with an acetyl group of acetyl coenzyme A. The reaction is catalyzed by a hepatic drug-metabolizing enzyme called acetyltransferase. It was further established that humans may acetylate the drug rapidly or slowly, depending largely on genetically controlled differences in acetyltransferase activity. Clinically, people who are rapid acetylators may need larger-than-usual doses to achieve therapeutic effects, and people who are slow acetylators may need smaller-than-usual doses to avoid toxic effects. In addition, several genetic variations have been identified in subgroups of the cytochrome P-450 drug-metabolizing system. Specific variations may influence any of the chemical processes by which drugs are metabolized.

Another example of genetic variation in drug metabolism includes people who lack the plasma pseudocholinesterase enzyme that normally inactivates succinylcholine, a potent muscle relaxant used in major surgical procedures. These people may experience prolonged paralysis and apnea if given succinylcholine. Still another example includes people with deficient glucose-6-phosphate dehydrogenase, an enzyme normally found in red blood cells and other body tissues. These people may develop hemolytic anemia when given antimalarial drugs, sulfonamides, analgesics, antipyretics, and other drugs.

### Pharmacoanthropology

*Pharmacoanthropology* is a recently developed area of study that is concerned with racial and ethnic differences in responses to drugs. For the most part, available drug information has been derived from clinical drug trials with white male subjects, and few, if any, subjects of other ethnic groups are included. Interethnic variations became evident when drugs and dosages developed for white people produced unexpected responses, including toxicity, when given to other ethnic populations.

One common interethnic variation is that African-Americans are less responsive to some antihypertensive drugs than white people. For example, angiotensin-converting enzyme (ACE) inhibitors and beta-adrenergic blocking drugs are less effective as single-drug therapy. Generally, African-American hypertensive patients respond better to diuretics or calcium channel-blockers than to ACE inhibitors and beta-blockers. Another interethnic variation is that Asians generally require much smaller doses of some commonly used drugs, including beta-blockers and several psychotropic drugs (*e.g.*, alprazolam, an antianxiety agent, and haloperidol, an antipsychotic). Some documented interethnic variations are included in later chapters.

## Gender

Except during pregnancy and lactation, gender has been considered a minor influence on drug action. Almost all research studies related to drugs have involved male subjects, and clinicians have extrapolated the findings to female patients. Several reasons have been advanced for excluding women in clinical drug trials, including the risks to a fetus if a woman becomes pregnant and the greater complexity in sample size and data analysis. However, because differences between males and females in responses to drug therapy are being identified, the need to include women in drug studies is evident.

Some gender-related differences in responses to drugs may stem from hormonal fluctuations in women during the menstrual cycle. Although this area has received little attention in research studies and clinical practice, altered responses have been demonstrated in some women taking clonidine, an antihypertensive; lithium, a mood-stabilizing agent; phenytoin, an anticonvulsant; propranolol, a beta-adrenergic blocking drug used in the management of hypertension, angina pectoris, and migraine; and antidepressants. For example, women with clinical depression may need higher doses of antidepressant medications premenstrually, when symptoms may exacerbate, and lower doses during the rest of the menstrual cycle.

Another example is that women with schizophrenia require lower dosages of antipsychotic medications than men. If given the higher doses required by men, women are likely to develop adverse drug reactions.

## Pathologic conditions

Pathologic conditions may alter pharmacokinetic processes. All pharmacokinetic processes are decreased in cardiovascular disorders characterized by decreased blood flow to tissues, such as hypotension, shock, low plasma volume, and congestive heart failure. In addition, absorption of oral drugs is decreased with vomiting, diarrhea, intestinal malabsorption, and other gastrointestinal disorders. Distribution is altered in malnutrition, liver or kidney disease, and other conditions that decrease the number of plasma proteins providing drug-binding sites. Metabolism is decreased in severe liver disease; it may be increased in conditions that generally increase body metabolism, such as hyperthyroidism and fever. Excretion is decreased in severe kidney disease.

## Psychological considerations

Psychological considerations influence individual responses to drug administration, although specific mechanisms are unknown. An example is the "placebo re-

sponse." A placebo is a pharmacologically inactive substance, such as sugar or sodium chloride solution. Placebos are used in clinical drug trials to compare the medication being tested with a "dummy" medication. Interestingly, recipients often report both therapeutic and adverse effects from placebos.

Attitudes and expectations related to drugs in general, a particular drug, or a placebo influence client response. They also influence compliance or willingness to carry out the prescribed drug regimen, especially with long-term drug therapy.

## Adverse effects of drugs

As used in this book, the term *adverse effects* refers to any undesired responses to drug administration, as opposed to *therapeutic effects*, which are desired responses. Most drugs produce a mixture of therapeutic and adverse effects; all drugs can produce adverse effects. Adverse effects may be common or rare, mild or severe and life-threatening, localized or widespread, depending on the drug and the person taking it.

Some adverse effects occur with usual therapeutic doses of drugs; others are more likely to occur and to be more severe with high doses. Some of the factors influencing the incidence and severity of adverse effects are as follows:

1. *Gastrointestinal effects* (anorexia, nausea, vomiting, constipation, diarrhea) are among the most common adverse reactions to drugs. These occur with many oral drugs from local irritation of the gastrointestinal tract and with drugs that stimulate the vomiting center in the medulla oblongata, whatever the route of administration. Some drugs also cause bleeding or ulceration (notably aspirin and nonsteroidal anti-inflammatory agents).
2. *Hematologic effects* (blood coagulation disorders, bleeding disorders, bone marrow depression, anemias, leukopenia, agranulocytosis, thrombocytopenia) are relatively common and potentially life-threatening. They are associated in particular with antineoplastic drugs but may occur with others as well.
3. *Hepatotoxicity* (hepatitis, hepatic necrosis, biliary tract obstruction) is relatively rare but potentially life-threatening. Because most drugs are metabolized by the liver, the liver is especially susceptible to drug-induced injury. Commonly used hepatotoxic drugs include acetaminophen (Tylenol), chlorpromazine (Thorazine), halothane (Fluothane), isoniazid (INH), methotrexate (Mexate), methyldopa (Aldomet), nitrofurantoin (Macrodantin), oxymetholone (Anadrol),

phenelzine (Nardil) and other MAO inhibitors, phenytoin (Dilantin), aspirin and other salicylates, and tetracycline (Achromycin). In the presence of drug- or disease-induced liver damage, the metabolism of many drugs is impaired. Consequently, drugs metabolized by the liver tend to accumulate in the body and cause adverse effects. Besides actual hepatotoxicity, many drugs produce abnormal values in liver function tests without producing clinical signs of liver dysfunction.

4. *Nephrotoxicity* (renal insufficiency or failure) occurs with several antimicrobial agents (*e.g.*, gentamicin and other aminoglycosides) and other drug classes. It is potentially serious because it may interfere with drug excretion, thereby causing drug accumulation and increased adverse effects.

5. *Hypersensitivity or allergy* may occur with almost any drug in susceptible clients. It is largely unpredictable and unrelated to dose. It occurs in those who have previously been exposed to the drug or a similar substance (antigen) and who have developed antibodies. When readministered, the drug reacts with the antibodies to cause cell damage and release of histamine and other intracellular substances. These substances produce reactions ranging from mild skin rashes to anaphylactic shock. Anaphylactic shock is a life-threatening hypersensitivity reaction characterized by respiratory distress and cardiovascular collapse. It occurs within a few minutes after drug administration and requires emergency treatment with epinephrine, antihistamines, and bronchodilator drugs. Some allergic reactions occur 1 to 2 weeks after the drug is given.

6. *Idiosyncrasy* refers to an unexpected reaction to a drug that occurs the first time the drug is given. These reactions are usually attributed to genetic characteristics that alter the person's drug-metabolizing enzymes.

7. *Drug dependence* may occur with mind-altering drugs, such as narcotic analgesics, sedative-hypnotic agents, antianxiety agents, and amphetamines. Dependence may be physiologic or psychological. Physiologic dependence produces unpleasant physical symptoms when the drug is withdrawn. Psychological dependence leads to excessive preoccupation with drugs and drug-seeking behavior. Drug dependence is discussed further in Chapter 15.

8. *Carcinogenicity* is the ability of a substance to cause cancer. Several drugs are carcinogens, including some hormones and anticancer drugs. Carcinogenicity apparently results from drug-induced alterations in cellular DNA.

9. *Teratogenicity* is the ability of a substance to cause abnormal fetal development when given to pregnant women. Drug groups considered teratogenic include analgesics, diuretics, antihistamines, antibiotics, antiemetics, and others.

## Tolerance and cross-tolerance

Drug *tolerance* is a situation in which the body becomes accustomed to a particular drug over time so that larger doses must be given to produce the same effects. Tolerance may be acquired to the pharmacologic action of many drugs, especially narcotic analgesics, barbiturates, alcohol, and other CNS depressants. Tolerance to pharmacologically related drugs is called *cross-tolerance*. For example, a person who regularly drinks large amounts of alcohol becomes able to ingest even larger amounts before becoming intoxicated: This is tolerance to alcohol. If the person is then given sedative-type drugs or a general anesthetic, larger-than-normal doses are usually required to produce a pharmacologic effect: this is cross-tolerance.

Tolerance and cross-tolerance are usually attributed to activation of drug-metabolizing enzymes in the liver, which accelerate metabolism and excretion of the drug. They also are attributed to a decrease in the sensitivity of drug-receptor sites to the drug and to a decrease in the number of receptor sites. Rapid development of tolerance after only a few doses of a drug is called *tachyphylaxis*.

### Review and Application Exercises

1. What are some factors that decrease absorption of an oral drug?
2. Drug dosage is a major determinant of both therapeutic and adverse drug effects. How can you use this knowledge in monitoring a client's response to drug therapy?
3. Does protein binding speed up or slow down drug distribution to sites of action?
4. Are drugs equally distributed throughout the body? Why or why not?
5. What are the implications of hepatic enzyme induction and inhibition in terms of drug metabolism and elimination from the body?
6. For a drug in which biotransformation produces active metabolites, is drug action shortened or lengthened? What difference does this make in client care?
7. Which pharmacokinetic processes are likely to be impaired with severe cardiovascular disease and with severe renal disease?
8. What are the main elements of the receptor theory of drug action?

**9.** When drug-drug interactions occur, are drug actions increased or decreased?

**10.** Giving the same drug and dosage often results in differences in blood levels and other client responses. What are some reasons for individual differences in responses to drugs?

## Selected References

Guttendorf, R. J., & Wedlund, P. J. (1992). Genetic aspects of drug disposition and therapeutics. *Journal of Clinical Pharmacology, 32*, 107–117.

Guyton, A. C. (1991). *Textbook of medical physiology* (8th ed.). Philadelphia: W.B. Saunders.

Hamilton, J. A. (1992). Medical research: The forgotten 51%. In, *Medical and health annual 1992* (pp. 317–322). Chicago: Encyclopaedia Britannica.

Kallis, D. J., Berkhousen, M. C., & Hoff, R. P. (1990). Development of an adverse drug reaction reporting program self-study module for nursing personnel. *Hospital Pharmacy, 25*, 143–221.

Kaplowitz, N. (1992). Hepatic biotransformation. In W. N. Kelley (Ed.), *Textbook of internal medicine* (2nd ed.) (pp. 435–440). Philadelphia: J.B. Lippincott.

Kudzma, E. C. (1992). Drug response: All bodies are not created equal. *American Journal of Nursing, 92*, 49–50.

Mendoza, R., Smith, M. W., Poland, R. E., Lin, M., & Strickland, T. (1991). Ethnic psychopharmacology: The Hispanic and Native American perspective. *Psychopharmacology Bulletin, 27*(4), 449–461.

Meyer, U. A. (1992). Drugs in special patient groups: Clinical importance of genetics in drug effects. In K. L. Melmon, H. F. Morrelli, B. B. Hoffman, & D. W. Nierenberg (Eds.), *Clinical pharmacology: Basic principles in therapeutics* (3rd ed.) (pp. 875–894). New York: McGraw-Hill.

Pless, B. S., & Tatro, E. H. (1992). Cellular, homeostatic, and disease mechanisms. In L. O. Burrell (Ed.), *Adult nursing in hospital and community settings* (pp. 68–78). Norwalk, CT: Appleton & Lange.

Porth, C. M. (1990). *Pathophysiology: Concepts of altered health states* (3rd ed.). Philadelphia: J.B. Lippincott.

Ross, E. M. (1990). Pharmacodynamics: Mechanisms of drug action and the relationship between drug concentration and effect. In A. G. Gilman, T. W. Rall, A. S. Nies, & P. Taylor (Eds.), *The pharmacological basis of therapeutics* (8th ed.) (pp. 33–48). New York: Pergamon Press.

Rutledge, D. R. (1991). Are there beta-adrenergic receptor response differences between racial groups? *DICP, The Annals of Pharmacotherapy, 25*, 824–834.

Williams, L., Davis, J. A., & Lowenthal, D. T. (1993). The influence of food on the absorption and metabolism of drugs. *Medical Clinics of North America, 77*(4), 815–829.

Wood, A. J. J., & Zhou, H. H. (1991). Ethnic differences in drug disposition and responsiveness. *Clinical Pharmacokinetics, 20*(5), 350–373.

# CHAPTER 2

# Administering Medications

Drugs given for therapeutic purposes are usually called *medications*. Giving medications to clients is an important nursing responsibility, especially in agencies such as hospitals and long-term care facilities. Basic requirements for accurate drug administration are often called the "five rights": giving the right *drug*, in the right *dose*, to the right *client*, by the right *route*, at the right *time*. Each "right" requires knowledge, skills, and specific nursing interventions:

1. Right drug
   a. Interpret the physician's order accurately (*i.e.*, name of drug).
   b. If the drug is unfamiliar, seek information from an authoritative source.
   c. Read labels of drug containers accurately.
   d. Question the prescribing physician about the order if the name of the drug is unclear or if the drug seems inappropriate for the client's condition.
2. Right dose
   a. Interpret abbreviations accurately.
   b. Interpret measurements accurately.
   c. Calculate doses accurately.
   d. Measure doses accurately.
3. Right client
   a. Check identification bands on institutionalized clients.
   b. Verify identity of ambulatory clients.

4. Right route
   a. Use correct techniques for all routes of administration.
   b. Always use appropriate anatomic landmarks to identify sites for intramuscular (IM) injections.
   c. For intravenous (IV) medications, follow manufacturers' instructions for preparation and administration.
5. Right time
   a. Schedule to maximize therapeutic effects and minimize adverse effects.
   b. Omit or delay doses when indicated by the client's condition.

Drug administration in children is potentially more problematic than in most other clients. One reason is that many drugs are prepared in dosage forms and concentrations suitable for adults. This often requires dilution (which may change the drug's stability and compatibility), calculation, preparation, and administration of minute doses (which are more likely to be inaccurate and possibly toxic than standard doses). In addition, children have limited sites for administration of IV drugs, and several may be given through the same site. In many cases, the need for small volumes of fluid precludes extensive flushing between drugs (which may produce undesirable interactions with other drugs and IV solutions).

Anne Collins Abrams: CLINICAL DRUG THERAPY, Fourth Edition.
© 1995 J.B. Lippincott Company.

The rest of this chapter emphasizes general information needed to fulfill responsibilities related to drug administration.

## Medication systems

Each agency has a system for dispensing drugs. A widely used method is the unit-dose system, in which most drugs are dispensed in single-dose containers. Drug orders are checked by a pharmacist, who then places the indicated number of doses in the client's medication drawer at scheduled intervals. When a dose is due, the nurse removes the medication and takes it to the client. Unit-dose wrappings should be left in place until the medication is given at the client's bedside.

Advantages of the unit-dose system include spending less time preparing drugs for administration, being able to identify most drugs until they are administered to the client, and having to calculate fewer doses. The major disadvantage is having to reorder or otherwise obtain the needed dose when it is not available in the client's medication drawer. This may lead to delayed or omitted doses. Whatever dispensing system is used, each dose of a drug must be recorded on a medication sheet after administration.

Controlled drugs, such as narcotic analgesics, are usually kept as a stock supply in a locked drawer or cabinet and replaced as needed. Each dose is signed out on a special narcotic sheet and recorded on the client's medication sheet. Each nurse must comply with legal regulations and agency policies for dispensing and recording controlled drugs.

## Medication orders

Nurses administer medications from orders by licensed physicians and dentists. Drug orders should include the full name of the client; the generic or trade name of the drug; the dose, route, and frequency of administration; and the date, time, and signature of the prescribing physician.

For clients in a hospital or other health-care agency, written orders are safer and much preferred, but occasionally verbal or telephone orders are acceptable. These are written on the client's order sheet, signed by the person taking the order, and later countersigned by the physician. Once the order is written, a copy is sent to the pharmacy, where the order is recorded and the drug is dispensed to the appropriate patient care unit. In many institutions, pharmacy staff prepare computer-generated medication administration records (MAR) for each 24-hour period. The MAR is used to record each dose of a drug that is administered and becomes part of the client's permanent medical record.

For outpatients, the procedure is essentially the same for drugs to be given immediately. For drugs to be taken at home, written prescriptions are given. In addition to the previous information, a prescription should include the client's address, instructions for taking the drug (*e.g.,* dose and frequency), whether the prescription is to be labeled with the name of the drug, and whether the prescription can be refilled. Prescriptions for Schedule II controlled drugs cannot be refilled; a new prescription is required.

To interpret medication orders accurately, the nurse must know some commonly used abbreviations for routes, dosages, and times of drug administration. These are listed in Table 2-1. If the nurse cannot read the physician's order or if the order seems erroneous, he or she must question the order before giving the drug.

**TABLE 2-1.  COMMON ABBREVIATIONS**

### *Routes of Drug Administration*

| | |
|---|---|
| IM | intramuscular |
| IV | intravenous |
| OD | right eye |
| OS | left eye |
| OU | both eyes |
| PO | by mouth, oral |
| SC | subcutaneous |
| SL | sublingual |

### *Drug Dosages*

| | |
|---|---|
| cc | cubic centimeter |
| g | gram |
| gr | grain |
| gt | drop* |
| mg | milligram |
| ml | milliliter |
| oz | ounce |
| tbsp | tablespoon |
| tsp | teaspoon |

### *Times of Drug Administration*

| | |
|---|---|
| a.c. | before meals |
| ad lib | as desired |
| b.i.d. | twice daily |
| h.s. | bedtime |
| p.c. | after meals |
| PRN | when needed |
| q.d. | every day, daily |
| q4h | every four hours |
| q.i.d. | four times daily |
| q.o.d. | every other day |
| stat | immediately |
| t.i.d. | three times daily |

* drops = gtt.

# Drug preparations and dosage forms

Drug preparations and dosage forms vary according to chemical characteristics, purposes, and routes of administration. Some drugs are available in only one preparation or dosage form; others are available in several forms.

Dosage forms of systemic drugs include liquids, tablets, capsules, suppositories, and transdermal and pump delivery systems. Systemic liquids are given orally or parenterally. Those given by injection must be sterile.

Tablets and capsules are given orally. Tablets contain active drug plus binders, colorants, preservatives, and other substances. They are available in many shapes, sizes, and colors. Capsules usually contain a powder or liquid form of active drug enclosed in a gelatin capsule. Most tablets and capsules dissolve in the acid fluids of the stomach and are absorbed in the alkaline fluids of the upper small intestine. Some—called *enteric-coated tablets and capsules*—are coated with a substance that is insoluble in stomach acids. This delays dissolution until the medications reach the intestine, usually to avoid gastric irritation or to keep the drug from being destroyed by gastric acid. Tablets for sublingual or buccal administration must be specifically formulated for such use.

Several controlled-release dosage forms or drug delivery systems have been developed to allow less frequent administration and more consistent serum drug levels. Although sustained-release tablets and capsules have been available for some years, newer formulations and mechanisms of release continue to be developed. Transdermal formulations include systemically absorbed clonidine, estrogen, fentanyl, nitroglycerin, and scopolamine. Pump delivery systems may be external or implanted under the skin and refillable or long-acting without refills. Pumps are used to administer insulin, narcotic analgesics, antineoplastics, and other drugs.

Ointments, creams, and suppositories are applied topically to skin or mucous membranes. They are usually specifically formulated for the intended route of administration.

# Calculating drug dosages

Nurses in most practice settings are infrequently required to calculate drug doses because pharmacists usually perform necessary calculations prior to dispensing drugs. Still, when calculations are needed, the importance of accuracy cannot be overemphasized. Accuracy requires basic skills in mathematics, knowledge of common units of measurement, and methods of using data in performing calculations.

## COMMONLY USED SYSTEMS OF MEASUREMENT

The most commonly used system of measurement is the *metric system*, in which the meter is used for linear measure, the gram for weight, and the liter for volume. One milliliter (ml) equals one cubic centimeter (cc), and both equal one gram (g) of water. The *apothecary system*, now obsolete and rarely used, has units called grains, minims, drams, ounces, pounds, pints, and quarts. The *household system*, with units of drops, teaspoons, tablespoons, and cups, is infrequently used in health-care agencies but may be used at home. Table 2-2 lists equivalent measurements within and among these systems. Equivalents are approximate.

A few drugs are ordered and measured in terms of units (U) or milliequivalents. Units express biologic activity in animal tests (*i.e.*, the amount of drug required to produce a particular response). Units are unique for each drug. Concentrations of insulin, heparin, and penicillin are expressed in units. There is *no* relationship or correspondence between a unit of insulin, for example, and a unit of heparin. These drugs are usually ordered in the number of units per dose (*e.g.*, NPH insulin 30 units SC every morning or heparin 5000 units SC q12h) and labeled in number of units per milliliter (U 100 insulin contains 100 units/ml; heparin may have 1000, 5000, or 10,000 units/ml). Milliequivalents express ionic activity of a drug. Drugs such as potassium chloride are ordered and labeled in the number of milliequivalents per dose, tablet, or milliliter.

## MATHEMATICAL CALCULATIONS

Most physicians' drug orders and most drug labels are expressed in metric units of measurement. If the amount specified in the order is the same as that on the drug label, no calculations are required, and preparing the right dose is a simple matter. For example, if the order

## TABLE 2-2. EQUIVALENTS

| Metric | Apothecary | Household |
|---|---|---|
| 1 ml = 1 cc | = 15 or 16 minims | = 15 or 16 drops |
| 4 or 5 ml | = 1 fluid dram | = 1 tsp |
| 60 or 65 mg | = 1 gr | |
| 30 or 32 mg | = ½ gr | |
| 30 g = 30 ml | = 1 oz | = 2 tbsp |
| 250 ml | = 8 oz | = 1 cup |
| 454 g | = 1 lb | |
| 500 ml = 500 cc | = 16 oz = 1 pint | = 1 pint |
| 1 L = 1000 ml | = 32 oz = 1 quart | = 1 quart |
| 1000 μg* | = 1 mg | |
| 1000 mg | = 1 g | |
| 1000 g = 1 kg | = 2.2 lb | = 2.2 lb |
| 0.6 g = 600 mg or 650 mg | = 10 gr | |

* μg = microgram

reads "acetaminophen 325 mg PO" and the drug label reads "acetaminophen 325-mg tablets," it is clear that one tablet is to be given.

What happens if the order calls for a 650-mg dose and 325-mg tablets are available? The question is "how many 325-mg tablets are needed to give a dose of 650 mg?" In this case, the answer can be readily calculated mentally to indicate two tablets. This is a simple example that also can be used to illustrate mathematical calculations. This problem can be solved by several acceptable methods; the following formula is presented because of its relative simplicity for students lacking a more familiar method.

$$\frac{D}{H} = \frac{X}{V}$$

D = desired dose (dose ordered by the physician, often in mg)

H = on-hand or available dose (dose on the drug label, often in mg/tablet, capsule, or milliliter)

X = unknown (number of tablets, in this example)

V = unit (one tablet, here)

$$\frac{650 \text{ mg}}{325 \text{ mg}} = \frac{X \text{ tablets}}{1 \text{ tablet}}$$

Cross multiply:

$$325X = 650$$

$$X = \frac{650}{325} = 2 \text{ tablets}$$

What happens if the order and the label are written in different units? For example, the order may read "amoxicillin 0.5 g" and the label may read "amoxicillin 500 mg/capsule." To calculate the number of capsules needed for the dose, the first step is to convert 0.5 g to the equivalent number of mg, or convert 500 mg to the equivalent number of g. *Note that the desired or ordered dose and the available or label dose must be in the same units of measurement.* Using equivalents (*i.e.*, 1 g = 1000 mg) listed in Table 2-2, an equation can be set up as follows:

$$\frac{1 \text{ g}}{1000 \text{ mg}} = \frac{0.5 \text{ g}}{X \text{ mg}}$$

$$X = 0.5 \times 1000 = 500 \text{ mg}$$

The next step is to use the new information in the formula, which then becomes:

$$\frac{D}{H} = \frac{X}{V}$$

$$\frac{500 \text{ mg}}{500 \text{ mg}} = \frac{X \text{ capsules}}{1 \text{ capsule}}$$

$$500X = 500$$

$$X = \frac{500}{500} = 1 \text{ capsule}$$

The same procedure and formula can be used to calculate portions of tablets or dosages of liquids. These are illustrated in the following problems:

1. Order: 25 mg PO
   Label: 50-mg tablet

$$\frac{25 \text{ mg}}{50 \text{ mg}} = \frac{X \text{ tablet}}{1 \text{ tablet}}$$

$$50X = 25$$

$$X = \frac{25}{50} = 0.5 \text{ tablet}$$

2. Order: 25 mg IM
   Label: 50 mg in 1 cc

$$\frac{25 \text{ mg}}{50 \text{ mg}} = \frac{X \text{ cc}}{1 \text{ cc}}$$

$$50X = 25$$

$$X = \frac{25}{50} = 0.5 \text{ cc}$$

3. Order: 50 mg PO
   Label: 10 mg/cc

$$\frac{50 \text{ mg}}{10 \text{ mg}} = \frac{X \text{ cc}}{1 \text{ cc}}$$

$$10X = 50$$

$$X = \frac{50}{10} = 5 \text{ cc}$$

4. Order: Heparin 5000 units
   Label: Heparin 10,000 units/ml

$$\frac{5000 \text{ units}}{10{,}000 \text{ units}} = \frac{X \text{ ml}}{1 \text{ ml}}$$

$$10{,}000X = 5000$$

$$X = \frac{5000}{10{,}000} = 0.5 \text{ ml}$$

5. Order: KCl 20 mEq
   Label: KCl 10 mEq/5 ml

$$\frac{20 \text{ mEq}}{10 \text{ mEq}} = \frac{X \text{ ml}}{5 \text{ ml}}$$

$$10X = 100$$

$$X = \frac{100}{10} = 10 \text{ ml}$$

# Routes of administration

Routes of administration depend largely on drug characteristics, client characteristics, and desired responses. The major routes are oral, parenteral, and topical. Each has advantages, disadvantages, indications for use, and specific techniques of administration.

## ORAL ROUTE

The oral route of drug administration is most commonly used. It is simple, convenient, and relatively inexpensive, and it can be used by most people. The main disadvantages are rather slow drug action and possible irritation of gastrointestinal mucosa, which may produce adverse effects, such as anorexia, nausea, vomiting, diarrhea, and ulceration.

Drugs also may be given through tubes placed into the gastrointestinal tract, such as nasogastric or gastrostomy tubes. In people who cannot take drugs orally for prolonged periods, this route is usually preferable to injections.

## PARENTERAL ROUTES

The term parenteral refers to any route other than gastrointestinal (enteral) but is commonly used to indicate subcutaneous (SC), IM, and IV injections. Injections require special drug preparations, equipment, and techniques.

### Drugs for injection

Parenteral drugs must be prepared, packaged, and administered in ways to maintain sterility. Vials are closed glass or plastic containers with rubber stoppers through which a sterile needle can be inserted for withdrawing medication. Single-dose vials generally do not contain a preservative and must be discarded after a dose is withdrawn; multiple-dose vials contain a preservative and may be reused if aseptic technique is maintained.

Ampules are sealed glass containers, the tops of which must be broken off to allow insertion of a needle and withdrawal of the medication. Broken ampules and any remaining medication are discarded; they are no longer sterile and cannot be reused. When vials or ampules contain a powder form of the drug, a sterile solution of water or 0.9% sodium chloride must be added and the drug dissolved before withdrawal. Use a filter needle to withdraw the medication from an ampule because broken glass may need to be removed from the drug solution.

Many injectable drugs, including various concentrations of commonly used parenteral narcotic analgesics, are available in ready-to-use plastic or glass syringes with attached needles. These units are inserted into specially designed holders and used like other needle-syringe units.

### Equipment for injections

Sterile needles and syringes are used to contain, measure, and administer parenteral medications. They may be packaged together or separately. Needles are available in various gauges and lengths. The term *gauge* refers to lumen size, with larger numbers indicating smaller lumen sizes. For example, a 25-gauge needle is smaller than an 18-gauge needle. Choice of needle gauge and length depends on route of administration, viscosity of the solution to be given, and size of the client. Usually, a 25-gauge, $5/8$-inch needle is used for SC injections, and a 22- or 20-gauge, 1.5-inch needle is used for IM injections. Other needle sizes are available for special uses, such as intradermal injections. A recent technologic advance was the development of needleless systems (*i.e.*, a plastic cannula on the syringe instead of a needle and vials which can be entered with the cannula and then reseal themselves). These systems were developed because of the risk of injury and spread of bloodborne pathogens, such as the viruses that cause acquired immunodeficiency syndrome (AIDS) and hepatitis B. When needles are used, avoid recapping them and dispose of them appropriately.

Syringes also are available in various sizes, such as 1, 3, 5, 10, 20, and 50 ml. The 3-ml size is probably used most often. It is usually plastic and is available with or without an attached needle. Syringes are calibrated so that drug doses can be measured accurately. However, the calibrations vary according to the size and type of syringe.

Insulin and tuberculin syringes are used for specific purposes. Insulin syringes are calibrated to measure up to 100 units of insulin. Safe practice requires that *only* insulin syringes be used to measure insulin and that they be used for no other drugs. Tuberculin syringes have a capacity of 1 ml. They should be used for small doses of any drug because measurements are more accurate than with larger syringes.

### Subcutaneous route

The SC route involves injection of drugs under the skin. This route is used for a small volume (about 1 ml or less) of drug. Absorption is slower, and drug action is generally longer with SC injections than with IV or IM injections. The SC route is commonly used for only a few drugs. Many drugs cannot be given SC because they are

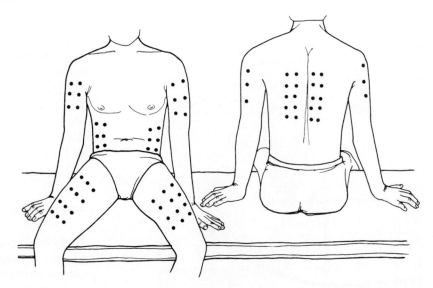

***FIGURE 2-1.*** Subcutaneous injection sites.

too irritating to SC tissues and may cause tissue necrosis and abscess formation. Insulin is a major drug that is given SC. Common sites for SC injections are the upper arms, abdomen, back, and thighs (Fig. 2-1).

## Intramuscular route

The IM route involves injection of drugs into certain muscles. This route is used for several drugs, usually in doses of 3 ml or less. Absorption is more rapid than from SC injections because muscle tissue has a greater blood supply. Site selection is especially important with IM injections because incorrect placement of the needle may damage blood vessels or nerves. Commonly used sites are the deltoid, dorsogluteal, ventrogluteal, and vastus lateralis. These sites must be selected by first identifying anatomic landmarks. The sites and anatomic landmarks are illustrated in Figures 2-2 through 2-5.

## Intravenous route

The IV route involves injection of a drug into the bloodstream. Drugs given intravenously act rapidly, and larger amounts can be given than by SC or IM injection. One way of giving drugs intravenously is to prepare the drug with a needle and syringe, insert the needle into a vein, and inject the drug. More often, however, drugs are given through an established IV line, intermittently or continuously. Direct injection is useful for emergency drugs, intermittent infusion is often used for antibiotics, and continuous infusion is used for potassium chloride and a few other drugs. The nurse should wear latex gloves to start IV infusions or when there is a risk of exposure to bloodborne pathogens, such as hepatitis B or the AIDS virus.

Drug administration is usually more comfortable and convenient for the client through an IV line. Disadvantages of this route include the time and skill required for venipuncture, the difficulty of maintaining IV lines, the greater potential for adverse reactions from rapid drug action, and possible complications of IV therapy (*i.e.*, bleeding, infection, and fluid overload).

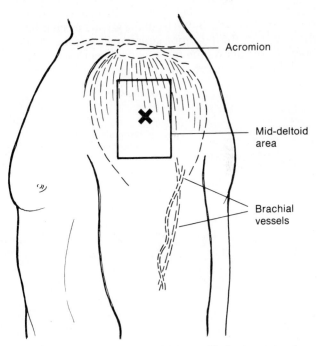

***FIGURE 2-2.*** Placement of the needle for insertion into the deltoid muscle. The area of injection is bounded by the lower edge of the acromion on the top to a point on the side of the arm opposite the axilla on the bottom. The side boundaries of the rectangular site are parallel to the arm and one third and two thirds of the way around the side of the arm.

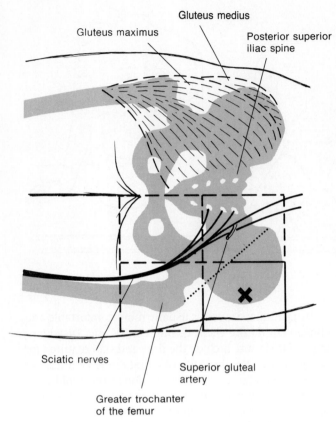

**FIGURE 2-3.** Proper placement of the needle for an IM injection into the dorsogluteal site. It is above and outside a diagonal line drawn from the greater trochanter of the femur to the posterior superior iliac spine. Notice how this site allows the nurse to avoid entering an area near the sciatic nerve and the superior gluteal artery.

## Other parenteral routes

Other parenteral routes include injection into layers of the skin (intradermal), injection into arteries (intra-arterial), injection into joints (intra-articular), and injection into cerebrospinal fluid (intrathecal). Nurses may administer drugs intradermally or intra-arterially (if an established arterial line is present); physicians administer intra-articular and intrathecal medications.

## TOPICAL ROUTES

Topical administration involves application of drugs to skin or mucous membranes. Application to mucous membranes includes drugs given by inhalation or instillation into the lungs, eyes, nose, and ears, as well as those inserted under the tongue (sublingual), into the cheek (buccal), and into the vagina or rectum.

An advantage of topical administration is that many of the drugs act locally where applied; therefore, the likelihood of systemic adverse reactions is decreased. (However, several drugs are given topically for systemic effects.) A disadvantage is that specific drug preparations must be used for the various routes. Thus, only dermatologic preparations are safe to use on skin, only ophthalmic drugs are used in the eyes, only a few drugs are given sublingually or buccally, and only vaginal or rectal preparations are given by those respective routes.

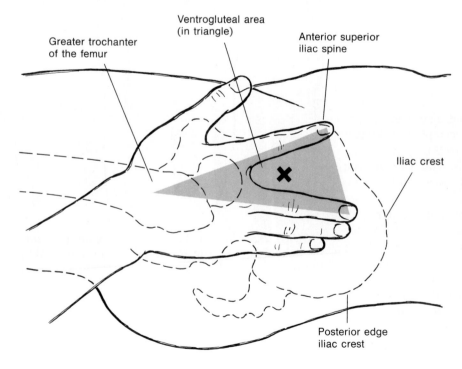

**FIGURE 2-4.** Placement of the needle for insertion into the ventrogluteal area. Notice how the nurse's palm is placed on the greater trochanter, and the index finger on the anterior superior iliac spine. The middle finger is spread posteriorly as far as possible along the iliac crest. The injection is made in the middle of the triangle formed by the nurse's fingers and the iliac crest.

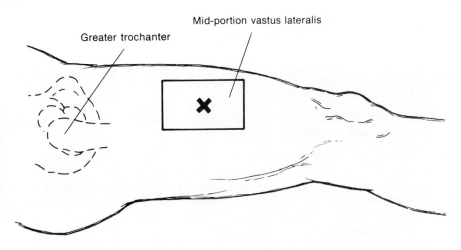

Greater trochanter

Mid-portion vastus lateralis

**FIGURE 2-5.** Placement of the needle for insertion into the vastus lateralis. It is generally easier to have the client lying on his or her back. However, the client may be sitting when using this site for IM injections. It is a suitable site for children when the nurse grasps the muscle in her hand to concentrate the muscle mass for injection.

## NURSING ACTIONS: DRUG ADMINISTRATION

| *Nursing Actions* | *Rationale/Explanation* |
|---|---|
| **1. Follow general rules for administering medications safely and effectively.** | |
| **a.** Prepare and give drugs in well-lighted areas, as free of interruptions and distractions as possible. | To prevent errors in selecting ordered drugs, calculating dosages, and identifying clients |
| **b.** Wash hands before preparing medications and, if needed, during administration. | To prevent infection and cross-contamination |
| **c.** Use sterile technique in preparing and administering injections. | To prevent infection. Sterile technique involves using sterile needles and syringes, using sterile drug solutions, not touching sterile objects to any unsterile objects, and cleansing injection sites with an antiseptic. |
| **d.** Read the medication administration record (MAR) carefully. Read the label on the drug container, and compare with the MAR in terms of drug, dosage or concentration, and route of administration. | For accurate drug administration. Most nursing texts instruct the nurse to read a drug label three times: when removing the container, while measuring the dose, and before returning the container. |
| **e.** Do not leave medications unattended. | To prevent accidental or deliberate ingestion by anyone other than the intended person. Also, to prevent contamination or spilling of medications. |
| **f.** Identify the client, preferably by comparing the identification wrist band to the medication sheet. | This is the best way to verify identity. Calling by name, relying on the name on a door or bed, and asking someone else are unreliable methods, although they must be used occasionally when the client lacks a name band. |
| **g.** Identify yourself, if indicated, and state your reason for approaching the client. For example, "I'm . . . I have your medication for you." | Explaining actions helps to decrease client anxiety and increase cooperation in taking prescribed medication. |
| **h.** Position the client appropriately for the intended route of administration. | To prevent complications, such as aspiration of oral drugs into the lungs |
| **i.** Provide water or other supplies as needed. | To promote comfort of the client and to ensure drug administration |
| **j.** Do not leave medications at the bedside as a general rule. Common exceptions are antacids, nitroglycerin, and eye medications. | To prevent omitting or losing the drug or hoarding of the drug by the client |

*(continued)*

**Nursing Actions**

**Rationale/Explanation**

**k.** Do not give a drug when signs and symptoms of toxicity are present. Notify the physician, and record that the drug was omitted and why.

Additional doses of a drug increase toxicity. However, drugs are not omitted without a careful assessment of the client's condition and a valid reason.

**l.** Record drug administration (or omission) as soon as possible and according to agency policies.

To maintain an accurate record of drugs received by the client

**m.** If it is necessary to omit a scheduled dose for some reason, the decision to give the dose later or omit it completely depends largely on the drug and frequency of administration. Generally, give drugs ordered once or twice daily at a later time. For others, omit the one dose, and give the drug at the next scheduled time.

Clients may be unable to take the drug at the scheduled time because of diagnostic tests or many other reasons. A temporary change in the time of administration—usually for one dose only—may be necessary to maintain therapeutic effects.

**n.** For medications ordered as needed (PRN), assess the client's condition; check the physician's orders or MAR for the name, dose, and frequency of administration; and determine the time of the most recently administered dose.

Administration of PRN medications is somewhat different from that of regularly scheduled drugs. Analgesics, antiemetics, and antipyretics are often ordered PRN.

**o.** For narcotics and other controlled substances, sign drugs out on separate narcotic records according to agency policies.

To meet legal requirements for dispensing controlled substances

**p.** If, at any time during drug preparation or administration, any question arises regarding the drug, the dose, or whether the client is supposed to receive it, check the original physician's order. If the order is not clear, call the physician for clarification before giving the drug.

To promote safety and prevent errors. The same procedure applies when the client questions drug orders at the bedside. For example, the client may state he has been receiving different drugs or different doses.

**2. For oral medications**
   **a.** With adults

   (1) To give tablets or capsules, open the unit-dose wrapper, place medication in a medicine cup, and give the cup to the client. For solutions, hold the cup at eye level, and measure the dosage at the bottom of the meniscus. For suspensions, shake or invert containers to mix the medication before measuring the dose.

To maintain clean technique and measure doses accurately. Suspensions settle on standing, and if not mixed, diluent may be given rather than the active drug.

   (2) Have the client in a sitting position when not contraindicated.

To decrease risks of aspirating medication into lungs. Aspiration may lead to difficulty in breathing and aspiration pneumonia.

   (3) Give before, with, or after meals as indicated by the specific drug.

Food in the stomach usually delays drug absorption and action. It also decreases gastric irritation, a common side effect of oral drugs. Giving drugs at appropriate times in relation to food intake can increase therapeutic effects and decrease adverse effects.

   (4) Give most oral drugs with a full glass (8 oz) of water or other fluid.

To promote dissolution and absorption of tablets and capsules. Also, to decrease gastric irritation by diluting drug concentration.

   **b.** With children, liquids or chewable tablets are usually given.

Children under 5 years of age are often unable to swallow tablets or capsules.

   (1) Measure and give liquids to infants with a dropper or syringe, placing medication on the tongue or buccal mucosa and giving slowly.

For accurate measurement and administration. Giving slowly decreases risks of aspiration.

## Nursing Actions

## Rationale/Explanation

(2) Medications are often mixed with juice, applesauce, or other vehicle.

To increase the child's ability and willingness to take the medication. If this is done, use a small amount, and be sure the child takes all of it; otherwise, less than the ordered dose is given.

**c.** Do not give oral drugs if the client is:

(1) NPO (receiving nothing by mouth)

Oral drugs and fluids may interfere with diagnostic tests or be otherwise contraindicated. Most drugs can be given after diagnostic tests are completed. If the client is having surgery, preoperative drug orders are cancelled. New orders are written postoperatively.

(2) Vomiting

Oral drugs and fluids increase vomiting. Thus, no benefit results from the drug. Also, fluid and electrolyte problems may result from loss of gastric acid.

(3) Excessively sedated or unconscious

To avoid aspiration of drugs into the lungs owing to impaired ability to swallow

**3. For medications given by nasogastric tube:**

**a.** Use a liquid preparation when possible. If necessary, crush a tablet or empty a capsule into about 30 ml of water and mix well. Do not crush enteric coated or sustained-release products, and do not empty sustained-release capsules.

Particles of tablets or powders from capsules may obstruct the tube lumen. Altering sustained-release products increases risks of overdosage and adverse effects.

**b.** Use a clean bulb syringe or other catheter-tipped syringe.

The syringe allows aspiration and serves as a funnel for instillation of medication and fluids into the stomach.

**c.** Before instilling medication, aspirate gastric fluid or instill 10 to 20 cc of air while listening with a stethoscope over the stomach.

To be sure the tube is in the stomach

**d.** Instill medication by gravity flow, and follow it with at least 50 ml of water. Do not allow the syringe to empty completely between additions.

Gravity flow is safer than applying pressure. Water "pushes" the drug into the stomach and rinses the tube, thereby maintaining tube patency. Additional water or other fluids may be given according to fluid needs of the client. Add fluids to avoid instilling air into the stomach unnecessarily with possible client discomfort.

**e.** Clamp off the tube from suction or drainage for at least 30 minutes.

To avoid removing the medication from the stomach

**4. For SC injections:**

**a.** Use only sterile drug preparations labeled or commonly used for SC injections.

Many parenteral drugs are too irritating to subcutaneous tissue for use by this route.

**b.** Use a 25-gauge, ⅝-inch needle for most SC injections.

This size needle is effective for most clients and drugs.

**c.** Select an appropriate injection site, based on client preferences, drug characteristics, and visual inspection of possible sites. In long-term therapy, such as with insulin, rotate injection sites. Avoid areas with lumps, bruises, or other lesions.

These techniques allow the client to participate in his or her care; avoid tissue damage and unpredictable absorption, which occur with repeated injections in the same location; and increase client comfort and cooperation.

**d.** Cleanse the site with an alcohol sponge.

To prevent infection

**e.** Tighten the skin or pinch a fold of skin and tissue between thumb and fingers.

Either is acceptable for most clients. If the client is obese, tightening the skin may be easier. If the client is very thin, the tissue fold may keep the needle from hitting bone.

*(continued)*

| *Nursing Actions* | *Rationale/Explanation* |
|---|---|
| **f.** .Hold the syringe like a pencil, and insert the needle quickly at a 45-degree angle. Use enough force to penetrate the skin and subcutaneous tissue in one smooth movement. | To give the drug correctly with minimal client discomfort |
| **g.** Release the skin so that both hands are free to manipulate the syringe. Pull back gently on the plunger (aspirate). If no blood enters the syringe, inject the drug. If blood is aspirated into the syringe, remove the needle, and reprepare the medication. | To prevent accidental injection into the bloodstream. Blood return in the syringe is an uncommon occurrence. |
| **h.** Remove the needle quickly and apply gentle pressure for a few seconds. | To prevent bleeding |
| **5. For IM injections:** | |
| **a.** Use only drug preparations labeled or commonly used for IM injections. Check label instructions for mixing drugs in powder form. | Some parenteral drug preparations cannot be given safely by the IM route. |
| **b.** Use a 1½-inch needle for most adults and a ⅝ to 1½-inch needle for children, depending on the size of the client. | A long needle is necessary to reach muscle tissue, which underlies subcutaneous fat. |
| **c.** Use the smallest gauge needle that will accommodate the medication. A 22 gauge is satisfactory for most drugs; a 20 gauge may be used for viscous medications. | To decrease tissue damage and client discomfort |
| **d.** Select an appropriate injection site, based on client preferences, drug characteristics, anatomic landmarks, and visual inspection of possible sites. Rotate sites if frequent injections are being given, and avoid areas with lumps, bruises, or other lesions. | To increase client comfort and participation and to avoid tissue damage. Identification of anatomic landmarks is mandatory for safe administration of IM drugs. |
| **e.** Cleanse the site with an alcohol sponge. | To prevent infection |
| **f.** Tighten the skin, hold the syringe like a pencil, and insert the needle quickly at a 90-degree angle. Use enough force to penetrate the skin and subcutaneous tissue into the muscle in one smooth motion. | To give the drug correctly with minimal client discomfort |
| **g.** Aspirate (see 4g, SC Injections). | |
| **h.** Remove the needle quickly and apply pressure for several seconds. | To prevent bleeding |
| **6. For IV injections:** | |
| **a.** Use only drug preparations that are labeled for IV use. | Others are not likely to be pure enough for safe injection into the bloodstream or are not compatible with the blood pH (7.35–7.45). |
| **b.** Check label instructions for the type and amount of fluid to use for dissolving or diluting the drug. | Some drugs require special preparation techniques to maintain solubility or pharmacologic activity. Most drugs in powder form can be dissolved in sterile water or sodium chloride for injection. Most drug solutions can be given with dextrose or dextrose and sodium chloride IV solutions. |
| **c.** Prepare drugs just before use, as a general rule. Also, add drugs to IV fluids just before use. | Some drugs are unstable in solution. In some agencies, drugs are mixed and added to IV fluids in the pharmacy. This is the preferred method because sterility can be better maintained. |

*(continued)*

## Nursing Actions

## Rationale/Explanation

**d.** For venipuncture and direct injection into a vein, apply a tourniquet, select a site in the arm, cleanse the skin with an antiseptic (*e.g.,* povidone-iodine or alcohol), insert the needle, and aspirate a small amount of blood into the syringe to be sure that the needle is in the vein. Remove the tourniquet, and inject the drug slowly. Remove the needle and apply pressure until there is no evidence of bleeding.

For safe and accurate drug administration with minimal risk to the client. The length of time required to give the drug depends on the specific drug and the amount. Slow administration, over several minutes, allows immediate discontinuation if adverse effects occur.

**e.** For administration by an established IV line:

(1) Check the infusion for patency and flow rate. Check the venipuncture site for signs of infiltration and phlebitis before each drug dose.

The solution must be flowing freely for accurate drug administration. If infiltration or phlebitis is present, do not give the drug until a new IV line is begun.

(2) For direct injection, cleanse an injection site on the IV tubing, insert the needle, and inject the drug slowly.

Most tubings have injection sites to facilitate drug administration.

(3) To use a volume control set, fill it with 50 to 100 ml of IV fluid, and clamp it so that no further fluid enters the chamber and dilutes the drug. Inject the drug into an injection site after cleansing the site with an alcohol sponge and infuse, usually in 1 hour or less. Once the drug is infused, add solution to maintain the infusion.

This method is used for administration of antibiotics on an intermittent schedule. Dilution of the drug decreases adverse effects.

(4) To use a "piggyback" method, add the drug to 50 to 100 ml of IV solution in a separate container. Attach the IV tubing and a needle. Insert the needle in an injection site on the main IV tubing after cleansing the site. Infuse the drug over 15 to 60 minutes, depending on the drug.

This method is also used for intermittent administration of antibiotics and other drugs. Whether a volume control or piggyback apparatus is used depends on agency policy and equipment available.

**f.** When more than one drug is to be given, flush the line between drugs. Do not mix drugs in syringes or in IV fluids unless the drug literature states that the drugs are compatible.

Physical and chemical interactions between the drugs may occur and cause precipitation, inactivation, or increased toxicity. Most nursing units have charts depicting drug compatibility, or information may be obtained from the pharmacy.

**7. For application to skin:**
Use drug preparations labeled for dermatologic use. Cleanse the skin, remove any previously applied medication, and apply the drug in a thin layer. For broken skin or open lesions, use sterile gloves, tongue blade, or cotton-tipped applicator to apply the drug.

To promote therapeutic effects and minimize adverse effects

**8. For instillation of eye drops:**
Use drug preparations labeled for ophthalmic use. Wash your hands, open the eye to expose the conjunctival sac, and drop the medication into the sac, not on the eyeball, without touching the dropper tip to anything. Provide a tissue for blotting any excess drug. If two or more eye drops are scheduled at the same time, wait 1 to 5 minutes between instillations.

Ophthalmic preparations must be sterile to avoid infection. Blot any excess drug from the inner canthus near the nose to decrease systemic absorption of the drug.

With children, prepare the medication, place the child in a head-lowered position, steady the hand holding the medication on the child's head, gently retract the lower lid, and instill the medication into the conjunctival sac.

Careful positioning and restraint to avoid sudden movements are necessary to decrease risks of injury to the eye.

*(continued)*

| *Nursing Actions* | *Rationale/Explanation* |
|---|---|
| **9. For instillation of nose drops and nasal sprays:**<br>Have the client hold his or her head back, and drop the medication into the nostrils. Give only as ordered.<br>    With children, place in a supine position with the head lowered, instill the medication, and maintain the position for 2 to 3 minutes. Then, place the child in a prone position. | When nose drops are used for rhinitis and nasal congestion accompanying the common cold, overuse results in a rebound congestion that may be worse than the original symptom. |
| **10. For instillation of ear medications:**<br>Open the ear canal by pulling the ear up and back for adults, down and back for children, and drop the medication on the side of the canal. | To straighten the canal and promote maximal contact between medication and tissue |
| **11. For rectal suppositories:**<br>Lubricate the end with a water-soluble lubricant, wear a glove or finger cot, and insert into the rectum the length of the finger. Place the suppository next to the mucosal wall. If the client prefers and is able, provide supplies for self-administration. | To promote absorption. Allowing self-administration may prevent embarrassment to the client. Be sure the client knows the correct procedure. |
| **12. For vaginal medications:**<br>Use gloves or an applicator for insertion. If an applicator is used, wash thoroughly with soap and water after each use. If the client prefers and is able, provide supplies for self-administration. | Some women may be embarrassed and prefer self-administration. Be sure the client knows the correct procedure. |

## Review and Application Exercises

1. When giving an oral medication, what are some interventions to aid absorption and hasten therapeutic effects?
2. What are advantages and disadvantages of the oral route and the IV route of drug administration?
3. For a client who receives all medications through a nasogastric feeding tube, which dosage forms are acceptable? Which are not acceptable and why?
4. Which dosage forms need to be kept sterile during administration?
5. What are some legal factors that influence a nurse's administration of medications?
6. When administering medications, what safety precautions are needed with various routes?
7. What safety precautions does the nurse need to practice consistently to avoid self-injury and exposure to bloodborne pathogens?

8. With a client who refuses an important medication, what approaches or interventions might persuade the client to take the medication? Would the same approach be indicated if the medication were a vitamin supplement or a laxative?

## Selected References

Bolinger, A. M., Murphy, V. A., & Bubica, G. (1992). General pediatric therapy. In M. A. Koda-Kimble & L. Y. Young (Eds.), *Applied therapeutics: The clinical use of drugs* (5th ed.) (pp. 77-1–77-24). Vancouver, WA: Applied Therapeutics.

(1993). *Drug facts and comparisons*. St. Louis: Facts and Comparisons.

Holder, C., & Alexander, J. (1990). A new and improved guide to IV therapy. *American Journal of Nursing, 90*, 43–47.

Kee, J. L., & Hayes, E. R. (1993). *Pharmacology: A nursing process approach*. Philadelphia: W.B. Saunders.

Swonger, A. K., & Matejski, M. P. (1991). *Nursing pharmacology: An integrated approach to drug therapy and nursing practice* (2nd ed.). Philadelphia: J.B. Lippincott.

# CHAPTER 3

# Nursing Process in Drug Therapy

Drug therapy involves the use of drugs to prevent or treat disease processes and manifestations. It may save lives, improve the quality of life, and otherwise benefit recipients. It also may cause harm because drugs may cause virtually any sign or symptom. Adverse effects and failure to achieve therapeutic effects may occur with correct use, but they are more likely to occur with incorrect use. Physicians, pharmacists, clients, and nurses all have important roles to play in the safe and effective use of drugs. For the nurse, drug therapy is one of many responsibilities in client care. To fulfill this responsibility, the nurse must be knowledgeable about pharmacology (drugs and their effects on the body), physiology (normal body functions), and pathophysiology (alterations in mental and physical functions due to disease processes) and must be adept at using all steps of the nursing process.

Chapter 1 included general information about drugs and human responses to drugs. Chapter 2 emphasized techniques of preparing and administering drugs safely and effectively. Although the importance of safe and accurate administration cannot be overemphasized, this is only one aspect of the nursing process in drug therapy. The nurse also must monitor responses to drug therapy, both therapeutic and adverse, and teach clients about drugs, both prescribed and over-the-counter. To help the nurse acquire knowledge and skills related to drug therapy, this chapter includes suggestions for studying pharmacology, legal responsibilities, nursing process guidelines, general principles of drug therapy, and general nursing actions.

## Using the prototype approach to study pharmacology

The beginning student of pharmacology is faced with a bewildering number and variety of drugs. This number can be greatly reduced by concentrating initial study on therapeutic classifications or groups of drugs and prototypes of those groups. For example, narcotic analgesics is one classification or group, and morphine is the prototype of that group. Morphine and other narcotic analgesics have many common characteristics, including the following:

1. They are used primarily to relieve pain.
2. They produce central nervous system (CNS) depression ranging from slight drowsiness to unconsciousness, depending on dose.
3. A major adverse reaction is respiratory depression (depression of the respiratory center in the medulla oblongata as part of the CNS depression). Thus, the nurse must check rate and depth of respiration.
4. They have a high potential for abuse and dependence; therefore, their use is regulated by narcotic laws and requires special records and procedures.
5. They must be used with caution in people who already have respiratory depression or an impaired level of consciousness.

Understanding these characteristics makes studying all other narcotic analgesics easier because other drugs are compared to morphine, especially in their ability to relieve pain and likelihood of causing respiratory depression.

Once you know the characteristics of the major drug groups, you must continue to study to add depth and scope to your drug knowledge. Almost all new or unfamiliar drugs fit into an established classification. For example, you may know that the unfamiliar drug is a thiazide diuretic. By recalling your knowledge of this drug classification, you have a base of information on which to build as you study the unfamiliar drug.

## GUIDELINES FOR EFFECTIVE STUDY

When learning about an individual drug, you must assimilate a large amount of data. Although some people try to memorize drug information, this is not an effective way to learn, retain, and apply drug knowledge. Some guidelines for effective study include the following:

1. *Try to understand how the drug acts in the body.* This allows you to predict therapeutic effects and to predict, prevent, or minimize adverse effects by early detection and treatment.
2. *Concentrate your study efforts on major characteristics.* These include the main indications for use, common and potentially serious adverse effects, conditions in which the drug is relatively or absolutely contraindicated, usual dosage ranges, and related nursing care needs.
3. *Compare the drug with a prototype when possible.* Relating the unknown to the known aids learning and retention of knowledge.
4. *Keep an authoritative, up-to-date drug reference readily available, preferably at work and home.* This is a much more reliable source of drug information than memory. Use the reference freely whenever you encounter an unfamiliar drug or when a question arises about a familiar one.
5. *Use your own words, when possible, when taking notes or writing drug information cards.* The mental processing required to put information in your own words aids learning and retention.
6. *Mentally practice applying drug knowledge in nursing care* by asking yourself, "What if I have a client who is receiving this drug? What must I do? For what must I observe? What if my client is an elderly person or a child?"

## Legal responsibilities of the nurse

Registered nurses are legally empowered, under state nurse practice acts, to give medications ordered by licensed physicians and dentists. In some states, nurse practitioners may prescribe medications.

*When giving medications, the nurse is legally responsible for safe and accurate administration* (right drug, right dose, right client, right route, and right time). This means the nurse may be held liable for *not* giving a drug or for giving a wrong drug or a wrong dose. Also, *the nurse is expected to have sufficient drug knowledge to recognize and question erroneous orders.* If, after questioning the prescribing physician and seeking information from other authoritative sources, the nurse considers that giving the drug is unsafe, the nurse must refuse to give the drug. The fact that a physician wrote an erroneous order does not excuse the nurse from legal liability if he or she carries out that order. The nurse also is legally responsible for actions delegated to people who are inadequately prepared for or legally barred from administering medications (such as nursing assistants).

The nurse is responsible for storing narcotics and other controlled substances in locked containers, administering them only to people for whom they are prescribed, recording each dose given on appropriate narcotic sheets and on the client's medication administration record, counting the amounts of each drug at the end of a work shift, and reporting any discrepancies to the proper authorities.

The nurse who follows safe practices in giving medications does not need to be excessively concerned about legal liability. The basic techniques and guidelines listed in Chapter 2 are aimed at safe and accurate preparation and administration; most errors result when these practices are not followed consistently.

Legal responsibilities in other aspects of drug therapy are less tangible and clear-cut. However, nurses are generally expected to observe clients for therapeutic and adverse effects and to teach clients safe and effective self-administration of drugs when indicated.

## *Applying the Nursing Process in Drug Therapy*

The nursing process is a systematic way of gathering information and using that information to plan and provide client care and to evaluate the outcomes of care. Knowledge and skill in the nursing process are required for drug therapy as in other aspects of client care. Each of the five steps of the nursing process is described and illustrated below.

### Assessment

The first step involves collecting data about client characteristics known to affect drug therapy. This can be done by observing and interviewing the client, interviewing family members or others involved in client care, completing a physical assessment, reviewing medical records for pertinent laboratory and diagnostic test reports, and other methods. Information is also sought about the ordered drugs, if needed. Data from all sources are then analyzed.

## Nursing diagnoses

These statements, as developed by the North American Nursing Diagnosis Association, describe client problems or needs and are based on assessment data. They should be individualized according to the client's condition and particular drug(s). Thus, the nursing diagnoses chosen and the number needed to reflect adequately the client's condition vary considerably. Because almost any nursing diagnosis may apply in specific circumstances, this text emphasizes those diagnoses that generally apply to any course of drug therapy. These and others may be used to guide the nursing care of clients in relation to their drug therapy.

## Planning/Goals

This step involves stating the expected outcomes of the prescribed drug therapy. As a general rule, goals should be stated in terms of client behavior, not nurse behavior.

## Interventions

This step involves implementing the planned activities. General interventions include preventing the need for drug therapy and using nondrug measures to increase safety and effectiveness. Specific interventions include actions needed once a drug is ordered (i.e., accurate administration, observing for therapeutic and adverse effects). In addition, teaching clients and family members is an important intervention in drug therapy.

## Evaluation

This step involves evaluating the client's status in relation to stated goals and expected outcomes. Some outcomes can be evaluated within a few minutes of drug administration (e.g., relief of acute pain following administration of an analgesic). Most, however, require much longer periods of time, often extending from hospitalization and direct observation by the nurse to self-care at home and occasional contact with a health-care provider.

With the current emphasis on outpatient treatment and short hospitalizations, the client is likely to experience brief contacts with many health-care providers rather than more extensive contacts with a few health-care providers. These factors, plus a client's usual reluctance to admit noncompliance, contribute to difficulties in evaluating outcomes of drug therapy. These difficulties can be managed by using appropriate techniques and criteria of evaluation.

Techniques include directly observing a client's status; interviewing the client, family members, or other health-care providers; and checking medication records and laboratory and diagnostic test reports. With outpatients, "pill counts" may be done to compare doses remaining with the number prescribed during a designated time. These techniques may be used with every contact with a client, if appropriate.

General criteria include progress toward stated outcomes, such as relief of symptoms, accurate administration, avoidance of preventable adverse effects, compliance with instructions, and others. Specific criteria indicate parameters that must be measured to evaluate responses to particular drugs (e.g., normal blood sugar with antidiabetic drugs or normal blood pressure with antihypertensive drugs, if these are realistic for the particular client).

Each step of the nursing process is more specifically illustrated below.

## Assessment

Initially (before drug therapy is started or on first contact), assess each client regarding age, weight, health status (especially cardiovascular, renal, and hepatic function), acute or chronic disease processes, and ability to function in usual activities of daily living. The effects of these client-related factors on drug therapy are discussed in Chapter 1.

Assess for previous and current use of prescription, nonprescription, and nontherapeutic (e.g., alcohol, caffeine, nicotine, cocaine, marijuana) drugs. A medication history (Box 3-1) is useful. Some specific questions and areas of assessment include:

- What are current drug orders?
- What does the client know about current drugs? Is teaching needed?
- What drugs has the client taken before? Include any drugs taken regularly, such as those taken for chronic illnesses (hypertension, diabetes mellitus, arthritis, and others). It may be helpful to ask specifically about corticosteroids, oral contraceptives, and other hormonal drugs because they may have long-lasting effects. It also may be helpful to ask about nonprescription (over-the-counter, or OTC) drugs for headache, colds, indigestion, or constipation, because some people do not think of OTC preparations as drugs
- Has the client ever had an allergic reaction to a drug? If so, what signs and symptoms occurred? This information is necessary because many people describe minor nausea and other symptoms as allergic reactions. Unless the reaction is further explored, the client may have therapy withheld inappropriately.
- What are the client's attitudes about drugs? Try to obtain information to help assess whether the client takes drugs freely or reluctantly, is likely to comply with a prescribed drug regimen, and is likely to abuse drugs.
- If long-term drug therapy is likely, can the client afford to buy medications?
- Can the client communicate his or her needs, such as requesting medication? Can he or she swallow oral medications? Are any other conditions present that influence drug therapy?
- In addition to nursing assessment data, use progress notes, laboratory reports, and other sources as they are available and relevant. As part of the initial assessment, obtain baseline data on measurements to be used in monitoring therapeutic or adverse effects. Specific data to be acquired depend on the medication and the client's condition. Laboratory tests of liver, kidney, and bone marrow function are often helpful because some drugs may damage these organs. Also, if liver or kidney damage exists, drug metabolism or excretion may be altered. More specific laboratory tests include serum potassium levels before diuretic therapy, culture and susceptibility studies before antimicrobial therapy, and blood clotting tests before anticoagulant therapy. Nonlaboratory data that may be relevant include vital signs, weight, and urine output.

After drug therapy is begun, continue to assess the client's response in relation to therapeutic and adverse effects, ability and willingness to take the drugs as prescribed, and other aspects of safe and effective drug therapy.

## BOX 3-1. MEDICATION HISTORY

Name _____ Age _____

Health problems, acute and chronic

Are you allergic to any medications?

If yes, describe specific effects or symptoms.

### Part 1: Prescription Medications

1. Do you take any prescription medications on a regular basis?

2. If yes, ask the following about each medication.
   Name                                    Dose
   Frequency                               Specific times
   How long taken                          Reason for use

3. Are you able to take this medicine pretty much as prescribed?

4. Does anyone else help you take your medications?

5. What information or instructions were you given when the medications were first prescribed?

6. Do you think the medication is doing what it was prescribed to do?

7. Have you had any problems that you attribute to the medication?

8. Do you take any prescription medications on an irregular basis?
   If yes, ask the following about each medication.
   Name                                    Reason
   Dose                                    How long taken
   Frequency

### Part 2: Nonprescription Medications
Do you take OTC medications?

| | | Medication | | |
|---|---|---|---|---|
| **Problem** | Yes/No | Name | Amount | Frequency |
| Pain | | | | |
| Headache | | | | |
| Sleep | | | | |
| Cold | | | | |
| Indigestion | | | | |
| Heartburn | | | | |
| Diarrhea | | | | |
| Constipation | | | | |
| Other | | | | |

### Part 3: Social Drugs

| | Yes/No | Amount |
|---|---|---|
| Coffee | | |
| Tea | | |
| Cola drinks | | |
| Alcohol | | |
| Tobacco | | |

## Nursing diagnoses

- Knowledge Deficit: Drug therapy regimen (*e.g.*, drug ordered, reason for use, expected effects, expected duration, and monitoring of response by health-care providers, including diagnostic tests and office visits)
- Knowledge Deficit: Safe and effective self-administration (when appropriate)
- High Risk for Injury: Adverse drug effects
- Noncompliance: Overuse
- Noncompliance: Underuse

## Planning/Goals

*The client will:*
- Receive or take drugs as prescribed
- Experience relief of signs and symptoms
- Avoid preventable adverse drug effects
- Avoid unnecessary drug ingestion
- Self-administer drugs safely and accurately
- Verbalize essential drug information
- Keep appointments for monitoring and follow-up

## Interventions

Use nondrug measures when appropriate to decrease the need for drugs, to enhance therapeutic effects, or to decrease adverse effects. General interventions include:
- Promoting healthful life-styles in terms of nutrition, fluids, exercise, rest, and sleep
- Handwashing and other measures to prevent infection
- Positioning
- Assisting to cough and deep breathe
- Ambulating
- Applying heat or cold
- Increasing or decreasing sensory stimulation
- Scheduling activities to allow periods of rest or sleep
- Recording vital signs, fluid intake, urine output, and other assessment data
- Implementing specific interventions indicated by a particular drug or the client's condition

*Teach clients:*
- Healthful life-style habits in relation to nutrition, exercise, rest, and sleep
- To avoid drug use when feasible and to use drugs cautiously when necessary
- Nondrug measures to prevent or relieve common health problems and prevent the need for drug therapy
- Nondrug measures to enhance beneficial effects and decrease adverse effects of drugs
- Not to take drugs prescribed for another person and not to share prescription drugs with anyone else. The likelihood of having the right drug in the right dose is extremely remote and the risk of adverse effects extremely high under such circumstances.
- To notify any physician or dentist of drugs being taken

## Evaluation

Observe and interview clients and check appropriate medical records about drug usage, compliance with prescribed therapy, relief of symptoms, adverse effects, and drug knowledge.

# General principles of drug therapy

## GENERAL GUIDELINES

1. *The goal of drug therapy should be to maximize beneficial effects and minimize adverse effects.*
2. *Expected benefits should outweigh potential adverse effects.* Thus, drugs generally should not be prescribed for trivial problems or problems for which nondrug measures are effective. Nondrug measures are generally safer than drug therapy.
3. *Drug therapy should be individualized.* Many variables influence a drug's effects on the human body. Failure to consider these variables may decrease therapeutic effects or increase risks of adverse effects to an unacceptable level.

## GENERAL DRUG SELECTION AND DOSAGE CONSIDERATIONS

Numerous factors must be considered when choosing a drug and dosage range for a particular client, including the following:

1. For the most part, use as few drugs in as few doses as possible. Minimizing the number of drugs and the frequency of administration increases client compliance with the prescribed drug regimen and decreases risks of serious adverse effects, including hazardous drug interactions. There are notable exceptions to this basic rule. For example, multiple drugs are commonly used to treat severe hypertension or serious infections.
2. Individual drugs allow greater flexibility and individualization of dosage than fixed-dose combinations. However, fixed-dose combinations are commonly used because they are convenient and may promote compliance. Individualization may be accomplished by giving separate drugs initially. Then, if established dosages are similar to those in a combination product, the combination product may be given.
3. The least amount of the least potent drug that will yield therapeutic benefit should be given to decrease adverse reactions. For example, if a mild non-narcotic and a strong narcotic analgesic are both ordered, give the non-narcotic drug if it is effective in relieving pain.
4. Recommended dosages are listed in amounts likely to be effective for most people, but they are only guidelines to be interpreted according to the client characteristics discussed previously. For example, clients with serious illnesses may require larger doses of some drugs than clients with milder illnesses and

clients with severe kidney disease often need much smaller than usual doses of renally excreted drugs.

5. Treatment with a particular drug can be started rapidly or slowly. If a drug has a long half-life and maximal therapeutic effects do not usually occur for several days or weeks, the physician may give a limited number of relatively large (loading) doses followed by a regular schedule of smaller (maintenance) doses. When drug actions are not urgent, therapy may be initiated with a maintenance dose.

6. Different salts of the same drug rarely differ pharmacologically. Hydrochloride, sulfate, and sodium salts are often used. Pharmacists and chemists choose salts on the basis of cost, convenience, solubility, and stability. For example, solubility is especially important with parenteral drugs, while taste is a factor with oral drugs.

## DRUG THERAPY IN CHILDREN

Drug therapy during infancy (1 month to 1 year) and childhood (approximately 1–12 years) requires special consideration because of the child's changing size, developmental level, and organ function. Physiologic differences alter drug pharmacokinetics (Table 3-1), and drug therapy is less predictable than in adults. Most drug use in children is empirical in nature because few studies have been done in that population. For many drugs, manufacturers' literature states that "safety and effectiveness for use in children have not been established." Neonates (birth to 1 month) are especially vulnerable to adverse drug effects because of their immature liver and kidney function (see Table 3-1). Neonatal therapeutics are discussed further in Chapter 70.

Most drugs given to adults also are given to children, and general principles, techniques of drug administration, and nursing process guidelines apply. Additional principles and guidelines include the following:

1. All aspects of pediatric drug therapy must be guided by the child's age, weight, and level of growth and development.

2. Choice of drug is often restricted because many drugs commonly used in adult drug therapy have not been sufficiently investigated to ensure safety and effectiveness in children.

3. Safe therapeutic dosage ranges are less well defined for children than for adults. Some drugs are not recommended for use in children, and therefore dosages have not been established. For many drugs, doses for children are extrapolated from those established for adults. When pediatric dosage ranges are listed in drug literature, these should be used. Often, however, they are expressed in amount of drug to be given per kilogram of body weight or square meter of body sur-

## TABLE 3-1. CHILDREN: PHYSIOLOGIC CHARACTERISTICS AND PHARMACOKINETIC CONSEQUENCES

| Physiologic Characteristics | Pharmacokinetic Consequences |
|---|---|
| Increased thinness and permeability of skin in neonates and infants | Increased absorption of topical drugs (*e.g.*, corticosteroids may be absorbed sufficiently to suppress adrenocortical function) |
| Immature blood-brain barrier in neonates and infants | Increased distribution of drugs into the central nervous system because myelinization (which creates the blood-brain barrier to the passage of drugs) is not mature until about 2 years of age |
| Increased percentage of body water (70% to 80% in neonates and infants, compared to 50% to 60% in children above 2 years of age and adults) | Usually increased volume of distribution in infants and young children, compared to adults. This would seem to indicate a need for larger doses. However, prolonged drug half-life and decreased rate of drug clearance may offset. The net effect is often a need for decreased dosage. |
| Altered protein binding until about 1 year of age, when it reaches adult levels | The amount and binding capacity of plasma proteins may be reduced. This may result in a greater proportion of unbound or pharmacologically active drug and greater risks of adverse drug effects. Dosage requirements may be decreased or modified by other factors. Drugs with decreased protein binding in neonates, compared with older children and adults, include ampicillin (Omnipen, others), diazepam (Valium), digoxin (Lanoxin), lidocaine (Xylocaine), nafcillin (Unipen), phenobarbital, phenytoin (Dilantin), salicylates (*e.g.*, aspirin), and theophylline (TheoDur). |
| Decreased glomerular filtration rate in neonates and infants, compared with older children and adults. Kidney function develops progressively during the first few months of life and is fairly mature by 1 year of age. | In neonates and infants, slowed excretion of drugs eliminated by the kidneys. Dosage of these drugs may need to be decreased, depending on the infant's age and level of growth and development. |
| Decreased activity of liver drug-metabolizing enzyme systems in neonates and infants | Decreased capacity for biotransformation of drugs. This results in slowed metabolism and elimination, with increased risks of drug accumulation and adverse effects. |
| Increased activity of liver drug-metabolizing enzyme systems in children | Increased capacity for biotransformation of some drugs. This results in a rapid rate of metabolism and elimination. For example, theophylline is cleared about 30% faster in a 7-year-old child than in an adult and about four times faster than in a neonate. |

face area, and the amount needed for a specific dose must be calculated as a fraction of the adult dose. The following methods are used for these calculations:

A. Clark's rule is based on weight and is used for children at least 2 years old.

$$\frac{\text{Weight (in pounds)}}{150} \times \text{adult dose} = \text{child's dose}$$

B. Calculating dosage based on body surface area is considered a more accurate method than those based on other characteristics. Body surface area, based on height and weight, is estimated using a nomogram (Fig. 3-1). Use the estimated body surface area in the following formula to calculate the child's dose:

$$\frac{\text{Body surface area (in square meters)}}{1.73 \text{ square meters } (m^2)} \times \text{adult dose} = \text{child's dose}$$

Dosages obtained from these calculations are approximate and *must* be individualized. These doses can be used initially and then increased or decreased according to the child's response.

4. Use the oral route of drug administration when possible. Try to obtain the child's cooperation; *never* force oral medications. Forcing may lead to aspiration.
5. If intramuscular injections are required in infants, use the thigh muscles because the deltoid muscles are quite small, and the gluteal muscles do not develop until the child is walking.
6. For safety, keep all medications in childproof con-

**Nomogram for Estimating the Surface Area of Infants and Young Children**

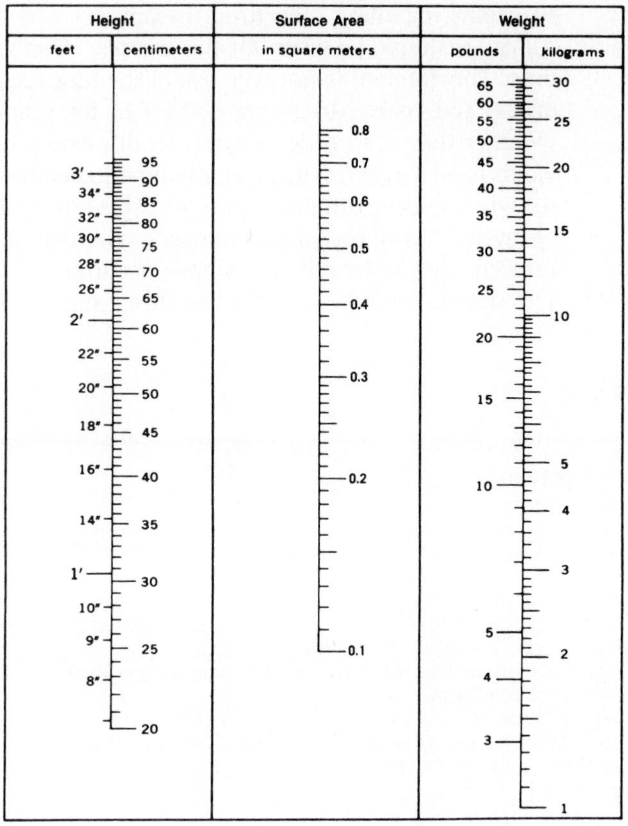


**Nomogram for Estimating the Surface Area of Older Children and Adults**

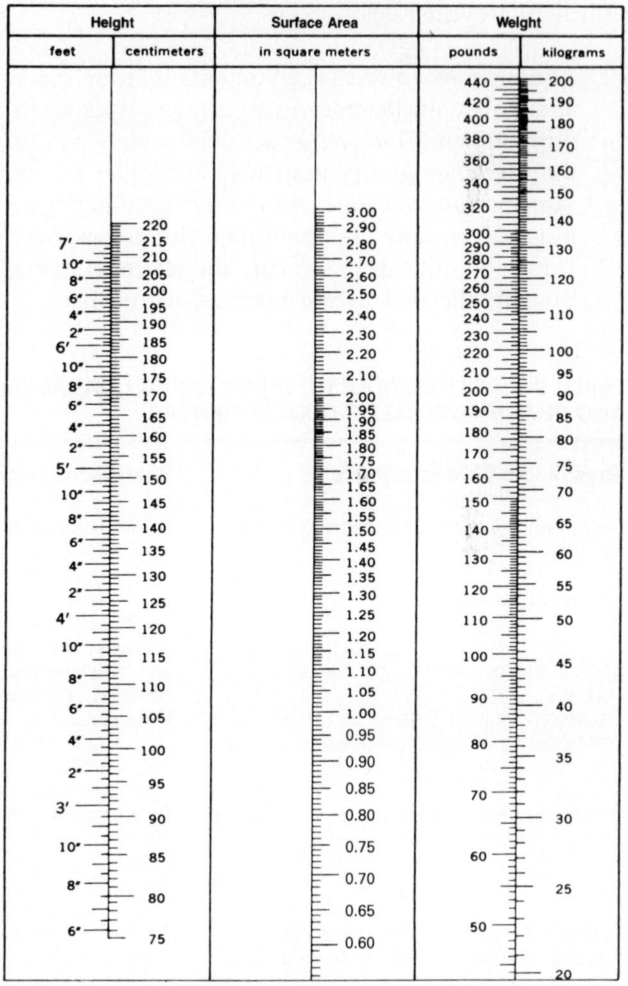


*FIGURE 3-1.* Body-surface nomograms. To determine the surface area of the client, draw a straight line between the point representing his or her height on the left vertical scale to the point representing weight on the right vertical scale. The point at which this line intersects the middle vertical scale represents the client's surface area in square meters. (Courtesy of Abbott Laboratories)

tainers, out of reach of children, and do not refer to medications as ''candy.''

## DRUG THERAPY IN OLDER ADULTS

Aging is a continuum; precisely when an individual becomes an older adult is not clearly established, but in this book people 65 years and older are categorized as ''older adults.'' In this population, general nursing process guidelines and principles of drug therapy apply. In addition, adverse effects are especially likely to occur due to physiologic changes associated with aging (Table 3-2), pathologic changes due to disease processes, multiple drug therapy for acute and chronic disorders, impaired memory and cognition, and difficulty in complying with drug orders. Overall, the goal of drug therapy may be ''care'' rather than ''cure,'' with efforts to prevent or control symptoms and maintain the client's ability to function in usual activities of daily living. Additional principles are listed below.

1. Although age in years is an important factor, older adults are quite heterogeneous in their responses to drug therapy. Thus, responses differ widely within the same age group. Responses also differ in the same person over time. Physiologic age (*i.e.*, organ function) is more important than chronologic age.
2. It may be difficult to separate the effects of aging from the effects of disease processes or drug therapy,

particularly long-term drug therapy. Symptoms attributed to aging or disease actually may be caused by medications. This occurs because older adults generally metabolize and excrete drugs less efficiently, and thus drugs are more likely to accumulate.

3. Medications—both prescription and nonprescription drugs—should be taken only when necessary.
4. Review current medications before prescribing new drugs; discontinue unnecessary drugs.
5. When drug therapy is required, the choice of drug should be based on the available drug information regarding effects in older adults.
6. The basic principle of giving the smallest effective number of drugs applies especially to older adults. A regimen of several drugs increases the incidence of adverse reactions and potentially hazardous drug interactions. Some studies have demonstrated that three or four drugs are all that can be self-administered effectively. Beyond three or four drugs, many older adults are unable or unwilling to follow instructions regarding their drug therapy.
7. All drugs should be given for the shortest effective time. This interval is not well established for most drugs, and many drugs are continued for years, whether they are needed or not. Health-care providers need to reassess drug regimens periodically to see whether drugs, dosages, or other aspects need to be revised. This is especially important when significant changes in health status have occurred.
8. The smallest number of effective doses should be

**TABLE 3-2.   OLDER ADULTS: PHYSIOLOGIC CHARACTERISTICS AND PHARMACOKINETIC CONSEQUENCES**

| Physiologic Characteristics | Pharmacokinetic Consequences |
| --- | --- |
| Decreased gastrointestinal secretions and motility | Slower absorption of oral drugs and delayed onset of action. However, total absorption may be increased because drug molecules have more contact with sites of absorption in the small intestine. |
| Decreased cardiac output | Slower absorption from sites of administration (*e.g.*, gastrointestinal tract, subcutaneous or muscle tissue). Decreased distribution to sites of action in tissues, with potential for delaying the onset and reducing the extent of therapeutic effects. |
| Decreased blood flow to the liver and kidneys | The resultant delays in metabolism and excretion may lead to drug accumulation and increased risks of adverse or toxic effects. |
| Decreased total body water and lean body mass per kg of weight; increased body fat | Water-soluble drugs (*e.g.*, ethanol, lithium) are distributed into a smaller area, with resultant higher plasma concentrations and higher risks of toxicity with a given dose. Fat-soluble drugs (*e.g.*, diazepam) are distributed to a larger area, accumulate in fat, and have a longer duration of action in the body. |
| Decreased serum albumin | Decreased availability of protein for binding and transporting drug molecules. This increases serum concentration of free, pharmacologically active drug, especially for those that are normally highly protein bound (*e.g.*, aspirin, warfarin). This may increase risks of adverse effects. However, the drug also may be metabolized and excreted more rapidly, thereby offsetting at least some of the risks. |
| Decreased blood flow to the liver; decreased number and activity of drug-metabolizing enzymes | Slowed metabolism and detoxification, with increased risks of drug accumulation and toxic effects |
| Decreased blood flow to the kidneys, decreased number of functioning nephrons, decreased glomerular filtration rate, and decreased tubular secretion | Impaired drug excretion, prolonged half-life, and increased risks of toxicity |

prescribed. This allows less disruption of usual activities and promotes compliance with the prescribed regimen.

9. When any drug is started, the dosage generally should be smaller than for younger adults. The dosage can then be increased or decreased according to response. If an increased dosage is indicated, increments should be smaller and made at longer intervals in older adults. This conservative, safe approach is sometimes called "start low, go slow."

10. Use nondrug measures to decrease the need for drugs and to increase their effectiveness or decrease their adverse effects. For example, insomnia is a common complaint among older adults. Preventing it (*e.g.*, by avoiding caffeine-containing beverages and excessive napping) is much safer than taking sedative-hypnotic drugs.

11. For people receiving long-term drug therapy at home, use measures to help them take drugs safely and effectively.
    A. If vision is impaired, label drug containers with large lettering for easier readability. A magnifying glass also may be useful.
    B. Be sure the client can open drug containers. For example, avoid childproof containers for an older adult with arthritic hands.
    C. Several devices may be used to schedule drug doses and decrease risks of omitting or repeating doses. These include written schedules, calendars, and charts. Also available are drug containers with doses prepared and clearly labeled as to the day and time each dose is to be taken. With the latter system, the client can tell at a glance whether a dose has been taken.
    D. Enlist family members or friends when necessary.

12. When a client develops new symptoms or becomes less able to function in usual activities of daily living, consider the possibility of adverse drug effects. Often, new signs and symptoms are attributed to aging or disease. They may then be ignored or treated by prescribing a new drug, when stopping or reducing the dose of an old drug is the indicated intervention.

## NURSING ACTIONS: MONITORING DRUG THERAPY

| Nursing Actions | Rationale/Explanation |
|---|---|
| **1. Prepare and administer drugs accurately (see Chap. 2)** | |
| **a.** Practice the five rights of drug administration (right *drug*, right *client*, right *dose*, right *route*, and right *time*). | These rights are ensured if the techniques described in Chapter 2 are consistently followed. The time may vary by about 30 minutes. For example, a drug ordered for 9 AM can be given between 8:30 AM and 9:30 AM. No variation is allowed in the other "rights." |
| **b.** Use correct techniques for different routes of administration. | For example, sterile equipment and techniques are required for injection of any drug. |
| **c.** Follow label instructions regarding mixing or other aspects of giving specific drugs. | Some drugs require specific techniques of preparation and administration. |
| **2. Observe for therapeutic effects** | Generally, the nurse should know the expected effects and when they are likely to occur. Specific observations depend on the specific drug or drugs being given. |
| **3. Observe for adverse effects** | All drugs are potentially harmful, although the incidence and severity of adverse reactions vary among drugs and clients. People most likely to suffer adverse reactions are those with severe liver or kidney disease, those who are very young or very old, those receiving several drugs, and those receiving large doses of any drug. Specific adverse effects for which to observe depend on the drugs being given. |

*(continued)*

| *Nursing Actions* | *Rationale/Explanation* |
|---|---|
| **4. Observe for drug interactions** | The nurse must be knowledgeable about common and potentially significant drug interactions. Also, because interactions may occur anytime the client is receiving two or more drugs concurrently, they should be considered as a possible cause of unexpected responses to drug therapy. |
| **5. Teach clients about their drug therapy**<br>**a.** General instructions | |
| (1) Take medications as directed. | Therapeutic effect greatly depends on taking medications correctly. Altering the dose or time may cause underdosage or overdosage. |
| (2) Do not start or stop drugs without consulting the physician. | Drug therapy is often a state of delicate balance. Altering this balance greatly increases risks of drug interactions, adverse effects, and loss of therapeutic effectiveness. |
| (3) Do not keep drugs for long periods. | The chemical composition of drugs tends to become altered over time. Manufacturers' drug labels often include a date after which the drug should be discarded. This information is not ordinarily included with prescription drugs dispensed to clients. Outdated drugs at best do no good and at worst may be harmful. |
| (4) Develop a routine for taking medications. For example, take them at the same time and place each day. | Having a routine helps clients remember to take medications as directed. |
| (5) Do not keep medications in the bathroom medicine cabinet. | Medications may deteriorate more rapidly owing to warmth and moisture. |
| (6) Never put several medications, such as different tablets, in one container | This is never a safe practice. The risk of taking the wrong medication or wrong dose is greatly increased if this is done. In addition, the drugs may interact chemically, altering drug composition. |
| (7) Take medication in a well-lighted area. | To allow reading the label to ensure that the drug taken is the one intended |
| (8) Keep all medications out of reach of children, and never refer to medications as ''candy.'' | To prevent accidental ingestion and poisoning |
| **b.** Instructions related to specific drugs | Many drugs are self-administered, and information is required to do this correctly, safely, and effectively. |
| (1) Name of the drug(s) | Knowledge of the drug name can be a safety measure, especially if the person has an allergic or other potentially serious adverse reaction or an overdose. It also may give the person a greater sense of control and responsibility regarding drug therapy. |
| (2) Purpose of the drug | People vary in the amount of drug information they want and need. For most, the purpose can be simply stated in terms of symptoms to be relieved or other expected benefits. |
| (3) Dosage schedule | This should be specific and as convenient as possible within the limitations imposed by the particular drugs. Working with the client to individualize drug therapy may help increase compliance with the prescribed regimen. |

## Nursing Actions

## Rationale/Explanation

| Nursing Actions | Rationale/Explanation |
|---|---|
| (4) Method of administration | Most people are accustomed to taking drugs orally, although they may need information about the amount or type of fluids to take with a particular drug or other instructions. For other routes of administration, instructions may need to be more specific and complete. Rectal suppositories and topical application of drugs to the eyes or skin are examples in which correct administration is essential to therapeutic effect. |
| (5) Adverse reactions or side effects to be reported | The goal is to provide needed information without causing unnecessary anxiety. Most drugs produce undesirable effects; some of these are minor, and others are potentially serious. Many people stop taking a drug rather than report adverse reactions. If reactions are reported, it may be possible to allow continued drug therapy by reducing dosage or by implementing other measures. The occurrence of severe reactions indicates that the drug should be stopped. In such cases the prescribing physician should be notified. |
| (6) Miscellaneous instructions, such as safety measures for taking certain drugs, storage, and others as indicated | |

## Review and Application Exercises

1. Why do nurses need to know the adverse effects of the drugs they give?
2. Given a newly assigned client, what information is needed about present and previous medications?
3. Try to anticipate questions a client might ask about a drug and rehearse possible answers, including drugs that are well-known to you and those that are not.
4. With children, what are some potential difficulties with drug administration, and how can they be prevented or minimized?
5. With older adults, what are some potential difficulties with drug administration and how can they be prevented or minimized?
6. For older adults, explain what is meant by "start low, go slow" and why it is a good approach to drug therapy.
7. Why is client teaching about drug therapy needed, and what information should generally be included?

## Selected References

Beare, P. G., & Myers, J. L. (Eds.) (1990). *Principles and practice of adult health nursing*. St. Louis: C.V. Mosby.

Bolinger, A. M., Murphy, V. A., & Bubica, G. (1992). General pediatric therapy. In M. A. Koda-Kimble & L. Y. Young (Eds.), *Applied therapeutics: The clinical use of drugs* (5th ed.) (pp. 77-1–77-24). Vancouver, WA: Applied Therapeutics.

Burrell, L. O., Jowers, L., Andersen, B. K., & Bailey, D. R. (1992). Contemporary nursing practice. In L. O. Burrell (Ed.), *Adult nursing in hospital and community settings*. Norwalk, CT: Appleton & Lange.

Bressler, R. (1993). Adverse drug reactions. In R. Bressler & M. D. Katz (Eds.), *Geriatric pharmacology* (pp. 41–61). New York: McGraw-Hill.

Horne, E., Nykamp, D., & Spruill, K. (1990). Dosing guidelines for common neonatal and pediatric drugs. *Hospital Pharmacy, 25*, 154–184.

Jinks, M. J., & Fuerst, R. H. (1992). Geriatric therapy. In M. A. Koda-Kimble & L. Y. Young (Eds.), *Applied therapeutics: The clinical use of drugs* (5th ed.) (pp. 79-1–79-19). Vancouver, WA: Applied Therapeutics.

Swonger, A. K., & Matejski, M. P. (1991). *Nursing pharmacology: An integrated approach to drug therapy and nursing practice* (2nd ed.). Philadelphia: J.B. Lippincott.

# Drugs Affecting the Central Nervous System

### CHAPTER 4

# Physiology of the Central Nervous System

The central nervous system (CNS), composed of the brain and spinal cord, is concerned mainly with higher intellectual functions, such as thought, learning, reasoning, and memory, and with muscle function, both skeletal and smooth. It coordinates a person's reactions to the constantly changing internal and external environment. Information on blood levels of oxygen and carbon dioxide, body temperature, and sensory stimuli is constantly fed into the CNS. The CNS processes that information and sends messages to body parts to adjust the environment toward homeostasis. More specific characteristics are reviewed below to aid understanding of drugs that act by altering CNS functions.

## Characteristics and functions of the CNS

### NEURONS, NEUROTRANSMITTERS, AND SYNAPTIC PHYSIOLOGY

The basic functional unit of the CNS is the nerve cell or neuron. *Neurons* are specialized cells that exhibit excitability (the ability to be stimulated) and conductivity (the ability to convey electrical impulses). Neurons in a chain do not touch each other; they are separated by a microscopic gap called a *synapse*. The electrical impulse arriving at the end of the first neuron (presynaptic fiber) causes small sacs (synaptic vesicles) to release *neurotransmitters*. Neurotransmitters are chemical substances that carry messages from one neuron to another. They are synthesized and stored in presynaptic nerve terminals. When released from synaptic vesicles, molecules of neurotransmitter cross the synapse, bind to receptor proteins in the cell membrane of the postsynaptic neuron, and excite or inhibit postsynaptic neurons, depending on whether the neuronal membrane contains excitatory or inhibitory receptors (Fig 4-1). These chemical synapses conduct the electrical signal in one direction, in contrast to electrical synapses that can transmit signals in more than one direction (*e.g.*, sympathetic nerves transmit impulses from one smooth muscle fiber to the next in visceral smooth muscle and from one cardiac muscle cell to another).

Most acute CNS responses are caused by small-molecule, rapidly acting neurotransmitters, such as acetylcholine, the amines (dopamine, epinephrine, norepinephrine, serotonin), and amino acids (aspartate, gamma-aminobutyric acid [GABA], glutamate, and glycine). These neurotransmitters usually act on postsynaptic neuron receptors to alter conduction of ions through channels in the cell membrane. For example, increased conduction of sodium causes excitation, and increased conduction of potassium or chloride causes inhibition. Sometimes, though, a neurotransmitter stimulates receptor-activated enzymes and alters cellular metabolism instead of opening ion channels. In addition, some receptors are located on presynaptic nerve terminals, such as alpha$_2$-adrenergic receptors. Additional characteristics of these neurotransmitters are summarized in Box 4-1.

Anne Collins Abrams: CLINICAL DRUG THERAPY, Fourth Edition.
© 1995 J.B. Lippincott Company.

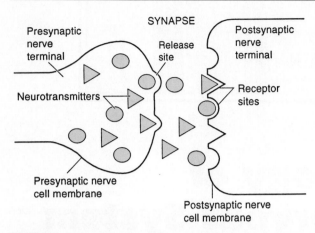

**FIGURE 4-1.** Neurotransmission in the central nervous system. Neurotransmitter molecules (*e.g.*, norepinephrine and acetylcholine), released by the presynaptic nerve, cross the synapse and bind with receptor proteins in the cell membrane of the postsynaptic nerve.

Most prolonged CNS responses are caused by large-molecule, slowly acting neurotransmitters, such as the neuropeptide hormones (adrenocorticotropic hormone [ACTH, or corticotropin], insulin, and others). Prolonged effects are thought to involve closure of calcium channels, changes in cellular metabolism, changes in activation or deactivation of specific genes in the cell nucleus, and alterations in the numbers of excitatory or inhibitory postsynaptic membrane receptors.

## Factors affecting neurotransmitters

The availability and function of synaptic neurotransmitters can be altered by several circumstances. One major factor is *synaptic fatigue*, in which synaptic transmission becomes progressively weaker during prolonged periods of excitation. Another major factor is the *number of receptors* in the cell membranes of presynaptic and postsynaptic nerve endings.

Receptors increase in numbers (usually called upgrading or upregulation) when there is underactivity at the synapse and decrease in numbers (downgrading or downregulation) when there is overactivity. It is believed that receptor proteins are constantly being formed by the endoplasmic reticulum–Golgi apparatus and inserted into presynaptic and postsynaptic membranes. If the synapses are overused and excessive amounts of neurotransmitter combine with receptor proteins, it is then postulated that many of the receptor proteins are inactivated and removed from the synaptic membrane. Thus, synaptic fatigue and downgrading or upgrading of receptors work with other control mechanisms of the nervous system to readjust abnormally stimulated or depressed nerve function toward normal function. Serious problems could occur with either excessive stimulation (*e.g.*, muscle cramps, convulsions, psychotic distur-

bances, hallucinations, tension) or depression (*e.g.*, decreased levels of consciousness, respiratory depression).

Other important factors include *acid-base imbalances* (acidosis decreases synaptic transmission, causing CNS depression; alkalosis increases synaptic transmission, causing CNS stimulation); *hypoxia*, which causes CNS depression (coma occurs within seconds without oxygen); and *drugs*, which may cause either CNS stimulation or depression.

Following their physiologic actions, neurotransmitters are rapidly deactivated and removed from the synapse by three mechanisms. These mechanisms are diffusion into surrounding body fluids, destruction by enzymes (*e.g.*, acetylcholine is degraded by cholinesterase; norepinephrine is metabolized by monamine oxidase and catecholomethyl transferase), and transportation back into the presynaptic nerve terminal (called reuptake) for reuse. The extent to which each mechanism is used varies with the type of neurotransmitter.

## ETIOLOGY AND PATHOPHYSIOLOGY OF PSYCHIATRIC SYMPTOMS

As discussed previously, neurotransmitters are chemical messengers that control neural function by exciting or inhibiting action potentials of nerve cells. Neurotransmitter abnormalities (*e.g.*, dysfunction of the neurons that normally produce neurotransmitters or altered postsynaptic response to neurotransmitters) are implicated in the etiology and pathophysiology of many psychiatric and CNS disorders. For example, *dopamine* abnormalities occur in psychosis and Parkinson's disease; *GABA* abnormalities occur in anxiety, hyperarousal states, and seizure disorders; *glutamate* has been implicated in the pathogenesis of epilepsy, stroke, and Huntington's disease; and *serotonin* abnormalities are thought to be involved in mental depression and sleep disorders.

Except for mental depression, most psychiatric symptoms result from CNS stimulation and usually involve physical and mental hyperactivity. Such hyperactivity reflects a wide range of observable behaviors and nonobservable thoughts and feelings. In most people, manifestations may include pleasant feelings of mild euphoria and high levels of enthusiasm, energy, and productivity. In people with psychiatric illnesses, such as anxiety or psychosis, manifestations include unpleasant feelings of tension, psychomotor agitation, nervousness, and decreased ability to rest and sleep, even when very tired. Many psychiatric disorders, therapeutic drugs, and drugs of abuse may cause varying degrees of CNS stimulation. Generally, the pathogenesis of excessive CNS stimulation may involve one or more of the following mechanisms:

1. Excessive amounts of excitatory neurotransmitters (*e.g.*, norepinephrine)

# BOX 4-1. SMALL-MOLECULE NEUROTRANSMITTERS

| *Excitatory Neurotransmitters* | *Characteristics* |
|---|---|
| Acetylcholine | • Located in many areas of the brain, including the motor cortex, basal ganglia, motor neurons that innervate skeletal muscle, preganglionic neurons of the autonomic nervous system (ANS), postganglionic neurons of the parasympathetic nervous system (PNS), and some postganglionic neurons of the sympathetic nervous system (SNS) |
| | • Exerts mainly excitatory effects at synapses and nerve-muscle junctions; (for inhibitory effects see below) |
| | • Associated with level of arousal, memory, motor conditioning, and speech |
| Aspartic acid | • An amino acid with neurotransmitter functions |
| Epinephrine | • A catecholamine synthesized in SNS nerve endings from the amino acid, tyrosine |
| | • Produced by postganglionic neurons in the adrenal medulla and comprises about 80% of the catecholamines released from adrenal glands. Adrenal synthesis of epinephrine is influenced by glucocorticoids from the adrenal cortex. Glucocorticoid hormones are transported from the cortex to the medulla where they stimulate SNS neurons to increase production of epinephrine by stimulating enzyme activity. Thus, any stress situation sufficient to evoke increased levels of glucocorticoids also increases epinephrine levels. |
| Glutamic acid (glutamate) | • An amino acid with neurotransmitter functions |
| | • Found throughout the brain in the cerebral cortex and presynaptic nerve endings of many sensory pathways |
| Norepinephrine | • Like dopamine and epinephrine, norepinephrine is a catecholamine synthesized from tyrosine. |
| | • Located in postganglionic SNS neurons that supply blood vessels and the adrenal medulla |
| | • Associated with mood, motor activity, regulation of arousal, and reward |

| *Inhibitory Neurotransmitters* | *Characteristics* |
|---|---|
| Acetylcholine | • See above |
| | • Effects mainly excitatory but exerts inhibitory effects at a few peripheral sites, such as organs supplied by the vagus nerves |
| Dopamine | • A catecholamine synthesized in SNS nerve endings and a precursor substance in the synthesis of norepinephrine and epinephrine. (Each step of production requires a different enzyme, and the type of neurotransmitter produced depends on the type of enzymes that are available in a nerve terminal.) |
| | • Located in the substantia nigra and basal ganglia of the brain and in renal and mesenteric blood vessels |
| | • Associated with aggression and stereotypic behaviors and vasodilation in renal and mesenteric blood vessels |
| Gamma-aminobutyric acid (GABA) | • Synthesized in the brain (cerebellum, basal ganglia, and cortex) and spinal cord |
| | • One of most common inhibitory neurotransmitters. It opposes the strongly excitatory effects of aspartate and glutamate. |
| Glycine | • An amino acid with neurotransmitter functions |
| | • Found in spinal cord synapses |
| Serotonin | • Derived from the amino acid tryptophan |
| | • Secreted by nuclei originating in brain stem and extending to many brain areas, especially the spinal cord and hypothalamus |
| | • Inhibits pain pathways in the spinal cord |
| | • Associated with mood, the sleep-wake cycle, sensory perception, and habituation |

2. Increased numbers or sensitivity of excitatory receptors
3. Insufficient amounts of inhibitory neurotransmitters (*e.g.*, GABA)
4. Decreased numbers or sensitivity of inhibitory receptors

## CEREBRAL CORTEX

The cerebral cortex is involved in all conscious processes, such as learning, memory, reasoning, verbalization, and voluntary body movements. Some parts of the cortex receive incoming nerve impulses and are called *sensory areas*; other parts send out impulses to peripheral structures and are called *motor areas*. Around the sensory and motor areas are the "association" areas, which occupy the greater portion of the cortex. These areas analyze the information received by the sensory areas and decide on the appropriate response. In some instances, the response may be to store the perception in memory; in others, it may involve stimulation of motor centers to produce movement or speech.

## THALAMUS

The thalamus receives impulses carrying sensations such as heat, cold, pain, and muscle position sense. These sensations produce only a crude awareness at the thalamic level. They are relayed to the cerebral cortex, where they are interpreted regarding location, quality, intensity, and significance.

## HYPOTHALAMUS

The hypothalamus has extensive neuronal connections with higher and lower levels of the CNS and the posterior pituitary gland. It also regulates the activity of the anterior pituitary. It constantly collects information about the internal environment of the body and helps to maintain homeostasis by making continuous adjustments in water balance, body temperature, hormone levels, arterial blood pressure, heart rate, gastrointestinal motility, and other body functions. The hypothalamus is stimulated or inhibited by nerve impulses from different portions of the nervous system and by concentrations of nutrients, electrolytes, water, and hormones in the blood. Specific functions include:

1. Producing oxytocin and antidiuretic hormone (ADH), which are then stored in the posterior pituitary gland and released in response to nerve impulses from the hypothalamus. Oxytocin initiates uterine contractions to begin labor and delivery and helps to release milk from breast glands during breast-feeding. ADH helps to maintain fluid balance by controlling water excretion. ADH secretion is controlled by the osmolarity of the extracellular fluid. When osmolarity is high, more ADH is secreted. This means that water is retained in the body to dilute the extracellular fluid and return it toward normal or homeostatic levels. When osmolarity is low, less ADH is secreted, and more water is excreted in the urine.
2. Regulating body temperature. When body temperature is elevated, sweating and dilation of blood vessels in the skin lower the temperature. When body temperature is low, sweating ceases and vasoconstriction occurs. When heat loss is decreased, the temperature is raised.
3. Assisting in regulation of arterial blood pressure by its effects on the vasomotor center. The vasomotor center in the medulla oblongata and pons maintains a state of partial contraction in blood vessels, a state called *vasomotor tone*. The hypothalamus can exert excitatory or inhibitory effects on the vasomotor center, depending on which portions of the hypothalamus are stimulated. When nerve impulses from the hypothalamus excite the vasomotor center, vasomotor tone or vasoconstriction is increased, and blood pressure is raised. When the impulses from the hypothalamus inhibit the vasomotor center, vasomotor tone or vasoconstriction is decreased, with the overall effect of relative vasodilation and lowering of arterial blood pressure.
4. Regulating anterior pituitary hormones, including thyroid-stimulating hormone, ACTH, and growth hormone. The hypothalamus secretes "releasing factors," which cause the anterior pituitary to secrete these hormones. There is a hypothalamic releasing factor for each hormone. The hypothalamic factor called prolactin-inhibiting factor inhibits secretion of prolactin, another anterior pituitary hormone.
5. Regulating food and water intake by the hypothalamic thirst, appetite, hunger, and satiety centers.

## MEDULLA OBLONGATA

The medulla oblongata contains groups of neurons that form the vital cardiac, respiratory, and vasomotor centers. For example, if the respiratory center is stimulated, respiratory rate and depth are increased. If the respiratory center is depressed, respiratory rate and depth are decreased. The medulla also contains reflex centers for coughing, vomiting, sneezing, swallowing, and salivating.

The medulla and pons varolii also contain groups of neurons from which originate cranial nerves 5 through 12. Together with the midbrain, these structures form the brain stem.

## RETICULAR ACTIVATING SYSTEM

The reticular activating system is a network of neurons that extends from the spinal cord through the medulla and pons to the thalamus and hypothalamus. It receives impulses from all parts of the body, evaluates the significance of the impulses, and decides which impulses to transmit to the cerebral cortex. It also excites or inhibits motor nerves that control both reflex and voluntary movement. Stimulation of these neurons produces wakefulness and mental alertness, while depression causes sedation and loss of consciousness.

## LIMBIC SYSTEM

The limbic system is an area of the brain that involves several structures, including the thalamus, hypothalamus, basal ganglia, hippocampus, amygdala, and septum. The function of the limbic system is to regulate emotions (e.g., pleasure, fear, anger, sadness) and behavior (e.g., aggression, laughing, crying). Many nerve impulses from the limbic system are transmitted through the hypothalamus; thus, physiologic changes in blood pressure, heart rate, respiration, and hormone secretion occur in response to the emotions.

## CEREBELLUM

The cerebellum, which is connected with motor centers in the cerebral cortex and basal ganglia, coordinates muscular activity. When several skeletal muscles are involved, some are contracted and some are relaxed for smooth, purposeful movements. It also helps to maintain balance and posture by receiving nerve impulses from the inner ear that produce appropriate reflex responses.

## BASAL GANGLIA

The basal ganglia are concerned with skeletal muscle tone and orderly activity. Normal function is influenced by dopamine, a neurotransmitter produced in the midbrain by a specific group of nerve cells called the *substantia nigra*. Degenerative changes in these cells cause dopamine to be released in decreased amounts. This process is a factor in the development of Parkinson's disease, which is characterized by rigidity and increased muscle tone.

## PYRAMIDAL AND EXTRAPYRAMIDAL SYSTEMS

The pyramidal and extrapyramidal systems are pathways out of the cerebral cortex. In the pyramidal or corticospinal tract, nerve fibers originate in the cerebral cortex, go down the brain stem to the medulla where the fibers cross, and continue down the spinal cord, where they end at various levels. Impulses are then carried from the spinal cord to skeletal muscle. Because the fibers cross in the medulla, impulses from the right side of the

cerebral cortex control skeletal muscle movement of the left side of the body, and impulses from the left control muscle movements of the right side. In the extrapyramidal system, fibers originate mainly in the premotor area of the cerebral cortex and travel to the basal ganglia and brain stem. The fibers are called extrapyramidal because they do not enter the medullary pyramids and cross over. Pyramidal and extrapyramidal systems intermingle in the spinal cord; disease processes affecting higher levels of the CNS involve both tracts.

## BRAIN METABOLISM

To function correctly, the brain must have an adequate and continuous supply of nutrients, especially oxygen, glucose, and thiamine. *Oxygen* is carried to the brain by the carotid and vertebral arteries. The brain requires more oxygen than any other organ. Cerebral cortex cells are very sensitive to lack of oxygen (hypoxia), and interruption of blood supply causes immediate loss of consciousness. Brain stem cells are less sensitive to hypoxia. People in whom hypoxia is relatively prolonged may survive, although they may have irreversible brain damage. *Glucose* is required as an energy source for brain cell metabolism. Hypoglycemia (low blood sugar) may cause mental confusion, dizziness, convulsions, loss of consciousness, and permanent damage to the cerebral cortex. *Thiamine* is required for production and use of glucose. Thiamine deficiency can reduce glucose use by about half and can cause degeneration of the myelin sheaths of nerve cells. Such degeneration in central neurons leads to a form of encephalopathy known as Wernicke-Korsakoff syndrome. Degeneration in peripheral nerves leads to polyneuritis and muscle atrophy, weakness, and paralysis.

## SPINAL CORD

The spinal cord is continuous with the medulla oblongata and extends downward through the vertebral column to the sacral area. The cord consists of 31 segments, each of which is the point of origin for a pair of spinal nerves. The cord functions as a pathway for conduction of impulses to and from the brain and as a center for reflex actions. Reflexes are involuntary responses to certain nerve impulses received by the spinal cord. Examples are the knee-jerk and pupillary reflexes.

# Classification of CNS drugs

Drugs affecting the CNS, sometimes called centrally active drugs, are broadly classified as depressants or stimulants. CNS depressant drugs (e.g., general anesthetics, narcotic analgesics, and sedative-hypnotics) produce a general depression of the CNS when given in sufficient dosages. Mild CNS depression is characterized by lack of interest in surroundings and inability to focus on a topic (short attention span). As depression progresses, there is drowsiness or sleep, decreased muscle tone, decreased ability to move, and decreased perception of sensations such as pain, heat, and cold. Severe CNS depression produces unconsciousness or coma, loss of reflexes, respiratory failure, and death.

CNS stimulants produce a variety of effects. Mild stimulation is characterized by wakefulness, mental alertness, and decreased fatigue. Increasing stimulation produces hyperactivity, excessive talking, nervousness, and insomnia. Excessive stimulation can cause convulsive seizures, cardiac arrhythmias, and death. Because it is difficult to avoid excessive, harmful CNS stimulation by these drugs, CNS stimulants are less useful for therapeutic purposes than are CNS depressants.

## Review and Application Exercises

1. Where are neurotransmitters synthesized and stored?
2. What events occur at the synapse between two nerve cells or a nerve cell and an effector cell (*e.g.*, in the heart, skeletal muscle, or other tissue)?
3. Once a neurotransmitter is released and acts on receptors, how are the remaining molecules inactivated?
4. What are the main functions of acetylcholine, dopamine, GABA, norepinephrine, and serotonin?
5. What part of the brain is concerned mainly with thoughts, reasoning, and learning?
6. What part of the brain contains vital respiratory and cardiovascular centers?

## Selected References

Bullock, B. L., & Rosendahl P. P. (1992). *Pathophysiology: Adaptations and alterations in function* (3rd ed.). Philadelphia: J.B. Lippincott.

Flannery, J. C. (1992). Overview of anatomy, physiology, and pathophysiology of the nervous system. In L. O. Burrell (Ed.), *Adult nursing in hospital and community settings* (pp. 830–863). Norwalk, CT: Appleton & Lange.

Guttman, M. (1992). Principles of neuropharmacology. In W. N. Kelley (Ed.), *Textbook of internal medicine* (2nd ed.) (pp. 2255–2258). Philadelphia: J.B. Lippincott.

Guyton, A. C. (1991). *Textbook of medical physiology* (8th ed.). Philadelphia: W.B. Saunders.

Porth, C. M. (1990). *Pathophysiology: Concepts of altered health states* (3rd ed.). Philadelphia: J.B. Lippincott.

Swonger, A. K., & Matejski, M. P. (1991). *Nursing pharmacology: An integrated approach to drug therapy and nursing practice* (2nd ed.). Philadelphia: J.B. Lippincott.

### CHAPTER 5

# Narcotic Analgesics and Narcotic Antagonists

Pain, the most common symptom prompting people to seek health care, is an unpleasant sensation that often indicates tissue damage and impels the person to remove the cause of the damage. In cancer, however, extensive tissue damage may occur before pain develops. Also, pain does not indicate the extent of tissue damage, and it may be reported when there is no evident cause. Narcotic analgesics are drugs that relieve moderate to severe pain. To aid understanding of drug actions, selected characteristics of pain are described.

## Pain

Pain occurs when free nerve endings (pain receptors or nociceptors) are stimulated by potentially harmful substances. Painful stimuli may be physical (*e.g.*, heat, cold, pressure) or chemical (*e.g.*, pain related to products of inflammation, including histamine and bradykinin). The skin, joint surfaces, arterial walls, and periosteum contain many pain receptors, while most internal organs, such as lung and uterine tissue, contain few. When pain receptors are stimulated, the sensation is carried to the CNS by sensory nerve fibers. In the CNS, the nerve impulse initiates reflex action in the spinal cord to cause rapid withdrawal from the painful stimulus or travels to the brain for analysis and determination of action needed. Pain is often described as acute or chronic and superficial or deep.

*Acute* pain demands the sufferer's attention and compels behavior to seek relief. It is often accompanied by anxiety and objective signs of discomfort, such as facial expressions of distress; moaning or crying; positioning to protect the affected part; tenderness, edema, skin color, or temperature changes in the affected part; and either restlessness and excessive movement or limited movement if movement increases pain.

*Chronic* pain, usually defined as pain of 6 months' duration, less urgently demands attention, may not be characterized by visible signs, and is often accompanied by depression and changes in personality, life-style, and functional ability. It may occur with or without evidence of tissue damage.

*Superficial* pain originates in the skin or closely underlying structures and is readily localized by the sufferer. Superficial pain or pain of low to moderate intensity usually stimulates the sympathetic nervous system and produces increased blood pressure, pulse, and respiration; dilated pupils; and increased skeletal muscle tension, such as rigid posture or clenched fists.

*Deep* pain originates in bones and abdominal or thoracic organs and produces a dull, aching sensation that is hard to localize. Deep or severe pain stimulates the parasympathetic nervous system and produces decreased blood pressure and pulse, nausea and vomiting, weakness, syncope, and possibly loss of consciousness.

## Description of narcotic analgesics

Narcotic analgesics are drugs that relieve moderate to severe pain by reducing perception of pain sensation, producing sedation, and decreasing the emotional up-

Anne Collins Abrams: CLINICAL DRUG THERAPY, Fourth Edition.

sets often associated with pain. Most of these analgesics are Schedule II drugs under federal narcotic laws and may lead to drug abuse and dependence. *Morphine* is the prototype of these analgesics and the standard by which others are measured. These drugs are often called opioids (drugs that act like morphine in the body).

Morphine and other opioids exert widespread pharmacologic effects, especially in the central nervous system (CNS) and the gastrointestinal (GI) system. These effects occur with usual doses and may be therapeutic or adverse, depending on the reason for use. CNS effects include analgesia, CNS depression ranging from drowsiness to sleep to unconsciousness, decreased mental and physical activity, respiratory depression, nausea and vomiting, and pupil constriction. Sedation and respiratory depression are major adverse effects and are potentially life-threatening. Most newer narcotic analgesics have been developed in an effort to find drugs as effective as morphine in relieving pain while causing less sedation, respiratory depression, and dependence. This effort has not been successful: *Equianalgesic doses of these drugs produce sedative and respiratory depressant effects comparable to those of morphine.*

In the GI system, narcotic analgesics slow motility and may cause smooth muscle spasms in the bowel, biliary tract, and urinary tract.

## MECHANISM OF ACTION

Opioids relieve pain by binding to opioid receptors on the cell membranes of specific neurons in the brain. Six major types of receptors have been identified; Table 5-1 summarizes the receptors and their effects. Narcotic analgesics and narcotic antagonists bind to different receptors to varying degrees, and their pharmacologic actions can be differentiated and classified on this basis. Opioid

receptors also bind with endogenous (produced by the body) pain-relieving substances called *enkephalins* and *endorphins*. These substances act like opioid drugs in the body. The word "endorphin" was coined from "endogenous morphine."

## INDICATIONS FOR USE

The main indication for use of opioids is to prevent or relieve acute or chronic pain. Specific conditions in which opioid drugs are used for analgesic effects include acute myocardial infarction, biliary colic, renal colic, burns and other traumatic injuries, and postoperative states. These drugs are usually given for chronic pain only when other measures and milder drugs are ineffective, as in terminal malignancy. Other clinical uses include:

1. Before and during surgery to promote sedation, decrease anxiety, facilitate induction of anesthesia, and decrease the amount of anesthesia required
2. Before and during invasive diagnostic procedures, such as angiograms and endoscopic examinations
3. During labor and delivery (obstetric analgesia)
4. Treating GI disorders, such as abdominal cramping and diarrhea
5. Treating acute pulmonary edema (morphine is used)
6. Treating severe, unproductive cough (codeine is generally used)

## CONTRAINDICATIONS FOR USE

These drugs are contraindicated or must be used very cautiously in people with respiratory depression, chronic lung disease, liver or kidney disease, prostatic hypertrophy, increased intracranial pressure, or hypersensitivity reactions to opiates and related drugs.

# Classifications and individual drugs

## AGONISTS

Narcotic agonists include morphine and morphine-like drugs. These agents have activity at mu, kappa, and possibly delta opioid receptors and thus produce prototypical narcotic effects.

**Morphine** is a naturally occurring opium alkaloid used mainly to relieve acute or chronic severe pain. It is a Schedule II narcotic that is given orally and parenterally. Client response depends on route and dosage. After intravenous (IV) injection, maximal analgesia and respiratory depression usually occur within 10 to 20 minutes.

**TABLE 5-1.  OPIATE RECEPTORS AND THEIR EFFECTS**

| Drug Group | Receptor | Effects |
|---|---|---|
| Agonists (*e.g.*, morphine) | Mu-1 | Analgesia |
|  | Mu-2 | Constipation |
|  |  | Euphoria |
|  |  | Physical dependence |
|  |  | Respiratory depression |
|  | Kappa | Analgesia |
|  |  | Miosis |
|  |  | Sedation |
|  | Delta? | Analgesia |
|  | Epsilon | Analgesia |
| Agonist/antagonists (*e.g.*, pentazocine) | Kappa | Analgesia |
|  |  | Miosis |
|  |  | Sedation |
|  | Sigma | Dysphoria |
|  |  | Hallucinations |
|  |  | Respiratory stimulation |
|  |  | Vasomotor stimulation |

After intramuscular (IM) injection, these effects occur in approximately 30 minutes. With subcutaneous (SC) injection, effects may be delayed up to 60 to 90 minutes.

Oral administration of morphine is becoming more common, usually for chronic pain associated with cancer. When given orally, much higher doses are required because a large proportion of each dose is metabolized in the liver and never reaches the systemic circulation. Concentrated solutions (*e.g.*, Roxanol, which contains 20 mg morphine/ml) and controlled-release tablets (*e.g.*, MS Contin, which contains 30 mg/tablet) have been developed for oral administration of these high doses. In some instances of severe pain that cannot be controlled by other methods, morphine is administered as a continuous IV infusion.

Morphine is primarily metabolized in the liver and excreted by the kidneys. Consequently, impaired liver and kidney function may cause prolonged drug action and accumulation with subsequent increased incidence and severity of adverse effects.

### Routes and dosage ranges

*Adults:* PO 10–30 mg q4h PRN or as ordered by physician

PO controlled-release tablets, 30 mg q8–12h or as ordered by physician

IM, SC 5–20 mg/70 kg q4h PRN

IV injection, 2.5–15 mg/70 kg, diluted in 5 ml water for injection and injected slowly, for approximately 5 min, PRN

IV continuous infusion, 0.1–1 mg/ml in 5% dextrose in water, by controlled infusion pump

Epidural injection, 5 mg/24 h; continuous infusion, 2–4 mg/24 h

Intrathecal injection, 0.2–1 mg/24 h

Rectal, 10–20 mg q4h or as ordered by physician

*Infants and children:* IM, SC 0.1–0.2 mg/kg (up to 15 mg) q4h

**Alfentanil** (Alfenta), **fentanyl** (Sublimaze), and **sufentanil** (Sufenta) are potent drugs with a short duration of action. They are most often used in anesthesia (see Chap. 14) as analgesic adjuncts or primary anesthetic agents in open-heart surgery or complicated neurologic and orthopedic procedures. Fentanyl also is used for preanesthetic medication, postoperative analgesia, and chronic pain that requires an opioid analgesic. A transdermal formulation (Duragesic) is used in the treatment of chronic pain. The active drug is deposited in the skin and slowly absorbed systemically. Thus, the skin patches have a slow onset of action (approximately 12–24 hours), but they last approximately 3 days. When a patch is removed, the drug continues to be absorbed from the skin deposits for 24 hours or longer.

Alfentanil

### Routes and dosage ranges

*Adults:* Analgesic adjunct in general anesthesia, IV initial dose 8–50 μg/kg; maintenance injection, 3–5 μg/kg; maintenance infusion, 0.5–1 μg/kg per minute

Anesthesia induction, IV injection 130–245 μg/kg over 3 min or IV infusion 50–75 μg/kg

Anesthesia maintenance, IV infusion 0.5–3 μg/kg per minute

Fentanyl

### Routes and dosage ranges

*Adults:* Preanesthetic, IM 0.05–0.1 mg 30–60 min before surgery

Analgesic adjunct to general anesthesia, IV total dose of 0.002–0.05 mg/kg, depending on type and length of surgical procedure

Adjunct to regional anesthesia, IM or slow IV (over 1–2 min) 0.05–0.1 mg PRN

Postoperative analgesia, IM 0.05–0.1 mg, repeat in 1–2 h if needed

General anesthesia, IV 0.05–0.1 mg/kg with oxygen and a muscle relaxant (maximum dose 0.15 mg/kg with open-heart surgery, other major surgeries, and complicated neurologic or orthopedic procedures)

Chronic pain, transdermal system 2.5–10 mg every 72 h

*Children under 12 years:* General anesthesia induction and maintenance, IV 1.7–3.3 mg/kg (20–30 μg/20–25 lb)

Sufentanil

### Routes and dosage ranges

*Adults:* Analgesic adjunct to general anesthesia, IV initial dose 1–8 μg/kg; maintenance, 10–25 μg PRN

General anesthesia IV induction, 8–30 μg/kg; maintenance, 25–50 μg PRN

*Children under 12 years:* General anesthesia, IV induction 10–25 μg with 100% oxygen; maintenance 25–50 μg PRN

**Codeine** is a naturally occurring opium alkaloid used for analgesic and antitussive effects. Codeine is similar to morphine but produces weaker analgesic and antitussive effects and milder adverse effects. Compared with other narcotic analgesics, codeine is more effective when given orally and is less likely to lead to abuse and dependence. Parenteral administration is more effective in relieving pain than oral administration, but onset (15–30 minutes) and duration of action (4–6 hours) are about the same. Larger doses are required for analgesic than for antitussive effects. Codeine is often given with aspirin or acetaminophen for additive analgesic effects.

### Routes and dosage ranges

*Adults:* PO, SC, IM 15–60 mg q4–6h PRN
    Cough, PO 10–20 mg q4h PRN
*Children:* PO, SC, IM 0.5 mg/kg q4–6h PRN
    Cough, PO 6–12 y, 5–10 mg q4–6h
    Cough, PO 2–6 y, 2.5–5 mg q4–6h

**Hydrocodone** (Codone) is similar to codeine. It may be given alone or with other ingredients for analgesic or antitussive effects. For example, Hydrocet and Vicodin are analgesic combinations containing hydrocodone 5 mg and acetaminophen 500 mg.

### Route and dosage ranges

*Adults:* PO 5–10 mg q6–8h
*Children:* PO 0.6 mg/kg per day in three or four divided doses

**Hydromorphone** (Dilaudid) is a semisynthetic derivative of morphine that has the same actions, uses, contraindications, and adverse effects as morphine. Hydromorphone is more potent on a milligram basis and is relatively more effective orally than morphine. Effects occur in 15 to 30 minutes, peak in 30 to 90 minutes, and last 4 to 5 hours.

### Routes and dosage ranges

*Adults:* PO 2–4 mg q4–6h PRN
    IM, SC, IV 1–1.5 mg q4–6h PRN (may be increased to 4 mg for severe pain)
    Rectal suppository 3 mg q6–8h

**Levorphanol** (Levo-Dromoran) is a synthetic drug that is chemically and pharmacologically related to morphine. It has the same uses and produces the same adverse effects, although some reports indicate a lower occurrence of nausea and vomiting. The average dose is probably equianalgesic with 10 mg of morphine. Maximal analgesia occurs 60 to 90 minutes after SC injection. Effects last 4 to 8 hours.

### Routes and dosage ranges

*Adults:* PO, SC 2–3 mg q4–6h PRN

**Meperidine** (Demerol) is a synthetic drug that is similar to morphine in pharmacologic actions. It is one of the most frequently prescribed narcotic analgesics. A parenteral dose of 80 to 100 mg is equivalent to 10 mg of morphine. Oral meperidine is only half as effective as a parenteral dose because approximately half is metabolized in the liver and never reaches the systemic circulation. Meperidine produces sedation and respiratory depression comparable to morphine. Meperidine differs from morphine as follows:

1. It has a shorter duration of action and requires more frequent administration. After parenteral administration, analgesia occurs in about 10 to 20 minutes, peaks in about 1 hour, and lasts about 2 to 4 hours.
2. It has little antitussive effect. However, excessive sedation with meperidine reduces the ability to cough effectively.
3. It causes less respiratory depression in the newborn when used for obstetric analgesia.
4. It causes less smooth muscle spasm and is preferred in renal and biliary colic.
5. With chronic use, toxic doses, or renal failure, meperidine may cause CNS stimulation characterized by tremors, hallucinations, and seizures. These effects are attributed to accumulation of a metabolite, normeperidine.

### Routes and dosage ranges

*Adults:* IM, IV, SC, PO 50–100 mg q2–4h
    Obstetric analgesia, IM, SC 50–100 mg q2–4h for three or four doses

**Methadone** (Dolophine) is a synthetic drug that has essentially the same pharmacologic actions as morphine. Compared to morphine, methadone has a longer duration of action and is relatively more effective when given orally. Analgesia occurs within 10 to 20 minutes after injection and 30 to 60 minutes after oral administration. Methadone is used for severe pain and in the detoxification and maintenance treatment of opiate addicts.

### Routes and dosage ranges

*Adults:* IM, SC 2.5–10 mg q3–4h PRN
    PO 5–20 mg q6–8h PRN

**Oxycodone** is a semisynthetic derivative of codeine used to relieve moderate pain. It is reportedly less potent and less likely to produce dependence than morphine but is more potent and more likely to produce dependence than codeine. It is a drug of abuse. Pharmacologic actions are similar to those of other narcotic analgesics. Oxycodone also is available in combination with aspirin (Percodan) and in combination with acetaminophen (Percocet, Tylox).

### Route and dosage range

*Adults:* PO 5 mg q6h PRN
*Children:* Not recommended for children under 12 years

**Oxymorphone** (Numorphan) is a semisynthetic derivative of morphine. Its actions, uses, and adverse effects are similar to those of morphine, except that it has little antitussive effect.

### Routes and dosage ranges

*Adults:* IM, SC 1–1.5 mg q4–6h PRN, IV 0.5 mg
q4–6h PRN
Rectal suppository, 5 mg q4–6h PRN
Obstetric analgesia, IM 0.5–1 mg

**Propoxyphene** (Darvon) is a synthetic drug chemically related to methadone. It is used for mild to moderate pain but is considered no more effective than 650 mg of aspirin or acetaminophen, with which it is usually given. Propoxyphene is abused (alone and with alcohol or other CNS depressant drugs), and deaths have occurred from overdoses. An overdose causes respiratory depression, excessive sedation, and circulatory failure. Despite these characteristics and recommendations against its usage, the drug continues to be prescribed. Propoxyphene is a Schedule IV drug.

Propoxyphene hydrochloride

#### Route and dosage range

*Adults:* PO 65 mg q4h PRN (maximal daily dose,
390 mg)
*Children:* Not recommended

Propoxyphene napsylate

#### Route and dosage range

*Adults:* PO 100 mg q4h PRN (maximal daily dose,
600 mg)
*Children:* Not recommended

## Agonists-antagonists

These agents have agonist activity at some receptors and antagonist activity at others. Because of their agonist activity, they are potent analgesics with a lower abuse potential than pure agonists; because of their antagonist activity, they may produce withdrawal symptoms in people with opiate dependence.

**Buprenorphine** (Buprenex) is a semisynthetic opioid with a long duration of action and a low incidence of causing physical dependence. These characteristics are attributed to its high affinity for and slow dissociation from mu receptors. With IM administration, analgesia onset occurs in 15 minutes, peaks in 60 minutes, and lasts 6 hours, approximately. It is highly protein bound (about 96%) and has an elimination half-life of 2 to 3 hours. It is metabolized in the liver, and clearance is related to hepatic blood flow. It is excreted mainly in feces.

### Routes and dosage ranges

*Adults:* IM or slow IV (over 2 min) 0.3 mg q6h PRN

**Butorphanol** (Stadol) is a synthetic agonist analgesic similar to morphine and meperidine in analgesic effects and ability to cause respiratory depression. It is used in moderate to severe pain and is given parenterally or topically to nasal mucosa by a metered spray (Stadol NS). After IM or IV administration, analgesia peaks in approximately 30 to 60 minutes. After nasal application, analgesia peaks within 1 to 2 hours. Butorphanol also has antagonist activity and therefore should not be given to people who have been receiving narcotic analgesics or who have narcotic dependence. Other adverse effects include drowsiness or sedation and nausea and vomiting. Butorphanol has not been established as a safe and effective drug for use in pregnancy, labor, delivery, or lactation or in children under 18 years of age.

### Routes and dosage ranges

*Adults:* IM, IV 1–4 mg q3–4h PRN
Nasal spray 1 mg (one spray in one nostril) q3–4h
PRN
*Children:* Not recommended

**Dezocine** (Dalgan) is a synthetic analgesic used for moderate to severe pain and given parenterally. It is similar to morphine in its effects. Onset of analgesia occurs within 15 minutes after IV administration and within 30 minutes after IM injection. Like other drugs in this group, dezocine may cause respiratory depression, sedation, nausea and vomiting, and other adverse effects. It also may cause allergic reactions, especially in people with asthma or allergy to sulfites because it contains metabisulfite.

### Routes and dosage ranges

*Adults:* IM 5–20 mg q3–6h PRN
IV 2.5–10 q2–4h PRN
*Children:* Not recommended

**Nalbuphine** (Nubain) is a synthetic analgesic used for moderate to severe pain and given parenterally. Onset, duration, and extent of analgesia and respiratory depression are comparable to those produced by morphine. Other adverse effects include sedation, sweating, headache, and psychotic symptoms, but these are reportedly minimal at doses of 10 mg or less.

### Routes and dosage ranges

*Adults:* IM, IV, SC 10 mg/70 kg of body weight q3–6h
PRN

**Pentazocine** (Talwin) is a synthetic analgesic drug of abuse and may produce physical and psychological drug dependence. It is a Schedule IV drug. Generally, pentazocine is used for the same clinical indications as other strong analgesics and causes similar adverse effects. Recommended doses for analgesia are less effective than usual doses of morphine or meperidine, but some people may tolerate pentazocine better than morphine or meperidine. Parenteral pentazocine usually produces analgesia within 10 to 30 minutes and lasts 2 to 3 hours. Adverse effects include hallucinations, bizarre dreams or nightmares, depression, nervousness, feelings of depersonalization, extreme euphoria, tissue damage with ulceration and necrosis or fibrosis at injection sites with long-term use, and respiratory depression.

Oral pentazocine tablets contain naloxone 0.5 mg, a narcotic antagonist that prevents the effects of pentazocine if the oral tablet is injected. It has no pharmacologic action if taken orally. Naloxone was added to prevent a method of abuse in which oral tablets of pentazocine and tripelennamine, an antihistamine, were dissolved and injected intravenously. The mixture caused such adverse effects as pulmonary emboli and stroke (from obstruction of blood vessels by talc and other insoluble ingredients in the tablets).

### Routes and dosage ranges

*Adults:* PO 50–100 mg q3–4h (maximal dose, 600 mg/d)

IM, SC, IV 30– 60 mg q3–4h (maximal dose, 360 mg/d)

*Children:* Not recommended for children under 12 years

## NARCOTIC ANTAGONISTS

Narcotic antagonists reverse the analgesic and depressant effects of narcotic agonists by displacing the agonists from their receptor sites. When an opiate cannot bind to receptor sites, it is "neutralized" and cannot exert its effects on body cells. Narcotic antagonists do not relieve the depressant effects of other drugs, such as sedative-hypnotics, antianxiety agents, and antipsychotic agents. *The chief clinical use of these drugs is to relieve the severe CNS and respiratory depression that occurs with narcotic overdose.* They produce withdrawal symptoms when given to opiate-dependent people.

**Naloxone** (Narcan) injection is the drug of choice in respiratory depression known or thought to be caused by a narcotic. Therapeutic effects occur within minutes after parenteral injection and last 1 to 2 hours. Naloxone has a shorter duration of action than narcotics, and repeated injections are usually needed. For a long-acting drug, such as methadone, injections may be needed for 2 to 3 days. Naloxone produces few adverse effects, and repeated injections can be given safely.

### Routes and dosage ranges

*Adults:* IV, IM, SC 0.1–0.4 mg, repeated IV q2–3 min PRN

*Children:* IV, IM, SC 0.01 mg/kg of body weight initially, repeated IV q2–3 min PRN

**Naltrexone** (Trexan) is structurally and pharmacologically similar to naloxone. It competes with narcotics for opioid receptor sites in the brain to prevent narcotic binding with receptors or displaces narcotics already occupying receptor sites. This action blocks euphoria, analgesia, and other physiologic effects of narcotics. Naltrexone is used in the maintenance of opiate-free states in opiate addicts. It is apparently effective in highly motivated, detoxified people. If given before the client is detoxified, acute withdrawal symptoms occur. Clients receiving naltrexone will not respond to analgesics if pain control is needed. The drug is recommended for use in conjunction with psychological and social counseling.

### Route and dosage range

*Adults:* PO 50 mg/day

## Nursing Process

### Assessment

Pain is a subjective experience (whatever the person says it is), and individuals display a wide variety of responses. Although pain thresholds (the point at which a stimulus produces a sensation of pain) are similar, people differ in their perceptions, behaviors, and tolerance of pain. Differences in pain perception may result from psychological components, especially when fatigue, anxiety, and other stressors are present along with the pain. Differences in behaviors may or may not indicate pain to observers, and overt signs and symptoms are not reliable indicators of the presence or extent of pain. Especially with chronic pain, overt signs and symptoms may be absent or minimal. Differences in tolerance of pain (the point at which an individual seeks relief) often reflect the person's concern about the meaning of the pain and the type or intensity of the painful stimulus. Thus, pain is a complex physiologic, psychological, and sociocultural phenomenon that must be thoroughly assessed if it is to be managed effectively.

The nurse needs to assess every client in relation to pain, initially to determine appropriate interventions and later to determine whether the interventions were effective in preventing or relieving pain. Although the client is usually the best source of data, other people may be questioned about the client's words and behaviors that indicate pain. This is especially important with young children. During assessment, keep in mind that acute pain may coexist or be superimposed on chronic pain. Specific assessment data usually include:

- *Location*. Determining location may assist in relieving pain or identifying its underlying cause. Ask the person to show you where it hurts, if possible, and whether the pain stays in one place or radiates to other parts of the body. The term *referred pain* is used when pain arising from tissue damage in one area of the body is felt in another area. Patterns of referred pain may be helpful in diagnosis. For example, pain of cardiac origin may radiate to the neck, shoulders, chest muscles, and down the arms, often on the left side. This form of pain usually results from myocardial ischemia due to atherosclerosis of coronary arteries. Stomach pain is usually referred to the epigastrium and may indicate gastritis or peptic ulcer. Gallbladder and bile duct pain is usually localized in the midepigastrium or right upper quadrant of the abdomen. Uterine pain is usually felt as abdominal cramping or low back pain. Deep or chronic pain is usually more difficult to localize than superficial or acute pain.

- *Intensity or severity*. Because pain is a subjective experience and cannot be objectively measured, assessment of severity is based on the client's description and the nurse's observations. It may help to ask the client to rank the pain as mild, moderate, or severe or to use a number scale, such as 0 (no pain) to 10 (severe pain).
- *Relationship to time, activities, and other signs and symptoms*. Specific questions include:
  - When did the pain start?
  - What activities were occurring when the pain started?
  - Does the pain occur with exercise or when at rest?
  - Do other signs and symptoms occur before, during, or after the pain?
  - Is this the first episode of this particular type of pain, or is this a repeated occurrence?
  - How long does the pain last?
  - What, if anything, decreases or relieves the pain?
  - What, if anything, aggravates the pain?
- *Other data*. For example, do not assume that postoperative pain is incisional and requires narcotic analgesics for relief. A person who has had abdominal surgery may have headache, musculoskeletal discomfort, or "gas pains." Also, restlessness may be caused by hypoxia rather than pain.

### Nursing diagnoses

- Pain
- High Risk for Impaired Gas Exchange related to sedation and decreased mobility
- High Risk for Injury related to sedation and decreased mobility
- Constipation related to slowed peristalsis
- High Risk for Altered Tissue Perfusion related to drug-induced decrease in cardiac output and blood pressure
- High Risk for Urinary Retention related to decreased bladder contractility
- Knowledge Deficit: Appropriate use of narcotic drugs
- High Risk for Noncompliance: Drug dependence related to overuse

### Planning/Goals

*The client will:*
- Avoid or be relieved of pain
- Use narcotic analgesics appropriately
- Avoid preventable adverse effects
- Be closely monitored for excessive sedation and respiratory depression
- Be able to perform activities of daily living when feasible

### Interventions

Use measures to prevent, relieve, or decrease pain when possible. General measures include those that promote optimal body functioning and those that prevent trauma, inflammation, infection, and other sources of painful stimuli. Specific measures include:
- Encourage pulmonary hygiene techniques (*e.g.*, coughing, deep breathing, and ambulation), to promote respiration

and prevent pulmonary complications, such as pneumonia and atelectasis.
- Use sterile technique when caring for wounds, urinary catheters, or IV lines.
- Use exercises, ambulation, and position changes to promote circulation.
- Handle any injured tissue very gently to avoid further trauma.
- Prevent bowel or bladder distention.
- Apply heat or cold.
- Use relaxation or distraction techniques.
- If a client is in pain on initial contact, try to relieve the pain as soon as possible. Once pain is controlled, plan with the client to avoid or manage future episodes.
- If a client is not in pain initially but anticipates surgery or an uncomfortable diagnostic procedure, plan with the client ways to minimize and manage discomfort.

*Teach clients:*
- Personalized methods of pain prevention
- Personalized methods of pain management
- That use of a narcotic analgesic for acute pain is acceptable and unlikely to lead to physical dependence (addiction)
- To use the least amount of the mildest drug that is likely to be effective in a particular situation
- *Preoperatively*:
  - How postoperative pain will be managed (*e.g.*, analgesics are usually given by injection for 2 or 3 days after surgery, then orally; analgesics may be ordered every 1 to 6 hours as needed and be nurse administered or patient controlled)
  - How to report pain or request pain medication.
  - That it is better to take adequate medication to control pain and be able to cough, deep breathe, and ambulate than to avoid medication and be unable to perform activities that promote recovery
- To avoid other CNS depressant drugs (*e.g.*, alcoholic beverages, antihistamines, sleeping pills) when taking narcotic analgesics as an outpatient and to report perceived adverse drug effects to a health-care provider

### Evaluation

- Ask clients about their levels of comfort or relief from pain.
- Observe behaviors that indicate the presence or absence of pain.
- Observe participation and ability to function in usual activities of daily living.
- Observe for presence or absence of sedation and respiratory depression.
- Observe for drug-seeking behavior (possibly indicating dependence).

## Principles of therapy

### THE NEED FOR EFFECTIVE PAIN MANAGEMENT

Numerous studies have indicated ineffective management of patients' pain, especially moderate to severe pain associated with surgery or cancer. Much of the difficulty has been attributed to inadequate or improper use of narcotic analgesics, including administering the wrong drug, prescribing inadequate dosage, or leaving long intervals between doses. Even when ordered appropriately, nurses or patients and family members may not administer the drugs effectively. Traditionally, concerns about respiratory depression, excessive sedation, drug dependence, and other adverse effects have contributed to reluctance and delay in administering narcotic analgesics. Also, many health care providers and patients have thought it desirable to take the least amount possible and only when pain is intolerable. Studies indicate that this approach allows alternating episodes of pain and relief, which contribute to anxiety, depression, and other emotional upsets from anticipation of pain recurrence.

During the past several years, a more humane approach to pain management has evolved. Basic assumptions of this approach are that no one should suffer pain needlessly; that pain occurs when the patient says it does and should be relieved by whatever means required, including pharmacologic and nonpharmacologic treatments; that doses of narcotics should be titrated to achieve maximum effectiveness and minimum toxicity; and that dependence rarely results from drugs taken for physical pain. Proponents of this view emphasize the need to assess and monitor all clients receiving narcotic analgesics.

## DRUG SELECTION

1. Morphine is often the drug of first choice for severe pain. It is effective, available in a variety of dosage strengths and forms, can be used short- or long-term, and its adverse effects are well known. In addition, it is a "non-ceiling" drug. This means that there is no upper limit to the dosage that can be given to clients who have developed tolerance to previous dosages. This characteristic is especially valuable in cancer patients with severe pain, because drug dosage can be increased and titrated to relieve pain when pain increases or tolerance develops. Thus, some patients have safely received extremely large doses. Hydromorphone, levorphanol, and methadone are other non-ceiling drugs.

   In contrast, meperidine and pentazocine are "ceiling" drugs of which doses cannot be increased sufficiently or titrated to relieve increasing pain without greatly increasing the incidence and severity of adverse effects. These drugs are not recommended for treatment of chronic cancer pain.
2. When more than one analgesic drug is ordered, use the least potent drug that is effective in relieving pain. For example, use non-narcotic analgesics, such as aspirin or acetaminophen, rather than a narcotic analgesic when feasible.
3. Non-narcotic analgesics may be alternated or given concurrently with narcotic analgesics, especially in chronic pain. This increases client comfort, reduces the likelihood of drug abuse and dependence, and decreases tolerance to pain-relieving effects of the narcotic analgesics.
4. In many instances, the drug preparation of choice may be one that combines a narcotic and a non-narcotic. The drugs act by different mechanisms and therefore produce greater analgesic effects. Commonly used examples are Tylenol #3 (acetaminophen 325 mg and codeine 30 mg/tablet) and Percocet (acetaminophen 325 mg and oxycodone 5 mg/tablet).

## ROUTE SELECTION

1. IV injection of a narcotic is usually preferred for rapid relief of acute pain. Small, frequent IV doses are often effective in relieving pain with minimal risk of serious adverse effects. This is especially advantageous during a serious illness or after surgery.

   A technique called patient-controlled analgesia allows self-administration. This device consists of a syringe of diluted drug connected to an IV line and infusion pump. The syringe delivers the dose when the patient pushes a button. The amount of drug delivered with each dose and the intervals between doses are preset and limited. Studies indicate that analgesia is more effective, patient satisfaction is high, and smaller amounts of drug are used than with conventional PRN administration.
2. Continuous IV infusion may be used to treat severe, chronic pain.
3. Two other routes of administration are used to manage acute pain. One route involves injection of narcotic analgesics directly into the CNS (epidural and intrathecal). The other involves the use of local anesthetics to provide regional analgesia. Both of these methods are effective in relieving pain, but they also increase risks of adverse effects and require special techniques and monitoring procedures for safe use.
4. Oral drugs are preferred when feasible, especially for long-term use; patients are often discharged from clinical settings on oral preparations.

## DOSAGE

Dosages of narcotic analgesics should be sufficient to relieve pain without causing unacceptable adverse effects. Thus, dosages should be individualized according to the type and severity of pain; the client's age, size, and health or illness status; whether the client has previously taken narcotics and developed drug tolerance; whether the client has progressive or worsening disease; and other characteristics that influence responses to pain. Guidelines include:

1. Small to moderate doses relieve constant, dull pain; moderate to large doses relieve intermittent, sharp pain caused by trauma or conditions affecting the viscera.
2. When a narcotic analgesic is ordered in variable amounts (such as 8–10 mg of morphine), give the smaller amount as long as it is effective in relieving pain.
3. Dosages of narcotic analgesics should be reduced for clients who also are receiving other CNS depressants, such as antipsychotic or antianxiety agents, barbiturates, or other sedative-hypnotic drugs.

## SCHEDULING

Narcotic analgesics may be given as needed, within designated time limits, or on a regular schedule. Traditionally, the drugs have often been scheduled every 4 to 6 hours PRN. Numerous studies have indicated that such a schedule is often ineffective in managing patients' pain. Because narcotic analgesics are used for moderate to severe pain, they should generally be scheduled to provide effective and consistent pain relief. Some guidelines for scheduling drugs include:

1. When analgesics are ordered PRN, have a clear-cut system by which the client reports pain or requests medication. The client should know that analgesic drugs have been ordered and will be given promptly when needed. If a drug cannot be given or if administration must be delayed, explain this to the client. In addition, offer or give the drug when indicated by the client's condition rather than waiting for the client to request medication.
2. In *acute pain*, narcotic analgesics are most effective when given parenterally and at the onset of pain. In *chronic, severe pain*, narcotic analgesics are most effective when given on a regular schedule.
3. When needed, analgesics should be given before coughing and deep-breathing exercises, dressing changes, and other therapeutic and diagnostic procedures.
4. Narcotics are not recommended for prolonged periods except for advanced malignant disease. Healthcare agencies usually have an automatic "stop order" for narcotics after 48 to 72 hours; this means that the drug is discontinued when the time limit expires if the physician does not reorder it.

## DRUG USE IN SPECIFIC SITUATIONS

### Malignant disease

When narcotic analgesics are required in the chronic pain associated with malignancy, the main consideration is client comfort, not preventing drug addiction. Effective treatment requires that pain be relieved and prevented from recurring. With disease progression and the development of drug tolerance, extremely large doses and frequent administration may be required. In addition to analgesics, other drugs or treatments may be used to increase client comfort. For example, tricyclic antidepressant drugs are thought to have analgesic effects, and laxatives may be needed to prevent constipation from the narcotics.

### Biliary, renal, or ureteral colic

When narcotic analgesics are used to relieve the acute, severe pain associated with various types of colic, an antispasmodic drug such as atropine may be needed as well. Narcotic analgesics may increase smooth muscle tone and cause spasm. Atropine does not have strong antispasmodic properties of its own in usual doses, but it apparently reduces the spasm-producing effects of narcotic analgesics.

### Postoperative use

When analgesics are used postoperatively, the goal is to relieve pain without excessive sedation so that clients can do deep-breathing exercises, cough, ambulate, and implement other measures to promote recovery.

### Burns

In severely burned people, use narcotic analgesics cautiously. A common cause of respiratory arrest in burned clients is excessive administration of analgesic drugs. Generally, agitation in a burned person should be interpreted as hypoxia or hypovolemia rather than pain, until proved otherwise. When narcotic analgesics are necessary, they are usually given IV in small doses. Drugs given by other routes are absorbed erratically in the presence of shock and hypovolemia.

## MANAGEMENT OF TOXICITY OR OVERDOSE

Acute toxicity or narcotic overdose can occur from therapeutic use or from abuse by drug-dependent people (see Chap. 15). The main goal of treatment is to restore and maintain adequate respiratory function. This can be accomplished by inserting an artificial airway, such as an endotracheal tube, and starting mechanical ventilation or by giving a narcotic antagonist, such as naloxone.

## USE IN CHILDREN

Other than reduced dosage, there are few guidelines about use of narcotic analgesics in children. There also are few guidelines about assessment and management of pain with other interventions.

1. Expressions of pain may differ according to age and developmental level. Infants may cry and have muscular rigidity and thrashing behavior. Preschoolers may behave aggressively or complain verbally of discomfort. School-aged children may express pain verbally or behaviorally, often with regression to behaviors used at younger ages. Adolescents may be reluctant to admit they are uncomfortable or need help.

2. Narcotic formulations specifically for children are not generally available. When children's doses are calculated from adult doses, the fractions and decimals that often result greatly increase the risk of a dosage error.

3. Narcotic rectal suppositories may be used more often in children than in adults. Although they may be useful when oral or parenteral routes are not indicated, there are disadvantages as well. One disadvantage is that drug absorption is erratic, and therefore the drug dose is unpredictable. Another disadvantage is that adult suppositories are sometimes cut in half or otherwise altered; this may lead to an unknown dose.

4. Narcotic effects in children may differ from those expected in adults because of physiologic and pharmacokinetic differences. Be alert for unusual signs and symptoms.

## USE IN OLDER ADULTS

Narcotic analgesics should be used very cautiously in older adults, generally for acute, severe pain or terminal cancer pain. They also should be given in smaller doses and at longer intervals because the duration of action may be longer. Older adults are especially sensitive to respiratory depression, excessive sedation, and other adverse effects.

# NURSING ACTIONS: NARCOTIC ANALGESICS

## *Nursing Actions*

## *Rationale/Explanation*

1. **Administer accurately**
   **a.** Check the rate, depth, and rhythm of respirations before each dose. If the rate is below 12 per minute, delay or omit the dose and report to the physician.

   Respiratory depression is a major adverse reaction to strong analgesics. Assessing respirations before each dose can help prevent or minimize potentially life-threatening respiratory depression.

   **b.** Have the client lie down to receive injections of narcotic analgesics and for at least a few minutes afterward.

   To prevent or minimize hypotension, nausea, and vomiting. These side effects are more likely to occur in the ambulatory client. Also, the client may be sedated enough to make ambulation hazardous without help.

   **c.** When injecting narcotic analgesics intravenously, give small doses; inject slowly over several minutes; and have narcotic antagonist drugs, artificial airways, and equipment for artificial ventilation readily available.

   Large doses or rapid intravenous injection may cause severe respiratory depression and hypotension.

   **d.** Give meperidine and pentazocine intramuscularly rather than subcutaneously.

   Subcutaneous injections of these drugs may cause pain, tissue irritation, and possible abscess. This reaction is more likely with long-term use.

   **e.** Put siderails up; instruct the client not to smoke or try to ambulate without help. Keep the call light within reach.

   To prevent falls or other injuries

2. **Observe for therapeutic effects**

   Therapeutic effects depend on the reason for use, usually for analgesic effects, sometimes for antitussive or antidiarrheal effects.

   **a.** A verbal statement of pain relief

   **b.** Decreased behavioral manifestations of pain or discomfort

   **c.** Sleeping

*(continued)*

## Nursing Actions

## Rationale/Explanation

**d.** Increased participation in usual activities of daily living, including social interactions with other people in the environment

**e.** Fewer and shorter episodes of nonproductive coughing when used for antitussive effects

Narcotic analgesics relieve cough by depressing the cough center in the medulla oblongata.

**f.** Lowered blood pressure, decreased pulse rate, slower and deeper respirations, and less dyspnea when morphine is given for pulmonary edema

Morphine may relieve pulmonary edema by causing vasodilation, which in turn decreases venous return to the heart and decreases cardiac work.

**g.** Decreased diarrhea when given for constipating effects

These drugs slow secretions and motility of the gastrointestinal tract. Constipation is usually an adverse effect. However, in severe diarrhea or with ileostomy, the drugs decrease the number of bowel movements and make the consistency more paste-like than liquid.

**3. Observe for adverse effects**
**a.** Respiratory depression—hypoxemia, restlessness, dyspnea, slow, shallow breathing, changes in blood pressure and pulse, decreased ability to cough

Respiratory depression is a major adverse effect of narcotic analgesics and results from depression of the respiratory center in the medulla oblongata. Respiratory depression occurs with usual therapeutic doses and increases in incidence and severity with large doses or frequent administration.

**b.** Hypotension

Hypotension stems from drug effects on the vasomotor center in the medulla oblongata that cause peripheral vasodilation and lowering of blood pressure. This is a therapeutic effect with pulmonary edema.

**c.** Excessive sedation—drowsiness, slurred speech, impaired mobility and coordination, stupor, coma

This is caused by depression of the CNS and is potentially life-threatening.

**d.** Nausea and vomiting

Narcotic analgesics stimulate the chemoreceptor trigger zone in the brain. Consequently, nausea and vomiting may occur with oral or parenteral routes of administration. They are more likely to occur with ambulation than with recumbency.

**e.** Constipation

This is caused by the drug's slowing effects on the gastrointestinal tract. Constipation may be alleviated by activity, adequate food and fluid intake, and regular administration of mild laxatives.

**4. Observe for drug interactions**
**a.** Drugs that *increase* effects of narcotic analgesics

(1) CNS depressants—alcohol, general anesthetics, antianxiety agents, tricyclic antidepressants, antihistamines, antipsychotic agents, barbiturates, and other sedative-hypnotic drugs

All these drugs alone, as well as the narcotic analgesics, produce CNS depression. When combined, additive CNS depression results. If dosage of one or more interacting drugs is high, severe respiratory depression, coma, and death may ensue.

(2) Diuretics

Orthostatic hypotension, an adverse effect of strong analgesics and diuretics, may be increased if the two drug groups are given concurrently.

(3) Monoamine oxidase (MAO) inhibitors

These drugs interfere with detoxification of some narcotic analgesics, especially meperidine. They may cause additive CNS depression with hypotension and respiratory depression or CNS stimulation with hyperexcitability and convulsions. If an MAO inhibitor is necessary, dosage should be reduced because the combination is potentially life-threatening.

(continued)

## Nursing Actions                          ## Rationale/Explanation

**b.** Drugs that *decrease* effects of narcotic analgesics

(1) Narcotic antagonists

These drugs reverse respiratory depression produced by narcotic analgesics. This is their only clinical use, and they should not be given unless severe respiratory depression is present. They do not reverse respiratory depression caused by other CNS depressants.

(2) Butorphanol, nalbuphine, and pentazocine

These analgesics are weak antagonists of narcotic analgesics, and they may cause withdrawal symptoms in people who have been receiving opiates or who are physically dependent on narcotic analgesics.

**5. Teach clients:**

**a.** Take only as prescribed. If desired effects are not achieved, report to the physician. Do not increase the dose, and do not take medication more often than prescribed.

Although these principles apply to all medications, they are especially important with analgesics because of potentially serious adverse reactions, including drug dependence, and because analgesics may mask or enable the client to tolerate pain for which medical attention is needed.

**b.** Do not drink alcohol or take other drugs without the physician's knowledge.

Alcohol and pain-relieving narcotics depress the nervous system; combining them can cause serious, even life-threatening problems. Numerous other drugs have depressant effects as well, and additive effects leading to excessive adverse reactions can result. For example, tranquilizers, sleeping pills, antihistamines, and cold remedies can all increase the risks of drug-induced problems that could be worse than the initial problem.

**c.** Do not drive a car or operate machinery when drowsy or dizzy or when vision is blurred from medication.

Automobiles and machinery should be operated only by fully alert people with good vision.

**d.** Do not smoke when drowsy from medication.

Smoking when less than alert is unsafe.

**e.** Stay in bed at least 30 to 60 minutes after receiving injection of an analgesic.

To prevent or minimize hypotension, nausea, and vomiting, which often occur with ambulation. Also, a sedated person is risking falls and traumatic injuries. An exception may be the person who has been receiving the drug for some time and who has developed tolerance to its sedative effects.

**f.** Do not object to having side rails up on the bed after an injection of analgesic.

Side rails promote safety by serving as a reminder to stay in bed or to call for assistance.

**g.** If not contraindicated, eat high-fiber foods, such as whole-grain cereals, fruits, and vegetables, drink 2 to 3 quarts of fluid daily, and be as active as tolerated.

To prevent or minimize constipation

## Review and Application Exercises

1. When assessing a client for pain, what are major guidelines?
2. What kinds of behaviors may indicate acute pain? Are similar behaviors associated with chronic pain?
3. What are some nonpharmacologic interventions for pain, and why should they be used instead of or along with analgesics?

4. What are the major adverse effects of narcotic analgesics? How does naloxone (Narcan) act to counteract adverse effects?
5. For a client who has had major surgery during the previous 24 to 72 hours, what type of analgesic is indicated? Why?
6. What are the potential differences in dosage between short-term (a few days) and long-term (weeks or months) administration of morphine?
7. Explain the rationale for using both narcotic an-

algesics and non-narcotic analgesics in the treatment of pain.

8. For a client with chronic cancer pain, what are advantages and disadvantages of using narcotic analgesics?

9. Why is meperidine (Demerol) not recommended for management of chronic cancer pain?

10. For a client with chronic cancer pain, should narcotic analgesics be given as needed or on a regular schedule? Why?

## Selected References

Acute Pain Management Guideline Panel (1992). *Acute pain management: Operative or medical procedures and trauma. Clinical practice guideline*. AHCPR Pub. No. 92-0032. Rockville, MD: Agency for Health Care Policy and Research, Public Health Service, U.S. Department of Health and Human Services for Health Care Policy and Research.

Curtis, S. M., & Curtis, R. L. (1990). Somatosensory function and pain. In C. M. Porth (Ed.), *Pathophysiology: Concepts of altered health states* (3rd ed.) (pp. 839–872). Philadelphia: J.B. Lippincott.

(1993). *Drug facts and comparisons*. St. Louis: Facts and Comparisons.

Guyton, A. C. (1991). *Textbook of medical physiology* (8th ed.). Philadelphia: W.B. Saunders.

Holdsworth, M., & Forman, W. B. (1993). Pain control. In R. Bressler & M. D. Katz (Eds.), *Geriatric pharmacology* (pp. 207–229). New York: McGraw-Hill.

Kee, J. L., & Hayes, E. R. (1993). *Pharmacology: A nursing process approach*. Philadelphia: W.B. Saunders.

Kelley, W. N. (Ed.) (1992). *Textbook of internal medicine* (2nd ed.). Philadelphia: J.B. Lippincott.

Koo, P. J., & Dube, J. E. (1992). Pain. In M. A. Koda-Kimble & L. Y. Young (Eds.), *Applied therapeutics: The clinical use of drugs* (5th ed.) (pp. 4-1–4-19). Vancouver, WA: Applied Therapeutics.

(1993). *Physicians' desk reference* (47th ed.). Montvale, NJ: Medical Economics Data.

Stanski, D. R., & Roizen, M. F. (1992). Analgesia and anesthesia. In K. L. Melmon, H. F. Morrelli, B. B. Hoffman, & D. W. Nierenberg (Eds.), *Clinical pharmacology: Basic principles in therapeutics* (3rd ed.) (pp. 721–737). New York: McGraw-Hill.

Wallace, K. G. (1992). Nursing management of adults in pain. In L. O. Burrell (Ed.), *Adult nursing in hospital and community settings* (pp. 177–207). Norwalk, CT: Appleton & Lange.

### CHAPTER 6

# Analgesic–Antipyretic– Anti-inflammatory and Related Drugs

## Description

The analgesic–antipyretic–anti-inflammatory drugs relieve pain, fever, and inflammation. Acetylsalicylic acid (ASA, aspirin) is the prototype of the group. Except for acetaminophen, the drugs in this group also are called nonsteroidal anti-inflammatory drugs (NSAIDs). Several NSAIDs are used primarily for their anti-inflammatory effects in rheumatic diseases, such as rheumatoid arthritis and gout. Acetaminophen (Tylenol and others) is not an NSAID because it does not have anti-inflammatory effects. It is included in this chapter because of its extensive use as an analgesic and antipyretic.

The other drugs included here are those used in the prevention and treatment of gout attacks and those used in the treatment of migraine. (The adrenocorticosteroids, the most potent anti-inflammatory drugs, are discussed in Chap. 24.) Most of these drugs inhibit the synthesis of prostaglandins, and both therapeutic and adverse effects are attributed primarily to this action. To understand the effects of these drugs, therefore, an understanding of prostaglandins, as well as of pain, fever, and inflammation, is needed.

## Prostaglandins

*Prostaglandins* are substances synthesized in the body from arachidonic acid, a free fatty acid released from the phospholipids in cell membranes in response to various physical, chemical, hormonal, bacterial, and other stimuli. They are produced in specific body tissues, where they exert their effects and are then rapidly inactivated. The specific type of prostaglandin produced depends on the tissue involved, the stimulus, the hormonal environment, and other factors. Table 6-1 lists several physiologically important prostaglandins and their effects.

Prostaglandins are found in most body tissues and help to regulate many cell functions, including the following:

1. In the inflammatory process, prostaglandins potentiate the pain and edema caused by bradykinin, histamine, and other substances released in areas of tissue damage.
2. They regulate smooth muscle in blood vessels, the gastrointestinal tract, respiratory system, and reproductive system.

Anne Collins Abrams: CLINICAL DRUG THERAPY, Fourth Edition.
© 1995 J.B. Lippincott Company.

**TABLE 6-1. PROSTAGLANDINS AND THEIR EFFECTS**

| Prostaglandin | Effects |
|---|---|
| $D_2$ | Bronchoconstriction |
| $E_2$ | Vasodilation |
| | Bronchodilation |
| | Increased activity of gastrointestinal (GI) smooth muscle |
| | Increased sensitivity to pain |
| | Increased body temperature |
| $F_2$ | Bronchoconstriction |
| | increased uterine contraction |
| | Increased activity of GI smooth muscle |
| $I_2$ (Prostacyclin) | Vasodilation |
| | Decreased platelet aggregation |
| Thromboxane $A_2$ | Vasoconstriction |
| | Increased platelet aggregation |

3. They protect gastrointestinal mucosa from the erosive effects of gastric acid.
4. They regulate renal blood flow and distribution.
5. They control platelet function.
6. They maintain a patent ductus arteriosus in the fetus.

## PAIN, FEVER, AND INFLAMMATION

*Pain* is the sensation of discomfort, hurt, or distress. It may be mild or severe, acute or chronic (see Chap. 5).

*Fever* is an elevation of body temperature above the normal range. Body temperature is controlled by a regulating center in the hypothalamus. Normally, there is a balance between heat production and heat loss so that a constant body temperature is maintained. When there is excessive heat production, mechanisms to increase heat loss are activated. As a result, blood vessels dilate, more blood flows through the skin, sweating occurs, and body temperature usually stays within normal range. When fever occurs, the heat-regulating center in the hypothalamus is reset so that it tolerates a higher body temperature. Fever may be produced by dehydration, inflammatory and infectious processes, some drugs, brain injury, or diseases involving the hypothalamus. Prostaglandin formation is stimulated by such circumstances and, along with bacterial toxins and other substances, prostaglandins act as pyrogens (fever-producing agents).

*Inflammation* is the normal body response to tissue damage from chemicals, microorganisms, trauma, foreign bodies, surgery, and ionizing radiation. It may occur in any tissue or organ. It is an attempt by the body to remove the damaging agent and repair the damaged tissue. The local manifestations of inflammation are redness, heat, edema, and pain. Redness and heat result from vasodilation and increased blood supply; edema results from leakage of blood plasma into the area; and pain is produced by the pressure of edema and secretions

on nerve endings and by chemical irritation of bradykinin, histamine, and other substances released by the damaged cells. Prostaglandins also are released and increase the pain and edema caused by other substances. Systemic manifestations of inflammation include leukocytosis, increased erythrocyte sedimentation rate, fever, headache, loss of appetite, lethargy or malaise, and weakness. Both local and systemic manifestations vary according to the cause and extent of tissue damage. Like pain, inflammation may be acute or chronic.

## Mechanism of action

Aspirin and NSAIDs inactivate cyclooxygenase (also called prostaglandin synthetase), the enzyme that initiates the formation of prostaglandins from arachidonic acid. This action prevents or inhibits prostaglandin formation and thereby prevents or inhibits its effects on body tissues. Although other factors may be involved, this antiprostaglandin effect is thought to be the primary mechanism of action for these drugs.

To relieve pain, the analgesic–antipyretic–anti-inflammatory drugs act peripherally to prevent sensitization of pain receptors to various chemical substances released by damaged cells. To relieve fever, the drugs act on the hypothalamus to decrease its response to pyrogens and reset the "thermostat" at a lower level. For inflammation, they prevent prostaglandins from increasing the pain and edema produced by bradykinin and other substances released by damaged cells. Although these drugs relieve symptoms and contribute greatly to the client's comfort and quality of life, they do not cure the underlying disorders that cause the symptoms.

The mechanism and extent of antiplatelet effects differ with aspirin and other NSAIDs. When aspirin is absorbed into the bloodstream, the acetyl portion dissociates, then binds irreversibly to platelet cyclooxygenase. This action prevents synthesis of thromboxane $A_2$ and thereby inhibits platelet aggregation. A small single dose (325 mg or less) irreversibly acetylates circulating platelets within a few minutes, and effects last for the life span of the platelets (7–10 days). Other NSAIDs bind reversibly with platelet cyclooxygenase so that antiplatelet effects occur only while the drug is present in the blood. Thus, aspirin has greater effects, but all the drugs inhibit platelet aggregation, cause hypoprothrombinemia, interfere with blood coagulation, and increase the risk of bleeding.

In addition to analgesic–antipyretic–anti-inflammatory and antiplatelet activity, aspirin and NSAIDs cause gastrointestinal bleeding and irritation and ulceration of gastric mucosa. Most of the newer drugs have been developed in an effort to retain the analgesic and anti-inflammatory properties of aspirin while decreasing the adverse effects. These efforts have been only partly successful.

## Indications for use

Despite many similarities, aspirin and other NSAIDs differ in their approved indications for use. Aspirin, a salicylate, has long been the drug of choice in many disorders characterized by pain, fever, or inflammation, and it may be used for one, two, or all three of these symptoms. It also is often prescribed for clients at high risk of myocardial infarction or stroke from thrombosis. This indication for use stems from its antiplatelet activity and resultant effects on blood coagulation (*i.e.*, decreased clot formation).

Acetaminophen, which differs chemically from aspirin, is commonly used as an aspirin substitute for pain and fever, but it lacks anti-inflammatory effects. It is increasingly used to relieve pain associated with osteoarthritis because the disease process is degenerative rather than inflammatory. Ibuprofen (Motrin and others) and other propionic acid derivatives were initially used as anti-inflammatory agents, but they are increasingly used as analgesics as well. Ketorolac (Toradol), which can be given orally and parenterally, is used only as an analgesic. Most of the other NSAIDs are considered too toxic to use as analgesics and antipyretics. They are used primarily in rheumatoid arthritis and other musculoskeletal disorders that do not respond to safer drugs.

Some commonly used drugs and their indications for use are summarized in Table 6-2.

## Contraindications for use

Contraindications to clinical use of these drugs include peptic ulcer disease, gastrointestinal or other bleeding disorders, history of hypersensitivity reactions, and impaired renal function. In people who are allergic to aspirin, nonaspirin NSAIDs also are contraindicated because hypersensitivity reactions may occur with any drugs that inhibit prostaglandin synthesis.

## Individual drugs

**Aspirin** is the prototype of the analgesic–antipyretic–anti-inflammatory drugs and is by far the most commonly used salicylate. Aspirin is effective in pain of low to moderate intensity, especially that involving the skin,

**TABLE 6-2. CLINICAL INDICATIONS FOR COMMONLY USED ANALGESIC–ANTIPYRETIC–ANTI-INFLAMMATORY DRUGS**

| Generic/Trade Name | Pain | Fever | Osteoarthritis | Rheumatoid Arthritis | Juvenile Rheumatoid Arthritis | Dysmenorrhea | Acute Painful Shoulder | Ankylosing Spondylitis | Bursitis | Gout | Tendinitis |
|---|---|---|---|---|---|---|---|---|---|---|---|
| **Acetaminophen** (Tylenol, others) | ✔ | ✔ | | | | | | | | | |
| **Acetylsalicylic Acid** (Aspirin) | ✔ | ✔ | ✔ | ✔ | ✔ | ✔ | ✔ | ✔ | ✔ | ✔ | ✔ |
| **Diclofenac** (Voltaren) | | | ✔ | ✔ | | | | ✔ | | | |
| **Diflunisal** (Dolobid) | ✔ | | ✔ | ✔ | | | | | | | |
| **Etodolac** (Lodine) | ✔ | | ✔ | | | | | | | | |
| **Fenoprofen** (Nalfon) | ✔ | | ✔ | ✔ | | | | | | | |
| **Flurbiprofen** (Ansaid) | | | ✔ | ✔ | | | | | | | |
| **Ibuprofen** (Motrin, others) | ✔ | ✔ | ✔ | ✔ | | ✔ | | | | ✔ | ✔ |
| **Indomethacin** (Indocin) | | | ✔ | ✔ | | | ✔ | ✔ | ✔ | ✔ | ✔ |
| **Ketoprofen** (Orudis) | ✔ | | ✔ | ✔ | | ✔ | | | ✔ | ✔ | ✔ |
| **Ketorolac** (Toradol) | ✔ | | | | | | | | | | |
| **Nabumetone** (Relafen) | | | ✔ | ✔ | | | | | | | |
| **Naproxen** (Naprosyn) | ✔ | | ✔ | ✔ | ✔ | ✔ | | ✔ | ✔ | ✔ | ✔ |
| **Piroxicam** (Feldene) | | | ✔ | ✔ | | | | | | | |
| **Sulindac** (Clinoril) | | | ✔ | ✔ | | | ✔ | ✔ | ✔ | ✔ | ✔ |
| **Tolmetin** (Tolectin) | | | ✔ | ✔ | ✔ | | | | | | |

muscles, joints, and other connective tissue. It is especially useful in disorders in which inflammation contributes to pain, such as rheumatoid arthritis. However, it does not relieve the underlying disease process that produces those symptoms.

Because aspirin is a nonprescription drug, it is a frequently used home remedy for headaches, colds, influenza and other respiratory infections, muscular aches, and fever. It also is prescribed by physicians for a variety of clinical conditions, often with codeine for additive analgesic effects. Other common conditions in which aspirin is used are dysmenorrhea, acute rheumatic fever, rheumatoid arthritis, and other musculoskeletal disorders.

Aspirin can be purchased in plain, chewable, enteric-coated, and effervescent tablets and rectal suppositories. It is not marketed in liquid form because it is unstable in solution. It also is available in combination with other analgesics, antacids, and antihistamines and is an ingredient in many nonprescription cold and allergy remedies.

### Routes and dosage ranges

*Adults:* Analgesia and antipyresis, PO 325–650 mg q4h PRN; usual single dose, 650 mg
  Anti-inflammatory effect, PO or rectal suppository 3.6–5.2 g/d in divided doses
  Myocardial infarction prophylaxis, PO 325 mg/d
  Rheumatic fever, PO up to 7.8 g/d in divided doses
  Transient ischemic attacks in men, PO 1300 mg/d in divided doses (650 mg twice a day or 325 mg four times per day)
*Children:* Analgesia and antipyresis, PO or rectal suppository 11 mg/kg six times per day or 16 mg/kg four times per day
  Anti-inflammatory effect, PO or rectal suppository 100–125 mg/kg per day in divided doses q4–6h. Reduce amount for long-term use.
  Rheumatic fever, PO or rectal suppository 3 g/d in divided doses

**Diflunisal** (Dolobid) is a salicylic acid derivative that differs chemically from aspirin. It is reportedly equal or superior to aspirin in mild to moderate pain, rheumatoid arthritis, and osteoarthritis. It differs from aspirin in that it has less antipyretic effect and causes less gastric irritation; its longer duration of action allows for twice-daily administration.

### Route and dosage ranges

*Adults:* Mild to moderate pain, PO 500–1000 mg initially, then 250–500 mg q8–12h
  Rheumatoid arthritis, osteoarthritis PO 500–1000 mg/d, in two divided doses, increased to a maximum of 1500 mg/d if necessary

**Acetaminophen** USP (Tylenol and others) is equal to aspirin in analgesic and antipyretic effects, but it lacks anti-inflammatory activity. Acetaminophen is a nonprescription drug commonly used as an aspirin substitute because it produces fewer adverse reactions than aspirin. More specifically, acetaminophen in usual therapeutic doses does not cause nausea, vomiting, or gastrointestinal bleeding, and it does not interfere with blood clotting. However, toxic doses produce potentially fatal liver necrosis, and usual therapeutic doses may cause or increase liver damage in alcoholics. Acetaminophen is available in tablet, liquid, and rectal suppository forms and is in numerous combination products marketed as analgesics and cold remedies. It is often prescribed with codeine or oxycodone (Percocet-5) for added analgesic effects.

### Routes and dosage ranges

*Adults:* PO, rectal suppository 325–650 mg q4–6h, or 1000 mg three to four times per day; maximum 4 g/d
*Children:* PO, rectal suppository 10 mg/kg or according to age as follows: 0–3 mo, 40 mg; 4–11 mo, 80 mg; 1–2 y, 120 mg; 2–3 y, 160 mg; 4–5 y, 240 mg; 6–8 y, 320 mg; 9–10 y, 400 mg; 11 y, 480 mg. Doses may be given q4h–6h to a maximum of five doses in 24 h.

**Fenoprofen** (Nalfon), **flurbiprofen** (Ansaid), **ibuprofen** (Motrin and others), **ketoprofen** (Orudis), and **naproxen** (Naprosyn, Anaprox) are propionic acid derivatives that are chemically and pharmacologically similar. In addition to their use as anti-inflammatory agents in rheumatoid arthritis, osteoarthritis, gout, tendinitis, and bursitis, they are used as analgesics in conditions not necessarily related to inflammation (*e.g.*, dysmenorrhea, episiotomy, minor trauma) and as antipyretics. For adults, ibuprofen is available with a prescription (300, 400, 600, and 800 mg tablets) and over-the-counter (200 mg tablets). For children, ibuprofen liquid suspension containing 100 mg/5 ml (Children's Advil, PediaProfen) is available with prescription. Although these drugs are usually better tolerated than aspirin, they are much more expensive and may cause all the adverse effects associated with aspirin and other prostaglandin inhibitors.

Fenoprofen

### Route and dosage ranges

*Adults:* Rheumatoid arthritis, osteoarthritis, PO 300–600 mg three to four times per day; maximum 3200 mg/d
  Mild to moderate pain, PO 200 mg q4–6h PRN
*Children:* Juvenile arthritis, PO 20–40 mg/kg per day, depending on severity of disease, in three or four divided doses
  Fever (ages 12 mo to 12 y), 5 mg/kg per dose for fever of 39.2°C (102.5°F) or less; 10 mg/kg per

dose for fever above 39.2°C. May be repeated every 8 hours if necessary to a maximum dose of 40 mg/kg per day

### Flurbiprofen

#### *Route and dosage ranges*

*Adults:* Rheumatoid arthritis, osteoarthritis, PO 200–300 mg/d in two, three, or four divided doses

### Ibuprofen

#### *Route and dosage ranges*

*Adults:* Rheumatoid arthritis, osteoarthritis, PO 300–600 mg three or four times per day; maximum 2400 mg/d

Mild to moderate pain, PO 200–400 mg q4–6h PRN

Primary dysmenorrhea, PO 400 mg q4h PRN

### Ketoprofen

#### *Route and dosage ranges*

*Adults:* Rheumatoid arthritis, osteoarthritis, PO 150–300 mg/d in three or four divided doses; maximum 300 mg/d

Mild to moderate pain, primary dysmenorrhea, PO 25–50 mg q6–8h PRN; maximum 300 mg/d

### Naproxen

#### *Route and dosage ranges*

*Adults:* Rheumatoid arthritis, osteoarthritis, ankylosing spondylitis, PO 250–375 mg twice a day

Acute gout, PO 750 mg initially, then 250 mg q8h until the attack subsides

Mild to moderate pain, primary dysmenorrhea, acute tendinitis and bursitis, PO 500 mg initially, then 250 mg q6–8h

### Naproxen sodium (Anaprox)

#### *Route and dosage ranges*

*Adults:* Rheumatoid arthritis, osteoarthritis, ankylosing spondylitis, PO 275 mg twice a day

Acute gout, PO 825 mg initially, then 275 mg q8h until the attack subsides

Mild to moderate pain, primary dysmenorrhea, acute tendinitis and bursitis, PO 550 mg initially, then 275 mg q6–8h

**Indomethacin** (Indocin), **sulindac** (Clinoril), and **tolmetin** (Tolectin) are acetic acid derivatives used for moderate to severe rheumatoid arthritis, osteoarthritis, ankylosing spondylitis, acute gouty arthritis, and acute, painful shoulder (bursitis, tendinitis). These drugs have potent anti-inflammatory effects but are associated with greater incidence and severity of adverse effects than aspirin and the propionic acid derivatives. Thus, they are not recommended for general use as analgesics or antipyretics. Uncommon but potentially serious adverse effects include gastrointestinal ulceration, bone marrow depression, hemolytic anemia, mental confusion, depression, and psychosis. These adverse effects are especially associated with indomethacin; the other drugs were developed in an effort to find equally effective but less toxic derivatives of indomethacin. Although adverse reactions occur less often with sulindac and tolmetin, they are still common.

In addition to the uses listed above, tolmetin is approved for treatment of juvenile rheumatoid arthritis, and intravenous indomethacin is approved for treatment of patent ductus arteriosus in premature infants. (The ductus arteriosus joins the pulmonary artery to the aorta in the fetal circulation. When it fails to close, blood is shunted from the aorta to the pulmonary artery, causing severe cardiopulmonary problems.)

Newer drugs related to this group are **etodolac** (Lodine), **ketorolac** (Toradol), and **nabumetone** (Relafen). Etodolac is used for pain and osteoarthritis and reportedly causes less gastric irritation, especially in older adults at high risk of gastrointestinal bleeding. Ketorolac is used only for pain, and although it can be given orally, its unique characteristic is that it can be given by injection. Parenteral ketorolac is reportedly comparable to morphine and other opiates in analgesic effectiveness for moderate or severe pain. However, hematomas and wound bleeding have been reported with postoperative use. Nabumetone is approved for treatment of rheumatoid arthritis and osteoarthritis.

### Etodolac

#### *Route and dosage ranges*

*Adults:* Osteoarthritis, PO 600–1200 mg/d in two to four divided doses; maximum dose, 1200 mg/d

Pain, PO 200–400 mg q6–8h PRN; maximum dose, 1200 mg/d

### Indomethacin

#### *Routes and dosage ranges*

*Adults:* PO, rectal suppository 75 mg/d initially, increased by 25 mg/d at weekly intervals to a maximum of 150–200 mg/d if necessary

Acute gouty arthritis, acute painful shoulder, PO 75–150 mg/d in three or four divided doses until pain and inflammation are controlled (about 3–5 d for gout, 7–14 d for painful shoulder), then discontinued

*Children:* Premature infants with patent ductus arteriosus, IV 0.2–0.3 mg/kg q12h for a total of three doses

## Ketorolac

### Routes and dosage ranges

*Adults:* PO 10 mg q4–6h for limited duration; maximum dose, 40 mg/d

IM 30–60 mg initially, then 15–30 mg q6h on a regular schedule or as needed to control pain, up to 5 days

## Nabumetone

### Route and dosage ranges

*Adults:* Osteoarthritis, rheumatoid arthritis, PO 1000–2000 mg/d in one or two doses. For long-term treatment, use the lowest effective dose.

## Sulindac

### Route and dosage ranges

*Adults:* PO 150–200 mg twice a day; maximum 400 mg/d

Acute gouty arthritis, acute painful shoulder, PO 200 mg twice a day until pain and inflammation are controlled (about 7–14 days), then discontinued

## Tolmetin

### Route and dosage ranges

*Adults:* PO 400 mg three times per day initially, increased to 1600 mg/d for osteoarthritis or 2000 mg/d for rheumatoid arthritis if necessary

*Children:* Rheumatoid arthritis, PO 20 mg/kg per day in three or four divided doses

**Diclofenac** (Voltaren) is chemically different but pharmacologically similar to other NSAIDs. It is indicated for use in rheumatoid arthritis, osteoarthritis, and ankylosing spondylitis.

### Route and dosage ranges

*Adults:* Rheumatoid arthritis, PO 150–200 mg/d in three or four divided doses

Osteoarthritis, PO 100–150 mg/d in three or four divided doses

Ankylosing spondylitis, PO 100–125 mg/d in three or four divided doses

**Piroxicam** (Feldene) is an oxicam NSAID that differs chemically from other agents but has similar pharmacologic properties. Approved for treatment of rheumatoid arthritis and osteoarthritis, it reportedly causes less gastrointestinal irritation than aspirin. Its long half-life allows for once-daily dosing, but optimal efficacy may not occur for 1 to 2 weeks.

### Route and dosage range

*Adults:* PO 20 mg/d

## LESS COMMONLY USED NSAIDS

**Meclofenamate** (Meclomen) and **mefenamic acid** (Ponstel) are fenamate NSAIDs that are used less often than most other agents because of frequent gastrointestinal and neurologic adverse effects.

## Meclofenamate

### Route and dosage ranges

*Adults:* Rheumatoid arthritis, osteoarthritis, PO 200–400 mg/d in three or four divided doses

## Mefenamic acid

### Route and dosage ranges

*Adults:* Acute pain, PO 500 mg initially, then 250 mg q6h PRN for no longer than 1 wk

Primary dysmenorrhea PO 500 mg at start of menses, then 250 mg q6h PRN for 2 or 3 days

*Children over 14 years:* Acute pain PO 500 mg initially, then 250 mg q6h PRN for no longer than 1 wk

## DRUGS USED IN GOUT AND HYPERURICEMIA

**Allopurinol** (Zyloprim) is used to prevent or treat hyperuricemia (high levels of uric acid in the blood), which occurs with gout and with antineoplastic drug therapy. Uric acid is formed by purine metabolism and an enzyme called xanthine oxidase. Allopurinol prevents formation of uric acid by inhibiting xanthine oxidase. It is especially useful in chronic gout characterized by tophi (deposits of uric acid crystals in the joints, kidneys, and soft tissues) and impaired renal function. The drug promotes resorption of urate deposits and prevents their further development. Acute attacks of gout may result when urate deposits are mobilized. These may be prevented by concomitant administration of colchicine until serum uric acid levels are lowered.

### Route and dosage ranges

*Adults:* Mild gout, PO 200–400 mg/d

Severe gout, PO 400–600 mg/d

Hyperuricemia in clients with renal insufficiency, PO 100–200 mg/d

Secondary hyperuricemia from anticancer drugs, PO 100–200 mg/d; maximum 800 mg/d

*Children:* Secondary hyperuricemia from anticancer drugs: under 6 y, PO 150 mg/d; 6–10 y, PO 300 mg/d

**Colchicine** is an anti-inflammatory drug that is effective only in gout. It has no analgesic or antipyretic effects. It is given to prevent or treat acute attacks of gout. In acute attacks, it is the drug of choice for relieving joint pain and edema. Colchicine decreases inflammation by decreasing movement of leukocytes into body tissues containing urate crystals.

### Routes and dosage ranges

*Adults:* Acute attacks, PO 0.5 mg q1h until pain is relieved or toxicity (nausea, vomiting, diarrhea) occurs; 3-day interval between courses of therapy IV 1–2 mg initially, then 0.5 mg q3–6h until response is obtained; maximum total dose 4 mg Prophylaxis, PO 0.5–1 mg/d

**Probenecid** (Benemid) increases urinary excretion of uric acid. This uricosuric action is used therapeutically to treat hyperuricemia and gout. It is not effective in acute attacks of gouty arthritis but prevents hyperuricemia and tophi associated with chronic gout. Probenecid may precipitate acute gout until serum uric acid levels are within normal range; concomitant administration of colchicine prevents this effect. (Probenecid also is used with penicillin, most often in treating sexually transmitted diseases. It increases blood levels and prolongs the action of penicillin by decreasing the rate of urinary excretion.)

### Route and dosage ranges

*Adults:* PO 250 mg twice a day for 1 wk, then 500 mg twice a day
*Children over 2 years:* PO 40 mg/kg per day in divided doses

**Sulfinpyrazone** (Anturane) is a uricosuric agent similar to probenecid. It is not effective in acute gout but prevents or decreases tissue changes of chronic gout. Colchicine is usually given during initial sulfinpyrazone therapy to prevent acute gout.

### Route and dosage range

*Adults:* PO 100–200 mg twice a day, gradually increased over 1 wk to a maximum of 400–800 mg/d

## DRUGS USED IN MIGRAINE

**Ergotamine tartrate** (Ergomar) is an ergot alkaloid used only in the treatment of migraine. Migraine, which involves paroxysmal attacks of severe headache, vomiting, and increased sensitivity to light and sound, is attributed to dilation of the extracerebral cranial arteries. Ergot preparations relieve migraine by constricting the vascular smooth muscle of blood vessels in the brain. Ergotamine is most effective when given sublingually or by inhalation at the onset of headache. When given orally, ergotamine is erratically absorbed, and therapeutic effects may be delayed for 20 to 30 minutes.

Ergotamine is contraindicated during pregnancy and in the presence of severe hypertension, peripheral vascu-

lar disease, coronary artery disease, renal or hepatic disease, and severe infections.

### Routes and dosage ranges

*Adults:* PO 1–2 mg at onset of acute migraine attack, then 2 mg every 30 min, if necessary, to a maximum of 6 mg/24 h or 10 mg/wk SL
Inhalation, 0.36 mg (one inhalation) at onset of acute migraine, repeated in 5 min if necessary, to a maximum of 6 inhalations/24 h

**Ergotamine tartrate and caffeine** (Cafergot) is a commonly used antimigraine preparation. Caffeine reportedly increases absorption and vasoconstrictive effects of ergotamine. The combination product is available in oral tablets containing ergotamine 1 mg and caffeine 100 mg and in rectal suppositories containing ergotamine 2 mg and caffeine 100 mg.

### Routes and dosage ranges

*Adults:* PO 2 tablets at the onset of acute migraine, then 1 tablet every 30 min if necessary, up to 6 tablets per attack or 10 tablets/wk
Rectal suppository ½–1 suppository at the onset of acute migraine, repeated in 1 h if necessary, up to 2 suppositories per attack or 5 suppositories/wk
*Children:* PO ½–1 tablet initially, then ½ tablet every 30 min if necessary, up to a maximum of 3 tablets

**Dihydroergotamine mesylate** (DHE 45) is a semisynthetic derivative of ergotamine that is less toxic and less effective than the parent drug.

### Routes and dosage ranges

*Adults:* IM 1 mg at onset of acute migraine, repeated hourly if necessary to a total of 3 mg
IV 1 mg, repeated if necessary after 1 h; maximum dose 2 mg. Do not exceed 6 mg/wk

**Methysergide** (Sansert) is an ergot derivative used only for prophylaxis of migraine; it is ineffective in acute migraine attacks. The drug is indicated only when migraine attacks are frequent or severe and for no longer than 4 consecutive months because of fibrosis in the aorta, heart, and lungs. Usage has declined because of adverse effects.

### Route and dosage range

*Adults:* PO 4–8 mg/d in divided doses

**Sumatriptan** (Imitrex) increases serotonin in the brain and relieves acute migraine attacks by causing arterial vasoconstriction. Because of its vasoconstrictive properties, sumatriptan is contraindicated in patients with ischemic heart disease or uncontrolled hypertension. The drug produces fewer adverse effects than ergot alkaloids, and those that occur, including discomfort at injection sites, anxiety, dizziness, and drowsiness, are usually mild and of short duration.

### Routes and dosage ranges

*Adults:* PO 100 mg as a single dose
SC 6 mg as a single dose; maximum dose, 12 mg/d

## Nursing Process

### Assessment

- Assess for signs and symptoms of pain, such as location, severity, duration, and factors that cause or relieve the pain (see Chap. 5).
- Assess for fever (thermometer readings above 99.6°F or 37.3°C are usually considered fever). Hot, dry skin; flushed face; reduced urine output; and concentrated urine may accompany fever if the person also is dehydrated.
- Assess for inflammation. Local signs are redness, heat, edema, and pain or tenderness; systemic signs include fever, elevated white blood cell count (leukocytosis), and weakness.
- With arthritis or other musculoskeletal disorders, assess for limitations in activity and mobility.
- Ask about use of over-the-counter analgesic, antipyretic, or anti-inflammatory drugs.
- Ask about allergic reactions to aspirin or NSAIDs.
- Assess for history of peptic ulcer disease, gastrointestinal bleeding, or kidney disorders.

### Nursing diagnoses

- Pain
- Chronic pain
- Activity Intolerance related to pain and impaired physical mobility
- Impaired Physical Mobility related to pain and inflammation
- High Risk for Injury related to adverse drug effects (gastrointestinal bleeding, renal insufficiency)
- Knowledge Deficit: Comparative characteristics of over-the-counter and prescription drugs for pain, fever, and inflammation
- Knowledge Deficit: Therapeutic and adverse effects of commonly used drugs
- Knowledge Deficit: Correct usage of over-the-counter drugs for pain, fever, and inflammation

### Planning/Goals

*The client will:*
- Experience relief of discomfort with minimal adverse drug effects
- Experience increased mobility and activity tolerance
- Inform health-care providers if taking aspirin or an NSAID regularly
- Self-administer the drugs safely
- Verbalize signs and symptoms of adverse drug effects to be reported to health-care providers
- Avoid overuse of the drugs

- Use measures to prevent accidental ingestion or overdose, especially in children

### Interventions

Implement measures to prevent or minimize pain, fever, and inflammation:
- **Diagnosis and treatment of the underlying condition are very important**. Measures aimed at relief of the disorder, such as prevention or treatment of infections and improvement of the blood supply, may be helpful in alleviating symptoms.
- **Institute treatment measures as soon as they seem indicated**. Timing depends on thorough assessment and the ability to recognize early signs and symptoms. When drug therapy seems indicated, it generally should not be delayed any longer than necessary. With pain, for example, early treatment may prevent severe pain and allow the use of milder analgesic drugs. Other measures that may be used instead of or along with drug therapy include positioning, hygienic care, heat or cold applications, rest or exercise, and distraction or relaxation techniques. Assess response to various therapeutic approaches as carefully as initial signs and symptoms.

*Teach clients:*
- To inform any health-care provider if they are taking aspirin, ibuprofen, or other NSAIDs regularly
- That with inflammatory disorders, such as arthritis, improvement may take 1 to 2 weeks
- That if one drug is not effective, another one may work because people vary in responses to the drugs
- That because fever is one way the body fights infection, drug therapy may not be needed unless the fever is high or is accompanied by other uncomfortable signs and symptoms
- That aspirin is as effective as the more costly prescription NSAIDs
- That the main advantage of other NSAIDs over aspirin is decreased gastrointestinal upset
- To avoid over-the-counter products containing aspirin (*e.g.*, Alka-Seltzer, Anacin, Arthritis Pain Formula, Excedrin, Midol, Vanquish) and buffered (*e.g.*, Ascriptin, Bufferin) or coated (*e.g.*, Ecotrin) forms of aspirin when taking aspirin or NSAIDs regularly
- To avoid aspirin for approximately 2 weeks before and after major surgery or dental work to decrease the risk of excessive bleeding
- That acetaminophen is an effective aspirin substitute for pain or fever but not for inflammation or preventing heart attack or stroke
- That there are many trade names of over-the-counter preparations of acetaminophen, and most contain 500 mg of drug per tablet or capsule. In addition, many over-the-counter analgesics and cold remedies contain acetaminophen. Thus, all consumers should read product labels carefully to avoid duplicate sources and potential overdoses. Overuse may cause life-threatening liver damage.
- To avoid over-the-counter products containing ibuprofen (*e.g.*, Advil and others) when taking any prescription NSAID. Acetaminophen may be taken safely if needed for pain or fever.
- Correct scheduling and administration techniques to minimize risk of adverse effects

### Evaluation

- Interview and observe regarding relief of symptoms.
- Interview and observe regarding mobility and activity levels.
- Interview and observe regarding safe, effective usage of the drugs.
- Select drugs appropriately.

## Principles of therapy

### GUIDELINES FOR THERAPY WITH ASPIRIN

When pain, fever, or inflammation is present, aspirin is often the drug of choice, and its usefulness extends across a wide range of clinical conditions. Because it is a non-prescription drug and is widely available, people tend to underestimate its effectiveness. Like any other drug, aspirin must be used appropriately to maximize therapeutic benefits and minimize adverse reactions. Some guidelines for correct usage include the following:

1. For *pain*, aspirin is useful alone when the discomfort is of low to moderate intensity. For more severe pain, aspirin may be combined with a narcotic or given between narcotic doses for better analgesia or to allow lower doses of the narcotic. Aspirin and narcotic analgesics act by different mechanisms, so such usage is rational. Aspirin with codeine is especially effective. Aspirin may be used with other narcotics in clients who can take oral medications. For acute pain, aspirin is taken when the pain occurs and is often effective within a few minutes. For chronic pain, a regular schedule of administration, such as every 4 to 6 hours, is more effective.
2. For *fever*, aspirin is usually the drug of choice if drug therapy is indicated. However, aspirin may delay diagnosis of conditions in which fever and its patterns of occurrence are significant.
3. For *inflammation*, aspirin is useful in both short- and long-term therapy. It is especially useful in conditions characterized by pain and inflammation, such as rheumatoid arthritis.
4. Aspirin is usually the drug of choice when salicylate therapy is indicated. Sodium salicylate may be used for people who are hypersensitive to aspirin, but it is less effective, produces similar adverse reactions, and may be contraindicated because of its sodium content. Choline salicylate and a few other preparations are advertised as producing fewer gastrointestinal adverse reactions but seem to offer no particular advantage over aspirin.
5. For most purposes, plain aspirin tablets are preferred. Enteric-coated tablets are more slowly absorbed and therefore take longer to exert their therapeutic effects.

They may be better tolerated for long-term use of high doses in rheumatoid arthritis, however. Rectal suppositories are sometimes used when oral administration is contraindicated.

6. Aspirin dosage depends mainly on the condition being treated. Lower doses are needed when there is a low serum albumin level because a larger proportion of the dose is free to exert pharmacologic activity. Larger doses are needed for anti-inflammatory effects than for analgesic and antipyretic effects.
7. To decrease risks of toxicity, plasma salicylate levels should be measured periodically when large doses of aspirin are given for anti-inflammatory effects. Chronic administration of large doses saturates a major metabolic pathway, thereby slowing drug elimination, prolonging serum half-life, and causing drug accumulation.
8. Salicylate intoxication may occur with an acute overdose or chronic use of therapeutic doses. Manifestations of salicylism include nausea, vomiting, fever, fluid and electrolyte deficiencies, tinnitus, decreased hearing, visual changes, drowsiness, confusion, hyperventilation, and others. Severe central nervous system dysfunction (*e.g.*, delirium, stupor, coma, and seizures) indicates life-threatening toxicity. In children, metabolic acidosis develops rapidly and may be present on initial contact. In adults, metabolic acidosis develops more slowly and with severe overdosage.

In mild salicylism, stopping the drug or reducing the dose is usually sufficient. In severe salicylate overdose, treatment is symptomatic and aimed at preventing further absorption from the gastrointestinal tract, increasing urinary excretion, and correcting fluid, electrolyte, and acid-base imbalances. When the drug is still thought to be in the gastrointestinal tract, emesis, gastric lavage, and activated charcoal, or a combination of these, help to reduce absorption. Intravenous sodium bicarbonate produces an alkaline urine in which salicylates are more rapidly excreted, and hemodialysis effectively removes salicylates from the blood. Intravenous fluids are indicated when high fever or dehydration is present. The specific content of intravenous fluids depends on serum electrolyte and acid-base status.

### GUIDELINES FOR THERAPY WITH ACETAMINOPHEN

Acetaminophen is an effective aspirin substitute for treatment of pain and fever when aspirin is contraindicated or not tolerated. It may be the drug of choice for children with febrile illness (because of the association of aspirin with Reye's syndrome), elderly adults with impaired renal function (because aspirin may cause further impairment), and pregnant women (because aspirin is associated with several maternal and fetal disorders).

Probably the major drawback to acetaminophen is liver damage. Factors related to identification and treatment of hepatotoxicity include the following:

1. Acute hepatic failure may occur with a single large dose, usually about 10 to 15 g, but it has been reported with 6 g. Acute acetaminophen poisoning may be characterized by cyanosis, anemia, pancytopenia, jaundice, fever, vomiting, and central nervous system stimulation with excitement and delirium followed by vascular collapse, convulsions, coma, and death. Early symptoms (within 24 hours after ingestion) are nonspecific (*e.g.*, anorexia, nausea, vomiting). Peak hepatotoxicity occurs in 3 to 4 days, and recovery occurs in 7 to 8 days.
2. If overdose is detected soon after ingestion, activated charcoal can be given to inhibit absorption. However, the specific antidote is acetylcysteine (Mucomyst), a mucolytic agent given by inhalation in respiratory disorders (see Chap. 52). For acetaminophen poisoning, it is given orally. It combines with a toxic metabolite and decreases hepatotoxicity if given within 24 hours of acetaminophen ingestion.
3. Hepatotoxicity also occurs with chronic ingestion of acetaminophen (5–8 g/d for several weeks or 3–4 g/d for 1 year) and short-term ingestion of usual therapeutic doses in alcoholics.

## GUIDELINES FOR THERAPY WITH NSAIDS

Most NSAIDs are prescription drugs used primarily for analgesic and anti-inflammatory effects in arthritis and other musculoskeletal disorders. However, several are approved for more general use as an analgesic or antipyretic. Ibuprofen is widely used for all these purposes and is available by prescription and over the counter. Although NSAIDs may be no more effective than aspirin, they may cause fewer gastrointestinal adverse effects than aspirin and thus may be better tolerated by some clients. These drugs are much more expensive than aspirin.

NSAIDs inhibit platelet activity only while drug molecules are in the bloodstream, not for the life of the platelet (about 7–10 days) as aspirin does. Thus, they are *not* prescribed therapeutically for antiplatelet effects.

## GUIDELINES FOR TREATING RHEUMATOID ARTHRITIS AND RELATED DISORDERS

The primary goals of treatment are to control pain and inflammation and to minimize immobilization and disability. Rest, exercise, physical therapy, and drugs are used to attain these goals. None of these measures prevents joint destruction or related pathologic conditions.

Aspirin relieves pain and inflammation, and it is inexpensive, an important factor in the long-term treatment of chronic musculoskeletal disorders. Dosage should be individualized to relieve symptoms, maintain therapeutic salicylate blood levels, and minimize adverse effects. Regular administration of aspirin every 4 to 6 hours usually produces a therapeutic serum salicylate level of 15 to 25 mg/100 ml. For people who cannot take aspirin because of peptic ulcer disease, bleeding disorders, and other contraindications, another NSAID is usually ordered. The choice of a specific drug is largely empirical; one person may respond better to one NSAID than another. A drug may be given for 2 or 3 weeks on a trial basis. If therapeutic benefits occur, the drug may be continued; if no benefits seem evident or toxicity occurs, another drug may be tried.

Ibuprofen and other propionic acid derivatives are often used because they are associated with fewer gastrointestinal adverse effects than most other NSAIDs. However, they do cause significant toxicity in some cases and are quite expensive for long-term use. Indomethacin is effective, but its usage is limited because of toxicity. Generally, newer NSAIDs offer few clear-cut advantages over older ones.

Several other drugs also may be used to treat rheumatoid arthritis. These include adrenal corticosteroids and the disease-modifying antirheumatic drugs, such as gold, hydroxychloroquine (Plaquenil), penicillamine (Cuprimine, Depen), azathioprine (Imuran), cyclophosphamide (Cytoxan), and methotrexate. These drugs have anti-inflammatory or immunosuppressant effects and may cause significant toxicity. Until recently, they were used in clients who do not respond to the NSAIDs. Now they are being used more often in early rheumatoid arthritis with the goal of slowing tissue damage, which the NSAIDs are unable to do.

## GUIDELINES FOR PERIOPERATIVE USE OF ASPIRIN AND OTHER NSAIDS

Aspirin should generally be avoided for at least 2 weeks before and after surgery. This precaution is indicated because aspirin increases the risk of bleeding. Most other NSAIDs should be discontinued approximately 3 days before surgery; nabumetone (Relafen) and piroxicam (Feldene) have long half-lives and need to be discontinued approximately 1 week preoperatively. Postoperatively, especially after relatively minor procedures, such as dental extractions and episiotomies, several of the drugs are used to relieve pain. Caution is needed because of increased risks of bleeding, and the drugs should not be given if there are other risk factors for bleeding. In addition, ketorolac (Toradol), the only injectable NSAID, has been used in more extensive surgeries. Although the drug has several advantages over narcotic analgesics, bleeding and hematomas may occur.

## USE OF ASPIRIN, ACETAMINOPHEN, AND NSAIDS IN CHILDREN

*Acetaminophen* is usually the drug of choice for pain or fever in children. Ibuprofen also may be given for fever. Aspirin is not recommended because of its association with Reye's syndrome, a life-threatening illness characterized by encephalopathy, hepatic damage, and other serious problems. Reye's syndrome usually occurs after a viral infection, such as influenza B or chickenpox, during which aspirin was given for fever. For children with juvenile rheumatoid arthritis, aspirin, ibuprofen, or tolmetin is preferred because these drugs have been tested more extensively in children. Pediatric indications for use and dosages have not been established for most of the other drugs.

## USE OF ASPIRIN, ACETAMINOPHEN, AND NSAIDS IN OLDER ADULTS

*Acetaminophen* is generally safe in recommended doses unless liver damage is present. *Aspirin* is generally safe in the small doses prescribed for prevention of myocardial infarction and stroke (antiplatelet effects). *Aspirin* and *NSAIDs* are probably safe in therapeutic doses for occasional use as an analgesic or antipyretic. However, older adults have a high incidence of musculoskeletal disorders (*e.g.*, rheumatoid arthritis and osteoarthritis), and aspirin or an NSAID is often prescribed. Long-term use of the relatively high doses required for anti-inflamma-

tory effects increases the risk of serious gastrointestinal bleeding. Small doses, gradual increments, and taking the drug with food or a full glass of water may decrease gastrointestinal effects. Older adults also may be more likely than younger adults to develop nephrotoxicity with NSAIDs.

## GUIDELINES FOR TREATING HYPERURICEMIA AND GOUT

Opinions differ regarding treatment of asymptomatic hyperuricemia. Some authorities do not think drug therapy is indicated, while others think that lowering serum uric acid levels may prevent joint inflammation and renal calculi. Allopurinol, probenecid, or sulfinpyrazone may be given for this purpose. Colchicine also should be given for several weeks to prevent acute attacks of gout while serum uric acid levels are being lowered. During initial administration of these drugs, a high fluid intake (to produce about 2000 ml of urine per day) and alkaline urine are recommended to prevent renal calculi. Urate crystals are more likely to precipitate in acid urine.

## GUIDELINES FOR TREATING MIGRAINE

For treatment of migraine and similar disorders, ergot preparations should be given at the onset of headache, and the client should lie down in a quiet, darkened room. Help the client identify and avoid precipitating factors when possible. The newer drug, sumatriptan, may be preferred because it is effective and reportedly causes fewer adverse effects than ergot preparations.

---

# NURSING ACTIONS: ANALGESIC–ANTIPYRETIC-ANTI-INFLAMMATORY AND RELATED DRUGS

| *Nursing Actions* | *Rationale/Explanation* |
|---|---|
| **1. Administer accurately**<br>**a.** Give aspirin and other nonsteroidal anti-inflammatory drugs (NSAIDs) with a full glass of water or other fluid and with or just after food. | To decrease gastric irritation. Even though food delays absorption and decreases peak plasma levels of some of the drugs, it is probably safer to give them with food. |
| **b.** Give antimigraine preparations at the onset of headache. | To prevent development of more severe symptoms |
| **c.** Give methysergide with meals. | To decrease nausea and vomiting |
| **2. Observe for therapeutic effects**<br>**a.** When drugs are given for pain, observe for decreased or absent manifestations of pain. | Pain relief is usually evident within 30 to 60 minutes. |

## Nursing Actions

## Rationale/Explanation

**b.** When drugs are given for fever, record temperature every 2 to 4 hours, and observe for a decrease.

**c.** When drugs are given for arthritis and other inflammatory disorders, observe for decreased pain, edema, redness, heat, and stiffness of joints. Also observe for increased joint mobility and exercise tolerance.

With aspirin, improvement is usually noted within 24 to 48 hours. With most of the nonsteroidal anti-inflammatory drugs, 1 to 2 weeks may be required before beneficial effects become evident.

**d.** When colchicine is given for acute gouty arthritis, observe for decreased pain and inflammation in involved joints.

Therapeutic effects occur within 4 to 12 hours after intravenous colchicine administration and 24 to 48 hours after oral administration. Edema may not decrease for several days.

**e.** When allopurinol, probenecid, or sulfinpyrazone is given for hyperuricemia, observe for normal serum uric acid level (about 2–8 mg/100 ml).

Serum uric acid levels usually decrease to normal range within 1 to 3 weeks.

**f.** When the above drugs are given for chronic gout, observe for decreased size of tophi, absence of new tophi, decreased joint pain and increased joint mobility, and normal serum uric acid levels.

**g.** When ergot preparations are given in migraine headache, observe for relief of symptoms.

Therapeutic effects are usually evident within 15 to 30 minutes.

**3. Observe for adverse effects**
  **a.** With analgesic–antipyretic–anti-inflammatory and antigout agents, observe for:

    (1) *Gastrointestinal problems*—anorexia, nausea, vomiting, diarrhea, bleeding, ulceration

These are common reactions, more likely with aspirin, indomethacin, piroxicam, sulindac, tolmetin, colchicine, and sulfinpyrazone and less likely with acetaminophen, diflunisal, etodolac, fenoprofen, ibuprofen, and naproxen. A prostaglandin called misoprostol (Cytotec) may be given concurrently with aspirin and other NSAIDs to prevent gastric ulcers (see Chap. 63).

    (2) *Hematologic problems*—petechiae, bruises, hematuria, melena, epistaxis, and bone marrow depression (leukopenia, thrombocytopenia, anemia)

Bone marrow depression is more likely to occur with colchicine.

    (3) *Central nervous system effects*—headache, dizziness, fainting, ataxia, insomnia, confusion, drowsiness

These effects are relatively common with indomethacin and may occur with most of the other drugs, especially with high dosages.

    (4) *Skin rashes, dermatitis*

    (5) *Hypersensitivity reactions* with dyspnea, bronchospasm, skin rashes

These effects may simulate asthma in people who are allergic to aspirin and aspirin-like drugs.

    (6) *Tinnitus, blurred vision*

Tinnitus (ringing or roaring in the ears) is a classic sign of aspirin overdose (salicylate intoxication). It occurs with NSAIDs as well, especially with overdosage.

    (7) *Nephrotoxicity*—decreased urine output, increased blood urea nitrogen (BUN), increased serum creatinine, hyperkalemia, retention of sodium and water with resultant edema

More likely to occur in people with preexisting renal impairment, especially when fluid intake is decreased or fluid loss is increased. Elderly adults are at greater risk because of decreased renal blood flow and increased incidence of congestive heart failure and diuretic therapy. Renal damage is usually reversible when the drug is discontinued.

    (8) *Cardiovascular and hepatic effects*

These are not common with usual therapeutic doses, but all vital organs may be adversely affected with overdoses.

*(continued)*

| *Nursing Actions* | *Rationale/Explanation* |
|---|---|
| **b.** With antimigraine preparations, observe for: | |
| (1) *Nausea, vomiting, diarrhea* | These drugs have a direct effect on the vomiting center of the brain and stimulate contraction of gastrointestinal smooth muscle. |
| (2) *Symptoms of ergot poisoning* (ergotism)—coolness, numbness, and tingling of the extremities, headache, vomiting, dizziness, thirst, convulsions, weak pulse, confusion, angina-like chest pain, transient tachycardia or bradycardia, muscle weakness and pain, cyanosis, gangrene of the extremities | The ergot alkaloids are highly toxic; poisoning may be acute or chronic. Acute poisoning is rare; chronic poisoning is usually a result of overdosage. Circulatory impairments may result from vasoconstriction and vascular insufficiency. Large doses also damage capillary endothelium and may cause thrombosis and occlusion. Gangrene of extremities rarely occurs with usual doses unless peripheral vascular disease or other contraindications are also present. |
| (3) *Hypertension* | Blood pressure may rise as a result of generalized vasoconstriction induced by the ergot preparation. |
| (4) *Hypersensitivity reactions*—local edema and pruritus, anaphylactic shock | Allergic reactions are relatively uncommon. |
| (5) With *methysergide*—inflammation followed by fibrosis in some body tissues. Retroperitoneal fibrosis can lead to urinary tract obstruction; fibrosis of lung tissue can lead to pulmonary complications. Cardiac valves and major arteries also may be affected by fibrotic thickening. | These growths usually regress if symptoms are detected and the drug discontinued. The client is examined frequently during long-term therapy. A drug-free interval of several weeks is recommended between courses of therapy. |
| **4. Observe for drug interactions** | |
| **a.** Drugs that *increase* effects of aspirin and other NSAIDs: | |
| (1) Acidifying agents (*e.g.*, ascorbic acid) | Acidify urine and thereby decrease the urinary excretion rate of salicylates |
| (2) Alcohol | Increases gastric irritation and occult blood loss |
| (3) Anticoagulants, oral | Increase risk of bleeding substantially. People taking anticoagulants should not take aspirin or aspirin-containing products. |
| (4) Codeine, other narcotic analgesics, and some related analgesics such as methotrimeprazine (Levoprome) and pentazocine (Talwin) | Additive analgesic effects because of different mechanisms of action. Aspirin can be used with these drugs to provide adequate pain relief without excessive doses and sedation, in many cases. |
| (5) Corticosteroids (*e.g.*, prednisone) | Additive gastric irritating and ulcerogenic effects |
| **b.** Drugs that *decrease* effects of aspirin and other NSAIDs: | |
| (1) Alkalinizing agents (*e.g.*, sodium bicarbonate) | Increase rate of renal excretion |
| (2) Misoprostol (Cytotec) | This drug, a prostaglandin, was developed specifically to prevent aspirin and NSAID-induced gastric ulcers. |
| **c.** Drugs that *increase* effects of indomethacin: | |
| (1) Anticoagulants, oral | Increase risk of gastrointestinal bleeding. Indomethacin causes gastric irritation and is considered an ulcerogenic drug. |
| (2) Corticosteroids | Increase ulcerogenic effect |
| (3) Salicylates | Increase ulcerogenic effects |

## Nursing Actions

## Rationale/Explanation

(4) Heparin

Increases risk of bleeding. These drugs should not be used concurrently.

**d.** Drugs that *decrease* effects of indomethacin
Antacids

Delay absorption from the gastrointestinal tract

**e.** Drugs that *decrease* effects of allopurinol, probenecid, and sulfinpyrazone:

(1) Alkalinizing agents (*e.g.,* sodium bicarbonate)

Decrease risks of renal calculi from precipitation of uric acid crystals. Alkalinizing agents are recommended until serum uric acid levels return to normal.

(2) Colchicine

Decreases attacks of acute gout. Recommended for concurrent use until serum uric acid levels return to normal.

(3) Diuretics

Decrease uricosuric effects

(4) Salicylates

Mainly at salicylate doses less than 2 g/d, decrease uricosuric effects of probenecid and sulfinpyrazone but do not interfere with the action of allopurinol. Salicylates are uricosuric at doses greater than 5 g/d.

**f.** Drugs that *increase* effects of ergot preparations
Vasoconstrictors (*e.g.,* ephedrine, epinephrine, phenylephrine)

Additive vasoconstriction with risks of severe, persistent hypertension and intracranial hemorrhage

**5. Teach clients:**

**a.** With analgesic–antipyretic–anti-inflammatory and antigout agents:

(1) Take the drugs with a full glass of liquid and food

To decrease stomach irritation and upset

(2) Drink 2½ to 3 quarts of fluid daily if not contraindicated

To decrease gastric irritation. With long-term use of aspirin, an adequate fluid intake also is needed to prevent precipitation of salicylate crystals in the urinary tract. With allopurinol, probenecid, and sulfinpyrazone, fluids are needed to help prevent precipitation of urate crystals and formation of urate kidney stones. Fluid intake is especially important initially when serum uric acid levels are high and large amounts of uric acid are being excreted in the urine.

(3) Report signs of bleeding (nose bleed, vomiting blood, bruising, blood in urine or stools), difficulty in breathing, skin rash or hives, ringing in ears, dizziness, or severe stomach upset.

(4) Store aspirin in a closed child-proof container and keep out of reach of children. *Never* call aspirin "candy."

A closed container reduces exposure of the drug to moisture and air, which cause chemical breakdown. Aspirin that is deteriorating smells like vinegar (acetic acid). Special precautions are needed with children because aspirin ingestion is a common cause of drug poisoning in children.

(5) With colchicine for chronic gout, carry the drug, and start taking as directed (usually one pill every hour for several hours until relief is obtained or nausea, vomiting, and diarrhea occur) when joint pain starts.

To prevent or minimize an attack of gouty arthritis

**b.** With ergot preparations, report signs of vascular insufficiency, such as tingling sensation or coldness, numbness, or weakness of the extremities. Do not exceed recommended doses.

These are symptoms of ergot toxicity. To avoid potentially serious adverse reactions, do not exceed recommended doses.

## Review and Application Exercises

1. How do aspirin and other NSAIDs produce analgesic, antipyretic, anti-inflammatory, and anti-platelet effects?
2. What adverse effects occur with aspirin and other NSAIDs, especially with daily ingestion?
3. Compare and contrast uses and effects of aspirin and acetaminophen.
4. For a 6-year-old child with fever, would aspirin or acetaminophen be preferred? Why?
5. For a 50-year-old adult with rheumatoid arthritis, would aspirin, another NSAID, or acetaminophen be preferred? Why?
6. For a 75-year-old adult with osteoarthritis and a long history of "stomach trouble," would aspirin, another NSAID, or acetaminophen be preferred? Why?
7. What are some nursing interventions to decrease adverse effects of aspirin, other NSAIDs, and acetaminophen?
8. When teaching a client about home use of aspirin, other NSAIDs, and acetaminophen, what information needs to be included?
9. What is the rationale for using acetylcysteine in the treatment of acetaminophen toxicity?
10. What is the rationale for combining narcotic and non-narcotic analgesics in the treatment of moderate pain?

## Selected References

Albers, G. W., & Peroutka, S. J. (1992). Neurologic disorders. In K. L. Melmon, H. F. Morrelli, B. B. Hoffman, & D. W. Nierenberg (Eds.), *Clinical pharmacology: Basic principles in therapeutics* (3rd ed.) (pp. 309–337). New York: McGraw-Hill.

(1993). *Drug facts and comparisons*. St. Louis: Facts and Comparisons.

Empting-Koschorke, L. D., Hendler, N., Kolodny, A. L., & Kraus, H. (1990). Nondrug management of chronic pain. *Patient Care, 24,* 165–185.

Furst, D. E. (1990). Rheumatoid arthritis: Practical use of medications. *Postgraduate Medicine, 87,* 79–90.

Gall, E. P., & Higbee, M. (1993). Pharmacologic therapy of rheumatic diseases. In R. Bressler & M. D. Katz (Eds.), *Geriatric pharmacology* (pp. 467–506). New York: McGraw-Hill.

Guyton, A. C. (1991). *Textbook of medical physiology* (8th ed.). Philadelphia: W.B. Saunders.

Jackson, C. G., & Williams, H. J. (1992). Current method of management of rheumatoid arthritis. *Comprehensive Therapy, 18*(12), 3–7.

Lindsley, C. B., & Waraday, B. A. (1990). Nonsteroidal antiinflammatory drugs: Renal toxicity. *Clinical Pediatrics, 29,* 10–13.

Nattel, S. (1992). Management of poisoning. In K. L. Melmon, H. F. Morrelli, B. B. Hoffman, & D. W. Nierenberg (Eds.), *Clinical pharmacology: Basic principles in therapeutics* (3rd ed.) (pp. 787–804). New York: McGraw-Hill.

(1993). *Physicians' Desk Reference*. Montvale, NJ: Medical Economics Data.

Reardon, E. V., & Clough, J. D. (1992). Drug therapy in the rheumatic diseases. *Comprehensive Therapy, 18*(11), 22–25.

Shlotzhauer, T. L., Lambert, R. E., & McGuire, J. L. (1992). Metabolic and degenerative disorders of connective tissue and bone. In K. L. Melmon, H. F. Morrelli, B. B. Hoffman, & D. W. Nierenberg (Eds.), *Clinical pharmacology: Basic principles in therapeutics* (3rd ed.) (pp. 486–504). New York: McGraw-Hill.

# CHAPTER 7

# Sedative-Hypnotics

## Description

Sedative drugs produce relaxation and decrease anxiety; hypnotic drugs produce sleep. The difference between the two types of drugs is one of degree and depends largely on dosage. Because these drugs generally depress the central nervous system (CNS), some are used as antianxiety, anticonvulsant, and anesthetic agents. The drugs discussed in this chapter are those used primarily to induce sleep.

## Sleep

Sleep is a recurrent period of decreased mental and physical activity during which the person is relatively unresponsive to sensory and environmental stimuli. Normal sleep allows rest, renewal of energy for performing activities of daily living, and alertness when awakening. When a person retires for sleep, there is an initial period of drowsiness or sleep latency, which lasts about 30 minutes. Once the person is asleep, cycles occur about every 90 minutes during the sleep period. During each cycle, the individual progresses from drowsiness (stage I) to deep sleep (stage IV). These stages are characterized by depressed body functions, nonrapid eye movements (non-REM), and nondreaming and are thought to be physically restorative. Stage IV is followed by a period of 5 to 20 minutes of rapid eye movements (REM), dreaming, and increased physiologic activity. REM sleep is thought to be mentally and emotionally restorative; REM deprivation can lead to serious psychological problems.

Insomnia, prolonged difficulty in going to sleep or staying asleep long enough to feel rested, is the most common sleep disorder. Insomnia has many causes, including such stressors as pain, anxiety, illness, changes in life-style or environment, and various drugs. Occasional sleeplessness is a normal response to many stimuli and is not usually harmful.

## Sedative-hypnotic drugs

Sedative-hypnotic drugs produce varying degrees of CNS depression ranging from drowsiness and mild sedation to sleep, anesthesia, respiratory depression, coma, and death. They are usually subclassified as barbiturates, benzodiazepines, and nonbarbiturate, nonbenzodiazepines. The individual sedative-hypnotic drugs are listed in Table 7-1.

### BARBITURATES

Barbiturates are the prototype sedative-hypnotic drugs, although they are infrequently used. All barbiturates have similar pharmacologic actions and differ primarily in onset and duration of action. They are usually described as ultrashort-, short-, intermediate-, and long-acting. The ultrashort-acting drugs are used mainly for anesthesia and are discussed in Chapter 14. Barbiturates are metabolized into water-soluble, inactive metabolites in the liver; the metabolites are excreted by the kidneys. Additional characteristics are described below.

Anne Collins Abrams: CLINICAL DRUG THERAPY, Fourth Edition.
© 1995 J.B. Lippincott Company.

## TABLE 7-1. SEDATIVE-HYPNOTICS

| Generic/Trade Name | Major Clinical Use | Routes and Dosage Ranges | | Remarks |
|---|---|---|---|---|
| | | *Adults* | *Children* | |

### Barbiturates

#### Short-acting

| Generic/Trade Name | Major Clinical Use | Adults | Children | Remarks |
|---|---|---|---|---|
| **Pentobarbital sodium** (Nembutal) | Hypnotic, preoperative sedation | *Sedative*: PO 30 mg 3–4 times daily; rectal 120–200 mg<br>*Hypnotic*: PO 100 mg; rectal 120–200 mg; IM 150–200 mg; IV 100 mg | *Sedative*: PO rectal 2 mg/kg per day in 4 divided doses<br>*Hypnotic*: IM 25–80 mg; rectal under 1 year, 30 mg; 1–4 years, 30 or 60 mg; 5–12 years, 60 mg; 12–14 years, 60 or 120 mg | Pentobarbital and secobarbital are Schedule II controlled substances. They lose effectiveness as hypnotics in about 2 weeks of continuous administration. Do not divide rectal suppositories. |
| **Secobarbital sodium** (Seconal) | Hypnotic, preoperative sedation | *Sedative*: PO rectal 120–200 mg<br>*Hypnotic*: PO 100 mg; rectal 120–200 mg; IV 50–250 mg; IM 100–200 mg | *Sedative*: PO, rectal 6 mg/kg per day in 3 divided doses<br>*Hypnotic*: IM 3–5 mg/kg; maximum dose, 100 mg | See pentobarbital |

#### Intermediate-acting

| Generic/Trade Name | Major Clinical Use | Adults | Children | Remarks |
|---|---|---|---|---|
| **Amobarbital sodium** (Amytal) | Hypnotic | *Sedative*: PO 50–300 mg daily in divided doses<br>*Hypnotic*: PO 65–200 mg; IM, IV 65–500 mg | *Sedative*: over 12 years, same as adult dosage; under 12 years, PO 2 mg/kg per day in 4 divided doses<br>*Hypnotic*: over 12 years, same as adult dosage | Schedule II drug |
| **Aprobarbital** (Alurate) | Sedative, hypnotic | *Sedative*: PO 40 mg 3 times daily<br>*Hypnotic*: PO 40–160 mg | | Schedule III drug |
| **Butabarbital sodium** (Butisol) | Sedative | *Sedative*: PO 50–120 mg/d in 3–4 divided doses<br>*Hypnotic*: PO 50–100 mg | *Sedative*: PO 2 mg/kg per day in 3 divided doses | Schedule IV drug |

#### Long-acting

| Generic/Trade Name | Major Clinical Use | Adults | Children | Remarks |
|---|---|---|---|---|
| **Mephobarbital** (Mebaral) | Anticonvulsant | PO 200 mg at bedtime to 600 mg daily in divided doses | *Over 5 years*: PO 32–64 mg 3–4 times daily<br>*Under 5 years*: PO 16–32 mg 3–4 times daily | Serum levels of phenobarbital can be used as guidelines for adjusting dosage because mephobarbital is metabolized to phenobarbital. |
| **Phenobarbital** (Luminal, others) | Sedative, anticonvulsant | *Sedative*: PO,IM,IV 30–120 mg daily in 2–3 divided doses<br>*Hypnotic*: PO,IM,IV 100–300 mg<br>*Anticonvulsant*: PO 100–300 mg daily in 2–3 divided doses | *Sedative*: PO, rectal 1–2 mg/kg per day in 2–3 divided doses<br>*Hypnotic*: PO 2–4 mg/kg<br>*Anticonvulsant*: PO 5 mg/kg per day in 2–3 divided doses | Schedule IV drug. Not likely to produce abuse or dependence with chronic administration of anticonvulsant doses. Therapeutic plasma levels in seizure disorders are usually 10–25 µg/ml. |

### Benzodiazepines

| Generic/Trade Name | Major Clinical Use | Adults | Children | Remarks |
|---|---|---|---|---|
| **Estazolam** (ProSom) | Hypnotic | PO 1–2 mg | Not recommended | Schedule IV |
| **Flurazepam** (Dalmane) | Hypnotic | PO 15–30 mg | Not recommended | Schedule IV |
| **Quazepam** (Doral) | Hypnotic | PO 7.5–15 mg | Not recommended | Schedule IV |
| **Temazepam** (Restoril) | Hypnotic | PO 15–30 mg | Not recommended | Schedule IV |
| **Triazolam** (Halcion) | Hypnotic | PO 0.125–0.25 mg | Not recommended | Schedule IV |

### Nonbarbiturate, Nonbenzodiazepines

| Generic/Trade Name | Major Clinical Use | Adults | Children | Remarks |
|---|---|---|---|---|
| **Chloral hydrate** | Sedative, hypnotic | *Sedative*: PO, rectal suppository 250 mg 3 times per day, after meals<br>*Hypnotic*: PO, rectal suppository 500–1000 mg at bedtime; maximum dose, 2 g/d | *Sedative*: PO, rectal suppository 25 mg/kg per day, in 3 or 4 divided doses<br>*Hypnotic*: PO, rectal suppository 50 mg/kg at bedtime; maximum single dose, 1 g | |
| **Ethchlorvynol** (Placidyl) | Hypnotic | PO 500 mg | Not recommended | |
| **Zolpidem** (Ambien) | Hypnotic | PO 10 mg | Not recommended | |

## Suppression of REM sleep

When barbiturates are given in hypnotic doses for insomnia, they alter normal sleep patterns by decreasing REM sleep and increasing non-REM sleep. Decreased REM sleep is followed by a compensatory increase in REM sleep when the drug is discontinued, as though the mind needs to make up the lost dreaming time. This REM rebound effect can occur even when barbiturates are used for only 3 or 4 days. With longer drug use, REM rebound may be severe and accompanied by vivid dreams, nightmares, restlessness, and frequent awakening.

Normal sleep patterns may not return for several weeks after a barbiturate is discontinued, especially if it is stopped abruptly. Some authorities think this promotes dependence and abuse of the drugs because people continue taking them to avoid REM rebound and prolonged changes in sleep patterns. Unless these effects are explained, clients may attribute their continued sleeping difficulties to physical, emotional, or environmental problems rather than to drug use.

## Enzyme induction

Barbiturates increase the liver's ability to metabolize themselves, several other drugs (*e.g.*, phenytoin, alcohol), and numerous substances that may be endogenous or administered as drugs (*e.g.*, adrenal corticosteroids, bile salts, sex hormones, vitamin K). They do so by stimulating liver cells to produce larger amounts of drug-metabolizing enzymes. Larger amounts of the enzymes allow larger amounts of a drug or other substance to be metabolized during a given period of time. This is one mechanism by which barbiturates produce tolerance and lose their effectiveness as sedative-hypnotics in approximately 2 weeks of daily use. This is also the basis for cross-tolerance with other CNS depressants and other important drug interactions because many drugs are metabolized by the same enzyme system in the liver. Barbiturate-induced enzyme induction apparently disappears a few weeks after the drug is discontinued.

## Dependence and abuse

Barbiturates have a high potential for dependence and abuse; see Chapter 15.

## BENZODIAZEPINES

The benzodiazepines include several drugs used for a variety of indications (see Chap. 8). When a hypnotic is deemed necessary, a benzodiazepine is preferred over a barbiturate because the benzodiazepines have a wider safety margin between therapeutic and toxic doses, are rarely lethal in overdose unless combined with another CNS depressant drug such as alcohol, do not significantly suppress REM sleep, do not cause induction of drug-metabolizing enzymes, are effective for approximately 4 weeks, and cause less dependence and abuse. However, they may cause excessive sedation, impairment of physical and mental activities, respiratory depression and other effects characteristic of CNS depressant drugs. They are also Schedule IV drugs and may cause abuse and dependence, especially with large doses, long-term use, or both. The drugs should not be stopped abruptly after long-term use because withdrawal symptoms occur and may be severe; instead, the drugs should be gradually tapered and discontinued.

Although sufficient doses of any benzodiazepine can induce sleep, the oral drugs promoted by manufacturers as hypnotics are **estazolam** (ProSom), **flurazepam** (Dalmane), **quazepam** (Doral), **temazepam** (Restoril), and **triazolam** (Halcion). All of the drugs are effective in treating insomnia and differ mainly in their serum half-lives and whether they produce active or inactive metabolites.

Flurazepam and quazepam are similar; the drugs and their active metabolites have long half-lives. Thus, they are more effective on the second or third night of administration and are more likely to cause residual sedation ("morning hangover"), which may last for several days after the drug is discontinued.

Estazolam, temazepam, and triazolam have shorter half-lives and inactive metabolites. Therefore, they are less likely to cause daytime sedation or accumulation. Triazolam has been removed from the market in several countries because of adverse effects, including psychiatric symptoms. In most studies, these effects occurred with larger doses than those currently recommended. None of these drugs is recomended for long-term use.

## NONBARBITURATES, NONBENZODIAZEPINES

Nonbarbiturate, nonbenzodiazepine hypnotics include **chloral hydrate**, **ethchlorvynol** (Placidyl), and **zolpidem** (Ambien). Chloral hydrate, the oldest sedative-hypnotic drug, is relatively safe, effective, and inexpensive in usual therapeutic doses. It reportedly does not suppress REM sleep. Tolerance develops after about 2 weeks of continual use. It is a drug of abuse and may cause physical dependence. Ethchlorvynol is infrequently used because it has most of the undesirable characteristics of the barbiturates, a high potential for abuse, and overdoses are difficult to manage. Zolpidem is a newer drug that is apparently as effective as the benzodiazepines but is more likely to cause adverse effects, such as excessive sedation and motor impairment. It is not recommended as a first-choice hypnotic.

In addition, several antihistamines (see Chap. 51) cause drowsiness and are used as hypnotics, although they are not FDA-approved for this purpose. Diphenhydramine (Benadryl) is used in hospitalized clients and is available over the counter. An antihistamine is the active ingredient in nonprescription sleep aids (*e.g.*, diphenhydramine in Compoz, Nytol, Sominex, Sleep-Eze; doxylamine in Unisom).

## Mechanism of action

Barbiturates produce CNS depression by inhibiting functions of nerve cells, such as electrical stimulation, depolarization, impulse transmission, and neurotransmitter release. Neurons in the reticular formation, which control cerebral cortex activity and level of arousal or wakefulness, are especially sensitive to the depressant effects of barbiturates. Benzodiazepines bind with specific receptors in the brain and increase the effects of gamma-aminobutyric acid, an inhibitory neurotransmitter.

## Indications for use

Clinical indications for use of sedative-hypnotic drugs include short-term treatment of insomnia and sedation prior to surgery or invasive diagnostic tests (*e.g.*, angiograms and endoscopies). Barbiturates also are used for their general anesthetic and anticonvulsant effects.

## Contraindications for use

Contraindications to sedative-hypnotic drugs include severe respiratory disorders, hypersensitivity reactions, a history of alcohol or drug abuse, and severe liver or kidney disease. In addition, barbiturates are contraindicated in acute intermittent porphyria (a rare hereditary metabolic disorder characterized by recurrent attacks of physical and mental disturbances).

## *Nursing Process*

### Assessment

- Assess the client's need for sedative-hypnotic drugs, including intensity and duration of symptoms.
- Try to identify factors contributing to insomnia. Some common ones are anxiety, excessive daytime sleep, too little exercise and activity, and excessive CNS stimulation from caffeine-containing beverages or drugs such as bronchodilators and nasal decongestants.

- Assess previous use of and response to sedative-hypnotic agents.
- Assess the client's usual mechanisms for coping with stress and insomnia.
- Assess the likelihood of drug abuse and dependence. People who abuse other drugs, including alcohol, are likely to abuse sedative-hypnotics.
- Once drug therapy is begun, assess the client's level of consciousness and functional ability before each dose so that excessive sedation can be avoided.

### Nursing diagnoses

- Sleep Pattern Disturbance: Insomnia related to one or more causes (*e.g.*, daytime sleep)
- High Risk for Injury related to depressed level of consciousness
- High Risk for Impaired Gas Exchange related to respiratory depression
- High Risk for Noncompliance: Overuse
- Knowledge Deficit: Drug effects and safe usage

### Planning/Goals

*The client will:*
- Experience decreased signs and symptoms of insomnia
- Use sedative-hypnotic drugs safely, avoiding adverse effects and nightly use
- Identify factors contributing to insomnia and act to eliminate or minimize them when feasible

### Interventions

Implement measures to decrease need for or increase effectiveness of sedative-hypnotic drugs, such as the following:
- Modify the environment to promote rest and sleep by reducing noise and light or by changing ventilation and temperature.
- Plan care to allow uninterrupted periods of rest and sleep when possible.
- Relieve symptoms that interfere with rest and sleep. Drugs such as analgesics for pain or antitussives for cough are usually safer and more effective than sedative-hypnotic drugs. Nondrug measures, such as positioning, exercise, and backrubs, may be helpful in relieving muscle tension and other discomforts. Allowing the client to verbalize concerns, providing information so that the client knows what to expect, or consulting other personnel (*e.g.*, social worker, chaplain) may be useful in decreasing anxiety.
- Assist the client to modify his or her life-style when indicated. Some changes that may help in promoting sleep include avoiding or limiting intake of caffeine-containing beverages, limiting intake of fluids during evening hours if nocturia interferes with sleep, avoiding daytime naps, having a regular schedule of rest and sleep periods, increasing physical activity, and not trying to sleep unless tired or drowsy.

### *Teach clients:*
- Nondrug measures to promote rest and sleep
- To avoid smoking, ambulating without help, driving a car, or operating machinery after taking a sedative-hypnotic. These activities may lead to falls or other injuries if undertaken while sedated.

- To avoid other CNS depressant drugs (*e.g.*, alcohol, antihistamines, narcotic analgesics, antianxiety drugs) while taking a sedative-hypnotic
- Not to take sedative-hypnotic drugs every night. These drugs lose their effectiveness in 2 to 4 weeks if taken nightly. They also cause sleep disturbances when withdrawn.

### Evaluation

- Interview and observe regarding decreased symptoms or increased rest and sleep.
- Observe for "morning hangover" or excessive daytime drowsiness.

## Principles of therapy

### DRUG SELECTION AND SCHEDULING TO ACHIEVE TREATMENT GOALS

The goal of treatment with sedative-hypnotic drugs is to relieve anxiety or sleeplessness without permitting sensory perception, responsiveness to the environment, or alertness to drop below safe levels. Guidelines to help meet this goal include the following:

1. Give the least amount of the least potent drug for the shortest time that will be effective. This basic principle applies especially to sedative-hypnotic drug therapy because abuse, dependence, overdose, and suicide are more likely to occur with large doses and prolonged use.
2. As a general rule, start with small doses and increase them only if necessary. Low doses are often adequate in people who are elderly or debilitated or who have liver or kidney disease.
3. Do not give sedative-hypnotic drugs every night unless necessary. Intermittent administration helps maintain drug effectiveness and decreases the risks of drug abuse and dependence. It also decreases disturbances of normal sleep patterns and REM rebound.
4. When sedative-hypnotic drugs are prescribed for outpatients, the prescription should limit the number of doses dispensed and the number of refills. This is one way of decreasing the risk of abuse, suicide, and other problems.
5. In chronic insomnia, no hypnotic drug has any real advantage over the others. They all lose their effectiveness in producing sleep after 1 to 2 weeks of daily use, except the benzodiazepines, which last about 4

weeks. It is not helpful to switch from one drug to another because cross-tolerance develops. To restore the sleep-producing effect, administration of the hypnotic drug must be interrupted for 1 to 2 weeks.

### MANAGEMENT OF BENZODIAZEPINE TOXICITY

Flumazenil (Romazicon) is a specific antidote to reverse the toxic effects of benzodiazepines. See Chapter 8 for additional information and recommended dosage ranges.

### USE IN CHILDREN

Sedative-hypnotic drugs are rarely indicated in children except for phenobarbital in seizure disorders. Of the benzodiazepines, only chlordiazepoxide (Librium) and diazepam (Valium) have been extensively used. Others do not have established dosages and are not recommended for use in children. As with other CNS depressant drugs, sedative-hypnotics may cause paradoxical CNS stimulation (excitement, irritability, hostility) in children.

### USE IN OLDER ADULTS

Sedative-hypnotic drugs should generally be avoided or minimized in older adults, despite frequent complaints of insomnia. Finding and treating the cause(s) and using nondrug measures to aid sleep are much safer, as discussed previously in this chapter. If a sedative-hypnotic is used, recommendations for safe use are as follows:

1. Shorter-acting benzodiazepines are preferred, because they are eliminated more rapidly and are therefore less likely to accumulate and increase adverse effects.
2. Dosages should be smaller than for younger adults.
3. The drugs should not be used every night or for longer than a few days.
4. Older adults should be monitored closely for excessive sedation, dizziness, ataxia, and confusion to prevent falls and other injuries.
5. The drugs should be tapered rather than discontinued abruptly to avoid withdrawal symptoms. Withdrawal symptoms may occur within 24 hours after stopping the short-acting drugs.

## NURSING ACTIONS: SEDATIVE-HYPNOTIC DRUGS

| *Nursing Actions* | *Rationale/Explanation* |
|---|---|
| **1. Administer accurately** | |
| **a.** Give oral sedative-hypnotic drugs with a glass of water or other fluid. | The fluid enhances dissolution and absorption of the drug for a quicker onset of action. |
| **b.** Prepare the client for sleep before giving hypnotic doses of any drug. | Most of these drugs cause drowsiness within 15 to 30 minutes. The client should be in bed when he or she becomes drowsy to increase the therapeutic effectiveness of the sedative-hypnotic and to decrease the likelihood of falls or other injuries. |
| **c.** Raise bedrails, and instruct client to stay in bed or ask for help if necessary to get out of bed. | To avoid falls and other injuries related to sedation and impaired mobility |
| **d.** Do not leave a dose of sedative-hypnotic drugs at the client's bedside. | There is a risk that the client will save the drugs and use them to commit suicide or inadvertently take an overdose. |
| **e.** Use the following special precautions when giving barbiturates parenterally: | |
| (1) Do not use any parenteral solutions that are cloudy or contain a precipitate. | |
| (2) Do not mix with any other drugs in the same syringe. | Many drugs form precipitates if mixed with barbiturates. |
| (3) For intramuscular administration, inject deeply into a large muscle mass. | To minimize tissue irritation |
| (4) For intravenous injection, inject *slowly*, and have equipment available for artificial ventilation. | The intravenous route is usually used only for anesthesia or to terminate acute convulsions. Check agency policy regarding administration of intravenous medications by nurses. |
| (5) When giving barbiturates parenterally, be very careful to avoid extravasation of the drug into surrounding tissues and accidental intra-arterial injection. | Parenteral barbiturate solutions are highly alkaline and irritating to tissues. Accidental injection into an artery causes severe vasoconstriction and ischemia and can cause gangrene of the extremity. Acute, severe pain, edema, redness, and obliteration of pulses beyond the injection site occur rapidly in the affected limb. |
| **2. Observe for therapeutic effects** | Therapeutic effects depend largely on the reason for use. The degree of drowsiness desired or tolerated could be different in a hospitalized person as compared with someone continuing work or other usual activities. |
| **a.** When a drug is given for mild sedation and antianxiety effects, the recipient appears relaxed, perhaps drowsy, but is easily aroused. | |
| **b.** When a drug is given for hypnotic effects, the recipient goes to sleep within about 30 minutes, does not awaken more than once or twice, and sleeps several hours. During this time, the person can be aroused easily if necessary. | |
| **c.** When an drug is given for anticonvulsant effect, lack of seizure activity is a therapeutic effect. | |
| **3. Observe for adverse effects** | |
| **a.** *Excessive sedation*—drowsiness, stupor, slurred speech, impaired mobility, impaired mental processes, coma | This is due to depressant effects on the central nervous system (CNS). The severity depends mostly on drug dosage and the degree of drug tolerance that has developed. It is more likely to occur when drug therapy is begun, and it usually decreases within a week. |

## Nursing Actions

## Rationale/Explanation

**b.** *Respiratory depression*—hypoxemia, restlessness, dyspnea, shallow breathing

This stems from depression of the respiratory center in the medulla oblongata. Respiratory failure is the usual cause of death in acute drug intoxication. If death is delayed, it is likely to be caused by hypostatic pneumonia or pulmonary edema.

**c.** *Shock*—hypotension, tachycardia

Shock probably results from hypoxia and depression of the vasomotor center in the brain.

**d.** *Chronic intoxication*—sedation, confusion, emotional lability, muscular incoordination, impaired mental processes, mental depression, gastrointestinal problems, weight loss

This is similar to chronic alcohol abuse.

**e.** *Withdrawal or abstinence syndrome*—anxiety, insomnia, restlessness, irritability, tremulousness, postural hypotension, seizures

This syndrome develops when the drugs are suddenly withdrawn in dependent people. These symptoms progressively increase in severity. They can be prevented or minimized by using a long-acting agent (*i.e.*, phenobarbital) and gradually tapering the dose.

**4. Observe for drug interactions**
　**a.** Drugs that *increase* effects of sedative-hypnotics:

　　(1) CNS depressants—alcohol, narcotic analgesics, antidepressants, antihistamines, phenothiazines, and other antipsychotic agents

All these drugs produce CNS depression when given alone. Any combination initially increases CNS depression and is potentially serious or even fatal. With long-term use, tolerance develops and CNS depression becomes less apparent. As a general rule, these drugs should not be given concurrently.

　　(2) Cimetidine

Prolongs elimination half-life and increases plasma concentrations of diazepam

　**b.** Drugs that *decrease* effects of sedative-hypnotics
　　Enzyme inducers (*e.g.*, barbiturates)

With chronic use, these drugs antagonize their own actions and the actions of other drugs metabolized in the liver. They increase the rate of drug metabolism and elimination from the body.

　**c.** Drugs that *increase* effects of barbiturates (in addition to those that increase effects of sedative-hypnotics in general):

　　(1) Acidifying agents (*e.g.*, ascorbic acid)

These agents increase absorption of barbiturates in the gastrointestinal tract and increase drug reabsorption in renal tubules (except for phenobarbital).

　　(2) Benzodiazepines (*e.g.*, diazepam)

May potentiate sedative and respiratory effects of barbiturates

　**d.** Drugs that *decrease* barbiturate effects
　　Alkalinizing agents (*e.g.*, sodium bicarbonate)

Increase renal excretion of phenobarbital

**5. Teach clients:**
　**a.** Take sedative-hypnotic drugs as prescribed. Do not increase the amount or frequency of administration.

This is especially important in view of drug dependence and other serious or life-threatening adverse reactions that can occur with these drugs. Risks of adverse reactions and habituation increase with prolonged use.

　**b.** Use nondrug measures to relax or go to sleep when possible.

Individuals vary greatly in what they find relaxing or sleep-inducing. For one person, it may be reading; for another, it may be watching television. It is advantageous for anyone to identify and use relaxation techniques rather than drugs.

　**c.** Store sedative-hypnotic drugs safely.

*(continued)*

| Nursing Actions | Rationale/Explanation |
|---|---|
| (1) Never keep at the bedside. | A person sedated by a previous dose may take additional doses if the drugs are within reach. |
| (2) Keep the drugs away from children and from adults who are confused or less than alert. | |
| **d.** When "sleeping pills" are discontinued, there may be increased dreaming or more frequent awakenings temporarily. | These effects are caused by withdrawal of the medication. They are *not* caused by the sleeping problem for which the medication was originally prescribed. Continuing the drug to avoid these effects aggravates the situation. This reaction is less likely with benzodiazepines. |
| **e.** As a general rule, take these drugs in the smallest effective dose for the shortest possible time. | To avoid abuse and dependence. |

## Review and Application Exercises

1. Why is sleep necessary? What functions does sleep fulfill?
2. What is the main difference between sedative drugs and hypnotic drugs?
3. What is the reticular activating system and how is it affected by sedative–hypnotic and other CNS depressant drugs?
4. What are the stages of CNS depression between alertness and coma?
5. What is drug dependence?
6. What are some mechanisms by which sedative-hypnotic drugs cause dependence, tolerance, cross-tolerance, and withdrawal symptoms?
7. Why are benzodiazepine hypnotics preferred over barbiturate hypnotics?
8. Why are nonpharmacologic interventions to promote relaxation and sleep usually preferred over sedative-hypnotic drugs?
9. What factors need to be considered when planning care for an older adult who often takes a "sleeping pill"?
10. For an ambulatory client beginning a prescription for a benzodiazepine hypnotic, what instructions need to be emphasized for safe, effective, and rational drug usage?

## Selected References

Crismon, M. L. (1992). Insomnia. In M. A. Koda-Kimble & L. Y. Young (Eds.), *Applied therapeutics: The clinical use of drugs* (5th ed.) (pp. 55-1–55-17). Vancouver, WA: Applied Therapeutics.

(1993). *Drug facts and comparisons.* St. Louis: Facts and Comparisons.

Fankhauser, M. P. (1993). Anxiolytic drugs and sedative-hypnotic agents. In R. Bressler & M. D. Katz (Eds.), *Geriatric pharmacology* (pp. 165–205). New York: McGraw-Hill.

Guyton, A. C. (1991). *Textbook of medical physiology* (8th ed.). Philadelphia: W.B. Saunders

Hollister, L. E. (1992). Psychiatric disorders. In K. L. Melmon, H. F. Morrelli, B. B. Hoffman, & D. W. Nierenberg (Eds.), *Clinical pharmacology: Basic principles in therapeutics* (3rd ed.) (pp. 338–380). New York: McGraw-Hill.

Kirkwood, C. K. (1992). Sleep disorders. In J. T. DiPiro, R. L. Talbert, P. E. Hayes, G. C. Yee, G. R. Matzke, & L. M. Posey (Eds.), *Pharmacotherapy: A pathophysiologic approach* (2nd ed.) (pp. 1110–1119). New York: Elsevier.

### CHAPTER 8

# Antianxiety Drugs

Antianxiety agents are central nervous system (CNS) depressants with sedative-hypnotic properties. They are commonly prescribed worldwide.

## Anxiety

*Anxiety* is difficult to define because it is mainly subjective, and terminology is inconsistent. It may be called apprehension, fear, nervousness, tension, worry, or other terms that denote an unpleasant feeling state. It occurs when a person perceives a situation as threatening to physical, emotional, social, or economic well-being. Causes of anxiety vary among people and even in the same person at different times. Many occur with everyday events associated with home, work, school, social activities, and chronic illness. Others occur episodically, such as an acute illness, death, divorce, loss of a job, starting a new job, or taking a test. Thus, anxiety is a normal response to a stressful situation and may be beneficial when it motivates the person toward constructive, problem-solving, coping activities.

However, when anxiety is severe or prolonged, it impairs the ability to function in usual activities of daily living. The American Psychiatric Association delineates anxiety disorders as medical diagnoses in the *Diagnostic and Statistical Manual*, third edition, revised, published in 1987. This classification includes phobias and panic, obsessive-compulsive, post-traumatic stress, and atypical anxiety disorders, as well as generalized anxiety disorder. *Generalized anxiety disorder* includes:

1. Excessive anxiety about two or more circumstances for 6 months or longer
2. Six of 18 symptoms related to motor tension (*e.g.*, muscle tension, restlessness, trembling, fatigue), overactivity of the autonomic nervous system (*e.g.*, dyspnea, palpitations, tachycardia, sweating, dry mouth, dizziness, nausea, diarrhea), and increased vigilance (feeling keyed up, startling easily, difficulty concentrating, irritability, insomnia)
3. Disease processes or other causative factors (*e.g.*, hyperthyroidism, excessive caffeine or other stimulants) ruled out

## Benzodiazepines

The benzodiazepines are by far the most commonly used drugs for treatment of anxiety disorders. Chlordiazepoxide (Librium) is the prototype of the group, although others are more frequently prescribed. When first marketed in about 1960, the benzodiazepines were thought to be effective in relieving emotional distress with minimal adverse effects. Compared to the barbiturates (see Chap. 7), which had been widely used previously, the benzodiazepines had a wider margin of safety between therapeutic and toxic doses and were rarely fatal, even in overdose, unless combined with other CNS depressant drugs, such as alcohol. They also were considered nonaddictive. Consequently, they were widely prescribed and were popular with physicians and clients.

However, within a few years it became evident that

the drugs were being abused and were causing physical and psychological dependence. Although the drugs are still widely used, it is recommended that they be prescribed more selectively and for shorter periods.

These drugs are highly lipid-soluble, widely distributed in body tissues, and extensively bound to plasma proteins. Most are metabolized in the liver and excreted in the urine. They are Schedule IV drugs under the Controlled Substances Act. They are well-absorbed with oral administration. Chlordiazepoxide, diazepam (Valium), lorazepam (Ativan), and midazolam (Versed) are available for parenteral use.

Pharmacologically, all the benzodiazepines have similar characteristics and produce the same effects. However, they differ in clinical uses because the manufacturers developed and promoted them for particular purposes. Some are approved for use only as hypnotics (see Chap. 7), for example, although a sufficient dose of any benzodiazepine produces sleep.

The drugs also differ in duration of action. Several (*e.g.*, chlordiazepoxide, diazepam, and clorazepate [Tranxene]) have long half-lives and produce pharmacologically active metabolites that also have long half-lives. As a result, these drugs require about 5 to 7 days to reach steady-state serum levels. Therapeutic effects (*e.g.*, decreased anxiety) and adverse effects (*e.g.*, sedation, ataxia) are more likely to occur after 2 or 3 days of therapy than initially. Such effects accumulate with chronic usage and persist for several days after the drugs are discontinued. The other drugs have short half-lives and produce inactive metabolites; thus their durations of action are much shorter, and they do not accumulate.

## MECHANISM OF ACTION

The benzodiazepines bind with a receptor complex in nerve cells of the brain; this receptor complex also has binding sites for gamma-aminobutyric acid (GABA), an inhibitory neurotransmitter (see Chap. 4). This GABA-benzodiazepine receptor complex regulates entry of chloride ions into the cell. When GABA binds to the receptor complex, chloride ions enter the cell and stabilize (hyperpolarize) the cell membrane so that it is less responsive to excitatory neurotransmitters, such as norepinephrine. Benzodiazepines bind at a different site on the receptor complex and facilitate the inhibitory effect of GABA to relieve anxiety, tension, nervousness, and so forth.

## INDICATIONS FOR USE

Major clinical uses of the benzodiazepines are as antianxiety, hypnotic, and anticonvulsant agents. They also are given for preoperative sedation, prevention of agitation and delirium tremens in acute alcohol withdrawal,

and other uses. Not all benzodiazepines are approved for all uses (see Chap. 7 for benzodiazepine hypnotics). Diazepam has been extensively studied and has more approved uses than others. Table 8-1 lists indications for use of individual benzodiazepines.

## CONTRAINDICATIONS FOR USE

Contraindications include severe respiratory disorders, severe liver or kidney disease, hypersensitivity reactions, and a history of drug abuse.

# Individual antianxiety drugs

## BENZODIAZEPINE ANTIANXIETY AGENTS

See Table 8-1.

## NONBENZODIAZEPINE ANTIANXIETY AGENTS

**Buspirone** (BuSpar) differs chemically and pharmacologically from other antianxiety drugs. Its mechanism of action is unclear, but it apparently interacts with serotonin and dopamine receptors in the brain. Compared to the benzodiazepines, buspirone lacks muscle relaxant and anticonvulsant effects, does not cause sedation or physical or psychological dependence, does not increase the CNS depression of alcohol and other drugs, and is not a controlled substance. Its only clinical indication for use is the short-term treatment of anxiety. Because therapeutic effects may be delayed for a few weeks, it is not considered beneficial for immediate effects or occasional (PRN) use.

Buspirone is rapidly absorbed following oral administration. Peak plasma levels occur within 45 to 90 minutes. It is metabolized by the liver to inactive metabolites, which are then excreted in the urine and feces. Its elimination half-life is 2 to 3 hours.

### Route and dosage range

*Adults:* PO 5 mg three times per day, increased by 5 mg/d at 2- to 3-day intervals if necessary
  Usual maintenance dose 20–30 mg/d in divided doses; maximum dose 60 mg/d

**Clomipramine** (Anafranil) is a tricyclic antidepressant (see Chap. 10) used for treatment of obsessive-compulsive disorder.

### Route and dosage range

*Adults:* PO 25 mg/d initially; increase to 100 mg/d during the first 2 weeks and to a maximum dose of 250 mg/d over several weeks if necessary

## TABLE 8-1. ANTIANXIETY BENZODIAZEPINES

| Generic/Trade Name | Clinical Indications | Half-life (h) | Metabolite(s) | Routes and Dosage Ranges |
|---|---|---|---|---|
| **Alprazolam** (Xanax) | Anxiety<br>Panic attacks | Short<br>(7–15) | Active | Adults: PO 0.25–0.5 mg 3 times daily; maximal dose, 4 mg daily in divided doses<br>Elderly or debilitated adults: 0.25 mg 2–3 times daily, increased gradually if necessary |
| **Chlordiazepoxide** (Librium) | Anxiety<br>Acute alcohol withdrawal | Long<br>(5–30) | Active | Adults: PO 15–100 mg daily, once at bedtime or in 3–4 divided doses. IM, IV 50–100 mg, maximal daily dose 300 mg; for short-term use<br>Elderly or debilitated adults: PO 5–10 mg 2–4 times daily<br>Children over 6 years: PO, IM 0.5 mg/kg per day in 3–4 divided doses<br>Children under 6 years: Not recommended |
| **Clonazepam** (Klonopin) | Seizure disorders | Long<br>(20–40) | Inactive | Adults: PO 0.5 mg 3 times daily, increased by 0.5–1 mg every 3 days until seizures are controlled or adverse effects occur. Maximal daily dose, 20 mg |
| **Clorazepate** (Tranxene) | Anxiety<br>Seizure disorders | Long<br>(30–100) | Active | Adults: PO 7.5 mg 3 times daily, increased by no more than 7.5 mg/wk. Maximal daily dose, 90 mg<br>Children 9–12 years: PO 7.5 mg 2 times daily, increased by no more than 7.5 mg/wk. Maximal daily dose, 60 mg<br>Children under 9 years: Not recommended |
| **Diazepam** (Valium) | Anxiety<br>Seizure disorders<br>Acute alcohol withdrawal<br>Muscle spasm<br>Preoperative sedation<br>Hypnotic | Long<br>(20–50) | Active | Adults: PO 2–10 mg 2–4 times daily; sustained release, PO 15–30 mg once daily; IM, IV 5–10 mg, repeated in 3–4 hours if necessary<br>Elderly or debilitated adults: PO 2–5 mg once or twice daily, increased gradually if needed and tolerated.<br>Children: PO 1–2.5 mg 3–4 times daily, increased gradually if needed and tolerated<br>Children over 30 days and under 5 years of age: Seizures IM, IV 0.2–0.5 mg/2–5 min to a maximum of 5 mg<br>Children 5 years or older: Seizures, IM, IV 1 mg/2–5 min to a maximum of 10 mg |
| **Halazepam** (Paxipam) | Anxiety | Short<br>(5–15) | Active | Adults: PO 20–40 mg 3–4 times daily |
| **Lorazepam** (Ativan) | Anxiety<br>Preoperative sedation | Short<br>(8–15) | Inactive | Adults: PO 2–6 mg/d in 2–3 divided doses. IM 0.05 mg/kg to a maximum of 4 mg. IV 2 mg, diluted with 2 ml of sterile water, sodium chloride, or 5% dextrose injection, injected over 1 minute or longer.<br>Elderly or debilitated adults: PO 1–2 mg/d in divided doses |
| **Midazolam** (Versed) | Preoperative sedation<br>Sedation prior to short diagnostic tests and endoscopic examinations<br>Induction of general anesthesia<br>Supplementation of nitrous oxide/oxygen anesthesia for short surgical procedures | Short<br>(1–12) | Active | Adults: Preoperative sedation, IM 0.05–0.08 mg/kg about 1 hour before surgery<br>Prediagnostic test sedation, IV 0.1–0.15 mg/kg or up to 0.2 mg/kg initially; maintenance dose, about 25% of initial dose. Reduce dose by 25% to 30% if a narcotic is also given.<br>Induction of anesthesia, IV 0.3–0.35 mg/kg initially, reduce dose as above for maintenance. Reduce initial dose to 0.15–0.3 mg/kg if a narcotic is also given. |
| **Oxazepam** (Serax) | Anxiety<br>Acute alcohol withdrawal | Short<br>(5–15) | Inactive | Adults: PO 30–120 mg daily in 3–4 divided doses<br>Elderly or debilitated adults: PO 30 mg daily in 3 divided doses, gradually increased to 45–60 mg daily if necessary |
| **Prazepam** (Centrax) | Anxiety | Long<br>(30–100) | Active | Adults: PO 20–40 mg daily in divided doses<br>Elderly or debilitated adults: PO 10–15 mg daily in divided doses |

Give in divided doses with food to minimize gastrointestinal upset; when the effective dose is established, give once daily at bedtime to minimize daytime sedation.

*Children and adolescents:* PO 25 mg/d initially; increase to 3 mg/kg or 100 mg, whichever is smaller, during the first 2 weeks and to 3 mg/kg or 200 mg, whichever is smaller, over several weeks if necessary. Give as with adults, above.

**Hydroxyzine** (Vistaril) is chemically different from the benzodiazepines but shares a number of their clinical indications, such as treatment of anxiety and preoperative sedation. When hydroxyzine is combined with narcotic analgesics, dosage of the analgesics must be reduced because hydroxyzine potentiates their sedative effects. In contrast to the benzodiazepines, hydroxyzine has antiemetic and antihistaminic effects that account for a large portion of its clinical usefulness. It is often used, for example, to relieve nausea and vomiting that occur after surgery and with motion sickness. Its antihistaminic effects have been useful in treating urticaria and other manifestations of allergic dermatoses. Hydroxyzine is not a controlled drug.

### Routes and dosage ranges

*Adults:* PO 75–400 mg/d in three or four divided doses

    Preoperative and postoperative and prepartum and postpartum sedation, IM 25–100 mg in a single dose

*Children:* PO 2 mg/kg per day in four divided doses

    Preoperative and postoperative sedation, IM 1 mg/kg in a single dose

**Meprobamate** (Equanil, Miltown) is an antianxiety agent that is chemically different from the benzodiazepines and hydroxyzine. It is also used as a muscle relaxant, but its effectiveness for that purpose is questionable. Meprobamate is a Schedule IV drug. Drug tolerance, abuse, dependence, and withdrawal symptoms occur with long-term use.

### Route and dosage range

*Adults:* PO 1.2–1.6 g daily in three or four divided doses; maximum dose 2.4 g/d

*Children over 6 years:* PO 25 mg/kg per day in two or three divided doses

*Children under 6 years:* Not recommended

## Nursing Process

### Assessment

Assess the client's need for antianxiety drugs. Manifestations of anxiety are more obvious with moderate or severe anxiety. Some guidelines for assessing anxiety include the following:

- What is the client's statement of the situation? Does he or she dwell on physical problems or symptoms as a cause of distress? Does the client describe himself or herself as worried, tense, or nervous? Is distress attributed to situational factors, such as illness, death of a friend or family member, divorce, or job stress? All these may indicate anxiety, but additional information is needed for verification.
- How does the stated problem affect the client's ability to function? Interview and observe the client to answer this question. Generally, try to determine to what extent the client is able to carry out usual activities of daily living. If he or she is overactive and agitated or underactive and withdrawn, productivity and the ability to function are likely to be impaired.
- Obtain a careful history of drugs taken previously and currently, especially the use of alcohol and sedative-hypnotic drugs. Also assess for use of CNS stimulants and anxiety-provoking drugs (*e.g.*, appetite suppressants, bronchodilators, nasal decongestants, excessive caffeine, cocaine).
- Try to identify factors that precipitate anxiety. For example, what does the client see as anxiety-provoking events? Is misinformation or lack of information a source of anxiety?
- Observe for behavioral manifestations of anxiety, such as psychomotor agitation, facial grimaces, tense posture, crying, and others.
- Observe for physiologic manifestations of anxiety. These may include increased blood pressure and pulse rate, increased rate and depth of respiration, increased muscle tension, and pale, cool skin.
- If behavioral or physiologic manifestations seem to indicate anxiety, try to determine whether this is actually the case. Because similar manifestations may indicate pain or other problems rather than anxiety, the observer's perceptions must be validated by the client before appropriate action can be taken.
- Identify coping mechanisms and support systems used in handling previous situations of stress and anxiety. These are very individualized. Reading, watching television, listening to music, or talking to a friend are examples. Some people are quiet and inactive, while others participate in strenuous activity. Some prefer to be alone, while others prefer being with a "significant other" or a group.

### Nursing diagnoses

- Ineffective Individual Coping related to need for antianxiety drug
- Knowledge Deficit: Appropriate use and effects of antianxiety drugs
- Knowledge Deficit: Nondrug measures for relieving stress and anxiety
- High Risk for Noncompliance: Overuse
- High Risk for Injury related to sedation and other adverse effects
- Alteration in Thought Processes related to confusion (especially in older adults)

### Planning/Goals

*The client will:*
- Feel more calm, relaxed, and comfortable
- Be monitored for excessive sedation and impaired mobility to prevent falls or other injuries (in health-care settings)

- Verbalize and demonstrate nondrug activities to reduce or manage stress
- Demonstrate safe, accurate drug usage
- Avoid preventable adverse effects, including abuse and dependence

### Interventions

Use nondrug measures to relieve anxiety or to enhance the effectiveness of antianxiety drugs.

- Support the client's usual coping mechanisms when feasible: Provide the opportunity for reading, exercising, or watching television; promote contact with significant others; or simply allow the client to be alone and uninterrupted for a while.
- Use interpersonal and communication techniques to help the client handle anxiety. The degree of anxiety and the clinical situation largely determine which techniques are appropriate. For example, staying with the client, showing interest, listening, and allowing him or her to verbalize his or her concerns may be sufficient to decrease anxiety.
- Providing information may be a therapeutic technique when anxiety is related to medical conditions. People vary in the amount and kind of information they desire, but generally the following topics should be included:
  - The overall treatment plan, including medical or surgical treatment, choice of outpatient care or hospitalization, expected length of treatment, and expected outcomes in terms of health and ability to function in activities of daily living
  - Specific diagnostic tests, including preparation, after-effects if any, and the way in which the client will be informed of results
  - Specific medication and treatment measures, including expected therapeutic results
  - What the client must do to carry out the plan of treatment. When offering information and explanations to clients, keep in mind that anxiety interferes with intellectual functioning. Thus, communication should be brief, clear, and repeated as necessary because clients may misunderstand or forget what is said.
- Modify the environment to decrease anxiety-provoking stimuli. Modifications may involve altering temperature, light, and noise levels or changing roommates.
- Use measures to increase physical comfort. These may include a wide variety of activities, such as positioning, assisting to bathe or ambulate, giving backrubs, or providing fluids of the client's choice.
- Consult with other services and departments on the client's behalf. For example, if financial problems were identified as causes of anxiety, social services may be able to help.
- When a benzodiazepine is used with diagnostic tests or minor surgery, provide instructions for postprocedure care to the client before the drug is administered or to family members, preferably in written form. Because the drugs cause anterograde amnesia, clients are unlikely to remember instructions given before the drug wears off.

### Teach clients:

- That antianxiety drugs help to relieve symptoms; they do not relieve underlying psychological problems
- That the drugs are recommended only for short-term use; that benzodiazepines may cause dependence
- To consider psychotherapy or other counseling if symptoms are prolonged or impair ability to function
- That all the benzodiazepines have similar characteristics and effects
- That drowsiness usually decreases within a few days after starting the drugs
- To avoid alcohol and other CNS depressant drugs (*e.g.*, antihistamines, sleeping pills, narcotic analgesics)
- To avoid driving a car, operating machinery, and other potentially hazardous tasks if alertness is impaired
- Not to abruptly stop taking benzodiazepines. They must be tapered gradually, under supervision of a health-care provider.

### Evaluation

- Decreased symptoms of anxiety and improved functioning in activities of daily living are observed.
- Excessive sedation and motor impairment are not observed.
- The client reports no serious adverse effects.
- Monitoring of prescriptions (*e.g.*, "pill counts") does not indicate excessive use.

## Principles of therapy

### GUIDELINES FOR RATIONAL USE OF ANTIANXIETY DRUGS

There are few clear-cut guidelines for using antianxiety drugs. Although still widely used, they are declining in popularity. One reason for this decreased use is their potential for producing drug abuse and physiologic and psychological dependence. These drugs have been extensively abused, often in combination with alcohol. A second reason is doubts about whether drug therapy is advisable for everyday stresses and anxiety: Some authorities believe such usage promotes reliance on drugs and decreases development of more healthful coping mechanisms.

Few problems develop with short-term use of antianxiety drugs unless an overdose is taken or other CNS depressant drugs are taken concurrently. Most problems occur with long-term use, especially of larger-than-usual doses. In some instances, however, withdrawal symptoms occur with therapeutic doses within 4 to 6 weeks. To minimize these problems, some recommendations include the following:

1. As a general rule, use antianxiety drugs only for people whose anxiety causes disability and interferes with job performance, interpersonal relationships, and other activities of daily living.
2. Give the drugs for short periods, such as 2 or 3 weeks, at the lowest effective dose.
3. Chronic anxiety states are probably more effectively treated with psychotherapy.
4. Chronic physical disorders, such as angina pectoris,

hypertension, and peptic ulcer disease, are more effectively treated with drugs specifically indicated for those conditions. The secondary effects claimed for antianxiety agents, such as muscle relaxant or antispasmodic effects, occur with any drug that depresses the CNS and are rarely significant with recommended doses.

5. Because anxiety often accompanies pain, antianxiety agents are sometimes used to manage pain. In the management of chronic pain, antianxiety drugs have not demonstrated a definite benefit. Anxiety about recurrence of pain is probably better controlled by adequate analgesia than by antianxiety drugs.

## DOSAGE

Dosage requirements of antianxiety agents vary among clients. The goal of drug therapy is to find the lowest effective dose that does not cause excessive daytime drowsiness. One way of doing this is to start with the smallest dose that is likely to be effective, then to evaluate the client's response and increase the dose only if necessary. Additional guidelines include the following:

1. Smaller-than-usual doses may be indicated in clients receiving cimetidine or several other drugs that decrease hepatic metabolism of most benzodiazepines (see drug interactions that increase effects, below) and elderly or debilitated clients. In the elderly, most benzodiazepines are metabolized more slowly, and half-lives are longer than in younger adults. Exceptions are oxazepam and lorazepam, of which half-lives and dosages are the same for elderly adults as for younger ones.
2. Larger-than-usual doses may be needed for clients who are severely anxious or agitated. Also, large doses are usually required to relax skeletal muscle, control muscle spasm, control seizures, and provide sedation before surgery, cardioversion, endoscopy, and angiography.
3. When antianxiety drugs are used with narcotic analgesics, the analgesic dose should be reduced initially and increased gradually to avoid excessive CNS depression.

## SCHEDULING

The benzodiazepines are often given in three or four daily doses. This is necessary for the short-acting agents, but there is no pharmacologic basis for multiple daily doses of the long-acting drugs. Because of their prolonged actions, all or most of the daily dose can be given at bedtime. This schedule promotes sleep, and there is usually enough residual sedation to maintain anti-anxiety effects throughout the next day. If necessary, one or two small supplemental doses may be given during the day.

## ASSESSMENT AND MANAGEMENT OF BENZODIAZEPINE WITHDRAWAL

Physical dependence on benzodiazepines is indicated by withdrawal symptoms when the drugs are stopped. Mild symptoms may occur in nearly half of the clients taking therapeutic doses for 6 to 12 weeks; severe symptoms are most likely to occur when high doses of a short-acting drug are taken regularly for more than 4 months and then abruptly discontinued. Common manifestations include increased anxiety, psychomotor agitation, insomnia, irritability, headache, tremor, and palpitations. Less common but more serious manifestations include confusion, abnormal perception of movement, depersonalization, psychosis, and seizures. Symptoms may occur within 24 hours of stopping a short-acting drug, such as alprazolam (Xanax), but usually occur 4 to 5 days after stopping a long-acting drug, such as diazepam.

To prevent withdrawal symptoms, the drug should be tapered in dose and gradually discontinued. Generally, reducing the dose by 10% to 25% every 1 or 2 weeks over 4 to 16 weeks is effective. However, the rate may need to be even slower with high doses or long-term use. Although the drugs have not been proven effective for more than 4 months of regular use, this period is probably exceeded quite often in clinical practice.

## USE OF ANTIDOTE FOR BENZODIAZEPINE TOXICITY

With mild toxicity, such as excessive drowsiness, omitting one or more doses or decreasing dosage is usually effective. With severe sedation or coma, maintaining respiratory and cardiovascular functions until the drug is metabolized and eliminated from the body is usually effective.

Flumazenil (Romazicon) is a specific antidote that competes with benzodiazepines for benzodiazepine receptors and reverses sedation, coma, and respiratory depression. The degree of reversal depends on the plasma concentration of the ingested benzodiazepine and the flumazenil dose and frequency of administration. The drug acts rapidly, with onset within 2 minutes and peak effects within 6 to 10 minutes. However, the duration of action is short (serum half-life is 60–90 minutes) compared to that of most benzodiazepines, so repeated doses are usually required. Clinical indications for use include benzodiazepine overdose and reversal of sedation following diagnostic or therapeutic procedures. Adverse effects include precipitation of acute benzodiazepine withdrawal symptoms, agitation, confusion, and seizures. Resedation and hypoventilation may occur if flumazenil is not given long enough to coincide with the duration of action of the benzodiazepine.

The drug should be injected into a freely flowing IV line in a large vein. Dosage recommendations vary with use. For reversal of conscious sedation or general anesthesia, the initial dose is 0.2 mg over 15 seconds, then 0.2 mg every 60 seconds, if necessary, to a maximum of 1.0 mg (total of five doses). For overdose, the initial dose is 0.2 mg over 30 seconds, wait 30 seconds, then 0.3 mg over 30 seconds, then 0.5 mg every 60 seconds up to a total dose of 3 mg if necessary for the client to reach the desired level of consciousness. Slow administration and repeated doses are recommended to awaken the client gradually and decrease the risks of causing acute withdrawal symptoms. If the client does not respond within 5 minutes of administering the total recommended dose, he or she should be reassessed for other causes of sedation.

## USE IN LIVER DISEASE

In the presence of liver disease (*e.g.*, cirrhosis, hepatitis), metabolism of most benzodiazepines is slowed, with resultant accumulation and increased risk of adverse effects. If a benzodiazepine is deemed necessary, oxazepam or lorazepam is preferred because liver disease does not significantly affect drug elimination.

## USE IN HYPOALBUMINEMIA

Benzodiazepines are highly bound to plasma proteins, especially those with long half-lives. If a benzodiazepine is given to clients with low serum albumin levels (*e.g.*, from malnutrition or liver disease), alprazolam or lorazepam is preferred because these drugs are less extensively bound to plasma proteins and less likely to cause adverse effects.

## USE IN CHILDREN

Children may have unanticipated or variable responses to antianxiety drugs, including paradoxical CNS stimulation and excitement rather than CNS depression and calming. The drugs should be used only when clearly indicated and in the lowest effective dose. Of the benzodiazepines, only chlordiazepoxide and diazepam have been extensively used in children. Others do not have established dosages and are not recommended.

## USE IN OLDER ADULTS

Most antianxiety drugs are metabolized and excreted more slowly in older adults, so the effects last longer from a given dose. Also, several of the benzodiazepines produce pharmacologically active metabolites, prolonging drug actions. Thus, the drugs may accumulate and increase adverse effects if dosages are not reduced. With benzodiazepines, short-acting drugs, such as alprazolam, lorazepam, and oxazepam (Serax), are preferred over the long-acting agents, such as chlordiazepoxide and diazepam.

The initial dose of any antianxiety drug should be small and increments made gradually, according to response, to decrease risks of adverse effects. Although hypotension is uncommon, the drugs should be used cautiously when a drop in blood pressure may cause cardiac complications. Other adverse effects include oversedation, dizziness, confusion, and impaired mobility, which may contribute to falls and other injuries unless clients are carefully monitored and safeguarded.

Benzodiazepines should be tapered rather than discontinued abruptly in older adults as in other populations. Withdrawal symptoms may occur within 24 hours of abruptly stopping short-acting drugs, but may not occur for several days after stopping long-acting agents.

# NURSING ACTIONS: ANTIANXIETY DRUGS

| *Nursing Actions* | *Rationale/Explanation* |
| --- | --- |
| **1. Administer accurately** | |
| **a.** If a client appears excessively sedated when a dose is due, omit the dose and record the reason. | To avoid excessive sedation and other adverse effects |
| **b.** When feasible, give larger proportions of the ordered daily dose at bedtime. | To promote sleep, minimize adverse reactions, and allow more nearly normal daytime activities |

*(continued)*

*Nursing Actions*                                             *Rationale/Explanation*

**c.** If given a choice, administer antianxiety agents orally when feasible.

These drugs are well absorbed from the gastrointestinal tract, and onset of action occurs within a few minutes. Chlordiazepoxide and diazepam are better absorbed with oral than with intramuscular administration. When injected intramuscularly, these drugs crystallize in muscle tissue and are slowly absorbed so that many hours may be required to achieve therapeutic concentrations in the blood.

**d.** Give intramuscular antianxiety agents deeply, into large muscle masses, such as the gluteus muscle of the hip. If repeated intramuscular injections are necessary, rotate injection sites.

These drugs are irritating to tissues and may cause pain at the injection site.

**e.** To give chlordiazepoxide parenterally, follow manufacturer's instructions for preparation of the solution.

This drug is dispensed in powder form because it is unstable in solution. Preparation and administration differ with intramuscular and intravenous routes.

**f.** To give diazepam intravenously:

These precautions are necessary to prevent apnea and minimize venous thrombosis, phlebitis, local irritation, edema, and vascular impairment due to the highly irritating effect of diazepam on body tissues.

(1) Inject slowly, at least 1 minute for each 5 mg (1 ml).

(2) Do not use small veins, such as wrist veins or those on the dorsum of the hand.

(3) Be very careful to avoid intra-arterial administration or extravasation into surrounding tissues.

(4) If not feasible to inject directly into a vein, it may be injected slowly through infusion tubing as close as possible to the venipuncture site.

(5) Have equipment available for respiratory assistance.

Apnea may occur.

**g.** To give midazolam intravenously, dilute the dose with 0.9% sodium chloride injection or 5% dextrose in water, and give slowly over 2 minutes.

Rapid IV injection may cause severe respiratory depression and apnea; dilution facilitates slow injection.

**h.** Do not mix chlordiazepoxide or diazepam with any other drug in a syringe or add to intravenous fluids.

Chlordiazepoxide is unstable in solution, and diazepam is physically incompatible with other drugs and solutions.

**i.** Midazolam may be mixed in the same syringe with morphine sulfate, meperidine, and atropine sulfate. It is also compatible with 5% dextrose in water, 0.9% sodium chloride, and lactated Ringer's intravenous solutions.

No apparent chemical or physical incompatibilities occur with these substances.

**j.** Hydroxyzine can be mixed in the same syringe with atropine, meperidine, and most other narcotic analgesics that are likely to be ordered at the same time for preoperative sedation. Give hydroxyzine orally and intramuscularly only.

Hydroxyzine is also very irritating to body tissues and causes pain with intramuscular injection. It is not given subcutaneously because of tissue irritation with pain, induration, and possible thrombus formation.

**2. Observe for therapeutic effects**

As with most other drugs, therapeutic effects depend on the reason for use. Observations of individual recipients of antianxiety drugs can be more accurate if the same nurse assesses the person before and after the drug is given.

**a.** When a drug is given for anxiety, observe for:

(1) Verbal statements, such as "less worried," "more relaxed," "resting better"

## Nursing Actions

## Rationale/Explanation

(2) Decrease or absence of behavioral manifestations of anxiety, such as rigid posture, facial grimaces, and crying

(3) Decrease or absence of physiologic manifestations of anxiety, such as elevated blood pressure, pulse, and respiration

**b.** When a drug is given for sedation or sleep, drowsiness should be apparent within a few minutes.

**c.** When diazepam is given intravenously for control of acute convulsive disorders, seizure activity should decrease or stop almost immediately.

**d.** When hydroxyzine is given for nausea and vomiting, absence of vomiting and verbal statements of relief indicate therapeutic effect.

**e.** When hydroxyzine is given for antihistaminic effects in skin disorders, observe for decreased itching and fewer statements of discomfort.

**3. Observe for adverse effects**
**a.** Oversedation—drowsiness, ataxia, fatigue, dizziness, respiratory depression, cognitive and memory impairment, psychomotor impairment, confusion

Most adverse reactions are caused by CNS depression. Drowsiness is the most common adverse effect, although the others also occur relatively often. They are more likely to occur with large doses or if the recipient is elderly, debilitated, or has liver disease that slows drug metabolism. Respiratory depression and apnea are most likely to occur with rapid intravenous administration of diazepam, chlordiazepoxide, or midazolam.

**b.** Hypotension

More likely to occur with rapid intravenous administration of diazepam or chlordiazepoxide

**c.** Pain and induration at injection site

These symptoms are caused by local irritation of tissues. They can be minimized by deep intramuscular injection into the large gluteal muscles or intravenous injection into a large vein.

**d.** Paradoxical excitement, anger, aggression, and hallucinations

This reaction is difficult to predict but may occur more often in clients who are more than 50 years of age and in those who are psychotic.

**e.** Skin rashes

**f.** With buspirone, the most common adverse effects are headache, dizziness, nausea, nervousness, fatigue, and excitement. Less frequent effects include dry mouth, chest pain, tachycardia, palpitations, drowsiness, confusion, and depression.

Buspirone is much less likely to cause sedation than other agents.

**4. Observe for drug interactions**
**a.** Drugs that *increase* effects of antianxiety agents:

(1) CNS depressants—alcohol, antidepressants, barbiturates and other sedative-hypnotics, narcotic analgesics, phenothiazines and other antipsychotics

These drugs cause additive CNS depression, sedation, and respiratory depression. Combinations of these drugs are hazardous and should be avoided. Alcohol with antianxiety drugs may cause respiratory depression, coma, and convulsive seizures. Although buspirone does not appear to cause additive CNS depression, concurrent use with other CNS depressants is best avoided.

*(continued)*

| *Nursing Actions* | *Rationale/Explanation* |
|---|---|
| (2) Cimetidine, disulfiram, fluoxetine, isoniazid, keto-conazole, metoprolol, omeprazole, oral contraceptives, propranolol, valproic acid | These drugs interfere with the hepatic metabolism of diazepam and other benzodiazepines. They do not affect elimination of oxazepam or lorazepam. |
| **b.** Drugs that *decrease* effects of antianxiety agents | |
| (1) CNS stimulants—adrenergic drugs (*e.g.*, ephedrine, pseudoephedrine, phenylpropanolamine), theophylline, caffeine | Adrenergic drugs are frequent components of over-the-counter cold remedies, decongestants, and appetite suppressants. |
| **5. Teach clients** | |
| **a.** Omit one or more doses if excessive drowsiness occurs. | To avoid falls and other injuries or adverse effects. These drugs may interfere with mental and physical functioning. |
| **b.** Use the drugs only when necessary—do not increase dosage, do not increase frequency of administration, and do not take for prolonged periods. | These drugs are frequently misused and abused. They can produce psychological and physiologic dependence, which may eventually cause worse problems than the original anxiety. |
| **c.** These drugs produce more beneficial effects and fewer adverse reactions when used in the smallest effective doses and for the shortest duration feasible in particular circumstances. | |
| **d.** Large amounts of coffee can cancel or decrease the sedative and antianxiety effects of these drugs. | Coffee contains caffeine, which is a stimulant. Cola beverages and tea also contain caffeine, although in lesser amounts. Other stimulant drugs, such as appetite suppressants, can also decrease the effects of these drugs. |
| **e.** With buspirone, expect little, if any, sedation. Relief of symptoms may be delayed for a few weeks. | To clarify expectations, especially if the client has previously taken sedative-type antianxiety agents |

## Review and Application Exercises

1. What is anxiety, and how may it be manifested?
2. What terms may an adult use to indicate anxiety? What terms would a preschool child use?
3. How do benzodiazepines act to relieve anxiety?
4. What are some nonpharmacologic interventions to decrease anxiety?
5. Why are benzodiazepines considered safer for use as antianxiety agents than barbiturates?
6. For what other purposes are benzodiazepines commonly used?
7. When assessing a client before giving an antianxiety benzodiazepine, what assessment data would cause you to omit the dose?
8. In terms of nursing care, what difference does it make whether a benzodiazepine is metabolized to active or inactive metabolites?
9. What are drug dependence, tolerance, and withdrawal symptoms in relation to the benzodiazepines?

## Selected References

American Psychiatric Association (1990). *Benzodiazepine dependence, toxicity, and abuse: A task force report*. Washington, DC: Author.

(1993). *Drug facts and comparisons*. St. Louis: Facts and Comparisons.

Fankhauser, M. P. (1993). Anxiolytic drugs and sedative-hypnotics. In R. Bressler & M. D. Katz (Eds.), *Geriatric pharmacology* (pp. 165–205). New York: McGraw-Hill.

Glod, C. A. (1992). Xanax: Pros and cons. *Journal of Psychosocial Nursing, 30*(6), 36–37.

Hartman, C. R., & Knight, M. (1990). Pharmacotherapy. In A. W. Burgess (Ed.), *Psychiatric nursing in the hospital and the community* (5th ed.) (pp. 374–424). Norwalk, CT: Appleton & Lange.

Hayes, P. E., & Kirkwood, C. K. (1992). Anxiety disorders. In J. T. DiPiro, R. L. Talbert, P. E. Hayes, G. C. Yee, G. R. Matzke, & L. M. Posey (Eds.), *Pharmacotherapy: A pathophysiologic approach* (2nd ed.) (pp. 1092–1109). New York: Elsevier.

Hollister, L. E. (1992). Psychiatric disorders. In K. L. Melmon, H. F. Morrelli, B. B. Hoffman, & D. W. Nierenberg (Eds.), *Clinical pharmacology: Basic principles in therapeutics* (3rd ed.) (pp. 338–380). New York: McGraw-Hill.

Jann, M. J. (1992). Anxiety. In M. A. Koda-Kimble & L. Y. Young (Eds.), *Applied therapeutics: The clinical use of drugs* (5th ed.) (pp. 54-1–54-21). Vancouver, WA: Applied Therapeutics.

Juergens, S. M. (1993). Problems with benzodiazepines in elderly patients. *Mayo Clinic Proceedings, 68*, 818–820.

# CHAPTER 9

# Antipsychotic Drugs

## Psychosis

Antipsychotic drugs are used mainly for the treatment of *psychosis*, a severe mental disorder characterized by disordered thought processes (disorganized and often bizarre thinking); blunted or inappropriate emotional responses; bizarre behavior ranging from hypoactivity to hyperactivity with agitation, aggressiveness, hostility, and combativeness; autism (self-absorption in which the person pays no attention to the environment or to other people); deterioration from previous levels of occupational and social functioning (poor self-care and interpersonal skills); hallucinations; and paranoid delusions. *Hallucinations* are sensory perceptions of people or objects that are not present in the external environment. More specifically, people see, hear, or feel (and occasionally taste or smell) stimuli that are not visible to external observers and are unable to distinguish between these false perceptions and reality. Hallucinations occur with delirium, dementias, schizophrenia, and other psychotic states. Those occurring in schizophrenia or bipolar affective disorder are usually auditory, those in delirium are usually visual or tactile, and those in dementias are usually visual. *Delusions* are false beliefs that persist in the absence of reason or evidence. Deluded people often believe that other people control their thoughts, feelings and behaviors or seek to harm them (paranoia). Delusions indicate severe mental illness. Although they are commonly associated with schizophrenia, delusions also occur with delirium, dementias, and other psychotic disorders.

Psychoses may be organic or functional. *Organic psychoses* are caused by physical disorders such as brain damage related to cerebrovascular disease, head injury, or chronic alcohol abuse. Fluid and electrolyte imbalances, adverse drug effects, and sensory deprivation or overload (*e.g.*, in intensive care units) also may cause episodes of psychotic behavior. *Functional psychoses*, of which schizophrenia is the most common, show no discernible organ pathology as a cause of symptoms. *Schizophrenia* is not a single disease; rather, it includes a variety of related disorders. Symptoms may begin gradually or suddenly, usually during adolescence or early adulthood. According to the American Psychiatric Association's *Diagnostic and Statistical Manual*, third edition, revised, overt psychotic symptoms must be present for 6 months before schizophrenia can be diagnosed. Thus, schizophrenia is a chronic illness, and this characteristic aids the differential diagnosis between schizophrenia and other psychotic states.

### ETIOLOGY

There is substantial evidence that psychoses result from increased dopamine activity in the brain. This etiology is supported by the determination that antipsychotic drugs exert their therapeutic effects by decreasing dopamine activity (*i.e.*, blocking dopaminergic receptors) and that drugs that increase dopamine levels in the brain (*e.g.*, bromocriptine, levodopa) can cause psychotic signs and symptoms. Another factor that increases the amount of dopamine available to bind with receptors is decreased activity of dopamine beta-hydroxylase. Because this enzyme normally converts dopamine to norepinephrine in adrenergic nerve endings, decreased activity results in larger amounts of dopamine. In addition to the increased amount of dopamine, dopamine receptors are apparently involved as well. Studies of dopamine receptor

Anne Collins Abrams: CLINICAL DRUG THERAPY, Fourth Edition.
© 1995 J.B. Lippincott Company.

binding demonstrate that schizophrenic patients have increased numbers of dopamine receptors, even if they have not received dopamine-blocking antipsychotic drugs.

In addition to dopamine, other neurotransmitters may be involved in the production of psychosis. One indication of such involvement is the wide variety of drugs that may cause psychosis, including adrenergics (increase norepinephrine), antidepressants (affect norepinephrine or serotonin), some anticonvulsants (increase the effects of gamma-aminobutyric acid), and others with unknown effects on neurotransmitters and receptors.

# Antipsychotic drugs

Antipsychotic drugs are derived from several chemical groups and are broadly categorized as phenothiazines and nonphenothiazines. Despite chemical differences, their pharmacologic actions and antipsychotic effectiveness are similar.

The largest and most frequently used group of antipsychotic drugs is the phenothiazines, of which chlorpromazine (Thorazine) is the prototype. The phenothiazines are well absorbed after oral and parenteral administration. They are distributed to most body tissues and reach high concentrations in the brain. They are metabolized in the liver and excreted in urine. Some metabolites have pharmacologic activity similar to that of the parent compound. These drugs do not cause physical or psychological drug dependence.

Phenothiazines exert many pharmacologic effects in the body, including central nervous system (CNS) depression, autonomic nervous system depression (antiadrenergic and anticholinergic effects), antiemetic effects, lowering of body temperature, hypersensitivity reactions, and others. They differ mainly in potency and adverse effects. Differences in potency are demonstrated by the fact that some phenothiazines (piperazine subgroup) are as effective in doses of a few milligrams as others (aliphatic and piperadine subgroups) are in doses of several hundred milligrams. All phenothiazines produce the same kinds of adverse effects, but the subgroups differ in incidence and severity of particular adverse effects.

Nonphenothiazine antipsychotic drugs represent several different chemical groups but are few in number. These drugs have pharmacologic actions, clinical uses, and adverse effects similar to those of the phenothiazines.

## MECHANISM OF ACTION

The antipsychotic drugs act primarily by occupying dopamine receptors in brain tissue, thereby decreasing the effects of dopamine. The drugs act within hours to decrease manifestations of hyperarousal (*e.g.*, anxiety, agitation, hyperactivity, insomnia, aggressive or combative behavior, hallucinations, and delusions). Several weeks or months may be required to eliminate thought disorder and increase socialization.

## INDICATIONS FOR USE

The major clinical indication for use of antipsychotic drugs is schizophrenia. The drugs also are used in other psychiatric disorders, but the indications are less clear. Thus, they are probably useful in chronic brain syndromes (relatively permanent organic impairments of cerebral function related to various disorders, such as brain tumor) to control hyperactivity, delusions, agitation, and other psychotic symptoms. They may be useful in the manic phase of bipolar affective disorder to control manic behavior until lithium, the drug of choice, becomes effective. They also may be used to treat psychotic symptoms induced by alcohol withdrawal. They are not generally used for depressive disorders but may occasionally be used to treat agitated depression.

Clinical indications not associated with psychiatric illness include prevention and treatment of nausea and vomiting and treatment of intractable hiccups. The drugs relieve nausea and vomiting by blocking dopamine receptors in the chemoreceptor trigger zone (CTZ). The CTZ is a group of neurons in the medulla oblongata that, when activated by physical or psychological stimuli, causes nausea and vomiting. The mechanism by which the drugs relieve hiccups is unclear.

## CONTRAINDICATIONS FOR USE

Because of their wide-ranging adverse effects, antipsychotic drugs may cause or aggravate a number of conditions. Thus, they are contraindicated in clients with liver damage, coronary artery disease, cerebrovascular disease, parkinsonism, bone marrow depression, severe hypotension or hypertension, coma, or severely depressed states. They should be used cautiously in seizure disorders, diabetes mellitus, glaucoma, prostatic hypertrophy, peptic ulcer disease, and chronic respiratory disorders.

# Individual antipsychotic drugs

## PHENOTHIAZINES

Commonly used phenothiazine antipsychotic drugs are listed in Table 9-1. **Promethazine** (Phenergan) is a phenothiazine that is not used clinically for antipsychotic effects but is often used for sedative, antiemetic, and antihistaminic effects.

**TABLE 9-1. PHENOTHIAZINE ANTIPSYCHOTIC DRUGS**

| Generic/Trade Name | Routes of Administration and Dosage Ranges | Major Side Effects (Incidence) | | | Remarks |
|---|---|---|---|---|---|
| | | Sedation | Extrapyramidal Reactions | Hypotension | |
| **Acetophenazine** (Tindal) | Adults: PO 60 mg daily in divided doses, may be gradually increased by 20 mg daily until therapeutic or adverse effects occur. Usual optimal dosage is 80–120 mg daily.<br>Elderly or debilitated adults: one-third to one-half usual adult dose<br>Children: 0.8–1.6 mg/kg per day in 3 divided doses (maximum, 80 mg daily) | Moderate | High | Low | 20 mg is equivalent to 100 mg of chlorpromazine. |
| **Chlorpromazine** (Thorazine) | Adults: PO 200–600 mg daily in divided doses. Dose may be increased by 100 mg daily q2–3 days until symptoms are controlled, adverse effects occur, or a maximum daily dose of 2 g is reached. IM 25–100 mg initially for acute psychotic symptoms, repeated in 1–4 hours PRN until control is achieved<br>Elderly or debilitated adults: PO one-third to one-half usual adult dose, increased by 25 mg daily q2–3 days if necessary. IM 10 mg q6–8h until acute symptoms are controlled<br>Children: PO IM 0.5 mg/kg q4–8h. Maximum IM dose, 40 mg daily in children below 5 years of age and 75 mg for older children | High | Moderate | Moderate to high | Sustained-release capsules and liquid concentrates are available. |
| **Fluphenazine decanoate and enanthate** (Prolixin decanoate; Prolixin enanthate) | Adults under 50 years: IM, SC 12.5 mg initially followed by 25 mg every 2 weeks. Dosage requirements rarely exceed 100 mg q2–6 weeks.<br>Adults over 50, debilitated clients, or clients with a history of extrapyramidal reactions: 2.5 mg initially followed by 2.5–5 mg q10–14 days<br>Children: No dosage established | Low to moderate | High | Low | |
| **Fluphenazine hydrochloride** (Prolixin, Permitil) | Adults: PO 2.5–10 mg initially, gradually reduced to maintenance dose of 1–5 mg (doses above 3 mg are rarely necessary). Acute psychosis: IM 1.25 mg initially, increased gradually to 2.5–10 mg daily in 3–4 divided doses<br>Elderly or debilitated adults: PO 1–2.5 mg daily; IM one-third to one-half the usual adult dose<br>Children: PO 0.75–10 mg daily in children 5 to 12 years. IM no dosage established | Low to moderate | High | Low | 2 mg of the oral hydrochloride salt is equivalent to 100 mg of chlorpromazine. |
| **Mesoridazine** (Serentil) | Adults and children over 12 years: PO 150 mg daily in divided doses initially, increased gradually in 50-mg increments until symptoms are controlled. Usual dose range, 100–400 mg. IM 25–175 mg daily in divided doses<br>Elderly and debilitated adults: one-third to one-half usual adult dose | High | Low | Moderate | 50 mg is equivalent to 100 mg of chlorpromazine. |

(continued)

**TABLE 9-1. PHENOTHIAZINE ANTIPSYCHOTIC DRUGS** *(Continued)*

| Generic/Trade Name | Routes of Administration and Dosage Ranges | Major Side Effects (Incidence) | | | Remarks |
|---|---|---|---|---|---|
| | | Sedation | Extrapyramidal Reactions | Hypotension | |
| | Children under 12 years: no dosage established | | | | |
| **Perphenazine** (Trilafon) | Adults: PO 16–64 mg daily in divided doses. Acute psychoses: IM 5–10 mg initially, then 5 mg q6h if necessary. Maximum daily dose, 15 mg for ambulatory clients and 30 mg for hospitalized clients<br>Elderly or debilitated adults: PO, IM one-third to one-half usual adult dose<br>Children: PO dosages not established, but the following amounts have been given in divided doses: Ages 1–6 years, 4–6 mg daily; 6–12 years, 6 mg daily; over 12 years, 6–12 mg daily | Low to moderate | High | Low | 8 mg is equivalent to 100 mg of chlorpromazine |
| **Prochlorperazine** (Compazine) | Adults: PO 10 mg 3–4 times daily, increased gradually (usual daily dose, 100–150 mg). IM 10–20 mg; may be repeated in 2–4 hours. Switch to oral form as soon as possible<br>Children over age 2 years: PO, rectal 2.5 mg 2–3 times daily. IM 0.06 mg/lb | Moderate | High | Low | 10 mg is equivalent to 100 mg of chlorpromazine. |
| **Promazine** (Sparine) | Adults: initially, 50–150 mg IM; maintenance, PO, IM 10–200 mg q4–6h<br>Children over 12 years: 10–25 mg q4–6h | Moderate | Moderate | Moderate | 200 mg is equivalent to 100 mg of chlorpromazine. |
| **Thioridazine** (Mellaril) | Adults: PO 150–300 mg daily in divided doses, gradually increased if necessary to a maximum daily dose of 800 mg<br>Elderly or debilitated adults: PO one-third to one-half the usual adult dose<br>Children 2 years and over: 1 mg/kg per day in divided doses. Maximum dose, 3 mg/kg per day<br>Children under 2 years: no dosage established | High | Low | Moderate | Thioridazine is probably the most frequently used antipsychotic drug. It differs from other phenothiazines by lacking antiemetic effects. It also has little, if any, effect on seizure threshold; 100 mg is equivalent to 100 mg of chlorpromazine. |
| **Trifluoperazine** (Stelazine) | Adults: Outpatients PO 2–4 mg daily in divided doses. Hospitalized clients, PO 4–10 mg daily in divided doses. Acute psychoses: IM 1–2 mg q4–5h, maximum of 10 mg daily<br>Elderly or debilitated adults: PO, IM one-third to one-half usual adult dose. If given IM, give at less frequent intervals than above.<br>Children 6 years or over: PO, IM 1–2 mg daily, maximum daily dose 15 mg<br>Children under 6 years: no dosage established | Moderate | High | Low | 5 mg is equivalent to 100 mg of chlorpromazine. |

## NONPHENOTHIAZINES

**Chlorprothixene** (Taractan) and **thiothixene** (Navane) are thioxanthenes chemically similar to phenothiazines. These potent and effective antipsychotic drugs are used clinically only for their antipsychotic effects, although they produce other effects similar to those of the phenothiazines. A 100-mg dose of chlorprothixene is therapeutically equivalent to 100 mg of chlorpromazine; a 4-mg dose of thiothixene is equivalent to 100 mg of chlorpromazine.

Chlorprothixene

### Routes and dosage ranges

*Adults:* Acute psychosis, PO, IM 75–200 mg/d in divided doses, increased to a maximal oral dose of 600 mg/d if necessary

*Elderly or debilitated adults:* PO, IM 30–100 mg daily in divided doses, reduced when symptoms have been controlled

*Children over 12 years:* PO, IM, same as adults

*Children 6–12 years:* PO 30–100 mg/d in divided doses; IM dosage not established

*Children under 6 years:* Dosage not established

Thiothixene

### Routes and dosage ranges

*Adults:* PO 6–10 mg/d in divided doses; maximum 60 mg/d

Acute psychosis, IM 8–16 mg/d in divided doses; maximum 30 mg/d

*Elderly or debilitated adults:* PO, IM one-third to one-half the usual adult dosage

*Children over 12 years:* Same as adults

*Children under 12 years:* Dosage not established

**Haloperidol** (Haldol) is a butyrophenone compound and the only drug of this group available for use in psychiatric disorders; a related drug, droperidol (Inapsine), is used in anesthesia and as an antiemetic. Haloperidol is a frequently used antipsychotic agent that is chemically different but pharmacologically similar to the phenothiazines. A potent, long-acting drug, it is readily absorbed following oral or intramuscular administration, metabolized in the liver, and excreted in urine and bile. Haloperidol may cause adverse effects similar to those of other antipsychotic drugs. Usually, it produces a relatively low incidence of hypotension and sedation and a high incidence of extrapyramidal effects.

Haloperidol is used as the initial drug for treating psychotic disorders or as a substitute in clients who are hypersensitive or refractory to the phenothiazines. It also is used for some conditions in which other antipsychotic drugs are not used, including mental retardation with hyperkinesia (abnormally increased motor activity), Tourette's syndrome (a rare disorder characterized by involuntary movements and vocalizations), and Huntington's disease (a rare genetic disorder that involves progressive psychiatric symptoms and involuntary movements). A 2-mg dose is therapeutically equivalent to 100 mg of chlorpromazine.

### Routes and dosage ranges

*Adults:* Acute psychosis, PO 1–15 mg/d initially in divided doses, gradually increased to 100 mg/d if necessary; usual maintenance dose, 2–8 mg daily, IM 2–10 mg q1–8h until symptoms are controlled (usually within 72 hours)

Chronic refractory schizophrenia, PO 6–15 mg/d; maximum 100 mg/d; dosage is reduced for maintenance, usually 15–20 mg/d

Tourette's syndrome, PO 6–15 mg/d; maximum 100 mg/d; usual maintenance dose, 9 mg/d

Mental retardation with hyperkinesia, PO 80–120 mg/d, gradually reduced to a maintenance dose of about 60 mg/d, IM 20 mg/d in divided doses, gradually increased to 60 mg/d if necessary. Oral administration should be substituted after symptoms are controlled.

*Elderly or debilitated adults:* Same as for children under 12 years

*Children over 12 years:* Acute psychosis, chronic refractory schizophrenia, Tourette's syndrome, mental retardation with hyperkinesia: dosage same as for adults

*Children under 12 years:* Acute psychosis, PO 0.5–1.5 mg/d initially, gradually increased in increments of 0.5 mg; usual maintenance dose, 2–4 mg/d. IM dosage not established.

Chronic refractory schizophrenia, dosage not established

Tourette's syndrome, PO 1.5–6 mg/d initially in divided doses; usual maintenance dose, about 1.5 mg/d

Mental retardation with hyperkinesia, PO 1.5 mg/d initially in divided doses, gradually increased to a maximum of 15 mg/d if necessary. When symptoms are controlled, dosage is gradually reduced to the minimum effective level. IM dosage not established.

**Loxapine** (Loxitane) and **clozapine** (Clozaril) are dibenzoxazepines pharmacologically similar to other antipsychotic drugs. They are recommended for use only in the treatment of schizophrenia, especially for clients who have not responded to other drugs. Clozapine does not cause the extrapyramidal effects (*e.g.*, acute dystonia, parkinsonism, akathisia, tardive dyskinesia) associated with most antipsychotic agents. However, there is a relatively high risk of agranulocytosis, a life-threatening decrease in white blood cells. Weekly white blood counts are recommended. Other adverse effects include sedation, orthostatic hypotension, and electrocardiographic (ECG) changes.

### Loxapine

#### *Route and dosage ranges*

***Adults and adolescents 16 years and older:*** PO 10 mg twice a day to a total of 50 mg/d in severe psychoses; usual maintenance dose 60–100 mg/d; maximum dose, 250 mg/d

***Elderly or debilitated adults:*** One-third to one-half the usual adult dosage

***Children under 16 years:*** Dosage not established

### Clozapine

#### *Route and dosage ranges*

***Adults:*** PO 50–900 mg/d
***Children:*** Dosage not established

**Molindone** (Moban) is an antipsychotic agent that differs chemically from other agents but has similar pharmacologic actions. A 20-mg dose is equivalent to 100 mg of chlorpromazine.

#### *Route and dosage range*

***Adults:*** PO 50–75 mg/d, increased gradually if necessary up to 225 mg/d, then reduced for maintenance; usual maintenance dose, 15–40 mg/d

***Elderly or debilitated adults:*** One-third to one-half the usual adult dosage

***Children under 12 years:*** Dosage not established

**Pimozide** (Orap) is an antipsychotic drug approved only for treatment of Tourette's syndrome in clients who fail to respond to haloperidol. Potentially serious adverse effects include tardive dyskinesia, major motor seizures, and sudden death.

#### *Route and dosage range*

***Adults:*** PO 1–2 mg/d in divided doses initially, increased if necessary; usual maintenance dose, about 10 mg/d; maximum dose, 20 mg/d

## *Nursing Process*

### Assessment

Assess mental health status, need for antipsychotic drugs, and response to drug therapy. There is a wide variation in response to drug therapy. Close observation of physical and behavioral reactions is necessary to evaluate effectiveness and to individualize dosage schedules. Accurate assessment is especially important when starting drug therapy and when increasing or decreasing dosage. Some assessment factors include the following:

- Interviewing the client and family members. Attempts to interview an acutely psychotic person are likely to yield little useful information, owing to the client's distorted perception of reality. The nurse may be able to assess level of orientation and delusional and hallucinatory activity. If possible, try to determine from family members or other people what the client was doing or experiencing when the acute episode began (*i.e.*, predisposing factors, such as increased environmental stress or crisis situation); whether this is a first or a repeated episode of psychotic behavior; whether the person has physical illnesses, takes any drugs, or uses alcohol; whether the client seems to be a hazard to himself or herself or others; and some description of preillness personality traits, level of social interaction, and ability to function in usual activities of daily living.
- Observing behavior for the presence or absence of psychotic symptoms, such as agitation, hyperactivity, combativeness, and bizarre behavior
- Obtaining baseline data to help monitor the client's response to drug therapy. Some authorities advocate initial and periodic laboratory tests of liver, kidney, and blood functions, as well as ECGs. Although such tests do not help greatly in preventing adverse reactions, they may assist in earlier detection and treatment of adverse reactions. Baseline blood pressure readings also may be helpful.
- Continuing assessment of responses to drug therapy and ability to function in activities of daily living, whether the client is hospitalized or receiving outpatient treatment

### Nursing diagnoses

- Alteration in Thought Processes related to the disease, especially during the first few weeks of antipsychotic drug therapy
- Self-care Deficit related to the disease process or drug-induced sedation
- Impaired Physical Mobility related to sedation
- High Risk for Decreased Cardiac Output related to cardiac arrhythmias and hypotension
- High Risk for Decreased Tissue Perfusion related to hypotension
- High Risk for Injury related to excessive sedation and movement disorders (extrapyramidal effects)
- High Risk for Violence: Self-Directed or Directed at Others
- High Risk for Noncompliance related to underuse of prescribed drugs
- Knowledge Deficit: Expected recurrence of symptoms and hospitalization if drug therapy is not continued in chronic schizophrenia

### Planning/Goals

*The client will:*

- Become less agitated within a few hours after drug therapy is started and less psychotic within a few days
- Be kept safe while sedated during early drug therapy
- Be cared for by staff in areas of nutrition, hygiene, exercise, and social interactions when unable to provide self-care
- Improve in ability to participate in self-care activities
- Avoid preventable adverse drug effects, especially those that impair safety

● Be assisted to take medications as prescribed and return for follow-up appointments with health-care providers

### Interventions

Use nondrug measures when appropriate to increase the effectiveness of drug therapy and to decrease adverse reactions.

● Obviously, drug therapy will not be effective if the client does not receive the medication as prescribed. For numerous reasons, many people are unable or unwilling to take medications as prescribed. Any nursing action aimed toward more accurate drug administration will increase the effectiveness of drug therapy.

    Specific nursing actions must be individualized to the particular client. Some general nursing actions that may be helpful include emphasizing the therapeutic benefits expected from drug therapy, answering questions or providing information about drug therapy and other aspects of the treatment plan, devising a schedule of administration times that is as convenient as possible for the client, and giving the drug in the form (*e.g.*, syrup, capsule) most acceptable to the client.
● Supervise ambulation to prevent falls or other injuries if the client is drowsy or elderly or has postural hypotension.
● Several measures help to prevent or minimize hypotension, such as having the client lie down for about an hour after an injection of antipsychotic medication or a large oral dose, applying elastic stockings, and instructing the client to change positions gradually, elevate legs when sitting, avoid standing for prolonged periods, and avoid hot baths. (Hot baths cause vasodilation and increase the incidence of hypotension.)
● Dry mouth and oral infections can be decreased by frequent brushing of the teeth, rinsing the mouth with water, or chewing sugarless gum or candy.
● The usual measures of increasing fluid intake, dietary fiber, and exercise can help prevent constipation.

*Teach clients and caretakers:*
● About the planned drug therapy regimen, including the desired therapeutic results and the length of time before therapeutic results can be expected. This is especially important to improve compliance in long-term drug therapy. Failure to take prescribed medications is a frequent reason for recurring episodes of acute illness and hospitalization.
● About the possible adverse effects of drug therapy. Emphasize those related to safety; for example, warn the client not to drive a car or operate machinery. Providing a detailed list of adverse effects is unnecessary and may confuse the client or increase anxiety. It may be helpful to note that drowsiness and impaired mental and motor activity are especially evident during the first 2 weeks of drug therapy but tend to decrease with time.
● To report unusual side effects and all physical illnesses, because changes in drug therapy may be indicated
● To avoid using *any* nonprescribed drugs, such as those available without prescription or those prescribed for another person, to prevent undesirable drug interactions. Alcohol and sleeping pills should be avoided because they may cause excessive drowsiness and decreased awareness of safety hazards in the environment.
● To consult the physician who prescribed the medication

before taking any drug prescribed by another physician, also to avoid undesirable drug interactions

### Evaluation

● Interview the client to determine the presence and extent of hallucinations and delusions.
● Observe behavior for decreased signs and symptoms. Document abilities and limitations in self-care.
● No injuries occur during drug therapy.

## Principles of therapy

### GOALS OF TREATMENT

Overall goals of treatment are to alleviate psychotic symptoms, increase the client's ability to cope with the environment, promote optimal functioning in self-care and activities of daily living, and prevent or shorten hospitalization. With drug therapy, clients often can participate in psychotherapy, group therapy, or other treatment modalities; return to community settings; and return to their preillness level of functioning.

### LIMITATIONS ON INDICATIONS FOR USE

The effectiveness of antipsychotic drug therapy depends on the accuracy of the diagnosis. Antipsychotic drugs are indicated for the treatment of schizophrenia and acute psychotic symptoms (*e.g.*, hallucinations; severe hyperactivity, agitation, and hostility) that pose a threat to the client or to others.

Despite recommendations that long-term use of antipsychotic drugs be reserved for treatment of major psychiatric illness, these drugs are often prescribed for relatively minor emotional disorders, such as nonpsychotic excitement, anxiety, or severe tension. Such use is not recommended for two reasons. First, benzodiazepine antianxiety drugs are better tolerated and more effective in most people. Second, antipsychotic drugs may produce dysphoria (feelings of depression or restlessness) in nonpsychotic clients. Therefore, if antipsychotic drugs are used at all for these conditions, they should be used only when other agents are ineffective, in small doses, and for short-term treatment.

### DRUG SELECTION

The physician's choice of a particular antipsychotic drug is largely empirical because clear-cut guidelines have not been established. Some general factors to consider include the client's age and physical condition, severity and duration of illness, frequency and severity of adverse effects produced by each drug, response to antipsychotic drugs in the past, subjective response to the drugs (such as the adverse reactions a person is willing to tolerate), supervision available, and the physician's experience with a particular drug. Some specific factors include the following:

1. Antipsychotic drugs are apparently equally effective regardless of the client's symptoms. Drugs producing greater sedation are often prescribed for agitated, overactive people, and drugs producing less sedation are prescribed for those who are apathetic and withdrawn.
2. Despite the similarities of antipsychotic drugs in therapeutic benefits and adverse effects, some clients who do not respond well to one type of antipsychotic drug may respond to another. Unfortunately, there is no way of predicting which drug is likely to be most effective for a particular client.
3. There is no logical basis for giving more than one antipsychotic agent at a time. There is no therapeutic advantage, and the risk of serious adverse reactions is increased.
4. If lack of therapeutic response requires that another antipsychotic drug be substituted for the one a client is currently receiving, this substitution must be done gradually; abrupt substitution may cause reappearance of symptoms. This can be avoided by gradually decreasing doses of the old drug while substituting equivalent doses of the new one.
5. Nonphenothiazine antipsychotic drugs are probably best used for clients with chronic schizophrenia whose symptoms have not been controlled by the phenothiazines and for clients with hypersensitivity reactions to the phenothiazines. Although adverse reactions to these agents are similar to those caused by phenothiazines, clients who are allergic to the phenothiazines can usually tolerate one of the other antipsychotic drugs.
6. Unless choice of a drug is dictated by the client's previous favorable response to a particular drug, the preferred drug should be available in both parenteral and oral forms for flexibility of administration.
7. Clients who are unable or unwilling to take daily doses of a maintenance antipsychotic drug may be given periodic injections of a long-acting form of fluphenazine.
8. Any person who has had an allergic or hypersensitivity reaction to an antipsychotic drug generally should not be given that drug again or any drug in the same chemical subgroup. Cross-sensitivity apparently occurs, and the likelihood of another allergic reaction is high.

## DOSAGE AND ADMINISTRATION

Dosage and route of administration must be individualized. Initial drug therapy for acute psychotic episodes usually requires high dosage, intramuscular administration, divided doses, and hospitalization. Symptoms are usually controlled within 48 to 72 hours, after which oral drugs can be given and dosage gradually reduced to the lowest effective amount. For maintenance therapy, drug dosages are usually much smaller, oral drugs are preferred, and a single bedtime dose is effective for most people. This schedule increases compliance with prescribed drug therapy, allows better nighttime sleep, and decreases hypotension and daytime sedation. Effective maintenance therapy requires close supervision and contact with the client and family members.

## DURATION OF THERAPY

In schizophrenia, antipsychotic drugs are usually given for years. There are no clear guidelines regarding duration of drug therapy. There is a high rate of relapse (acute psychotic reactions) in schizophrenic clients when drug therapy is discontinued, most often by clients who become unwilling or unable to continue their medication regimen.

## MANAGEMENT OF EXTRAPYRAMIDAL SYMPTOMS

For most people receiving antipsychotic drugs, concurrent antiparkinsonism drug therapy should be given only after extrapyramidal symptoms (*e.g.*, abnormal rigidity and muscle movements) occur. Such neuromuscular symptoms appear in less than half the clients taking antipsychotic drugs and are better handled by reducing dosage, if this does not cause recurrence of psychotic symptoms. If antiparkinsonism drugs are given, they should be gradually discontinued in about 3 months. Extrapyramidal symptoms do not usually recur despite continued administration of the same antipsychotic drug and the same dosage.

## ETHNIC OR GENETIC CONSIDERATIONS

People of Asian heritage may have higher serum drug levels than white people given comparable doses, probably because of slower metabolism and elimination of the drugs. A cautious approach to antipsychotic drug therapy in this population would be lower initial doses (about half the usual dosage of white people) and titration of later doses according to clinical response and serum drug levels. Note that most studies have been done with haloperidol and with a limited number of Asian subgroups. Thus, it cannot be assumed that all antipsychotic drugs and all people of Asian heritage respond the same.

## USE IN PERIOPERATIVE PERIODS

A major concern about giving antipsychotic drugs perioperatively is their potential for adverse interactions with other drugs. For example, the drugs potentiate the effects of general anesthetics and other CNS-depressant drugs that are often used before, during, and after surgery. As a result, risks of hypotension and excessive sedation are increased unless doses of other agents are reduced. If hypotension occurs and requires vasopressor drugs, phenylephrine (Neo-Synephrine) or norepinephrine (Levophed) should be used rather than epinephrine (Adrenalin) because antipsychotic drugs inhibit the vasoconstrictive (blood-pressure raising) effects of epinephrine.

## USE IN CHILDREN

Antipsychotic drugs are not generally recommended for children under 12 years of age. Thioridazine, prochlorperazine, trifluoperazine, and haloperidol may be used in children aged 2 to 12 years, but are not recommended for children under 2 years. Extrapyramidal symptoms are more likely to occur in children than adults.

## USE IN OLDER ADULTS

Antipsychotic drugs should be used cautiously in older adults. Before they are started, a thorough assessment is needed because psychiatric symptoms are often caused by organic disease or other drugs. If this is the case, treating the disease or stopping the offending drug(s) may cancel the need for an antipsychotic drug. When the drugs are required, dosage should be reduced by 30% to 50% and increased gradually if necessary. Once symptoms are controlled, dosage should be reduced to the lowest effective level. Adverse effects are likely to occur because of slowed drug metabolism. These include cardiovascular (hypotension, arrhythmias), sedative, and anticholinergic effects that may be especially dangerous in older adults. Tardive dyskinesia may occur with long-term use of antipsychotic drugs.

In addition, older adults are more likely to have problems in which the drugs are contraindicated (*e.g.*, severe cardiovascular disease, liver damage, parkinsonism) or must be used very cautiously (diabetes mellitus, glaucoma, prostatic hypertrophy, peptic ulcer disease, chronic respiratory disorders).

For older adults in long-term care facilities, there is concern that antipsychotic drugs may be overused to control agitated or disruptive behavior caused by non-psychotic disorders and for which other treatments are preferable. For example, clients with dementias may become agitated from environmental or medical problems. Alleviating such causes, when possible, is safer and more effective than administering antipsychotic drugs. Inappropriate use of the drugs exposes clients to adverse drug effects and does not resolve underlying problems. Because of the many implications for patient safety and welfare, the Health Care Financing Administration, a federal agency, established regulations for antipsychotic use in facilities paid with Medicare and Medicaid funds. These regulations include appropriate (*e.g.*, psychotic disorders, delusions, schizophrenia, and dementia and delirium that meet certain criteria) and inappropriate (*e.g.*, agitation not thought to indicate potential harm to the resident or others, anxiety, depression, uncooperativeness, wandering) indications.

## NURSING ACTIONS: ANTIPSYCHOTIC DRUGS

| *Nursing Actions* | *Rationale/Explanation* |
|---|---|
| **1. Administer accurately** | |
| **a.** When feasible, give oral antipsychotic drugs once daily, within 1 to 2 hours of bedtime. | Peak sedation occurs about 2 hours after administration and aids sleep. Hypotension, dry mouth, and other adverse reactions are less bothersome with this schedule. Although antipsychotic drugs are probably more often prescribed in two or three daily doses, their long duration of action usually allows once-daily dosage. |
| **b.** When preparing oral concentrated solutions or parenteral solutions, try to avoid contact with the solution. If contact is made, wash the area immediately. | These solutions are irritating to the skin and may cause contact dermatitis. |
| **c.** Mix liquid concentrates with at least 60 ml of fruit juice or water just before administration. | To mask the taste. If the client does not like juice or water, check the package insert for other diluents. Some of the drugs may be mixed with coffee, tea, milk, or carbonated beverages. |

*(continued)*

| Nursing Actions | Rationale/Explanation |
|---|---|
| **d.** For intramuscular injections: | |
| (1) Give only those preparations labeled for intramuscular use. | |
| (2) Do not mix any other drugs in the same syringe with antipsychotic drugs. | These drugs are physically incompatible with many other drugs, and a precipitate may occur. |
| (3) Change the needle after filling the syringe for injection. | Parenteral solutions of these drugs are highly irritating to body tissues. Changing needles helps to protect the tissues of the injection tract from unnecessary contact with the drug. |
| (4) Inject slowly and deeply into gluteal muscles. | Using a large muscle mass for the injection site decreases tissue irritation. |
| (5) Have the client lie down for 30 to 60 minutes after the injection. | To observe for adverse reactions. Orthostatic hypotension is likely if the client tries to ambulate. |
| **e.** Do not give antipsychotic drugs subcutaneously, except for fluphenazine decanoate and fluphenazine enanthate. | More tissue irritation occurs with subcutaneous administration than with intramuscular administration. |
| **f.** When parenteral fluphenazine is ordered, check the drug preparations very closely. | The hydrochloride solution of fluphenazine is given intramuscularly only. The decanoate and enanthate preparations (long-acting, sesame oil preparations) can be given intramuscularly or subcutaneously. |
| **2. Observe for therapeutic effects** | |
| **a.** When the drug is given for acute psychotic episodes, observe for decreased agitation, combativeness, and psychomotor activity. | The sedative effects of antipsychotic drugs are exerted within 48 to 72 hours. Sedation that occurs with treatment of acute psychotic episodes is a therapeutic effect. Sedation that occurs with treatment of nonacute psychotic disorders, or excessive sedation at any time, is an adverse reaction. |
| **b.** When the drug is given for acute or chronic psychosis, observe for decreased psychotic behavior, such as: | These therapeutic effects may not be evident for 3 to 6 weeks after drug therapy is begun. |
| (1) Decreased auditory and visual hallucinations | |
| (2) Decreased delusions | |
| (3) Continued decrease in or absence of agitation, hostility, hyperactivity, and other behavior associated with acute psychosis | |
| (4) Increased socialization | |
| (5) Increased ability in self-care activities | |
| (6) Increased ability to participate in other therapeutic modalities along with drug therapy. | |
| **c.** When the drug is given for antiemetic effects, observe for decreased or absent nausea or vomiting. | |
| **3. Observe for adverse effects** | |
| **a.** Excessive sedation—drowsiness, lethargy, fatigue, slurred speech, impaired mobility, and impaired mental processes | Excessive sedation is most likely to occur during the first few days of treatment of an acute psychotic episode, when large doses are usually given. Psychotic clients also seem sedated because the drug lets them catch up on psychosis-induced sleep deprivation. Sedation is more likely to occur in elderly or debilitated people. Tolerance to the drugs' sedative effects develops, and sedation tends to decrease with continued drug therapy. |

| Nursing Actions | Rationale/Explanation |
|---|---|
| **b.** Extrapyramidal reactions: | |
| (1) *Akathisia*—compulsive, involuntary restlessness and body movements | Akathisia is the most common extrapyramidal reaction, and it may occur about 5 to 60 days after the start of antipsychotic drug therapy. The motor restlessness may be erroneously interpreted as psychotic agitation necessitating increased drug dosage. This condition can sometimes be controlled by substituting an antipsychotic drug that is less likely to cause extrapyramidal effects or by giving an anticholinergic antiparkinson drug. |
| (2) *Parkinsonism*—loss of muscle movement (akinesia), muscular rigidity and tremors, shuffling gait, postural abnormalities, mask-like facial expression, hypersalivation, and drooling | These symptoms are the same as those occurring with idiopathic Parkinson's disease. They can be controlled with anticholinergic antiparkinson drugs, given along with the antipsychotic drug for about 3 months, then discontinued. This reaction may occur about 5 to 30 days after antipsychotic drug therapy is begun. |
| (3) *Dyskinesias* (involuntary, rhythmic body movements) and *dystonias* (uncoordinated, bizarre movements of the neck, face, eyes, tongue, trunk, or extremities) | These are less common extrapyramidal reactions, but they may occur suddenly, about 1 to 5 days after drug therapy is started, and be very frightening to affected people and health-care personnel. The movements are caused by muscle spasms and result in exaggerated posture and facial distortions. These symptoms are sometimes misinterpreted as seizures, hysteria, or other disorders. Antiparkinson drugs are given parenterally during acute dystonic reactions, but continued administration is not usually required. These reactions occur most often in younger people. |
| (4) *Tardive dyskinesia*—hyperkinetic movements of the face (sucking and smacking of lips, tongue protrusion, and facial grimaces) and choreiform movements of the trunk and limbs | This syndrome occurs after months or years of high-dose antipsychotic drug therapy. The drugs may mask the symptoms so that the syndrome is more likely to be diagnosed when dosage is decreased or the drug is discontinued for a few days. It occurs gradually and at any age but is more common in older people, women, and people with organic brain disorders. The condition is usually irreversible, and there is no effective treatment. Symptoms are not controlled and may be worsened by antiparkinson drugs. Low dosage and short-term use of antipsychotic drugs help prevent tardive dyskinesia; drug-free periods may aid early detection. |
| **c.** Antiadrenergic effects—hypotension, tachycardia, dizziness, faintness, and fatigue | Hypotension is potentially one of the most serious adverse reactions to the antipsychotic drugs. It is most likely to occur when the client assumes an upright position after sitting or lying down (orthostatic or postural hypotension), but it does occur in the recumbent position. It is caused by peripheral vasodilation. Orthostatic hypotension can be assessed by comparing blood pressure readings taken with the client in supine and standing positions.<br>Tachycardia occurs as a compensatory mechanism in response to hypotension and as an anticholinergic effect in which the normal vagus nerve action of slowing the heart rate is blocked. |
| **d.** Anticholinergic effects—dry mouth, dental caries, blurred vision, constipation, paralytic ileus, urinary retention | These atropine-like effects are common with therapeutic doses and increased with large doses of phenothiazines. |

*(continued)*

| *Nursing Actions* | *Rationale/Explanation* |
|---|---|
| **e.** Respiratory depression—slow, shallow breathing and decreased ability to breathe deeply, cough, and remove secretions from the respiratory tract | This stems from general central nervous system (CNS) depression, which causes drowsiness and decreased movement. It may cause pneumonia or other respiratory problems, especially in people with hypercarbia and chronic lung disease. |
| **f.** Endocrine effects—menstrual irregularities, possibly impotence and decreased libido in the male, weight gain | These apparently result from drug-induced changes in pituitary and hypothalamic functions. |
| **g.** Hypothermia or hyperthermia | Antipsychotic drugs may impair the temperature-regulating center in the hypothalamus. Hypothermia is more likely to occur. Hyperthermia occurs with high doses and warm environmental temperatures. |
| **h.** Hypersensitivity reactions: | |
| (1) *Cholestatic hepatitis*—may begin with fever and influenza-like symptoms followed in about 1 week by jaundice | Cholestatic hepatitis results from drug-induced edema of the bile ducts and obstruction of the bile flow. It occurs most often in women and after 2 to 4 weeks of receiving the drug. It is usually reversible if the drug is discontinued. |
| (2) *Blood dyscrasias*—leukopenia, agranulocytosis (fever, sore throat, weakness) | Some degree of leukopenia occurs rather often and does not seem to be serious. Agranulocytosis, on the other hand, occurs rarely but is life-threatening. Agranulocytosis is most likely to occur during the first 4 to 10 weeks of drug therapy, in women, and in older people. |
| (3) *Skin reactions*—photosensitivity, dermatoses | Skin pigmentation and discoloration may occur with exposure to sunlight. |
| **i.** Electrocardiogram (ECG) changes | The mechanism and clinical significance of ECG changes are not completely clear. However, some antipsychotic drugs, especially thioridazine, alter normal impulse conduction through the ventricles. There is probably increased risk of cardiac arrhythmias, which may be serious in a person with cardiovascular disease. |
| **j.** *Neuroleptic malignant syndrome*—fever (may be confused with heat stroke), muscle rigidity, agitation, confusion, delirium, dyspnea, tachycardia, respiratory failure, acute renal failure | A rare but potentially fatal reaction that may occur hours to months after initial drug use. Symptoms usually develop rapidly over 24 to 72 hours. Treatment includes stopping the antipsychotic drug, supportive care related to fever and other symptoms, and drug therapy (dantrolene, a skeletal muscle relaxant, and amantadine or bromocriptine, dopamine-stimulating drugs). |
| **4. Observe for drug interactions**<br>   **a.** Drugs that *increase* effects of antipsychotic drugs: | |
| (1) Anticholinergic drugs (*e.g.,* atropine) | Additive anticholinergic effects, especially with thioridazine |
| (2) Antidepressants, tricyclic | Potentiation of sedative and anticholinergic effects. Additive CNS depression, sedation, orthostatic hypotension, urinary retention, and glaucoma may occur unless dosages are decreased. Apparently these two drug groups inhibit the metabolism of each other, thus prolonging the actions of both groups if they are given concomitantly. |
| (3) Antihistamines | Additive CNS depression and sedation |
| (4) CNS depressants—alcohol, narcotic analgesics, antianxiety agents, barbiturates and other sedative-hypnotics | Additive CNS depression. Also, severe hypotension, urinary retention, seizures, severe atropine-like reactions, and others may occur, depending on which group of CNS depressant drugs is given. |

| *Nursing Actions* | *Rationale/Explanation* |
|---|---|
| (5) Propranolol (Inderal) | Additive hypotensive and ECG effects |
| (6) Thiazide diuretics, such as hydrochlorothiazide (HydroDIURIL) | Additive hypotension |
| (7) Lithium | Acute encephalopathy, including irreversible brain damage and dyskinesias, has been reported. |
| **b.** Drugs that *decrease* effects of antipsychotic drugs: | |
| (1) Antacids | Oral antacids, especially aluminum hydroxide and magnesium trisilicate, may inhibit gastrointestinal absorption of antipsychotic drugs. |
| (2) Barbiturates | By induction of drug-metabolizing enzymes in the liver |
| (3) Norepinephrine (Levophed), phenylephrine (Neo-Synephrine) | Antagonize the hypotensive effects of antipsychotic drugs |
| **5. Teach clients**<br>**a.** Do not take antacids with these drugs. If an antacid is needed, take it 1 hour before or 2 hours after the antipsychotic drug. | Antacids may decrease absorption of these drugs from the intestine. |
| **b.** Lie down for about an hour after receiving medication when drug therapy is started or after any injection. | To avoid low blood pressure, dizziness, and faintness, which may occur with standing |
| **c.** If dizziness and faintness occur on standing, they can be minimized by changing positions slowly and sitting on the bedside a few minutes before standing. Do not try to stand or walk when feeling dizzy. | To avoid falls or other injuries |
| **d.** Practice good oral hygiene measures, including dental checkups, thorough and frequent toothbrushing, drinking fluids, and frequent mouth rinsing. | Mouth dryness is a common side effect of these drugs. Although more annoying than serious for the most part, it can predispose to mouth infections, dental cavities, and ill-fitting dentures. |
| **e.** If skin reactions occur, stay out of sunlight or wear protective clothing and use sunscreen lotions. | Sensitivity to sunlight is an adverse reaction of these drugs. |
| **f.** Avoid exposure to excessive heat. | Fever (hyperthermia) and heat prostration may occur with high environmental temperatures. |

## Review and Application Exercises

1. How do antipsychotic drugs act to relieve psychotic symptoms?
2. What are some uses of antipsychotic drugs other than treatment of schizophrenia?
3. Do the phenothiazine, butyrophenone, and thioxanthene antipsychotic drugs differ significantly in therapeutic effects?
4. What are major adverse effects of antipsychotic drugs?
5. When instructing a client to lie down for awhile or to rise slowly from a sitting or lying position, which adverse effect of an antipsychotic drug is the nurse trying to prevent?
6. In a client receiving an antipsychotic drug, what appearances or behaviors would lead you to suspect an extrapyramidal reaction?
7. Describe potential difficulties in getting psychotic clients to take their drugs as prescribed and interventions to overcome the difficulties.
8. Are antipsychotic drugs likely to be overused and abused? Why or why not?
9. In an older client on an antipsychotic drug, what special safety measures are needed? Why?

## Selected References

Ballenger, J. C. (1992). Major psychiatric disorders. In W. N. Kelley (Ed.), *Textbook of internal medicine* (2nd ed.) (pp. 2197–2201). Philadelphia: J.B. Lippincott.

Blair, D. T., & Dauner, A. (1992). Extrapyramidal symptoms are serious side effects of the antipsychotic and other drugs. *Nurse Practitioner, 17*(11), 56–65.

Blair, D. T., & Dauner, A. (1993). Neuroleptic malignant syndrome: Liability in nursing practice. *Journal of Psychosocial Nursing, 3*(1), 5–12.

Crismon, M. L., & Dorson, P. G. (1992). Schizophrenia. In J. T. DiPiro, R. L. Talbert, P. E. Hayes, G. C. Yee, G. R. Matzke, & L. M. Posey (Eds.), *Pharmacotherapy: A pathophysiologic approach* (2nd ed.) (pp. 1020–1043). New York: Elsevier.

Druckenbrod, R. W., Rosen, J., & Cluxton, R. J., Jr. (1993). As-needed dosing of antipsychotic drugs: Limitations and guidelines for use in the elderly agitated patient. *The Annals of Pharmacotherapy, 27,* 645–648.

(1993). *Drug facts and comparisons.* St. Louis: Facts and Comparisons.

Ereshefsky, L., & Richards, A. L. (1992). Psychoses. In M. A. Koda-Kimble & L. Y. Young (Eds.), *Applied therapeutics: The clinical use of drugs* (5th ed.) (pp. 56-1–56-43). Vancouver, WA: Applied Therapeutics.

Gelenberg, A. J., & Katz M. D. (1993). Antipsychotic agents. In R. Bressler & M. D. Katz (Eds.), *Geriatric pharmacology* (pp. 375–408). New York: McGraw-Hill.

Harris, B. (1992). Psychopharmacology. In J. Haber, A. L. McMahon, P. Price-Hoskins, & B. F. Sideleau (Eds.), *Comprehensive psychiatric nursing* (4th ed.). St. Louis: C.V. Mosby.

Hartman, C. R., & Knight, M. (1990). Pharmacotherapy. In A. W. Burgess (Ed.), *Psychiatric nursing in the hospital and the community* (5th ed.) (pp 374–424). Norwalk, CT: Appleton & Lange.

Hollister, L. E. (1992). Psychiatric disorders. In K. L. Melmon, H. F. Morrelli, B. B. Hoffman, & D. W. Nierenberg (Eds.), *Clinical pharmacology: Basic principles in therapeutics* (3rd ed.) (pp. 338–380). New York: McGraw-Hill.

Hollister, L. E., & Csernansky, J. G. (1990). *Clinical pharmacology of psychotherapeutic drugs* (3rd ed.). New York: Churchill Livingstone.

Kudzma, E. C. (1992). Drug response: All bodies are not created equal. *American Journal of Nursing, 92,* 49–50.

Lauriello, J., & Dilip, V. J. (1992). Neuroleptic treatment of schizophrenia. *Comprehensive Therapy, 18*(1), 30–35.

Lin, K. M., & Shen, W. W. (1991). Pharmacotherapy for Southeast Asian psychiatric patients. *Journal of Nervous and Mental Disease, 179,* 346–350.

Medical Letter on Drugs and Therapeutics (1991). Adverse effects of psychiatric drugs. *33,* 43–50.

Mendoza, R., Smith, M. W., Poland, R. E., Lin, M., & Strickland, T. (1991). Ethnic psychopharmacology. *Psychopharmacology Bulletin, 27*(4), 449–461.

Ziring, B. (1993). Issues in the perioperative care of the patient with psychiatric illness. *Medical Clinics of North America, 77*(2), 443–452.

# CHAPTER 10

# Antidepressants

## Depression

Depression is an affective disorder often described as the most common mental illness. It is characterized by depressed mood, feelings of sadness, or emotional upset, and it occurs in all age groups. Numerous terms have been used to describe depression. Mild depression probably occurs in everyone as a normal response to life stresses and losses and usually does not require treatment; severe depression is a psychiatric illness and requires treatment. Depression also is categorized as unipolar, in which people of usually normal moods experience recurrent episodes of depression, and bipolar, in which episodes of depression alternate with episodes of mania.

### MAJOR DEPRESSION

The American Psychiatric Association's *Diagnostic and Statistical Manual*, third edition, revised, lists two major categories of depression. One category is *major depression*, which consists of a depressed mood plus at least five of the following symptoms:

Loss of energy
Fatigue
Indecisiveness
Difficulty thinking and concentrating
Loss of interest in appearance, work, and leisure and sexual activities
Inappropriate feelings of guilt and worthlessness
Loss of appetite and weight loss or excessive eating and weight gain

Sleep disorders (hypersomnia or insomnia)
Somatic symptoms (*e.g.*, constipation, headache, atypical pain)
Obsession with death, thoughts of suicide
Psychotic symptoms, such as hallucinations and delusions

### DYSTHYMIA

The other category is *dysthymia*, a chronically depressed mood or loss of interest in usual activities that is not severe enough or does not last long enough to meet the criteria for major depression. Dysthymia is further described as primary or secondary.

Primary (formerly called endogenous) depression cannot be related to an identifiable cause. Secondary (formerly called exogenous or reactive) depression may be precipitated by the following:

*Environmental stress* (*e.g.*, job loss or dissatisfaction, financial worries)
*Adverse life events* (*e.g.*, divorce, death of a family member or friend)
*Drugs* (alcohol; antiarrhythmics, such as lidocaine, procainamide, and tocainide; antihypertensive drugs, such as clonidine, methyldopa, and prazosin; beta-blockers; corticosteroids; opiates; and oral contraceptives)
*Concurrent disease states*, including endocrine disorders (hypothyroidism and hyperthyroidism, diabetes mellitus, adrenal insufficiency or excess), central nervous system (CNS) disorders (stroke, tumors, or other brain lesions; Parkinson's disease), cardio-

Anne Collins Abrams: CLINICAL DRUG THERAPY, Fourth Edition.
© 1995 J.B. Lippincott Company.

vascular disorders (myocardial infarction, congestive heart failure, hypertension), and miscellaneous disorders (rheumatoid arthritis, infectious disease, malnutrition)

Differentiating between major depression and dysthymia is difficult because symptoms are similar, and the main differences are the severity and duration of symptoms. *Seasonal affective disorder*, a type of depression that occurs during winter months, also has been described. Its classification and differentiation from major depression and dysthymia are unclear.

## ETIOLOGY

As with other CNS and psychiatric disorders, depression is attributed to neurotransmitter or receptor abnormalities, with much of the available information derived from studies about the actions of antidepressant drugs. The neurotransmitter hypothesis states that depression is associated with decreased amounts of neurotransmitters (serotonin and norepinephrine), while the receptor sensitivity concept emphasizes receptor response to neurotransmitters. Both concepts may be involved because antidepressant drugs block neurotransmitter reuptake within minutes to hours after single doses, but relief of depression occurs only after several weeks of drug therapy. For these reasons, long-term treatment with the drugs may produce adaptive changes in receptors, such as decreasing the responsiveness of postsynaptic beta-adrenergic receptors and increasing responsiveness of alpha-adrenergic and serotonergic receptors.

A third idea, called the dysregulation hypothesis, incorporates some of the receptor sensitivity concept but emphasizes impaired regulation of neurotransmitters rather than a simple increase or decrease in their activity. For example, differences in neurotransmission (*i.e.*, decreased receptor binding sites for neurotransmitters) have been demonstrated in people with major depression (compared with control subjects) and in depressed elderly people (compared with depressed middle-aged and nondepressed elderly people). Thus, older adults may be biologically predisposed to develop depression. This hypothesis proposes that antidepressant drugs restore the normal regulatory mechanisms. In addition, genetic factors are considered important in unipolar and bipolar affective disorders.

In bipolar disorder, periods of depression alternate with periods of mania, an excited state characterized by excessive CNS stimulation with physical and mental hyperactivity (*e.g.*, energetic and constant movement, decreased sleep, talkativeness, racing thoughts, short attention span, grandiose ideation). Hypomania is sometimes used to indicate a lesser state of CNS stimulation and hyperactivity than mania. Like depression, mania and hypomania may result from abnormal functioning of neurotransmitters or receptors, such as a relative excess of excitatory neurotransmitters (*e.g.*, norepinephrine) or a relative deficiency of inhibitory neurotransmitters (*e.g.*, serotonin and gamma-aminobutyric acid [GABA]). Drugs that stimulate the CNS can cause manic and hypomanic behaviors that are easily confused with schizophreniform psychoses.

# Antidepressant Drugs

Antidepressant drugs are used in the pharmacologic management of depressive disorders (also called mood or affective disorders). They are derived from several chemical groups. Older or first-generation antidepressants include the tricyclic antidepressants (TCAs) and the monoamine oxidase (MAO) inhibitors. Newer or second-generation drugs include serotonin enhancers and several other drugs, some of which differ chemically from the tricyclics but are similar in pharmacologic actions and antidepressant effectiveness. Other characteristics of these drugs and lithium, an antimanic agent used for bipolar affective disorder, are described in the following section.

## TRICYCLIC ANTIDEPRESSANTS

TCAs are chemically and pharmacologically similar drugs. They contain a triple-ring nucleus from which their name is derived. The drugs are structurally similar to phenothiazine antipsychotic agents (see Chap. 9) and have similar antiadrenergic and anticholinergic properties. They produce a relatively high incidence of sedation, orthostatic hypotension, cardiac arrhythmias, and other adverse effects, in addition to dry mouth and anticholinergic effects. TCAs are well absorbed after oral administration. However, first-pass metabolism by the liver results in blood-level variations of 10- to 30-fold among people given identical doses. Once absorbed, these drugs are widely distributed throughout body tissues and metabolized by the liver to active and inactive metabolites. Amitriptyline (Elavil) and imipramine (Tofranil) are commonly used TCAs.

## MONOAMINE OXIDASE INHIBITOR ANTIDEPRESSANTS

MAO inhibitors are well absorbed following oral administration and produce maximal inhibition of MAO within 5 to 10 days. However, clinical improvement in depression may require 2 to 3 weeks.

MAO inhibitors may interact with numerous foods

and drugs to produce hypertensive crisis (*i.e.*, severe hypertension, severe headache, fever, possible myocardial infarction, or intracranial hemorrhage). Foods that interact with MAO inhibitor drugs are those containing tyramine, a monoamine precursor of norepinephrine. Normally, tyramine is deactivated in the gastrointestinal tract and liver so that large amounts do not reach the systemic circulation. However, when deactivation of tyramine is blocked by MAO inhibitors, tyramine is absorbed systemically and transported to adrenergic nerve terminals, where it causes a sudden release of large amounts of norepinephrine. Hypertensive crisis may result. Several drugs also may interact with MAO inhibitors to cause hypertensive crisis. Foods and drugs to be avoided during (and 2 to 3 weeks after) drug therapy with MAO inhibiting agents are listed in Table 10-1.

## SEROTONIN REUPTAKE INHIBITORS

Serotonin reuptake inhibitors (SRIs) are as effective as TCAs and have a similar onset of action. They are well-absorbed with oral administration, undergo extensive first-pass metabolism in the liver, are highly protein bound (about 95%), and have a half-life of 24 to 72 hours, which may lead to accumulation with chronic administration. Fluoxetine also forms active metabolites with a half-life of 7 to 9 days. Thus, steady-state blood levels are achieved slowly, and drug effects decrease slowly when fluoxetine is discontinued. The drugs do not produce the sedation, anticholinergic effects, orthostatic hypotension, cardiac arrhythmias, and weight gain associated with TCAs. Their adverse effects include CNS stimulation (*e.g.*, anxiety, nervousness, insomnia), nausea, anorexia, weight loss, and a skin rash that some-

times requires stopping the drug. The currently available drugs in this group are given once daily.

## MISCELLANEOUS ANTIDEPRESSANTS

**Bupropion** (Wellbutrin) is chemically unrelated to other available antidepressants, and its mechanism of action is unknown. During premarketing studies, bupropion was found to increase the risk of seizures almost tenfold between daily doses of 450 and 600 mg. Plans for marketing were suspended, and further studies evaluated seizure potential. It was later marketed with warnings and precautions related to seizure activity. Seizures are most likely to occur with doses above 450 mg/d and in clients known to have a seizure disorder. Recommendations to prevent seizures are described in the section, Principles of Therapy.

After an oral dose, peak plasma levels are reached in approximately 2 hours. The average drug half-life is about 14 hours. The drug is metabolized in the liver and excreted primarily in the urine. Several metabolites are pharmacologically active. Dosage should be reduced with impaired hepatic or renal function. Acute episodes of depression usually require several months of drug therapy.

In addition to seizures, common adverse effects include agitation, dry mouth, insomnia, headache, nausea and vomiting, constipation, and tremor. The drug has CNS stimulating effects (excitement, increased motor activity, restlessness, agitation, insomnia, anxiety) that may require a sedative during the first few days of bupropion therapy. These effects may increase risks of abuse.

**Maprotiline** (Ludiomil) is a tetracyclic antidepressant that also has anxiolytic properties. It causes adverse effects similar to the TCAs and seems to have few, if any, advantages over the TCAs.

**Trazodone** (Desyrel) is a triazolopyridine derivative and represents a different chemical class of antidepressants. Oral trazodone is well absorbed, and peak plasma concentrations are obtained within 30 minutes to 2 hours. Trazodone is metabolized by the liver and excreted primarily by the kidneys. Although trazodone reportedly produces less anticholinergic activity than the TCAs, it causes a number of other adverse effects, including sedation, dizziness, edema, cardiac arrhythmias, and priapism (prolonged and painful penile erection).

## MOOD STABILIZING AGENT

**Lithium carbonate** (Eskalith) is a naturally occurring metallic salt used in the management of bipolar affective disorder. Lithium is more effective in the treatment and prevention of mania than in preventing depression. It is sometimes described as an "antimanic" drug.

Lithium is well absorbed after oral administration.

### TABLE 10-1. FOODS AND DRUGS TO BE AVOIDED DURING THERAPY WITH MAO INHIBITOR DRUGS

| Foods to Avoid | Drugs to Avoid |
| --- | --- |
| Aged cheese (*e.g.*, cheddar, Camembert, Stilton, Gruyere) | Amphetamines |
| Alcoholic beverages (beer, Chianti and other red wines) | Antiallergy and antiasthmatic drugs (*e.g.*, ephedrine, epinephrine, phenylpropanolamine, pseudoephedrine) |
| Avocados and guacamole dip | |
| Bananas | |
| Caffeine-containing beverages (coffee, tea, cola drinks) | Antidepressants (tricyclic antidepressants, serotonin reuptake inhibitors) |
| Chicken livers | |
| Chocolate (in large amounts) | Antihistamines (including over-the-counter cough and cold remedies) |
| Fava bean pods | |
| Figs (canned) | Antihypertensive drugs (*i.e.*, guanethidine, methyldopa) |
| Meat tenderizers | |
| Pickled herring | Levodopa |
| Raisins | Meperidine |
| Sour cream | |
| Soy sauce | |
| Yogurt | |

Peak serum levels occur in 1 to 3 hours after a dose of lithium, and steady-state concentrations are reached in 5 to 7 days. Because serum concentrations of lithium vary widely among clients with comparable doses, frequent monitoring of serum lithium concentration is required (see the section, Principles of Therapy below).

Lithium is not metabolized by the body; it is entirely excreted by the kidneys, so adequate renal function is a prerequisite for lithium therapy. Approximately 80% of a lithium dose is reabsorbed in the proximal renal tubules. The amount of reabsorption depends on the concentration of sodium in the proximal renal tubules. A deficiency of sodium causes more lithium to be reabsorbed and increases risk of lithium toxicity; excessive sodium intake causes more lithium to be excreted (*i.e.*, "lithium diuresis") and may lower serum lithium levels to nontherapeutic ranges.

Before lithium therapy is begun, baseline studies of renal, cardiac, and thyroid status should be obtained because adverse drug effects involve these organ systems. Baseline electrolyte studies are also necessary.

## MECHANISMS OF ACTION

The mechanisms by which most antidepressant drugs exert therapeutic effects are directly related to hypothesized causes of depression. That is, the drugs are thought to increase the amount of neurotransmitter (*e.g.*, norepinephrine, serotonin) available to stimulate receptors or to alter sensitivity (and possibly numbers) of the receptors.

After neurotransmitters are released from presynaptic nerve endings, they are normally inactivated by reuptake into the presynaptic nerve fiber that released them or metabolized by the enzyme MAO. The TCAs, maprotiline, and trazodone prevent reuptake of one or more neurotransmitters. The SRIs selectively inhibit the reuptake of serotonin into presynaptic nerve endings, thereby increasing the amount of serotonin in the synapse available to bind with receptor sites on postsynaptic neurons. The MAO inhibitors prevent the metabolism of neurotransmitter molecules. Apparently all of the currently available drugs decrease the sensitivity of receptors, especially postsynaptic beta-adrenergic receptors, with chronic use.

The exact mechanism by which lithium exerts therapeutic effects is unknown. However, it is known to affect the synthesis, release, and reuptake of several neurotransmitters in the brain, including acetylcholine, dopamine, GABA, and norepinephrine. For example, the drug may increase the activity of GABA, an inhibitory neurotransmitter. It also stabilizes postsynaptic receptor sensitivity to neurotransmitters, probably by competing with calcium, magnesium, potassium, and sodium ions for binding sites.

## INDICATIONS FOR USE

Antidepressant drug therapy may be indicated if depressive symptoms persist at least 2 weeks, impair social relationships or work performance, and occur independently of life events. In addition, TCAs may be used in children and adolescents in the management of enuresis, involuntary urination ("bed-wetting") resulting from a physical or psychological disorder. A TCA may be given after physical causes (*e.g.*, urethral irritation, excessive intake of fluids) have been ruled out.

## CONTRAINDICATIONS FOR USE

Antidepressant drugs are contraindicated or must be used with caution in clients with acute schizophrenia; mixed mania and depression; suicidal tendencies; severe renal, hepatic, or cardiovascular disease; narrow-angle glaucoma; and seizure disorders.

# Individual antidepressants

See Table 10-2 for names, routes, and dosage ranges of individual antidepressants.

## *Nursing Process*

### Assessment

Assess the client's condition in relation to depressive disorders.
- Identify clients at risk for current or potential depression. Areas to assess include health status, family and social relationships, and work status. Severe or prolonged illness, impaired interpersonal relationships, inability to work, and job dissatisfaction may precipitate depression. Depression also occurs without a specific, discernible cause.
- Observe for the signs and symptoms of depression listed above. Manifestations may occur in any client, not just those who have or are suspected of having psychiatric illness. Clinical manifestations are nonspecific and vary in severity. For example, fatigue and insomnia may be caused by a variety of disorders and range from mild to severe. When symptoms are present, try to determine their frequency, duration, and severity.
- When a client appears depressed or has a history of depression, assess for suicidal thoughts and behaviors. Statements indicating a detailed plan, accompanied by the intent, ability, and method for carrying out the plan, place the client at high risk for suicide.
- Identify the client's usual coping mechanisms for stressful situations. Coping mechanisms vary widely among people, and behavior that may be helpful to one client may not be helpful to another. For example, one person may prefer being alone or having decreased contact with family and

### TABLE 10-2. ANTIDEPRESSANT AGENTS

| Generic/Trade Name | Routes and Dosage Ranges | |
| --- | --- | --- |
| | *Adults* | *Children* |
| ***Tricyclic Antidepressants*** | | |
| **Amitriptyline** (Elavil, Endep, others) | PO 75–100 mg daily in divided doses, gradually increased to 150–300 mg daily if necessary. Maintenance dose, 50–100 mg once daily at bedtime.<br>IM 80–120 mg daily in 4 divided doses<br>*Older adults:* PO 10 mg 3 times daily and 20 mg at bedtime | Adolescents, PO 10 mg 3 times daily and 20 mg at bedtime<br>Enuresis in children aged 5–14 years: PO 25 mg once daily at bedtime |
| **Amoxapine** (Asendin) | PO 50 mg 3 times daily, increased to 100 mg 3 times daily on the third day. Maintenance dose may be given in a single dose at bedtime. | Not recommended for children under age 16 years |
| **Desipramine** (Pertofrane, Norpramin) | PO 75 mg daily in divided doses, gradually increased to a maximum of 200–300 mg daily if necessary<br>*Older adults:* PO 25–50 mg daily in divided doses, gradually increased to 100 mg daily if necessary | Not recommended |
| **Doxepin** (Sinequan, Adapin) | PO 75–150 mg daily, gradually increased to a maximum of 300 mg daily if necessary | Not recommended |
| **Imipramine** (Tofranil) | PO 75 mg daily in 3 divided doses, gradually increased to a maximum of 300 mg daily if necessary. Maintenance dose, 75–150 mg daily<br>*Older adults:* PO 30–40 mg daily in divided doses, increased to 100 mg daily if necessary | Enuresis: PO 25–50 mg 1 hour before bedtime |
| **Nortriptyline** (Aventyl, Pamelor) | PO 40 mg daily in divided doses, gradually increased to 100–150 mg daily if necessary | Enuresis: PO 25 mg once daily at bedtime |
| **Protriptyline** (Vivactil) | PO 15 mg daily in divided doses, increased to 60 mg daily if necessary | |
| **Trimipramine maleate** (Surmontil) | PO 75–100 mg daily, gradually increased to 300 mg daily if necessary | |
| ***Monoamine Oxidase Inhibitor Antidepressants*** | | |
| **Isocarboxazid** (Marplan) | PO 30 mg daily in divided doses. Maintenance dose, up to 20 mg daily | Dosage not established |
| **Phenelzine** (Nardil) | PO 60 mg daily in 3 divided doses, increased to 90 mg daily if necessary | Dosage not established |
| **Tranylcypromine** (Parnate) | PO 20 mg daily in 2 divided doses in the morning and afternoon for 2 weeks, then adjusted according to client's response. Maximal daily dose, 30 mg | Dosage not established |
| ***Serotonin Reuptake Inhibitor Antidepressants*** | | |
| **Fluoxetine** (Prozac) | PO 20 mg once daily in the morning, increased after several weeks if necessary. Divide doses larger than 20 mg, and give morning and noon; maximum daily dose, 80 mg. | Dosage not established |
| **Paroxetine** (Paxil) | PO 20 mg once daily in the morning, increased after 3–4 weeks if necessary; maximum dose, 50 mg daily (40 mg for older adults). | Dosage not established |
| **Sertraline** (Zoloft) | PO 50 mg once daily morning or evening, increased at 1 week or longer intervals to a maximum daily dose of 200 mg | Dosage not established |
| ***Miscellaneous Antidepressants*** | | |
| **Bupropion** (Wellbutrin) | PO 100 mg twice daily, increased to 100 mg 3 times daily if necessary. Maximal single dose, 150 mg | Dosage not established |
| **Maprotiline** (Ludiomil) | PO 75 mg daily in single or divided doses, increased to a maximum dose of 300 mg daily if necessary | Not recommended for children under age 18 years |
| **Trazodone** (Desyrel) | PO 100–300 mg daily, increased to a maximum dose of 600 mg daily if necessary | |
| ***Mood-Stabilizing Agent*** | | |
| **Lithium carbonate** (Eskalith) | Bipolar disorder (formerly called manic-depressive disorder), PO 900–1200 mg daily in divided doses, gradually increased in 300-mg increments if necessary, according to serum lithium levels and client's response | Not FDA-approved for use in children under 12 years but sometimes given PO 300–900 mg or 30 mg/kg per day, in divided doses |

friends, whereas another may find increased contact desirable.

### Nursing diagnoses

- Dysfunctional Grieving, related to loss (of health, ability to perform usual tasks, job, significant other, and so forth)
- Self-Care Deficit related to fatigue and self-esteem disturbance with depression or sedation with antidepressant drugs
- Sleep Pattern Disturbance related to depression
- Impaired Physical Mobility related to sedation
- Alteration in Thought Processes related to confusion (especially in older adults)
- Knowledge Deficit: Effects and appropriate usage of antidepressant drugs
- High Risk for Decreased Cardiac Output related to cardiac arrhythmias and hypotension
- High Risk for Altered Tissue Perfusion related to hypotension
- High Risk for Injury related to sedation
- High Risk for Violence: Self-Directed or Directed at Others

### Planning/Goals

*The client will:*

- Experience improvement of mood and depressive state
- Receive or self-administer the drugs correctly
- Be kept safe while sedated during early drug therapy
- Be assessed regularly for suicidal tendencies. If present, caretakers will implement safety measures.
- Be cared for by staff in areas of nutrition, hygiene, exercise, and social interactions when unable to provide self-care
- Resume self-care and other usual activities
- Avoid preventable adverse drug effects

### Interventions

Use measures to prevent or decrease severity of depression. General measures include supportive psychotherapy and reduction of environmental stress. Specific measures include the following:

- Support the client's usual mechanism for handling stressful situations, when feasible. Helpful actions may involve relieving pain or insomnia, scheduling rest periods, and increasing or decreasing socialization with other people.
- Call the client by name, encourage self-care activities, allow him or her to participate in goal setting and decision making, and praise efforts to accomplish tasks. These actions help to promote a positive self-image.
- When signs and symptoms of depression are observed, initiate treatment before depression becomes severe. Institute suicide precautions for clients at risk. These usually involve close observation, often on a one-to-one basis, and removal of potential weapons from the environment. For clients hospitalized on medical-surgical units, a transfer to a psychiatric unit may be needed.

*Teach clients and caretakers:*

- To take antidepressant drugs as directed to maximize therapeutic benefits and minimize adverse effects. Do not alter doses when symptoms subside. TCAS and MAO inhibitors are usually given for several months; lithium therapy may be lifelong.
- That therapeutic effects (*i.e.*, relief of symptoms) may not occur for 2 or 3 weeks after drug therapy is started. If clients do not know that therapeutic effects are delayed, they may think the drug is ineffective and stop taking it prematurely.
- Not to take any other drugs without the physician's knowledge, including over-the-counter cold remedies. Potentially serious drug interactions may occur with prescription or nonprescription drugs.
- To tell any other physician, surgeon, or dentist consulted about the antidepressant drugs being taken. Potentially serious adverse effects or drug interactions may occur if certain other drugs are prescribed.

### Evaluation

- Observe for behaviors indicating lessened depression.
- Interview regarding feelings and mood.
- Observe and interview regarding adverse drug effects.
- Observe and interview regarding suicidal thoughts and behaviors.

# Principles of therapy

## DRUG SELECTION

The choice of an antidepressant depends on two major factors: the type and severity of depression and a drug's effectiveness and adverse effects. Because the available drugs seem similarly effective, adverse effects may be a major determinant.

Guidelines for choosing a drug include the following:

1. The SRIs are overtaking the TCAs as drugs of first choice. These drugs are effective and generally produce fewer and milder adverse effects.
2. For many years, a TCA was the primary drug of choice for most depressed clients. There is little basis for choosing one TCA over another, but some clients may tolerate or respond better to one TCA than to another.
   a. Initial selection of a specific TCA may be based on the client's previous response or susceptibility to adverse effects. For example, if a client (or a close family member) responded well to a particular drug in the past, that is probably the drug of choice for repeated episodes of depression. The response of family members to individual drugs may be significant because there is a strong genetic component to depression and drug response.
   b. The first two TCAs developed (imipramine and amitriptyline) are the most commonly prescribed agents. If therapeutic effects do not occur within 4 weeks, the TCA probably should be discontinued or changed.
3. MAO inhibitors are considered second-line drugs for treatment of depression because of their potential

interactions with other drugs and certain foods. An MAO inhibitor is most likely to be prescribed when the client does not respond to other antidepressant drugs or when electroconvulsive therapy is refused or contraindicated.

4. Bupropion also is effective but has potentially serious adverse effects, especially with larger-than-recommended doses. Thus, its role in the treatment of depression is still being defined by clinical usage.

5. Lithium is the primary drug of choice for clients with bipolar disorder. When used therapeutically, lithium is effective in controlling mania in about 65% to 80% of clients. When used prophylactically, the drug decreases the frequency and intensity of manic cycles. Carbamazepine (Tegretol), an anticonvulsant, may be as effective as lithium as a mood stabilizing agent. It is often used in clients who do not respond to lithium, althought it is not FDA-approved for that purpose.

## DOSAGE AND ADMINISTRATION

Dosage of antidepressant drugs should be individualized according to clinical response. Antidepressant drug therapy is usually initiated with small, divided doses that are gradually increased (every 2 to 3 days) until therapeutic or adverse effects occur. Specific guidelines for dosage include the following:

1. With SRIs, therapy is begun with once daily, oral administration of the manufacturer's recommended dosage. Dosage may be increased after 3 or 4 weeks if depression is not relieved. As with most other drugs, smaller dosages may be indicated in older adults and clients taking multiple medications.

2. With TCAs, therapy is begun with small doses, which are increased to the desired dose over 1 to 2 weeks. Minimal effective doses are about 150 mg/d of imipramine or its equivalent. TCAs can be administered once or twice daily because they have long elimination half-lives. Once dosage is established, TCAs are often given once daily at bedtime. This regimen is effective and well tolerated by most clients. Elderly clients may experience fewer adverse reactions if divided doses are continued.

3. With bupropion, seizures are more likely to occur with large single doses, large total doses, and large or abrupt increases in dosage. Recommendations to avoid these risk factors are:
   a. Give the drug in equally divided doses, preferably at least 6 hours apart.
   b. Single doses are usually 100 mg; the maximal single dose is 150 mg.
   c. The recommended initial dose is 200 mg, gradually increased to 300 mg. If no clinical improve-

ment occurs after several weeks of 300 mg/d, dosage may be increased to 450 mg, the maximal daily dose.
   d. The recommended maintenance dose is the lowest amount that maintains remission.

4. With lithium therapy, dosage should be based on serum lithium levels, control of symptoms, and occurrence of adverse effects. Serum levels are required because therapeutic doses are only slightly lower than toxic doses and because clients vary widely in rates of lithium absorption and excretion. Consequently, a dose that is therapeutic in one client may be toxic or lethal in another. Lower doses are indicated for older adults and for any clients with conditions that impair lithium excretion (*e.g.*, diuretic drug therapy, dehydration, low-salt diet, renal impairment, decreased cardiac output).

When lithium therapy is being initiated, serum drug concentration should be measured two or three times weekly in the morning, 12 hours after the last dose of lithium. For most clients, the therapeutic range of serum levels is 0.5 to 1.2 mEq/L (SI units, 0.5–1.2 mmol/L). Serum lithium levels should not exceed 1.5 mEq/L because the risk of serious toxicity is increased at higher levels.

Once symptoms of mania are controlled, lithium doses should be lowered, and serum lithium levels should be measured at least every 3 months during long-term maintenance therapy.

## DURATION OF DRUG THERAPY

Guidelines for duration of antidepressant and lithium therapy are not well established, and there are differences of opinion. However, evidence seems to be accumulating that long-term maintenance therapy may be desirable. One argument for this approach is that depression tends to relapse or recur, and successive episodes often are more severe and more difficult to treat.

Maintenance therapy for depression requires close supervision and periodic reassessment of the client's condition and response. With TCAs for acute depression, maintenance therapy has usually consisted of low doses for about 3 to 6 months after recovery, followed by gradual tapering of the dose and drug discontinuation. However, recent studies indicate that full therapeutic doses (if clients can tolerate the adverse effects) for up to 5 years are effective in preventing recurrent episodes. Long-term effects (beyond 2–4 months) of SRIs have not been studied. Long-term therapy is the usual practice with lithium, because of a high recurrence rate if the drug is discontinued. When lithium is discontinued, most often because of adverse effects or a client's lack of adherence to the prescribed regimen, gradually tapering the dose over 2 to 4 weeks delays recurrence of symptoms.

## ASSESSMENT AND MANAGEMENT OF TOXICITY

Antidepressant drugs are highly toxic and potentially lethal when taken in large doses. Toxicity is most likely to occur in depressed clients who intentionally ingest large amounts of drug in suicide attempts and in young children who accidentally gain access to improperly stored medication containers. Measures to prevent acute poisoning from drug overdose include dispensing only a few days' supply (*i.e.*, 5–7 days) to clients with suicidal tendencies and storing the drugs in places inaccessible to young children. General measures to treat acute poisoning include early detection of signs and symptoms, stopping the drug, and instituting treatment if indicated. Specific measures include the following:

1. Overdosage of TCAs: Symptoms occur about 1 to 4 hours after drug ingestion and consist primarily of CNS depression and cardiovascular effects (*e.g.*, nystagmus, tremor, restlessness, seizures, hypotension, arrhythmias, and myocardial depression). Death usually results from cardiac, respiratory, and circulatory failure.

   Management of TCA toxicity consists of gastric lavage and administration of activated charcoal to reduce drug absorption, administration of cathartics to increase drug excretion, establishing and maintaining a patent airway, continuous electrocardiographic (ECG) monitoring of comatose clients or those with respiratory insufficiency or wide QRS intervals, administration of intravenous fluids and vasopressors for severe hypotension, and intravenous administration of phenytoin or a parenteral benzodiazepine (*e.g.*, diazepam, lorazepam) if seizures occur.

2. Overdosage of MAO inhibitors: Symptoms occur 12 hours or longer after drug ingestion and consist primarily of adrenergic effects (*e.g.*, tachycardia, increased rate of respiration, agitation, tremors, convulsive seizures, sweating, heart block, hypotension, delirium, and coma). Management consists of forced diuresis, acidification of urine, or hemodialysis to remove the drug from the body.

3. Overdosage of SRIs: Symptoms include nausea, vomiting, agitation, restlessness, hypomania, and other signs of CNS stimulation. Management includes symptomatic and supportive treatment, such as maintaining an adequate airway and ventilation and administering activated charcoal.

4. Overdosage of bupropion: Symptoms include agitation and other mental status changes, nausea and vomiting, and seizures. General treatment measures include hospitalization, decreasing absorption (*e.g.*, inducing vomiting and giving activated charcoal to conscious clients), and supporting vital functions. If seizures occur, an intravenous benzodiazepine (*e.g.*, lorazepam) is the drug of first choice.

5. Lithium overdose: Toxic manifestations occur with serum lithium levels above 2.5 mEq/L and include nystagmus, tremors, oliguria, confusion, impaired consciousness, visual or tactile hallucinations, choreiform movements, convulsions, coma, and death. Treatment involves supportive care to maintain vital functions, including correction of fluid and electrolyte imbalances. With severe overdoses, hemodialysis is the preferred treatment, because it removes lithium from the body.

## USE IN PERIOPERATIVE PERIODS

Antidepressants must be used very cautiously, if at all, perioperatively because of the risk of serious adverse effects and adverse interactions with anesthetics and other commonly used drugs. MAO inhibitors are contraindicated and should be discontinued at least 10 days before elective surgery. TCAs should be discontinued several days before elective surgery and resumed several days postoperatively. Lithium should be stopped 1 to 2 days before surgery and resumed when full oral intake of food and fluids is allowed. Lithium may prolong effects of anesthetic and neuromuscular blocking drugs.

## USE IN CHILDREN

In children, any antidepressant drug should be used only when clearly indicated and then very cautiously.

TCAs are not recommended for use in children under 12 years of age except for short-term treatment of enuresis in children over 6 years. With imipramine, the most commonly used drug, dosage should not exceed 2.5 mg/kg per day. ECG changes have occurred in children taking higher doses; the significance of the changes in terms of cardiac function is unknown. Effectiveness for enuresis may decrease with continued use, and no residual benefits continue once the drug is stopped. Common adverse effects include sedation, fatigue, nervousness, and sleep disorders.

Safety and effectiveness have not been established for amoxapine (Asendin) in children under 16 years, MAO inhibitors in children under 16 years, and SRIs, bupropion, and maprotiline in children under 18 years. Lithium is not FDA-approved for use in children under 12 years of age, but it has been used to treat bipolar disorder and aggressiveness. Children normally excrete lithium more rapidly than adults. As with adults, initial doses should be relatively low and gradually increased according to regular measurements of serum drug levels.

## USE IN OLDER ADULTS

Tricyclic and related antidepressants should be given in small doses initially and gradually increased over several weeks, if necessary, to achieve therapeutic effects. Initial and maintenance doses should be small because the drugs are metabolized and excreted more slowly than in younger adults. Dosage should be decreased by 30% to 50% to avoid serious adverse reactions. Impaired compensatory mechanisms make older adults more likely to experience anticholinergic effects, confusion, hypotension, and sedation. MAO inhibitors may be more likely to cause hypertensive crises in older adults because cardiovascular, renal, and hepatic functions are often diminished. The SRIs produce similar adverse effects in older adults as in younger adults. Although their effects in older adults are not well-delineated, SRIs may be eliminated more slowly, and smaller or less frequent doses may be prudent. With lithium, initial doses should generally be low and increased gradually, according to regular measurements of serum drug levels.

## NURSING ACTIONS: ANTIDEPRESSANTS

| *Nursing Actions* | *Rationale/Explanation* |
|---|---|
| **1. Administer accurately**<br>Give lithium with or just after meals. | To decrease gastric irritation and nausea |
| **2. Observe for therapeutic effects**<br>**a.** With tricyclic antidepressants (TCAs) and monoamine oxidase (MAO) inhibitors, observe for statements of feeling better or being less depressed; increased appetite, physical activity, and interest in surroundings; improved sleep patterns; improved appearance; decreased anxiety; decreased somatic complaints. | Therapeutic effects usually do not occur for 2 to 3 weeks after drug therapy is started. |
| **b.** With lithium, observe for decreases in manic behavior and mood swings. | Therapeutic effects do not occur until approximately 7 to 10 days after therapeutic serum drug levels are attained. In severe mania, an antipsychotic drug is usually given to control behavior until the lithium takes effect. |
| **3. Observe for adverse effects**<br>**a.** With TCAs, observe for:<br><br>(1) Dry mouth, constipation, blurred vision, tachycardia, orthostatic hypotension, drowsiness, dizziness, excessive sweating, weight gain<br><br>(2) Urinary retention, fainting, tremor, nausea, cardiac arrhythmias<br><br>(3) Confusion, delirium, seizures, skin rash, agranulocytosis, cholestatic jaundice, impotence, transition to mania in clients with bipolar disorder. | Most adverse effects result from anticholinergic or antiadrenergic activity. Symptoms listed in (1) commonly occur, especially when TCA therapy is initiated. Symptoms listed in (2) occur less frequently, and those listed in (3) rarely occur. |
| **b.** With bupropion, observe for seizure activity, central nervous system (CNS) stimulation (agitation, insomnia, hyperactivity, hallucinations, delusions), headache, nausea and vomiting, and weight loss. | Adverse effects are most likely to occur if recommended doses are exceeded. |
| **c.** With serotonin reuptake inhibitors (SRIs), observe for headache, nervousness, sedation, insomnia, nausea, diarrhea, dry mouth, constipation, skin rash, palpitations, and dyspnea. | Although numerous adverse effects may occur, they are usually less serious than those occurring with other antidepressants. Compared to the TCAs, SRIs are less likely to cause significant sedation, hypotension, and cardiac arrhythmias but are more likely to cause nausea, nervousness, and insomnia. |
| **d.** With MAO inhibitors, observe for hypotension, dizziness, increased incidence of angina, dry mouth, blurred vision, constipation, urinary retention, hypoglycemia. | Anticholinergic effects are common. Hypoglycemia results from a drug-induced reduction in blood sugar. |

*(continued)*

| *Nursing Actions* | *Rationale/Explanation* |
|---|---|
| **e.** With lithium, observe for: | Most clients who take lithium experience adverse effects. Symptoms listed in (1) are common, occur at therapeutic serum drug levels (0.8–1.2 mEq/L) and usually subside during the first few weeks of drug therapy. Symptoms listed in (2) occur at higher serum drug levels (1.5–2.5 mEq/L). Nausea may be decreased by giving lithium with meals. Propranolol (Inderal), 20–120 mg daily, may be given to control tremors. Severe or persistent adverse effects may be managed by decreasing lithium dosage, omitting a few doses, or discontinuing the drug temporarily. Toxic symptoms occur at serum drug levels above 2.5 mEq/L. |
| (1) Metallic taste, hand tremors, nausea, polyuria, polydipsia, diarrhea, muscular weakness, fatigue, edema, and weight gain | |
| (2) More severe nausea and diarrhea, vomiting, ataxia, incoordination, dizziness, slurred speech, blurred vision, tinnitus, muscle twitching and tremors, increased muscle tone. | |
| (3) Leukocytosis | Lithium mobilizes white blood cells (WBCs) from bone marrow to the blood stream. Maximum increase in WBC occurs in 7 to 10 days. The drug has been given therapeutically for this effect in cancer patients with neutropenia, but studies do not indicate decreased infections. |
| **4. Observe for drug interactions**<br>**a.** Drugs that increase effects of TCAs | |
| (1) Antiarrhythmics (*e.g.*, quinidine, disopyramide, procainamide) | Additive effects on cardiac conduction, increasing risk of heart block |
| (2) Antihistamines, atropine, and other drugs with anticholinergic effects | Additive anticholinergic effects (*e.g.*, dry mouth, blurred vision, urinary retention, constipation) |
| (3) Antihypertensives | Additive hypotension |
| (4) Cimetidine, fluoxetine | Increase risks of toxicity by decreasing hepatic metabolism and increasing blood levels of TCAs |
| (5) CNS depressants (*e.g.*, alcohol, benzodiazepine antianxiety and hypnotic agents, narcotic analgesics) | Additive sedation and CNS depression |
| (6) Urinary alkalizers (*e.g.*, sodium bicarbonate) | Decrease excretion of TCAs |
| **b.** Drugs that *decrease* effects of TCAs: | |
| (1) Barbiturates, chloral hydrate, nicotine (cigarette smoking) | These drugs decrease blood levels of TCAs by increasing the rate of hepatic metabolism of the antidepressant agent. |
| (2) Urinary acidifiers (*e.g.*, ascorbic acid) | Increase excretion of TCAs |
| **c.** Drugs that *increase* effects of MAO inhibitors: | |
| (1) Anticholinergic drugs (*e.g.*, atropine, antipsychotic agents, TCAs) | Additive anticholinergic effects |
| (2) Adrenergic agents (*e.g.*, epinephrine, isoproterenol, phenylephrine), alcohol (some beers and wines), guanethidine, levodopa, meperidine | Hypertensive crisis may occur. |
| **d.** Drugs that *increase* effects of lithium: | |
| (1) Angiotensin-converting enzyme inhibitors (*e.g.*, captopril) | These drugs decrease renal clearance of lithium and thus increase serum lithium levels. |
| (2) Diuretics (*e.g.*, ethacrynic acid, furosemide, hydrochlorothiazide) | Increase neurotoxicity and cardiotoxicity of lithium by increasing excretion of sodium and potassium and thereby decreasing excretion of lithium |
| (3) Nonsteroidal anti-inflammatory drugs (NSAIDs) | These drugs decrease renal clearance of lithium and thus increase serum levels and risks of lithium toxicity. |
| (4) Phenothiazines | Increased risk of hyperglycemia |

## Nursing Actions

## Rationale/Explanation

| | |
|---|---|
| (5) Potassium iodide, TCAs | Increased risk of hypothyroidism |
| (6) TCAs | May increase antidepressant effects of lithium and are sometimes given in combination with lithium for this purpose. These drugs also may precipitate a manic episode. |
| e. Drugs that *decrease* effects of lithium: Acetazolamide (Diamox), sodium bicarbonate, sodium chloride (in excessive amounts), drugs with a high sodium content (*e.g.*, carbenicillin, ticarcillin), theophylline compounds | Increase excretion of lithium |

**5. Teach clients**

**a.** With TCAs, report urinary retention, fainting, irregular heart beat, seizures, restlessness, and mental confusion.

These are potentially serious adverse drug effects. The physician may be able to alter drug therapy and decrease adverse effects.

**b.** With MAO inhibitors:

(1) Report severe headache to the physician.

Severe headache may be a symptom of a serious adverse effect.

(2) Avoid the foods and drugs listed in Table 10-1.

Severe hypertension and intracranial hemorrhage may occur.

**c.** With lithium:

(1) Do not alter dietary salt intake.

Deceased salt intake (*e.g.*, low-salt diet) increases risk of adverse effects from lithium. Increased intake may decrease therapeutic effects.

(2) Drink 2 to 3 quarts of fluids daily; avoid excessive intake of caffeine-containing beverages.

Dehydration increases lithium toxicity; caffeine has a diuretic effect.

(3) Minimize activities that cause excessive perspiration.

Loss of salt in sweat increases risk of adverse effects from lithium.

(4) Report for measurements of lithium blood levels as instructed, and do not take the morning dose of lithium until the blood sample has been obtained.

Regular measurements of blood lithium levels are necessary for safe and effective lithium therapy. Accurate measurement of serum drug levels requires that blood be drawn 12 hours after the previous dose of lithium.

## Review and Application Exercises

1. During an initial assessment of any client, what kinds of appearances or behaviors may indicate depression?
2. Is antidepressant drug therapy indicated for most episodes of temporary sadness? Why or why not?
3. What are the major groups of antidepressant drugs?
4. How do the drugs act to relieve depression?
5. When a client begins antidepressant drug therapy, why is it important to explain that relief of depression may not occur for 2 to 3 weeks?
6. What are common adverse effects of TCAs, and how may they be minimized?
7. What is the advantage of giving a TCA at bedtime rather than early morning?
8. For a client taking an MAO inhibitor, what information would you provide for preventing a hypertensive crisis?
9. How do the SRIs differ from TCAs?
10. What are common adverse effects of lithium, and how may they be minimized?

## Selected References

Ballenger, J. C. (1992). Major psychiatric disorders. In W. N. Kelley (Ed.), *Textbook of internal medicine* (2nd ed.) (pp. 2197–2201). Philadelphia: J.B. Lippincott.

Blazer, D. G. (1992). Depression in late life. In W. N. Kelley (Ed.),

*Textbook of internal medicine* (2nd ed.) (pp. 2414–2416). Philadelphia: J.B. Lippincott.

Bressler, R. (1993). Depression. In R. Bressler & M. D. Katz (Eds.), *Geriatric pharmacology* (pp. 329–373). New York: McGraw-Hill.

Brown, C. S., & Bryant, S. G. (1992). Major depressive disorders. In M. A. Koda-Kimble & L. Y. Young (Eds.), *Applied therapeutics: The clinical use of drugs* (5th ed.) (pp. 57-1–57-18). Vancouver, WA: Applied Therapeutics.

Cole, J. O., & Bodkin, J. A. (1990). Antidepressant drug side effects. *Journal of Clinical Psychiatry, 51*(Suppl.), 21–26.

Depression Guideline Panel (1993). *Clinical practice guideline: Depression in primary care, 2: Treatment of major depression.* Rockville, MD: U.S. Department of Health and Human Services, Public Health Service, Agency for Health Care Policy and Research; AHCPR publication no. 93-0551.

(1993). *Drug facts and comparisons.* St. Louis: Facts and Comparisons.

Faedda, G. L., Tondo, L., Baldessarini, R. J., Suppes, T., & Tohen, M. (1993). Outcome after rapid vs gradual discontinuation of lithium treatment in bipolar disorders. *Archives of General Psychiatry, 50,* 448–455.

Fankhauser, M. P. (1992). Bipolar disorder. In J. T. DiPiro, R. L. Talbert, P. E. Hayes, G. C. Yee, G. R. Matzke, & L. M. Posey (Eds.), *Pharmacotherapy: A pathophysiologic approach* (2nd ed.) (pp. 1044–1064). New York: Elsevier.

Harris, B. (1992). Psychopharmacology. In J. Haber, A. L. McMahon, P. Price-Hoskins, & B. F. Sideleau (Eds.), *Comprehensive psychiatric nursing* (4th ed.). St. Louis: C.V. Mosby.

Hartman, C. R., & Knight, M. (1990). Pharmacotherapy. In A. W. Burgess (Ed.), *Psychiatric nursing in the hospital and the community* (5th ed.) (pp. 374–424). Norwalk, CT: Appleton & Lange.

Hollister, L. E. (1992). Psychiatric disorders. In K. L. Melmon, H. F. Morrelli, B. B. Hoffman, & D. W. Nierenberg (Eds.), *Clinical pharmacology: Basic principles in therapeutics* (3rd ed.) (pp. 338–380). New York: McGraw-Hill.

Hollister, L. E., & Csernansky, J. G. (1990). *Clinical pharmacology of psychotherapeutic drugs* (3rd ed.). New York: Churchill Livingstone.

Kupfer, D. J., Frank, E., Perel, J. M., Cornes, C., Mallinger, A. G., Thase, M. E., McEachran, A. B., & Grochocinski, V. J. (1992). Five-year outcome for maintenance therapies in recurrent depression. *Archives of General Psychiatry, 49,* 769–773.

Nattel, S. (1992). Management of poisoning. In K. L. Melmon, H. F. Morrelli, B. B. Hoffman, & D. W. Nierenberg (Eds.), *Clinical pharmacology: Basic principles in therapeutics* (3rd ed.) (pp. 787–804). New York: McGraw-Hill.

Shearer, S. L., & Adams, G. K. (1993). Nonpharmacologic aids in the treatment of depression. *American Family Physician, 47,* 435–441.

Skowron, D. M., & Stimmel, G. L. (1992). Antidepressants and the risk of seizures. *Pharmacotherapy, 12*(1), 18–22.

Weber, S. S., Saklad, S. R., & Kastenholz, K. V. (1992). Bipolar affective disorders. In M. A. Koda-Kimble & L. Y. Young (Eds.), *Applied therapeutics: The clinical use of drugs* (5th ed.) (pp. 58-1–58-17). Vancouver, WA: Applied Therapeutics.

Wells, B. G., & Hayes, P. E. (1992). Depressive disorders. In J. T. DiPiro, R. L. Talbert, P. E. Hayes, G. C. Yee, G. R. Matzke, & L. M. Posey (Eds.), *Pharmacotherapy: A pathophysiologic approach* (2nd ed.) (pp. 1065–1083). New York: Elsevier.

Ziring, B. (1993). Issues in the perioperative care of the patient with psychiatric illness. *Medical Clinics of North America, 77*(2), 443–452.

### CHAPTER 11

# Anticonvulsants

## Seizure disorders

Anticonvulsant drugs are used to treat seizure disorders. The terms seizure and convulsion are often used interchangeably, although they are not the same. A *seizure* involves a brief episode of abnormal electrical activity in nerve cells of the brain that may or may not be accompanied by visible changes in appearance or behavior. A *convulsion* is a common, tonic-clonic type of seizure characterized by spasmodic contractions of involuntary muscles.

Seizures may occur as single events in response to hypoglycemia, fever, electrolyte imbalances, overdoses of numerous drugs (*e.g.,* cocaine, isoniazid, lidocaine, lithium, phenothiazine antipsychotic drugs, theophylline), and withdrawal of alcohol or sedative-hypnotic drugs. In these instances, treatment of the underlying problem alone or with temporary use of an anticonvulsant drug may relieve the seizures.

### EPILEPSY

When seizures occur in a chronic, recurrent pattern, the disorder is called *epilepsy*, and drug therapy is usually required. Epilepsy is characterized by abnormal and excessive electrical discharges of nerve cells. It is diagnosed by clinical signs and symptoms of seizure activity and by the presence of abnormal brain wave patterns on the electroencephalogram (EEG). The cause of most cases of epilepsy is unknown. When epilepsy begins in infancy, causes include developmental defects, metabolic disease, or birth injury. When it begins in adulthood, it is usually caused by an acquired brain disorder, such as head injury, disease or infection of the brain and spinal cord, cerebrovascular accident (stroke), metabolic disorder, primary or metastatic brain tumor, or other recognizable neurologic disease.

Epilepsy is classified as partial and generalized seizures. *Partial* or *focal seizures* begin in a specific area of the brain and produce symptoms ranging from simple motor and sensory manifestations to more complex abnormal movements and bizarre behavior. Movements are usually automatic, repetitive, and inappropriate to the situation, such as chewing, swallowing, or aversive movements. Behavior is sometimes so bizarre that the person is diagnosed as psychotic or schizophrenic.

*Generalized seizures* are bilateral and symmetric and have no discernible point of origin in the brain. The most common type is the tonic-clonic or major motor seizure, formerly called grand mal seizures. The tonic phase involves sustained contraction of skeletal muscles; abnormal postures, such as opisthotonos; and absence of respiration, during which the person becomes cyanotic. The clonic phase is characterized by rapid rhythmic and symmetric jerking movements of the body. Tonic-clonic seizures are sometimes preceded by an aura, a brief warning, such as a flash of light or a specific sound.

Another type of generalized seizure is the absence seizure, characterized by abrupt alterations in consciousness that last only a few seconds. The person may have a blank, staring expression with or without blinking of the eyelids, twitching of the head or arms, and other motor movements. Other types of generalized seizures include the myoclonic type (contraction of a muscle or group of muscles) and the akinetic type (absence of movement). Some people are subject to mixed seizures.

*Status epilepticus* is usually a life-threatening emergency characterized by generalized tonic-clonic convul-

Anne Collins Abrams: CLINICAL DRUG THERAPY, Fourth Edition.
© 1995 J.B. Lippincott Company.

sions occurring at close intervals. The client does not regain consciousness between seizures, and hypotension, hypoxia, and cardiac arrhythmias may occur. There is a high risk of permanent brain damage and death unless prompt, appropriate treatment is instituted.

In a person taking medications for a diagnosed seizure disorder, the most common cause of status epilepticus is abruptly stopping anticonvulsant drugs. In other clients, whether they are known to have a seizure disorder or not, causes of status epilepticus include brain trauma or tumors, systemic or central nervous system (CNS) infections, alcohol withdrawal, and overdoses of drugs, such as cocaine, lidocaine, theophylline, and many others.

# Anticonvulsant drugs

Anticonvulsant drugs (also called antiepileptic drugs or AEDs), which belong to several different chemical groups, can control seizure activity but do not cure the underlying disorder. Long-term administration is usually required.

Most anticonvulsant drugs can be taken orally and are absorbed through the intestinal mucosa. The degree of absorption depends on drug solubility and other chemical or enzymatic conversions in the gastrointestinal tract. After absorption, the drugs pass through the liver and undergo transformation by liver enzymes, during which some of the drug is inactivated. All anticonvulsant drugs are metabolized in the liver.

Clinical usage of AEDs has changed during recent years, mostly as a result of research studies. One change is from polytherapy (multiple AEDs) to monotherapy (a single AED) in many cases. This change resulted from evidence that polytherapy greatly increases risks of adverse effects with little increase in therapeutic effects. Another change involves increased usage of some AEDs (*e.g.*, carbamazepine, valproate) and decreased usage of phenobarbital and primidone. Carbamazepine and valproate are as effective as other AEDs when used appropriately. Although serious adverse effects can occur with these drugs, they are considered uncommon. Phenobarbital and primidone are used less often because they produce sedation and cognitive impairment. Phenytoin, ethosuximide, and some benzodiazepines (see Chap. 8) continue to be widely used.

The focus of this chapter is the AEDs named above. Several other drugs are available but are rarely used because of lack of efficacy, serious adverse effects, or both. These drugs, which include mephenytoin (Mesantoin), ethotoin (Peganone), methsuximide (Celontin), phensuximide (Milontin), paramethadione (Paradione), and trimethadione (Tridione) will not be discussed further.

## MECHANISM OF ACTION

Anticonvulsant drugs have similar antiseizure properties, but the precise mechanism and site of action are unclear. It is thought that the drugs act in two ways to control seizure activity. First, they may act directly on abnormal neurons to decrease neuronal excitability and responsiveness to stimuli. Consequently, the seizure threshold is raised, and seizure activity is decreased. Second, and more commonly, they prevent the spread of impulses to normal neurons surrounding the abnormal ones. This helps to prevent or minimize seizures by confining excessive electrical activity to a small portion of the brain.

The drugs' ability to reduce the responsiveness of normal neurons to stimuli may be related to alterations in the activity of sodium, potassium, calcium, and magnesium ions at the cell membrane. Such ionic activity is necessary for normal conduction of nerve impulses, and changes engendered by the anticonvulsant drugs result in stabilized, less responsive cell membranes.

## INDICATIONS FOR USE

The major clinical indication for anticonvulsant drugs is prevention or treatment of seizure activity, especially the chronic recurring seizures of epilepsy. Indications for particular drugs depend on the types of seizures involved.

In addition to maintenance treatment of epilepsy, anticonvulsant drugs also are used to stop acute convulsions and status epilepticus. The drug of choice for this purpose is an intravenous (IV) benzodiazepine, such as diazepam (Valium) or lorazepam (Ativan). Once acute seizure activity is controlled, a longer-acting drug, such as phenytoin, is given to prevent recurrence. Anticonvulsant drugs also are used prophylactically in people with brain trauma from injury or surgery.

## CONTRAINDICATIONS FOR USE

Anticonvulsants are contraindicated or must be used with caution in clients with CNS depression. Phenytoin, ethosuximide, and carbamazepine are contraindicated with hepatic or renal damage and bone marrow depression (*e.g.*, leukopenia, agranulocytosis). Valproic acid is contraindicated with liver disease. Felbamate is contraindicated in clients who have experienced hypersensitivity reactions to the drug.

# Individual anticonvulsant drugs

**Felbamate** (Felbatol), a new anticonvulsant drug, is approved for treatment of partial seizures in adults and partial or generalized seizures in children with Lennox-

Gastaut syndrome (an uncommon seizure disorder that usually occurs in mentally retarded young children with febrile illnesses). In adults, the drug is used alone or in combination with other anticonvulsants; in children, it is used in combination regimens.

Felbamate is well absorbed following oral administration, is about 25% protein bound, and is eliminated in the urine as unchanged drug and metabolites. Adverse effects are reportedly mild to moderate in severity with the most common symptoms being gastrointestinal (anorexia, nausea, vomiting) or CNS (dizziness, drowsiness, headache, and insomnia) in nature in both adults and children.

When adding felbamate to other anticonvulsant drugs, dosage of the other drugs must be reduced 20% to minimize adverse effects.

### Route and dosage ranges

*Adults (14 years and older):* Monotherapy, PO 1200 mg daily in three or four divided doses, increased in 600-mg increments every 2 weeks up to 3600 mg daily

Adjunctive therapy, PO 1200 mg daily in three or four divided doses initially, with dosage of other anticonvulsants reduced by 20%; increased in 1200-mg increments weekly to 3600 mg daily. Additional reductions in dosage of other anticonvulsants may be necessary as dosage of felbamate is increased.

*Children:* Adjunctive therapy, PO 15 mg/kg per day in three or four divided doses, with dosage of other anticonvulsants reduced by 20%; increased in 15 mg/kg per day increments at weekly intervals to 45 mg/kg per day, with additional reductions in dosage of other anticonvulsants

**Phenytoin** (Dilantin) is one of the oldest and most widely used anticonvulsant drugs. It is effective for generalized tonic-clonic and some partial seizures, such as psychomotor seizures. Phenytoin is often the initial drug of choice, especially in adults. It is also used to prevent seizures in people who have had brain surgery or brain injury. Phenytoin is ineffective in absence, myoclonic, or akinetic seizures. The drug also is used occasionally to treat cardiac arrhythmias.

The rate at which phenytoin is metabolized varies, but the average half-life is approximatley 18 to 24 hours. The clinical significance of this relatively long half-life is that phenytoin can be given once or twice daily and that, when it is started at usual maintenance doses, a steady-state concentration in plasma is not reached for about 7 to 21 days. The therapeutic serum level is 5 to 20 μg/ml (SI units 40–80 μmol/L). Concentrations at or above the upper therapeutic range may be associated with clinical signs of toxicity.

### Routes and dosage ranges

*Adults:* PO 100 mg three times daily initially; 300 mg (long-acting) once daily as maintenance
IV 100 mg every 6–8 hours; maximum 50 mg/min
*Children:* PO 4–7 mg/kg per day in divided doses; maximum dose, 300 mg daily

## BARBITURATES

**Phenobarbital** is a long-acting barbiturate that has been widely used alone or combined with another anticonvulsant drug, most often phenytoin. It is most effective in generalized tonic-clonic epilepsy and temporal lobe and other partial seizures. It is less effective in absence seizures and in myoclonic and akinetic epilepsy, but it is sometimes helpful because generalized tonic-clonic seizures may complicate other types of seizures. It also may be used to treat status epilepticus.

Sedation and cognitive impairment commonly occur with phenobarbital and are the main reasons for the drug's declining clinical usage. CNS depression and other adverse effects associated with barbiturates may occur, but drug dependence and barbiturate intoxication are unlikely with usual antiepileptic doses. Because phenobarbital has a long half-life, it takes about 2 to 3 weeks to reach therapeutic serum levels and about 3 to 4 weeks to reach a steady-state concentration. Serum drug levels of 15 to 40 μg/ml (SI units 65–172 μmol/L) are considered in the therapeutic range; higher concentrations are often accompanied by signs and symptoms of toxicity.

**Mephobarbital** (Mebaral) is another long-acting barbiturate used clinically in seizure disorders, usually in children who become hyperactive or hyperexcitable with phenobarbital. For further discussion and anticonvulsant dosages of barbiturates, see Chapter 7.

## BENZODIAZEPINES

**Clonazepam** (Klonopin) may be used alone or with other anticonvulsant drugs in myoclonic or akinetic seizures. It is possibly effective in generalized tonic-clonic and psychomotor seizures. Its effectiveness in absence seizures is variable, but it may be helpful in some clients who do not respond to ethosuximide. Tolerance to anticonvulsant effects develops with long-term use.

Clonazepam has a long half-life and may require weeks of continued administration to achieve therapeutic serum levels. As occurs with other benzodiazepines, clonazepam produces physical dependence and withdrawal symptoms. Because of its long half-life, withdrawal symptoms may appear several days after administration is stopped. Abrupt withdrawal may precipitate seizure activity or status epilepticus. For more discussion of benzodiazepines, see Chapter 8.

### Route and dosage ranges

*Adults:* PO 1.5 mg/d, increased by 0.5 mg/d every 3–7 days if necessary; maximum dose, 20 mg/d

*Children:* PO 0.01–0.03 mg/kg per day, increased by 0.25–0.5 mg/d every 3–7 days if necessary; maximum dose, 0.2 mg/kg per day

**Clorazepate** (Tranxene) is used for anxiety, acute alcohol withdrawal, and adjunctive therapy in the management of partial seizures.

### Route and dosage ranges

*Adults:* Seizures, PO initially no more than 7.5 mg 3 times per day, increased by no more than 7.5 mg/wk; maximum dose, 90 mg/d

*Children 9–12 years:* Seizures, PO initially no more than 7.5 mg twice a day, increased by no more than 7.5 mg/wk; maximum dose, 60 mg/d

**Diazepam** is widely used as an antianxiety or sedative agent. In seizure disorders, it is often used to terminate acute convulsive seizures, especially the life-threatening seizures of status epilepticus. The drug has a short duration of action and must be given in repeated doses. In status epilepticus, it is followed with a long-acting anticonvulsant, such as phenytoin.

### Route and dosage ranges

*Adults:* Acute convulsive seizures, status epilepticus, IV 5–10 mg at no more than 2 mg/min; repeat every 5–10 min if needed; maximum dose, 30 mg. If necessary, repeat regimen in 2–4 h; maximum dose, 100 mg/24 hr.

*Children:* Acute convulsive seizures, status epilepticus, IV (slowly as above), IM 2–5 mg in a single dose; repeat dose in 2–4 h if necessary

**Lorazepam** also is used to terminate acute seizures or status epilepticus. Compared to diazepam, lorazepam is similar in effectiveness, rapid onset of action (about 3 minutes), and adverse effects. However, it has less lipid solubility and tissue binding, so the effects of a single dose last longer.

### Route and dosage ranges

*Adults:* Acute convulsive seizures, status epilepticus, IV 2–10 mg, diluted in an equal amount of sterile water for injection, 0.9% sodium chloride injection, or 5% dextrose in water and injected over 2 min

## MISCELLANEOUS ANTICONVULSANT DRUGS

**Carbamazepine** (Tegretol) is related chemically to the tricyclic antidepressants and pharmacologically to phenytoin. It is used mainly for psychomotor, generalized tonic-clonic, and mixed seizures. It is ineffective for absence, myoclonic, or akinetic seizures. The therapeutic range of serum drug levels is about 4 to 12 μg/ml (SI units, 17–51 μmol/L).

Carbamazepine is contraindicated in clients with previous bone marrow depression or hypersensitivity to carbamazepine or tricyclic antidepressants or clients who are receiving monoamine oxidase (MAO) inhibitors. MAO inhibitors should be discontinued at least 14 days before carbamazepine is started. Carbamazepine also is used to treat facial pain associated with trigeminal neuralgia (tic douloureux).

### Route and dosage ranges

*Adults:* Epilepsy, PO 200 mg twice a day initially, increased gradually to 600–1200 mg if needed in three or four divided doses

Trigeminal neuralgia, PO 200 mg/d initially, increased gradually to 1200 mg if necessary

*Children:* PO 200 mg twice a day initially, gradually increased to 20–30 mg/kg per day if necessary to control seizures

**Ethosuximide** (Zarontin) is the anticonvulsant of choice for absence seizures. It also may be effective in myoclonic and akinetic epilepsy but is usually ineffective in psychomotor and generalized tonic-clonic seizures. Ethosuximide may be used with other anticonvulsants for treatment of mixed seizures. The therapeutic range of serum drug levels is about 40 to 80 μg/ml, and about 5 days of drug administration are necessary to reach a steady-state serum concentration.

### Route and dosage ranges

*Adults:* PO initially 500 mg/d, increased by 250 mg at weekly intervals until seizures are controlled or toxicity occurs; maximum dose, about 1500 mg/d

*Children:* PO initially 250 mg/d, increased as above; maximum dose, about 750–1000 mg/d

**Primidone** (Mysoline) is used for generalized tonic-clonic, psychomotor or partial seizures, alone or with other anticonvulsants. Because it produces marked sedation, primidone is an alternative rather than a primary drug. Excessive sedation is minimized by increasing dosage gradually. Sedation decreases with continued administration of the drug.

Primidone is converted to two metabolites, phenobarbital and phenylethylmalonamide (PEMA). The parent drug and both metabolites exert anticonvulsant effects. Therefore, measurements of plasma drug levels should include all three chemicals. The therapeutic ranges are phenobarbital, 10 to 20 μg/ml; primidone, 5 to 10 μg/ml; and PEMA, 7 to 15 μg/ml.

### Route and dosage ranges

*Adults:* PO 500–1500 mg/d in divided doses

*Children:* PO 5–20 mg/kg per day

**Valproic acid** (Depakene) is used to treat absence and mixed seizures. It is chemically unrelated to other anticonvulsant drugs and produces a much lower incidence of adverse effects. Though uncommon, potentially serious adverse effects include hepatotoxicity and pancreatitis. The drug's mechanism of action is unknown. Therapeutic plasma levels are about 50 to 100 µg/ml (SI units 350–700 µmol/L).

Derivatives of valproic acid include sodium valproate and divalproex sodium (Depakote). Divalproex sodium contains equal parts of valproic acid and sodium valproate. Dosages of all formulations are expressed in valproic acid equivalents.

### Route and dosage ranges

*Adults:* PO 1000–3000 mg/d in divided doses
*Children:* PO 15–30 mg/kg per day

## Nursing Process

### Assessment

Assess client status in relation to seizure activity and other factors:
- If the client has a known seizure disorder and is taking anticonvulsant drugs, helpful assessment data can be obtained by interviewing the client. Some questions and guidelines include the following:
  - How long has the client had the seizure disorder?
  - How long has it been since seizure activity occurred, or what is the frequency of seizures?
  - Does any particular situation or activity seem to cause a seizure?
  - Does an aura warn of an impending seizure?
  - How does the seizure affect the client? For example, what parts of the body are involved? Does he or she lose consciousness? Is he or she drowsy and tired afterward?
  - Which anticonvulsant drugs are taken? How do they affect the client? How long has the client taken the drugs? Is the currently ordered dosage the same as that which the client has been taking? Does the client usually take the drugs as prescribed, or does he or she find it difficult to do so?
  - What other drugs are taken? This includes both prescription and nonprescription drugs, as well as those taken regularly or periodically. This information is necessary because many drugs interact with anticonvulsant drugs to decrease seizure control or increase drug toxicity.
  - What is the client's attitude toward the seizure disorder? Clues to attitude may include terminology, willingness or reluctance to discuss the seizure disorder, compliance or rejection of drug therapy, and others.
- Check reports of serum drug levels for abnormal values.
- People without previous seizure activity may develop seizure disorders with brain surgery, head injury, hypoxia, hypoglycemia, drug overdosage (CNS stimulants, such as amphetamines, or local anesthetics, such as lidocaine),

and withdrawal from CNS depressants, such as alcohol and barbiturates.
- To observe and record seizure activity accurately, note location (localized or generalized); specific characteristics of abnormal movements or behavior; duration; concomitant events, such as loss of consciousness and loss of bowel or bladder control; and postseizure behavior.
- Assess for risk of status epilepticus. Specific risk factors include recent changes in anticonvulsant drug therapy, chronic alcohol ingestion, use of drugs known to cause seizures, and infection.

### Nursing diagnoses

- Ineffective Individual Coping related to anger or denial of the disease process and need for long-term drug therapy
- Self-Esteem Disturbance related to having a seizure disorder
- Impaired Social Interaction related to perceived stigma of epilepsy
- Knowledge Deficit: Disease process
- Knowledge Deficit: Drug effects
- High Risk for Injury: Trauma related to ataxia, drowsiness, confusion
- High Risk for Injury: Seizure activity
- High Risk for Noncompliance: Underuse of medications

### Planning/Goals

*The client will:*
- Take medications as prescribed
- Experience control of seizures
- Avoid adverse drug effects
- Verbalize knowledge of the disease process and treatment regimen
- Avoid discontinuing anticonvulsant medications abruptly
- Keep follow-up appointments with health-care providers

### Interventions

Use measures to minimize seizure activity. Guidelines include the following:
- Help the client identify conditions under which seizures are likely to occur. These precipitating factors, to be avoided or decreased when possible, may include ingestion of alcoholic beverages or stimulant drugs, such as amphetamines; fever; severe physical or emotional stress; and sensory stimuli, such as flashing lights and loud noises.
- Teach the client such health-promotion measures as getting enough rest and exercise and eating a balanced diet.
- Help the client comply with prescribed drug therapy by:
  - Teaching the client and family members about the seizure disorder and the plan for treatment, including drugs
  - Involving the client in decision making when possible
  - Informing the client and family that seizure control is not gained immediately when drug therapy is started. The goal is to avoid unrealistic expectations and excessive frustration while drugs and dosages are being changed in an effort to determine the best combination for the client.
  - Discussing social and economic factors that promote or prevent compliance
- To protect a client experiencing a generalized tonic-clonic seizure:

- Place a pillow or piece of clothing under the head if injury could be sustained from the ground or floor.
- Place a padded tongue depressor, rolled washcloth, or something similar between the teeth to protect the jaws and the tongue. Do not use spoons or similar objects that can be aspirated or increase mouth trauma. If the teeth are clenched tightly, do not try to force them open to insert something. Teeth may be broken off and aspirated.
- Do not restrain the client's movements; fractures may result.
- Loosen tight clothing, especially around the chest, to promote respiration.
- When convulsive movements stop, turn the client to one side so that accumulated secretions can drain from the mouth and the throat. The cyanosis, abnormal movements, and loss of consciousness that characterize a generalized tonic-clonic seizure can be quite alarming to witnesses. Most of these seizures, however, subside within 3 or 4 minutes, and the person starts responding and regaining normal skin color. If the person has one seizure after another (status epilepticus), has trouble breathing or continued cyanosis, or has sustained an injury, further care is needed, and a physician should be notified immediately.
- When risk factors for seizures, especially status epilepticus, are identified, try to prevent or minimize their occurrence.

*Teach clients:*
- To take drugs as prescribed. This is extremely important. These drugs must be taken regularly to maintain blood levels adequate to control seizure activity. At the same time, additional doses must not be taken because of increased risks of serious adverse reactions. Also, these drugs must not be stopped abruptly, or seizures are likely to result.
- To report any difficulties with drug therapy to the prescribing physician or other health-care worker. These difficulties include seizure activity, excessive drowsiness, or other adverse effects. The physician may be able to adjust dosage or time of administration to relieve the problem.
- Not to drive a car, operate machinery, or perform other activities requiring physical and mental alertness when drowsy from anticonvulsant drugs. Drowsiness, sedation, decreased physical coordination, and decreased mental alertness increase the likelihood of injury.
- Not to take other drugs without the physician's knowledge and to inform any other physician or dentist about taking anticonvulsant drugs. There are many potential drug interactions in which the effects of the anticonvulsant drug or other drugs may be altered when drugs are given concomitantly.
- To carry adequate identification, such as a card or a Medic-Alert device, that contains pertinent medical information. This is necessary for rapid and appropriate treatment in the event of a seizure, accidental injury, or other emergency situation.

**Evaluation**
- Interview and observe for decrease or absence of seizure activity.
- Interview and observe for avoidance of adverse drug effects, especially those that impair safety.

# Principles of therapy

## DRUG SELECTION

With drug therapy for epilepsy, the goal is control of seizure activity without severe adverse drug effects. To meet this goal, therapy must be individualized.

1. The choice of drugs is determined largely by the type of seizure. Therefore, an accurate diagnosis is essential before drug therapy is started. For generalized convulsive and focal seizures, phenytoin, carbamazepine, phenobarbital, and valproic acid are effective. For absence seizures, ethosuximide is the drug of choice; clonazepam and valproic acid also are effective. For mixed seizures, a combination of drugs is usually necessary.

   Because most types of seizures can be treated effectively by a variety of drugs, adverse effects of drugs are being increasingly considered an important factor in drug selection. Numerous studies have documented cognitive and psychomotor impairment with the sedating anticonvulsants (*e.g.*, phenobarbital, phenytoin), so carbamazepine and valproic acid are increasingly used. However, carbamazepine and valproic acid may cause other potentially serious adverse effects. Other factors influencing drug choice include drug cost and client willingness to comply with the prescribed regimen.

2. Monotherapy or use of a single drug is recommended when possible. Advantages of monotherapy include better seizure control, fewer adverse drug effects, fewer drug-drug interactions, lower costs, and usually greater client compliance. If adequate doses of a single drug do not control seizures, alternative interventions include reassessing the client for type of seizure or compliance with the prescribed drug therapy, adding a second drug, or substituting another anticonvulsant drug. When substituting, the second drug should be added and allowed to reach therapeutic blood levels before the first drug is gradually decreased in dosage and discontinued.

## DRUG DOSAGE

1. Generally, larger doses are needed for a single drug than for multiple drugs, for people with a large body mass (assuming normal liver and kidney function), and in cases involving trauma, surgery, and emotional stress.
2. Smaller doses are usually required when liver disease is present and when multiple drugs are being given.
3. For most drugs, initial doses are relatively low; doses are gradually increased until seizures are controlled or adverse effects occur.
4. When phenytoin is used, larger doses may be needed

for intramuscular (IM) injection because the drug is deposited in tissues and complete absorption requires about 5 days. The IM route is also very painful. However, phenytoin can be given IM if necessary, preferably for 1 week or less. When substituted for oral phenytoin, the IM dose is 50% larger than the previous oral dose. When oral administration is resumed, the oral dose is about half the dose taken before use of IM phenytoin. This dose can be gradually increased over several days, using serum drug levels as a guide, until the previous oral maintenance dose is reached. If clients are given full oral doses as soon as IM injections are stopped, toxicity may occur because phenytoin is still being absorbed into the bloodstream from injection sites.

## MONITORING DRUG THERAPY

1. The effectiveness of drug therapy is evaluated primarily by client response in terms of therapeutic or adverse effects. Measuring serum drug levels may be helpful in validating drug dosages, assessing client compliance with the prescribed drug therapy regimen, and documenting toxicity or adverse drug effects. Serum drug levels must be interpreted in relation to clinical responses because there are wide variations among individuals receiving similar doses, probably owing to differences in hepatic metabolism. That is, doses should not be increased or decreased solely to maintain a certain serum drug level.

2. Most anticonvulsant drugs have the potential for causing blood, liver, and kidney disorders. For this reason, it is usually recommended that baseline blood studies (complete blood count, platelet count) and liver function tests (e.g., bilirubin, serum protein, aspartate aminotransferase) be performed before drug therapy starts and periodically thereafter.

3. When drug therapy fails to control seizures, there are several possible reasons. Probably the most frequent one is client failure to take the anticonvulsant drug as prescribed. Other common causes include incorrect diagnosis of the type of seizure, use of the wrong drug for the type of seizure, inadequate drug dosage, and too-frequent changes or premature withdrawal of drugs (changing or withdrawing a drug before serum concentration has reached therapeutic levels and before the response can be evaluated properly). Additional causes may include drug overdoses (e.g., theophylline) and severe electrolyte imbalances (e.g., hyponatremia).

## DURATION AND DISCONTINUATION OF THERAPY

Anticonvulsant drug therapy was formerly thought to be lifelong. Now, however, drugs may be discontinued for some clients, usually after a seizure-free period of at least 2 years. Although opinions differ about whether, when, and how the drugs should be discontinued, studies indicate that medications can be stopped in approximately two-thirds of patients whose epilepsy is completely controlled with drug therapy. Advantages of discontinuation include avoiding adverse drug effects and decreasing health care costs; disadvantages include recurrence of seizures, with possible status epilepticus. Even if drugs cannot be stopped completely, periodic attempts to decrease the number or dosage of drugs are probably desirable to minimize adverse reactions. Discontinuing drugs, changing drugs, or changing dosage must be done gradually over 2 to 3 months for each drug and with close medical supervision because sudden withdrawal or dosage decreases may cause status epilepticus. Only one drug should be reduced in dosage or gradually discontinued at a time.

## DRUG THERAPY FOR STATUS EPILEPTICUS

An IV benzodiazepine (e.g., diazepam, lorazepam, or midazolam) is the drug of first choice for rapid control of tonic-clonic seizures. However, seizures often recur within 15 to 20 minutes unless the benzodiazepine is repeated or another, longer-acting drug is given (e.g., IV phenytoin). Because there is a risk of significant respiratory depression with IV benzodiazepines, personnel and supplies for emergency resuscitation must be readily available.

## USE IN CHILDREN

Oral drugs are absorbed slowly and inefficiently in newborns. If an anticonvulsant drug is necessary during the first 7 to 10 days of life, IM phenobarbital is effective. Metabolism and excretion also are delayed during the first 2 weeks of life, but rates become more rapid than those of adults by 2 to 3 months of age. In infants and children, oral drugs are rapidly absorbed and have shorter half-lives. This produces therapeutic serum drug levels earlier in children than in adults. Rates of metabolism and excretion also are increased. Consequently, children require higher doses per kilogram of body weight than adults. The rapid rate of drug elimination persists until about 6 years of age, then decreases until it stabilizes around the adult rate by 10 to 14 years of age. These drugs must be used cautiously to avoid excessive sedation and interference with learning and social development.

## USE IN OLDER ADULTS

Anticonvulsants should be used cautiously in older adults because liver and kidney functions may not be sufficient to metabolize and excrete the drugs. With impaired elimination, the drugs are more likely to accumulate and cause toxic effects unless dosage is reduced.

## NURSING ACTIONS: ANTICONVULSANT DRUGS

| *Nursing Actions* | *Rationale/Explanation* |
| --- | --- |

**1. Administer accurately**

**a.** Give on a regular schedule, about the same time each day.

To maintain therapeutic blood levels of drugs.

**b.** Give oral anticonvulsant drugs after meals or with a full glass of water or other fluid.

Most anticonvulsant drugs cause some gastric irritation, nausea, or vomiting. Taking the drugs with food or fluid helps to decrease gastrointestinal side effects.

**c.** To give phenytoin:

(1) Shake oral suspensions of the drug vigorously before pouring, and always use the same measuring equipment.

When a drug preparation is called a *suspension*, it means that particles of drug are suspended or floating in water or other liquid. On standing, drug particles settle to the bottom of the container. Shaking the container is necessary to achieve a uniform distribution of drug particles in the liquid vehicle. If the contents are not mixed well every time a dose is given, the liquid vehicle will be given initially, and the concentrated drug will be given later. That is, underdosage will occur at first, and little if any therapeutic benefit will result. Overdosage will follow, and the risks of serious toxicity are greatly increased. Using the same measuring container ensures consistent dosage. Calibrated medication cups or measuring teaspoons or tablespoons are acceptable. Regular household teaspoons and tablespoons used for eating and serving are *not* acceptable because sizes vary widely.

(2) Do not mix parenteral phenytoin in the same syringe with any other drug.

Phenytoin solution is highly alkaline (pH approximately 12) and physically incompatible with other drugs. A precipitate occurs if mixing is attempted.

(3) Give phenytoin as an undiluted IV bolus injection at a rate not exceeding 50 mg/min, then flush the IV line with normal saline or dilute in 50 to 100 ml of normal saline (0.9% NaCl) and administer over approximately 30 to 60 minutes. If "piggybacked" into a primary IV line, the primary IV solution must be normal saline or the line must be flushed with normal saline before and after administration of phenytoin. An in-line filter is recommended.

Phenytoin cannot be diluted or given in IV fluids other than normal saline because it precipitates within minutes. Slow administration and dilution decrease local venous irritation from the highly alkaline drug solution. Rapid administration must be avoided because it may produce myocardial depression, hypotension, cardiac arrhythmias, and even cardiac arrest.

(4) Give IM phenytoin deeply into a large muscle mass, and rotate injection sites.

Phenytoin is absorbed slowly when given IM and causes local tissue irritation. Correct administration helps to increase absorption and decrease pain.

**d.** To give carbamazepine and phenytoin suspensions by nasogastric (NG) feeding tube, dilute with an equal amount of water, and rinse the NG tube before and after administration.

Absorption is slow and decreased, possibly because of drug adherence to the NG tube. Dilution and tube irrigation decrease such adherence.

**2. Observe for therapeutic effects**

**a.** When the drug is given on a long-term basis to prevent seizures, observe for a decrease or absence of seizure activity.

Therapeutic effects begin later with anticonvulsant drugs than with most other drug groups because the anticonvulsant drugs have relatively long half-lives. Optimum therapeutic benefits of phenytoin occur about 7 to 10 days after drug therapy is started. Those of phenobarbital occur in about 2 weeks; those of ethosuximide, in about 5 days.

## Nursing Actions

## Rationale/Explanation

**b.** When the drug is given to stop an acute convulsive seizure, seizure activity usually slows or stops within a few minutes.

Diazepam is the drug of choice for controlling an acute convulsion because it acts rapidly. Even when given IV, phenytoin and phenobarbital do not act for several minutes.

**3. Observe for adverse effects**

**a.** CNS effects—drowsiness, sedation, ataxia, diplopia, nystagmus

These effects are common, especially during the first week or two of drug therapy.

**b.** Gastrointestinal effects—anorexia, nausea, vomiting

These common effects of oral drugs can be reduced by taking the drugs with food or a full glass of water.

**c.** Skin disorders—rash, urticaria, exfoliative dermatitis, Stevens-Johnson syndrome (a severe reaction accompanied by headache, arthralgia, and other symptoms in addition to skin lesions)

These may occur with almost all the anticonvulsant drugs. Some are mild; some are potentially serious but rare. Most skin reactions are apparently caused by hypersensitivity or idiosyncratic reactions and are usually sufficient reason to discontinue the drug.

**d.** Blood dyscrasias—anemia, leukopenia, thrombocytopenia, agranulocytosis

Most anticonvulsant drugs produce decreases in the levels of folic acid, which may progress to megaloblastic anemia. The other disorders indicate bone marrow depression and are potentially life-threatening. They do not usually occur with phenytoin, phenobarbital, or primidone but may infrequently occur with most other anticonvulsant drugs.

**e.** Respiratory depression

This is not likely to be a significant adverse reaction except when a depressant drug, such as diazepam or a barbiturate, is given IV to control acute seizures, such as status epilepticus. Even then, respiratory depression can be minimized by avoiding overdosage and rapid administration.

**f.** Liver damage—hepatitis symptoms, jaundice, abnormal liver function tests

Hepatic damage may occur with phenytoin, and fatal hepatotoxicity has been reported with valproic acid.

**g.** Gingival hyperplasia

Occurs often with phenytoin, especially in children. It may be prevented or delayed by vigorous oral hygiene or treated surgically by gingivectomy.

**h.** Hypocalcemia

May occur when anticonvulsant drugs are taken in high doses and over long periods

**i.** Lymphadenopathy resembling malignant lymphoma

This reaction has occurred with several anticonvulsant drugs, most often with phenytoin and other hydantoins.

**4. Observe for drug interactions**

**a.** Drugs that *increase* effects of anticonvulsants:

(1) CNS depressants

Additive CNS depression

(2) Other anticonvulsants

Additive or synergistic effects

**b.** Drugs that *decrease* effects of anticonvulsants:

(1) Tricyclic antidepressants (TCAs), antipsychotic drugs

These drugs may lower the seizure threshold and precipitate seizures. Dosage of anticonvulsant drugs may need to be increased.

(2) Barbiturates and other enzyme inducers

These drugs inhibit themselves and other anticonvulsant drugs by activating liver enzymes and accelerating the rate of drug metabolism.

*(continued)*

## *Nursing Actions*

## *Rationale/Explanation*

**c.** Additional drugs that alter effects of phenytoin:

(1) Alcohol (acute ingestion), allopurinol, amiodarone, benzodiazepines, chloramphenicol, chlorpheniramine, cimetidine, disulfiram, fluconazole, ibuprofen, isoniazid, metronidazole, miconazole, omeprazole, phenothiazine antipsychotic drugs, salicylates, TCAs, and trimethoprim increase effects.

These drugs increase phenytoin toxicity by inhibiting hepatic metabolism of phenytoin or by displacing it from plasma protein binding sites.

(2) Alcohol (chronic ingestion), antacids, antineoplastics, folic acid, loxapine, nitrofurantoin, pyridoxine, rifampin, sucralfate, and theophylline decrease effects.

These drugs decrease effects of phenytoin by decreasing absorption, accelerating metabolism, or by unknown mechanisms.

(3) Phenobarbital has variable interactions with phenytoin.

Phenytoin and phenobarbital have complex interactions with unpredictable effects. Interactions are considered separately because the two drugs are often used at the same time. Although phenobarbital induces drug metabolism in the liver and may increase the rate of metabolism of other anticonvulsant drugs, its interaction with phenytoin differs. Phenobarbital apparently decreases serum levels of phenytoin and perhaps its half-life. Still, the anticonvulsant effects of the two drugs together are greater than those of either drug given alone. The interaction apparently varies with dosage, route, time of administration, the degree of liver enzyme induction already present, and other factors. Thus, whether a significant interaction will occur in a client is unpredictable. Probably the most important clinical implication is that close observation of the client is necessary when either drug is being added or withdrawn.

**d.** Additional drugs that alter effects of carbamazepine:

(1) Cimetidine, erythromycin, isoniazid, and valproic acid increase effects.

These drugs inhibit hepatic drug metabolizing enzymes, thereby increasing blood levels of carbamazepine.

(2) Alcohol, phenytoin, phenobarbital, and primidone decrease effects.

These drugs increase activity of hepatic drug metabolizing enzymes, thereby decreasing blood levels of carbamazepine.

**e.** Additional drugs that alter effects of valproate:

(1) Chlorpromazine, cimetidine, and salicylates increase effects.

These drugs decrease clearance and increase blood levels of valproic acid.

**f.** Interactions with phenobarbital:

(1) Valproic acid

May increase plasma levels of phenobarbital as much as 40%, probably by inhibiting liver-metabolizing enzymes

(2) Other drugs

Many drugs interact with the barbiturates, the drug group of which phenobarbital is a member. These drug interactions are listed in Chapter 7.

**g.** Interactions with clonazepam, clorazepate, lorazepam, and diazepam

These drugs are benzodiazepines, which are discussed in Chapter 8.

**5. Teach clients and parents of children**

**a.** Take anticonvulsant drugs with food or a full glass of fluid.

To avoid nausea, vomiting, and gastric distress, which are adverse reactions to most of these drugs

**b.** When taking phenytoin:

(1) Ask for the same brand and form of the drug when renewing prescriptions.

There may be differences in drugs produced by different manufacturers. These differences, such as how fast and how completely the drug is absorbed into the bloodstream, influence seizure control and likelihood of adverse reactions.

## *Nursing Actions*

## *Rationale/Explanation*

| | |
|---|---|
| (2) If taking or giving a liquid preparation of phenytoin, always mix thoroughly and use the same size medicine cup or measuring spoon. Do not use household teaspoons or tablespoons. | This is necessary to ensure accurate and consistent dosage. Household spoons vary widely in size, and using them leads to inaccurate dosages. |

## Review and Application Exercises

1. For a client with a newly developed seizure disorder, why is it important to verify the type of seizure by EEG before starting anticonvulsant drug therapy?
2. What are the indications for use of the major AEDs?
3. What are the major adverse effects of commonly used AEDs, and how can they be minimized?
4. What are the advantages and disadvantages of treatment with a single drug and of treatment with multiple drugs?
5. Which of the benzodiazepines (antianxiety agents and hypnotics) are used as anticonvulsants?
6. What are the advantages of carbamazepine and valproic acid in comparison with the benzodiazepines, phenytoin, and phenobarbital?
7. What is the treatment of first choice for an acute convulsion or status epilepticus?
8. Why is it important when teaching clients to emphasize that none of the AEDs should be stopped abruptly?

## Selected References

Albers, G. W., & Peroutka, S. J. (1992). Neurologic disorders. In K. L. Melmon, H. F. Morrelli, B. B. Hoffman, & D. W. Nierenberg (Eds.), *Clinical pharmacology: Basic principles in therapeutics* (3rd ed.) (pp. 309–337). New York: McGraw-Hill.

Armstrong, E. P. (1993). Epilepsy. In R. Bressler & M. D. Katz (Eds.), *Geriatric pharmacology* (pp. 289–308). New York: McGraw-Hill.

Asconape, J. J., Penry, J. K., Dreifuss, F. E., Riela, A., & Mirza, W. (1993). Valproate-associated pancreatitis. *Epilepsia, 34*(1), 177–183.

Bader, M. K. (1993). A case study of two methods of administering phenytoin enterally and the subsequent serum phenytoin levels in head-injured patients. *Journal of Neuroscience Nursing, 25*(1), 57–58.

Cascino, G. D. (1993). Antiepileptic drug management in patients with seizure disorders. *Hospital Formulary, 28,* 154–172.

Delgado-Escueta, A. V. (1992). Approach to the patient with seizures. In W. N. Kelley (Ed.), *Textbook of internal medicine* (2nd ed.) (pp. 2311–2317). Philadelphia: J.B. Lippincott.

Dilorio, C., Faherty, B., & Manteuffel, B. (1993). Learning needs of persons with epilepsy: A comparison of perceptions of persons with epilepsy, nurses and physicians. *Journal of Neuroscience Nursing, 25*(1), 22–29.

(1993). *Drug facts and comparisons.* St. Louis: Facts and Comparisons.

Farwell, J. R., Lee, Y. J., Hirtz, D. G., Sulzbacher, S. I., Ellenber, J. H., & Nelson, K. B. (1990). Phenobarbital for febrile seizures: Effects on intelligence and on seizure recurrence. *New England Journal of Medicine, 322,* 364–369.

Garnett, W. R. (1992). Epilepsy. In J. T. DiPiro, R. L. Talbert, P. E. Hayes, G. C. Yee, G. R. Matzke, & L. M. Posey (Eds.), *Pharmacotherapy: A pathophysiologic approach* (2nd ed.) (pp. 879–903). New York: Elsevier.

Guttman, M. (1992). Principles of neuropharmacology. In W. N. Kelley (Ed.), *Textbook of internal medicine* (2nd ed.) (pp. 2255–2259). Philadelphia: J.B. Lippincott.

Guyton, A. C. (1991). *Textbook of medical physiology* (8th ed.). Philadelphia: W.B. Saunders.

Lott, R. S. (1992). Seizure disorders. In M. A. Koda-Kimble & L. Y. Young (Eds.), *Applied therapeutics: The clinical use of drugs* (5th ed.) (pp. 63-1–63-22). Vancouver, WA: Applied Therapeutics.

Meador, K. J., Loring, D. W., Abney, O. L., Allen, M. E., Moore, E. E., Zamrini, E. Y., & King, D. W. (1993). Effects of carbamazepine and phenytoin on EEG and memory in healthy adults. *Epilepsia, 34*(1), 153–157.

Porth, C. M. (1990). *Pathophysiology: Concepts of altered health states* (3rd ed.) (pp. 963–966). Philadelphia: J.B. Lippincott.

Ramsay, R. E. (1993). Treatment of status epilepticus. *Epilepsia, 34*(Suppl. 1), S71–S81.

So, E. L. (1993). Update on epilepsy. *Medical Clinics of North America, 77*(1), 203–214.

### CHAPTER 12

# Antiparkinson Drugs

## Parkinson's disease

Parkinson's disease is a chronic, progressive, degenerative disorder of the central nervous system (CNS) characterized by abnormalities in movement and posture (tremor, bradykinesia, joint and muscular rigidity). It occurs equally in men and women, usually between 50 and 80 years of age. The cause of classic parkinsonism is unknown. Signs and symptoms of the disease also may occur with other CNS diseases or trauma and with the use of antipsychotic drugs.

The basal ganglia in the brain normally contain substantial amounts of dopamine, an inhibitory neurotransmitter, and acetylcholine, an excitatory neurotransmitter. The correct balance of dopamine and acetylcholine is important in regulating posture, muscle tone, and voluntary movement. People with Parkinson's disease suffer an imbalance in these neurotransmitters, resulting in a functional and absolute decrease in brain dopamine and a relative increase in acetylcholine. Other neurotransmitters (*e.g.*, norepinephrine, serotonin) may be involved as well, but their roles have not been elucidated.

## Antiparkinson drugs

Drugs used in Parkinson's disease act to increase levels of dopamine (dopaminergic agents) or inhibit the actions of acetylcholine (anticholinergic agents) in the brain. Thus, the drugs help adjust the balance of neurotransmitters.

### DOPAMINERGIC DRUGS

Levodopa, carbidopa, amantadine, bromocriptine, pergolide, and selegiline increase dopamine concentrations in the brain and exert dopaminergic activity, directly or indirectly. Levodopa is the mainstay of drug therapy for classic or idiopathic parkinsonism. Carbidopa is used only in conjunction with levodopa. The other four drugs are used as adjunctive agents, usually with levodopa.

### ANTICHOLINERGIC DRUGS

Anticholinergic drugs are discussed in Chapter 21 and listed in Table 12-1. They are described here only in relation to their use in the treatment of Parkinson's disease. Only anticholinergic drugs that are centrally active (*i.e.*, penetrate the blood-brain barrier) are useful in treating parkinsonism. Trihexyphenidyl (Artane) is often used. Atropine and scopolamine are centrally active but are not used because of a high incidence of adverse reactions. Synthetic anticholinergic-antispasmodic drugs sometimes used in the treatment of gastrointestinal disorders do not penetrate the blood-brain barrier and thus are ineffective in Parkinson's disease.

In addition to the primary anticholinergic drugs, a phenothiazine (ethopropazine) and two antihistamines (diphenhydramine and orphenadrine) are used for parkinsonism because of their strong anticholinergic effects.

### MECHANISMS OF ACTION

Dopaminergic drugs increase the amount of dopamine in the brain by different mechanisms. Amantadine increases dopamine release and decreases dopamine re-

Anne Collins Abrams: CLINICAL DRUG THERAPY, Fourth Edition.
© 1995 J.B. Lippincott Company.

### TABLE 12-1. ANTICHOLINERGIC ANTIPARKINSON DRUGS

| Generic/Trade Name | Routes and Dosage Ranges (Adults) |
| --- | --- |
| *Primary Agents* | |
| **Benztropine** (Cogentin) | PO 0.5–1 mg at bedtime initially, gradually increased to 4–6 mg daily if necessary |
| **Biperiden** (Akineton) | Parkinsonism, PO 2 mg 3–4 times daily |
| | Drug-induced extrapyramidal reaction, PO 2 mg 1–3 times daily, IM 2 mg repeated q30 minutes if necessary to a maximum of 8 mg in 24 hours |
| **Procyclidine** (Kemadrin) | PO 5 mg twice daily initially, gradually increased to 5 mg 3–4 times daily if necessary |
| **Trihexyphenidyl** (Artane) | PO 1–2 mg daily initially, gradually increased up to 12–15 mg daily, until therapeutic or adverse effects occur |
| | Drug-induced extrapyramidal reactions, PO 1 mg initially, gradually increased to 5–15 mg daily if necessary |
| *Secondary Agents* | |
| **Diphenhydramine hydrochloride** (Benadryl) | PO 25 mg 3 times daily, gradually increased to 50 mg 4 times daily if necessary |
| | Drug-induced extrapyramidal reactions, IM, IV 10–50 mg; maximal single dose, 100 mg; maximal daily dose, 400 mg |
| | Children: Drug-induced extrapyramidal reactions, IM 5 mg/kg per day; maximal daily dose, 300 mg |
| **Ethopropazine hydrochloride** (Parsidol) | PO 50 mg once or twice daily initially, gradually increased to a maximal daily dose of 600 mg if necessary |
| **Orphenadrine hydrochloride** (Disipal) | PO 50 mg 3 times daily initially, gradually increased up to 250 mg daily if necessary and tolerated |

uptake by presynaptic nerve fibers. Bromocriptine and pergolide are dopamine agonists that directly stimulate postsynaptic dopamine receptors. Levodopa is a precursor substance that enters the brain rapidly and is converted to dopamine. Selegiline blocks the enzyme (monoamine oxidase B, or MAO B) that normally inactivates dopamine. Anticholinergic drugs decrease the effects of acetylcholine. This decreases the apparent excess of acetylcholine in relation to the amount of dopamine.

## INDICATIONS FOR USE

A common indication for use is idiopathic or acquired parkinsonism (*e.g.*, postencephalitic). Levodopa, pergolide, and selegiline are used only for parkinsonism; carbidopa is used only to decrease peripheral biotransformation of levodopa. Most of the other drugs have additional uses. For example, amantadine is also used to prevent and treat influenza A viral infections. Bromocriptine is also used in the treatment of amenorrhea and galactorrhea associated with hyperprolactinemia and for suppression of postpartal lactation.

Anticholinergic drugs are used in idiopathic parkinsonism to decrease salivation, spasticity, and tremors. They are used primarily for people who have minimal symptoms, who cannot tolerate levodopa, or in combination with other antiparkinson drugs. Anticholinergic agents also are used to relieve symptoms of parkinsonism that can occur with the use of antipsychotic drugs. If used for this purpose, a course of therapy of about 3 months is recommended, because symptoms usu-

ally subside by then even if the antipsychotic drug is continued.

## CONTRAINDICATIONS FOR USE

Levodopa is contraindicated in clients with narrow-angle glaucoma, hemolytic anemia, severe angina pectoris, transient ischemic attacks, a history of melanoma or undiagnosed skin disorders and in clients who are taking MAO inhibitor drugs. In addition, levodopa must be used with caution in clients with severe cardiovascular, pulmonary, renal, hepatic, or endocrine disorders. Bromocriptine and pergolide are ergot derivatives and therefore contraindicated in people who are hypersensitive to ergot alkaloids or who have uncontrolled hypertension. Selegiline is contraindicated in hypersensitive people.

Anticholinergic drugs are contraindicated in clients with glaucoma, gastrointestinal obstruction, prostatic hypertrophy, urinary bladder neck obstruction, and myasthenia gravis. The drugs must be used cautiously in clients with cardiovascular disorders (*e.g.*, tachycardia, arrhythmias, hypertension) and liver or kidney disease.

## Individual antiparkinson drugs

### DOPAMINERGIC AGENTS

**Levodopa** (Larodopa) is the most effective drug available for the treatment of Parkinson's disease. It relieves all major symptoms of parkinsonism, especially bradykinesia and rigidity. Although levodopa does not alter the underlying disease process, it may improve a client's quality of life.

Levodopa acts to replace dopamine in the basal ganglia of the brain. Dopamine cannot be used for replacement therapy because it does not enter the brain in sufficient amounts. Levodopa, in contrast, readily penetrates the CNS and is converted to dopamine by the enzyme L-aromatic amino acid decarboxylase. The concentration of decarboxylase is greater in peripheral tissues than in the brain. Consequently, most levodopa is biotransformed in peripheral tissues, and large amounts are required to obtain therapeutic levels of dopamine in the brain unless carbidopa also is given. Levodopa and carbidopa are often given together in a fixed-dose formulation called Sinemet, which is available in three dosages: 10 mg carbidopa/100 mg levodopa, 25 mg carbidopa/100 mg levodopa, and 25 mg carbidopa/250 mg levodopa.

Levodopa is well absorbed from the small intestine after oral administration and has a short serum half-life (1–3 hours). Absorption is decreased by delayed gastric emptying, hyperacidity of gastric juice, and competition with amino acids (from digestion of protein foods) for sites of absorption in the small intestine. Levodopa is metabolized to 30 or more metabolites, some of which are pharmacologically active and probably contribute to drug toxicity; the metabolites are excreted primarily in the urine, usually within 24 hours.

Because of side effects and recurrence of parkinsonian symptoms after a few years of levodopa therapy, levodopa is often reserved for clients with significant symptoms and functional disabilities. In addition to treating Parkinson's disease, levodopa also may be useful in other CNS disorders in which symptoms of parkinsonism occur (*e.g.*, juvenile Huntington's chorea, chronic manganese poisoning). Levodopa relieves only parkinsonian symptoms in these conditions.

Levodopa is ineffective in drug-induced extrapyramidal reactions and should not be used for this purpose.

### Route and dosage range

*Adults:* PO 0.5–1 g/d initially in three or four divided doses, increased gradually by increments of 100–500 mg/d, every 3–7 d. The rate of dosage increase depends primarily on the client's tolerance of adverse effects, especially nausea and vomiting. Average daily maintenance dose is 3–6 g/d; maximum dose is 8 g/d. Dosage must be reduced when carbidopa is also given (see carbidopa, below). Therapeutic effects may be increased and adverse effects decreased by frequent administration of small doses.

**Carbidopa** (Lodosyn) inhibits the enzyme L-aromatic amino acid decarboxylase. As a result, less levodopa is decarboxylated in peripheral tissues, more levodopa reaches the brain where it is decarboxylated to dopamine, and much smaller doses of levodopa can be given. Carbidopa does not penetrate the blood-brain barrier. A levodopa-carbidopa fixed-dose combination product (Sinemet) is available (see levodopa, above).

### Route and dosage range

*Adults:* PO initially levodopa 400 mg and carbidopa 40 mg/d in divided doses. This dosage can be gradually increased if necessary to a daily maximum of 2000 mg of levodopa and 200 mg of carbidopa. When carbidopa is added to a regimen of levodopa, the levodopa should be withheld at least 8 h before Sinemet therapy is begun, and dosage should be about 25% of the previous levodopa dosage.

**Amantadine** (Symmetrel) is a synthetic antiviral agent initially used to prevent infection from influenza A virus. Amantadine increases release and inhibits reuptake of dopamine in the brain, thereby increasing dopamine levels. The drug relieves symptoms rapidly, within 1 to 5 days, but it loses efficacy with about 6 to 8 weeks of continuous administration. Consequently, it is usually given for 2- to 3-week periods during initiation of drug therapy with longer-acting agents (*e.g.*, levodopa) or when symptoms worsen. Amantadine is often given in conjunction with levodopa. Compared with other antiparkinson drugs, amantadine is considered less effective than levodopa but more effective than anticholinergic agents.

Amantadine is well absorbed from the gastrointestinal tract and has a relatively long duration of action. It is excreted unchanged in the urine. Dosage must be reduced with impaired renal function to avoid drug accumulation.

### Route and dosage range

*Adults:* PO 100 mg twice a day

**Bromocriptine** (Parlodel) and **pergolide** (Permax) are ergot derivatives that directly stimulate dopamine receptors in the brain. They are used in the treatment of idiopathic or postencephalitic Parkinson's disease, with levodopa-carbidopa, to prolong effectiveness and allow reduced dosage of levodopa. Pergolide has a longer duration of action than bromocriptine and may be effective in some patients who are unresponsive to bromocriptine. Adverse effects are similar for the two drugs.

Bromocriptine

### Route and dosage range

*Adults:* PO 1.25 mg twice a day with meals, increased by 2.5 mg/d every 2–4 wk if necessary for therapeutic benefit. Reduce dose gradually if severe adverse effects occur.

Pergolide

### Route and dosage range

*Adults:* PO 0.05–0.1 mg/d at bedtime, increased by 0.05–0.15 mg every 3 d to a maximum dose of 6 mg/d if necessary

**Selegiline** (Eldepryl), also called deprenyl, increases dopamine in the brain by inhibiting its metabolism by MAO B. MAO has long been known as an important enzyme. In recent years, two types have been differentiated. MAO A metabolizes catecholamines, such as norepinephrine, serotonin, and tyramine; MAO B metabolizes dopamine. Within the brain, most MAO activity is due to type B. The drug's ability to inhibit MAO B selectively may not be evident at higher doses. Selegiline is added when clients experience decreased responsiveness with levodopa-carbidopa. Its addition aids symptom control and allows the dosage of levodopa-carbidopa to be reduced. Overall, therapeutic effects are limited in extent and duration.

### Route and dosage range

*Adults:* PO 5 mg twice daily, morning and noon

## Nursing Process

### Assessment

Assess for signs and symptoms of Parkinson's disease and drug-induced extrapyramidal reactions. These may include the following, depending on the severity and stage of progression:
- Slow movements (bradykinesia) and difficulty in changing positions, assuming an upright position, eating, dressing, and other self-care activities
- Stooped posture
- Accelerating gait with short steps
- Tremor at rest (*e.g.,* "pill rolling" movements of fingers)
- Rigidity of arms, legs, and neck
- Mask-like, immobile facial expression
- Speech problems (*e.g.,* low volume, monotonous tone, rapid, difficult to understand)
- Excessive salivation and drooling
- Dysphagia
- Excessive sweating
- Constipation from decreased intestinal motility
- Mental depression from self-consciousness and embarrassment over physical appearance and activity limitations. The intellect is usually intact until the late stages of the disease process.

### Nursing diagnoses

- Self-Care Deficit: Total, related to tremors and impaired motor function
- Impaired Physical Mobility related to alterations in balance and coordination
- Body Image Disturbance related to disease and disability

- Knowledge Deficit: Safe usage and effects of antiparkinson drugs
- Alteration in Thought Processes related to impaired mentation
- Altered Nutrition: Less than Body Requirements related to difficulty in chewing and swallowing food
- High Risk for Injury: Dizziness, hypotension related to adverse drug effects

### Planning/Goals

*The client will:*
- Experience relief of excessive salivation, muscle rigidity, spasticity, and tremors
- Experience improved motor function, mobility, and self-care abilities
- Experience improvement of self-concept and body image
- Increase knowledge of the disease process and drug therapy
- Take medications as instructed
- Avoid falls and other injuries from the disease process or drug therapy

### Interventions

Use measures to assist the client and family in coping with symptoms and maintaining function. These include the following:
- Provide physical therapy for heel-to-toe gait training, widening stance to increase balance and base of support, other exercises.
- Encourage ambulation and frequent changes of position, assisted if necessary.
- Help with active and passive range-of-motion exercises.
- Encourage self-care as much as possible. Cutting meat, opening cartons, frequent small meals, and allowing privacy during mealtime may be helpful. If the client has difficulty chewing or swallowing, chopped or soft foods may be necessary. Velcro-type fasteners or zippers are easier to handle than buttons. Slip-on shoes are easier to manage than laced ones.
- Spend time with the client and encourage socialization with other people. Victims of Parkinson's disease tend to become withdrawn, isolated, and depressed.
- Schedule rest periods. Tremor and rigidity are aggravated by fatigue and emotional stress.
- Provide facial tissues if drooling is a problem.

*Teach clients:*
- Not to take other drugs without the physician's knowledge and consent. This is necessary to avoid adverse drug interactions. Prescription and nonprescription drugs may interact with antiparkinson drugs to increase or decrease effects.
- To avoid driving an automobile or operating other potentially hazardous machinery if vision is blurred or drowsiness occurs with levodopa
- To change positions slowly, especially when assuming an upright position, and to wear elastic stockings if needed

### Evaluation

- Interview and observe for relief of symptoms.
- Interview and observe for increased mobility and participation in activities of daily living.
- Interview and observe regarding correct usage of medications.

# Principles of therapy

## GOAL OF TREATMENT

The goal of antiparkinson drug therapy is to control symptoms and improve the client's ability to perform activities of daily living.

## DRUG SELECTION AND DOSAGE

The choice of antiparkinson drug depends on the type of parkinsonism (idiopathic or drug-induced) and the severity of symptoms.

1. Anticholinergic agents may be the drugs of choice for early idiopathic parkinsonism, when symptoms are relatively mild, and for drug-induced symptoms. These agents are most effective in decreasing salivation and tremor.
2. Levodopa and carbidopa are the drugs of choice in idiopathic parkinsonism when bradykinesia and rigidity are prominent symptoms.
3. Combination drug therapy may be preferred for many clients. Two advantages of combination therapy are better control of symptoms and reduced dosage of individual drugs. Anticholinergic drugs may be given with levodopa alone or with a levodopa-carbidopa combination. Amantadine, bromocriptine pergolide, and selegiline are usually used as adjuncts to levodopa-carbidopa.

## DRUG DOSAGE

The dosage of antiparkinson drugs is highly individualized. The general rule is to start with a low initial dose and gradually increase dosage until therapeutic effects, adverse effects, or maximum drug dosage is achieved. Optimal dosage may not be established for 6 to 8 weeks with levodopa. When combinations of drugs are used, dosage adjustments of individual components are sometimes necessary. When levodopa is added to a regimen of anticholinergic drug therapy, for example, the anticholinergic drug need not be discontinued or reduced in dosage. However, when carbidopa is given with levodopa, the dosage of levodopa must be reduced by about 75%. Dosage of levodopa-carbidopa is also reduced when adjunctive dopaminergic drugs are added.

## USE IN CHILDREN

Safety and effectiveness for use in children have not been established for most antiparkinson drugs, including the centrally acting anticholinergics (all ages), levodopa (under 12 years), and bromocriptine (under 15 years).

Because parkinsonism is a degenerative disorder of adults, antiparkinson drugs are most likely to be used for other purposes in children. Amantadine, for influenza A prevention or treatment, is not recommended for neonates or infants under 1 year old but may be given to children 9 to 12 years old.

## USE IN OLDER ADULTS

When amantadine is given to older adults, dosage may need to be reduced. Because about 90% of a dose is excreted unchanged in the urine and renal function is usually decreased in older adults, there is a risk of accumulation and toxicity. Dosage reduction is recommended for people with creatinine clearance under 80 ml/min.

Anticholinergic drugs may cause dry mouth, tachycardia, urinary retention, blurred vision, mental confusion, and delirium. They also decrease sweating and the ability to adapt to high environmental temperatures; consequences may be fever or heat stroke. Fever may occur in any age group, but heat stroke is more likely to occur in older adults, especially with cardiovascular disease, strenuous activity, and high environmental temperatures.

When centrally active anticholinergics, such as trihexyphenidyl and benztropine (Cogentin) are given for Parkinson's disease, mental confusion, agitation, hallucinations, and psychotic-like symptoms may occur. Dosage should be carefully regulated and supervised.

In addition to the primary anticholinergic agents, many other drugs have significant anticholinergic activity. These include many antihistamines (histamine-1 receptor antagonists), tricyclic antidepressants, and phenothiazine antipsychotic drugs.

# NURSING ACTIONS: ANTIPARKINSON DRUGS

| *Nursing Actions* | *Rationale/Explanation* |
|---|---|
| **1. Administer accurately**<br>**a.** Give levodopa and bromocriptine with or just after food intake. | To prevent or reduce anorexia, nausea, and vomiting |
| **b.** Give selegiline in the morning and at noon. | To decrease central nervous system (CNS) stimulating effects that may interfere with sleep if the drug is taken in the evening |
| **2. Observe for therapeutic effects**<br>**a.** With anticholinergic agents, observe for decreased tremor, salivation, drooling, and sweating. | Decreased salivation and sweating are therapeutic effects when these drugs are used in Parkinson's disease, but they are adverse effects when the drugs are used in other disorders. |
| **b.** With levodopa, observe for improvement in mobility, balance, posture, gait, speech, handwriting, and self-care ability. Drooling and seborrhea may be abolished, and mood may be elevated. | Therapeutic effects are usually evident within 2 to 3 weeks, as dosage approaches 2 to 3 g/d, but may not reach optimum levels for 6 months. |
| **3. Observe for adverse effects**<br>**a.** With anticholinergic drugs, observe for atropine-like effects, such as: | |
| (1) Tachycardia and palpitations | These effects may occur with usual therapeutic doses but are not likely to be serious except in people with underlying heart disease. |
| (2) Excessive CNS stimulation (tremor, restlessness, confusion, hallucinations, delirium) | This effect is most likely to occur with large doses of trihexyphenidyl (Artane) or benztropine (Cogentin). It may occur with levodopa. |
| (3) Sedation and drowsiness | These are most likely to occur with benztropine. The drug has antihistaminic and anticholinergic properties, and sedation is attributed to the antihistamine effect. |
| (4) Constipation, impaction, paralytic ileus | These effects result from decreased gastrointestinal motility and muscle tone. They may be severe because decreased intestinal motility and constipation also are characteristics of Parkinson's disease; thus, additive effects may occur. |
| (5) Urinary retention | This reaction is caused by loss of muscle tone in the bladder and is most likely to occur in elderly men who have enlarged prostate glands. |
| (6) Dilated pupils (mydriasis), blurred vision, photophobia | Ocular effects are due to paralysis of accommodation and relaxation of the ciliary muscle and the sphincter muscle of the iris. |
| **b.** With levodopa, observe for:<br>(1) Anorexia, nausea, and vomiting | These symptoms usually disappear after a few months of drug therapy. They may be minimized by giving levodopa with food, gradually increasing dosage, administering smaller doses more frequently, or adding carbidopa so that dosage of levodopa can be reduced. |
| (2) Orthostatic hypotension—check blood pressure in both sitting and standing positions q4h while the client is awake. | This effect is common during the first few weeks but usually subsides eventually. It can be minimized by arising slowly from supine or sitting positions and by wearing elastic stockings. |

*(continued)*

| Nursing Actions | Rationale/Explanation |
|---|---|
| (3) Cardiac arrhythmias (tachycardia, premature ventricular contractions) and increased myocardial contractility | Levodopa and its metabolites stimulate beta-adrenergic receptors in the heart. People with preexisting coronary artery disease may need a beta-adrenergic blocking agent (*e.g.*, propranolol) to counteract these effects. |
| (4) Dyskinesia—involuntary movements that may involve only the tongue, mouth, and face or the whole body | Dyskinesia eventually develops in most people who take levodopa. It is related to duration of levodopa therapy rather than dosage. Carbidopa may heighten this adverse effect, and there is no way to prevent it except by decreasing levodopa dosage. Many people prefer dyskinesia to lowering drug dosage and subsequent return of the parkinsonism symptoms. |
| (5) CNS stimulation—restlessness, agitation, confusion, delirium | This is more likely to occur with levodopa-carbidopa combination drug therapy. |
| (6) Abrupt swings in motor function (on–off phenomenon) | This fluctuation may indicate progression of the disease process. It often occurs after long-term levodopa use. |
| **c.** With amantadine, observe for: | |
| (1) CNS stimulation—insomnia, hyperexcitability, ataxia, dizziness, slurred speech, mental confusion, hallucinations | Compared with other antiparkinson drugs, amantadine produces few adverse effects. The ones that occur are mild, transient, and reversible. However, adverse effects increase if daily dosage exceeds 200 mg. |
| (2) Livedo reticularis—patchy, bluish discoloration of skin on the legs | This is a benign but cosmetically unappealing condition. It usually occurs with long-term use of amantadine and disappears when the drug is discontinued. |
| **d.** With bromocriptine and pergolide observe for: | |
| (1) Nausea | These symptoms are usually mild and can be minimized by starting with low doses and increasing the dose gradually until the desired effect is achieved. If adverse effects do occur, they usually disappear with a decrease in dosage. |
| (2) Confusion and hallucinations | |
| (3) Hypotension | |
| **e.** With selegiline, observe for: | |
| (1) CNS effects—agitation, ataxia, bradykinesia, confusion, dizziness, dyskinesias, hallucinations, insomnia | |
| (2) Nausea, abdominal pain | |
| **4. Observe for drug interactions** | |
| **a.** Drugs that *increase* effects of anticholinergic drugs: Antihistamines, disopyramide (Norpace, an antiarrhythmic agent), phenothiazines, thioxanthene agents, and tricyclic antidepressants | These drugs have anticholinergic properties and produce additive anticholinergic effects. |
| **b.** Drugs that *decrease* effects of anticholinergic drugs: Cholinergic agents | These drugs counteract the inhibition of gastrointestinal motility and tone, which is a side effect of anticholinergic drug therapy. |
| **c.** Drugs that *increase* effects of levodopa: | |
| (1) Amantadine, anticholinergic agents, bromocriptine, carbidopa, pergolide, selegiline | These drugs are often used in combination for treatment of Parkinson's disease. |
| (2) Tricyclic antidepressants | These drugs potentiate levodopa effects and increase the risk of cardiac arrhythmias in people with heart disease. |

## Nursing Actions

## Rationale/Explanation

(3) MAO-A inhibitors, including isocarboxazid (Marplan), phenelzine (Nardil), and tranylcypromine (Parnate)

The combination of a catecholamine precursor (levodopa) and MAO-A inhibitors that decrease metabolism of catecholamines can result in excessive amounts of dopamine, epinephrine, and norepinephrine. Heart palpitations, headache, hypertensive crisis, and stroke may occur. Levodopa and MAO-A inhibitors should *not* be given concurrently. Also, levodopa should not be started within 3 weeks after an MAO-A inhibitor is discontinued. Effects of MAO-A inhibitors persist for 1 to 3 weeks after their discontinuation.

These effects are unlikely to occur with selegiline, an MAO-B inhibitor, which more selectively inhibits the metabolism of dopamine. However, selectivity may be lost at doses higher than the recommended 10 mg/d. Selegiline is used with levodopa.

d. Drugs that *decrease* effects of levodopa:

(1) Anticholinergics

Although anticholinergics are often given with levodopa for increased antiparkinson effects, they also may decrease effects of levodopa by delaying gastric emptying. This causes more levodopa to be metabolized in the stomach and decreases the amount available for absorption from the intestine.

(2) Alcohol, antianxiety agents (*e.g.*, diazepam [Valium] and probably other benzodiazepines), antiemetics, antipsychotic agents (phenothiazines, butyrophenones, thioxanthenes)

The mechanisms by which most of these drugs decrease effects of levodopa are not clear. Phenothiazines block dopamine receptors in the basal ganglia.

(3) Oral iron preparations

Iron binds with levodopa and reduces levodopa absorption, possibly as much as 50%.

(4) Pyridoxine (vitamin $B_6$)

Pyridoxine stimulates decarboxylase, the enzyme that converts levodopa to dopamine. As a result, more levodopa is metabolized in peripheral tissues, and less reaches the CNS, where antiparkinson effects occur. This interaction does not occur when carbidopa is given with levodopa.

e. Drugs that decrease effects of dopaminergic antiparkinson drugs

(1) Antipsychotic drugs

(2) Metoclopramide

These drugs are dopamine antagonists and therefore inhibit the effects of dopamine agonists.

5. **Teach clients**

a. Excessive mouth dryness can be minimized by maintaining an adequate fluid intake (2000–3000 ml daily if not contraindicated) and using sugarless chewing gum and hard candies.

Both anticholinergics and levodopa may cause mouth dryness. This is usually a therapeutic effect in Parkinson's disease. However, excessive mouth dryness (xerostomia) causes discomfort and dental caries.

b. Limit intake of alcohol and high-protein foods (*e.g.*, meat, poultry, fish, milk, eggs, cheese, nuts). Do not take multivitamin preparations that contain vitamin $B_6$.

Alcohol, protein, and vitamin $B_6$ decrease the therapeutic effects of levodopa alone but not the effects of levodopa-carbidopa in combination. Larobec is a multivitamin preparation available without vitamin $B_6$.

c. Report adverse effects.

Adverse effects can often be reduced by changing drugs or dosages. However, some adverse effects usually must be tolerated for control of disease symptoms.

## Review and Application Exercises

1. Which neurotransmitter is deficient in idiopathic and drug-induced parkinsonism?
2. How do the antiparkinson drugs act to alter the level of the deficient neurotransmitter?
3. What are the advantages and disadvantages of the various drugs used to treat parkinsonism?
4. What are the major adverse effects of antiparkinson drugs, and how can they be minimized?
5. What is the rationale for combining carbidopa with levodopa?

## Selected References

Albers, G. W., & Peroutka, S. J. (1992). Neurologic disorders. In K. L. Melmon, H. F. Morrelli, B. B. Hoffman, & D. W. Nierenberg, (Eds.), *Clinical pharmacology: Basic principles in therapeutics* (3rd ed.) (pp. 309–337). New York: McGraw-Hill.

(1993). *Drug facts and comparisons.* St. Louis: Facts and Comparisons.

Flaherty, J. F. (1992). Parkinson's disease. In M. A. Koda-Kimble & L. Y. Young (Eds.), *Applied therapeutics: The clinical use of drugs* (5th ed.) (pp. 62-1–62-14). Vancouver, WA: Applied Therapeutics.

Guttman, M. (1992). Principles of neuropharmacology. In W. N. Kelley (Ed.), *Textbook of internal medicine* (2nd ed.) (pp. 2255–2259). Philadelphia: J.B. Lippincott.

Montgomery, E. B., & Lipsy, R. J. (1993). Treatment of Parkinson's disease. In R. Bressler & M. D. Katz (Eds.), *Geriatric pharmacology.* New York: McGraw-Hill.

Siemers, E. (1992). Recent progress in the treatment of Parkinson's disease. *Comprehensive Therapy, 18*(9), 20–24.

Tsui, J. K., & Calne, D. B. (1992). Approach to the patient with abnormal movements and posture, including cerebellar ataxia. In W. N. Kelley (Ed.), *Textbook of internal medicine* (2nd ed.) (pp. 2321–2323). Philadelphia: J.B. Lippincott.

### CHAPTER 13

# Skeletal Muscle Relaxants

## Skeletal muscle relaxants

Skeletal muscle relaxants are used to decrease muscle spasm or spasticity that occurs in certain neurologic and musculoskeletal disorders. (Neuromuscular blocking agents used as adjuncts to general anesthesia for surgery are discussed in Chapter 14.)

*Muscle spasm* is sudden movement that may involve alternating contraction and relaxation (clonic) or sustained contraction (tonic). Muscle spasm may occur with musculoskeletal trauma or inflammation (*e.g.*, sprains, strains, bursitis, arthritis). It is also encountered with acute or chronic low back pain, a common condition that is primarily a disorder of posture.

*Spasticity* involves increased muscle tone or contraction, which produces stiff, awkward movements. Spasticity results from neurologic disorders, such as cerebral palsy, stroke, paraplegia, spinal cord injury, and multiple sclerosis.

### MECHANISM OF ACTION

Almost all skeletal muscle relaxants are centrally active agents. Pharmacologic action is probably caused by general depression of the central nervous system (CNS) but may result from blockage of nerve impulses that cause increased muscle tone and contraction. It is unclear whether relief of pain results from sedative effects, muscular relaxation, or a placebo effect. In addition, although parenteral administration of some drugs (*e.g.*, diazepam [Valium], methocarbamol [Robaxin]) relieves pain associated with acute musculoskeletal trauma or inflammation, it is uncertain whether oral administration of usual doses exerts a beneficial effect in acute or chronic disorders. Dantrolene (Dantrium) is the only skeletal muscle relaxant that acts peripherally on the muscle itself.

### INDICATIONS FOR USE

Skeletal muscle relaxants are recommended for use primarily as adjuncts to other treatment measures. Occasionally, parenteral agents are given to facilitate various orthopedic procedures and examinations. In spastic disorders, skeletal muscle relaxants are not generally indicated for use only to relieve spasticity. However, they may be indicated when spasticity causes severe pain or inability to tolerate physical therapy, sit in a wheelchair, or participate in self-care activities of daily living (eating, dressing, and so forth). Drugs should not be given if they cause excessive muscle weakness and impair rather than facilitate mobility and function.

Dantrolene also is indicated for prevention and treatment of malignant hyperthermia, a rare but life-threatening complication of anesthesia characterized by hypercarbia, metabolic acidosis, skeletal muscle rigidity, fever, and cyanosis. For preoperative prophylaxis in people with previous episodes of malignant hyperthermia, the drug is given orally for 1 to 2 days before surgery. For intraoperative malignant hyperthermia, the drug is given intravenously. Postoperatively, following occurrences, the drug is given orally for 1 to 3 days to prevent recurrence of symptoms.

Anne Collins Abrams: CLINICAL DRUG THERAPY, Fourth Edition.
© 1995 J.B. Lippincott Company.

## CONTRAINDICATIONS FOR USE

Most skeletal muscle relaxants cause CNS depression and have the same contraindications as other CNS depressants. They should be used cautiously in the presence of impaired renal or hepatic function, respiratory depression, and in clients who need to be alert for activities of daily living (*i.e.*, driving a car, operating potentially hazardous machinery). Orphenadrine and cyclobenzaprine have high levels of anticholinergic activity and therefore should be used cautiously with glaucoma, urinary retention, cardiac arrhythmias, or tachycardia.

Individual skeletal muscle relaxants are listed in Table 13-1.

## Nursing Process

### Assessment

Assess for muscle spasm and spasticity.
- With muscle spasm, assess for:
  - **Pain**. This is a prominent symptom of muscle spasm and is usually aggravated by movement. Try to determine the location as specifically as possible, as well as the intensity, duration, and precipitating factors (*i.e.*, traumatic injury, strenuous exercise).
  - **Accompanying signs and symptoms**, such as bruises (ecchymoses), edema, or signs of inflammation (redness, heat, edema, tenderness to touch).
- With spasticity, assess for pain and impaired functional ability in self-care (*e.g.*, eating, dressing). In addition, severe spasticity interferes with physical therapy exercises to maintain joint and muscle mobility.

### Nursing diagnoses

- Pain related to muscle spasm
- Impaired Physical Mobility related to spasm and pain
- Self-Care Deficit related to spasm and pain
- Knowledge Deficit: Nondrug measures to relieve muscle spasm, pain, and spasticity
- Knowledge Deficit: Safe usage and effects of skeletal muscle relaxants
- High Risk for Injury: Dizziness, sedation related to CNS depression

### Planning/Goals

*The client will:*
- Experience relief of pain and spasm
- Experience improved motor function

### TABLE 13-1.  SKELETAL MUSCLE RELAXANTS

| Generic/Trade Name | Routes and Dosages Ranges | |
| --- | --- | --- |
| | *Adults* | *Children* |
| **Baclofen** (Lioresal) | PO 5 mg 3 times daily initially, increased to 10 mg 3 times daily after 3 days, then gradually increased further if necessary; maximal dose, 20 mg 4 times daily<br>Dosage must be reduced in the presence of impaired renal function | Under age 12 years, not recommended |
| **Carisoprodol** (Rela, Soma) | PO 350 mg 4 times daily | Age 5 years and over, PO 25 mg/kg per day in 4 divided doses |
| **Chlorphenesin** (Maolate) | PO 800 mg 3 times daily until desired effect attained, then 400 mg 4 times daily or less for maintenance as needed | Dosage not established |
| **Chlorzoxazone** (Paraflex) | PO 250–750 mg 3 or 4 times daily | PO 20 mg/kg per day in 3 or 4 divided doses |
| **Cyclobenzaprine** (Flexeril) | PO 10 mg 3 times daily. Maximal recommended duration, 3 weeks; maximal recommended dose, 60 mg daily | |
| **Dantrolene** (Dantrium) | PO 25 mg daily initially, gradually increased weekly (by increments of 50–100 mg/d) to a maximal dose of 400 mg daily in 4 divided doses | PO 1 mg/kg per day initially, gradually increased to a maximal dose of 3 mg/kg 4 times daily, not to exceed 400 mg daily |
| | Preoperative prophylaxis of malignant hyperthermia: PO 4–8 mg/kg per day in 3–4 divided doses for 1 or 2 days before surgery<br>Intraoperative malignant hyperthermia: IV push 1 mg/kg initially, continued until symptoms are relieved or a maximum total dose of 10 mg/kg has been given<br>Postcrisis follow-up treatment: PO 4–8 mg/kg per day in 4 divided doses for 1–3 days | Same as adult |
| **Diazepam** (Valium) | PO 2–10 mg 3 or 4 times daily<br>IM, IV 5–10 mg repeated in 3–4 hours if necessary | PO 0.12–0.8 mg/kg per day in 3 or 4 divided doses<br>IM, IV 0.04–0.2 mg/kg in a single dose, not to exceed 0.6 mg/kg within an 8-hour period |
| **Metaxalone** (Skelaxin) | PO 800 mg 3 or 4 times daily for not more than 10 consecutive days | |
| **Methocarbamol** (Robaxin) | PO 1.5–2 g 4 times daily for 48–72 hours, reduced to 1.0 g 4 times daily for maintenance<br>IM 500 mg q8h<br>IV 1–3 g daily at a rate not to exceed 300 mg/minute (3 ml of 10% injection). Do not give IV more than 3 days. | PO, IM, IV 60–75 mg/kg per day in 4 divided doses |
| **Orphenadrine citrate** (Norflex) | PO 100 mg twice daily<br>IM, IV 60 mg twice daily | |

- Increase self-care abilities in activities of daily living
- Take medications as instructed
- Use nondrug measures appropriately
- Be safeguarded when sedated from drug therapy

### Interventions

*Use adjunctive measures for muscle spasm and spasticity:*

- Physical therapy (massage, moist heat, exercises)
- Bed rest for acute muscle spasm
- Relaxation techniques
- Correct posture and lifting techniques (*e.g.*, stooping rather than bending to lift objects, holding heavy objects close to the body, and *not* lifting excessive amounts of weight)
- Regular exercise programs and use of warm-up exercises. Strenuous exercise performed on an occasional basis (*e.g.*, weekly or monthly) is more likely to cause acute muscle spasm.

*Teach clients:*

- How to use nondrug measures, such as exercises and applications of heat and cold, to decrease muscle spasm and spasticity
- Not to attempt activities that require mental alertness or physical coordination (*e.g.*, driving an automobile, operating potentially dangerous machinery) if drowsy from medication
- Not to take other drugs without the physician's knowledge, including nonprescription drugs. The major risk occurs with concurrent use of alcohol, antihistamines, sleeping aids, or other drugs that cause drowsiness.

### Evaluation

- Interview and observe for relief of symptoms.
- Interview and observe regarding correct usage of medications and nondrug therapeutic measures.

## Principles of therapy

### GOAL OF TREATMENT

The goal of treatment is to relieve pain, muscle spasm, and muscle spasticity without impairing the ability to perform self-care activities of daily living.

### DRUG SELECTION

Choice of a skeletal muscle relaxant depends primarily on the disorder being treated:

1. For acute muscle spasm and pain, a drug that can be given parenterally (*e.g.*, diazepam, methocarbamol) is usually the drug of choice.
2. Parenteral agents are preferred for orthopedic procedures because they have greater sedative and pain-relieving effects.
3. Baclofen (Lioresal) is approved for treatment of spasticity in people with multiple sclerosis. It is variably effective, and its clinical usefulness may be limited by adverse reactions. Baclofen is not recommended for pregnant women or children under 12 years of age.
4. None of the skeletal muscle relaxants has been established as safe for use during pregnancy and lactation.
5. Many of the skeletal muscle relaxants have not been established as safe for use in children. Choice of drug should be limited to those with established pediatric dosages.

### USE IN CHILDREN

For most of the drugs, safety and effectiveness for use in children 12 years and younger have not been established. The drugs should be used only when clearly indicated, for short periods of time, when close supervision is available for monitoring drug effects (especially sedation), and when mobility and alertness are not required.

### USE IN OLDER ADULTS

Any CNS depressant or sedating drugs should be used cautiously in older adults. Risks of falls, mental confusion, and other adverse effects are generally higher in older adults because of impaired drug metabolism and excretion.

---

## NURSING ACTIONS: SKELETAL MUSCLE RELAXANTS

| *Nursing Actions* | *Rationale/Explanation* |
|---|---|
| **1. Administer accurately**<br>**a.** Give baclofen, chlorphenesin, chlorzoxazone, metaxalone with milk or food. | To decrease gastrointestinal distress |
| **b.** Do not mix parenteral diazepam in a syringe with any other drugs. | Diazepam is physically incompatible with other drugs. |

*(continued)*

| Nursing Actions | Rationale/Explanation |
|---|---|
| **c.** Inject IV diazepam directly into a vein or the injection site nearest the vein (during continuous IV infusions) at a rate of about 2 mg/min. | Diazepam may cause a precipitate if diluted. Avoid contact with IV solutions as much as possible. A slow rate of injection minimizes the risks of respiratory depression and apnea. |
| **d.** Avoid extravasation with IV diazepam, and inject IM diazepam deeply into a gluteal muscle. | To prevent or reduce tissue irritation |
| **e.** With IV methocarbamol, inject or infuse slowly. | Rapid administration may cause bradycardia, hypotension, and dizziness. |
| **f.** With IV methocarbamol, have the client lie down during and at least 15 minutes after administration. | To minimize orthostatic hypotension and other adverse drug effects |
| **g.** Avoid extravasation with IV methocarbamol, and give IM methocarbamol deeply into a gluteal muscle. (Dividing the dose and giving two injections is preferred.) | Parenteral methocarbamol is a hypertonic solution that is very irritating to tissues. Thrombophlebitis may occur at IV injection sites, and sloughing of tissue may occur at sites of extravasation or IM injections. |
| **2. Observe for therapeutic effects**<br>**a.** When the drug is given for acute muscle spasm, observe for: | Therapeutic effects usually occur within 30 minutes after IV injection of diazepam or methocarbamol. |
| (1) Decreased pain and tenderness | |
| (2) Increased mobility | |
| (3) Increased ability to participate in activities of daily living | |
| **b.** When the drug is given for spasticity in chronic neurologic disorders, observe for: | |
| (1) Increased ability to maintain posture and balance | |
| (2) Increased ability for self-care (*e.g.,* eating and dressing) | |
| (3) Increased tolerance for physical therapy and exercises | |
| **3. Observe for adverse effects**<br>**a.** With centrally active agents, observe for: | |
| (1) Drowsiness and dizziness | These are the most common adverse effects. |
| (2) Blurred vision, lethargy, flushing | These effects occur more often with IV administration of drugs. They are usually transient. |
| (3) Nausea, vomiting, abdominal distress, constipation or diarrhea, ataxia, areflexia, flaccid paralysis, respiratory depression, tachycardia, hypotension | These effects are most likely to occur with large oral doses. |
| (4) Hypersensitivity—skin rash, pruritus | The drug should be discontinued if hypersensitivity reactions occur. Serious allergic reactions (*e.g.,* anaphylaxis) are rare. |
| (5) Psychological or physical dependence with diazepam and other antianxiety agents | Most likely to occur with long-term use of large doses |
| **b.** With a peripherally active agent (dantrolene), observe for: | Adverse effects are usually transient. |
| (1) Drowsiness, fatigue, lethargy, weakness, nausea, vomiting | These effects are the most common. |
| (2) Headache, anorexia, nervousness | Less common effects |

| *Nursing Actions* | *Rationale/Explanation* |
|---|---|
| (3) Hepatotoxicity | This potentially serious adverse effect is most likely to occur in people more than 35 years of age who have taken the drug 60 days or longer. Women over 35 who take estrogens have the highest risk. Hepatotoxicity can be prevented or minimized by administering the lowest effective dose, monitoring liver enzymes (aspartate aminotransfersase [AST], alanine aminotransferase [ALT]) during therapy, and discontinuing the drug if no beneficial effects occur within 45 days. |
| **4. Observe for drug interactions**<br>**a.** Drugs that *increase* effects of skeletal muscle relaxants: | |
| (1) CNS depressants (alcohol, antianxiety agents, antidepressants, antihistamines, antipsychotic drugs, sedative-hypnotics) | Additive CNS depression with increased risks of excessive sedation and respiratory depression or apnea |
| (2) MAO inhibitors | May potentiate effects by inhibiting metabolism of muscle relaxants |
| **5. Teach clients**<br>**a.** Take the drugs with milk or food. | To avoid nausea and gastric irritation |
| **b.** Do not stop drugs abruptly. Dosage should be decreased gradually, especially with baclofen, carisoprodol, and cyclobenzaprine. | Abrupt withdrawal of baclofen may cause hallucinations; abrupt withdrawal of the other drugs may cause headache, nausea, and malaise. |

## Review and Application Exercises

1. How do skeletal muscle relaxants act to relieve spasm and pain?
2. What are indications for use of skeletal muscle relaxants?
3. What are contraindications for use of these drugs?
4. What are major adverse effects of these drugs, and how may they be minimized?
5. What are some nonpharmacologic interventions to use instead of or along with the drugs?

## Selected References

Bullock, B. L. (1992). Normal and altered functions of the muscular system. In B. L. Bullock & P. P. Rosendahl (Eds.), *Pathophysiology: Adaptations and alterations in function* (3rd ed.) (pp. 838–850). Philadelphia: J.B. Lippincott.

(1993). *Drug facts and comparisons.* St. Louis: Facts and Comparisons.

Guyton, A. C. (1991). *Textbook of medical physiology* (8th ed.). Philadelphia: W.B. Saunders.

Shlafer, M. (1993). *The nurse, pharmacology and drug therapy: A prototype approach* (2nd ed.). Redwood City, CA: Addison-Wesley.

# CHAPTER 14

# Anesthetics

Anesthesia means loss of sensation with or without loss of consciousness. Anesthetic drugs are given to prevent pain and promote relaxation during surgery, childbirth, and some diagnostic tests and treatments. They interrupt the conduction of painful nerve impulses from a site of injury to the brain. The two basic types of anesthesia are general and regional.

## General anesthesia

General anesthesia is a state of profound central nervous system (CNS) depression, during which there is complete loss of sensation, consciousness, pain perception, and memory. It has three components: hypnosis, analgesia, and muscle relaxation. Several different drugs are usually combined to produce desired levels of these components without excessive CNS depression. This so-called balanced anesthesia also allows lower dosages of potent general anesthetics.

The four stages of general anesthesia are analgesia (I), excitement and hyperactivity (II), surgical anesthesia (III), and medullary paralysis (IV). General anesthesia is administered so that stage III anesthesia is maintained as long as necessary, and stage IV is avoided. Spontaneous breathing stops with stage IV; death follows unless the anesthetic is discontinued and resuscitative measures are undertaken. These stages were described in relation to ether, an older anesthetic that is now obsolete, and may not be discernible with newer agents. Knowing the stages is important for the nurse because people recovering from anesthesia progress through the same stages in reverse. Thus, analgesia or hyperactivity may extend into the postanesthesia recovery period.

General anesthesia is usually induced with an ultra–short-acting barbiturate given intravenously (IV) and is maintained with a gas mixture of an anesthetic agent and oxygen given by inhalation. The IV agent produces a rapid loss of consciousness, is not explosive, and provides a pleasant induction and recovery. Its rapid onset of action is attributed to rapid circulation to the brain and accumulation in the neuronal tissue of the cerebral cortex. Duration of action is also very short with a single dose but can be prolonged with continuous IV infusion. These drugs also may be used alone for anesthesia during brief diagnostic tests or surgical procedures.

Inhalation anesthetics vary in the degree of CNS depression produced and thereby vary in the rate of induction, anesthetic potency, degree of muscle relaxation, and analgesic potency. CNS depression is determined by the concentration of the drug in the CNS. Drug concentration, in turn, depends on the rate at which the drug is transported from the alveoli to the blood, transported past the blood-brain barrier to reach the CNS, redistributed by the blood to other body tissues, and eliminated by the lungs. Depth of anesthesia can be regulated readily by varying the concentration of the inhaled anesthetic gas. General inhalation anesthetics should be given only by specially trained people, such as anesthesiologists and nurse anesthetists, and only with appropriate equipment.

## Regional anesthesia

Regional anesthesia involves loss of sensation and motor activity in localized areas of the body. It is induced by application or injection of local anesthetic drugs. The

Anne Collins Abrams: CLINICAL DRUG THERAPY, Fourth Edition.
© 1995 J.B. Lippincott Company.

drugs act to decrease the permeability of nerve cell membranes to ions. This action stabilizes the cell membrane, prevents initiation and transmission of nerve impulses, and therefore prevents the cells from responding to pain impulses and other sensory stimuli.

Regional anesthesia is usually categorized according to the site of application. The area anesthetized may be the site of application, or it may be distal to the point of injection. Specific types of anesthesia attained with local anesthetic drugs include the following:

1. Topical or surface anesthesia involves applying local anesthetic agents to skin or mucous membrane. Such application makes sensory receptors unresponsive to pain, itching, and other stimuli. Local anesthetics for topical use are usually ingredients of various ointments, solutions, or lotions designed for use at particular sites. For example, preparations are available for use on eyes, ears, nose, oral mucosa, perineum, hemorrhoids, and skin.
2. Infiltration involves injecting the local anesthetic solution directly into or very close to the area to be anesthetized.
3. Peripheral nerve block involves injecting the anesthetic solution into the area of a larger nerve trunk or a nerve plexus at some access point along the course of a nerve distant from the area to be anesthetized.
4. Field block anesthesia involves injecting the anesthetic solution around the area to be anesthetized.
5. Spinal anesthesia involves injecting the anesthetic agent into the cerebrospinal fluid, usually in the lumbar spine. The anesthetic blocks sensory impulses at the root of peripheral nerves as they enter the spinal cord. Spinal anesthesia is especially useful for surgery involving the lower abdomen and legs.

    The body area anesthetized is determined by the level to which the drug solution rises in the spinal canal. This, in turn, is determined by the site of injection, the position of the client, and the specific gravity, amount, and concentration of the injected solution.

    Solutions of local anesthetic drugs used for spinal anesthesia are either hyperbaric or hypobaric. *Hyperbaric* or heavy solutions are diluted with dextrose, have a higher specific gravity than cerebrospinal fluid, and gravitate toward the head when the person is tilted in a head-down position. *Hypobaric* or light solutions are diluted with distilled water, have a lower specific gravity than cerebrospinal fluid, and gravitate toward the lower (caudal) end of the spinal canal when the person is tilted in a head-down position.
6. Epidural or caudal anesthesia involves injecting the anesthetic into the epidural space. In lumbar epidural anesthesia, the injection is usually made between the second lumbar and the first sacral vertebrae to avoid injuring the spinal cord, which ends at the first lumbar vertebra in 95% of people. In caudal anesthesia, the drug solution is injected into the caudal canal through the sacral area. Epidural or caudal anesthesia is used most often in obstetrics during labor and delivery and occasionally in surgery of the perineal or rectal areas.

Generally, the area anesthetized is determined by the site of injection (lumbar or caudal), the position of the client, the volume and concentration of the anesthetic solution, the age of the client, whether the client is pregnant, and the extent of arteriosclerosis. A smaller area is anesthetized if the recipient is in a sitting position. A larger area is anesthetized if high volumes and high concentrations of drug solutions are used, if the client is a child or is elderly, if the client is pregnant and at full term, and if occlusive arterial disease is present.

The extent and duration of anesthesia produced by injection of local anesthetics depend on several factors. Generally, large amounts, high concentrations, or injections into highly vascular areas (*e.g.*, head and neck, intercostal and paracervical sites) produce rapid peak plasma levels. Duration depends on the chemical characteristics of the drug used and the rate at which it leaves nerve tissue. When a vasoconstrictor drug, such as epinephrine, has been added, onset and duration of anesthesia are prolonged owing to slowed absorption of the anesthetic agent.

## Adjuncts to anesthesia

Several nonanesthetic drugs are used as adjuncts or supplements to anesthetic drugs. Most are discussed elsewhere and are described here only in relation to anesthesia. Drug groups include antianxiety agents (see Chap. 8), sedative-hypnotics (see Chap. 7), anticholinergics (see Chap. 21), and narcotic analgesics (see Chap. 5). The neuromuscular blocking agents are described in this chapter.

### ANTIANXIETY AGENTS AND SEDATIVE-HYPNOTICS

*Antianxiety agents* and *sedative-hypnotics* are given to decrease anxiety, promote rest, and increase client safety by allowing easier induction of anesthesia and smaller doses of anesthetic agents. These drugs are often given the night before to aid sleep and 1 or 2 hours before the scheduled procedure. Hypnotic doses are usually given for greater sedative effects. Some commonly used drugs are diazepam (Valium), promethazine (Phenergan), and hydroxyzine (Vistaril).

## ANTICHOLINERGICS

*Anticholinergic drugs* are given to prevent excessive activity of the parasympathetic nervous system (vagal stimulation). Vagal stimulation occurs with some inhalation anesthetics, such as halothane and cyclopropane; with succinylcholine, a commonly used muscle relaxant; and with surgical procedures in which there is manipulation of the pharynx, trachea, peritoneum, stomach, intestine, or other viscera and procedures in which pressure is exerted on the eyeball. If not blocked by anticholinergic drugs, vagal stimulation may cause excessive bradycardia, hypotension, and cardiac arrest. Useful drugs are atropine and glycopyrrolate (Robinul).

Anticholinergic drugs also have been widely used to decrease secretions in the respiratory tract. Because newer inhalation anesthetics produce less respiratory tract irritation and fewer secretions, anticholinergic drugs are not routinely indicated. However, the drugs may be useful with bronchoscopy or head and neck surgery.

## NARCOTIC ANALGESICS

*Narcotic analgesics*, such as morphine and meperidine (Demerol), induce relaxation and pain relief in the pre-anesthetic period. These drugs potentiate the CNS depression produced by other drugs, and less anesthetic agent is required. Morphine and fentanyl may be given in anesthetic doses in certain circumstances.

## NEUROMUSCULAR BLOCKING AGENTS

*Neuromuscular blocking agents* cause muscle relaxation, the third component of general anesthesia, and allow usage of smaller amounts of anesthetic agent. Artificial ventilation is necessary because these drugs paralyze muscles of respiration as well as other skeletal muscles. The drugs do not cause sedation; therefore, unless the recipients are unconscious, they can see and hear environmental activities and conversations.

There are two types of neuromuscular blocking agents: depolarizing and nondepolarizing. Succinylcholine is the only commonly used depolarizing drug. Like acetylcholine, the drug combines with cholinergic receptors at the motor endplate to produce depolarization and muscle contraction initially. Repolarization and further muscle contraction are then inhibited as long as an adequate concentration of drug remains at the receptor site.

Muscle paralysis is preceded by muscle spasms, which may damage muscles. Injury to muscle cells may cause postoperative muscle pain and release potassium into the circulation. If hyperkalemia develops, it is usually mild and insignificant but may cause cardiac arrhythmias or even cardiac arrest in some situations. Succinylcholine is normally deactivated by plasma pseudocholinesterase. There is no antidote except reconstituted fresh frozen plasma that contains pseudocholinesterase.

Nondepolarizing neuromuscular blocking agents also are called competitive blocking agents, curariform drugs, and antidepolarizing agents. They prevent acetylcholine from acting at neuromuscular junctions. Consequently, the nerve cell membrane is not depolarized, the muscle fibers are not stimulated, and skeletal muscle contraction does not occur. The prototype drug is tubocurarine, the active ingredient of curare, a naturally occurring plant alkaloid that causes skeletal muscle relaxation or paralysis. Most of the newer drugs are synthetic preparations. Anticholinesterase drugs, such as neostigmine (Prostigmin; see Chap. 20), are antidotes and are often used to reverse muscle paralysis.

# Individual anesthetic agents

General anesthetics are listed in Table 14-1, neuromuscular blocking agents in Table 14-2, and local anesthetics in Table 14-3.

# *Nursing Process*

### Preoperative assessment

- Assess nutritional status.
- Assess use of prescription and nonprescription drugs, especially those taken within the past 3 days. Ask if corticosteroids have been taken within the past 3 months.
- Ask about drug allergies. If use of local or regional anesthesia is anticipated, ask if the client has ever had an allergic reaction to a local anesthetic.
- Assess for risk factors for complications of anesthesia and surgery (cigarette smoking, obesity, limited exercise or activity, chronic cardiovascular, respiratory, renal, or other disease processes).
- Assess the client's understanding of the intended procedure, attitude toward anesthesia and surgery, and degree of anxiety and fear.
- Assess ability and willingness to participate in postoperative activities to promote recovery.
- Assess vital signs, laboratory data, and other data as indicated to establish baseline measurements for monitoring changes.

### Postoperative assessment

- During the immediate postoperative period, assess vital signs and respiratory and cardiovascular function every 5 to 15 minutes until reactive and stabilizing.
- Continue to assess vital signs, fluid balance, and laboratory and other data.

## TABLE 14-1. GENERAL ANESTHETICS

| Generic/Trade Name | Characteristics | Remarks |
|---|---|---|
| *General Inhalation Anesthetics* | | |
| **Cyclopropane** | Explosive, flammable gas; wide margin of safety; good analgesia and muscle relaxation; rapid induction and recovery; minimal myocardial depression; ventricular arrhythmias are uncommon unless ventilation is inadequate or adrenergic drugs are given | Used less often since newer nonexplosive and nonflammable agents have been developed |
| **Desflurane** (Suprane) | Similar to isoflurane | Used for induction and maintenance of general anesthesia |
| **Enflurane** (Ethrane) | Nonexplosive, nonflammable volatile liquid; similar to halothane but may produce better analgesia and muscle relaxation; sensitizes heart to catecholamines—increases risks of cardiac arrhythmias; renal or hepatic toxicity not reported | A frequently used agent |
| **Halothane** (Fluothane) | Nonexplosive, nonflammable volatile liquid<br>Advantages:<br>1. Produces rapid induction with little or no excitement; rapid recovery with little excitement or nausea and vomiting<br>2. Does not irritate respiratory tract mucosa; therefore does not increase saliva and tracheobronchial secretions<br>3. Depresses pharyngeal and laryngeal reflexes, which decreases risk of laryngospasm and bronchospasm<br>Disadvantages:<br>1. Depresses contractility of the heart and vascular smooth muscle, which causes decreased cardiac output, hypotension, and bradycardia<br>2. Circulatory failure may occur with high doses.<br>3. Causes cardiac arrhythmias. Bradycardia is common; ventricular arrhythmias are uncommon unless ventilation is inadequate.<br>4. Sensitizes heart to catecholamines; increases risk of cardiac arrhythmias<br>5. Depresses respiration and may produce hypoxemia and respiratory acidosis (hypercarbia)<br>6. Depresses functions of the kidneys, liver, and immune system<br>7. May cause jaundice and hepatitis<br>8. May cause malignant hyperthermia | Halothane has largely been replaced by newer agents with increased efficacy, decreased adverse effects, or both.<br>It may be used in "balanced" anesthesia with other agents. Although quite potent, it may not produce adequate analgesia and muscle relaxation at a dosage that is not likely to produce significant adverse effects. Therefore, nitrous oxide is given to increase analgesic effects; a neuromuscular blocking agent is given to increase muscle relaxation; and an IV barbiturate is used to produce rapid, smooth induction, after which halothane is given to maintain anesthesia. |
| **Isoflurane** (Forane) | Similar to halothane in action; less likely to cause cardiovascular depression and ventricular arrhythmias than halothane. Isoflurane may cause malignant hyperthermia but apparently does not cause hepatotoxicity. | Used for induction and maintenance of general anesthesia |
| **Methoxyflurane** (Penthrane) | Nonexplosive, nonflammable volatile liquid; similar to halothane in most respects but is more analgesic when inhaled at low concentrations, has slower induction and recovery, does not sensitize the heart to catecholamines, and causes renal damage and failure. Renal failure is dose related and increases with drug concentration and length of time administered. It is attributed to metabolites of methoxyflurane. | Usage as a general anesthetic is limited because of renal toxicity. It is used in dentistry, childbirth, or other procedures in which small amounts can be given for brief periods. This does not allow enough accumulation of the drug or its metabolites to cause renal damage. |
| **Nitrous oxide** | Nonexplosive gas; good analgesic, weak anesthetic; one of oldest and safest anesthetics; causes no appreciable damage to vital organs unless hypoxia is allowed to develop and persist; administered with oxygen to prevent hypoxia; rapid induction and recovery. Note: nitrous oxide is an incomplete anesthetic; that is, by itself, it cannot produce stage III anesthesia. | Often used in "balanced" anesthesia with intravenous barbiturates, neuromuscular blocking agents, narcotic analgesics, and more potent inhalation anesthetics, such as halothane. It is safer for prolonged surgical procedures (see "Characteristics"). It is used alone for analgesia in dentistry, obstetrics, and brief surgical procedures. |
| *General Intravenous Anesthetics* | | |
| **Alfentanil** (Alfenta) | Opioid analgesic-anesthetic related to fentanyl and sufentanil. Rapid acting. | May be used as a primary anesthetic or an analgesic adjunct in balanced anesthesia. |
| **Etomidate** (Amidate) | A nonanalgesic hypnotic used for induction and maintenance of general anesthesia | May be used with nitrous oxide and oxygen in maintenance of general anesthesia for short operative procedures such as uterine dilation and curettage. |

*(continued)*

**TABLE 14-1.  GENERAL ANESTHETICS** *(Continued)*

| Generic/Trade Name | Characteristics | Remarks |
|---|---|---|
| **Fentanyl and droperidol combination** (Innovar) | Droperidol (Inapsine) is related to the antipsychotic agent haloperidol. It produces sedative and antiemetic effects. Fentanyl citrate (Sublimaze) is a very potent narcotic analgesic whose actions are similar to those of morphine but of shorter duration. Innovar is a fixed-dose combination of the two drugs. Additional doses of fentanyl are often needed because its analgesic effect lasts about 30 minutes while droperidol's effects last 3–6 hours. | Either drug may be used alone, but they are most often used together for neurolept-analgesia and combined with nitrous oxide for neuroleptanesthesia. Neuroleptanalgesia is a state of reduced awareness and reduced sensory perception during which a variety of diagnostic tests or minor surgical procedures can be done, such as bronchoscopy and burn dressings. Neuroleptanesthesia can be used for major surgical procedures. Consciousness returns rapidly, but respiratory depression may last 3–4 hours into the postoperative recovery period. |
| **Ketamine** (Ketalar) | Rapid-acting, nonbarbiturate anesthetic; produces marked analgesia, sedation, immobility, amnesia, and a lack of awareness of surroundings (called dissociative anesthesia); may be given IV or IM; awakening may require several hours; during recovery, unpleasant psychic symptoms may occur, including dreams and hallucinations; vomiting, hypersalivation, and transient skin rashes also may occur during recovery. | Used most often for brief surgical, diagnostic, or therapeutic procedures. It also may be used to induce anesthesia. If used for major surgery, it must be supplemented by other general anesthetics. It is generally contraindicated in individuals with increased intracranial pressure, severe coronary artery disease, hypertension, or psychiatric disorders. Hyperactivity and unpleasant dreams occur less often with children than adults. |
| **Methohexital sodium** (Brevital) | An ultra–short-acting barbiturate similar to thiamylal and thiopental | See thiamylal, thiopental, below. |
| **Midazolam** (Versed) | Short-acting benzodiazepine. May cause respiratory depression, apnea, death with IV administration. Smaller doses are needed if other CNS depressants (*e.g.*, narcotic analgesics, general anesthetics) are given concurrently. | Given IM for preoperative sedation. Given IV for conscious sedation during short endoscopic or other diagnostic procedures; induction of general anesthesia; and maintenance of general anesthesia with nitrous oxide and oxygen for short surgical procedures |
| **Propofol** (Diprivan) | A rapid-acting hypnotic used with other agents in balanced anesthesia. May cause hypotension, apnea, and other signs of CNS depression. Recovery is rapid, occurring within minutes after the drug is stopped. | Given by IV bolus or infusion for induction or maintenance of general anesthesia. |
| **Sufentanil** (Sufenta) | A synthetic opioid analgesic-anesthetic related to fentanyl. Compared to fentanyl, it is more potent and faster-acting and may allow a more rapid recovery. | May be used as a primary anesthetic or an analgesic adjunct in balanced anesthesia |
| **Thiamylal sodium** **Thiopental sodium** (Surital, Pentothal) | Ultra–short-acting barbiturates, used almost exclusively in general anesthesia; excellent hypnotics but do not produce significant analgesia or muscle relaxation; given IV by intermittent injection or by continuous infusion of a dilute solution | Thiopental is commonly used. A single dose produces unconsciousness in less than 30 seconds and lasts 20–30 minutes. Usually given to induce anesthesia. It is used alone only for brief procedures. For major surgery, it is usually supplemented by inhalation anesthetics and muscle relaxants. |

- Assess for signs of complications (*e.g.*, fluid and electrolyte imbalance, respiratory problems, thrombophlebitis, wound infection).

### Nursing diagnoses

- High Risk for Injury: Trauma related to impaired sensory perception and impaired physical mobility from anesthetic
- High Risk for Injury: CNS depression with premedications and general anesthetics
- Pain related to operative procedure
- Decreased Cardiac Output related to effects of anesthetics, other medications, and surgery
- Impaired Gas Exchange related to effects of anesthetics, other medications, and surgery
- Anxiety or Fear related to anticipated surgery and possible outcomes

### Planning/Goals

*The client will:*
- Receive sufficient emotional support and instruction to facilitate a smooth preoperative and postoperative course
- Be protected from injury and complications while self-care ability is impaired
- Have emergency supplies and personnel available if needed
- Have postoperative discomfort managed appropriately

### Interventions

Preoperatively, assist the client to achieve optimal conditions for surgery. Some guidelines include the following:
- Provide foods and fluids to improve or maintain nutritional status (*e.g.*, those high in protein, vitamin C and other vitamins, and electrolytes to promote healing).

## TABLE 14-2. NEUROMUSCULAR BLOCKING AGENTS (SKELETAL MUSCLE RELAXANTS)

| Generic/Trade Name | Characteristics | Uses |
| --- | --- | --- |
| *Depolarizing Type* | | |
| **Succinylcholine** (Anectine) | Short-acting after single dose; action can be prolonged by repeated injections or continuous IV infusion. Malignant hyperthermia may occur. | All types of surgery and brief procedures, such as endoscopy and endotracheal intubation |
| *Nondepolarizing Type* | | |
| **Atracurium** (Tracrium) | Intermediate-acting* | Adjunct to general anesthesia |
| **Doxacurium** (Nuromax) | Long-acting* | Adjunct to general anesthesia |
| **Gallamine** (Flaxedil) | Long-acting* | Adjunct to general anesthesia |
| **Metocurine** (Metubine) | Long-acting; more potent than tubocurarine* | Adjunct to general anesthesia |
| **Mivacurium** (Mivacron) | Short-acting* | Adjunct to general anesthesia |
| **Pancuronium** (Pavulon) | Long-acting* | Mainly during surgery after general anesthesia has been induced; occasionally to aid endotracheal intubation or mechanical ventilation |
| **Pipecuronium** (Arduan) | Long-acting* | Adjunct to general anesthesia; only recommended for procedures expected to last 90 minutes or longer |
| **Tubocurarine** | Long-acting; the prototype of nondepolarizing drugs* | Adjunct to general anesthesia; occasionally to facilitate mechanical ventilation |
| **Vecuronium** (Norcuron) | Intermediate-acting* | Adjunct to general anesthesia; to facilitate endotracheal intubation and mechanical ventilation |

* All of the nondepolarizing agents may cause hypotension; effects of the drugs can be reversed by neostigmine (Prostigmin).

- Assist to maintain exercise and activity, when feasible. This helps to promote respiratory and cardiovascular function and decreases anxiety.
- Explain the expected course of events of the perioperative period (*e.g.*, specific preparations for surgery, close observation and monitoring during postanesthesia recovery, approximate length of stay).
- Teach clients measures to facilitate recovery postoperatively (*e.g.*, coughing and deep-breathing exercises, leg exercises and early ambulation, maintaining fluid balance and urine output). Some of these will initially be performed or assisted by staff; others are best performed by the client when able.
- Explain how pain will be managed postoperatively. This is often a major source of anxiety.

Postoperatively, the major focus is to maintain a safe environment and vital functions. Specific interventions include:

- Observe and record vital signs, level of consciousness, respiratory and cardiovascular status, wound status, and elimination frequently until sensory and motor functions return, then at least daily until discharge.
- Maintain intravenous infusions. Monitor the site and amount and type of fluids. If potential problems are identified (*e.g.*, hypovolemia or hypervolemia), intervene to prevent their becoming actual problems.
- Give pain medication appropriately as indicated by the client's condition.
- Help the client to turn, cough, deep breathe, exercise legs, ambulate, and perform other self-care activities until he or she can perform them independently.
- Use sterile technique in wound care.
- Teach clients about the effects of narcotic analgesics on gastrointestinal and urinary functions.

- Teach clients ways to prevent postoperative complications, including respiratory and wound infections.
- Initiate discharge planning for a smooth transition to home care.

**Evaluation**

- Observe for absence of injury and complications (*e.g.*, no fever or other signs of infection).
- Observe for improved ability in self-care activities.
- The client states that pain has been managed satisfactorily.

## Principles of therapy

1. Principles for using adjunctive drugs (antianxiety agents, anticholinergics, narcotic analgesics) are the same when these drugs are given preoperatively as at other times. They are usually ordered by an anesthesiologist and sometimes by the surgeon. Many drugs are available for use as anesthetics and adjunctive agents. The anesthesiologist is usually responsible for choosing particular drugs, and the choice depends on several factors. Some client-related factors include age; the specific procedure to be performed and its anticipated duration; the client's physical condition, including severity of illness, presence of chronic diseases, and any other drugs being given; and the client's mental status. Severe anxiety, for example, may be a contraindication for regional anesthesia,

## TABLE 14-3.  LOCAL ANESTHETICS

| Generic/Trade Name | Characteristics | Clinical Uses |
|---|---|---|
| **Benzocaine** (Americaine) | Poorly water soluble and poorly absorbed; thus, anesthetic effects are relatively prolonged, and systemic absorption is minimal; available in many prescription and nonprescription preparations, including aerosol sprays, throat lozenges, rectal suppositories, lotions, and ointments | Topical anesthesia of skin and mucous membrane to relieve pain and itching of sunburn, other minor burns and wounds, skin abrasions, earache, hemorrhoids, sore throat, and other conditions. Caution: may cause hypersensitivity reactions. |
| **Bupivacaine** (Marcaine) | Given by injection; has a relatively long duration of action; may produce systemic toxicity | Regional anesthesia by infiltration, nerve block, and epidural anesthesia during childbirth. It is not used for spinal anesthesia. |
| **Butamben** (Butesin) | Applied topically to skin only | Used mainly in minor burns and skin irritations |
| **Chloroprocaine** (Nesacaine) | Chemically and pharmacologically related to procaine, but its potency is greater and duration of action is shorter; rapidly metabolized and less likely to cause systemic toxicity than other local anesthetics; given by injection | Regional anesthesia by infiltration, nerve block, and epidural anesthesia |
| **Cocaine** | One of the oldest local anesthetics; a naturally occurring plant alkaloid; readily absorbed through mucous membranes; a Schedule II controlled substance with high potential for abuse, largely because of euphoria and other CNS stimulatory effects; produces psychic dependence and tolerance with prolonged use; too toxic for systemic use | Topical anesthesia of ear, nose, and throat |
| **Dibucaine** (Nupercaine, Nupercainal) | Potent agent; onset of action slow but duration relatively long; rather high incidence of toxicity | Topical or spinal anesthesia |
| **Dyclonine** (Dyclone) | Rapid onset of action and duration comparable to procaine; absorbed through skin and mucous membrane | Topical anesthesia in otolaryngology |
| **Etidocaine** (Duranest) | A derivative of lidocaine that is more potent and more toxic than lidocaine; long duration of action | Regional nerve blocks and epidural anesthesia |
| **Lidocaine** (Xylocaine) | Given topically and by injection; more rapid in onset, intensity, and duration of action than procaine, also more toxic; acts as an antiarrhythmic drug by decreasing myocardial irritability. One of the most widely used local anesthetic drugs. | Topical anesthesia and regional anesthesia by local infiltration, nerve block, spinal, and epidural anesthesia. It also is used intravenously to prevent or treat cardiac arrhythmias (see Chap. 55). (Caution: do not use preparations containing epinephrine for arrhythmias.) |
| **Mepivacaine** (Carbocaine) | Chemically and pharmacologically related to lidocaine; action slower in onset and longer in duration than lidocaine; effective only in large doses; not used topically | Infiltration, nerve block, and epidural anesthesia |
| **Pramoxine** (Tronothane) | Not injected or applied to nasal mucosa because it irritates tissues | Topical anesthesia for skin wounds, dermatoses, hemorrhoids, endotracheal intubation, sigmoidoscopy |
| **Prilocaine** (Citanest) | Pharmacologically similar to lidocaine with about the same effectiveness but slower onset, longer duration, and less toxicity because it is more rapidly metabolized and excreted | Regional anesthesia by infiltration, nerve block, and epidural anesthesia |
| **Procaine** (Novocaine) | Most widely used local anesthetic for many years, but it has largely been replaced by lidocaine and other newer drugs. It is rapidly metabolized, which increases safety but shortens duration of action. | Regional anesthesia by infiltration, nerve block, and spinal anesthesia. Not used topically. |
| **Proparacaine** (Alcaine) | Causes minimal irritation of the eye but may cause allergic contact dermatitis of the fingers | Topical anesthesia of the eye for tonometry and for removal of sutures, foreign bodies, and cataracts |
| **Tetracaine** (Pontocaine) | Applied topically or given by injection | Topical and spinal anesthesia mainly; can be used for local infiltration or nerve block |

and the client may require larger doses of preanesthetic sedative-type medication.

a. General anesthesia can be used for almost any surgical, diagnostic, or therapeutic procedure. If a medical disorder of a vital organ system (cardiovascular, respiratory, renal) is present, it should be corrected before anesthesia is induced when possible. General anesthesia and major surgical procedures have profound effects on normal body functioning. When alterations due to other disorders are also involved, the risks of anesthesia and surgery are greatly increased.

b. Regional or local anesthesia is usually safer than general anesthesia because it produces fewer systemic effects. For example, spinal anesthesia is often the anesthesia of choice for surgery involving the lower abdomen and lower extremities, especially in people who are elderly or have chronic lung disease. A major advantage of spinal anesthesia is that it causes less CNS and respiratory depression.

2. Anesthetics should be given *only* by people with special training in correct usage. This applies especially to general anesthetics and neuromuscular blocking

agents, but it is also important with local anesthetics when they are injected. In addition, general and local anesthetics should be given only in locations where personnel, equipment, and drugs are available for emergency use or cardiopulmonary resuscitation.

3. Choice of a local anesthetic drug depends mainly on the reason for use or the type of regional anesthesia desired. Lidocaine is one of the most widely used, and it is available in topical and injectable forms.

## GUIDELINES FOR ADMINISTRATION OF A LOCAL ANESTHETIC

When local anesthetic solutions are injected, some guidelines for safe use include the following:

1. Local anesthetic solutions must not be injected into blood vessels because of the high risk of serious adverse reactions involving the cardiovascular and central nervous systems. To prevent accidental injection into a blood vessel, needle placement must be verified by aspirating before injecting the local anesthetic solution. If blood is aspirated into the syringe, another injection site must be selected.

2. Local anesthetics given during labor cross the placenta and may depress muscle strength, muscle tone, and rooting behavior in the newborn. Apgar scores are usually normal. If excessive amounts are used, in paracervical block, for example, local anesthetics may cause fetal bradycardia, increased movement, and expulsion of meconium before birth and marked depression after birth. Dosage used for spinal anesthesia during labor is too small to depress the fetus or the newborn.

3. For spinal or epidural anesthesia, use only local anesthetic solutions that have been specifically prepared for spinal anesthesia and are in single-dose containers. Multiple-dose containers are not used because of the risk of injecting contaminated solutions.

4. Use of local anesthetic solutions containing epinephrine requires some special considerations, such as the following:

   a. This combination of drugs should not be used for nerve blocks in areas supplied by end arteries (fingers, ears, nose, toes, penis) because it may produce ischemia and gangrene.

   b. This combination should not be given IV or in excessive dosage because the local anesthetic and epinephrine can cause serious systemic toxicity, including cardiac arrhythmias.

   c. This combination should not be used with inhalation anesthetic agents that increase myocardial sensitivity to catecholamines. Severe ventricular arrhythmias may result.

   d. These drugs should probably not be used in people who have severe cardiovascular disease or hyperthyroidism.

   e. If used in obstetrics, the concentration of epinephrine should be no greater than 1:200,000 because of the danger of producing vasoconstriction in uterine blood vessels. Such vasoconstriction may cause decreased placental circulation, decreased intensity of uterine contractions, and prolonged labor.

For topical anesthesia of mucous membranes of the nose, mouth, pharynx, larynx, trachea, bronchi, and urethra, local anesthetics are effective but should be given in reduced dosage. Because drug absorption from these areas is rapid, no more than one fourth to one-third of the dose used for infiltration should be given to minimize systemic adverse reactions.

## NURSING ACTIONS: ANESTHETIC DRUGS

| *Nursing Actions* | *Rationale/Explanation* |
|---|---|
| **1. Administer accurately** | Drug administration in relation to anesthesia refers primarily to preanesthetic or postanesthetic drugs because physicians, dentists, and nurse anesthetists administer anesthetic drugs. |
| **a.** Schedule the administration of preanesthetic medications so that their peak effects are reached at the optimal time, if possible. | Timing is important. It is probably better if these medications are administered so that peak sedative effects occur before administration of anesthetics to avoid excessive central nervous system (CNS) depression. If they are given too early, the client may be sedated longer than necessary, and the risk of postanesthetic respiratory and circulatory complications is increased. Also, the medication effects may wear off |

*(continued)*

| *Nursing Actions* | *Rationale/Explanation* |
|---|---|
| | before induction of anesthesia. If they are given too late, the client may suffer needless anxiety and not be relaxed and drowsy when anesthesia is being initiated. Preanesthetic medications are often ordered "on call" rather than for a specific time, and the client may or may not become sedated before being transported to the surgery suite. |
| **b.** When a combination of two or three preanesthetic medications is ordered, do *not* mix in the same syringe and give as one injection unless the drugs are known to be compatible and the total volume is about 2 ml. | A precipitate may develop, or one of the drugs may be inactivated or altered when combined. Although larger amounts are sometimes given, probably no more than 2 to 3 ml should be given intramuscularly (IM) for both drug absorption and client comfort. About 1¼ ml (20 minims) is the upper limit for subcutaneous injections. |
| (1) Morphine and meperidine (Demerol) mix with promethazine (Phenergan) and hydroxyzine (Vistaril) and may be combined in the same syringe. | These are commonly used drugs. |
| (2) Atropine and scopolamine mix with all the above drugs. A common order is for meperidine, promethazine, and atropine. These can be mixed if the total volume is not excessive. | |
| (3) Glycopyrrolate (Robinul) is often ordered instead of atropine or scopolamine. It is compatible with morphine, meperidine, Innovar, and hydroxyzine. | |
| (4) Do *not* mix injectable pentobarbital (Nembutal) or other barbiturates with any other drug. | Parenteral barbiturates are physically incompatible with other parenteral drugs. |
| (5) If there is any doubt about the compatibility of a drug combination, *do not mix.* Instead, give two or more injections if necessary. | |
| **c.** If assisting a physician in injecting a local anesthetic solution, show the drug container to the physician and verbally verify the name of the drug, the percentage concentration, and whether the solution is plain or contains epinephrine. | Although the physician is responsible for drugs he or she administers, the nurse often assists by obtaining and perhaps holding the drug vial while the physician aspirates drug solution into a syringe.<br><br>    Accuracy of administration is essential so that adverse reactions can be avoided or treated appropriately if they do occur. The incidence of adverse reactions increases with the amount and concentration of local anesthetic solution injected. Also, adverse reactions to epinephrine may occur. |
| **d.** Have drugs and equipment for resuscitation readily available in any location where local anesthetics are given. | |
| **e.** When applying local anesthetics for topical or surface anesthesia, be certain to use the appropriate preparation of the prescribed drug. | Most preparations are used in particular conditions or bodily locations. For example, lidocaine viscous is used only as an oral preparation for anesthesia of the mouth and throat. Other preparations are used only on the skin. |
| **2. Observe for therapeutic effects** | Therapeutic effects depend on the type of drug and the reason for use. |
| **a.** When adjunctive drugs are given for preanesthetic medication, observe for relaxation, drowsiness, and relief of pain. | Depending on dose and client condition, these effects are usually evident within 20 to 30 minutes after the drugs are given. |

| *Nursing Actions* | *Rationale/Explanation* |
|---|---|
| **b.** When local anesthetic drugs are applied for surface anesthesia, observe for relief of the symptom for which the drug was ordered, such as sore mouth or throat, pain in skin or mucous membrane, and itching of hemorrhoids. | Relief is usually obtained within a few minutes. Ask the client if the symptom has been relieved, and if not, assess the situation to determine whether further action is needed. |
| **3. Observe for adverse effects** | Serious adverse effects are most likely to occur during and within a few hours after general anesthesia and major surgery. During general anesthesia, the anesthesiologist monitors the client's condition constantly to prevent, detect, or treat hypoxia, hypotension, cardiac arrhythmias, and other problems. The nurse observes for adverse effects in the preanesthetic and postanesthetic periods. |
| **a.** With preanesthetic drugs, observe for excessive sedation. | The often-used combination of a narcotic analgesic and a sedative-type drug produces additive CNS depression. |
| **b.** After general anesthesia, observe for: | |
| (1) Excessive sedation—delayed awakening, failure to respond to verbal or tactile stimuli | The early recovery period is normally marked by a progressive increase in alertness, responsiveness, and movement. |
| (2) Respiratory problems—laryngospasm, hypoxia, hypercarbia | Laryngospasm may occur after removal of the endotracheal tube used to administer general anesthesia. Hypoxia and hypercarbia indicate inadequate ventilation and may result from depression of the respiratory center in the medulla oblongata, prolonged paralysis of respiratory muscles with muscle relaxant drugs, or retention of respiratory tract secretions due to a depressed cough reflex. |
| (3) Cardiovascular problems—hypotension, tachycardia and other cardiac arrhythmias, fluid and electrolyte imbalances | Vital signs are often unstable during the early recovery period and therefore need to be checked frequently. Extreme changes must be reported to the surgeon or the anesthesiologist. These problems are most likely to occur while general anesthesia is being administered and progressively less likely as the patient recovers or awakens. |
| (4) Other problems—restlessness, nausea, and vomiting. With ketamine, unpleasant dreams or hallucinations also may occur. | Restlessness may be caused by the anesthetic, pain, or hypoxia and should be assessed carefully before action is taken. For example, if caused by hypoxia but interpreted as being caused by pain, administration of analgesics would aggravate hypoxia. |
| **c.** After regional anesthesia, observe for: | |
| (1) CNS stimulation at first (hyperactivity, excitement, seizure activity) followed by CNS depression | These symptoms are more likely to occur with large doses, high concentrations, injections into highly vascular areas, or accidental injection into a blood vessel. |
| (2) Cardiovascular depression—hypotension, arrhythmias | Local anesthetics depress myocardial contractility and the cardiac conduction system. These effects are most likely to occur with high doses. Doses used for spinal or epidural anesthesia usually have little effect on cardiovascular function. |
| (3) Headache and urinary retention with spinal anesthesia | Headache is more likely to occur if the person does not lie flat for 8 to 12 hours after spinal anesthesia is given. Urinary retention may occur in anyone but is more likely in older men with enlarged prostate glands. |

*(continued)*

| *Nursing Actions* | *Rationale/Explanation* |
|---|---|
| **4. Observe for drug interactions** | For interactions involving preanesthetic medications, see Antianxiety Drugs (Chap. 8), Anticholinergic Drugs (Chap. 21), Narcotic Analgesics (Chap. 5), and Sedative-Hypnotics (Chap. 7). |
| **a.** Drugs that *increase* effects of general anesthetic agents: | |
| (1) Antibiotics—bacitracin, colistimethate, aminoglycosides (gentamicin and related drugs), polymyxin B, viomycin | These antibiotics inhibit neuromuscular transmission. When they are combined with general anesthetics, additive muscle relaxation occurs with increased likelihood of respiratory paralysis and apnea. |
| (2) Antihypertensives | Additive hypotension, shock, and circulatory failure may occur. |
| (3) Catecholamines—dopamine, epinephrine, isoproterenol, levarterenol | Increased likelihood of cardiac arrhythmias. Halothane, cyclopropane, and a few rarely used general anesthetics sensitize the myocardium to the effects of catecholamines. If they are combined, ventricular tachycardia or ventricular fibrillation may occur. Such a combination is contraindicated. |
| (4) CNS depressants—alcohol, antianxiety agents, anticonvulsants, antidepressants, antihistamines, antipsychotics, barbiturates, narcotic analgesics, sedative-hypnotics | CNS depressants include many different drug groups and hundreds of individual drugs. Some are used therapeutically for their CNS depressant effects; others are used mainly for other purposes, and CNS depression is a side effect. Any combination of these drugs with each other or with general anesthetic agents produces additive CNS depression. Extreme caution must be used to prevent excessive CNS depression. |
| (5) Corticosteroids | Additive hypotension may occur during and after surgery owing to adrenocortical atrophy and reduced ability to respond to stress. For clients who have been receiving corticosteroids, most physicians recommend administration of hydrocortisone before, during, and, in decreasing doses, after surgery. |
| (6) Monoamine oxidase (MAO) inhibitors—isocarboxazid, isoniazid, procarbazine, tranylcypromine, and others | Additive CNS depression. These drugs should be discontinued at least 10 days to 3 weeks before elective surgery. If emergency surgery is required, clients taking MAO inhibitors should not be given general anesthesia. Although they may be given spinal anesthesia, there is increased risk of hypotension. They should not be given local anesthetic solutions to which epinephrine has been added. |
| (7) Muscle relaxants—succinylcholine, tubocurarine, others | Additive relaxation of skeletal muscles. These drugs are given for this therapeutic effect so that smaller amounts of general anesthetics may be given. |
| **b.** Drugs that *decrease* effects of general anesthetics: | Few drugs actually decrease effects of general anesthetics. When clients are excessively depressed and develop hypotension, cardiac arrhythmias, respiratory depression, and other problems, the main treatment is stopping the anesthetic and supporting vital functions rather than giving additional drugs. Effects of general inhalation anesthetics decrease rapidly once administration is discontinued. Effects of IV anesthetics decrease more slowly. |
| (1) Alcohol | Alcohol is a CNS depressant, and acute ingestion has an additive CNS depressant effect with general anesthetic agents. With chronic ingestion, however, tolerance to the |

| *Nursing Actions* | *Rationale/Explanation* |
|---|---|
| | effects of alcohol and general anesthetics develops; that is, larger amounts of general anesthetic agents are required in clients who have developed tolerance to alcohol. |
| (2) Atropine | Atropine is often given as preanesthetic medication to prevent reflex bradycardia, which may occur with halothane, cyclopropane, and other general anesthetics. |
| **c.** Drugs that *increase* effects of local anesthetics: | |
| (1) Cardiovascular depressants—general anesthetics, propranolol (Inderal) | Additive depression and increased risk of hypotension and arrhythmias |
| (2) CNS depressants | Additive CNS depression with high doses |
| (3) Epinephrine | Epinephrine is often used in dental anesthesia to prolong anesthetic effects by delaying systemic absorption of the local anesthetic drug. It is contraindicated for this use, however, in clients with hyperthyroidism or severe heart disease or those receiving adrenergic blocking agents such as guanethidine (Ismelin) for hypertension. |
| (4) Succinylcholine (Anectine) | Apnea may be prolonged by the combination of a local anesthetic agent and succinylcholine. |
| **d.** Drugs that *decrease* effects of local anesthetics: | These are seldom necessary or desirable. If overdosage of local anesthetics occurs, treatment is mainly symptomatic and supportive. |
| Succinylcholine (Anectine) | This drug may be given to treat acute convulsions resulting from toxicity of local anesthetic drugs. |
| **e.** Drugs that *increase* effects of neuromuscular blocking agents (muscle relaxants): | |
| (1) Aminoglycoside antibiotics (*e.g.*, gentamicin), colistin (Coly-Mycin) and related antibiotics | Additive neuromuscular blockade, apnea, and respiratory depression |
| (2) Diuretics, potassium-losing (*e.g.*, furosemide, hydrochlorothiazide) | Diuretics that produce hypokalemia potentiate skeletal muscle relaxants. |
| (3) General anesthetics | Additive muscle relaxation |
| (4) Local anesthetics | Prolong apnea from succinylcholine |
| (5) MAO inhibitors | Additive respiratory depression |
| (6) Narcotic analgesics | Additive respiratory depression |
| (7) Procainamide (Pronestyl) and quinidine | Additive neuromuscular blockade |
| **f.** Drugs that *decrease* effects of neuromuscular blocking agents: Anticholinesterase drugs (*e.g.*, neostigmine) | These drugs often are used to reverse the effects of the nondepolarizing agents. (They do not reverse the effects of succinylcholine and may potentiate them instead.) |
| **5. Teach clients** | |
| **a.** With preanesthetic, sedative-type medications: | The medications cause drowsiness and relaxation. |
| (1) Stay in bed with siderails up. | Lying quietly helps the drugs to act. Activities are generally unsafe unless another person is available to provide assistance. |
| (2) Use call light if help is needed. | |

*(continued)*

*Nursing Actions*                          *Rationale/Explanation*

(3) Do not smoke.

**b.** With local anesthetics applied topically:

(1) Use the drug preparation only on the part of the body for which it was prescribed.

Most preparations are specifically made to apply on certain areas, and they cannot be used effectively and safely on other body parts.

(2) Use the drug only for the condition for which it was prescribed.

For example, a local anesthetic prescribed to relieve itching may aggravate an open wound.

(3) Apply local anesthetics to clean areas. If needed, wash skin areas or take a sitz bath to cleanse the perineal area.

To enhance drug effectiveness. The drug must have direct contact with the affected area.

(4) Do *not* apply more often than directed.

Local irritation, skin rash, and hives can develop.

(5) With spray preparations, do not inhale vapors, spray near food, or store near any heat source.

(6) Use local anesthetic preparations for only a short period. If the condition for which it is being used persists, report the condition to the physician.

(7) Inform dentists or other physicians if allergic to any local anesthetic drug.

To prevent further reactions. Allergic reactions are rare, but if they have occurred, another type of local anesthetic can usually be substituted safely.

## Review and Application Exercises

1. When assessing a client before, during, or after general anesthesia, what are important factors to consider?
2. What are major adverse effects of general anesthetics and neuromuscular blocking agents?
3. What interventions are needed to ensure client safety during recovery from general anesthesia?
4. When assessing a client before, during, or after local or regional anesthesia, what are important factors to consider?
5. What are major adverse effects of local anesthetic agents?
6. What interventions are needed to ensure client safety during recovery from local or regional anesthesia?

## Selected References

(1993). *Drug facts and comparisons*. St. Louis: Facts and Comparisons.

Guyton, A. C. (1991). *Textbook of medical physiology* (8th ed.). Philadelphia: W.B. Saunders.

Jowers, L., & Burrell, L. O. (1992). Nursing management of adults needing preoperative care. In L. O. Burrell (Ed.), *Adult nursing in hospital and community settings* (pp. 291–303). Norwalk, CT: Appleton & Lange.

Jowers, L., & Burrell, L. O. (1992). Nursing management of adults needing postoperative care. In L. O. Burrell (Ed.), *Adult nursing in hospital and community settings* (pp. 316–338). Norwalk, CT: Appleton & Lange.

Shlafer, M. (1993). *The nurse, pharmacology and drug therapy: A prototype approach* (2nd ed.). Redwood City, CA: Addison-Wesley.

Smith, C. L., & Clayton, G. (1992). Nursing management of adults needing intraoperative care. In L. O. Burrell (Ed.), *Adult nursing in hospital and community settings* (pp. 304–315). Norwalk, CT: Appleton & Lange.

Swonger, A. K., & Matejski M. P. (1991). *Nursing pharmacology: An integrated approach to drug therapy and nursing practice* (2nd ed.). Philadelphia: J.B. Lippincott.

# CHAPTER 15

# Alcohol and Other Drug Abuse

## Abuse and dependence

Abuse of alcohol and other drugs is a significant health, social, economic, and legal problem. As used here, the term *drug abuse* is defined as self-administration of a drug for prolonged periods or in excessive amounts to the point of producing physical or psychological dependence and reduced ability to function as a productive member of society. Most drugs of abuse are those that affect the central nervous system (CNS) and alter the state of consciousness. These include prescription and nonprescription and legal and illegal drugs. *Alcohol is the primary drug of abuse worldwide.* Also commonly abused are other CNS depressants, such as narcotic analgesics, antianxiety agents, sedative-hypnotics; CNS stimulants, such as amphetamines and cocaine; and other mind-altering drugs, such as lysergic acid diethylamide (LSD) and marijuana. Multiple drugs are often abused concomitantly.

Many terms are used to describe alcohol and drug abuse. In this context, alcohol abuse is synonymous with alcoholism, problem drinking, and other terms that denote excessive use of and preoccupation with alcohol. Similarly, drug abuse is considered synonymous with drug dependence, drug addiction, or other terms denoting excessive or inappropriate use of a mind-altering drug.

Drug dependence involves compulsive drug-seeking behavior. *Psychological dependence* involves feelings of satisfaction and pleasure from taking the drug. These feelings, perceived as extremely desirable by the drug-dependent person, contribute to acute intoxication, development and maintenance of drug abuse patterns, and return to drug-taking behavior after periods of abstinence.

*Physical dependence* involves physiologic adaptation to chronic use of a drug so that unpleasant and uncomfortable signs and symptoms occur when the drug is stopped or its action is antagonized by another drug. The withdrawal or abstinence syndrome produces specific manifestations according to the type of drug and does not occur as long as adequate dosage is maintained. Attempts to avoid withdrawal symptoms reinforce psychological dependence and promote continuing drug use and relapses to drug-taking behavior. Tolerance is often an element of drug dependence, and increasing doses are therefore required to obtain psychological effects or avoid physical withdrawal symptoms. A person may be dependent on more than one drug.

Why does drug dependence occur? One view is that drugs act on centers in the hypothalamus to produce pleasure and euphoria or to decrease discomfort or pain.

Some influencing factors include a person's psychological and physiologic characteristics, environmental or circumstantial characteristics, and characteristics of the drug itself, including amount, frequency, and route of administration. Peer pressure seems to be an important factor in initial and continuing drug ingestion. A genetic factor seems evident in alcohol abuse: Studies indicate that children of abusers are at risk of becoming abusers themselves, even if reared away from the abusing parent.

Anne Collins Abrams: CLINICAL DRUG THERAPY, Fourth Edition.
© 1995 J.B. Lippincott Company.

# Types of drug dependence

## ALCOHOL-TYPE DEPENDENCE

1. Alcohol-type dependence is usually characterized by consumption of alcohol in excess of the limits accepted by the person's culture, at times considered inappropriate by that culture, and to the extent that physical health and social relationships are impaired. Psychological dependence, physical dependence, and tolerance are prominent characteristics.
2. It is similar to barbiturate or benzodiazepine-type dependence. Signs and symptoms of intoxication and withdrawal are similar for alcohol and barbiturates. Cross-tolerance develops with these drugs.
3. Signs and symptoms of alcohol withdrawal or abstinence include tremors, sweating, nausea, tachycardia, fever, hyperreflexia, postural hypotension, and if severe, convulsions and delirium. Delirium tremens (DTs), the most serious form of alcohol withdrawal, is characterized by confusion, disorientation, delusions, visual hallucinations, and other signs of acute psychosis. The intensity of the alcohol withdrawal syndrome probably varies with the duration and amount of alcohol ingestion.
4. Alcohol dependence can cause as much harm to a person as any other type of drug dependence. Alcohol impairs thinking, judgment, and psychomotor coordination. These impairments lead to poor work performance, accidents, and disturbed relationships with other people. Conscious control of behavior is lost, and exhibitionism, aggressiveness, and assaultiveness often result. Alcohol causes severe organic damage and mental problems.
5. Alcohol dependence can cause a great deal of damage to other people. Some problems commonly associated with alcohol abuse include automobile accidents, child and spouse abuse, job absenteeism, inability to keep a job, and loss of productivity.

## AMPHETAMINE-TYPE DEPENDENCE

1. Amphetamines produce stimulation and euphoria, effects often sought by drug users. The user may increase the amount and frequency of administration to reach or continue the state of stimulation. Similar to the production of "crack" cocaine, methamphetamine may be chemically treated to produce potent crystals (called "ice"), which are then heated and the vapors smoked or inhaled. Psychological effects of amphetamines are similar to those produced by cocaine and are largely dose-related. Small amounts produce mental alertness, wakefulness, and increased energy. Large amounts, especially if taken intravenously (IV), may produce psychotic behavior (*e.g.,* hallucinations and paranoid delusions). Tolerance develops to amphetamines.
2. Amphetamines or related stimulant drugs mask underlying problems (such as fatigue or depression), and withdrawal allows these conditions to emerge in an exaggerated form. Exhaustion and depression probably reinforce the compulsion to continue using the drug.
3. Related drugs that produce amphetamine-type drug dependence include methylphenidate (Ritalin) and phenmetrazine (Preludin).
4. Nonmedical use of these drugs is apparently increasing. Users take them alone or to counteract the effects of alcohol or barbiturates. In the latter case, these drugs are part of a pattern of polydrug use in which CNS depressants, such as alcohol or barbiturates ("downers"), are alternated with CNS stimulants, such as amphetamines ("uppers").

## BARBITURATE AND BENZODIAZEPINE-TYPE DEPENDENCE

1. Drugs that produce dependence of this type include the barbiturates and benzodiazepine antianxiety and sedative-hypnotic agents.
2. It resembles alcohol-type dependence in symptoms of intoxication and withdrawal. It is also characterized by strong physical and psychological dependence. Tolerance and cross-tolerance develop with these drugs.
3. Signs and symptoms of withdrawal include anxiety, tremors and muscle twitching, progressive weakness, dizziness, distorted visual perceptions, nausea and vomiting, insomnia, weight loss, postural hypotension, generalized tonic-clonic (grand mal) seizures, and delirium that resembles the DTs of alcoholism or a major psychotic episode. Convulsions are more likely to occur during the first 48 hours of withdrawal and delirium after 48 to 72 hours.

## MARIJUANA (CANNABIS)-TYPE DEPENDENCE

1. The amount of psychoactive (mind-altering) substance in a cannabis preparation varies according to specific characteristics of the plant, the place and circumstances of its growth, the age of the harvested material, its preparation, and the storage method used.
2. Cannabis preparations are usually smoked. Hashish, a secretion from the plant's flowers, also is taken orally in candies, cookies, and beverages. Effects appear sooner with smoking; larger amounts are required to produce effects when the drug is taken orally. Specific effects of cannabis preparations de-

pend on the dose to some extent but also on the user's personality, expectations, and physical condition and on the environment in which the drug is used. Low-to-moderate doses usually produce euphoria, sensory and perceptual changes, decreased sense of identity and reality, visual and sometimes auditory hallucinations, increased pulse rate, and decreased muscle strength. These symptoms may be followed by sedation and sleep. Regular smoking for a prolonged period produces inflammatory and other changes in the respiratory tract.

3. Tolerance and psychic dependence do not usually develop with occasional use but may occur with chronic use; physical dependence rarely occurs.

## COCAINE-TYPE DEPENDENCE

1. Cocaine is a CNS stimulant that induces euphoria, excitement, hallucinations, and strong psychic dependence. The CNS effects are attributed to the drug's ability to prevent reuptake of the catecholamine neurotransmitters, norepinephrine and dopamine. The euphoria is brief and often leads to drug ingestion every few minutes as long as the drug is available. Cocaine is not thought to produce physical dependence, although fatigue, depression, and drowsiness occur as drug effects dissipate.

2. It is usually taken by sniffing drug crystals into the nose, where it is rapidly absorbed.

3. "Crack" is a widely used form of cocaine. It is prepared by altering cocaine hydrochloride with chemicals and heat to form rock-like formations of cocaine base. The process removes impurities and results in a very potent drug. When the drug is heated and the vapors inhaled, crack produces intense feelings of euphoria within a few seconds. It reportedly can cause psychological dependence with one use.

## HALLUCINOGEN (LSD)-TYPE DEPENDENCE

1. There are many hallucinogenic drugs, including LSD, peyote, phencyclidine (PCP), and psilocybin (obtained from a type of mushroom).

2. Drugs producing this type of dependence cause mood changes, anxiety, distorted visual and other sensory perceptions, hallucinations, delusions, depersonalization, pupil dilation, elevated body temperature, and elevated blood pressure.

3. Tolerance develops, but there is no apparent physical dependence or abstinence syndrome. Psychological dependence probably occurs but is usually not intense. Users may prefer one of these drugs, but they apparently do without or substitute another drug if the one they favor is unavailable.

4. A major danger with these drugs is their ability to impair judgment and insight, which can lead to panic reactions in which users may try to injure themselves (*e.g.*, by running into traffic).

## OPIATE (MORPHINE)-TYPE DEPENDENCE

1. These drugs produce tolerance and high degrees of psychological and physical dependence. Most other drugs that produce dependence do so with prolonged usage of large doses, but morphine-like drugs produce dependence with repeated administration of small doses. This characteristic is especially significant in medical usage of these potent analgesics because it implies that dependence may be induced by usual therapeutic dosages and initiated by the first dose given.

2. Effects of narcotic drugs vary according to dosage, route of administration, and physical and mental characteristics of the user. They usually produce euphoria, sedation, analgesia, apathy, lethargy, respiratory depression, postural hypotension, vasodilation, pupil constriction (miosis), and decreased gastrointestinal tract motility with constipation.

3. Opiate-type drugs produce a characteristic withdrawal syndrome. With morphine, withdrawal symptoms begin within a few hours of the last dose, reach peak intensity in 24 to 48 hours, and subside spontaneously. The more severe symptoms usually disappear within 10 days, but some residual symptoms may persist much longer.

4. The abstinence syndrome varies in time of onset, peak intensity, and duration, depending on the specific drug involved. If a narcotic antagonist, such as naloxone (Narcan), is given, withdrawal symptoms occur rapidly and are more intense but of shorter duration.

5. Withdrawal produces a wide array of signs and symptoms, including anxiety; restlessness; generalized body aches; insomnia; yawning; lacrimation; rhinorrhea; perspiration; pupil dilation (mydriasis); piloerection (goose flesh); hot flushes; nausea and vomiting; diarrhea; elevation of body temperature, respiratory rate, and systolic blood pressure; abdominal and other muscle cramps; dehydration; anorexia; and weight loss.

## VOLATILE SOLVENT (INHALANT)—TYPE DEPENDENCE

1. Some general inhalation anesthetics, such as nitrous oxide, have been used to the point of producing this type of dependence. More recently, however, volatile solvents, such as acetone, toluene, and gasoline, have been used. These solvents are constituents of various

products, including some types of glue, plastic cements, and aerosol sprays.

2. These substances are most often abused by preadolescents and adolescents who squeeze glue into a plastic bag, for example, and sniff the fumes. Suffocation sometimes occurs when the sniffer loses consciousness while the bag covers the face.

3. These substances depress the CNS and produce symptoms somewhat comparable to acute intoxication with alcohol, including initial mild euphoria followed by ataxia, confusion, and disorientation. Some substances in gasoline and toluene also may produce symptoms similar to those produced by the hallucinogens, including euphoria, hallucinations, recklessness, and loss of self-control. Large doses may cause convulsions, coma, and death.

   Substances containing gasoline, benzene, or carbon tetrachloride are especially likely to cause serious damage to the liver, kidneys, and bone marrow.

4. These substances produce psychological dependence, and some produce tolerance. There is some question about whether physical dependence occurs. If it does occur, it is considered less intense than the physical dependence associated with alcohol, barbiturates, and opiates.

## Selected individual drugs of abuse

Many drugs are abused for their mind-altering properties. Most of these have clinical usefulness and are discussed individually elsewhere in this text: Antianxiety Drugs (Chap. 8), Narcotic Analgesics and Narcotic Antagonists (Chap. 5), Sedative-Hypnotics (Chap. 7), and Central Nervous System Stimulants (Chap. 16). The individual drugs of abuse included here are those that are commonly abused but have little, if any, clinical usefulness. Except for alcohol, they are illegal.

### ALCOHOL (ETHANOL)

*Alcohol*, a CNS depressant drug, is the most abused drug in the world. It is legal and readily available, and its use is accepted in most societies. There is no clear-cut dividing line between use and abuse, but rather a continuum of progression over several years.

When an alcoholic beverage is ingested orally, a portion of the alcohol is inactivated in the stomach (by the enzyme gastric alcohol dehydrogenase) and not absorbed systemically. Women have less enzyme activity than men and therefore absorb about 30% more alcohol than men when comparable amounts are ingested according to weight and size. As a result, women are especially vulnerable to adverse effects of alcohol, including more rapid intoxication from smaller amounts of alcohol and earlier development of hepatic cirrhosis and other complications of alcohol abuse.

In men and women, alcohol is absorbed partly from the stomach but mostly from the upper small intestine. It is rapidly absorbed when the stomach and small intestine are empty. Food delays absorption by diluting the alcohol and delaying gastric emptying. Once absorbed, alcohol is quickly distributed to all body tissues, partly because it is lipid soluble and crosses cell membranes easily. The alcohol concentration in the brain rapidly approaches that in the blood, and CNS effects usually occur within a few minutes. These effects depend on the amount ingested, how rapidly it was ingested, whether the stomach was empty, and other factors. Generally, effects with acute intoxication progress from a feeling of relaxation to impaired mental and motor functions to stupor and sleep. Excited behavior may occur, due to depression of the cerebral cortex, which normally controls behavior. The person may seem more relaxed, talkative, and outgoing or more impulsive and aggressive because inhibitions have been lessened.

The major factor affecting the duration of the CNS effects of ingested alcohol is the rate at which alcohol is metabolized in the body. Between 90% and 95% of alcohol is oxidized in the liver to acetaldehyde, a substance that can be used for energy or converted to fat and stored. When metabolized to acetaldehyde, alcohol no longer exerts depressant effects on the CNS. Although the rate of metabolism differs with acute ingestion or chronic intake and some other factors, it is generally about 10 ml/h. This is the amount of alcohol contained in about ⅔ oz of whiskey, 3 to 4 oz of wine, or 8 to 12 oz of beer. *Alcohol is metabolized at the same rate regardless of the amount present in body tissues.* Efforts to find drugs or procedures to increase the rate of metabolism and thereby reverse the effects of alcohol have been unsuccessful.

Chronic alcohol abuse leads to alcoholism, a progressive illness that usually develops over 5 to 20 years. Alcoholism occurs in all ages and socioeconomic groups.

Alcohol exerts profound metabolic and physiologic effects on all organ systems. Some of these effects are evident with acute alcohol intake, while others become evident with chronic intake of substantial amounts.

### Central and peripheral nervous system effects

1. Sedation ranging from drowsiness to coma
2. Impaired mental processes, such as memory and learning
3. Impaired motor coordination: ataxia or staggering gait, altered speech patterns, poor task performance, hypoactivity or hyperactivity

4. Mental depression, anxiety, insomnia
5. Impaired interpersonal relationships
6. Brain damage
7. Polyneuritis and Wernicke-Korsakoff syndrome, which are attributed to thiamine deficiency

## Hepatic effects

1. Chronic alcohol ingestion induces drug-metabolizing enzymes in the liver and thereby increases the rate of metabolism of itself and several other drugs. This mechanism probably accounts for the development of tolerance to alcohol and cross-tolerance with other drugs. Once liver damage occurs, however, drug metabolism is slowed, and drugs metabolized by the liver may accumulate and produce toxic effects.
2. The liver decreases use and increases production of lactate, leading to accumulation of lactic acid in the blood. This in turn leads to lactic acidosis, decreased renal excretion of uric acid, and secondary hyperuricemia.
3. Lipid use is decreased and production increased, leading to hyperlipidemia and fatty liver. Fatty liver may be a precursor to hepatic cirrhosis and hepatitis.
4. Hepatomegaly occurs due to accumulation of fat and protein.
5. Severe liver injury is characterized by necrosis and inflammation (alcoholic hepatitis) or by fibrous bands of scar tissue that alter structure and function (cirrhosis). Cirrhosis is irreversible.
6. Liver damage from ethanol was formerly attributed to the malnutrition accompanying alcoholism rather than to direct toxic effects of ethanol on the liver, but this view has largely been disproved. The entire progression of liver damage, from early and mild to late and severe, is apparently caused by ethanol itself or to the metabolic changes produced by ethanol. The incidence of liver disease correlates with the amount of alcohol consumed; it does not correlate with dietary deficiencies.

## Gastrointestinal effects

1. Slowed gastric emptying time with large concentrations of alcohol
2. Increased intestinal motility, which probably contributes to the diarrhea that often occurs with alcoholism
3. Damage to the epithelial cells of the intestinal mucosa, which alters structure and function of the cells and may produce inflammatory reactions
4. Multiple nutritional deficiencies, including protein and water-soluble vitamins, such as thiamine, folic acid, and vitamin $B_{12}$

5. Pancreatic disease, which contributes to malabsorption of fat, nitrogen, and vitamin $B_{12}$
6. All the above factors probably contribute to the malabsorption that often occurs in alcoholism.

## Cardiovascular effects

1. Changes in cardiac metabolism and function, apparently due to toxic effects of alcohol on myocardial cells
2. Alcoholic cardiomyopathy, which includes signs and symptoms of cardiomegaly, rales, edema, dyspnea, third and fourth heart sounds, and a cardiac murmur. Electrocardiographic changes include indications of left ventricular hypertrophy, abnormal T waves, and conduction disturbances.
3. Effects on coronary blood flow and myocardial contractility are controversial. Some studies have shown increased coronary blood flow, although others have shown decreased flow or no change. Similarly, some investigators report depressed left ventricular contractility, but others do not. The different results may be caused by different levels of alcohol in the blood.

## Hematologic effects

1. Bone marrow depression due to alcohol or associated conditions, such as malnutrition, infection, and liver disease
2. Several types of anemia result from abnormalities in red blood cells. *Megaloblastic anemia* is caused by folic acid deficiency. Folic acid deficiency is caused, in turn, by alcohol ingestion or inadequate dietary intake in most instances, but gastrointestinal bleeding, hypersplenism, hemolysis, and infection also may contribute. *Sideroblastic anemia* (sideroblasts are precursors of red blood cells) is probably the result of nutritional deficiency. Low-grade *hemolytic anemia* results from abnormalities in the structure of red blood cells and from a shortened life span of red blood cells. *Iron deficiency anemia* is usually caused by gastrointestinal bleeding. Other causes of anemia in people who abuse alcohol include hemodilution, chronic infection, and fatty liver and bone marrow failure associated with cirrhosis.
3. Thrombocytopenia and decreased platelet aggregation due to folic acid deficiency, hypersplenism, and other factors
4. Decreased numbers and impaired function of white blood cells, which lead to decreased resistance to infection. Granulocytopenia sometimes occurs with intoxication in the absence of infection; paradoxical granulocytopenia may occur in alcoholics with severe bacterial infection. The mechanism by which

granulocytopenia occurs is unknown. Ethanol also may lower resistance to infection by decreasing the ability of leukocytes to migrate to an area of inflammation or infection. Other factors that probably contribute to lowered resistance include cigarette smoking, depression of cough, and impaired closure of the epiglottis.

## Endocrine effects

1. Increased release of cortisol and catecholamines and decreased release of aldosterone from the adrenal glands
2. Hypogonadism, gynecomastia, and feminization in men with cirrhosis due to decreased secretion of male sex hormones
3. Degenerative changes in the anterior pituitary gland and decreased secretion of antidiuretic hormone from the posterior pituitary
4. Hypoglycemia due to impaired glucose synthesis or hyperglycemia due to glycogenolysis

## Skeletal effects

1. Impaired growth and development. This has been most apparent in children born to alcoholic mothers. Fetal alcohol syndrome is characterized by low birth weight and length and by birth defects, such as cleft palate and cardiac septal defects. Impairment of growth and motor development persists in the postnatal period, and mental retardation becomes apparent.
2. Decreased bone density, osteoporosis, and increased susceptibility to fractures
3. Osteonecrosis due to obstructed blood supply
4. Skeletal system effects, including altered calcium and phosphorus metabolism. Hypocalcemia often occurs with alcoholism because of poor dietary intake of calcium, impaired absorption, and increased urinary and sometimes fecal losses. Hypocalcemia leads to release of parathyroid hormone, which in turn leads to bone resorption and decreased skeletal mass. Alcohol-induced losses of magnesium often accompany hypocalcemia and may further stimulate parathormone secretion and bone resorption. Hypophosphatemia is often observed in chronic alcoholism and is most likely caused by inadequate dietary intake of phosphorus.

## Muscular effects

1. Alcoholic cardiomyopathy produced by chronic damage to the myocardium
2. Myopathy, usually classified as subclinical, acute, or chronic. Elevated creatine phosphokinase is common with chronic alcoholism and may occur with no other manifestations of myopathy. Acute myopathy may involve acute pain, tenderness, and edema similar to deep vein thrombosis, and it may be accompanied by hyperkalemia. Chronic myopathy may involve muscle weakness, atrophy, and episodes of acute myopathy associated with a drinking spree.

## Drug interactions

Many drug interactions of potential clinical significance involve alcohol and other drugs. Alcohol increases or decreases the effects of several other drugs, and other drugs often increase or decrease the effects of alcohol. The interactions are frequently encountered and are complex. In relation to alcohol intake, drug interactions may differ depending on acute or chronic ingestion and if chronic, how much and for how long.

*Acute ingestion* tends to inhibit drug-metabolizing enzymes. This slows the metabolism rate of some drugs, thereby increasing their effects and the likelihood of toxicity. *Chronic ingestion* tends to induce metabolizing enzymes. This increases the rate of metabolism and decreases drug effects. Note, however, that long-term ingestion of large amounts of alcohol causes liver damage and impaired ability to metabolize drugs.

Because so many variables influence the incidence and significance of alcohol's interactions with other drugs, it is difficult to predict interactions in particular people. Generally, clinically significant interactions are likely to include the following:

1. Alcohol interacts with other general depressants of the CNS to produce additive CNS depression, sedation, respiratory depression, impaired mental and physical functioning, and other effects. These depressant drug groups include the sedative-hypnotics, narcotic analgesics, antianxiety agents, antipsychotic agents, general anesthetics, and tricyclic antidepressants (TCAs).

    Combining alcohol with barbiturates, benzodiazepines, or TCAs may be lethal and should be avoided. Chronic ingestion of large amounts of alcohol produces a cross-tolerance with barbiturates and general anesthetics. This means, for example, that the alcoholic client requires larger doses of these drugs when barbiturates are given during alcohol withdrawal syndromes or when a general anesthetic is given for a surgical procedure.
2. Alcohol has a vasodilating effect and thus increases the hypotensive effects of most antihypertensive drugs.
3. Alcohol potentiates hypoglycemic effects of oral antidiabetic drugs.
4. Alcohol's interaction with oral anticoagulants varies. Chronic ingestion of alcohol tends to decrease the effects of anticoagulants by inducing drug-metaboliz-

ing enzymes in the liver and increasing their rate of metabolism. However, if chronic ingestion has caused liver damage, metabolism of the oral anticoagulants may be slowed. This increases the risk of excessive anticoagulant effect and bleeding. Acute ingestion also increases the risk of bleeding.

5. Alcohol interacts with disulfiram (Antabuse) to produce symptoms such as flushing, dyspnea, hypotension, tachycardia, nausea, and vomiting (see Treatment of Alcohol Abuse under the section Principles of Therapy, below). A disulfiram-like reaction also may occur with other drugs, such as chloramphenicol (Chloromycetin), furazolidone (Furoxone), griseofulvin (Fulvicin), chlorpropamide (Diabinese), tolbutamide (Orinase), and metronidazole (Flagyl).

## COCAINE AND CRACK

Cocaine is a popular drug of abuse. It produces powerful CNS stimulation by preventing reuptake of neurotransmitters (*e.g.*, norepinephrine), which increases and prolongs neurotransmitter effects. Cocaine is commonly inhaled (snorted) through the nose; "crack," a strong, inexpensive, and extremely addicting form, is heated and the vapors inhaled. Acute use of cocaine or "crack" produces euphoria, tachycardia, increased blood pressure, and restlessness followed by depression, fatigue, and drowsiness as drug effects wear off. Hypersensitivity or overdosage can cause cardiac arrhythmias, convulsions, myocardial infarction, respiratory failure, stroke, and death, even in young, healthy adults and even with initial exposure. Chronic use produces numerous physiologic effects, as listed below:

### Central nervous system effects

1. Excessive CNS stimulation (*e.g.*, anxiety, hyperactivity, irritability, insomnia)
2. Anorexia and weight loss
3. Psychosis with paranoid delusions and hallucinations that may be indistinguishable from schizophrenia
4. Seizures

### Cardiovascular effects

1. Arrhythmias
2. Acute myocardial infarction
3. Stroke
4. Rupture of the aorta

### Respiratory effects

1. Ulceration and perforation of the nasal septum
2. Rhinitis, rhinorrhea
3. Pulmonary edema

### Gastrointestinal effects

1. Nausea
2. Weight loss
3. Intestinal ischemia, possibly gangrene

### Genitourinary effects

1. Delayed orgasm for men and women
2. Difficulty in maintaining erection

## HEROIN

*Heroin* is a semisynthetic derivative of morphine and is the opiate most widely used for illicit purposes. It is a potent analgesic and produces rapid, intense euphoria with IV injection. A Schedule I drug in the United States, it is not used therapeutically. It is used medically in other countries; in England, it is an ingredient in Brompton's solution (a combination of drugs used to relieve pain in terminally ill clients). Heroin produces psychological and physical dependence and tolerance within a few weeks of continued abuse. Like other opiates, heroin causes severe respiratory depression with overdose and produces a characteristic abstinence syndrome.

## MARIJUANA AND OTHER CANNABIS PREPARATIONS

Marijuana and other cannabis preparations are obtained from *Cannabis sativa*, the hemp plant, which grows in most parts of the world, including the entire United States. Marijuana and hashish are the two cannabis preparations used in the United States. Marijuana is obtained from leaves and stems; hashish, prepared from plant resin, is five to ten times as potent as commonly available marijuana. These cannabis preparations contain several related compounds called *cannabinoids*. Delta-9-tetrahydrocannabinol ($\Delta$-9-THC) is thought to be the active ingredient, but metabolites and other constituents also may exert pharmacologic activity.

Cannabis preparations are difficult to classify. Some people call them depressants, some call them stimulants, and others label them as mind-altering, hallucinogenic, psychotomimetic, or unique in terms of fitting into drug categories. It is also difficult to predict the effects of these drugs. Many factors apparently influence a person's response. One factor is the amount of active ingredients, which varies with the climate and soil where the plants are grown and with the method of preparation. Other factors include dose, route of administration, personality variables, and the environment in which the drug is taken.

Marijuana can be taken orally but is more often smoked and inhaled through the lungs. It is more potent and more rapid in its actions when inhaled. Low doses seem to be mildly intoxicating and similar to small amounts of alcohol. Large doses can produce panic reactions and hallucinations similar to acute psychosis. Many adverse reactions have been reported with marijuana use, including impaired ability to drive an automobile; chronic bronchitis and emphysema with prolonged, heavy use; chromosomal abnormalities; and impairments of cell metabolism, immune responses, and endocrine gland function. The first two reactions seem relatively well documented and accepted; the others are still being evaluated.

Except for dronabinol (Marinol), marijuana and other cannabis preparations are illegal and not used therapeutically in the United States. Dronabinol is Δ-9-THC, the main psychoactive ingredient of marijuana. It is used to treat nausea and vomiting associated with anticancer drugs (see Chap. 67). The risks of abuse are high, and the drug may cause physical and psychological dependence. It is a Schedule II controlled drug.

Cannabinoids are being investigated for possible use in glaucoma and for bronchodilating effects in asthma. The highly refined drugs used in research studies bear little resemblance to the cannabis preparations generally available to drug abusers.

## HALLUCINOGENS

*LSD* is a synthetic derivative of lysergic acid, a compound in ergot and some varieties of morning glory seeds. It is very potent, and small doses can alter normal brain functioning. LSD is usually distributed as a soluble powder and ingested in capsule, tablet, or liquid form. The exact mechanism of action is unknown, and effects cannot be predicted accurately. Generally, LSD alters sensory perceptions, supposedly enhancing their intensity; alters thought processes; impairs most intellectual functions, such as memory and problem-solving ability; distorts perception of time and space; and produces sympathomimetic reactions, including increased blood pressure, heart rate, body temperature, and pupil dilation. Adverse reactions include self-injury and possibly suicide, violent behavior, psychotic episodes, "flashbacks" (a phenomenon characterized by psychological effects and hallucinations that may recur days, weeks, or months after the drug is taken), and possible chromosomal damage resulting in birth defects.

*Mescaline* is an alkaloid of the peyote cactus. It is the least active of the commonly used psychotomimetic agents, but users are apparently attracted by the vivid visual hallucinations and psychic effects. As with LSD, mescaline produces hallucinations, impairs memory and problem-solving ability, and produces sympathomimetic changes, such as increased blood pressure and pulse and pupil dilation. It is usually ingested in the form of a soluble powder or capsule.

*PCP* emerged as a leading street drug during the late 1970s. Originally developed for use as an anesthetic, it produced excitement, visual disturbances, delirium, and hallucinations and was never approved for use in humans. It is used as a veterinary anesthetic. Cheap, widely available, and easily synthesized, it is usually distributed in liquid or crystal form and can be ingested, inhaled, or injected. It is usually sprayed or sprinkled on marijuana or herbs and smoked.

PCP produces profound psychological and physiologic effects, including a state of intoxication similar to that produced by alcohol; altered sensory perceptions; impaired thought processes; impaired motor skills; psychotic reactions; sedation and analgesia; eye disorders, such as nystagmus and diplopia; and pressor effects that can cause hypertensive crisis, cerebral hemorrhage, convulsions, coma, and death. Death from overdose also has occurred as a result of respiratory depression. Bizarre murders, suicides, and self-mutilations have been attributed to the schizophrenic reaction induced by PCP, especially in high doses. The drug also produces flashbacks.

Probably because it is cheap and readily available, PCP is often sold as LSD, mescaline, cocaine, or THC. It is also added to low-potency marijuana without the user's knowledge. Consequently, the drug user may experience severe and unexpected reactions, including death.

## *Nursing Process*

### Assessment

Assess clients for signs of alcohol and other drug abuse, including abuse of prescription drugs, such as antianxiety agents, narcotics, and sedative-hypnotics. Nurses and other health-care providers are considered at high risk for substance abuse, at least partly because of drug accessibility.

Some general screening-type questions are appropriate for any initial nursing assessment. The overall purpose of these questions is to determine whether a current or potential problem exists and whether additional information is needed. Some clients may refuse to answer or will give answers that contradict other assessment data. Denial of excessive drinking and of problems resulting from alcohol use is a prominent characteristic of alcoholism; it may be an important factor in other types of drug abuse as well. Useful information includes each specific drug, the amount, the frequency of administration, and the duration of administration. If answers to general questions reveal problem areas, such as long-term use of alcohol or psychotropic drugs, more specific questions can be formulated to assess the scope and depth of the problem. It may be especially difficult to obtain needed information about illegal "street drugs," most of which have numerous, frequently changed names. For nurses who often encounter substance abusers, efforts to keep up with drug names and terminology may be helpful.

- Interview the client regarding alcohol and drug use to help determine immediate and long-term nursing needs. For example, information may be obtained that would indicate the likelihood of a withdrawal reaction, the risk of increased or decreased effects of a variety of drugs, and the client's susceptibility to drug abuse. People who abuse one drug are likely to abuse others. These and other factors aid effective planning of nursing care.

- Assess behavior that may indicate drug abuse, such as alcohol on the breath, altered speech patterns, staggering gait, hyperactivity or hypoactivity, and other signs of excessive CNS depression or stimulation. Impairments in work performance and in interpersonal relationships also may be behavioral clues.
- Assess for disorders that may be caused by alcohol or drug abuse. These disorders may include infections, liver disease, accidental injuries, and psychiatric problems of anxiety or depression. These disorders may be caused by other factors, of course, and are nonspecific.
- Check laboratory reports, when available, for abnormal liver function tests, indications of anemia, abnormal white blood cell counts, abnormal electrolytes (hypocalcemia, hypomagnesemia, and acidosis are common in alcoholics), and alcohol and drug levels in the blood.

### Nursing diagnoses

- Ineffective Individual Coping related to reliance on alcohol or other drugs
- High Risk for Injury: Adverse drug effects
- High Risk for Violence related to altered thought processes, impaired judgment, and impulsive behavior
- Altered Nutrition: Less than Body Requirements related to drug effects and drug-seeking behavior
- Altered Thought Processes related to use of psychoactive drugs
- High Risk for Injury: Infection, hepatitis, acquired immunodeficiency syndrome related to use of contaminated needles and syringes for IV drugs

### Planning/Goals

- Safety will be maintained for clients impaired by alcohol and drug abuse.
- Information will be provided regarding drug effects and treatment resources.
- The client's efforts toward stopping drug usage will be recognized and reinforced.

### Interventions

- Administer prescribed drugs correctly during acute intoxication or withdrawal.
- Decrease environmental stimuli for the person undergoing drug withdrawal.
- Record vital signs; cardiovascular, respiratory, and neurologic functions; mental status; and behavior at regular intervals.
- Support use of resources for stopping drug abuse (psychotherapy, treatment programs).
- Teach nondrug techniques for coping with stress and anxiety.

### Evaluation

- Observe for improved behavior (*e.g.*, less impulsiveness, improved judgment and thought processes, commits no injury to self or others).

- Observe for use or avoidance of nonprescribed drugs while hospitalized.
- Interview to determine the client's insight into personal problems stemming from drug abuse.
- Verify enrollment in a treatment program.

## Principles of therapy

### PREVENTION OF ALCOHOL AND OTHER DRUG ABUSE

Use measures to prevent development of alcohol and drug abuse. Although there are difficulties in trying to prevent. conditions for which causes are not known, some of the following community-wide and individual measures may be helpful:

1. Decrease the supply or availability of commonly abused drugs. Most efforts at prevention have tried to reduce the supply of drugs. For example, laws designate certain drugs as illegal and provide penalties for possession or use of these drugs. Other laws regulate circumstances in which legal drugs, such as narcotic analgesics and barbiturates, may be used. Also, laws regulate the sale of alcoholic beverages.
2. Decrease the demand for drugs. Because this involves changing attitudes, it is likely to be very difficult but more effective in the long run. Many current attitudes seem to promote drug use, misuse, and abuse, including:
   a. The widespread belief that a drug is available for every mental and physical discomfort and should be taken in preference to tolerating even minor discomfort. Consequently, society has a permissive attitude toward taking drugs, and this attitude is probably perpetuated by physicians who are quick to prescribe drugs and nurses who are quick to administer them. Of course, there are many appropriate uses of drugs, and clients certainly should not be denied their benefits. The difficulties emerge when there is excessive reliance on drugs as chemical solutions to problems that are not amenable to chemical solutions.
   b. The widespread acceptance and use of alcohol. In some groups, every social occasion is accompanied by alcoholic beverages of some kind.
   c. The apparently prevalent view that drug abuse refers only to the use of illegal drugs and that using prescription drugs, however inappropriately, does not constitute drug abuse.
   d. The acceptance and use of illegal drugs in certain subgroups of the population. This is especially prevalent in high school and college students. Efforts to change attitudes and decrease demand for drugs can be made through education and

counseling about such topics as drug effects and nondrug ways to handle the stresses and problems of daily life.

3. Each person must take personal responsibility for drinking alcoholic beverages and taking mind-altering drugs. Initially, conscious, voluntary choices are made to drink or not to drink, to take a drug or not to take it. This period varies somewhat, but drug dependence develops in most instances only after prolonged use. When mind-altering drugs are prescribed for a legitimate reason, the client must use them in prescribed doses and preferably for a short time.

4. Physicians can help prevent drug abuse by prescribing drugs appropriately, prescribing mind-altering drugs in limited amounts and for limited periods, using nondrug measures when they are likely to be effective, educating clients about the drugs prescribed for them, participating in drug education programs, and recognizing, as early as possible, clients who are abusing or are likely to abuse drugs.

5. Nurses can help prevent drug abuse by administering drugs appropriately, using nondrug measures when possible, teaching clients about drugs prescribed for them, and participating in drug education programs.

6. Parents can help prevent drug abuse in their children by minimizing their own use of drugs and by avoiding heavy cigarette smoking. Children are more likely to use illegal drugs if their parents have a generally permissive attitude about drug taking, if either parent takes mind-altering drugs regularly, and if either parent is a heavy cigarette smoker.

7. Pregnant women should avoid alcohol and drugs in any form because of potentially harmful effects on the fetus.

## TREATMENT MEASURES FOR ALCOHOL AND DRUG ABUSE

Treatment measures for alcohol and drug abuse have not been especially successful. Even people who have been institutionalized and achieved a drug-free state for prolonged periods are apt to resume their drug-taking behavior when released from the institution. So far, voluntary groups, such as Alcoholics Anonymous and Narcotics Anonymous, have been more successful than health professionals in dealing with drug abuse. Health professionals are more likely to be involved in acute situations, such as intoxication or overdose, withdrawal syndromes, or various medical-surgical conditions. As a general rule, treatment depends on the type, extent, and duration of drug-taking behavior and the particular situation for which treatment is needed. Some general management principles include the following:

1. Psychological rehabilitation efforts should be part of any treatment program for a drug-dependent person.

Several approaches may be useful, including psychotherapy, voluntary groups, and other types of emotional support and counseling.

2. Drug therapy is relatively limited in treating drug dependence for several reasons. First, specific antidotes are available only for benzodiazepines (flumazenil) and opioid narcotics (naloxone). Second, there is a high risk of substituting one abused drug for another. Third, there are significant drawbacks to giving CNS stimulants to reverse effects of CNS depressants, and vice versa. Despite these drawbacks, however, there are some clinical indications for drug therapy. These include disulfiram as deterrent therapy in chronic alcohol abuse, methadone maintenance in treating heroin-type drug dependence, treatment of symptoms during acute drug toxicity or overdose, and treatment of withdrawal syndromes.

3. General care of clients with drug overdose is primarily symptomatic and supportive. The aim of treatment is usually to support vital functions, such as respiration and circulation, until the drug is metabolized and eliminated from the body. For example, respiratory depression from an overdose of a CNS depressant drug may be treated by inserting an artificial airway and mechanical ventilation. Removal of some drugs can be hastened by hemodialysis or hemoperfusion.

## TREATMENT OF ALCOHOL DEPENDENCE

*Treatment of alcohol abuse* can be divided into treatment of chronic alcoholism, acute intoxication, and withdrawal syndromes.

### Chronic alcoholism

*Chronic alcohol abuse* is a progressive illness. Therefore, early recognition and treatment are desirable. They also are quite difficult, at least partly because denial is a prominent characteristic of alcoholism. The alcohol-dependent person is unlikely to seek treatment for alcohol abuse until an acute situation forces the issue. He or she is likely, however, to seek treatment for numerous other disorders, such as nervousness, anxiety, depression, insomnia, and gastroenteritis. Thus, health professionals may recognize alcohol abuse in its early stages if they are aware of indicative assessment data.

If the first step of treatment is recognition or diagnosis of alcohol abuse, the second step is probably confronting the client with evidence of alcohol abuse and trying to elicit cooperation. Unless the client admits that alcohol abuse is a problem and agrees to participate in a treatment program, success is highly unlikely. The client may fail to make return visits or may seek treatment elsewhere. If the client agrees to treatment, the two primary approaches are psychological counseling and drug therapy.

1. Short-term drug therapy involves use of drugs to control nervousness, insomnia, and other symptoms and to prevent withdrawal symptoms. For example, antianxiety drugs, such as diazepam (Valium) or chlordiazepoxide (Librium), may be given. The primary purpose of such drug therapy is to help the client participate in rehabilitation programs. Long-term use of these drugs should be avoided because they also may be abused, and the client may simply be trading one type of drug abuse for another. These drugs can be gradually reduced in dosage and discontinued without precipitating withdrawal symptoms.

2. Long-term drug therapy may involve use of the deterrent drug *disulfiram*. Normally, alcohol is metabolized in the liver to acetaldehyde, acetaldehyde is metabolized to acetate by the enzyme aldehyde dehydrogenase, and acetate is metabolized to carbon dioxide and water. Disulfiram blocks the action of aldehyde dehydrogenase and allows acetaldehyde to accumulate. If alcohol is then ingested, signs and symptoms occur that include flushing of the face, dyspnea, hypotension, tachycardia, nausea and vomiting, syncope, vertigo, blurred vision, headache, and confusion. Severe reactions include respiratory depression, cardiovascular collapse, cardiac arrhythmias, myocardial infarction, congestive heart failure, unconsciousness, convulsions, and death. The severity of the reaction varies but is usually proportional to the amounts of alcohol and disulfiram taken. The duration of the reaction varies from a few minutes to several hours, as long as alcohol is present in the blood. Ingestion of prescription and over-the-counter medications that contain alcohol may cause a reaction in the disulfiram-treated alcoholic.

Disulfiram alone may produce adverse reactions of drowsiness, fatigue, impotence, headache, and dermatitis. These are more likely to occur during the first 2 weeks of treatment, after which they usually subside. Disulfiram also interferes with the metabolism of barbiturates, coumarin anticoagulants, phenytoin, and alcohol. Concurrent use of disulfiram and these drugs may increase blood levels of the drugs and increase their toxicity. Because of these reactions, disulfiram must be given only with the client's full consent, cooperation, and knowledge.

## Acute intoxication

*Acute intoxication with alcohol* does not usually require treatment. If the client is hyperactive and combative, a sedative-type drug may be given. The client must be closely observed because sedatives potentiate alcohol, and excessive CNS depression may occur. If the client is already sedated and stuporous, he or she can be allowed to sleep off the alcohol effects. If the client is comatose, supportive measures are indicated. For example, respiratory depression may require insertion of an artificial airway and mechanical ventilation.

## Withdrawal symptoms

*Abstinence or withdrawal from alcohol* is characterized by increased excitability of the nervous system, including sensory and motor stimulation. Withdrawal of mild to moderate severity is characterized by tremors, restlessness, agitation, insomnia, and other signs and symptoms. Withdrawal syndromes of greater severity include the above signs and symptoms plus seizures, hallucinations, and DTs.

Benzodiazepine antianxiety agents are usually the drugs of choice for treating alcohol withdrawal syndromes. They provide adequate sedation and have a significant anticonvulsant effect. Seizures require treatment if they are repeated or continuous. Anticonvulsant drugs need not be given for more than a few days unless the person has a preexisting seizure disorder. Other treatment measures include vitamins, nutritional therapy, and symptomatic measures.

## TREATMENT OF VARIOUS TYPES OF DEPENDENCE

### Barbiturate or benzodiazepine-type abuse

*Treatment of barbiturate or benzodiazepine-type abuse* (*e.g.*, barbiturates and benzodiazepine antianxiety and sedative-hypnotic agents) can be divided into treatment of overdose and withdrawal syndromes.

**Overdose.** *Overdose* of these drugs produces intoxication similar to that produced by alcohol. There may be a period of excitement and emotional lability followed by progressively increasing signs of CNS depression, such as impaired mental function, muscular incoordination, and sedation. Treatment is unnecessary for mild overdose if vital functions are adequate. The client usually sleeps off the effects of the drug. The rate of recovery depends primarily on the amount of drug ingested and its rate of metabolism.

More severe overdoses cause excessive CNS depression and impair vital functions. Respiratory depression and coma usually occur. There is no antidote for barbiturate overdose; treatment is symptomatic and supportive. The goals of treatment are to maintain vital functions until the drug is metabolized and eliminated from the body. Insertion of an artificial airway and mechanical ventilation often is necessary. Gastric lavage may help if started within about 3 hours of drug ingestion. If the person is comatose, a cuffed endotracheal tube should be inserted and the cuff inflated before lavage to prevent aspiration. Diuresis helps to eliminate the drugs and can be induced by IV fluids or diuretic drugs. Hemodialysis is effective in removing most of these drugs. It is most likely to be used in shock, failure to respond to other treatment measures, or the presence of a potentially fatal serum drug level. Hypotension and shock are usually treated with IV fluids rather than vasopressor drugs, but the drugs may be used if necessary.

Until recently, these treatments also were used for benzodiazepine overdoses and may still be needed in some cases (*e.g.*, overdoses involving multiple drugs). However, a specific antidote is now available to reverse sedation, coma, and respiratory depression. Flumazenil (Romazicon) competes with benzodiazepines for benzodiazepine receptors. The drug has a short duration of action, and repeated IV injections are usually needed. Recipients must be closely observed because symptoms of overdose may recur when the effects of a dose of flumazenil subside and because the drug may precipitate acute withdrawal symptoms (*e.g.*, agitation, confusion, seizures) in benzodiazepine abusers. See Chapter 8 for additional information, including dosage.

**Withdrawal Symptoms.** *Treatment of withdrawal* may involve administration of phenobarbital to relieve acute signs and symptoms, followed by gradually reduced doses until it can be discontinued entirely. Barbiturate and benzodiazepine withdrawal syndromes can be life-threatening. The person may experience cardiovascular collapse, generalized tonic-clonic (grand mal) seizures, and acute psychotic episodes. These can be prevented by gradually withdrawing the offending drug. If they do occur, each situation requires specific drug therapy and supportive measures. Withdrawal reactions should be supervised and managed by experienced people, such as health-care professionals or staff at detoxification centers.

## Opiate-type dependence

*Treatment of opiate-type dependence* can be divided into treatment of overdose and withdrawal or abstinence syndromes.

**Overdose.** *Overdosage* is likely to produce severe respiratory depression and coma, because opiates produce respiratory depression in varying degrees, depending largely on dosage. Insertion of an endotracheal tube and mechanical ventilation often are required. Drug therapy consists of a narcotic antagonist such as naloxone to reverse the effects of the opiate. Giving a narcotic antagonist can precipitate immediate withdrawal symptoms. Also, if there is no apparent response to the narcotic antagonist, the signs and symptoms may be caused by

depressant drugs other than opiates. In addition to profound respiratory depression, pulmonary edema, hypoglycemia, pneumonia, cellulitis, and other infections often accompany narcotic overdose and require specific treatment measures.

**Withdrawal.** *Signs and symptoms of withdrawal* from opiates and related drugs can be reversed immediately by giving the drug producing the dependence. Therapeutic withdrawal, which is more comfortable and safer, can be managed by gradually reducing dosage over several days. An alternative method that has been somewhat successful is treating opiate-type drug dependence by methadone maintenance. This method involves daily administration of a single oral dose. Proponents say that methadone blocks euphoria produced by heroin, acts longer, and thereby reduces preoccupation with drug seeking and drug taking. This allows a more nearly normal life-style for the client. Also, because methadone is usually furnished free, the heroin addict does not commit crimes to obtain drugs. However, close supervision is required. Opponents of methadone maintenance programs say this method only substitutes one type of drug dependence for another.

A newer treatment modality is naltrexone (Trexan), a narcotic antagonist that prevents opiates from occupying receptor sites and thereby prevents their physiologic effects. Used to maintain opiate-free states in the opiate addict, it is recommended for use in conjunction with psychological counseling to promote client motivation and compliance.

## Amphetamine-type abuse

*Treatment of amphetamine-type abuse* is mainly concerned with overdosage because these drugs supposedly do not produce physical dependence and withdrawal, at least in the sense that alcohol, opiates, and sedative-hypnotic drugs do. Because amphetamines delay gastric emptying, gastric lavage may be helpful even if several hours have passed since drug ingestion. The client is likely to be hyperactive, agitated, and hallucinating (toxic psychosis) and may have tachycardia, fever, and other symptoms. Symptomatic treatment includes sedation, lowering of body temperature, and administration of an antipsychotic drug. Sedative-type drugs must be used with great caution, however, because depression and sleep usually follow amphetamine use, and these after-effects can be aggravated by sedative administration.

## Cocaine abuse

*Treatment of cocaine abuse* is largely symptomatic. Thus, agitation and hyperactivity may be treated with a benzodiazepine sedative-type drug; psychosis may be treated with haloperidol or other antipsychotic agent; and cardiac arrhythmias may be treated with usual antiarrhythmic drugs and so forth. Initial detoxification and long-term treatment are best accomplished in centers or units that specialize in substance abuse disorders.

## Review and Application Exercises

1. Why is it important to assess each client in relation to alcohol or other substance abuse?
2. What are signs and symptoms of overdose with alcohol, benzodiazepine antianxiety or hypnotic agents, cocaine, and opiates?
3. What are general interventions for treatment of drug overdoses?
4. What are specific antidotes for opiate and benzodiazepine overdoses, and how are they administered?
5. Which commonly abused drugs may produce life-threatening withdrawal reactions if stopped abruptly?
6. How can severe withdrawal syndromes be prevented, minimized, or safely managed?
7. What are the advantages of treating substance abuse disorders in centers established for that purpose?

## Selected References

Benowitz, N. L. (1992). Substance abuse: Dependence and treatment. In K. L. Melmon, H. F. Morrelli, B. B. Hoffman, & D. W. Nierenberg (Eds.), *Clinical pharmacology: Basic principles in therapeutics* (3rd ed.) (pp. 763–786). New York: McGraw-Hill.

Buchanan, J. F., Joe, G., & McKinney, H. E., Jr. (1992). Alcohol abuse. In M. A. Koda-Kimble & L. Y. Young (Eds.), *Applied therapeutics: The clinical use of drugs* (5th ed.) (pp. 60-1–60-14). Vancouver, WA: Applied Therapeutics.

Buchanan, J. F., McKinney, H. E., Jr., Hayner, G. N., & Inaba, D. S. (1992). Drug abuse. In M. A. Koda-Kimble & L. Y. Young (Eds.), *Applied therapeutics: The clinical use of drugs* (5th ed.) (pp. 59-1–59-29). Vancouver, WA: Applied Therapeutics.

Bullock, B. L., & Rosendahl, P. P. (1992). *Pathophysiology: Adaptations and alterations in function* (3rd. ed.). Philadelphia: J.B. Lippincott.

Dusek, D. E., & Girdano, D. A. (1993). *Drugs: A factual account* (5th ed.). New York: McGraw-Hill.

Langston, J. W., & Finnegan, K. T. (1992). Approach to the patient with substance abuse. In W. N. Kelley (Ed.), *Textbook of internal medicine* (2nd ed.) (pp. 2298–2302). Philadelphia: J.B. Lippincott.

Li, T. K. (1992). Approach to the patient with alcoholism. In W. N. Kelley (Ed.), *Textbook of internal medicine* (2nd ed.) (pp. 2297–2298). Philadelphia: J.B. Lippincott.

Porth, C. M. (1990). *Pathophysiology: Concepts of altered health states* (3rd ed.) (pp. 1036–1038). Philadelphia: J.B. Lippincott.

Shore, F. & Gugino, H. S. (1992). Nursing management of adults with substance abuse. In L. O. Burrell (Ed.), *Adult nursing in hospital and community settings* (pp. 260–289). Norwalk, CT: Appleton & Lange.

### CHAPTER 16

# Central Nervous System Stimulants

## Uses

Many drugs stimulate the central nervous system (CNS), but only a few are used therapeutically, and their indications for use are limited. Two disorders treated with CNS stimulants are narcolepsy and attention deficit-hyperactivity disorder (ADHD; formerly called attention deficit disorder and hyperkinetic syndrome).

*Narcolepsy* is a rare disorder characterized by periodic "sleep attacks" in which the victim has an uncontrollable feeling of drowsiness and goes to sleep at any place or any time. In addition to excessive daytime drowsiness and fatigue, nighttime sleep patterns are disturbed. The hazards of suddenly going to sleep in unsafe environments restrict activities of daily living.

*ADHD* occurs in children and is characterized by hyperactivity, a short attention span, difficulty completing assigned tasks or schoolwork, restlessness, and impulsive behavior.

## Types of stimulants

Most CNS stimulants act by facilitating initiation and transmission of nerve impulses that excite other cells. The drugs are somewhat selective in their actions at lower doses but tend to involve the entire CNS at higher doses. The major groups of CNS stimulants are amphetamines and related drugs, analeptics, and xanthines.

*Amphetamines* produce mood elevation or euphoria, increase mental alertness and capacity for work, decrease fatigue and drowsiness, and prolong wakefulness. Larger doses, however, tend to produce signs of excessive CNS stimulation, such as restlessness, hyperactivity, agitation, nervousness, difficulty in concentrating on a task, and confusion. Overdoses can produce convulsions and psychotic behavior. Amphetamines also stimulate the sympathetic nervous system, resulting in increases in heart rate and blood pressure, mydriasis, slowed gastrointestinal motility, and other symptoms.

These drugs produce tolerance and psychological dependence. They are Schedule II drugs under the Controlled Substances Act, and prescriptions for them are nonrefillable. These drugs are widely sold on the street and commonly abused. (See Chap. 15 for amphetamine-type drug dependence.)

*Analeptics* stimulate respiration but do not reverse the effects of CNS depressant drugs. A major drawback to their clinical use is that doses sufficient to stimulate respiration often cause convulsive seizures. Respiratory depression can be more safely and effectively treated with endotracheal intubation and mechanical ventilation than with analeptic drugs.

*Xanthines* stimulate the cerebral cortex, increasing mental alertness and decreasing drowsiness and fatigue. Other effects include myocardial stimulation with increased cardiac output and heart rate, diuresis, and increased secretion of pepsin and hydrochloric acid. Large doses can impair mental and physical functions by pro-

Anne Collins Abrams: CLINICAL DRUG THERAPY, Fourth Edition.
© 1995 J.B. Lippincott Company.

ducing restlessness, nervousness, anxiety, agitation, insomnia, and cardiac arrhythmias.

# Central nervous system stimulants

## INDICATIONS FOR USE

Amphetamines are used in the treatment of narcolepsy, ADHD, and obesity. Use of the drugs as appetite suppressants is discussed in Chapter 30. Methylphenidate is indicated only for ADHD and narcolepsy. Analeptics may be used occasionally to treat respiratory depression. Caffeine (a xanthine) is often an ingredient in nonprescription analgesics and stimulants (*e.g.*, No-Doz). Caffeine and sodium benzoate is occasionally used as a respiratory stimulant in neonates.

## CONTRAINDICATIONS FOR USE

CNS stimulants cause cardiac stimulation and thus are contraindicated in clients with cardiovascular disease (*e.g.*, angina, arrhythmias, hypertension) that is likely to be aggravated by the drugs. They also are contraindicated in clients with anxiety or agitated states, glaucoma, or hyperthyroidism. They are generally contraindicated in clients with a history of drug abuse.

# Individual CNS stimulants

## AMPHETAMINES AND RELATED DRUGS

Amphetamine, dextroamphetamine (Dexedrine), and methamphetamine (Desoxyn) are closely related drugs that share characteristics of the amphetamines as a group. They are more important as drugs of abuse than as therapeutic agents.

### Amphetamine and dextroamphetamine

#### Route and dosage ranges

*Adults:* Narcolepsy, PO 5–60 mg/d in divided doses
*Children over 6 years:* Narcolepsy, PO 5 mg/d to start therapy; raise by 5 mg/wk to effective dose
    ADHD, PO 5 mg 1–2 times a day initially, increased by 5 mg/d at weekly intervals until optimal response is obtained (usually no greater than 40 mg/d). Do not initiate dosage with a long-acting preparation.
*Children 3–5 years:* ADHD, PO 2.5 mg/d initially, increased by 2.5 mg/d at weekly intervals until optimal response is obtained. Do not initiate dosage with a long-acting preparation.

### Methamphetamine

#### Route and dosage ranges

*Adults:* Narcolepsy, same as amphetamine
*Children over 6 years:* Narcolepsy, no dosage established
    ADHD, same as amphetamine
*Children under 6 years:* No dosage established

**Methylphenidate** (Ritalin) is chemically related to amphetamines and used to treat ADHD in children and narcolepsy in adults. The drug has actions and adverse effects similar to those produced by amphetamines. As a CNS stimulant, methylphenidate is considered less potent than amphetamines and more potent than caffeine. Methylphenidate is a Schedule II drug because it produces psychic dependence and is a drug of abuse.

#### Route and dosage ranges

*Adults:* Narcolepsy, PO 10–60 mg/d in two or three divided doses (average dose 20–30 mg/d)
*Children 6 years or older:* ADHD, PO 5 mg twice a day initially, increased by 5–10 mg at weekly intervals to a maximum of 60 mg/d

**Pemoline** (Cylert) differs chemically from amphetamines and methylphenidate but exerts similar pharmacologic actions. A Schedule IV controlled drug, it is used only in treating ADHD in children.

#### Route and dosage range

*Children over 6 years:* PO 37.5 mg/d initially in the morning; increase by 18.75 mg at weekly intervals until desired response is obtained; maximum dose 112.5 mg/d

## ANALEPTIC AGENT

**Doxapram** (Dopram) has limited clinical usefulness as a respiratory stimulant. Although it does increase tidal volume and respiratory rate, it also increases oxygen consumption and carbon dioxide production. Limitations include a short duration of action (5–10 minutes after a single IV dose) and therapeutic dosages near or overlapping those that produce convulsions. Mechanical ventilation is safer and more effective in relieving respiratory depression from depressant drugs or other causes. Doxapram is occasionally used by anesthesiologists and pulmonary specialists.

#### Route and dosage range

*Adults:* IV 0.5–1.5 mg/kg of body weight in single or divided doses; IV continuous infusion 5 mg/min initially, decreased to 2.5 mg/min or more. Dose by infusion should not exceed 3 g.

## XANTHINES

**Caffeine** is commercially prepared from tea leaves. Pharmaceutical preparations include an oral preparation and a solution for injection. Caffeine is usually prescribed as caffeine citrate for oral use and caffeine and sodium benzoate for parenteral use because these forms are more soluble than caffeine itself. Caffeine has limited therapeutic usefulness. It is an ingredient in some nonprescription analgesic preparations (Anacin, A.P.C., Excedrin, Vanquish) and may increase analgesia. It is also an ingredient in nonprescription stimulant (antisleep) preparations (*e.g.*, No-Doz). It is sometimes combined with an ergot alkaloid to treat migraine headaches (*e.g.*, Cafergot). Caffeine and sodium benzoate is used as a respiratory stimulant in neonatal apnea unresponsive to other therapies.

Most caffeine is consumed in beverages, such as coffee, tea, cocoa, and cola drinks. One cup of coffee contains about 100 to 150 mg of caffeine, analgesic preparations contain 30 to 60 mg, and antisleep preparations contain 100 to 200 mg. Thus, the stimulating effects of caffeine can be obtained as readily with coffee as with a drug preparation. Caffeine produces tolerance to its stimulating effects, and psychological dependence or habituation occurs.

**Theophylline** and theophylline salts are xanthine derivatives used therapeutically in the treatment of respiratory disorders, such as asthma and bronchitis. In these conditions, the desired effect is bronchodilation and improvement of breathing; CNS stimulation is then an adverse reaction. For additional information, see Chapter 50.

## *Nursing Process*

### Assessment

- Assess use of stimulant and depressant drugs (prescribed, over-the-counter, or street drugs).
- Assess for conditions that would be aggravated by CNS stimulants.
- Assess the client's behavior carefully. For example, assess behavior of a child with possible ADHD as specifically and thoroughly as possible; some authorities believe that this condition is diagnosed more often than it actually occurs and that stimulant drugs are prescribed unnecessarily. Also, assess behavior of any client receiving amphetamines or methylphenidate for signs of tolerance and abuse.

### Nursing diagnoses

- Sleep Pattern Disturbance related to hyperactivity, nervousness, insomnia
- High Risk for Injury: Adverse drug effects (excessive cardiac and CNS stimulation, drug dependence)
- Knowledge Deficit: Drug effects on children and adults
- High Risk for Noncompliance: Overuse of drug

### Planning/Goals

*The client will:*
- Take drugs safely and accurately
- Improve attention span and task performance and decrease hyperactivity (for children with ADHD)
- Have fewer sleep episodes during normal waking hours (for clients with narcolepsy)

### Interventions

- For a child receiving CNS stimulants, assist parents in scheduling drug holidays to help prevent drug dependence and stunting of growth.
- Teach parents to give drugs on school days or when high levels of attention and task performance are required.
- Teach clients to avoid other CNS stimulants, including caffeine.
- Teach clients to avoid doses within 6 to 8 hours of bedtime to avoid interference with sleep.
- Record weight at least weekly.
- Teach clients about their nutritional needs while receiving these drugs.
- Teach clients about their drug therapy.

### Evaluation

- Reports of improved behavior and academic performance from parents and teachers of children with ADHD
- Reports of decreased inappropriate sleep episodes with narcolepsy

## Principles of therapy

1. Counseling and psychotherapy are recommended along with drug therapy for clients with narcolepsy and ADHD. With narcolepsy, for example, clients must be informed about the risks of driving an automobile and other activities. With ADHD, parental counseling is indicated. For example, parents may be overmedicating the child in an effort to eliminate hyperactivity completely. If this is the case, they should be advised not to exceed the prescribed dosage. Other parents may fear that the child will become addicted if therapy is continued. They can be reassured that drug dependence does not occur with recommended dosages.
2. Stimulant drugs are often misused and abused by people who want to combat fatigue and delay sleep, such as long-distance drivers, students, and athletes. Use of amphetamines or other stimulants for this purpose is not justified. These drugs are dangerous for drivers and those involved in similar activities, and they have no legitimate use in athletics.
3. When an amphetamine or methylphenidate is prescribed, giving the smallest effective dose and limiting the number of doses obtained with one prescription will decrease the likelihood of drug dependence.

4. Analeptics are not indicated for most clients with depression of the CNS or the respiratory system. Anesthesiologists, if they use analeptic drugs at all, use them only in carefully selected circumstances and with great caution. Doxapram generally should not be used to stimulate ventilation in clients with drug-induced coma or exacerbations of chronic lung disease. Respiration can be more effectively and safely controlled with mechanical ventilation than with drugs.

## USE IN CHILDREN

CNS stimulants are not recommended for ADHD in children under 6 years of age or as anorexiants in children under 12 years. When used, dosage should be carefully monitored to avoid excessive CNS stimulation. Effects of long-term use are unknown, although suppression of weight and height have been reported. Growth should be monitored at regular intervals during drug therapy. In children with psychosis or Tourette's syndrome, CNS stimulants may exacerbate symptoms.

## USE IN OLDER ADULTS

CNS stimulants should be used cautiously in older adults. As with most other drugs, slowed metabolism and excretion increase risks of accumulation and toxicity. Older adults are likely to experience anxiety, nervousness, insomnia, and mental confusion from excessive CNS stimulation. In addition, older adults often have cardiovascular disorders (*e.g.*, angina, arrhythmias, hypertension) that may be aggravated by the cardiac-stimulating effects of the drugs.

# NURSING ACTIONS: CENTRAL NERVOUS SYSTEM STIMULANTS

| *Nursing Actions* | *Rationale/Explanation* |
|---|---|
| **1. Administer accurately**<br>If possible, give amphetamines and methylphenidate at least 6 hours before bedtime. | To avoid interference with sleep |
| **2. Observe for therapeutic effects** | Therapeutic effects depend on the reason for use. |
| **a.** Fewer "sleep attacks" with narcolepsy | |
| **b.** Improved task performance with attention deficit disorder | |
| **c.** Increased mental alertness and decreased fatigue | |
| **3. Observe for adverse effects** | Adverse effects may occur with acute or chronic ingestion of excessive amounts of coffee and with other forms of central nervous system (CNS) stimulant drugs. |
| **a.** Excessive CNS stimulation—hyperactivity, nervousness, insomnia, anxiety, tremors, convulsions, psychotic behavior | These reactions are more likely to occur with large doses. |
| **b.** Cardiovascular effects—tachycardia, other arrhythmias, hypertension | These reactions are caused by the sympathomimetic effects of the drugs. |
| **c.** Gastrointestinal effects—anorexia, weight loss, nausea, diarrhea, constipation | |
| **4. Observe for drug interactions**<br>**a.** Drugs that *increase* effects of amphetamines: | |
| (1) Alkalinizing agents (sodium bicarbonate, antacids, some diuretics) | Drugs that increase the alkalinity of the gastrointestinal tract increase intestinal absorption of amphetamines, and urinary alkalinizers decrease urinary excretion. Increased absorption and decreased excretion serve to potentiate drug effects. |

*(continued)*

| *Nursing Actions* | *Rationale/Explanation* |
|---|---|
| (2) Monoamine oxidase (MAO) inhibitors | Potentiate amphetamines by slowing drug metabolism. These drugs thereby increase the risks of headache, subarachnoid hemorrhage, and other signs of a hypertensive crisis. A variety of neurologic toxic effects and malignant hyperpyrexia may occur. The combination may cause death. |
| **b.** Drugs that *decrease* effects of amphetamines: | |
| (1) Acidifying agents | Urinary acidifying agents (*e.g.*, ammonium chloride) increase urinary excretion and lower blood levels of amphetamines. Decreased absorption and increased excretion serve to decrease drug effects. |
| (2) Antipsychotic agents | Decrease or antagonize the excessive CNS stimulation produced by amphetamines. Chlorpromazine (Thorazine) or haloperidol (Haldol) is sometimes used in treating amphetamine overdose. |
| **c.** Drugs that *increase* effects of doxapram: | |
| (1) MAO inhibitors; sympathomimetic or adrenergic drugs (*e.g.*, epinephrine, norepinephrine) | Synergistic vasopressor effects may occur. |
| **d.** Drugs that *decrease* effects of doxapram: | |
| (1) Barbiturates | These CNS depressant drugs (sedative-hypnotics) may be used to manage excessive CNS stimulation caused by doxapram overdosage. |
| **5. Teach clients** **a.** Take amphetamines and methylphenidate only as prescribed by a physician. | These drugs have a high potential for abuse. The risks of drug dependence are lessened if the drugs are taken correctly. |
| **b.** Do not take stimulant drugs to delay fatigue and sleep. | Fatigue and sleep are normal "resting" mechanisms for the body. |
| **c.** Get adequate rest and sleep. | This is a much safer and more effective way to function than preventing rest and sleep by taking drugs or drinking large amounts of coffee or other caffeine-containing beverages. |
| **d.** Prevent nervousness, anxiety, tremors, and insomnia from excessive caffeine intake by decreasing consumption of coffee and other caffeine-containing beverages or by drinking decaffeinated coffee, tea, and cola. | Brewed coffee generally has a larger amount of caffeine than instant coffee, tea, and other beverages. |

## Review and Application Exercises

1. What kinds of behaviors may indicate narcolepsy?
2. What kinds of behaviors may indicate ADHD?
3. What is the rationale for treating narcolepsy and ADHD with CNS stimulants?
4. What are major adverse effects of CNS stimulants, and how may they be minimized?
5. Why is it important that children taking CNS stimulants for ADHD have drug-free periods when feasible?

## Selected References

Bolinger, A. M., Murphy, V. A., & Bubica, G. (1992). General pediatric therapy. In M. A. Koda-Kimble & L. Y. Young (Eds.), *Applied therapeutics: The clinical use of drugs* (5th ed.) (pp. 77-1–77-24). Vancouver, WA: Applied Therapeutics.

Crismon, M. L. (1992). Insomnia. In M. A. Koda-Kimble & L. Y. Young (Eds.), *Applied therapeutics: The clinical use of drugs* (5th ed.) (pp. 55-1–55-17). Vancouver, WA: Applied Therapeutics.

(1993). *Drug facts and comparisons*. St. Louis: Facts and Comparisons.

Shlafer, M. (1993). *The nurse, pharmacology and drug therapy: A prototype approach* (2nd ed.). Redwood City, CA: Addison-Wesley.

Swonger, A. K., & Matejski M. P. (1991). *Nursing pharmacology: An integrated approach to drug therapy and nursing practice* (2nd ed.). Philadelphia: J.B. Lippincott.

# Drugs Affecting the Autonomic Nervous System

### CHAPTER 17

# Physiology of the Autonomic Nervous System

## The autonomic nervous system

The autonomic nervous system (ANS) is a branch of the nervous system regulated mainly by centers in the hypothalamus, brain stem, and spinal cord. These centers serve to alter and integrate activities of the ANS. The ANS automatically, without conscious thought or effort, regulates many body functions. These functions can be described broadly as mechanisms designed to maintain a constant internal environment (homeostasis), to respond to stress or emergencies, and to repair body tissues.

Autonomic nerve impulses are transmitted to body tissues through two major subdivisions of the ANS: the *sympathetic nervous system* (SNS) and the *parasympathetic nervous system* (PNS). More specifically, nerve impulses are carried through *preganglionic fibers, ganglia*, and *postganglionic fibers*. Preganglionic impulses travel from the central nervous system to ganglia (cell bodies of postganglionic fibers located outside the brain and spinal cord); postganglionic impulses travel from ganglia to effector tissues of the heart, blood vessels, glands, other visceral organs, and smooth muscle. Motor nerves of the ANS innervate all body structures except skeletal muscle, which is innervated by the somatic nerves.

Nerve impulses in the ANS are transmitted by acetylcholine and norepinephrine (see Chap. 4). Acetylcholine is synthesized from acetylcoenzyme A and choline and released at preganglionic fibers of both the SNS and PNS and at postganglionic fibers of the PNS. The nerve fibers that secrete acetylcholine are called *cholinergic fibers*. Norepinephrine is synthesized from the amino acid tyrosine by a series of enzymatic conversions that also produce dopamine and epinephrine (*i.e.*, tyrosine → dopamine → norepinephrine → epinephrine). Norepinephrine is the end-product except in the adrenal medulla where most of the norepinephrine is converted to epinephrine. Norepinephrine is released at postganglionic fibers of the SNS. Nerve fibers secreting norepinephrine are called *adrenergic fibers*.

Acetylcholine and norepinephrine act on body organs and tissues to cause parasympathetic or sympathetic effects, respectively. Stimulation of both systems causes excitatory effects in some organs but inhibitory effects in others. However, most organs are predominantly controlled by one system. Also, when the sympathetic system excites a particular organ, the parasympathetic system often inhibits it. For example, sympathetic stimulation of the heart causes an increased rate and force of myocardial contraction. Parasympathetic stimulation decreases rate and force of contraction, thereby resting the heart.

### THE SYMPATHETIC NERVOUS SYSTEM

The SNS is stimulated by physical or emotional stress, such as strenuous exercise or work, pain, hemorrhage, intense emotions, and temperature extremes. Increased capacity for vigorous muscle activity in response to a perceived threat, whether real or imaginary, is often called the "fight or flight" reaction. Specific body responses include:

1. Increased arterial blood pressure and cardiac output
2. Increased blood flow to the brain, heart, and skeletal muscles; decreased blood flow to viscera and organs not needed for "fight or flight"
3. Increased rate of cellular metabolism—increased oxygen consumption and carbon dioxide production
4. Increased breakdown of muscle glycogen for energy
5. Increased blood sugar
6. Increased mental activity and ability to think clearly
7. Increased muscle strength
8. Increased rate of blood coagulation
9. Increased rate and depth of respiration
10. Pupil dilation to aid vision

These responses are protective mechanisms designed to help the person cope with the stress or get away from it. The intensity and duration of responses depend on the amounts of norepinephrine and epinephrine present. Norepinephrine and epinephrine are naturally occurring catecholamines that function as neurotransmitters and hormones. Norepinephrine is synthesized in adrenergic nerve endings. As a neurotransmitter, norepinephrine is secreted when adrenergic nerve endings are stimulated. It exerts intense but brief effects. Then it is taken up again by the nerve endings and reused as a neurotransmitter, or it is metabolized by monoamine oxidase (MAO). As a hormone, norepinephrine is secreted by the adrenal medulla, along with epinephrine, in response to sympathetic nerve stimulation. These hormones are secreted into the bloodstream and transported to all body tissues. They are continually present in arterial blood in amounts that vary according to the degree of stress present and the ability of the adrenal medulla to respond to stimuli. The circulating hormones exert the same effects as those caused by direct stimulation of the SNS. However, these effects last longer because the hormones are removed from the blood more slowly. These hormones are metabolized mainly in the liver by the enzymes MAO and catecholomethyl transferase.

When norepinephrine and epinephrine act on body cells that respond to adrenergic or sympathetic nerve stimulation, they interact with two distinct adrenergic receptors, alpha and beta. Norepinephrine acts mainly on alpha receptors; epinephrine acts on both alpha and beta receptors. These receptors have been further subdivided into alpha$_1$, alpha$_2$, beta$_1$, and beta$_2$ receptors.

Cellular events following stimulation of adrenergic receptors are thought to include the following mechanisms:

*Alpha$_1$ receptors.* The binding of adrenergic substances to receptor proteins in the cell membrane of smooth muscle cells is thought to open ion channels, allow calcium ions to move into the cell, and produce muscle contraction.

*Alpha$_2$ receptors.* When norepinephrine in the synaptic cleft stimulates presynaptic alpha$_2$ receptors, less norepinephrine is released by subsequent nerve impulses. Calcium seems to be required for neurotransmitter release from storage vesicles. Thus, in this instance, calcium may be prevented from entering the presynaptic nerve cell.

*Beta$_1$ and beta$_2$ receptors.* Stimulation of these receptors stimulates activity of adenylate cyclase, an enzyme in cell membranes. Adenylate cyclase, in turn, stimulates formation of cyclic adenosine monophosphate (cAMP). The cAMP can initiate any of several different intracellular actions, with specific actions depending on the type of cell.

The number and the binding activity of receptors may be altered. These phenomena are most clearly understood with beta receptors. For example, when chronically exposed to high concentrations of substances that stimulate their function, the receptors decrease in number and become less efficient in stimulating adenylate cyclase. The resulting decrease in beta-adrenergic responsiveness is called desensitization or downregulation of receptors.

Conversely, when chronically exposed to substances that block their function, the receptors may increase in number and become more efficient in stimulating adenylate cyclase. The resulting increase in beta-adrenergic responsiveness (called hypersensitization or upregulation) may lead to an exaggerated response when the blocking substance is withdrawn.

The types of adrenergic receptors, their locations, and their effects on body tissues are summarized in Table 17-1.

## TABLE 17-1.  ADRENERGIC RECEPTORS

| Type | Location | Effects of Stimulation |
| --- | --- | --- |
| Alpha$_1$ | Blood vessels | Vasoconstriction |
| | Gastrointestinal (GI) tract | Inhibition |
| | Uterus | Contraction |
| | Eye | Blinking, mydriasis |
| Alpha$_2$ | Presynaptic adrenergic nerve endings | Inhibits release of norepinephrine |
| | Platelets | Aggregation |
| Beta$_1$ | Heart | Increased heart rate, force of contraction, automaticity, and rate of AV conduction |
| | Adipose tissue | Lipolysis |
| Beta$_2$ | Bronchioles | Bronchodilation |
| | Arterioles of skeletal muscle | Vasodilation |
| | GI tract | Decreased motility and tone |
| | Liver | Glycogenolysis, gluconeogenesis |
| | Urinary bladder | Relaxed detrusor muscle |
| | Pregnant uterus | Relaxation |

## THE PARASYMPATHETIC NERVOUS SYSTEM

Functions stimulated by the PNS are often described as resting, reparative, or vegetative functions. They include digestion, excretion, cardiac deceleration, anabolism, and near vision.

About 75% of all parasympathetic nerve fibers are in the vagus nerves. These nerves supply the thoracic and abdominal organs; their branches go to the heart, lungs, esophagus, stomach, small intestine, the proximal half of the colon, the liver, gallbladder, pancreas, and the upper portions of the ureters. Other parasympathetic fibers supply pupillary sphincters and ciliary muscles; lacrimal, nasal, submaxillary, and parotid glands; descending colon and rectum; lower portions of the ureters and bladder; and genitalia.

Specific body responses to parasympathetic stimulation include:

1. Dilation of blood vessels in the skin; no particular effect on systemic blood vessels
2. Decreased heart rate and force of myocardial contraction
3. Increased secretion of digestive enzymes and motility of the gastrointestinal tract
4. Constriction of bronchi
5. Increased glandular secretions generally
6. Constricted pupils
7. No apparent effects on blood coagulation, blood sugar, mental activity, or muscle strength

These responses are brief (milliseconds) because acetylcholine is rapidly split into acetate ion and choline by acetylcholinesterase, an enzyme present in the nerve ending and on the surface of the receptor organ.

## Characteristics of autonomic drugs

Many drugs are used clinically because of their ability to stimulate or block activity of the SNS or PNS. Drugs that stimulate activity act like endogenous neurotransmitter substances; drugs that block activity prevent the action of both endogenous substances and stimulating drugs.

Drugs that act on the ANS generally affect the entire body rather than certain organs and tissues. Drug effects depend on which branch of the ANS is involved and whether it is stimulated or inhibited by drug therapy. Thus, knowledge of the physiology of the ANS is required if drug effects are to be understood and predicted. In addition, it is becoming increasingly important to understand receptor activity and consequences of stimulation or inhibition. More drugs are being developed to stimulate or inhibit particular subtypes of receptors. This is part of the continuing effort to design drugs that act more selectively on particular body tissues and decrease adverse effects on other body tissues. For example, drugs (*e.g.*, terbutaline) have been developed to stimulate $beta_2$ receptors in the respiratory tract and produce bronchodilation (a desired effect) with decreased stimulation of $beta_1$ receptors in the heart (an adverse effect).

The terminology used to describe autonomic drugs is often confusing because different terms are used to refer to the same phenomenon. Thus, *sympathomimetic, adrenergic,* and *alpha- and beta-adrenergic agonists* are used to describe a drug that has the same effects on the human body as stimulation of the SNS. *Parasympathomimetic, cholinomimetic,* and *cholinergic* are used to describe a drug that has the same effects on the body as stimulation of the PNS. There are also drugs that oppose or block stimulation of these systems. *Sympatholytic, antiadrenergic,* and *alpha- and beta-adrenergic blocking* drugs inhibit sympathetic stimulation. *Parasympatholytic, anticholinergic,* and *cholinergic blocking* drugs inhibit parasympathetic stimulation. This book uses the terms *adrenergic, antiadrenergic, cholinergic,* and *anticholinergic.*

## Review and Application Exercises

1. What are the major differences between the sympathetic and parasympathetic branches of the ANS?
2. What are the major SNS and PNS neurotransmitters?
3. What are the locations and functions of SNS receptors?
4. What is meant when drugs are described as adrenergic, sympathomimetic, antiadrenergic, sympatholytic, cholinergic, or anticholinergic?

## Selected References

Flannery, J. C. (1992). Overview of anatomy, physiology, and pathophysiology of the nervous system. In L. O. Burrell (Ed.), *Adult nursing in hospital and community settings* (pp. 831–863). Norwalk, CT: Appleton & Lange.

Guyton, A. C. (1991). *Textbook of medical physiology* (8th ed.). Philadelphia: W.B. Saunders.

Halter, J. B. (1992). Structure and function of the autonomic nervous system. In W. N. Kelley (Ed.), *Textbook of internal medicine* (2nd ed.) (pp. 2145–2150). Philadelphia: J.B. Lippincott.

Porth, C. M., & Curtis, R. L. (1990). Normal and altered autonomic nervous system function. In C. M. Porth (Ed.), *Pathophysiology: Concepts of altered health states* (3rd ed.) (pp. 873–892). Philadelphia: J.B. Lippincott.

Shlafer, M. (1993). *The nurse, pharmacology and drug therpay: A prototype approach* (2nd ed.). Redwood City, CA: Addison-Wesley.

Swonger, A. K., & Matejski, M. P. (1991). *Nursing pharmacology: An integrated approach to drug therapy and nursing practice* (2nd ed.). Philadelphia: J.B. Lippincott.

# CHAPTER 18

# Adrenergic Drugs

## Description and uses

Adrenergic (sympathomimetic) drugs produce effects similar to those produced by stimulation of the sympathetic nervous system (see Chap. 17). Major effects include vasoconstriction (alpha-adrenergic receptors), cardiac stimulation ($beta_1$-adrenergic receptors), and bronchodilation ($beta_2$-receptors).

The drugs discussed in this chapter are epinephrine, ephedrine, isoproterenol, and phenylephrine. Because epinephrine and ephedrine stimulate both alpha- and beta-adrenergic receptors, these drugs have widespread effects on body tissues and multiple clinical uses. Isoproterenol stimulates beta-adrenergic receptors (both $beta_1$ and $beta_2$) and is used in the treatment of several clinical conditions. Phenylephrine stimulates alpha-adrenergic receptors and is used to induce vasoconstriction in several conditions.

Other adrenergic drugs act mainly on specific adrenergic receptors or are given topically to produce more selective effects. These drugs have relatively restricted clinical indications and are discussed more extensively elsewhere (Drugs Used in Hypotension and Shock, Chap. 57; Bronchodilating and Antiasthmatic Drugs, Chap. 50; Nasal Decongestants, Antitussives, Mucolytics, and Cold Remedies, Chap. 52; and Drugs Used in Ophthalmic Conditions, Chap. 68). Table 18-1 provides an overview of commonly used adrenergic drugs in relation to adrenergic receptor activity and clinical use.

## MECHANISM OF ACTION

Adrenergic drugs stimulate adrenergic receptors on cell membranes. This leads to a series of intracellular events

that result in characteristic physiologic and pharmacologic effects. For further discussion, see Chapter 17.

## INDICATIONS FOR USE

Clinical indications for the use of adrenergic drugs stem mainly from their effects on the heart, blood vessels, and bronchi. They are often used as emergency drugs in the treatment of acute cardiovascular, respiratory, and allergic disorders. In hypotension and shock, they may be given as cardiac stimulants and vasopressor agents. (Vasopressors cause the muscles of capillaries and arteries to contract; contraction increases the resistance of vessels to the flow of blood, resulting in an increase in blood pressure.) In bronchial asthma and other obstructive pulmonary diseases, the drugs are given as bronchodilators to relieve bronchoconstriction and bronchospasm. In allergic disorders, the drugs are given for vasoconstricting or decongestant effects to relieve edema in the respiratory tract, skin, and other tissues. Other clinical uses include topical application to skin and mucous membranes for vasoconstriction and hemostatic effects, to the eyes for vasoconstriction (decongestant) and mydriasis (pupil dilation), and to nasal mucosa for decongestant effects in upper respiratory infections or allergic disorders.

## CONTRAINDICATIONS FOR USE

Contraindications for using adrenergic drugs include cardiac arrhythmias, angina pectoris, hypertension, hyperthyroidism, and narrow-angle glaucoma. They should be used with caution in hemorrhagic or hypovolemic shock as second-line agents if adequate fluid volume replacement does not restore sufficient blood pressure and circulation to maintain organ perfusion.

## TABLE 18-1. ADRENERGIC DRUGS

| Generic/Trade Name | Major Clinical Uses |
|---|---|
| ***Alpha and Beta Activity*** | |
| **Dopamine** (Intropin) | Hypotension and shock |
| **Epinephrine** (Adrenalin) | Allergic reactions, cardiac arrest, hypotension and shock, local vasoconstriction, bronchodilation, cardiac stimulation, ophthalmic conditions |
| **Ephedrine** | Bronchodilation, cardiac stimulation, nasal decongestion |
| ***Alpha Activity*** | |
| **Levarterenol** (Levophed) | Hypotension and shock |
| **Metaraminol** (Aramine) | Hypotension and shock |
| **Methoxamine** (Vasoxyl) | Hypotension and shock |
| **Naphazoline hydrochloride** (Privine) | Nasal decongestion |
| **Oxymetazoline hydrochloride** (Afrin) | Nasal decongestion |
| **Phenylephrine** (Neo-Synephrine) | Hypotension and shock, nasal decongestion, ophthalmic conditions |
| **Phenylpropanolamine hydrochloride** (Propagest, Dexatrim) | Nasal decongestion, appetite suppression |
| **Propylhexedrine** (Benzedrex) | Nasal decongestion |
| **Tetrahydrozoline hydrochloride** (Tyzine, Visine) | Nasal decongestion, local vasoconstriction in the eye |
| **Tuaminoheptane** (Tuamine) | Nasal decongestion |
| **Xylometazoline hydrochloride** (Otrivin) | Nasal decongestion |
| ***Beta Activity*** | |
| **Albuterol** (Proventil) | Bronchodilation |
| **Bitolterol** (Tornalate) | Bronchodilation |
| **Dobutamine** (Dobutrex) | Cardiac stimulation |
| **Isoproterenol** (Isuprel) | Bronchodilation, cardiac stimulation |
| **Isoetharine** (Bronkosol) | Bronchodilation |
| **Metaproterenol** (Alupent) | Bronchodilation |
| **Pirbuterol** (Maxair) | Bronchodilation |
| **Terbutaline** (Brethine) | Bronchodilation |

# Individual adrenergic drugs

**Epinephrine** (Adrenalin) is the prototype of adrenergic drugs. When given systemically, the effects may be therapeutic or adverse, depending on the reason for use and route of administration. Specific effects include:

1. Increased systolic blood pressure due primarily to increased force of myocardial contraction and vasoconstriction in skin, mucous membranes, and kidneys
2. Vasodilation and increased blood flow to skeletal muscles, heart, and brain
3. Vasoconstriction in peripheral blood vessels. This allows shunting of blood to the heart and brain, with increased perfusion pressure in the coronary and cerebral circulations. This action is thought to be the main beneficial effect in cardiac arrest and cardiopulmonary resuscitation (CPR).
4. Increased heart rate and possibly arrhythmias due to stimulation of conducting tissues in the heart. A reflex bradycardia may occur when blood pressure is raised.
5. Relaxation of gastrointestinal smooth muscle
6. Relaxation or dilation of bronchial smooth muscle
7. Increased glucose, lactate, and fatty acids in the blood due to metabolic effects
8. Inhibition of insulin secretion
9. Miscellaneous effects, including increased total leukocyte count, increased rate of blood coagulation, and decreased intraocular pressure in wide-angle glaucoma. When given locally, the main effect is vasoconstriction.

Epinephrine stimulates both alpha and beta receptors. As the prototype of adrenergic drugs, effects and clinical indications for epinephrine are the same as for adrenergic drugs. In addition, epinephrine is the adrenergic drug of choice for relieving the acute bronchospasm and laryngeal edema of anaphylactic shock, the most life-threatening allergic reaction. Epinephrine is used in cardiac arrest for its cardiac stimulant and peripheral vasoconstrictive effects. It also is added to local anesthetics for vasoconstrictive effects to slow absorption and prolong action of the local anesthetic drug.

Epinephrine is not given orally because it is destroyed by enzymes in the gastrointestinal tract and liver. It may be given by inhalation, injection, or topical application. Numerous epinephrine solutions are available for various uses and routes of administration. Solutions vary widely in the amount of drug contained. These must be used correctly to avoid potentially serious hazards to recipients. Epinephrine is the active ingredient in over-the-counter (OTC) inhalation products for asthma (Asthma Nefrin, Asthma-Meter Mist, Micro Nefrin, Primatene Mist, Bronkaid Mist, and others). These products are very hazardous if used incorrectly.

**Sus-Phrine** is an aqueous suspension of epinephrine that is given subcutaneously only. Some of the epinephrine is in solution and acts rapidly; some is suspended in crystalline form for slower absorption and relatively prolonged activity.

*Epinephrine injection, 1:1000 (1 mg/ml) aqueous solution*

### Routes and dosage ranges

***Adults:*** IM, SC 0.1–0.5 ml q2h if necessary; IV 1 ml diluted to 10 ml with sodium chloride injection; final concentration 1:10,000 (0.1 mg/ml)
Intracardiac, 0.1–0.2 ml
***Children:*** SC 0.01 ml/kg q4h if necessary

Epinephrine inhalation, 1:100 (1%)
aqueous solution

### Route and dosage ranges

*Adults:* Oral inhalation by aerosol, nebulizer, or intermittent positive pressure breathing machine. This is not a preferred route of administration for epinephrine.

Epinephrine nasal solution, 1:1000 solution

### Routes and dosage ranges

*Adults:* Topical application to nasal mucosa, 1–2 drops per nostril q4–6h
  Topical application to skin and mucous membranes for hemostasis, nasal solution diluted to 1:50,000–1:2000

Sus-phrine injection, 1:200 suspension

### Route and dosage ranges

*Adults:* SC only, 0.1 ml initially, maximum dose 0.3 ml; do not repeat for at least 6 h
*Children:* SC 0.005 ml/kg, maximum dose 0.15 ml

**Ephedrine** is an adrenergic drug that acts by stimulating alpha and beta receptors and causing release of norepinephrine. Ephedrine can be given orally, and its actions are less potent but longer lasting than those of epinephrine. Ephedrine produces more central nervous system (CNS) stimulation than other adrenergic drugs. It is often used in treatment of bronchial asthma to prevent bronchospasm, but it is less effective than epinephrine for acute bronchospasm and respiratory distress. Ephedrine is a common ingredient in OTC asthma tablets (Bronkaid, Primatene, and others). The tablets contain about 24 mg of ephedrine and 100 to 130 mg of theophylline, a xanthine bronchodilator. Other clinical uses include shock associated with spinal or epidural anesthesia, Stokes-Adams syndrome (sudden attacks of unconsciousness caused by heart block), allergic disorders, nasal congestion, and eye disorders.

**Pseudoephedrine** (Sudafed) is a related drug with similar actions. It is used for bronchodilating and nasal decongestant effects. Formerly a prescription drug, pseudoephedrine is now available OTC.

Ephedrine

### Route and dosage ranges

*Adults:* Asthma, PO 25–50 mg q4h
  Hypotension, SC, IM 25–50 mg; IV 20 mg; do not exceed 150 mg/24 h
  Mydriasis, eye drops of 0.1% solution
  Nasal congestion, nose drops of 0.5%, 1%, or 3% solutions; PO 25–50 mg q4h
*Children 6–12 years:* PO 6.25–12.5 mg q4–6h
*Children 2–6 years:* PO 0.3–0.5 mg/kg q4–6h

Pseudoephedrine

### Route and dosage ranges

*Adults:* PO 60 mg three or four times a day
*Children 6–12 years:* PO 30 mg q6h
*Children 2–6 years:* PO 15 mg q6h

**Isoproterenol** (Isuprel) is a synthetic catecholamine that acts on beta-adrenergic receptors. Its main actions are to stimulate the heart, dilate blood vessels in skeletal muscle, and relax bronchial smooth muscle. It is well absorbed when given by injection or as an aerosol. However, absorption is unreliable with sublingual and oral preparations, and their use is not recommended. Isoproterenol is used clinically as a bronchodilator in respiratory conditions characterized by bronchospasm and as a cardiac stimulant in heart block and cardiogenic shock. Too-frequent use may lead to tachyphylaxis and a reversal of bronchodilating effects.

### Routes and dosage ranges

*Adults:* Bradycardia and heart block, IV 1–2 mg (5–10 ml of 1:5000 solution), diluted in 5% dextrose injection, infused at 0.5–5 μg/min initially, then changed according to heart rate as indicated by continuous electrocardiogram monitoring
  Hypotension and shock, IV 1–2 mg (5–10 ml of 1:5000 solution) diluted in 5% dextrose injection, infused at 1–10 μg/min
  Bronchospasm during anesthesia, IV 0.01–0.02 mg or 0.5–1 ml of diluted solution initially (1 ml of 1:5000 solution, diluted to 10 ml with sodium chloride or 5% dextrose injection for a final concentration of 1:50,000), repeated PRN
  Bronchodilation, inhalation by nebulizer, 5–15 deep inhalations of a mist of 1:200 solution, repeated in 10–30 min if necessary; by oxygen aerosol, up to 0.5 ml of 1:200 solution or 0.3 ml of 1:100 solution with oxygen flow at 4 L/min for 15–20 min; by measured-dose inhalers (Mistometer, Medihaler), 1 or 2 inhalations (second inhalation is given 2–5 min after first). These treatments should generally be given no more often than q4h.
  Sublingual tablets, 10–15 mg three or four times a day, maximum 60 mg/d; not a recommended route because absorption is unpredictable
*Children:* Bronchodilation, inhalation, generally the same as above, with adult supervision; sublingual, 5–10 mg three or four times a day, maximum 30 mg/day (not a preferred route because of erratic absorption)

**Phenylephrine** (Neo-Synephrine and others) is a synthetic drug that acts on alpha-adrenergic receptors to produce vasoconstriction with little cardiac stimulation. It is given to raise blood pressure in hypotension and shock. Compared with epinephrine, phenylephrine produces longer-lasting elevation of blood pressure (20–50 min with injection). When given systemically, phenylephrine produces a reflex bradycardia; this effect may be used therapeutically to relieve paroxysmal atrial tachycardia. Other uses include local application for nasal decongestant and mydriatic effects. Various preparations are available for different uses. Phenylephrine is often an ingredient in mixtures used for symptoms of the common cold and allergic rhinitis, both prescription and nonprescription.

### Routes and dosage ranges

*Adults:* Hypotension and shock, IM, SC 5–10 mg; IV 0.25–0.5 mg diluted in sodium chloride injection and given slowly, or 10 mg diluted in 500 ml 5% dextrose injection and infused slowly, according to blood pressure readings

Orthostatic hypotension, PO 20 mg three times per day

Nasal congestion, nasal solutions of 0.125%, 0.25%, 0.5%, or 1.0%

Mydriasis, ophthalmic solutions of 2.5% or 10%

## Nursing Process

### Assessment

Assess the client's status in relation to the following conditions:

- **Allergic disorders**. It is standard procedure to question a client about allergies on initial contact or admission to a health-care agency. If the client reports a previous allergic reaction, try to determine what caused it and what specific symptoms occurred. It may be helpful to ask if swelling, breathing difficulty, or hives (urticaria) occurred. With anaphylactic reactions, severe respiratory distress (from bronchospasm and laryngeal edema) and profound hypotension (from vasodilation) may occur.
- **Asthma**. If the client is known to have asthma, assess the frequency of attacks, the specific signs and symptoms experienced, the precipitating factors, the actions taken to obtain relief, and the use of bronchodilators or other medications on a long-term basis. With acute bronchospasm, respiratory distress is clearly evidenced by loud, rapid, gasping, wheezing respirations. Acute asthma attacks or bronchoconstriction may be precipitated by exposure to allergens or respiratory infections. When available, check arterial blood gas reports for the adequacy of oxygen–carbon dioxide gas exchange. Hypoxemia ($\downarrow$ pO$_2$), hypercarbia ($\uparrow$ pCO$_2$), and acidosis ($\downarrow$ pH) may occur with acute bronchospasm.
- **Chronic obstructive pulmonary disorders**. Emphysema and chronic bronchitis are characterized by bronchoconstriction and dyspnea with exercise or at rest. Check arterial blood gas reports when available. Hypoxemia, hypercarbia, and acidosis are likely with chronic bronchoconstriction. Acute bronchospasm may be superimposed on the chronic bronchoconstrictive disorder, especially with a respiratory infection.

- **Cardiovascular status**. Assess for conditions that are caused or aggravated by adrenergic drugs (*e.g.*, hypertension, tachyarrhythmias).

### Nursing diagnoses

- Impaired Gas Exchange related to bronchoconstriction
- Altered Tissue Perfusion related to hypotension and shock or vasoconstriction with drug therapy
- Altered Nutrition: Less than Body Requirements related to anorexia
- Sleep Pattern Disturbance: Insomnia, nervousness
- High Risk for Noncompliance: Overuse
- High Risk for Injury related to cardiac stimulation (arrhythmias, hypertension)
- Knowledge Deficit: Drug effects and safe usage

### Planning/Goals

*The client will:*
- Receive drugs accurately
- Experience relief of symptoms for which adrenergic drugs are given
- Comply with instructions for safe drug usage
- Demonstrate knowledge of accurate self-administration and adverse drug effects to be reported
- Avoid preventable adverse drug effects

### Interventions

Use measures to prevent or minimize conditions for which adrenergic drugs are required:
- Decrease exposure to allergens. Allergens include cigarette smoke, foods, drugs, air pollutants, plant pollens, insect venoms, and animal dander. Specific allergens must be determined for each person.
- For people with chronic lung disease, use measures to prevent respiratory infections. These include measures to aid removal of respiratory secretions, such as adequate hydration, ambulation, deep breathing and coughing exercises, and chest physiotherapy (percussion and postural drainage). Immunizations with pneumococcal pneumonia vaccine (a single dose) and influenza vaccine (annually) are also recommended.
- When administering substances known to produce hypersensitivity reactions (penicillin and other antibiotics, allergy extracts, vaccines, local anesthetics), observe the recipient carefully for at least 30 minutes after administration. Have adrenergic and other emergency drugs and equipment readily available in case a reaction occurs.

*Teach clients:*
- To use these drugs only as directed. The potential for abuse is high, especially for the client with asthma or other chronic lung disease who is seeking relief from labored breathing. Some of these drugs are often prescribed for long-term use, but excessive use does not increase therapeutic effects. Instead, it increases the incidence and severity of adverse reactions and causes tolerance and decreased benefit from usual doses.
- To take no other medications without the physician's knowledge and approval. Many OTC cold remedies and appetite suppressants contain adrenergic drugs. Use of these along with prescribed adrenergic drugs can result in overdose and serious cardiovascular or CNS problems. In addition, adrenergic drugs interact with numerous other drugs to in-

crease or decrease effects; some of these interactions may be life-threatening.

### Evaluation

- Observe for increased blood pressure and improved tissue perfusion when a drug is given for hypotension and shock or anaphylaxis.
- Interview and observe for improved breathing and arterial blood gas reports when a drug is given for bronchoconstriction or anaphylaxis.
- Interview and observe for decreased nasal congestion.

## Principles of therapy

### DRUG SELECTION AND ADMINISTRATION

Choice of drug, dosage, and route of administration depends largely on the reason for use. Epinephrine, injected IV or subcutaneously, is the drug of choice in anaphylactic shock. Isoproterenol by oral inhalation is often effective for producing bronchodilation. Adrenergic drugs are given IV only for emergencies, such as cardiac arrest, severe arterial hypotension, circulatory shock, and anaphylactic shock. No standard doses of individual adrenergic drugs are always effective; the dosage must be individualized according to the client's response. This is especially true in emergencies, but it also applies to long-term usage.

### USE IN SPECIFIC SITUATIONS

Because adrenergic drugs are often used in crises, they must be readily available in all health-care settings (e.g., hospitals, long-term care facilities, physicians' offices). All health-care personnel should know where emergency drugs are stored.

### Anaphylaxis

Epinephrine is the first drug of choice for treatment of anaphylaxis. It relieves bronchospasm, laryngeal edema, and hypotension. In conjunction with its alpha (vasoconstriction) and beta (cardiac stimulation, bronchodilation) effects, epinephrine acts as a physiologic antagonist of histamine and other bronchoconstricting and vasodilating substances released during anaphylactic reactions.

Victims of anaphylaxis who have been taking beta-adrenergic blocking drugs (e.g. propranolol [Inderal]) do not respond as readily to epinephrine as those not taking a beta-blocker. Larger doses of epinephrine and large amounts of IV fluids may be required.

### Cardiopulmonary resuscitation

Epinephrine is one of the first drugs administered during CPR. Its most important action is constriction of peripheral blood vessels. This shunts blood to the central circulation and increases blood flow to the heart and brain. It is also given for ventricular fibrillation, ventricular tachycardia, and asystole. In asystole, it stimulates electrical and mechanical activity to produce myocardial contraction. This effect is also thought to result from its vasoconstrictive action.

### Hypotension and shock

In hypotension and shock, initial efforts involve identifying and treating the cause when possible. Such treatments include blood transfusions, fluid and electrolyte replacement, and treatment of infection. If these measures are ineffective in raising blood pressure enough to maintain tissue perfusion, vasopressor drugs may be used. The usual goal of vasopressor drug therapy is to maintain tissue perfusion and a systolic blood pressure of at least 80 to 100 mm Hg.

### USE IN CHILDREN

Guidelines for safe and effective use of adrenergic drugs in children are not well established. Children are very sensitive to drug effects, including cardiac and CNS stimulation, and recommended doses generally should not be exceeded.

The main use of **epinephrine** in children is for treatment of bronchospasm due to asthma or allergic reactions. Parenteral epinephrine may cause syncope when given to asthmatic children.

Parenteral *terbutaline* is not recommended for use. Oral terbutaline is not recommended for children under 12 years of age.

With **albuterol** (Proventil), safety and effectiveness have not been established for tablets in children under 12 years or for the syrup formulation in children under 2 years. Albuterol, **bitolterol** (Tornalate), and **metaproterenol** (Alupent) have not been established as safe and effective for inhalation in children under 12 years.

**Isoproterenol** is rarely given parenterally, but if given, the first dose should be about half that of an adult, and later doses should be based on the response to the first dose. When given by inhalation, dosage for children is about the same as dosage for adults.

**Phenylephrine** is most often used to relieve congestion of the upper respiratory tract. Doses must be carefully measured. Rebound nasal congestion occurs with overuse.

**Phenylpropanolamine** and **pseudoephedrine** are common ingredients in OTC cold remedies. Dosage guidelines should be followed carefully, and the drugs should be inaccessible to young children. Phenylpropanolamine also is the active ingredient in OTC appetite suppressants. These should not be used for weight reduction in children.

## USE IN OLDER ADULTS

Adrenergic drugs stimulate the heart to increase rate and force of contraction and blood pressure. Older adults often have chronic cardiovascular conditions (*e.g.*, angina, arrhythmias, congestive heart failure, coronary artery disease, hypertension, peripheral vascular disease) that are aggravated by the drugs. Adrenergics are often prescribed as bronchodilators and decongestants in older adults. Therapeutic doses increase the workload of the heart and may cause symptoms of impaired cardiovascular function; overdoses may cause severe car-

diovascular dysfunction, including life-threatening arrhythmias.

The drugs also cause CNS stimulation. With therapeutic doses, anxiety, restlessness, nervousness, and insomnia often occur in older adults. Overdoses may cause hallucinations, convulsions, CNS depression, and death.

Adrenergics are ingredients in OTC asthma remedies, cold remedies, and nasal decongestants. Cautious use of these preparations is required for older adults. They should not be taken concurrently with prescription adrenergic drugs because of the high risk of overdose and toxicity.

Ophthalmic preparations of adrenergic drugs also should be used cautiously. For example, **phenylephrine** is used as a vasoconstrictor and mydriatic. Applying larger-than-recommended doses to the normal eye or usual doses to the traumatized, inflamed, or diseased eye may result in enough systemic absorption of the drug to cause increased blood pressure and other adverse effects.

## NURSING ACTIONS: ADRENERGIC DRUGS

| *Nursing Actions* | *Rationale/Explanation* |
|---|---|
| **1. Administer accurately**<br>**a.** Check package inserts or other references if not absolutely sure about the preparation or concentration and method of administration for an adrenergic drug. | The many different preparations and concentrations available for various routes of administration increase the risk of medication error unless extreme caution is used. Preparations for intravenous, subcutaneous, inhalation, ophthalmic, or nasal routes must be used by the designated route only. |
| **b.** To give epinephrine subcutaneously, use a tuberculin syringe, aspirate, and massage the injection site. | The tuberculin syringe is necessary for accurate measurement of the small doses usually given (often less than 0.5 ml). Aspiration is necessary to avoid inadvertent IV administration of the larger, undiluted amount of drug intended for subcutaneous use. Massaging the injection site accelerates drug absorption and thus relief of symptoms. |
| **c.** Give Sus-Phrine subcutaneously only, and shake well before using (both vial and syringe). | Sus-Phrine is a suspension preparation of epinephrine, and suspensions must not be given IV. Rotating or shaking the container ensures that the medication is evenly distributed throughout the suspension. |
| **d.** For inhalation, be sure to use the correct drug concentration, and use the nebulizing device properly. | Inhalation medications are often administered by clients themselves or by respiratory therapists if intermittent positive pressure breathing (IPPB) is used. The nurse may need to demonstrate and supervise self-administration initially. |
| **e.** Do *not* give epinephrine and isoproterenol at the same time or within 4 hours of each other. | Both of these drugs are potent cardiac stimulants, and the combination could cause serious cardiac arrhythmias. However, they have synergistic bronchodilating effects, and doses can be alternated and given safely if the drugs are given no more closely together than 4 hours. |

*(continued)*

| *Nursing Actions* | *Rationale/Explanation* |
|---|---|
| **f.** For IV injection of epinephrine, dilute 1 ml of 1:1000 solution to a total volume of 10 ml with sodium chloride injection, or use a commercial preparation of 1:10,000 concentration. Use parenteral solutions of epinephrine only if clear. | Dilution increases safety of administration. A solution that is brown or contains a precipitate should not be used. Discoloration indicates chemical deterioration of epinephrine. |
| **g.** For IV infusion of isoproterenol and phenylephrine: | |
| (1) Administer in an intensive care unit when possible. | These drugs are given IV in emergencies, during which the client's condition must be carefully monitored. Frequent recording of blood pressure and pulse and continuous electrocardiographic monitoring are needed. |
| (2) Use only clear drug solutions. | A brownish color or precipitate indicates deterioration, and such solutions should not be used. |
| (3) Dilute the drugs in 500 ml of 5% dextrose injection. Do not add the drug until ready to use. | A 5% dextrose solution is compatible with the drugs. Mixing solutions when ready for use helps to ensure drug stability. Note that drug concentration varies with the amount of drug and the amount of dextrose solution to which it is added. |
| (4) Use an infusion device to regulate flow rate accurately. | Flow rate usually requires frequent adjustment according to blood pressure measurements. An infusion device helps to regulate drug administration, so wide fluctuations in blood pressure are avoided. |
| (5) Use a ''piggyback'' IV apparatus. | Only one bottle contains an adrenergic drug, and it can be regulated or discontinued without disruption of the primary IV line. |
| (6) Start the adrenergic drug solution slowly and increase flow rate according to the client's response (*e.g.*, blood pressure, color, mental status). Slow or discontinue gradually as well. | To avoid abrupt changes in circulation and blood pressure. |
| **h.** When giving adrenergic drugs as eye drops or nose drops, do not touch the dropper to the eye or nose. | Contaminated droppers can be a source of bacterial infection. |
| **2. Observe for therapeutic effects** | These depend on the reason for use. |
| **a.** When the drug is used as a bronchodilator, observe for absence or reduction of wheezing, less labored breathing, and decreased rate of respirations. | Indicates prevention or relief of bronchospasm. Acute bronchospasm is usually relieved within 5 minutes by injected or inhaled epinephrine or inhaled isoproterenol. |
| **b.** When epinephrine is given in anaphylactic shock, observe for decreased tissue edema and improved breathing and circulation. | Epinephrine injection usually relieves laryngeal edema and bronchospasm within 5 minutes and lasts for about 20 minutes. |
| **c.** When isoproterenol or phenylephrine is given in hypotension and shock, observe for increased blood pressure, stronger pulse, and improved urine output, level of consciousness, and color. | These are indicators of improved circulation. |
| **d.** When a drug is given nasally for decongestant effects, observe for decreased nasal congestion and ability to breathe though the nose. | The drugs act as vasoconstrictors to reduce engorgement of nasal mucosa. |
| **e.** When given as eye drops for vasoconstrictor effects, observe for decreased redness. When giving for mydriatic effects, observe for pupil dilation. | |

## Nursing Actions

## Rationale/Explanation

**3. Observe for adverse effects**

Adverse effects depend to some extent on the reason for use. For example, cardiovascular effects are considered adverse reactions when the drugs are given for bronchodilation. Adverse effects occur with usual therapeutic doses and are more likely to occur with higher doses.

**a.** Cardiovascular effects—cardiac arrhythmias, hypertension

Tachycardia and hypertension are common; if severe or prolonged, myocardial ischemia or heart failure may occur. Premature ventricular contractions and other serious arrhythmias may occur. Propranolol (Inderal) or another beta-blocker may be given to decrease heart rate and hypertension resulting from overdosage of adrenergic drugs. Phentolamine (Regitine) may be used to decrease severe hypertension.

**b.** Excessive CNS stimulation—nervousness, anxiety, tremor, insomnia

These effects are more likely to occur with ephedrine or high doses of other adrenergic drugs. Sometimes, a sedative-type drug is given concomitantly to offset these effects.

**c.** Rebound nasal congestion, rhinitis, possible ulceration of nasal mucosa.

These effects occur with excessive use of nasal decongestant drugs.

**4. Observe for drug interactions**
  **a.** Drugs that *increase* effects of adrenergic drugs:

Most of these drugs increase incidence or severity of adverse reactions.

  (1) Anesthetics, general (halothane, cyclopropane)

Increased risk of cardiac arrhythmias. Potentially hazardous.

  (2) Anticholinergics (*e.g.,* atropine)

Increased bronchial relaxation. Also increased mydriasis and therefore contraindicated with narrow-angle glaucoma.

  (3) Antidepressants, tricyclic (*e.g.,* amitriptyline [Elavil])

Increased pressor response with intravenous epinephrine

  (4) Antihistamines

May increase pressor effects

  (5) Cocaine

Increases pressor and mydriatic effects by inhibiting uptake of norepinephrine by nerve endings. Cardiac arrhythmias, convulsions, and acute glaucoma may occur.

  (6) Digitalis

Sympathomimetics, especially beta-adrenergics like epinephrine and isoproterenol, increase the likelihood of cardiac arrhythmias due to ectopic pacemaker activity.

  (7) Doxapram (Dopram)

Increased pressor effect

  (8) Ergot alkaloids (*e.g.,* Gynergen)

Increased vasoconstriction. Extremely high blood pressure may occur. There also may be decreased perfusion of fingers and toes.

  (9) Monoamine oxidase (MAO) inhibitors (*e.g.,* isocarboxazid [Marplan])

Contraindicated. The combination may cause death. When these drugs are given concurrently with adrenergic drugs, there is danger of cardiac arrhythmias, respiratory depression, and acute hypertensive crisis with possible intracranial hemorrhage, convulsions, coma, and death. Effects of MAO inhibitors may not occur for several weeks after treatment is started and may last up to 3 weeks after the drug is stopped. Every client taking MAO inhibitors should be warned against taking any other medication without the advice of a physician or pharmacist.

*(continued)*

## Nursing Actions

## Rationale/Explanation

(10) Methylphenidate (Ritalin)

Increased pressor and mydriatic effects. The combination may be hazardous in glaucoma.

(11) Thyroid preparations (e.g., Synthroid)

Increased adrenergic effects, resulting in increased likelihood of arrhythmias

(12) Xanthines (in caffeine-containing substances, such as coffee, tea, cola drinks; theophylline)

Synergistic bronchodilating effect. Sympathomimetics with CNS-stimulating properties (e.g., ephedrine, isoproterenol) may produce excessive CNS stimulation with cardiac arrhythmias, emotional disturbances, and insomnia.

(13) Beta-adrenergic blocking agents (e.g., propranolol [Inderal])

May augment hypertensive response to epinephrine (see also b[4] below)

**b.** Drugs that *decrease* effects of adrenergics:

(1) Anticholinesterases (e.g., neostigmine [Prostigmin], pyridostigmine [Mestinon]) and other cholinergic drugs

Decrease mydriatic effects of adrenergics; thus, the two groups should not be given concurrently in ophthalmic conditions

(2) Antihypertensives (e.g., methyldopa [Aldomet])

Generally antagonize pressor effects of adrenergics, which act to increase blood pressure while antihypertensives act to lower it

(3) Antipsychotic drugs (e.g., haloperidol [Haldol], chlorpromazine [Thorazine])

Block the vasopressor action of epinephrine. Therefore, epinephrine should not be used to treat hypotension induced by these drugs.

(4) Beta-adrenergic blocking agents (e.g., propranolol [Inderal])

Decrease bronchodilating effects of adrenergics and may exacerbate asthma. Contraindicated with asthma.

(5) Phentolamine (Regitine)

Antagonizes vasopressor effects of adrenergics

**5. Teach clients**
 **a.** Inhaled solutions of isoproterenol may turn saliva and sputum pink.

This harmless discoloration is caused by the medication, not by bleeding.

**b.** Report adverse reactions, such as fast pulse, palpitations, chest pain.

So that drug dosage can be reevaluated and therapy changed if needed

**c.** Report if previously effective dose becomes ineffective.

This may indicate that drug tolerance has developed. This is more likely to occur with long-term use of ephedrine and isoproterenol for bronchodilation. Tolerance can be prevented or treated by discontinuing the individual drug for a few days or by substituting another adrenergic drug.

**d.** For clients receiving intravenous adrenergic drugs for cardiac stimulation or vasopressor effects, explain the necessity for cardiac monitoring, frequent checks of flow rate, blood pressure, urine output, and so on.

An explanation may help decrease anxiety in a seriously ill patient. He or she should know that these measures increase the safety and benefits of drug therapy rather than indicate the presence of a critical condition.

## Review and Application Exercises

1. How do adrenergic drugs act to relieve symptoms of acute bronchospasm, anaphylaxis, cardiac arrest, hypotension and shock, and nasal congestion?
2. Which adrenergic receptors are stimulated by administration of epinephrine?
3. Why is it important to have epinephrine and other adrenergic drugs readily available in all health care settings?

4. Which adrenergic drug is the first drug of choice to treat acute anaphylactic reactions?
5. Why is inhaled epinephrine not a drug of first choice for long-term treatment of asthma and other bronchoconstrictive disorders?
6. What are major adverse effects of adrenergic drugs?
7. Why are clients with cardiac arrhythmias, angina pectoris, hypertension, or diabetes mellitus especially likely to experience adverse reactions to adrenergic drugs?

8. For a client who reports frequent use of OTC asthma remedies and cold remedies, what teaching is needed to increase client safety?
9. Mentally rehearse nursing interventions for various emergency situations (*i.e.*, anaphylaxis, acute respiratory distress, cardiac arrest) in terms of medications and equipment needed and how to obtain them promptly.

## Selected References

Brater, C. (1992). Clinical pharmacology of cardiovascular drugs. In W. N. Kelley (Ed.), *Textbook of internal medicine* (2nd ed.) (pp. 315–335). Philadelphia: J.B. Lippincott.

(1993). *Drug facts and comparisons*. St. Louis: Facts and Comparisons.

Gotz, V. P. (1992). Chronic obstructive airways disease. In M. A. Koda-Kimble & L. Y. Young (Eds.), *Applied therapeutics: The clinical use of drugs* (5th ed.) (pp. 16-1–16-17). Vancouver, WA: Applied Therapeutics.

Guyton, A. C. (1991). *Textbook of medical physiology* (8th ed.). Philadelphia: W.B. Saunders.

Halter, J. B. (1992). Structure and function of the autonomic nervous system. In W. N. Kelley (Ed.), *Textbook of internal medicine* (2nd ed.) (pp. 2145–2150). Philadelphia: J.B. Lippincott.

Kelly, H. W. (1992). Asthma. In M. A. Koda-Kimble & L. Y. Young (Eds.). *Applied therapeutics: The clinical use of drugs* (5th ed.) (pp. 15-1–15-24). Vancouver, WA: Applied Therapeutics.

Lindell, K. O., & Mazzocco, M. C. (1990). Breaking bronchospasm's grip with MDIs. *American Journal of Nursing, 90,* 34–39.

Paré, P. D., & Montaner, J. S. (1992). Asthma. In W. N. Kelley (Ed.), *Textbook of internal medicine* (2nd ed.) (pp. 1707–1714). Philadelphia: J.B. Lippincott.

Petty, T. L. (1992). Chronic obstructive pulmonary disease. In W. N. Kelley (Ed.), *Textbook of internal medicine* (2nd ed.) (pp. 1717–1722). Philadelphia: J.B. Lippincott.

Porth, C. M. (1990). *Pathophysiology: Concepts of altered health states* (3rd ed.). Philadelphia: J.B. Lippincott.

Spitzer, W. O., Suissa, S., Ernst P., Horwitz, R. I., Habbick, B., & Cockcroft, J. (1992). Beta-agonists and the risk of death and near death from asthma. *New England Journal of Medicine, 326,* 501–506.

Swonger, A. K., & Matejski, M. P. (1991). *Nursing pharmacology: An integrated approach to drug therapy and nursing practice* (2nd ed.) Philadelphia: J.B. Lippincott.

### CHAPTER 19

# Antiadrenergic Drugs

## Description

Antiadrenergic drugs (also called adrenergic blocking or sympatholytic agents) block the effects of sympathetic nerve stimulation and adrenergic drugs. Centrally active antiadrenergic drugs (*e.g.*, clonidine, methyldopa) and ganglionic blocking agents (*e.g.*, guanethidine) are used almost exclusively in the treatment of hypertension. These drugs are discussed in Chapter 58. Peripherally active antiadrenergic agents (alpha- and beta-adrenergic blocking agents) are used for various clinical purposes. A basal level of sympathetic tone is necessary to maintain normal body functioning, including regulation of blood pressure, blood glucose, and stress response. Therefore, the goal of antiadrenergic drug therapy is to suppress pathologic stimulation, not the normal, physiologic response to activity, stress, and other stimuli.

### MECHANISM OF ACTION

These drugs act by occupying alpha and beta receptor sites in tissues and organs innervated by the sympathetic nervous system. By doing so, they prevent catecholamines and other sympathomimetic amines from occupying these sites and exerting their stimulating action. Thus, blocking agents can prevent the action of naturally occurring (endogenous) or externally administered (exogenous) catecholamines, such as epinephrine, norepinephrine, isoproterenol, and other adrenergic agents.

*Alpha-adrenergic blocking agents* occupy alpha-adrenergic receptor sites in smooth muscles and glands innervated by sympathetic nerve fibers. These drugs act primarily in the skin, mucosa, intestines, and kidneys to prevent alpha-mediated vasoconstriction. Specific effects include dilation of arterioles and veins, increased local blood flow, decreased blood pressure, constriction of pupils, and increased motility of the gastrointestinal tract.

*Beta-adrenergic blocking agents* occupy beta-adrenergic receptor sites and prevent the receptors from responding to sympathetic nerve impulses, circulating catecholamines, and beta-adrenergic drugs (Fig. 19-1). Specific effects include:

1. Decreased heart rate (negative chronotropy)
2. Decreased force of myocardial contraction (negative inotropy)
3. Decreased cardiac output at rest and with exercise
4. Slowed conduction through the atrioventricular (AV) node
5. Decreased automaticity of ectopic pacemakers
6. Decreased blood pressure in supine and standing positions
7. Bronchoconstriction from blockade of $beta_2$ receptors in bronchial smooth muscle. This effect occurs primarily in people with asthma or other chronic lung diseases with a bronchospastic component.
8. Less effective metabolism of glucose (decreased glycogenolysis) when needed by the body, especially in people who are taking beta-blocking agents along with antidiabetic drugs. These people may experience more severe and prolonged hypoglycemia. In addition, early symptoms of hypoglycemia (*e.g.*,

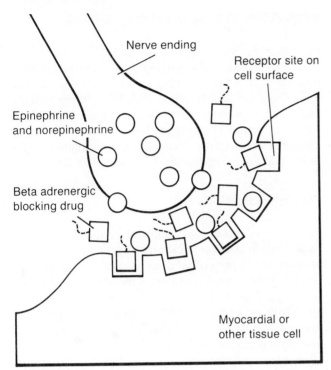

**FIGURE 19-1.** Beta-adrenergic blocking agents prevent epinephrine and norepinephrine from occupying receptor sites on cell membranes. This action alters cell functions normally stimulated by epinephrine and norepinephrine, according to the number of receptor sites occupied by the beta-blocking drugs. (Adapted by J. Harley from Encyclopedia Britannica Medical and Health Annual. Chicago, Encyclopedia Britannica, 1983)

tachycardia) may be blocked, delaying recognition of the hypoglycemia.

## INDICATIONS FOR USE

### Alpha-adrenergic blocking drugs

Clinical uses of these drugs are limited. Doxazosin, prazosin, and terazosin are used in the treatment of hypertension and are discussed further in Chapter 58. Phenoxybenzamine and phentolamine are not used as antihypertensive drugs except in hypertension caused by excessive catecholamines. Excessive catecholamines may result from overdosage of adrenergic drugs or from pheochromocytoma, a rare tumor of the adrenal medulla that secretes epinephrine and norepinephrine and causes hypertension, tachycardia, and cardiac arrhythmias. Although the treatment of choice for pheochromocytoma is surgical excision, alpha-adrenergic blocking drugs are useful adjuncts. They are given before and during surgery, usually in conjunction with beta-blockers. Alpha-blockers also are used in vascular diseases charac-

terized by vasospasm, such as Raynaud's disease and frostbite.

## Beta-adrenergic blocking drugs

Clinical indications for use of beta-blocking agents are mainly cardiovascular disorders (*i.e., angina pectoris, cardiac tachyarrhythmias, hypertension*, and *myocardial infarction*) and glaucoma. In angina, beta-blockers decrease myocardial contractility, cardiac output, heart rate, and blood pressure. These effects decrease myocardial oxygen demand (cardiac workload), especially in response to activity, exercise, and stress. In arrhythmias, drug effects depend on the sympathetic tone of the heart (that is, the degree of adrenergic stimulation of the heart that the drug must block or overcome). The drugs slow the sinus rate and prolong conduction through the AV node, thereby slowing the ventricular response rate to supraventricular tachyarrhythmias.

In hypertension, the actions by which the drugs lower blood pressure are unclear. Possible mechanisms include reduced cardiac output, inhibition of renin, and inhibition of sympathetic nervous system stimulation in the brain. However, the drugs effective in hypertension do not consistently demonstrate these effects (that is, a drug may lower blood pressure without reducing cardiac output or inhibiting renin, for example). Following myocardial infarction, the drugs help to protect the heart from reinfarction and decrease mortality rates over several years. A possible mechanism is preventing or decreasing the incidence of catecholamine-induced arrhythmias.

In glaucoma, the drugs reduce intraocular pressure by binding to beta-adrenergic receptors in the ciliary body of the eye and decreasing formation of aqueous humor.

Propranolol (Inderal) is the prototype of beta-adrenergic blocking agents. It is also the oldest, most widely used, and most extensively studied beta-blocker. In addition to its use in the treatment of hypertension, arrhythmias, angina pectoris, and myocardial infarction, propranolol is used in hypertrophic obstructive cardiomyopathies, in which it improves exercise tolerance; pheochromocytoma, in which it decreases tachycardia and arrhythmias but must be used along with an alpha-adrenergic blocking agent; hyperthyroidism, in which it decreases heart rate, cardiac output, and tremor; and prevention of migraine headaches by an unknown mechanism (it is not helpful in acute attacks of migraine). The drug also relieves palpitation and tremor associated with anxiety, but it is not approved for clinical use as an antianxiety drug.

## CONTRAINDICATIONS FOR USE

Alpha-adrenergic blocking agents are contraindicated in angina pectoris, myocardial infarction, and stroke. Beta-adrenergic blocking agents are contraindicated in bradycardia, heart block, congestive heart failure, and asthma and other allergic or pulmonary conditions characterized by bronchoconstriction.

# Individual antiadrenergic drugs

## ALPHA-ADRENERGIC BLOCKING DRUGS

**Phenoxybenzamine** (Dibenzyline) blocks alpha₁-adrenergic receptor sites to decrease blood pressure and increase blood flow to the skin, mucosa, and viscera. Thus, it may be used to aid arterial blood flow in peripheral vasospastic disorders, such as Raynaud's disorder and frostbite. It also may be given for hypertension resulting from pheochromocytoma, either during the perioperative period or during long-term treatment of clients who are not candidates for surgical excision. Phenoxybenzamine is long-acting; effects of a single dose persist for 3 to 4 days.

### Route and dosage range

*Adults:* PO 10 mg daily initially, gradually increased by 10 mg every 4 days until therapeutic effects are obtained or adverse effects become intolerable; optimum dosage level usually reached in 2 weeks; usual maintenance dose 20–60 mg/d

**Phentolamine** (Regitine) blocks alpha₁ and alpha₂ receptor sites. It dilates arteries and veins to decrease peripheral vascular resistance and decrease venous return to the heart. It generally has the same action, uses, and adverse effects as phenoxybenzamine. In addition, certain unique characteristics make it more useful clinically than phenoxybenzamine. Phentolamine is short-acting; effects last only a few hours and can be reversed by an alpha-adrenergic stimulant drug, such as levarterenol (Levophed). It is recommended for intravenous administration before and during surgical excision of pheochromocytoma. Phentolamine also can be used to prevent tissue necrosis from extravasation of potent vasoconstrictors (*e.g.,* levarterenol, dopamine) into subcutaneous tissues.

### Routes and dosage ranges

*Before and during surgery:* IV, IM 5–20 mg as needed to control blood pressure
*Prevention of tissue necrosis:* IV 10 mg in each liter of IV solution containing a potent vasoconstrictor
*Treatment of extravasation:* SC 5–10 mg in 10 ml saline, infiltrated into the area within 12 hours

## BETA-ADRENERGIC BLOCKING DRUGS

Sixteen beta-blocking agents are currently marketed in the United States. Although they produce similar effects, they differ in several characteristics, including clinical indications for use, receptor selectivity, intrinsic sympathomimetic activity, membrane-stabilizing ability, lipid solubility, routes of excretion, routes of administration, and duration of action. Characteristics of subgroups and individual drugs are described below and in Table 19-1.

### Clinical indications

Twelve beta-blockers are approved for the treatment of hypertension. A beta-blocker may be used alone or with another antihypertensive drug, such as a diuretic. Labetalol (Normodyne, Trandate) is the only beta-blocking agent approved for treatment of hypertensive emergencies. Only atenolol (Tenormin), metoprolol (Lopressor), nadolol (Corgard), and propranolol are approved as antianginal agents; only acebutolol (Sectral), esmolol (Brevibloc), propranolol, and sotalol (Betapace) are approved as antiarrhythmic agents. Atenolol, metoprolol, propranolol, and timolol (Blocadren) are used to prevent myocardial infarction or reinfarction. Betaxolol (Betoptic, Kerlone), carteolol (Cartrol, Ocupress), and timolol (Timoptic) are used for hypertension and glaucoma; levobunolol (Betagan) and metipranolol (OptiPranolol) are used only for glaucoma.

### Receptor selectivity

Carteolol, levobunolol, metipranolol, penbutolol (Levatol), nadolol, pindolol (Visken), propranolol, sotalol, and timolol are nonselective beta-blockers. The term *nonselective* indicates that the drugs block both beta₁ (cardiac) and beta₂ (mainly smooth muscle in the bronchi and blood vessels) receptors. Blockade of beta₂ receptors is associated with adverse effects, such as bronchoconstriction and interference with glycogenolysis.

Acebutolol, atenolol, betaxolol, bisoprolol (Zebeta), esmolol, and metoprolol are "cardioselective" agents. This means that they have more effect on beta₁ receptors than on beta₂ receptors. As a result, they may cause less bronchospasm, less impairment of glucose metabolism, and less peripheral vascular insufficiency. These drugs are preferred when beta-blockers are needed by clients with asthma or other bronchospastic pulmonary disorders, with diabetes mellitus, and with peripheral vascular disorders. Note, however, that cardioselectivity is lost at higher doses, because most organs have both beta₁ and beta₂ receptors rather than one or the other exclusively.

Labetalol is a unique drug that blocks alpha₁ receptors to cause vasodilation and beta₁ and beta₂ receptors to

## TABLE 19-1.  BETA-ADRENERGIC BLOCKING AGENTS

| Generic/Trade Name | Clinical Indications | Routes and Dosage Ranges |
| --- | --- | --- |

*Nonselective blocking agents*

| Generic/Trade Name | Clinical Indications | Routes and Dosage Ranges |
| --- | --- | --- |
| **Carteolol** (Cartrol, Ocupress) | Hypertension<br>Glaucoma | PO: Initially, 2.5 mg once daily, gradually increased to a maximum daily dose of 10 mg if necessary. Usual maintenance dose, 2.5–5 mg once daily. Extend dosage interval to 48 hours for a creatinine clearance of 20–60 ml/min and to 72 hours for a creatinine clearance below 20 ml/min.<br>Topically to affected eye, 1 drop twice daily |
| **Levobunolol** (Betagan) | Glaucoma | Topically to each eye, 1 drop once or twice daily |
| **Metipranolol** (OptiPranolol) | Glaucoma | Topically to affected eye(s), 1 drop twice daily |
| **Penbutolol** (Levatol) | Hypertension | PO 20 mg, once daily |
| **Propranolol** (Inderal) | Hypertension<br>Angina pectoris<br>Cardiac arrhythmias<br>Myocardial infarction<br>Hypertrophic obstructive cardiomyopathy<br>Migraine prophylaxis<br>Thyrotoxicosis<br>Pheochromocytoma | Hypertension, PO 40 mg twice daily, gradually increased to 160–480 mg daily in divided doses; maximal daily dose, 960 mg<br>Angina pectoris, dysrhythmias, PO 10–30 mg in divided doses, q4–6h<br>Migraine prophylaxis, PO 40 mg daily in divided doses<br>Life-threatening arrhythmias, IV 1–3 mg at a rate not to exceed 1 mg/min with electrocardiographic and blood pressure monitoring |
| **Nadolol** (Corgard) | Hypertension<br>Angina pectoris | Hypertension, PO 40 mg once daily initially, gradually increased. Usual daily maintenance dose, 80–320 mg<br>Angina, PO 40 mg once daily initially, increased by 40–80 mg at 3- to 7-day intervals. Usual daily maintenance dose, 80–240 mg |
| **Pindolol** (Visken) | Hypertension | PO 5 mg twice daily initially, increased by 10 mg every 3–4 weeks, to a maximal daily dose of 60 mg |
| **Sotalol** (Betapace) | Cardiac arrhythmias | PO 80–160 mg twice daily |
| **Timolol** (Blocadren, Timoptic) | Hypertension<br>Myocardial infarction<br>Glaucoma | Hypertension, PO 10 mg twice daily initially, increased at 7-day intervals to a maximum of 60 mg/d in 2 divided doses; usual maintenance dose, 20–40 mg daily<br>Myocardial infarction, PO 10 mg twice daily<br>Glaucoma, topically to eye, 1 drop of 0.25% or 0.5% solution (Timoptic) in each eye twice daily. |

*Cardioselective blocking agents*

| Generic/Trade Name | Clinical Indications | Routes and Dosage Ranges |
| --- | --- | --- |
| **Acebutolol** (Sectral) | Hypertension<br>Ventricular arrhythmias | Hypertension, PO 400 mg daily in 1 or 2 doses; usual maintenance dose, 400–800 mg daily<br>Arrhythmias, PO 400 mg daily in 2 divided doses; usual maintenance dose, 600–1200 mg daily |
| **Atenolol** (Tenormin) | Hypertension<br>Angina pectoris<br>Myocardial infarction | Hypertension, PO 50–100 mg daily<br>Angina, PO 50–100 mg daily, increased to 200 mg daily if necessary<br>Myocardial infarction, IV 5 mg over 5 minutes, then 5 mg 10 minutes later, then 50 mg PO 10 minutes later, then 50 mg 12 hours later. Thereafter, PO 100 mg daily, in 1 or 2 doses, for 6–9 days or until discharge from hospital |
| **Betaxolol** (Betoptic, Kerlone) | Glaucoma<br>Hypertension | Topically to each eye, 1 drop twice daily<br>Hypertension, PO 10–20 mg daily |
| **Bisoprolol** (Zebeta) | Hypertension | PO 5–20 mg once daily |
| **Esmolol** (Brevibloc) | Supraventricular tachy-arrhythmias | IV 50–200 μg/kg per minute; average dose, 100 μg/kg per minute, titrated to effect with close monitoring of client's condition |
| **Metoprolol** (Lopressor) | Hypertension<br>Myocardial infarction | Hypertension, PO 100 mg daily in single or divided doses, increased at 7-day or longer intervals; usual maintenance dose, 100–450 mg daily<br>Myocardial infarction, early treatment, IV 5 mg every 2 minutes for total of 3 doses (15 mg), then 50 mg PO q6h for 48 hours, then 100 mg PO twice daily. MI, late treatment, PO 100 mg twice daily, at least 3 months, up to 1–3 years |

*Alpha-beta blocking agent*

| Generic/Trade Name | Clinical Indications | Routes and Dosage Ranges |
| --- | --- | --- |
| **Labetalol** (Trandate, Normodyne) | Hypertension, including hypertensive emergencies | PO 100 mg twice daily<br>IV 20 mg over 2 minutes then 40–80 mg every 10 minutes until desired blood pressure achieved or 300 mg given<br>IV infusion 2 mg/min (*e.g.*, add 200 mg of drug to 250 ml 5% dextrose solution for a 2 mg/3 ml concentration) |

cause all the effects of the nonselective agents. Both alpha- and beta-adrenergic blocking actions contribute to its antihypertensive effects, but it is unclear whether labetalol has any definite advantage over other beta-blockers. It may cause less bradycardia but more postural hypotension than other beta-blocking agents, and it may cause less reflex tachycardia than other vasodilators.

### Intrinsic sympathomimetic activity

Drugs with this characteristic (*i.e.*, acebutolol, carteolol, penbutolol, and pindolol) have a chemical structure similar to, but not exactly like, catecholamines. As a result, they can block the receptor and bind with a few stimulating receptor sites. Consequently, these drugs are less likely to cause bradycardia and may be useful for clients experiencing bradycardia with other beta-blockers.

### Membrane stabilizing activity

Several beta-blockers have a membrane-stabilizing effect sometimes described as quinidine-like (*i.e.*, producing myocardial depression). Because the doses required to produce this effect are much higher than those used for therapeutic effects, this characteristic is considered clinically insignificant.

### Lipid solubility

The more lipid-soluble beta-blockers were thought to penetrate the central nervous system (CNS) more extensively and cause adverse effects, such as confusion, depression, hallucinations, and insomnia. The validity of this viewpoint is being questioned. Some clinicians state that this characteristic is important only in terms of drug usage and excretion in certain disease states. Thus, a water-soluble, renally excreted beta-blocker may be preferred in clients with liver disease, and a lipid-soluble, hepatically metabolized drug may be preferred in clients with renal disease.

### Routes of elimination

Most beta-blocking agents are metabolized in the liver. Atenolol, carteolol, nadolol, and an active metabolite of acebutolol are excreted by the kidneys, and dosage must be reduced in the presence of renal failure.

### Routes of administration

Most beta-blockers can be given orally. Atenolol, esmolol, labetalol, metoprolol, and propranolol also can be given intravenously, and ophthalmic solutions are applied topically to the eye. Betaxolol, carteolol, and timolol are available in oral and ophthalmic forms.

### Duration of action

Acebutolol, atenolol, bisoprolol, carteolol, penbutolol, and nadolol have long serum half-lives and can usually be given once daily. Labetalol, metoprolol, pindolol, sotalol, and timolol are usually given twice daily. Propranolol required administration several times daily until development of a sustained-release capsule allowed once-daily dosing.

## *Nursing Process*

### Assessment
- Assess the client's condition in relation to disorders in which antiadrenergic drugs are used; that is, check blood pressure for elevation and pulse for tachycardia or arrhythmia, and determine the presence or absence of chest pain, migraine headache, or hyperthyroidism. If the client reports or medical records indicate one or more of these disorders, assess for specific signs and symptoms.
- Assess for conditions that contraindicate the use of antiadrenergic drugs.
- Assess vital signs to establish a baseline for later comparisons.
- Assess for use of prescription and nonprescription drugs that are likely to increase or decrease effects of antiadrenergic drugs.

### Nursing diagnoses
- Decreased Cardiac Output related to drug-induced postural hypotension (alpha- and beta-blockers) and congestive heart failure (beta-blockers)
- Impaired Gas Exchange related to drug-induced bronchoconstriction with beta-blockers
- Sexual Dysfunction in males related to impotence and decreased libido
- Fatigue related to decreased cardiac output
- High Risk for Noncompliance related to adverse drug effects or inadequate understanding of drug therapy regimen
- High Risk for Injury, falls, or other trauma related to hypotension, dizziness
- Knowledge Deficit: Drug effects and safe usage

### Planning/Goals

*The client will:*
- Receive drugs accurately
- Experience relief of symptoms for which antiadrenergic drugs are given
- Comply with instructions for safe drug usage
- Avoid stopping beta-blockers abruptly
- Demonstrate knowledge of accurate self-administration and adverse drug effects to be reported
- Avoid preventable adverse drug effects

## Interventions

Use measures to prevent or decrease the need for antiadrenergic drugs. Because the sympathetic nervous system is stimulated by physical and emotional stress, efforts to decrease stress may indirectly decrease the need for drugs to antagonize sympathetic effects. Such efforts may include the following:

- Helping the client to stop or decrease cigarette smoking. Nicotine stimulates the CNS and the sympathetic nervous system to cause tremors, tachycardia, and elevated blood pressure.
- Teaching measures to relieve pain, anxiety, and other stresses
- Counseling regarding relaxation techniques
- Helping the client avoid temperature extremes
- Helping the client avoid excessive caffeine in coffee or other beverages
- Helping the client develop a reasonable balance between rest, exercise, work, and recreation
- Recording vital signs at regular intervals in hospitalized clients to monitor for adverse effects of beta-blockers
- Helping with activity or ambulation as needed to prevent injury from dizziness

### Teach clients:

- Stress management techniques (*e.g.*, relaxation, imagery)
- Not to take other drugs without the physician's knowledge and consent. Many drugs may interact to increase or decrease effects of the antiadrenergic drug.
- To inform any health-care provider from whom treatment is sought when taking drugs
- Not to stop taking beta-blocking drugs abruptly. To avoid serious problems, they must be tapered and discontinued gradually, with supervision.
- How to count pulse rate
- To record pulse rate daily and take the record to appointments with health-care providers

## Evaluation

- Observe for decreased blood pressure when beta-blockers are given for hypertension.
- Interview regarding decreased chest pain when beta-blockers are given for angina.
- Interview and observe for signs and symptoms of adverse drug effects (congestive heart failure, bronchoconstriction).
- Interview regarding knowledge and usage of drugs.

# Principles of therapy

## ALPHA-ADRENERGIC BLOCKING DRUGS

1. When phenoxybenzamine is given on a long-term basis, dosage must be carefully individualized. Because the drug is long-acting and accumulates in the body, dosage is small initially and gradually increased at intervals of about 4 days. Several weeks may be required for full therapeutic benefit, and drug effects persist for several days after the drug is discontinued.

2. If circulatory shock develops from overdosage or hypersensitivity, levarterenol can be given to overcome the blockade of alpha-adrenergic receptors in arterioles and to raise blood pressure. Epinephrine is contraindicated because it stimulates both alpha- and beta-adrenergic receptors, with a result of increased vasodilation and hypotension.

## BETA-ADRENERGIC BLOCKING DRUGS

1. For most people, a nonselective beta-blocker that can be taken on a convenient schedule, once or twice daily, is acceptable. For others, the choice of a beta-blocking agent depends largely on the client's condition and response to the drugs. For example, cardioselective drugs are preferred for clients with pulmonary disorders and diabetes mellitus; a drug with intrinsic sympathomimetic activity may be preferred for those who experience significant bradycardia with beta-blockers lacking this property.

2. Dosage of beta-blocking agents must be individualized because of wide variations in plasma levels from comparable doses. Variations are attributed to initial metabolism in the liver, the extent of binding to plasma proteins, and the degree of beta-adrenergic stimulation that the drugs must overcome. Generally, low doses should be used initially and increased gradually until therapeutic or adverse effects occur. Adequacy of dosage or extent of beta blockade can be assessed by determining whether the heart rate increases in response to exercise.

3. When a beta-blocker is used to prevent myocardial infarction, it should be started as soon as the client is hemodynamically stable after a definite or suspected acute myocardial infarction. The drug should be continued at least 3 months and possibly 1 to 3 years.

4. Beta-blocking drugs should not be discontinued abruptly. Long-term beta blockade produces increased sensitivity to catecholamines when the drugs are discontinued. There is a risk of severe hypertension, angina, arrhythmias, and myocardial infarction. Instead, the dosage should be tapered and gradually discontinued to allow beta-adrenergic receptors to return to predrug density and sensitivity. Although an optimal tapering period has not been defined, some authorities recommend decreasing dosage over at least 10 days to 30 mg/d of propranolol or an equivalent amount of other drugs. This dosage should be continued at least 2 weeks before the drug is stopped completely.

5. Opinions differ regarding use of beta-blockers before anesthesia and major surgery. On one hand, the drugs block arrhythmogenic properties of some general inhalation anesthetics; on the other hand, there is a risk of excessive myocardial depression. If feas-

ible, the drug may be tapered gradually and discontinued before surgery. If the drug is continued, the lowest effective dosage should be given. If emergency surgery is necessary, the effects of beta-blockers can be reversed by administration of beta-receptor stimulants, such as dobutamine or isoproterenol.

6. If bradycardia occurs, atropine can be given to increase heart rate. Digitalis and diuretics can be given for congestive heart failure. Vasopressor agents can be given to raise the blood pressure, and bronchodilator drugs can be given to relieve bronchospasm.

7. In the presence of hepatic disease (*e.g.*, cirrhosis) or impaired blood flow to the liver (*e.g.*, reduced cardiac output from any cause), dosage of propranolol, metoprolol, and timolol should be substantially reduced because these drugs are extensively metabolized in the liver. Atenolol or nadolol is preferred in liver disease because both are eliminated primarily by the kidneys.

8. In renal failure, dosage of acebutolol, atenolol, carteolol, and nadolol must be reduced because they are eliminated mainly through the kidneys. Dosage of acebutolol and nadolol should be reduced if creatinine clearance is under 50 ml/min; dosage of atenolol should be decreased if creatinine clearance is under 35 ml/min.

With carteolol, the same amount is given per dose, but the interval between doses is extended to 48 hours for a creatinine clearance of 20 to 60 ml/min and to 72 hours for a creatinine clearance below 20 ml/min.

## GENETIC OR ETHNIC CONSIDERATIONS

Most studies involve adults with hypertension and compare drug therapy responses between African-American and white people. Findings indicate that monotherapy with alpha$_1$-blockers and the combined alpha–beta blocker is equally effective in the two groups. However, monotherapy with beta-blockers is less effective in African-Americans than in whites. When beta-blockers are used in African-Americans, they should generally be part of a multidrug treatment regimen, and higher doses may be required.

Several studies indicate that Asian people achieve higher blood levels of beta-blockers with given doses and generally need much smaller doses than white people. This increased sensitivity to the drugs may result from slower metabolism and excretion.

## USE IN CHILDREN

Beta-adrenergic blocking agents are used in children for disorders similar to those occurring in adults. However, safety and effectiveness have not been established, and manufacturers of most of the drugs do not recommend pediatric use or doses. The drugs are probably contraindicated in young children with resting heart rates below 60 beats per minute.

When a beta-blocker is given, general guidelines include the following:

1. Dosage should be adjusted for body weight.
2. Monitor responses closely. Children are more sensitive to adverse drug effects than adults.
3. If given to infants (up to 1 year old) with immature liver function, blood levels may be higher and accumulation is more likely even when doses are based on weight.
4. When monitoring responses, remember that heart rate and blood pressure vary among children according to age group and level of growth and development. They also differ from those of adults.
5. Children are more likely to have asthma than adults. Thus, they may be at greater risk of drug-induced bronchoconstriction.

Propranolol is probably the most frequently used beta-blocker in children. Intravenous administration is not recommended. The drug is given orally for hypertension, and dosage should be individualized. The usual dosage range is 2 to 4 mg/kg per day in two equal doses. Dosage calculated from body surface area is not recommended because of excessive blood levels of drug and greater risk of toxicity. As with adults, dosage should be tapered gradually over 2 to 4 weeks. The drug should not be stopped abruptly.

Safety and effectiveness of other systemic beta-blockers have not been established. These drugs include acebutolol, atenolol, bisoprolol, carteolol, esmolol, labetalol, metoprolol, nadolol, pindolol, sotalol, and timolol.

## USE IN OLDER ADULTS

Beta-adrenergic blocking agents are commonly used in older adults for angina, arrhythmias, hypertension, and glaucoma. With hypertension, beta-blockers are not recommended for monotherapy because older adults may be less responsive than younger adults. Thus, the drugs are probably most useful as second drugs (with diuretics) in clients who require multidrug therapy and clients who also have angina pectoris or another disorder for which a beta-blocker is indicated.

Whatever the circumstances for using beta-blockers in older adults, use them cautiously and monitor responses closely. Older adults are likely to have disorders that place them at high risk of adverse drug effects, such as congestive heart failure and other cardiovascular conditions, renal or hepatic impairment, and chronic pulmonary disease. Thus, they may experience bradycardia, bronchoconstriction, and hypotension to a greater degree than younger adults. Dosage generally should be reduced because of decreased hepatic blood flow and subsequent slowing of drug metabolism. As with other populations, beta-blockers should be tapered in dosage and discontinued gradually to avoid myocardial ischemia and other potentially serious adverse cardiovascular effects.

## NURSING ACTIONS: ANTIADRENERGIC DRUGS

| Nursing Actions | Rationale/Explanation |
|---|---|
| **1. Administer accurately** | |
| **a.** With alpha-adrenergic blocking agents: | |
| (1) Reconstitute parenteral phentolamine (5 mg/1 ml sterile water for injection) at the time it is to be used. | The reconstituted solution should not be stored. |
| (2) To treat extravasation of levarterenol or dopamine, phentolamine, 5–10 mg, may be diluted in 10 ml of sodium chloride injection and injected subcutaneously around the area of extravasation. | This should be done as soon as extravasation is detected. It may prevent tissue necrosis if done within 12 hours. |
| **b.** With beta-adrenergic blocking agents: | |
| (1) Check blood pressure and pulse frequently, especially when dosage is being increased. It is probably best to omit the drug and report to the physician if systolic pressure is below 100 mm Hg and resting pulse rate is below 60. | To monitor therapeutic effects and the occurrence of adverse reactions. Some clients with heart rates between 50 and 60 beats per minute may be continued on a beta-blocker if they do not develop hypotension or escape arrhythmias. |
| (2) See Table 19-1 and manufacturers' literature regarding intravenous administration. | Specific instructions vary with individual drugs. |
| **2. Observe for therapeutic effects** | |
| **a.** With alpha-adrenergic blocking agents: | |
| (1) In pheochromocytoma, observe for decreased pulse rate, blood pressure, sweating, palpitations, and blood sugar. | Because symptoms of pheochromocytoma are caused by excessive sympathetic nervous system stimulation, blocking stimulation with these drugs produces a decrease or absence of symptoms. |
| (2) In Raynaud's disease or frostbite, observe affected areas for improvement in skin color and skin temperature and in the quality of peripheral pulses. | These conditions are characterized by vasospasm, which diminishes blood flow to the affected part. The drugs improve blood flow by vasodilation. |
| **b.** With beta-adrenergic blocking drugs: | |
| (1) When given in hypertension, observe for lowering of blood pressure toward normal ranges. | |
| (2) When given in tachyarrhythmias, observe for slowing of heart rate. | |
| (3) When given in angina pectoris, observe for decreased chest pain and increased exercise tolerance. | |
| **3. Observe for adverse effects** | Adverse effects are usually extensions of therapeutic effects. |
| **a.** With alpha-blocking agents: | |
| (1) Hypotension | Hypotension may range from transient postural hypotension to a more severe hypotensive state resembling shock. |

*(continued)*

## Nursing Actions

## Rationale/Explanation

(2) Tachycardia

Tachycardia occurs as a reflex mechanism to increase blood supply to body tissues in hypotensive states.

**b.** With beta-blocking agents:

(1) Bradycardia and heart block

These are extensions of the therapeutic effects, which slow conduction of electrical impulses through the AV node, particularly in clients with compromised cardiac function.

(2) Congestive heart failure—edema, dyspnea, fatigue

Caused by reduced force of myocardial contraction

(3) Bronchospasm—dyspnea, wheezing

Caused by drug-induced constriction of bronchi and bronchioles. It is much more likely to occur in people with bronchial asthma or other obstructive lung disease.

(4) Fatigue and dizziness, especially with activity or exercise

These symptoms occur because the usual sympathetic nervous system stimulation in response to activity or stress is blocked by drug action.

(5) CNS effects—depression, insomnia, vivid dreams, and hallucinations

The mechanism by which these effects are produced is unknown. Depression is particularly likely to occur in clients with a history of mood alterations.

**4. Observe for drug interactions**
   **a.** Drugs that *alter* effects of alpha-adrenergic blocking agents:

(1) Epinephrine

Epinephrine *increases* the hypotensive effects of alpha-adrenergic blocking agents and should not be given to treat shock caused by phenoxybenzamine or phentolamine. Because epinephrine stimulates both alpha- and beta-adrenergic receptors, the net effect is vasodilation and a further drop in blood pressure.

(2) Levarterenol

Levarterenol *decreases* effects of alpha-adrenergic blocking agents and is the drug of choice for treating shock caused by overdosage of or hypersensitivity to phenoxybenzamine or phentolamine.

**b.** Drugs that *increase* effects of beta-adrenergic blocking agents (*e.g.,* propranolol, nadolol):

(1) Alpha-adrenergic blocking drugs

Synergistic effects to prevent excessive hypertension before and during surgical excision of pheochromocytoma

(2) Chlorpromazine, cimetidine, furosemide

Increase plasma levels by slowing hepatic metabolism

(3) Digitalis

Additive bradycardia, heart block

(4) Hydralazine, prazosin

Synergistic antihypertensive effects. Clients who do not respond to beta-blockers or vasodilators alone may respond well to the combination. Also, beta-blockers prevent reflex tachycardia, which usually occurs with vasodilator antihypertensive drugs. *Note:* prazosin produces relatively little tachycardia compared to hydralazine.

(5) Phenytoin

Potentiates cardiac depressant effects of propranolol

(6) Quinidine

The combination may be synergistic in treating cardiac arrhythmias. However, additive cardiac depressant effects also may occur (bradycardia, negative inotropy, decreased cardiac output).

| Nursing Actions | Rationale/Explanation |
|---|---|
| (7) Verapamil, intravenous | The combination of intravenous verapamil and intravenous propranolol causes additive bradycardia and hypotension. |
| **c.** Drugs that *decrease* effects of beta-adrenergic blocking agents: | |
| (1) Atropine | Increases heart rate and may be used to counteract excessive bradycardia caused by propranolol and other beta-blocking agents |
| (2) Isoproterenol | Stimulates beta-adrenergic receptors and therefore antagonizes effects of beta-blocking agents. Isoproterenol also can be used to counteract excessive bradycardia. |
| **5. Teach clients**<br>**a.** With alpha-adrenergic blocking agents: | |
| (1) The adverse reactions of palpitations, weakness, and dizziness usually disappear with continued use. However, they may recur with conditions promoting vasodilation (exercise, dosage increase, ingesting alcohol or a large meal). | These are symptoms of postural hypotension and reflex tachycardia. |
| (2) If the above reactions occur, sit down or lie down immediately and flex arms and legs. Change positions slowly, especially from supine to standing. | To prevent falls and injuries due to postural hypotension |
| **b.** With beta-adrenergic blocking agents: | |
| (1) Take oral propranolol or metoprolol with food. | To enhance absorption |
| (2) Take the drug at the same time each day. | To maintain therapeutic blood levels and adequate blockade of beta-adrenergic receptors |
| (3) Count pulse daily; report to health-care provider if under 50 for several days in succession. | To determine if drug therapy regimen needs to be altered to avoid more serious adverse effects |
| (4) Report weight gain (more than 2 pounds within a week), ankle edema, shortness of breath, or excessive fatigue. | These are signs of congestive heart failure. If they occur, the drug will be stopped. |
| (5) Report fainting spells, excessive weakness, or difficulty in breathing. | Beta-blocking drugs decrease the usual adaptive responses to exercise or stress. Syncope may result from hypotension or bradycardia and heart block. Occurrence will probably indicate stopping or decreasing the dose of the drug. |

## Review and Application Exercises

1. What are the main mechanisms by which beta-blockers relieve angina pectoris?
2. How are beta-blockers throught to be "cardio-protective" in preventing repeat myocardial infarctions?
3. What are some noncardiovascular indications for use of propranolol?
4. What are the main differences between cardio-selective and nonselective beta-blockers?
5. Why are cardioselective beta-blockers preferred for clients with asthma or diabetes mellitus?
6. List at least five adverse effects of beta-blockers.
7. Explain the drug effects that contribute to each adverse reaction.
8. What signs, symptoms, or behaviors would lead you to suspect adverse drug effects?
9. Do the same adverse effects occur with beta-blocker eye drops that occur with systemic drugs? If so, how may they be prevented or minimized?

**10.** What information needs to be included in teaching clients about beta-blocker therapy?

**11.** What is the risk of abruptly stopping a beta-blocker drug rather than tapering the dose and gradually discontinuing, as recommended?

## Selected References

Auricchio, R. J. (1992). Cardiac arrhythmias. In M. A. Koda-Kimble & L. Y. Young, (Eds.), *Applied therapeutics: The clinical use of drugs* (5th ed.) (pp.10-1–10-40). Vancouver, WA: Applied Therapeutics.

Beare, P. G., & Myers, J. L. (Eds.) (1990). *Principles and practice of adult health nursing.* St. Louis: C.V. Mosby.

Brater, C. (1992). Clinical pharmacology of cardiovascular drugs. In W. N. Kelley (Ed.), *Textbook of internal medicine* (2nd ed.) (pp. 315–335). Philadelphia: J.B. Lippincott.

Byington, R. P., & Furbey, C. D. (1990). Beta blockers during and after myocardial infarction. In G. S. Francis & J. S. Alpert (Eds.), *Modern coronary care* (pp 511–539). Boston: Little, Brown.

(1993). *Drug facts and comparisons.* St. Louis: Facts and Comparisons.

Gollub, S. B. (1993). Combination medical therapy in the treatment of angina pectoris. *Hospital Formulary, 28,* 34–44.

Guyton, A. C. (1991). *Textbook of medical physiology* (8th ed.). Philadelphia: W.B. Saunders.

Hawkins, D. W., Bussey, H. I., & Prisant, L. M. (1992). Hypertension. In J. T. DiPiro, R. L. Talbert, P. E. Hayes, G. C. Yee, G. R. Matzke, & L. M. Posey (Eds.), *Pharmacotherapy: A pathophysiologic approach* (2nd ed.) (pp. 139–159). New York: Elsevier.

Joint National Committee on Detection, Evaluation, and Treatment of High Blood Pressure (1993). The Fifth Report. *Archives of Internal Medicine, 153,* 154–183.

May, D. B., Young, L. Y., & Wiser, T. H. (1992). Essential hypertension. In M. A. Koda-Kimble & L. Y. Young (Eds.), *Applied therapeutics: The clinical use of drugs* (5th ed.) (pp.7-1–7-32). Vancouver, WA: Applied Therapeutics.

(1993). New drug approved for life-threatening arrhythmias. *FDA Medical Bulletin, 23*(1), 5.

Porth, C. M., & Curtis, R. L. (1990). Normal and altered autonomic nervous system function. In C. M. Porth (Ed.), *Pathophysiology: Concepts of altered health states.* Philadelphia: J.B. Lippincott.

Raehl, C. L., & Nolan, P. E. (1992). Angina pectoris. In M. A. Koda-Kimble & L. Y. Young (Eds.), *Applied therapeutics: The clinical use of drugs* (5th ed.) (pp. 11-1–11-24). Vancouver, WA: Applied Therapeutics.

Rutledge, D. R. (1991). Are there beta-adrenergic response differences between racial groups? *DICP, The Annals of Pharmacotherapy, 25,* 824–834.

Steinwandt, S. M., Abadi, A. H., & Rutledge, D. R. (1993). Focus on bisoprolol. *Hospital Formulary, 28,* 453–464.

Wood, A. J. J., & Zhou, H. H. (1991). Ethnic differences in drug disposition and responsiveness. *Clinical Pharmacokinetics, 20*(5), 350–373.

# CHAPTER 20

# Cholinergic Drugs

## Description

Cholinergic drugs, also called parasympathomimetics and cholinomimetics, stimulate the parasympathetic nervous system in the same manner as acetylcholine. Some drugs act directly to stimulate cholinergic receptors; others act indirectly by slowing acetylcholine metabolism at autonomic nerve synapses and terminals.

Acetylcholine is formed from choline, an amino-alcohol involved in carbohydrate, fat, and protein metabolism. The enzyme necessary for formation of acetylcholine is choline acetylase; the enzyme necessary for its metabolism is acetylcholinesterase. Acetylcholinesterase rapidly splits acetylcholine into inactive acetate and choline, which are then released into the systemic circulation.

### MECHANISMS OF ACTION AND EFFECTS

*Direct-acting cholinergic drugs* are synthetic derivatives of choline. These drugs are able to exert their therapeutic effects because they are highly resistant to metabolism or breakdown by acetylcholinesterase. Their action is longer than the action of acetylcholine. They have widespread systemic effects when they combine with receptors in cardiac muscle, smooth muscle, and glands. Specific effects include:

1. Decreased heart rate, vasodilation, and unpredictable changes in blood pressure
2. Increased tone and contractility in gastrointestinal smooth muscle, relaxation of sphincters, increased salivary gland and gastrointestinal secretions
3. Increased tone and contractility of smooth muscle (detrusor) in the urinary bladder and relaxation of the sphincter
4. Increased tone and contractility of bronchial smooth muscle
5. Increased respiratory secretions
6. Constriction of pupils and contraction of ciliary muscle

*Indirect-acting cholinergic* or *anticholinesterase drugs* act at the neuromuscular junction by decreasing metabolism of acetylcholine. These agents compete with acetylcholine for attachment sites on the enzyme acetylcholinesterase. This prolongs the effect of acetylcholine by preventing inactivation of acetylcholine in the synaptic cleft. Acetylcholine is then able to accumulate and stimulate receptors. The longer period of acetylcholine activity decreases skeletal muscle weakness, improves contractility of skeletal and smooth muscle, and restores other physiologic responses. Anticholinesterase drugs have parasympathetic, sympathetic, and somatic effects. They stimulate skeletal muscle and increase the strength of muscle contraction. This effect is used therapeutically to treat myasthenia gravis, an autoimmune neuromuscular disorder characterized by inadequate acetylcholine activity and resultant skeletal muscle weakness.

### INDICATIONS FOR USE

Cholinergic drugs have limited but varied uses. A direct-acting drug, bethanechol, is used to treat urinary retention. The anticholinesterase agents are used in diagnosis and treatment of myasthenia gravis and to reverse the action of nondepolarizing neuromuscular blocking agents (*e.g.*, tubocurarine and related drugs) used in surgery. The drugs do not reverse the neuromuscular blockade produced by depolarizing agents, such as succinylcholine (Anectine). Several drugs have been used to treat glaucoma (see Chap. 68), but such usage has declined.

## CONTRAINDICATIONS FOR USE

These drugs are contraindicated in urinary or gastrointestinal tract obstruction, asthma, peptic ulcer disease, coronary artery disease, hyperthyroidism, pregnancy, and inflammatory abdominal conditions.

## Individual cholinergic drugs

### DIRECT-ACTING CHOLINERGICS

**Bethanechol** (Urecholine) is a synthetic derivative of choline with relatively specific effects on smooth muscle of the urinary tract. It is used to relieve urinary retention. Because the drug produces smooth-muscle contractions, it should not be used in obstructive conditions. Because oral bethanechol is not well absorbed from the gastrointestinal tract, oral doses are much larger than subcutaneous doses. Because severe adverse effects may occur with intramuscular or intravenous administration, the drug is not given by these routes.

#### Routes and dosage ranges

*Adults:* PO 10–30 mg two to four times per day; maximum dose 120 mg/d, SC 2.5–5 mg three or four times per day
*Children:* PO 0.2 mg/kg of body weight three times per day, SC 0.05 mg/kg of body weight three times per day

### INDIRECT-ACTING CHOLINERGICS (ANTICHOLINESTERASES)

**Neostigmine** (Prostigmin) is the prototype and the most widely used anticholinesterase agent. It is used for long-term treatment of myasthenia gravis and as an antidote for tubocurarine and other nondepolarizing skeletal muscle relaxants used in surgery. Neostigmine is poorly absorbed from the gastrointestinal tract; consequently, oral doses are much larger than parenteral doses. When it is used for long-term treatment of myasthenia gravis, resistance to its action may occur, and larger doses may be required.

#### Routes and dosage ranges

*Adults:* Myasthenia gravis, PO 15–30 mg q4h while awake
    Exacerbation of myasthenia gravis, IM, SC 0.25–2 mg q2–3h
    Prevention and treatment of urinary retention, IM, SC 0.25–0.5 mg q4–6h (up to 2 or 3 days)
*Children:* Myasthenia gravis, PO 0.3–0.6 mg/kg q3–4h while awake
    Exacerbation of myasthenia gravis, IM, SC 0.01–0.04 mg/kg q2–3h

**Edrophonium** (Tensilon) is a very short-acting cholinergic drug used only to diagnose myasthenia gravis, to differentiate between myasthenic crisis and cholinergic crisis, and to reverse the neuromuscular blockade produced by nondepolarizing skeletal muscle relaxants. It is given intramuscularly or intravenously by a physician who remains in attendance. Atropine, an antidote, and life-support equipment, such as respirators and endotracheal tubes, must be available when the drug is given.

#### Routes and dosage ranges

*Adults:* Diagnosis of myasthenia gravis, IV 2–4 mg initially; may be repeated and increased up to a total dose of 10 mg if no response is elicited by smaller amounts after 45 seconds; or IM 10 mg as a single dose
    Differential diagnosis of myasthenic crisis or cholinergic crisis, IV 1–2 mg
*Children:* Diagnosis of myasthenia gravis, IV 0.2 mg/kg
    Diagnosis in infants, IM 0.1 mg/kg

**Ambenonium** (Mytelase) is used therapeutically only for treatment of myasthenia gravis. It has the longest duration of action of indirect-acting agents. It is used less frequently than neostigmine and pyridostigmine. It may be useful in clients who are allergic to bromides, however, because the other drugs are both bromide salts. Ambenonium may increase respiratory secretions to a lesser degree than other anticholinesterase drugs and therefore may be useful for myasthenic clients on respirators.

#### Route and dosage range

*Adults:* PO 5 mg initially, increased to 10–30 mg q3–4h while awake. Dosage varies considerably, depending on client; dosage range, 5–75 mg/d
*Children:* PO 0.1 mg/kg of body weight initially, increased if necessary to 0.4 mg/kg q4h while awake

**Physostigmine salicylate** (Antilirium) is sometimes used as an antidote for overdosage of anticholinergic drugs ("atropine poisoning"), including tricyclic antidepressants. However, its potential for causing serious adverse effects limits its usefulness. Some preparations of physostigmine are used in glaucoma.

### Routes and dosage ranges

*Adults:* IV, IM 0.5–2 mg; give slowly IV, no faster than 1 mg/min

**Pyridostigmine** (Mestinon) is similar to neostigmine in actions, uses, and adverse effects. It may have a longer duration of action than neostigmine. Pyridostigmine is the maintenance drug of choice for clients with myasthenia gravis. An added advantage is the availability of a slow-release form, which is effective for 8 to 12 hours. When this form is taken at bedtime, the client does not have to take other medication during the night and does not awaken too weak to swallow.

### Routes and dosage ranges

*Adults:* PO 60–120 mg q3–4h when awake; maximal single dose, 180 mg; or one Timespan tablet (180 mg) at bedtime. Up to 1500 mg daily may be necessary.

IM (exacerbations of myasthenia gravis or when oral administration is contraindicated) 2 mg

*Children:* PO 1–2 mg/kg of body weight q3–4h when awake

Newborns whose mothers have myasthenia gravis, IM 0.05–0.15 mg/kg

## Nursing Process

### Assessment

Assess the client's condition in relation to disorders for which cholinergic drugs are used:

- In clients known to have myasthenia gravis, assess for muscle weakness. This may be manifested by ptosis (drooping) of the upper eyelid and diplopia (double vision) caused by weakness of the eye muscles. More severe disease may be indicated by difficulty in chewing, swallowing, and speaking; accumulation of oral secretions, which the client may be unable to expectorate or swallow; decreased skeletal muscle activity, including impaired chest expansion; and eventual respiratory failure.
- In clients with possible urinary retention, check for bladder distention and time and amount of previous urination, and assess fluid intake.

### Nursing diagnoses

- Altered Urinary Elimination: Incontinence
- Ineffective Breathing Patterns related to bronchoconstriction
- Ineffective Airway Clearance related to increased respiratory secretions
- Self-Care Deficit related to muscle weakness
- Knowledge Deficit: Drug administration and effects

### Planning/Goals

*The client will:*
- Verbalize or demonstrate correct drug administration
- Improve in self-care abilities

- Regain usual patterns of urinary elimination
- Maintain effective oxygenation of tissues
- Report adverse drug effects
- For clients with myasthenia gravis, at least one family member will verbalize or demonstrate correct drug administration, symptoms of too much or too little drug, and emergency care procedures.

### Interventions

- Use measures to prevent or decrease the need for cholinergic drugs. Ambulation, adequate fluid intake, and judicious use of narcotic analgesics or other sedative-type drugs help to prevent postoperative urinary retention. In myasthenia gravis, muscle weakness is aggravated by exercise and improved by rest. Therefore, scheduling activities to avoid excessive fatigue and to allow adequate rest periods may be beneficial.
- Before giving cholinergic drugs for bladder atony and urinary retention, be sure there is no obstruction in the urinary tract.
- For long-term use, assist clients and families to establish a schedule of drug administration that best meets the client's needs.
- With myasthenia gravis, recommend that one or more family members be trained in cardiopulmonary resuscitation.

### Teach clients and family:
- That when the drugs are taken for urinary retention, they usually act within about 60 minutes. Therefore, bathroom facilities need to be nearby.
- That with long-term use (*e.g.*, hypotonic bladder or myasthenia gravis), the client should wear a MedicAlert identification device with the name of the drug
- Signs and symptoms of underdosage and overdosage
- How to inject atropine intramuscularly

### Evaluation

- Observe and interview about the adequacy of urinary elimination.
- Observe abilities and limitations in self-care.
- Question the client and at least one family member of clients with myasthenia gravis about correct drug usage, symptoms of underdosage and overdosage, and emergency care procedures.

## Principles of therapy

### USE IN MYASTHENIA GRAVIS

Guidelines for the use of anticholinesterase drugs in myasthenia gravis include the following:

1. Drug dosage should be increased gradually until maximal benefit is obtained. Larger doses are often required with increased physical activity, with emotional stress, with infections, and sometimes premenstrually.
2. Some clients with myasthenia gravis cannot tolerate

optimal doses of anticholinesterase drugs unless atropine is given to decrease the severity of adverse reactions. However, atropine should be given only if necessary because it may mask the sudden increase of side effects. This increase is the first sign of overdose.

3. Drug dosage in excess of the amount needed to maintain muscle strength and function can produce a cholinergic crisis. A cholinergic crisis is characterized by excessive stimulation of the parasympathetic nervous system. If early symptoms are not treated, hypotension and respiratory failure may occur. At high doses, anticholinesterase drugs weaken rather than strengthen skeletal muscle contraction because excessive amounts of acetylcholine accumulate at motor endplates and reduce nerve impulse transmission to muscle tissue.

   a. *Treatment for cholinergic crisis* includes withdrawal of anticholinesterase drugs, administration of atropine, and measures to maintain respiration. Endotracheal intubation and mechanical ventilation may be necessary owing to profound skeletal muscle weakness (including muscles of respiration), which is not counteracted by atropine.

   b. *Differentiating myasthenic crisis from cholinergic crisis* may be difficult because both are characterized by respiratory difficulty or failure. It is necessary to differentiate between them, however, because they require *opposite* treatment measures. Myasthenic crisis requires more anticholinesterase drug, whereas cholinergic crisis requires discontinuing any anticholinesterase drug the person has been receiving. The physician may be able to make an accurate diagnosis from signs and symptoms and when they occur in relation to medication; that is, signs and symptoms having their onset within about 1 hour after a dose of anticholinesterase drug are more likely to be caused by cholinergic crisis (too much drug). Signs and symptoms beginning 3 hours or more after a drug dose are more likely to be caused by myasthenic crisis (too little drug).

   c. If the differential diagnosis cannot be made on the basis of signs and symptoms, the client can be intubated, mechanically ventilated, and observed closely until a diagnosis is possible. Still another way to differentiate between the two conditions is for the physician to inject a small dose of edrophonium intravenously. If the edrophonium causes a dramatic improvement in breathing, the diagnosis is myasthenic crisis; if it makes the patient even weaker, the diagnosis is cholinergic crisis. Note, however, that edrophonium or any other pharmacologic agent should be administered only after endotracheal intubation and controlled ventilation have been instituted.

4. Some people develop partial or total resistance to anticholinesterase drugs after taking them for months or years. Therefore, do not assume that drug therapy that is effective initially will continue to be effective over the long-term course of the disease.

## ANTIDOTE TO CHOLINERGIC AGENTS

Atropine, an anticholinergic drug, is a specific antidote to cholinergic agents. The drug and equipment for injection should be readily available whenever cholinergic drugs are given.

## USE IN CHILDREN

Bethanechol is occasionally used, but safety and effectiveness for children under 8 years old have not been established. Neostigmine is used to treat myasthenia gravis and to reverse neuromuscular blockade following general anesthesia but is not recommended for urinary retention. Other indirect-acting cholinergic drugs are used only in the treatment of myasthenia gravis. Precautions and adverse effects are the same for children as for adults.

## USE IN OLDER ADULTS

Indirect-acting cholinergic drugs may be used in myasthenia gravis or overdoses of atropine and other centrally acting anticholinergic drugs (*e.g.,* those used for parkinsonism). Older adults are more likely to experience adverse drug effects because of age-related physiologic changes and superimposed pathologic conditions.

# NURSING ACTIONS: CHOLINERGIC DRUGS

| *Nursing Actions* | *Rationale/Explanation* |
|---|---|
| **1. Administer accurately**<br>**a.** Give oral bethanechol before meals. | If given after meals, nausea and vomiting may occur because the drug stimulates contraction of muscles in the gastrointestinal (GI) tract. |
| **b.** Give parenteral bethanechol by the subcutaneous route *only*. | Intramuscular and intravenous injections may cause acute, severe hypotension and circulatory failure. Cardiac arrest may occur. |
| **c.** With pyridostigmine and other drugs for myasthenia gravis, give at regularly scheduled intervals. | For consistent blood levels and control of symptoms |
| **2. Observe for therapeutic effects**<br>**a.** When the drug is given for postoperative hypoperistalsis, observe for bowel sounds, passage of flatus through the rectum, or a bowel movement. | These are indicators of increased gastrointestinal muscle tone and motility. |
| **b.** When bethanechol or neostigmine is given for urinary retention, micturition usually occurs within about 60 minutes. If it does not, urinary catheterization may be necessary. | |
| **c.** When the drug is given in myasthenia gravis, observe for increased muscle strength as shown by:<br><br>(1) Decreased or absent ptosis of eyelids<br><br>(2) Decreased difficulty with chewing, swallowing, and speech<br><br>(3) Increased skeletal muscle strength, increased tolerance of activity, less fatigue | With neostigmine, onset of action is 2–4 hours after oral administration and 10–30 minutes after injection. Duration is about 3–4 hours. With pyridostigmine, onset of action is about 30–45 minutes after oral use, 15 minutes after intramuscular (IM) injection, and 2–5 minutes after intravenous (IV) injection. Duration is about 4–6 hours. The long-acting form of pyridostigmine lasts 8–12 hours. |
| **3. Observe for adverse effects** | Adverse effects occur with usual therapeutic doses but are more likely with large doses. They are caused by stimulation of the parasympathetic nervous system (PNS). |
| **a.** Respiratory effects—increased secretions, bronchospasm, respiratory failure | |
| **b.** Gastrointestinal effects—nausea and vomiting, diarrhea, increased peristalsis, abdominal cramping, hypersalivation. | |
| **c.** Cardiovascular effects—arrhythmias, bradycardia, hypotension | These may be detected early by regular assessment of blood pressure and heart rate. |
| **d.** Other effects—increased frequency and urgency of urination, increased sweating, miosis, skin rash | Skin rashes are most likely to occur from formulations of neostigmine or pyridostigmine that contain bromide. |
| **4. Observe for drug interactions**<br>**a.** Drugs that *decrease* effects of cholinergic agents:<br><br>(1) Anticholinergic drugs (*e.g.*, atropine) | Antagonize effects of cholinergic drugs (miosis, increased tone and motility in smooth muscle of the GI tract, bronchi and urinary bladder, bradycardia). Atropine is the specific antidote for overdosage with cholinergic drugs. |
| (2) Antihistamines | Most antihistamines have anticholinergic properties that antagonize effects of cholinergic drugs. |

*(continued)*

| *Nursing Actions* | *Rationale/Explanation* |
|---|---|
| **5. Teach clients with myasthenia gravis and at least one responsible family member to:** | Cholinergic drugs are not prescribed for long-term therapeutic use except for clients with myasthenia gravis, certain types of hypotonic bladder disorders, and glaucoma. |
| **a.** Take drugs as directed on a regular schedule. | To maintain consistent blood levels and control of symptoms. Underdosage will not relieve muscle weakness enough for adequate function; overdosage can cause severe, even life-threatening reactions. |
| **b.** Record symptoms of myasthenia and effects of drug therapy, especially when drug therapy is initiated and medication doses are being titrated. | Clients vary widely in the amounts of medication required. The physician usually aims for the lowest effective dose to minimize adverse drug reactions. Information provided by the client can allow the physician to prescribe more effectively. |
| **c.** Rest between activities; do not carry on activities to the point of extreme fatigue or exhaustion. | Although the dose of medication may be increased during periods of increased activity, spacing activities is probably more desirable to obtain optimal benefit from the drug while avoiding adverse reactions. |
| **d.** Have atropine readily available. | Atropine (0.6 mg IM or IV) is a specific antidote for overdosage with cholinergic drugs. |
| **e.** Report increased muscle weakness or recurrence of myasthenic symptoms to the physician. | Drug dosage may need to be increased or other alterations made in treatment. |
| **f.** Report adverse reactions, including abdominal cramps, diarrhea, excessive oropharyngeal secretions, difficulty in breathing, and muscle weakness. | These are signs of drug overdosage (cholinergic crisis) and require immediate discontinuation of drugs and treatment by the physician. Respiratory failure can result if this condition is not recognized and treated appropriately. |

## Review and Application Exercises

1. What are the actions of cholinergic drugs?
2. Which neurotransmitter is involved in cholinergic (parasympathetic) stimulation?
3. When a cholinergic drug is given to treat myasthenia gravis, what is the expected effect?
4. Is a cholinergic drug the usual treatment of choice for gastric or urinary bladder atony or hypotonicity? Why or why not?
5. What are adverse effects of cholinergic drugs?
6. What drug is an antidote for an overdose of a cholinergic drug?

## Selected References

Beare, P. G., & Myers, J. L. (Eds.) (1990). *Principles and practice of adult health nursing* (pp. 1164–1170). St Louis: C.V. Mosby.

(1993). *Drug facts and comparisons.* St. Louis: Facts and Comparisons.

Flannery, J. C. (1992). Nursing management of adults with degenerative neurologic disorders. In L. O. Burrell (Ed.), *Adult nursing in hospital and community settings* (pp. 1026–1064). Norwalk, CT: Appleton & Lange.

Guttman, M. (1992). Principles of neuropharmacology. In W. N. Kelley (Ed.), *Textbook of internal medicine* (2nd ed.) (pp. 2255–2259). Philadelphia: J.B. Lippincott.

Porth, C. M., & Curtis, R. L. (1990). Normal and altered autonomic nervous system function. In C. M. Porth (Ed.), *Pathophysiology: Concepts of altered health states* (3rd ed.) (pp. 873–892). Philadelphia: J.B. Lippincott.

### CHAPTER 21

# Anticholinergic Drugs

## Description

Anticholinergic drugs, also called cholinergic blocking and parasympatholytic agents, block the action of acetylcholine on the parasympathetic nervous system (PNS). This drug class includes belladonna alkaloids, their derivatives, and many synthetic substitutes. The prototype drug is *atropine*, an alkaloid of the potato plant family.

### MECHANISM OF ACTION AND EFFECTS

These drugs act by occupying receptor sites at parasympathetic nerve endings, thereby leaving fewer receptor sites free to respond to acetylcholine. Parasympathetic response is absent or decreased, depending on the number of receptors blocked by anticholinergic drugs and the underlying degree of parasympathetic activity.

Anticholinergic drugs have widespread effects on the body, including smooth muscle relaxation, decreased glandular secretions, and mydriasis. Specific effects on body tissues and organs include:

1. *Central nervous system (CNS) stimulation followed by depression*, which may result in coma and death. This is most likely to occur with large doses of anticholinergic drugs that cross the blood-brain barrier (atropine, scopolamine, and antiparkinson agents).
2. *Decreased cardiovascular response to parasympathetic (vagal) stimulation that slows heart rate*. Atropine is the anticholinergic drug most used for its cardiovascular effects. Usual clinical doses may produce a slight and temporary decrease in heart rate; moderate to large doses (0.5–1 mg) increase heart rate. This effect may be therapeutic in bradycardia or an adverse effect in other types of heart disease. Atropine usually has little or no effect on blood pressure. Large doses cause facial flushing due to dilation of blood vessels in the neck.
3. *Bronchodilation and decreased respiratory tract secretions*. Bronchodilating effects result from blocking the bronchoconstrictive effects of acetylcholine.
4. *Antispasmodic effects in the gastrointestinal tract due to decreased muscle tone and motility*. The drugs have little inhibitory effect on acidity and amount of gastric secretions, at least in usual doses, and insignificant effects on pancreatic and intestinal secretions.
5. *Mydriasis and cycloplegia in the eye*. Normally, anticholinergics do not change intraocular pressure, but with glaucoma, they may increase intraocular pressure. When the pupil is fully dilated, photophobia may be bothersome, and reflexes to light and accommodation may disappear.
6. *Miscellaneous effects* include decreased secretions from salivary and sweat glands; relaxation of ureters, urinary bladder, and the detrusor muscle; and relaxation of smooth muscle in the gallbladder and bile ducts.

The clinical usefulness of anticholinergic drugs has been limited by their far-reaching actions. Consequently, numerous synthetic drugs have been developed in an effort to increase selectivity of action on particular body

Anne Collins Abrams: CLINICAL DRUG THERAPY, Fourth Edition.
© 1995 J.B. Lippincott Company.

tissues, especially to retain the antispasmodic and anti-secretory effects of atropine while eliminating its adverse effects. This effort has been less than successful: All the synthetic drugs produce atropine-like adverse effects when given in sufficient dosage.

One group of synthetic drugs is used for antispasmodic effects in gastrointestinal disorders (Table 21-1). They are quaternary ammonium compounds, which do not readily cross the blood-brain barrier. They are therefore less likely to cause CNS effects than the natural alkaloids, which readily enter the CNS.

Another group of synthetic drugs includes centrally active anticholinergics used in the treatment of Parkinson's disease (see Chap. 12). They balance the relative cholinergic dominance that causes the movement disorders associated with parkinsonism.

## INDICATIONS FOR USE

Clinical indications for use of anticholinergic drugs include gastrointestinal, genitourinary, ophthalmic and respiratory disorders, bradycardia, and Parkinson's disease. They also are used preoperatively and prior to bronchoscopy.

Gastrointestinal disorders in which anticholinergics have been used include peptic ulcer disease, gastritis, pylorospasm, diverticulitis, ileitis, and ulcerative colitis. These conditions are often characterized by excessive gastric acid and abdominal pain due to increased motility and spasm of gastrointestinal smooth muscle. In

peptic ulcer disease, more effective drugs have been developed, and anticholinergics are rarely used. The drugs are weak inhibitors of gastric acid secretion even in maximal doses (which usually produce intolerable adverse effects). Although they do not heal peptic ulcers, they may relieve abdominal pain by relaxing gastrointestinal smooth muscle.

Anticholinergics may be helpful in treating irritable colon or colitis, but they may be contraindicated in chronic inflammatory disorders (e.g., diverticulitis, ulcerative colitis) or acute intestinal infections (e.g., bacterial, viral, amebic). Other drugs are used to decrease diarrhea and intestinal motility in these conditions.

In genitourinary disorders, anticholinergic drugs may be given for their antispasmodic effects on smooth muscle. In infections such as cystitis, urethritis, and prostatitis, the drugs decrease the frequency and pain of urination. The drugs are also given to increase bladder capacity in enuresis, paraplegia, or neurogenic bladder.

In ophthalmology, anticholinergic drugs are applied topically for mydriatic and cycloplegic effects to aid examination or surgery. They are also used to treat some inflammatory disorders. Anticholinergic preparations used in ophthalmology are discussed further in Chapter 68.

In respiratory disorders characterized by bronchoconstriction (i.e., asthma, chronic bronchitis), atropine or ipratropium (Atrovent) may be given by inhalation for bronchodilating effects (see Chap. 50).

In cardiology, atropine may be given to increase heart

**TABLE 21-1. SYNTHETIC ANTICHOLINERGIC-ANTISPASMODICS USED IN GASTROINTESTINAL DISORDERS**

| Generic/Trade Name | Routes and Dosage Ranges | |
| --- | --- | --- |
| | **Adults** | **Children** |
| **Anisotropine methylbromide** (Valpin) | PO 50 mg 3 times daily | Dosage not established |
| **Clidinium bromide** (Quarzan) | PO 2.5–5 mg 3–4 times daily<br>Geriatric: PO 2.5 mg TID before meals | Dosage not established |
| **Dicyclomine hydrochloride** (Bentyl) | PO, IM 10–20 mg 3–4 times daily | PO, IM 10 mg 3–4 times daily<br>Infants: 5 mg 3–4 times daily |
| **Glycopyrrolate** (Robinul) | PO 1–2 mg 3 times daily initially, 1 mg 2 times daily for maintenance<br>IM, IV, SC 0.1–0.2 mg 3–4 times daily at 4-hour intervals | Dosage not established |
| **Isopropamide chloride** (Darbid) | PO 5–10 mg q12h | Not recommended for children under 12 years |
| **Mepenzolate bromide** (Cantil) | PO 25 mg 4 times daily with meals and at bedtime, increased gradually to 50 mg if necessary | Dosage not established |
| **Methantheline bromide** (Banthine) | PO 50–100 mg q6h initially, reduced to 25–50 mg q6h for maintenance<br>IM 50 mg q6h | PO, IM 6 mg/kg per day in 4 divided doses |
| **Oxyphencyclimine bromide** (Daricon) | PO 10 mg 2 times daily (morning and at bedtime), gradually increased to 50 mg if no adverse effects | Dosage not established |
| **Propantheline bromide** (Pro-Banthine) | PO 15 mg 3 times daily before meals and 30 mg at bedtime<br>IM, IV 30 mg q6h | PO 1.5 mg/kg per day in 4 divided doses |
| **Tridihexethyl** (Pathilon) | PO 25–50 mg 3 or 4 times daily, before meals and at bedtime | Dosage not established |

rate in bradycardia and heart block characterized by hypotension and shock.

In Parkinson's disease, anticholinergic drugs are given for their central effects in decreasing salivation, spasticity, and tremors. They are used mainly in clients who have minimal symptoms, who do not respond to levodopa, or who cannot tolerate levodopa because of adverse reactions or contraindications. An additional use of anticholinergic drugs is to relieve parkinson-like symptoms that occur with antipsychotic drugs.

Preoperatively, anticholinergics are given to prevent vagal stimulation and potential bradycardia, hypotension, and cardiac arrest. They are also given to reduce respiratory tract secretions, especially in head and neck surgery and bronchoscopy.

## CONTRAINDICATIONS FOR USE

Contraindications to the use of anticholinergic drugs include any condition characterized by symptoms that would be aggravated by the drugs. Some of these are prostatic hypertrophy, glaucoma, tachyarrhythmias, myocardial infarction, and congestive heart failure unless bradycardia is present. They should not be given in hiatal hernia or other conditions contributing to reflux esophagitis because the drugs delay gastric emptying, relax the cardioesophageal sphincter, and increase esophageal reflux.

# Individual anticholinergic drugs

## BELLADONNA ALKALOIDS AND DERIVATIVES

**Atropine** is the prototype of anticholinergic drugs. It produces the same effects and has the same clinical indications for use and the same contraindications as those described above. In addition, it is used as an antidote for an overdose of cholinergic drugs and exposure to insecticides that have cholinergic effects.

Atropine is a naturally occurring belladonna alkaloid that can be extracted from the belladonna plant or prepared synthetically. It is usually prepared as atropine sulfate, a salt that is very soluble in water. It is well absorbed from the gastrointestinal tract and distributed throughout the body. It crosses the blood-brain barrier to enter the CNS, where large doses produce stimulant effects, and toxic doses produce depressant effects. Atropine is also absorbed systemically when applied locally to mucous membranes. The drug is rapidly excreted in the urine. Pharmacologic effects are of short duration except for ocular effects, which may last for several days.

### Routes and dosage ranges

*Adults:* Gastrointestinal disorders, PO, SC 0.3–1.2 mg q4–6h

Preoperatively, IM 0.4–0.6 mg in a single dose 45–60 min before anesthesia

Bradyarrhythmias, IV 0.4–1 mg q1–2h PRN

Bronchoconstriction, 0.025 mg/kg diluted with 3–5 ml saline and given by nebulizer three or four times per day

Topically to eye, one drop of 1% or 2% ophthalmic solution

*Children:* Gastrointestinal disorders, SC 0.01 mg/kg of body weight q4–6h

Preoperatively, IM 0.4 mg for children 3–14 years, less for younger children and infants

Bradyarrhythmias, IV 0.01–0.03 mg/kg of body weight

Bronchoconstriction, 0.05 mg/kg diluted with 3–5 ml saline and given by nebulizer three or four times per day

Topically to eye, one drop of 0.5% or 1% ophthalmic solution

**Belladonna tincture** is a mixture of alkaloids in an aqueous-alcohol solution. It is most often used in gastrointestinal disorders for antispasmodic effect. It is an ingredient in several drug mixtures.

### Route and dosage range

*Adults:* PO 0.6–1 ml three or four times per day

*Children:* PO 0.03 ml/kg per day in three or four divided doses

**Homatropine methylbromide** (Homapin) is a semisynthetic derivative of atropine used as eye drops to produce mydriasis and cycloplegia. Homatropine is sometimes preferable to atropine because ocular effects do not last as long.

### Route and dosage ranges

*Adults:* Topically to eye, 1 drop of 5% ophthalmic solution every 5 min for two or three doses for refraction; 1 drop of 2% to 5% solution two or three times per day for uveitis

**Hyoscyamine** (Anaspaz) is a belladonna alkaloid used in gastrointestinal and genitourinary disorders characterized by spasm, increased secretion, and increased motility. It has the same effects as other atropine-like drugs.

### Routes and dosage ranges

*Adults:* PO 0.125–0.25 mg q4–6h until symptoms are controlled; IM, SC, IV 0.25–0.5 mg q4–6h until symptoms are controlled

*Children:* PO 0.062–0.125 mg q4–6h for children 2–10 years; half this dosage for children under 2 years

**Methscopolamine** (Pamine) is a belladonna derivative used occasionally to treat peptic ulcer disease. It lacks the central action of scopolamine and is less potent and longer-acting than atropine.

### Route and dosage ranges

*Adults:* PO 2.5–5 mg four times per day
*Children:* PO 0.2 mg/kg/day in four divided doses

**Scopolamine** is very similar to atropine and has the same uses and adverse reactions for the most part; more specifically, scopolamine has similar peripheral effects but different central effects. When given parenterally, scopolamine depresses the CNS and usually causes drowsiness, euphoria, relaxation, amnesia, and sleep. Some over-the-counter sleeping pills contain small amounts of scopolamine. Effects of scopolamine appear more quickly and disappear more readily than those of atropine. Scopolamine also is used in motion sickness. It is available as oral tablets and as a transdermal adhesive disc that is placed behind the ear. The disc (Transderm-V) protects against motion sickness for 72 hours.

### Routes and dosage ranges

*Adults:* Preoperatively, IM 0.4 mg
  Motion sickness, PO 0.25–0.8 mg 1 hour before travel; transdermally 1 disc q72h
  Mydriasis, topically to the eye, 1 drop of 0.2% to 0.25% ophthalmic solution, repeated PRN
*Children:* Preoperatively, 6 months–3 years, IM 0.1–0.15 mg; 3–6 years, IM 0.15–0.2 mg; 6–12 years, 0.2–0.3 mg
  Mydriasis, same as for adults

## SYNTHETIC ANTICHOLINERGICS USED IN PARKINSON'S DISEASE

**Trihexyphenidyl** (Artane) is usually the anticholinergic drug of choice for treatment of parkinsonism. It is also effective in treating extrapyramidal reactions caused by antipsychotic drugs. Trihexyphenidyl relieves smooth muscle spasm by a direct action on the muscle and by inhibiting the PNS. The drug supposedly has fewer side effects than atropine, but about half the recipients report mouth dryness, blurring of vision, and other side effects common to anticholinergic drugs. Trihexyphenidyl requires the same precautions as other anticholinergic drugs and is contraindicated in glaucoma. **Biperiden** (Akineton) and **procyclidine** (Kemadrin) are chemical derivatives of trihexyphenidyl and have similar actions, uses, and adverse effects.

Trihexyphenidyl

### Route and dosage ranges

*Adults:* Parkinsonism, PO 2 mg two or three times per day initially, gradually increased until therapeutic effects or severe adverse effects occur
  Drug-induced extrapyramidal reactions, PO 1 mg initially, gradually increased to 5–15 mg/d in divided doses

Biperiden

### Routes and dosage ranges

*Adults:* Parkinsonism, PO 2 mg three or four times per day
  Drug-induced extrapyramidal reactions, IM 2 mg, repeated q30 min if necessary; maximum of four consecutive doses in 24 hours
*Children:* Drug-induced extrapyramidal reactions, IM 0.04 mg/kg, repeated as above if necessary

Procyclidine

### Route and dosage ranges

*Adults:* Parkinsonism, PO 5 mg twice daily initially, gradually increased to 5 mg three or four times per day if necessary
  Drug-induced extrapyramidal reactions, PO 2–2.5 mg three times per day, gradually increased to 10–20 mg/d if necessary

**Benztropine** (Cogentin) is a synthetic drug with both anticholinergic and antihistaminic effects. Its anticholinergic activity approximates that of atropine. A major clinical use is to treat acute dystonic reactions caused by antipsychotic drugs and to prevent their recurrence in clients receiving long-term antipsychotic drug therapy. It also may be given in small doses to supplement other antiparkinson drugs. In full dosage, adverse reactions are common.

### Routes and dosage ranges

*Adults:* PO 0.5–1 mg at bedtime, initially, gradually increased to 4–6 mg/d if required and tolerated
  Drug-induced extrapyramidal reactions PO, IM, IV 1–4 mg once or twice per day

## URINARY ANTISPASMODICS

**Flavoxate** (Urispas) was developed specifically to counteract spasm in smooth muscle tissue of the urinary tract. It has anticholinergic, local anesthetic, and analgesic effects. Thus, the drug relieves dysuria, urgency, frequency, and pain with genitourinary infections, such as cystitis and prostatitis.

### Route and dosage range

*Adults and children over 12:* PO 100–200 mg three or four times per day. Reduce dose when symptoms improve.
*Children under 12 years:* Dosage not established

**Oxybutynin** (Ditropan) has direct antispasmodic effects on smooth muscle and anticholinergic effects. It increases bladder capacity and decreases frequency of voiding in clients with neurogenic bladder.

### Route and dosage range

*Adults:* PO 5 mg two or three times per day; maximum dose 5 mg four times per day
*Children over 5 years:* PO 5 mg twice a day; maximum dose 5 mg three times per day

## Nursing Process

### Assessment

- Assess the client's condition in relation to disorders for which anticholinergic drugs are used (that is, check for bradycardia or heart block, diarrhea, dysuria, abdominal pain, and other disorders). If the client reports or medical records indicate a specific disorder, assess for signs and symptoms of that disorder (*e.g.*, Parkinson's disease).
- Assess for disorders in which anticholinergic drugs are contraindicated (*e.g.*, glaucoma, prostatic hypertrophy, reflux esophagitis).
- Assess use of other drugs with anticholinergic effects, such as antihistamines (histamine-1 receptor antagonists [see Chap. 51], antipsychotic agents, and tricyclic antidepressants).

### Nursing diagnoses

- Altered Urinary Elimination: Decreased bladder tone and urine retention
- Constipation related to slowed gastrointestinal function
- Altered Thought Processes: Confusion, disorientation, especially in older adults
- Knowledge Deficit: Drug effects and accurate usage
- High Risk for Injury related to drug-induced blurred vision and photophobia
- High Risk for Noncompliance related to adverse drug effects

### Planning/Goals

*The client will:*
- Receive or self-administer the drugs correctly
- Experience relief of symptoms for which anticholinergic drugs are given
- Be assisted to avoid or cope with adverse drug effects on vision, thought processes, and bowel and bladder elimination

### Interventions

Use measures to decrease the need for anticholinergic drugs. For example, with peptic ulcer disease, teach the client to avoid factors known to increase gastric secretion and gastroin-testinal motility (alcohol; cigarette smoking; caffeine-containing beverages, such as coffee, tea, and cola drinks; ulcerogenic drugs, such as aspirin). Late evening snacks also should be avoided because increased gastric acid secretion occurs about 90 minutes after eating and may cause pain and awakening from sleep. Although milk is traditionally an ulcer food, it contains protein and calcium, which promote acid secretion, and is a poor buffer of gastric acid. Thus, drinking large amounts of milk should be avoided.

### Teach clients:
- Not to take other drugs without the physician's knowledge. In addition to prescribed antidepressants, antihistamines and antipsychotic drugs with anticholinergic properties, over-the-counter sleeping pills and antihistamines have anticholinergic effects. Taking any of these concurrently could cause overdosage or excessive anticholinergic effects.
- Measures to minimize risks of heat exhaustion and heat stroke:
  - Wear light, cool clothing in warm climates or environments.
  - Maintain fluid and salt intake if not contraindicated.
  - Limit exposure to direct sunlight.
  - Limit physical activities.
  - Take frequent cool baths.
  - Ensure adequate ventilation, with fans or air conditioners if necessary.
  - Avoid alcoholic beverages.

### Evaluation

- Interview and observe in relation to safe, accurate drug administration.
- Interview and observe for relief of symptoms for which the drugs are given.
- Interview and observe for adverse drug effects.

## Principles of therapy

### USE IN SPECIFIC CONDITIONS

### Renal or biliary colic

Atropine is sometimes given with morphine or meperidine to relieve the severe pain of renal or biliary colic. It acts mainly to decrease the spasm-producing effects of the narcotic analgesics. It has little antispasmodic effect on the involved muscles and is not used alone for this purpose.

### Preoperative use in clients with glaucoma

Glaucoma is usually listed as a contraindication for anticholinergic drugs because the drugs impair outflow of aqueous humor and may cause an acute attack of glaucoma (increased intraocular pressure). However, anticholinergic drugs can be given safely preoperatively to clients with open-angle glaucoma (80% of clients with primary glaucoma) if they are receiving miotic drugs, such as pilocarpine. If anticholinergic preoperative medication is needed in clients predisposed to angle closure, the hazard of causing acute glaucoma can be minimized by also giving pilocarpine eye drops and acetazolamide (Diamox).

## Gastrointestinal disorders

When anticholinergic drugs are given for gastrointestinal disorders, larger doses may be given at bedtime to prevent pain and awakening during sleep.

## Parkinsonism

When these drugs are used in parkinsonism, small doses are given initially and gradually increased. This regimen decreases adverse reactions.

## Extrapyramidal reactions

When used in drug-induced extrapyramidal reactions (parkinson-like symptoms), these drugs should be prescribed only if symptoms occur. Anticholinergic drugs are used to treat extrapyramidal reactions; they are not used routinely to prevent extrapyramidal reactions because less than half the clients taking antipsychotic drugs experience such reactions. Most drug-induced reactions last about 3 months and do not recur if anticholinergic drugs are discontinued at that time. (An exception is tardive dyskinesia, which does not respond to anticholinergic drugs and may be aggravated by them.)

## Treatment of atropine or anticholinergic overdosage

Overdosage of atropine or other anticholinergic drugs produces the usual pharmacologic effects in a severe and exaggerated form. Physostigmine salicylate (Antilirium) is a specific antidote. It is usually given intravenously at a slow rate of injection. Adult dosage is 2 mg (no more than 1 mg/min); child dosage is 0.5 to 1 mg (no more than 0.5 mg/min). Rapid administration may cause bradycardia, hypersalivation (with subsequent respiratory distress), and seizures. Repeated doses may be given if life-threatening arrhythmias, convulsions, or coma occur. Diazepam (Valium) or a similar drug may be given for excessive CNS stimulation (delirium, excitement). Cardiopulmonary resuscitative measures are used if excessive depression of the CNS causes coma and respiratory failure.

## USE IN CHILDREN

Systemic anticholinergics, including atropine, glycopyrrolate (Robinul), and scopolamine are given to chil-

dren of all ages for essentially the same effects as for adults. The antispasmodic agents are also used. Flavoxate is not recommended for children under 12 years, and oxybutynin is not recommended for children under 5 years.

The drugs cause the same adverse effects in children as in adults. However, they may be more severe because children are especially sensitive to the drugs. Facial flushing is common in children, and a skin rash may occur.

Ophthalmic anticholinergic drugs are used for cycloplegia and mydriasis prior to eye examinations and surgical procedures. They should be used only with close medical supervision. Cyclopentolate (Cyclogyl) and tropicamide (Mydriacyl) have been associated with behavioral disturbances and psychotic reactions in children. Tropicamide also has been associated with cardiopulmonary collapse.

## USE IN OLDER ADULTS

Anticholinergic drugs are given for the same purposes as in younger adults. In addition to the primary anticholinergic drugs, many others that are commonly prescribed for older adults have high anticholinergic activity. These include many antihistamines (histamine-1 receptor antagonists), tricyclic antidepressants, and antipsychotic drugs.

Older adults are especially likely to have significant adverse reactions because of slowed drug metabolism and the frequent presence of several disease processes. Some common adverse effects and suggestions for reducing their impact are:

1. *Blurred vision.* The client may need help with ambulation, especially with stairs or other potentially hazardous environments. Remove obstacles and hazards when possible.
2. *Confusion.* Provide whatever assistance is needed to prevent falls and other injuries.
3. *Heat stroke.* Help to avoid precipitating factors, such as strenuous activity and high environmental temperatures.
4. *Constipation.* Encourage or assist with an adequate intake of high-fiber foods and fluids and adequate exercise when feasible.
5. *Urinary retention.* Encourage adequate fluid intake and avoid high doses of the drugs. Men should be examined for prostatic hypertrophy.
6. *Hallucinations and other psychotic symptoms.* These are most likely to occur with the centrally active anticholinergics given for Parkinson's disease or drug-induced extrapyramidal effects, such as trihexyphenidyl or benztropine. Dosage of these drugs should be carefully regulated and supervised.

# NURSING ACTIONS: ANTICHOLINERGIC DRUGS

| *Nursing Actions* | *Rationale/Explanation* |
|---|---|
| **1. Administer accurately** | |
| **a.** For gastrointestinal disorders, give most oral anticholinergic drugs about 30 minutes before meals and at bedtime. | To allow the drugs to reach peak antisecretory effects by the time ingested food is stimulating gastric acid secretion. Bedtime administration helps prevent awakening with abdominal pain. |
| **b.** When given preoperatively, parenteral preparations of atropine can be mixed in the same syringe with several other common preoperative medications, such as meperidine (Demerol), morphine, oxymorphone (Numorphan), and promethazine (Phenergan). | The primary reason for mixing medications in the same syringe is to decrease the number of injections and thus decrease client discomfort. Note, however, that extra caution is required when mixing drugs to be sure that the dosage of each drug is accurate. Also, if any question exists regarding compatibility with another drug, it is safer not to mix the drugs, even if two or three injections are required. |
| **c.** When applying topical atropine solutions or ointment to the eye, be sure to use the correct concentration and blot any excess from the inner canthus. | Atropine ophthalmic preparations are available in several concentrations (usually 1%, 2%, and 3%). Excess medication should be removed so that the drug will not enter the nasolacrimal (tear) ducts and be absorbed systemically through the mucous membrane of the nasopharynx or be carried to the throat and swallowed. |
| **d.** If propantheline is to be given intravenously, dissolve the 30-mg dose of powder in no less than 10 ml of sterile water for injection. | Parenteral administration is reserved for clients who cannot take the drug orally. |
| **e.** Instruct clients to swallow oral propantheline tablets, not to chew them. | The tablets have a hard sugar coating to mask the bitter taste of the drug. |
| **f.** Parenteral glycopyrrolate can be given through the tubing of a running intravenous infusion of physiologic saline or lactated Ringer's solution. | |
| **2. Observe for therapeutic effects** | Therapeutic effects depend primarily on the reason for use. Thus, a therapeutic effect in one condition may be a side effect or an adverse reaction in another condition. |
| **a.** When a drug is given for *peptic ulcer disease* or other gastrointestinal disorders, observe for decreased abdominal pain. | Relief of abdominal pain is due to the smooth muscle relaxant or antispasmodic effect of the drug. |
| **b.** When the drug is given for *diagnosing or treating eye disorders*, observe for pupil dilation (mydriasis) and blurring of vision (cycloplegia). | Note that these ocular effects are side effects when the drugs are given for problems not related to the eyes. |
| **c.** When the drug is given for *symptomatic bradycardia*, observe for increased pulse rate. | These drugs increase heart rate by blocking action of the vagus nerve. |
| **d.** When the drug is given for *urinary tract disorders*, such as cystitis or enuresis, observe for decreased frequency of urination. When the drug is given for *renal colic due to stones*, observe for decreased pain. | Anticholinergic drugs decrease muscle tone and spasm in the smooth muscle of the ureters and urinary bladder. |
| **e.** When the centrally acting anticholinergics are given for *Parkinson's disease*, observe for decrease in tremor, salivation, and drooling. | Decreased salivation is a therapeutic effect with parkinsonism but an adverse reaction in most other conditions. |
| **3. Observe for adverse effects** | These depend on reasons for use and are dose related. |

(*continued*)

| *Nursing Actions* | *Rationale/Explanation* |
|---|---|
| **a.** Tachycardia | Tachycardia may occur with usual therapeutic doses because anticholinergic drugs block vagal action, which normally slows heart rate. Tachycardia is not likely to be serious except in clients with underlying heart disease. For example, in clients with angina pectoris, prolonged or severe tachycardia may increase myocardial ischemia to the point of causing an acute attack of angina (chest pain) or even myocardial infarction. In clients with congestive heart failure, severe or prolonged tachycardia can increase the workload of the heart to the point of causing acute heart failure or pulmonary edema. |
| **b.** Excessive central nervous system (CNS) stimulation, (tremor, restlessness, confusion, hallucinations, delirium) followed by excessive CNS depression (coma, respiratory depression) | These effects are more likely to occur with large doses of atropine because atropine crosses the blood-brain barrier. Large doses of trihexyphenidyl (Artane) also may cause CNS stimulation. |
| **c.** Sedation and amnesia with scopolamine or benztropine (Cogentin) | This may be a therapeutic effect but becomes an adverse reaction if severe or if the drug is given for another purpose. Benztropine has anticholinergic and antihistaminic properties. Apparently, drowsiness and sedation are caused by the antihistaminic component. |
| **d.** Constipation or paralytic ileus | These effects are the result of decreased gastrointestinal motility and muscle tone. Constipation is more likely with large doses or parenteral administration. Paralytic ileus is not likely unless the drugs are given to clients who already have decreased gastrointestinal motility. |
| **e.** Decreased oral and respiratory tract secretions, which cause mouth dryness and thick respiratory secretions | Mouth dryness is more annoying than serious in most cases and is caused by decreased salivation. However, clients with chronic lung disease, who usually have excessive secretions, tend to retain them with the consequence of frequent respiratory tract infections. |
| **f.** Urinary retention | This reaction is caused by loss of bladder tone and is most likely to occur in elderly men with enlarged prostate glands. Thus, the drugs are generally contraindicated with prostatic hypertrophy. |
| **g.** Hot, dry skin; fever; heat stroke | These effects are due to decreased sweating and impairment of the normal heat loss mechanism. Fever may occur with any age group. Heat stroke is more likely to occur with cardiovascular disease, strenuous physical activity, and high environmental temperatures, especially in elderly people. |
| **h.** Ocular effects—mydriasis, blurred vision, photophobia | These are adverse effects when anticholinergic drugs are given for conditions not related to the eyes. |
| **4. Observe for drug interactions**<br>**a.** Drugs that *increase* effects of anticholinergic drugs: Antihistamines, disopyramide, phenothiazines, thioxanthene agents, and tricyclic antidepressants | These drugs have anticholinergic properties and produce additive anticholinergic effects. |
| **b.** Drugs that *decrease* effects of anticholinergic drugs: Cholinergic drugs | These drugs counteract the inhibition of gastrointestinal motility and tone induced by atropine. They are sometimes used in atropine overdose. |
| **5. Teach clients**<br>**a.** Mouth dryness commonly occurs. Use sugarless chewing gum and hard candy if not contraindicated. | To relieve mouth dryness |

| *Nursing Actions* | *Rationale/Explanation* |
|---|---|
| **b.** The importance of dental hygiene (*e.g.*, regular brushing of teeth) | Dental caries and loss of teeth may result from drug-induced xerostomia (dry mouth from decreased saliva production). This is more likely to occur with long-term use of these drugs. |
| **c.** Blurring of vision is also common. Avoid potentially hazardous activities (*e.g.*, driving a car or operating machinery) when this occurs. | To prevent injury |
| **d.** Dark glasses can be worn outdoors in strong light. | To reduce sensitivity to light (photophobia) |

## Review and Application Exercises

1. How do anticholinergic drugs exert their therapeutic effects?
2. What are indications for use and contraindications for anticholinergic drugs?
3. What is the effect of anticholinergic drugs on heart rate, and what is the mechanism for this effect?
4. Under what circumstances is it desirable to administer atropine preoperatively and why?
5. What are adverse effects of anticholinergic drugs?
6. What treatment measures are indicated for a client with an overdose of a drug with anticholinergic effects?
7. Name two other commonly used drug groups that have anticholinergic effects?
8. What nursing observations and interventions are needed to increase client safety and comfort during anticholinergic drug therapy?

## Selected References

Burrell, L. O. (1992). *Adult nursing in hospital and community settings.* Norwalk, CT: Appleton & Lange.

(1993). *Drug facts and comparisons.* St. Louis: Facts and Comparisons.

Gotz, V. P. (1992). Chronic obstructive airways disease. In M. A. Koda-Kimble & L. Y. Young (Eds.), *Applied therapeutics: The clinical use of drugs* (5th ed.) (pp. 16-1–16-17). Vancouver, WA: Applied Therapeutics.

Guttman, M. (1992). Principles of neuropharmacology. In W. N. Kelley (Ed.), *Textbook of internal medicine* (2nd ed.) (pp. 2255–2259). Philadelphia: J.B. Lippincott.

Guyton, A. C. (1991). *Textbook of medical physiology* (8th ed.). Philadelphia: W.B. Saunders.

Kelly, H. W. (1992). Asthma. In M. A. Koda-Kimble & L. Y. Young (Eds.), *Applied therapeutics: The clinical use of drugs* (5th ed.) (pp.15-1–15-24). Vancouver, WA: Applied Therapeutics.

Porth, C. M., & Curtis, R. L. (1990). Normal and altered autonomic nervous system function. In C. M. Porth (Ed.), *Pathophysiology: Concepts of altered health states* (3rd ed.) (pp. 873–892). Philadelphia: J.B. Lippincott

Shlafer, M. (1993). *The nurse, pharmacology, and drug therapy: A prototype approach.* Redwood City, CA: Addison-Wesley.

# Drugs Affecting the Endocrine System

### CHAPTER 22

# Physiology of the Endocrine System

## The endocrine system

The major organs of the endocrine system are the hypothalamus, pituitary, thyroid, parathyroids, pancreas, adrenals, ovaries, and testes. These tissues function through *hormones*, chemical substances that are synthesized and secreted into body fluids by one group of cells and have physiologic effects on other body cells. Most hormones from the traditional endocrine glands are secreted into the bloodstream and act on distant organs.

In addition to the major endocrine organs, numerous other tissues produce hormones. These are secreted into tissue fluids and act locally on nearby cells, as in the following examples:

Gastrointestinal mucosa produces hormones that are important in the digestive process (*e.g.*, gastrin, enterogastrone, secretin, and cholecystokinin).

The kidneys produce erythropoietin, a hormone that stimulates the bone marrow to produce red blood cells.

White blood cells produce cytokines that function as messengers among leukocytes in inflammatory and immune processes.

Most body tissues produce prostaglandins, which have a variety of physiologic effects.

Neoplastic disease also may produce hormones. In endocrine tissues, neoplasms may be an added source of the hormone normally produced by the organ. In non-endocrine tissues, various hormones may be produced.

For example, lung tumors may produce corticotropin, antidiuretic hormone, or parathyroid hormone; kidney tumors may produce parathyroid hormone. The usual effects are those of excess hormone secretion.

The focus of this chapter is the traditional endocrine organs and their hormones. Specific organs are discussed in the following chapters; some general characteristics of the endocrine system and hormones are described below.

## Endocrine system–nervous system interactions

The endocrine system works in harmony with the nervous system to regulate body functions. Generally, the nervous system regulates rapid muscular and sensory activities by secreting substances that act as neurotransmitters, circulating hormones, and local hormones (*e.g.*, norepinephrine, epinephrine). The endocrine system regulates slow metabolic activities by secreting hormones that control cellular metabolism, transport of substances across cell membranes, and other functions (*e.g.*, reproduction, growth and development, secretion).

The main connecting link between the nervous system and the endocrine system is the hypothalamus, which responds to nervous system stimulation by producing hormones. Thus, secretion of almost all hormones from the pituitary gland is controlled by the hypothalamus. Special nerve fibers originating in the hypothalamus and ending in the posterior pituitary gland control secretions of the posterior pituitary. The hypothalamus secretes hormones called *releasing* and *inhibitory factors*, which regulate functions of the anterior pituitary. The anterior pituitary, in turn, secretes corticotropin (ACTH), a hormone that stimulates functions of the adrenal cortex. This complex interrelationship is often referred to as the *hypothalamic-pituitary-adrenocortical* axis. It functions by a *negative feedback* system, in which hormone secretion is stimulated when hormones are needed and inhibited when they are not needed. The hypothalamic-pituitary-thyroid axis also functions by a negative feedback mechanism.

# General characteristics of hormones

Hormones are extremely important in regulating body activities. Their normal secretion and function help to maintain the internal environment and determine response and adaptation to the external environment. Hormones participate in complex interactions with other hormones and nonhormone chemical substances in the body to influence every aspect of life. Although hormones are usually studied individually, virtually all endocrine functions are complex processes that are influenced by more than one hormone. Abnormal secretion and function of hormones, even minor alterations, can affect physical well-being and in some cases, thought processes and emotional stability. Malfunction of an endocrine organ is usually associated with hyposecretion, hypersecretion, or inappropriate secretion of its hormones. Any malfunction can produce serious disease or death.

Although hormones circulating in the bloodstream reach essentially all body cells, some (*e.g.*, growth hormone, thyroid hormone) affect almost all cells, while others affect specific "target" tissues (*e.g.*, corticotropin stimulates the adrenal cortex, and ovarian hormones affect the endometrial lining of the uterus).

## HORMONE ACTION AT THE CELLULAR LEVEL

Once hormone molecules reach a responsive cell, they bind with receptors in the cell membrane (*e.g.*, catecholamines and protein hormones) or inside the cell (*e.g.*, steroid and thyroid hormones). The main target organs for a given hormone contain large numbers of receptors and therefore have a higher concentration of hormone than the circulating blood. Receptors on the plasma membrane are constantly being synthesized and degraded so that the number of receptors may change within hours. Receptor affinity for binding with hormone molecules probably changes as well.

After binding occurs, the resulting hormone-receptor complex initiates intracellular biochemical reactions, depending on the particular hormone and the type of cell. The most widely accepted theory of hormone action at the cellular level is that the hormone serves as a "first messenger" to the cell, and the hormone-receptor complex activates a "second messenger." The second messenger then activates intracellular structures to produce characteristic cellular functions and products.

Two major second messengers are cyclic adenosine monophosphate (cAMP) and calcium. cAMP is formed by the action of the enzyme adenyl cyclase on adenosine triphosphate, a component of all cells and the main source of energy for cellular metabolism. The amount of intracellular cAMP is increased by hormones that activate adenyl cyclase (*e.g.*, the pituitary hormones, calcitonin, glucagon, parathyroid hormone) and decreased by hormones that inactivate adenyl cyclase (*e.g.*, angiotensin, somatostatin). cAMP is degraded by phosphodiesterase enzymes. Calcium is the second messenger for angiotensin II, a strong vasoconstrictor that participates in control of arterial blood pressures and for gonadotropin-releasing hormone. The postulated sequence of events is that hormone binding to receptors increases intracellular calcium. The calcium binds with an intracellular regulatory protein called calmodulin. The calcium-calmodulin complex activates protein kinases, which then regulate contractile structures of the cell, cell membrane permeability, and intracellular enzyme activity. Second messengers for insulin, prolactin, and other hormones are thought to exist but are not yet identified.

## MAJOR HORMONES AND THEIR GENERAL FUNCTIONS

1. Anterior pituitary hormones are growth hormone (also called somatotropin), corticotropin, thyroid-stimulating hormone, follicle-stimulating hormone, luteinizing hormone, and prolactin. Most of these hormones function by stimulating secretion of other hormones.

2. Posterior pituitary hormones are antidiuretic hormone (ADH or vasopressin) and oxytocin. ADH helps maintain fluid balance; oxytocin stimulates uterine contractions during childbirth.

3. Adrenal cortex hormones, commonly called corticosteroids, include the glucocorticoids, such as cortisol, and the mineralocorticoids, such as aldosterone. Glucocorticoids influence carbohydrate storage, exert anti-inflammatory effects, suppress corticotropin secretion, and increase protein catabolism. Mineralocorticoids help regulate electrolyte balance, mainly by promoting sodium retention and po-

tassium loss. The adrenal cortex also produces sex hormones. Adrenal medulla hormones are epinephrine and norepinephrine (see Chap. 18).

4. Thyroid hormones include triiodothyronine ($T_3$ or liothyronine) and tetraiodothyronine ($T_4$ or thyroxine). These hormones regulate the metabolic rate of the body and greatly influence growth and development.

5. Parathyroid hormone, also called parathormone or PTH, regulates calcium and phosphate metabolism.

6. Pancreatic hormones are insulin and glucagon, which regulate the metabolism of glucose, lipids, and proteins.

7. Ovarian hormones (female sex hormones) are estrogens and progesterone. Estrogens promote growth of specific body cells and development of most secondary sexual characteristics in females. Progesterone helps prepare the uterus for pregnancy and the mammary glands for lactation.

8. Testicular hormone (male sex hormone) is testosterone, which regulates development of masculine characteristics.

9. Placental hormones are chorionic gonadotropin, estrogen, progesterone, and human placental lactogen, all of which are concerned with reproductive functions.

# General characteristics of hormonal drugs

1. Hormone preparations given for therapeutic purposes include natural hormones from human or animal sources and synthetic hormones. Many of the most important hormones have been synthesized, and these preparations may have more potent and prolonged effects than the naturally occurring hormones.

2. Hormones are given for physiologic or pharmacologic effects. Physiologic use involves giving small doses as a replacement or substitute for the amount ordinarily secreted by a normally functioning endocrine gland. Such usage is indicated only when a gland cannot secrete an adequate amount of hormone. Examples of physiologic use include insulin administration in diabetes mellitus and adrenal corticosteroid administration in Addison's disease. Pharmacologic use in-

volves relatively large doses for effects greater than physiologic effects. For example, adrenal corticosteroids are widely used for anti-inflammatory effects in endocrine and nonendocrine disorders.

3. Hormones are powerful drugs that produce widespread therapeutic and adverse effects.

4. Administration of one hormone may alter effects of other hormones. These alterations result from the complex interactions among hormones.

5. Hormonal drugs are more often given for disorders resulting from endocrine gland hypofunction than for those related to hyperfunction.

## Review and Application Exercises

1. How do hormones function in maintaining homeostasis?
2. What is the connection between the nervous system and the endocrine system?
3. What is meant by a negative feedback system?
4. Because classic hormones are secreted into blood and circulated to essentially all body cells, why do they not affect all body cells?
5. What are the functions and characteristics of the pituitary gland?

## Selected References

Granner, D. K. (1992). Mechanisms of hormone action. In W. N. Kelley (Ed.), *Textbook of internal medicine* (2nd ed.) (pp. 1922–1927). Philadelphia: J.B. Lippincott.

Gray, D. P. (1990). Mechanisms of hormonal regulation. In K. L. McCance & S. E. Huether, *Pathophysiology: The biologic basis for disease in adults and children* (pp. 564–593). St. Louis: C.V. Mosby.

Guyton, A. C. (1991). *Textbook of medical physiology* (8th ed.). Philadelphia: W.B. Saunders.

Hancock, M. R. (1992). Overview of anatomy, physiology, and pathophysiology of the endocrine system. In L. O. Burrell (Ed.), *Adult nursing in hospital and community settings*. Norwalk, CT: Appleton & Lange.

Porth, C. M. (1990). *Pathophysiology: Concepts of altered health states* (3rd ed.) (pp. 1067–1074). Philadelphia: J.B. Lippincott.

Wilson, J. D., & Foster, D. W. (1992). Hormones and hormone action. In J. D. Wilson & D. W. Foster (Eds.), *Williams textbook of endocrinology* (8th ed.) (pp. 1–8). Philadelphia: W.B. Saunders.

### CHAPTER 23

# Hypothalamic and Pituitary Hormones

## Description

The hypothalamus and pituitary gland (hypophysis) interact to control most metabolic functions of the body and to maintain homeostasis. They are anatomically connected by the hypophyseal stalk. The hypothalamus controls secretions of the pituitary gland. The pituitary gland, in turn, regulates secretions or functions of other body tissues, called "target" tissues. The pituitary gland is actually two glands, each with different structures and functions. The anterior pituitary (adenohypophysis) is composed of different types of glandular cells that synthesize and secrete different hormones. The posterior pituitary (neurohypophysis) is anatomically an extension of the hypothalamus and is composed largely of nerve fibers. It does not manufacture any hormones itself but stores and releases hormones synthesized in the hypothalamus.

### HYPOTHALAMIC HORMONES

The hypothalamus produces a releasing hormone (also called factor) or an inhibiting hormone that corresponds to each of the major hormones of the anterior pituitary gland. Specifically, they are:

1. *Corticotropin-releasing hormone*, which causes release of corticotropin in response to stress and threatening stimuli.
2. *Growth hormone-releasing factor*, which causes release

of growth hormone in response to low blood levels of the hormone.

3. *Growth hormone release-inhibiting hormone* (somatostatin), which inhibits release of growth hormone.
4. *Thyrotropin-releasing hormone* (TRH), which causes release of thyroid-stimulating hormone (TSH or thyrotropin) in response to stress, such as exposure to cold.
5. *Gonadotropin-releasing hormone* (GnRH), which causes release of follicle-stimulating hormone (FSH) and luteinizing hormone (LH).
6. *Prolactin-releasing factor*, which is active during lactation after childbirth.
7. *Prolactin-inhibitory factor* (PIF), which is active at times other than during lactation.
8. *Melanocyte-stimulating hormone releasing factor*, which stimulates release of melanocyte stimulating hormone.
9. *Melanocyte-stimulating hormone inhibiting factor*, which inhibits release of melanocyte-stimulating hormone.

### PITUITARY HORMONES

The anterior pituitary gland produces seven hormones. Two of these, growth hormone and prolactin, act directly on their target tissues; the other five act indirectly by stimulating target tissues to produce other hormones.

1. *Corticotropin*, also called adrenocorticotropic hormone (ACTH), stimulates the adrenal cortex to produce adrenocorticosteroids. Secretion is controlled by the hypothalamus and by plasma levels of cortisol,

Anne Collins Abrams: CLINICAL DRUG THERAPY, Fourth Edition.
© 1995 J.B. Lippincott Company.

the major adrenocorticosteroid. When plasma levels are adequate for body needs, the anterior pituitary does not release corticotropin (negative feedback mechanism).

2. *Growth hormone*, also called somatotropin, stimulates growth of all body tissues that are capable of responding. It promotes an increase in cell size and number, largely by affecting metabolism of carbohydrate, protein, fat, and bone tissue. Deficient growth hormone in children produces dwarfism, a condition marked by severely decreased linear growth and frequently, severely delayed mental, emotional, dental, and sexual growth as well. Excessive growth hormone in preadolescent children produces gigantism, marked by heights of 8 or 9 ft if untreated. Excessive growth hormone in adults produces acromegaly.

3. *Thyrotropin*, also called TSH, regulates secretion of thyroid hormones. Thyrotropin secretion is controlled by a negative feedback mechanism in proportion to metabolic needs. Thus, increased thyroid hormones in body fluids inhibit secretion of thyrotropin by the anterior pituitary and of TRH by the hypothalamus.

4. *FSH*, one of the gonadotropins, stimulates functions of sex glands. It is produced by the anterior pituitary gland of males and females beginning at puberty. FSH acts on the ovaries in a cyclical fashion during the reproductive years, stimulating growth of ovarian follicles. These follicles then produce estrogen, which prepares the endometrium for implantation of a fertilized ovum. FSH acts on the testes to stimulate the production and growth of sperm (spermatogenesis), but it does not stimulate secretion of male sex hormones.

5. *LH* (also called *interstitial cell-stimulating hormone*), is another gonadotropin that stimulates hormone production by the gonads of both sexes. LH is important in the maturation and rupture of the ovarian follicle (ovulation). After ovulation, LH acts on the cells of the collapsed sac to produce the corpus luteum, which then produces progesterone during the last half of the menstrual cycle. When blood progesterone levels rise, a negative feedback effect is exerted on hypothalamic and anterior pituitary secretion of gonadotropins. Decreased pituitary secretion of LH causes the corpus luteum to die and stop producing progesterone. Lack of progesterone causes slough and discharge of the endometrial lining as menstrual flow. (Of course, if the ovum has been fertilized and attached to the endometrium, menstruation does not occur.)

  In males, LH stimulates the Leydig's cells in the spaces between the seminiferous tubules. These cells then secrete androgens, mainly testosterone.

6. *Prolactin* plays a part in milk production by nursing mothers. It is not usually secreted in nonpregnant women because of the hypothalamic hormone PIF. During late pregnancy and lactation, various stimuli, including suckling, inhibit the production of PIF, and thus prolactin is synthesized and released.

7. *Melanocyte-stimulating hormone* plays a role in skin pigmentation, but its function in humans is not clearly delineated.

The posterior pituitary gland stores and releases two hormones that are actually synthesized by nerve cells in the hypothalamus:

1. *Antidiuretic hormone* (ADH), also called vasopressin. It functions to regulate water balance. When ADH is secreted, it makes renal tubules more permeable to water. This allows water in renal tubules to be reabsorbed into the plasma and so conserves body water. In the absence of ADH, little water is reabsorbed, and large amounts are lost in the urine.

  ADH is secreted when body fluids become concentrated (high amounts of electrolytes in proportion to the amount of water) and when blood volume is low. In the first instance, ADH causes reabsorption of water, dilution of extracellular fluids, and restoration of normal osmotic pressure. In the second instance, ADH raises blood volume and arterial blood pressure toward homeostatic levels.

2. *Oxytocin*, which functions in childbirth and lactation. It initiates uterine contractions at the end of gestation to induce childbirth, and it causes milk to move from breast glands to nipples so the infant can obtain the milk by suckling.

## Therapeutic limitations

There are few approved clinical uses for hypothalamic hormones and pituitary hormones. Drug formulations of some hypothalamic hormones are relatively new, and clinical experience with their uses and effects is limited. There are several reasons why pituitary hormones are not used extensively. First, other effective agents are available for some potential uses. When there is a deficiency of target gland hormones (*e.g.*, adrenocorticosteroids, thyroid hormones, male or female sex hormones), it is usually more convenient and effective to administer those hormones than the anterior pituitary hormones that stimulate their secretion. Second, some pituitary hormones must be obtained from natural sources, which tends to be inconvenient and relatively expensive. For example, corticotropin, thyrotropin, and ADH are obtained from the pituitary glands of domestic animals slaughtered for food; gonadotropins are obtained from the urine of pregnant or menopausal women. A third reason for the infrequent use of pituitary hormones is that most conditions in which pituitary hormones are indicated are uncommon.

Despite their limitations, pituitary hormones perform important functions when indicated for clinical use.

# Individual hormonal agents

## HYPOTHALAMIC HORMONES

**Gonadorelin acetate** (Lutrepulse), gonadorelin hydrochloride (Factrel), and nafarelin (Synarel) are synthetic equivalents of GnRH. The acetate salt is used to induce ovulation in women with hypothalamic amenorrhea. The hydrochloride salt is used in diagnostic tests of gonadotropic functions of the anterior pituitary. Nafarelin is used in the treatment of endometriosis. For specific instructions regarding administration, consult current literature from the drug manufacturer.

### Gonadorelin acetate

**Route and dosage range**

*Adults:* IV using special pump 5 μg every 90 min for about 21 days

### Gonadorelin hydrochloride

**Route and dosage range**

*Adults:* SC, IV 100 μg

### Nafarelin

**Route and dosage range**

*Adults:* One spray (200 μg) in one nostril in the morning and one spray in the other nostril in the evening (total daily dose, 400 μg), starting between the second and fourth days of the menstrual cycle

**Protirelin** (Thypinone, Relefact) is a synthetic equivalent of natural TRH. It is used for diagnostic tests of thyroid, pituitary, and hypothalamic function. For specific test methodology and interpretation, consult the drug manufacturers' instructions.

**Routes and dosage ranges**

*Adults:* IV 200–500 μg, injected over 15–30 sec, with patient supine and remaining supine for at least 15 min

*Children, 6–16 years of age:* 7 μg/kg, up to a maximum dose of 500 μg

*Infants and children up to 6 years of age:* Dosage not established

## ANTERIOR PITUITARY HORMONES

**Corticotropin** (ACTH, Acthar) is obtained from pituitary glands of cattle and hogs, then purified and standardized. Corticotropin is composed of 39 amino acids, 24 of which exert the characteristic physiologic effects. Because it is a protein substance, corticotropin is destroyed by proteolytic enzymes in the digestive tract and must therefore be given parenterally. Corticotropin has a short duration of action and must be administered frequently. There are, however, repository preparations (Cortrophin-Gel, Cortrophin-Zinc) that are slowly absorbed, have a longer duration of action, and can be given once daily.

Corticotropin is given to stimulate synthesis of hormones by the adrenal cortex (glucocorticoids, mineralocorticoids, sex hormones). It is not effective unless the adrenal cortex can respond. Adrenocortical response is variable, and dosage of corticotropin must be individualized. When corticotropin therapy is being discontinued, dosage is gradually reduced to avoid the steroid withdrawal syndrome characterized by muscle weakness, fatigue, and hypotension. Corticotropin is also used in laboratory tests of adrenal function.

**Cosyntropin** (Cortrosyn) is a synthetic drug with biologic activity similar to that of corticotropin. It is used as a diagnostic test in suspected adrenal insufficiency.

### Corticotropin

**Routes and dosage ranges**

*Adults:* Therapeutic use, IM, SC 20 units four times per day

Diagnostic use, IM 40–80 units daily for 1–3 days; IV 10–25 units in 500 ml of 5% dextrose or 0.9% sodium chloride solution, infused over 8 hours once a day. A continuous infusion with 40 units q12h for 48 hours may also be used.

### Cortrophin-gel

**Route and dosage range**

*Adults:* Therapeutic use, IM 40–80 units q24–72h
Diagnostic use, IM 40–80 units/d for 1–3 d

### Cosyntropin

**Routes and dosage ranges**

*Adults:* Diagnostic use, IM, IV 0.25 mg (equivalent to 25 units ACTH)

**Growth hormone** is synthesized from bacteria by recombinant DNA technology. Two forms are available. Somatropin (Humatrope) contains the same number and sequence of amino acids as pituitary-derived human growth hormone. Somatrem (Protropin) is the same except it contains one additional amino acid, methionine. The drugs are therapeutically equivalent to endogenous growth hormone produced by the pituitary gland. The only clinical use of the drugs is for children whose growth is impaired by a deficiency of endogenous growth hormone. The drugs are ineffective when impaired growth results from other causes or after puberty, when epiphyses of the long bones have closed. Dosage should be individualized according to response. Excessive administration can cause excessive growth (gigantism).

## Somatrem

### Route and dosage range

*Children:* IM, up to 0.1 mg/kg three times per week

## Somatropin

### Route and dosage range

*Children:* IM, up to 0.06 mg/kg three times per week

**Human chorionic gonadotropin** (HCG [Follutein]) is a placental hormone obtained from the urine of pregnant women. In men, HCG produces physiologic effects similar to those of the naturally occurring LH. HCG is used clinically to evaluate the ability of the Leydig's cells to produce testosterone and to treat cryptorchidism (undescended testicle) in preadolescent boys. Excessive doses or prolonged administration can lead to sexual precocity, edema, and breast enlargement caused by oversecretion of testosterone and possibly estrogen. In women, HCG is used in combination with menotropins to induce ovulation in the treatment of infertility.

### Route and dosage ranges

*Adults and preadolescent boys:* Cryptorchidism and hypogonadism in males, IM 500–4000 units two or three times per week for several weeks
To induce ovulation, IM 5000–10,000 units in one dose, 1 day after treatment with menotropins

**Menotropins** (Pergonal), a gonadotropin preparation obtained from the urine of postmenopausal women, contains both FSH and LH. It is usually combined with HCG to induce ovulation in the treatment of infertility caused by lack of pituitary gonadotropins.

### Route and dosage range

*Adults:* IM 1 ampule (75 units FSH and 75 units LH) daily for 9–12 days, followed by HCG to induce ovulation

**Thyrotropin** (Thytropar) is obtained from the anterior pituitary glands of cattle. It is used as a diagnostic agent to distinguish between primary hypothyroidism (caused by a thyroid disorder) and secondary hypothyroidism (caused by pituitary malfunction). If thyroid hormones in serum are elevated after the administration of thyrotropin, then the hypothyroidism is secondary to inadequate pituitary function. Thyrotropin must be used cautiously in clients with coronary artery disease, congestive heart failure, or adrenocortical insufficiency.

### Routes and dosage ranges

*Adults:* IM, SC 10 units daily for 1–3 days, followed by $^{131}$I in 18–24 h. Thyroid uptake of iodine is measured 24 h after iodine administration. Accumulation is greater in hypopituitarism than in primary hypothyroidism.

## POSTERIOR PITUITARY HORMONES

**Desmopressin acetate** (DDAVP, Stimate) is a synthetic analogue of ADH. A major clinical use is the treatment of neurogenic diabetes insipidus, a disorder characterized by a deficiency of ADH and the excretion of large amounts of dilute urine. Diabetes insipidus may be idiopathic, hereditary, or acquired as a result of trauma, surgery, tumor, infection, or other conditions that impair the function of the hypothalamus or posterior pituitary. Parenteral desmopressin is also used as a hemostatic in clients with hemophilia A or mild-to-moderate von Willebrand's disease (type 1). The drug is effective in controlling spontaneous or trauma-induced bleeding and intraoperative and postoperative bleeding when given 30 minutes before the procedure.

### Routes and dosage ranges

*Adults:* Diabetes insipidus, intranasally 0.1–0.4 ml/d, usually in two divided doses
Hemophilia A, von Willebrand's disease, IV 0.3 μg/kg in 50 ml sterile saline, infused over 15–30 min
*Children 3 months–2 years:* Diabetes insipidus, intranasally 0.05–0.3 ml/d in one or two doses
*Children weighing over 10 kg:* Hemophilia A, von Willebrand's disease, same as adult dosage
*Children weighing 10 kg or less:* Hemophilia A, von Willebrand's disease, IV 0.3 μg/kg in 10 ml of sterile saline

**Lypressin** is a synthetic vasopressin that has several advantages over the natural product. Because it is free of oxytocin impurity and foreign proteins, it is less likely to produce allergic reactions and other side effects than vasopressin, which is derived from animal sources. Lypressin is also advantageous in that it is given intranasally rather than by injection. It is used only for controlling the excessive water loss of diabetes insipidus caused by inadequate function of the posterior pituitary gland.

### Route and dosage range

*Adults:* Intranasal spray, 1 or 2 sprays to one or both nostrils, three or four times per day

**Vasopressin** (Pitressin) is available as an extract derived from animal pituitary glands and as a synthetic preparation. The synthetic preparation is preferred because it contains no oxytocin. Until lypressin was developed, vasopressin was the most widely used drug for diabetes insipidus caused by hypofunction of the posterior pituitary gland. Vasopressin has a short duration of action (a few hours). This short action is sometimes an advantage (for example, when acutely ill patients require precise control of fluid balance after brain surgery or trauma), but it is a disadvantage when long-term treatment of diabetes insipidus is necessary. Vasopressin tannate is a long-acting oil suspension that also must be injected; its effects last 1 to 3 days. Vasopressin has a vasoconstrictor effect and is used in the treatment of bleeding esophageal varices.

Vasopressin

### Routes and dosage ranges

*Adults:* IM, SC, intranasally on cotton pledgets, 0.25–0.5 ml (5–10 units) two or three times per day

*Children:* IM, SC, intranasally on cotton pledgets, 0.125–0.5 ml (2.5–10 units) three or four times per day

**Oxytocin** (Pitocin) is a synthetic drug that exerts the same physiologic effects as the posterior pituitary hormone. Thus, it promotes uterine contractility and is used clinically to induce labor and in the postpartum period to control bleeding. Oxytocin must be used only when clearly indicated and when the recipient can be supervised by well-trained personnel. It is usually given in a hospital.

### Routes and dosage ranges

*Adults:* Induction of labor, IV 1-ml ampule (10 units) in 1000 ml of 5% dextrose injection (10 units/1000 ml = 10 milliunits/ml), infused at 0.2–2 milliunits/min initially, then regulated according to frequency and strength of uterine contractions

Prevention or treatment of postpartum bleeding, IV 10–40 units in 1000 ml of 5% dextrose injection, infused at 125 ml/h (40 milliunits/min) or 0.6–1.8 units (0.06–0.18 ml) diluted in 3–5 ml sodium chloride injection and injected slowly IM 0.3–1 ml (3–10 units)

## Nursing Process

### Assessment

Assess for disorders for which hypothalamic and pituitary hormones are given:
- For children with impaired growth, assess height and weight (actual and in comparison with growth charts) and diagnostic x-ray reports of bone age.
- For clients with diabetes insipidus, assess baseline blood pressure, weight, fluid intake to urine output ratio, urine specific gravity, and laboratory reports of serum electrolytes.

### Nursing diagnoses
- Knowledge Deficit: Drug administration and effects
- Altered Growth and Development
- Anxiety related to multiple injections
- High Risk for Injury: Adverse drug effects

### Planning/Goals

*The client will:*
- Experience relief of symptoms without serious adverse effects
- Take or receive the drug accurately
- Comply with procedures for monitoring and follow-up

### Interventions
- For children receiving growth hormone, assist the family to set reasonable goals for increased height and weight and to comply with accurate drug administration and follow-up procedures (periodic x-rays to determine bone growth and progress toward epiphyseal closure, recording height and weight at least weekly).
- For clients with diabetes insipidus, teach them to weigh themselves daily, monitor their fluid intake and urine output for approximately equal amounts, or to check urine specific gravity daily (should be at least 1.015) and replace fluids accordingly.

### Evaluation
- Interview and observe for compliance with instructions for taking the drug(s).
- Observe for relief of symptoms for which pituitary hormones were prescribed.

## Principles of therapy

1. Hypothalamic hormones are rarely used in most clinical practice settings, and guidelines for their usage are still being developed. Generally, the drugs should be prescribed by physicians who are knowledgeable about endocrinology and administered according to current manufacturers' literature.
2. Most drug therapy with pituitary hormones is given to replace or supplement naturally occurring hormones in situations involving inadequate function

of the pituitary gland (hypopituitarism). Conditions resulting from excessive amounts of pituitary hormones (hyperpituitarism) are more often treated with surgery or irradiation.

3. Diagnosis of suspected pituitary disorders should be as complete and as specific as possible. This promotes more specific and more effective treatment measures, including drug therapy.

4. Even though manufacturers recommend corticotropin for treatment of diseases that respond to glucocorticoids, corticotropin is less predictable and less convenient than glucocorticoids and has no apparent advantages over them.

5. Dosage of any pituitary hormone must be individualized because responsiveness of affected tissues varies.

## NURSING ACTIONS: HYPOTHALAMIC AND PITUITARY HORMONES

| Nursing Actions | Rationale/Explanation |
|---|---|
| **1. Administer accurately**<br>Read the manufacturer's instructions and drug labels carefully before drug preparation and administration. | These hormone preparations are given infrequently and often require special techniques of administration. |
| **2. Observe for therapeutic effects** | Therapeutic effects vary widely, depending on the particular pituitary hormone given and the reason for use. |
| **a.** With gonadorelin, observe for ovulation or decreased symptoms of endometriosis and absence of menstruation. | Therapeutic effects depend on the reason for use. Note that different formulations are used to stimulate ovulation and treat endometriosis. |
| **b.** With corticotropin, therapeutic effects stem largely from increased secretion of adrenal cortex hormones, especially the glucocorticoids, and include anti-inflammatory effects (see Chap. 24). | Corticotropin is usually not recommended for the numerous nonendocrine inflammatory disorders that respond to glucocorticoids. Administration of glucocorticoids is more convenient and effective than administration of corticotropin. |
| **c.** With chorionic gonadotropin and menotropins given in cases of female infertility, ovulation and conception are therapeutic effects. | |
| **d.** With chorionic gonadotropins given in cryptorchidism, the therapeutic effect is descent of the testicles from the abdomen to the scrotum. | |
| **e.** With growth hormone, observe for increased skeletal growth and development. | Indicated by appropriate increases in height and weight |
| **f.** With antidiuretics (desmopressin, lypressin, and vasopressin), observe for decreased urine output, increased urine-specific gravity, decreased signs of dehydration, decreased thirst. | These effects indicate control of diabetes insipidus. |
| **g.** With oxytocin given to induce labor, observe for the beginning or the intensifying of uterine contractions. | |
| **h.** With oxytocin given to control postpartum bleeding, observe for a firm uterine fundus and decreased vaginal bleeding. | |
| **3. Observe for adverse effects**<br>**a.** With gonadorelin, observe for headache, nausea, light-headedness, and local edema, pain and pruritus after subcutaneous injections. | Systemic reactions occur infrequently. |
| **b.** With protirelin, observe for hypotension, nausea, headache, lightheadedness, anxiety, drowsiness. | Although adverse effects occur in about 50% of patients, they are usually minor and of short duration. |

(continued)

| *Nursing Actions* | *Rationale/Explanation* |
|---|---|
| **c.** With corticotropin, observe for sodium and fluid retention, edema, hypokalemia, hyperglycemia, osteoporosis, increased susceptibility to infection, myopathy, behavioral changes. | These adverse reactions are generally the same as those produced by adrenal cortex hormones. Severity of adverse reactions tends to increase with dosage and duration of corticotropin administration. |
| **d.** With human chorionic gonadotropin given to preadolescent boys, observe for sexual precocity, breast enlargement, and edema. | Sexual precocity results from stimulation of excessive testosterone secretion at an early age. |
| **e.** With growth hormone, observe for mild edema, headache, localized muscle pain, weakness, hyperglycemia. | Adverse effects are not common. Another adverse effect may be development of antibodies to the drug, but this does not prevent its growth-stimulating effects. |
| **f.** With menotropins, observe for symptoms of ovarian hyperstimulation, such as abdominal discomfort, weight gain, ascites, pleural effusion, oliguria, and hypotension. | Adverse effects can be minimized by frequent pelvic examinations to check for ovarian enlargement and by laboratory measurement of estrogen levels. Multiple gestation (mostly twins) is a possibility and is related to ovarian overstimulation. |
| **g.** With desmopressin, observe for headache, nasal congestion, nausea, and occasionally a slight increase in blood pressure. A more serious adverse reaction is water retention and hyponatremia. | Adverse reactions usually occur only with high dosages and tend to be relatively mild. Water intoxication (headache, nausea, vomiting, confusion, lethargy, coma, convulsions) may occur with any antidiuretic therapy if excessive fluids are ingested. |
| **h.** With lypressin, observe for headache and congestion of nasal passages, dyspnea and coughing (if the drug is inhaled), and water intoxication if excessive amounts of lypressin or fluid are taken. | Adverse effects are usually mild and occur infrequently with usual doses. |
| **i.** With vasopressin, observe for water intoxication; allergic reactions; chest pain, myocardial infarction, increased blood pressure; abdominal cramps, nausea, and diarrhea. | Adverse reactions to vasopressin are likely to be more widespread and to occur more often than reactions to the synthetic agents, desmopressin and lypressin. With high doses, vasopressin constricts blood vessels, especially coronary arteries, and stimulates smooth muscle of the gastrointestinal tract. Special caution is necessary in clients with heart disease, asthma, or epilepsy. |
| **j.** With oxytocin, observe for excessive stimulation or contractility of the uterus, uterine rupture, and cervical and perineal lacerations. | Severe adverse reactions are most likely to occur when oxytocin is given to induce labor and delivery. |
| **4. Observe for drug interactions**<br>**a.** Drugs that *decrease* effects of protirelin (*i.e.*, TSH response):<br>     Aspirin (2 g or more per day), glucocorticoids (pharmacologic doses), levodopa, thyroid hormones | |
| **b.** Drugs that *increase* effects of vasopressin: | |
| (1) General anesthetics, chlorpropamide (Diabinese) | Potentiate vasopressin |
| (2) Ganglionic blocking agents (*e.g.*, trimethaphan [Arfonad]) | Markedly increase the pressor effects of vasopressin |
| **c.** Drugs that *decrease* effects of vasopressin:<br><br>Lithium | Inhibits the renal tubular reabsorption of water normally stimulated by vasopressin |
| **d.** Drugs that *increase* effects of oxytocin:<br><br>(1) Estrogens | With adequate estrogen levels, oxytocin increases uterine contractility. When estrogen levels are low, the effect of oxytocin is reduced. |

| *Nursing Actions* | *Rationale/Explanation* |
|---|---|
| (2) Vasoconstrictors or vasopressors (*e.g.*, ephedrine, epinephrine, norepinephrine) | Severe, persistent hypertension with rupture of cerebral blood vessels may occur because of additive vasoconstrictor effects. This is a potentially lethal interaction and should be avoided. |
| **5. Teach clients** | |
| **a.** Take the drug as directed. | To increase therapeutic effects and decrease potentially serious adverse reactions |
| **b.** Report adverse effects. | The drug may need to be discontinued or reduced in dosage. |
| **c.** With corticotropin: | |
| (1) Follow a low-sodium, high-potassium diet. | To decrease sodium retention and potassium loss |
| (2) Weigh regularly. | Weight gain may indicate fluid retention. Edema may occur. |
| (3) Avoid exposure to infections, when possible. | Corticotropin increases susceptibility to infections. |
| (4) Follow instructions when the drug is being discontinued. | Corticotropin is gradually reduced in dosage to avoid symptoms such as fatigue, muscle weakness, and hypotension, which may occur with abrupt withdrawal. |
| (5) Test urine for glycosuria. | This is probably not indicated for all clients but may be helpful in those who have family histories of diabetes mellitus or who are obese. Corticotropin may cause hyperglycemia, activate latent diabetes mellitus, or aggravate existing diabetes mellitus. |
| **d.** With antidiuretics: | |
| (1) Reduce fluid intake when starting an antidiuretic drug. | To avoid water intoxication |
| (2) Regulate dosage in accordance with physician's instructions and with occurrence of excessive urination and thirst. | The purpose of the drugs is to control symptoms of diabetes insipidus. The amount of drug necessary to achieve this purpose varies among clients. |

## Review and Application Exercises

1. What hormones are secreted by the hypothalamus and pituitary, and what are their functions?
2. What are the functions and clinical uses of ADH, growth hormone, and oxytocin?
3. What are adverse effects of the hypothalamic and pituitary hormones used in clinical practice?

## Selected References

Bolinger, A. M., Murphy, V. A., & Bubica, G. (1992). General pediatric therapy. In M. A. Koda-Kimble & L. Y. Young (Eds.), *Applied therapeutics: The clinical use of drugs* (5th ed.) (pp. 77-1–77-24). Vancouver, WA: Applied Therapeutics.

(1993). *Drug facts and comparisons*. St. Louis: Facts and Comparisons.

Guyton, A. C. (1991). *Textbook of medical physiology* (8th ed.). Philadelphia: W.B. Saunders.

Porth, C. M. (1990). *Pathophysiology: Concepts of altered health states* (3rd ed.). Philadelphia: J.B. Lippincott.

### CHAPTER 24

# Corticosteroids

Corticosteroids, also called adrenocorticosteroids, are hormones produced by the adrenal cortex. These hormones are extremely important in maintaining homeostasis when secreted in normal amounts. Disease results from inadequate or excessive secretion. Exogenous corticosteroids are used as drugs in a variety of endocrine and nonendocrine disorders. Few other drug groups produce such profound therapeutic benefits or adverse reactions as the corticosteroids. Consequently, their use must be carefully regulated and their effects closely monitored. To understand the effects of corticosteroids used as drugs, one needs to understand physiologic effects and other characteristics of the endogenous hormones.

## Endogenous corticosteroids

The adrenal cortex produces about 30 steroid hormones, which are divided into glucocorticoids, mineralocorticoids, and adrenal sex hormones. Glucocorticoids have important roles in inflammatory and immune responses and in the metabolism of carbohydrates, proteins, and fats. Mineralocorticoids are important in maintaining fluid and electrolyte balance. The adrenal sex hormones are secreted in small amounts and are considered relatively unimportant in the normal functioning of the body.

Chemically, all corticosteroids are derived from cholesterol and all have similar chemical formulas. Despite their similarities, however, very slight differences in structure cause them to have different functions.

## SECRETION OF CORTICOSTEROIDS

Corticosteroid secretion is controlled by the hypothalamus, anterior pituitary, and adrenal cortex (the hypothalamic-pituitary-adrenal, or HPA, axis). Various stimuli (*e.g.*, low plasma levels of corticosteroids, pain, anxiety, trauma, illness, anesthesia) activate the system. These stimuli cause the hypothalamus to secrete corticotropin-releasing hormone (CRH). CRH stimulates the anterior pituitary to secrete corticotropin, and corticotropin stimulates the adrenal cortex to secrete corticosteroids.

The rate of corticosteroid secretion is usually maintained within relatively narrow limits but changes according to need. When plasma corticosteroid levels rise to an adequate level, secretion of corticosteroids slows or stops. The mechanism by which the hypothalamus and anterior pituitary are informed that no more corticosteroids are currently needed is called a *negative feedback mechanism*.

This negative feedback mechanism is normally very important, but it does not work during stressful situations; that is, during stress, it does not prevent further production of corticosteroids when blood levels are already adequate or high. For example, the rate of secretion accelerates rapidly, and the amount of corticosteroids, especially cortisol, may be as much as 10 times the normal amount during periods of stress. Inhibition of the negative feedback mechanism results from increased sympathetic nervous system (SNS) activity that stimulates the hypothalamus to release CRH and leads to continued corticosteroid secretion. Thus, the stress response activates both the SNS and corticosteroid secretion, and the synergistic interaction of cortisol with epinephrine and norepinephrine increases the person's

Anne Collins Abrams: CLINICAL DRUG THERAPY, Fourth Edition.
© 1995 J.B. Lippincott Company.

ability to respond to stress. However, when corticosteroid secretion is excessive and prolonged, body tissues are damaged.

Corticosteroids are secreted directly into the bloodstream and have a plasma half-life of about 1½ hours. They are metabolized primarily in the liver to water-soluble products, which are then rapidly excreted in the urine. Major secretory products can be measured in the urine. For example, measurement of 17-hydroxycorticosteroids in urine gives an estimate of cortisol production, and measurement of 17-ketosteroids gives an estimate of androgen (male sex hormone) secretion.

Metabolism is slowed by severe hepatic disease, and excretion is slowed by renal disease. In these conditions, corticosteroids may accumulate and cause signs and symptoms of hypercortism.

## GLUCOCORTICOIDS

The term *corticosteroids* actually means all secretions of the adrenal cortex, but it is most often used to designate the glucocorticoids. Glucocorticoids include cortisol, corticosterone, and cortisone. *Cortisol* accounts for at least 95% of glucocorticoid activity, and about 15 to 25 mg is secreted daily. Corticosterone has a small amount of activity, and about 1.5 to 4 mg is secreted daily. *Cortisone* has little activity and is secreted in minute quantities. *Glucocorticoids* are secreted cyclically, with the largest amount being produced in the early morning and the smallest amount during the evening hours (in people with a normal day–night schedule). At the cellular level, glucocorticoids account for most of the effects ascribed to the corticosteroids as a group, including the following:

1. Effects on carbohydrate metabolism
   a. *Stimulated formation of glucose (gluconeogenesis) by causing the breakdown of protein into amino acids.* The amino acids are then transported to the liver, where they are acted on by enzymes that convert them to glucose. The glucose is then returned to the circulation for use by body tissues or storage in the liver as glycogen.
   b. *Moderate decrease in cell use of glucose* (anti-insulin effect) by an unknown mechanism.
   c. *Increased production and decreased use of glucose,* which promote higher levels of glucose in the blood (hyperglycemia) and may lead to diabetes mellitus. These actions also increase the amount of glucose stored as glycogen in the liver, skeletal muscles, and other tissues.
2. Effects on protein metabolism
   a. *Increased breakdown of protein into amino acids* (catabolic effect). They further increase the rate at which amino acids are transported to the liver and converted into glucose.
   b. *Decreased rate at which new proteins are formed* from dietary and other amino acids (antianabolic effect).
   c. Both the increased breakdown of cell protein and decreased protein synthesis produce protein depletion in virtually all body cells except those of the liver. Thus, glycogen stores in the body are increased, while protein stores are decreased.
3. Effects on lipid metabolism
   a. *Increased breakdown of adipose tissue into fatty acids* in much the same way as they increase catabolism of protein into amino acids. These fatty acids are transported in the plasma and used as a source of energy by body cells.
   b. *Stimulated oxidation of fatty acids within body cells.*
4. Effects on inflammatory and immune responses
   a. *Suppressed inflammatory response.* Inflammation is the normal bodily response to tissue damage and involves three stages. First, a large amount of plasma-like fluid leaks out of capillaries into the damaged area and becomes clotted. Second, leukocytes migrate into the area. Third, tissue healing occurs, largely by growth of fibrous scar tissue. Normal or physiologic amounts of glucocorticoids probably do not significantly affect inflammation and healing, but large amounts of glucocorticoids inhibit all three stages of the inflammatory process.

   More specifically, corticosteroids stabilize lysosomal membranes (and thereby prevent the release of inflammatory proteolytic enzymes), decrease capillary permeability (and thereby decrease leakage of fluid and proteins into the damaged tissue), inhibit the accumulation of neutrophils and macrophages at sites of inflammation (and thereby impair phagocytosis of pathogenic microorganisms and waste products of cellular metabolism), and inhibit production of inflammatory chemicals, such as interleukin-1, prostaglandins, and leukotrienes by injured cells.
   b. *Suppressed immune response.* The immune system normally protects the body from foreign invaders, and several immune responses overlap inflammatory responses, including phagocytosis. In addition, the immune response stimulates the production of antibodies and activated lymphocytes to destroy the foreign substance. Glucocorticoids decrease the numbers of circulating lymphocytes and eosinophils, decrease the rate of lymphocyte conversion into antibodies, and decrease amounts of lymphoid tissue. These effects influence immune and allergic responses and help to account for the immunosuppressive and antiallergic actions of the glucocorticoids.
5. Effects on the nervous system
   a. Physiologic levels help to *maintain normal nerve excitability*; increased or pharmacologic amounts

decrease nerve excitability, slow activity in the cerebral cortex, and alter brain wave patterns.

   b. *Suppressed secretion of CRH by the hypothalamus and of corticotropin by the anterior pituitary gland.* This results in suppression of further glucocorticoid secretion by the adrenal cortex.

6. Effects on the musculoskeletal system
   a. *Maintenance of muscle strength* when present in physiologic amounts but muscle atrophy (from protein breakdown) when present in excessive amounts.
   b. *Inhibition of bone formation and growth and increased bone breakdown.* Glucocorticoids also decrease intestinal absorption and increase renal excretion of calcium. These effects contribute to bone demineralization (osteoporosis) in adults and to decreased linear growth in children.

7. Effects on the respiratory system
   a. *Maintenance of open airways.* Glucocorticoids do not have direct bronchodilating effects, but they probably play a role in maintaining responsiveness to the bronchodilating effects of endogenous catecholamines, such as epinephrine.
   b. *Stabilize mast cells* and other cells to inhibit the release of bronchoconstrictive and inflammatory substances, such as histamine.

8. Effects on the gastrointestinal system
   a. *Decreased viscosity of gastric mucus.* This effect may decrease protective properties of the mucus and contribute to the development of peptic ulcer disease.

9. Effects on fluid and electrolyte balance
   a. *Retention of sodium and water.*
   b. *Excretion of potassium and calcium.*

## MINERALOCORTICOIDS

Mineralocorticoids play a vital role in maintaining fluid and electrolyte balance. *Aldosterone* is the main mineralocorticoid and is responsible for 95% of mineralocorticoid activity. Characteristics and physiologic effects of mineralocorticoids, especially aldosterone, include the following:

1. The overall physiologic effects are to conserve sodium and water and eliminate potassium. Aldosterone increases sodium reabsorption from kidney tubules, and water is reabsorbed along with the sodium. When sodium is conserved, another cation must be excreted to maintain electrical neutrality of body fluids; potassium, not sodium, is the cation excreted. This is the only potent mechanism for controlling the concentration of potassium ions in extracellular fluids.

2. Secretion of aldosterone is controlled by several fac-

tors, most of which are related to kidney function. Generally, secretion is increased when the potassium level of extracellular fluid is high, the sodium level of extracellular fluid is low, the renin-angiotensin system of the kidneys is activated, or the anterior pituitary gland secretes corticotropin.

3. Inadequate secretion of aldosterone causes hyperkalemia, hyponatremia, and extracellular fluid volume deficit (dehydration). Hypotension and shock may result from decreased cardiac output. Absence of mineralocorticoids causes death.

4. Excessive secretion of aldosterone produces hypokalemia, hypernatremia, and extracellular fluid volume excess (water intoxication). Edema and hypertension may result.

## ADRENAL SEX HORMONES

The adrenal cortex secretes male (androgens) and female (estrogens and progesterone) sex hormones. The adrenal sex hormones are relatively insignificant compared with those produced by the testes and ovaries. Adrenal androgens, secreted continuously in small quantities by both men and women, are responsible for most of the physiologic effects exerted by the adrenal sex hormones. They increase protein synthesis (anabolism), which increases the mass and strength of muscle and bone tissue; they affect development of male secondary sex characteristics; and they increase hair growth and libido in women. Excessive secretion of adrenal androgens in women causes masculinizing effects (*e.g.,* hirsutism, acne, breast atrophy, deepening of the voice, and amenorrhea). Female sex hormones are secreted in small amounts and normally exert few physiologic effects. Excessive secretion may produce feminizing effects in men (*e.g.,* breast enlargement, decreased hair growth, voice changes).

## Disorders of the adrenal cortex

Disorders of the adrenal cortex involve increased or decreased production of corticosteroids, especially cortisol as the primary glucocorticoid and aldosterone as the primary mineralocorticoid. These disorders include:

1. *Primary adrenocortical insufficiency (Addison's disease)* is associated with destruction of the adrenal cortex by disorders such as tuberculosis, cancer, or hemorrhage; with atrophy of the adrenal cortex caused by autoimmune disease or excessive and prolonged administration of exogenous corticosteroids; and with surgical excision of the adrenal glands. In this condition, there is inadequate production of both cortisol and aldosterone.

2. *Secondary adrenocortical insufficiency,* produced by inadequate secretion of corticotropin, is most often caused by prolonged administration of corticosteroids. This condition is largely a glucocorticoid deficiency. Mineralocorticoid secretion is not significantly impaired.

3. *Congenital adrenogenital syndromes and adrenal hyperplasia* result from deficiencies in one or more enzymes required for cortisol production. Low plasma levels of cortisol lead to excessive corticotropin secretion, which then leads to excessive adrenal secretion of androgens and hyperplasia.

4. *Androgen-producing tumors* of the adrenal cortex, which are usually benign, produce masculinizing effects.

5. *Adrenocortical hyperfunction* (Cushing's disease) may result from excessive corticotropin or a primary adrenal tumor. Adrenal tumors may be benign or malignant. Benign tumors often produce one corticosteroid normally secreted by the adrenal cortex, but malignant tumors often secrete several corticosteroids.

6. *Hyperaldosteronism* is a rare disorder caused by adenoma or hyperplasia of the adrenal cortex cells that produce aldosterone. It is characterized by hypokalemia, hypernatremia, hypertension, thirst, and polyuria.

## Exogenous corticosteroids (glucocorticoids)

When corticosteroids are administered from sources outside the body, they are given for replacement, therapeutic, or diagnostic purposes. When given to replace or substitute for the endogenous hormones, they are given in relatively small doses to correct a deficiency state, and their purpose is to restore normal function. When given for therapeutic purposes, they are given in relatively large doses to exert pharmacologic effects. Drug effects involve extension of the physiologic effects of endogenous corticosteroids and new effects that do not occur with small, physiologic doses. The most frequently desired effects are anti-inflammatory, immunosuppressive, antiallergic, and antistress. These are glucocorticoid effects. Mineralocorticoid and androgenic effects are usually considered adverse reactions.

All adrenal corticosteroids are commercially available for use as drugs, as are many synthetic derivatives. The newer corticosteroids have been developed by chemically altering the basic steroid molecule in efforts to increase therapeutic effects while minimizing adverse effects. These efforts have been most successful in decreasing mineralocorticoid activity. Despite considerable progress, however, synthetic corticosteroids can produce all the adverse reactions associated with the natural corticosteroids.

Exogenous corticosteroids are palliative. They control many symptoms but do not cure the underlying disease process. In chronic disorders, for example, they may enable a client to continue the usual activities of daily living and delay disability. However, the disease may continue to progress. Long-term use of corticosteroids inevitably produces adverse effects.

Exogenous corticosteroids have widely different actions on body tissues and fluids, so a specific effect may be considered therapeutic in one client but adverse in another. For example, an increased blood sugar level is therapeutic for the client with adrenocortical insufficiency or an islet cell adenoma of the pancreas, but this is an adverse reaction for most clients, especially for those with diabetes mellitus. In addition, some clients respond more favorably or develop adverse reactions more readily than others taking equivalent doses. This is partially caused by individual differences in the rate at which corticosteroids are metabolized.

Administration of exogenous corticosteroids suppresses the HPA axis. This decreases secretion of corticotropin, which in turn causes atrophy of the adrenal cortex and decreased production of endogenous adrenal corticosteroids. Daily administration of physiologic doses (about 20 mg of hydrocortisone or its equivalent) or administration of pharmacologic doses (more than 20 mg of hydrocortisone or its equivalent) for about 2 weeks suppresses the HPA axis. Recovery may take 6 months or longer after corticosteroids are discontinued. During that time, the client's ability to respond to stress is impaired unless supplemental corticosteroids are given.

Hydrocortisone, the exogenous equivalent of endogenous cortisol, is the prototype of corticosteroid drugs. When a new corticosteroid is developed, it is compared with hydrocortisone to determine its potency in producing anti-inflammatory and antiallergic responses, increasing deposition of liver glycogen, and suppressing secretion of corticotropin.

Exogenous mineralocorticoid drugs are infrequently used for therapeutic purposes. Even with adrenocortical insufficiency in Addison's disease or adrenalectomy, many physicians prefer to use a glucocorticoid with high mineralocorticoid activity rather than separate drugs.

### MECHANISMS OF ACTION AND OTHER CHARACTERISTICS OF GLUCOCORTICOID DRUGS

Glucocorticoids are by far the largest subgroup of corticosteroids, and they account for almost all clinical usage of corticosteroid drugs. Specific characteristics of the glucocorticoids include the following:

1. Like endogenous glucocorticoids, exogenous drug molecules act at the cellular level by binding to glucocorticoid receptors in target tissues. The receptors are small proteins located in intracellular cytoplasm. The drug-receptor complex then moves to the cell nucleus where it influences genetically controlled aspects of cellular synthesis. Because the genes vary in different types of body cells, glucocorticoid effects also vary, depending on the specific cells being targeted.

2. Pharmacologic effects sought from glucocorticoid drugs are largely antiallergic, anti-inflammatory, antistress, and immunosuppressive. The mechanisms by which glucocorticoids produce these effects are not clearly understood but may include:

   a. Strengthening or stabilizing biologic membranes. This inhibits capillary permeability and thus prevents leakage of fluid into the injured area and development of edema. It further inhibits release of bradykinin, histamine, lysosomal enzymes, and perhaps other substances that normally cause vasodilation and tissue irritation.

   b. Impaired ability of phagocytic cells to migrate into the injured area from the blood

   c. Interference with lymphocyte function and antibody production

   d. Shrinkage of lymphoid tissues

   e. Decreased growth of new capillaries, fibroblasts, and collagen

3. Important differences among glucocorticoid drugs are duration of action, relative glucocorticoid potency, and relative mineralocorticoid potency. Anti-inflammatory potency of the various glucocorticoids is approximately equal when the drugs are given in equivalent doses. Mineralocorticoid activity is intermediate to high in the older drugs, cortisone and hydrocortisone, and low in newer agents.

4. Many glucocorticoid preparations are available for use in different clinical problems, and routes of administration vary. Several of these drugs can be given by more than one route; others can be given only orally or topically. For intramuscular (IM) or intravenous (IV) injections, sodium phosphate or sodium succinate salts are used because they are most soluble in water. For intra-articular or intralesional injections, acetate salts are used because they have low solubility in water and provide prolonged local action.

## INDICATIONS FOR USE

Corticosteroids are used to treat many different disorders that have few characteristics in common and produce a vast array of clinical signs and symptoms. Corticosteroid preparations applied topically in ophthalmic and dermatologic disorders are discussed in Chapters 68 and 69,

respectively. The corticosteroids discussed in this chapter are primarily those given systemically, topically to nasal and oral mucosa, or by local injection in potentially serious or disabling disorders. Individual corticosteroids are listed in Table 24-1. These disorders are as follows:

1. *Allergic* disorders, such as allergic reactions to drugs, serum and blood transfusions, and dermatoses with an allergic component

2. *Collagen* disorders, such as systemic lupus erythematosus, scleroderma, and periarteritis nodosa. Collagen is the basic structural protein of connective tissue, tendons, cartilage, and bone, and it is therefore present in almost all body tissues and organ systems. The collagen disorders are characterized by inflammation of various body tissues. Signs and symptoms depend on which body tissues or organs are affected and the severity of the inflammatory process.

3. *Dermatologic* disorders, such as pemphigus, exfoliative dermatitis, and severe psoriasis

4. *Endocrine* disorders, such as adrenocortical insufficiency and congenital adrenal hyperplasia. Corticosteroids are given to replace or substitute for the natural hormones (both glucocorticoids and mineralocorticoids) in cases of insufficiency and to suppress corticotropin when excess secretion causes adrenal hyperplasia. These conditions are rare and account for only a small percentage of corticosteroid usage.

5. *Gastrointestinal* disorders, such as ulcerative colitis and regional enteritis (Crohn's disease)

6. *Hematologic* disorders, such as idiopathic thrombocytopenic purpura or acquired hemolytic anemia

7. *Liver* disorders characterized by edema, such as cirrhosis and ascites

8. *Neoplastic* disease, such as acute and chronic leukemias, Hodgkin's disease, other lymphomas, and multiple myeloma. The effectiveness of corticosteroids in these conditions probably stems from their ability to suppress lymphocytes and other lymphoid tissue.

9. *Neurologic* conditions, such as cerebral edema, brain tumor, and myasthenia gravis

10. *Ophthalmic* disorders, such as optic neuritis, sympathetic ophthalmia, and chorioretinitis

11. *Organ or tissue transplants and grafts* (*e.g.*, kidney, heart, liver, others). Corticosteroids suppress cellular and humoral immune responses (see Chap. 45) and help prevent rejection of transplanted tissue. Drug therapy is continued as long as the transplanted tissue is in place (usually lifelong).

12. *Renal* disorders characterized by edema, such as the nephrotic syndrome

13. *Respiratory* disorders, such as asthma, status asthmaticus, chronic obstructive pulmonary disease

## TABLE 24-1. CORTICOSTEROIDS*

| Generic/Trade Name | Routes and Dosage Ranges | Anti-inflammatory Dose Equivalent to 20 mg of Hydrocortisone (mg) | Mineralocorticoid Activity | Duration of Action (h) |
|---|---|---|---|---|
| *Glucocorticoids* | | | | |
| **Beclomethasone** Oral inhalation (Beclovent, Vanceril) | Adults: 2 oral inhalations (84 μg) 3–4 times daily (maximal daily dose is 20 inhalations or 840 μg) Children 6–12 years: 1–3 oral inhalations (42–84 μg) 3–4 times daily (maximal daily dose is 10 inhalations or 420 μg) | | | |
| Nasal inhalation (Beconase, Vancenase) | Adults and children 12 years or older: 1 nasal inhalation (42 μg) in each nostril 2–4 times daily (total dose 168–336 μg/d) Children 6–12 years: 1 nasal inhalation in each nostril 3 times daily (252 μg/d) Children <6 years: Not recommended | | | |
| **Betamethasone** (Celestone) | Adults: PO 6–7.2 mg daily initially, depending on the disease being treated, gradually reduced to lowest effective maintenance dose | 0.6 | Low | 48 |
| **Betamethasone acetate and sodium phosphate** (Celestone Soluspan) | Adults: IM 1–2 ml (3–6 mg each of betamethasone acetate and betamethasone sodium phosphate) Intra-articular injection 0.25–2 ml Soft-tissue injection 0.25–1.0 ml | | | |
| **Cortisone** (Cortone) | Chronic adrenocortical insufficiency, PO 15–30 mg daily Congenital adrenal hyperplasia, PO 15–50 mg daily Anti-inflammatory effects, PO 25–50 mg daily for mild, chronic disorders; 125–300 mg daily in 4 or more doses for acute, life-threatening disease Anti-inflammatory effects, IM 75–300 mg daily for serious disease | 25 | High | 12 |
| **Dexamethasone** (Decadron) | PO 0.75–9 mg daily in 2–4 doses. Dosages in higher ranges are used for serious disease (leukemia, pemphigus) | 0.75 | Low | 48 |
| **Dexamethasone acetate** | IM 8–16 mg (1–2 ml) in single dose, repeated every 1–3 weeks if necessary Intralesional 0.8–1.6 mg (0.1–0.2 ml) Intra-articular or soft-tissue injection, 4–16 mg (0.5–2 ml), repeated every 1–3 weeks if necessary | | | |
| **Dexamethasone sodium phosphate** | IM, IV 0.5–9 mg, depending on severity of the disease Intra-articular, soft-tissue injection 0.2–6 mg, depending on size of affected area or joint | | | |
| (Decadron Turbinaire) (Decadron Respihaler) | Intranasal, 2 sprays in each nostril 2–3 times daily 2–3 inhalations 3–4 times daily | | | |
| **Dexamethasone/lidocaine** (Decadron with Xylocaine) | Soft-tissue injection, 0.5–0.75 ml | | | |
| **Flunisolide** Oral inhalation (Aerobid) | Adults: 2 oral inhalations (500 μg) twice daily Children 6–15 years: Same as adults | | | |
| Nasal inhalation (Nasalide) | Adults: 2 sprays (50 μg) in each nostril 2 times daily (total dose 200 μg/d); maximal daily dose is 8 sprays in each nostril (400 μg/d) Children 6–14 years: 1 spray (25 μg) in each nostril 3 times daily or 2 sprays (50 μg) in each nostril 2 times daily (total dose 150–200 μg/d); maximal daily dose 4 sprays in each nostril (200 μg/d) | | | |
| **Hydrocortisone** (Hydrocortone, Cortef) | Chronic adrenocortical insufficiency, PO 10–20 mg daily in 3–4 doses Chronic nonfatal diseases, PO 20–40 mg daily in 3–4 doses Congenital adrenal hyperplasia, PO 10–30 mg daily in 3–4 doses Chronic, potentially fatal diseases, PO 60–120 mg daily in 3–4 doses Acute, nonfatal diseases, PO 60–120 mg daily in 3–4 doses | 20 | Intermediate | 18 |

(continued)

**TABLE 24-1.  CORTICOSTEROIDS\*** *(Continued)*

| Generic/Trade Name | Routes and Dosage Ranges | Anti-inflam-matory Dose Equivalent to 20 mg of Hydrocortisone (mg) | Mineralo-corticoid Activity | Duration of Action (h) |
|---|---|---|---|---|
| | Acute life-threatening diseases, PO 100–240 mg daily in at least 4 divided doses | | | |
| | Disorders other than shock, IV 100–500 mg initially, repeated if necessary | | | |
| | Intra-articular injections, 5–50 mg depending on size of joint | | | |
| | Soft-tissue injection, 25–75 mg | | | |
| | Rectally, one enema (100 mg) nightly for 21 days or until an optimal response is obtained | | | |
| **Methylprednisolone** (Medrol) | PO 4–48 mg daily initially, gradually reduced to lowest effective level | 4 | Low | 18–36 |
| **Methylprednisolone sodium succinate** (Solu-Medrol) | IM 40–120 mg as needed | | | |
| | IV 100–250 mg q4–6h for shock; 10–40 mg as needed for other conditions | | | |
| | Intra-articular and soft-tissue injection, 4–80 mg as needed, depending on size of the affected area | | | |
| | Intralesional injection, 20–60 mg | | | |
| | Rectally, 40 mg as retention enema 3–7 times weekly for 2 or more weeks | | | |
| **Prednisolone** (Sterane, Delta-Cortef) | PO 5–60 mg daily initially, adjusted for maintenance | 5 | Intermediate | 18–36 |
| **Prednisolone acetate** (Fernisolone, others) | IM 4–60 mg daily initially, adjusted for maintenance | | | |
| | Intra-articular or soft-tissue injection, 4–60 mg daily, depending on the disease | | | |
| **Prednisolone sodium phosphate** (Hydeltrasol) | IM 4–60 mg daily initially, adjusted for maintenance | | | |
| | Emergencies, IV 20–100 mg, repeated if necessary, to a maximal daily dose of 400 mg. When the client's condition improves, 10–20 mg in single doses may be given. | | | |
| | Intra-articular or soft-tissue injection, 2–30 mg from once every 3–5 days to once every 2–3 weeks | | | |
| **Prednisolone sodium succinate** (Meticortelone soluble) | IM 4–60 mg daily initially, adjusted for maintenance | | | |
| | Emergencies, IV 20–100 mg, repeated if necessary to a maximal daily dose of 480 mg. When the client's condition improves, 10–20 mg in single doses may be given. | | | |
| **Prednisolone tebutate** (Hydeltra-TBA) | Intra-articular or soft-tissue injection, 4–60 mg daily, depending on the disease | | | |
| **Prednisone** (Deltasone) | PO 5–60 mg daily initially, reduced for maintenance | 5 | Intermediate | 18–30 |
| **Triamcinolone** (Aristocort, Kenacort) | PO 4–48 mg daily initially; dosage reduced for maintenance | 4 | Low | 18–36 |
| **Triamcinolone acetonide** (Kenalog-40) | IM (deep) 2.5–60 mg daily, depending on the disease. When the client's condition improves, dosage should be reduced and oral therapy instituted when feasible. | | | |
| | Intra-articular or intrabursal injection, 2.5–15 mg every 1–8 weeks depending on the size of the joint and the disease being treated | | | |
| | Soft-tissue injection, 5–48 mg | | | |
| Oral inhalation (Azmacort) | Adults: 2 oral inhalations (200 µg) 3 times daily | | | |
| | Children: 1–2 oral inhalations (100–200 µg) 3 times daily | | | |
| Nasal inhalation (Nasacort) | Adults and children >12 years: 2 sprays (110 µg) in each nostril once daily (total dose 220 µg/d). May increase to maximal daily dose of 440 µg. | | | |
| **Triamcinolone diacetate** (Aristocort diacetate, Kenacort diacetate) | PO 4–48 mg daily initially; dosage reduced for maintenance | | | |
| | IM (deep) 20–80 mg initially | | | |
| | Intra-articular injection, 2.5–80 mg every 1–8 weeks, depending on size of joint or affected area | | | |
| | Soft-tissue injection, 5–48 mg | | | |
| **Triamcinolone hexacetonide** (Aristospan) | Intra-articular injection, 2.5–80 mg every 1–8 weeks, depending on size of joint or affected area | | | |
| *Mineralocorticoid* | | | | |
| **Fludrocortisone** (Florinef) | Chronic adrenocortical insufficiency, PO 0.05–0.1 mg daily | | | |
| | Salt-losing adrenogenital syndromes, PO 0.1–0.2 mg daily | | | |

\* Ophthalmic and dermatologic preparations are discussed in Chapters 68 and 69, respectively

(COPD), and inflammatory disorders of nasal mucosa (rhinitis). In asthma, corticosteroids increase the number of beta-adrenergic receptors and increase or restore responsiveness of beta receptors to beta-adrenergic bronchodilating drugs. In asthma, COPD, and rhinitis, the drugs decrease mucus secretion and inflammation.

14. *Rheumatic* disorders, such as ankylosing spondylitis, acute and chronic bursitis, acute gouty arthritis, rheumatoid arthritis, and some types of osteoarthritis.

15. *Shock*. Corticosteroids are clearly indicated only for shock resulting from adrenocortical insufficiency (addisonian crisis); their use in other types of shock is controversial. Maximal levels of corticosteroids are already being produced in hemorrhagic or cardiogenic shock and in other forms of severe stress, and giving exogenous corticosteroids probably has little therapeutic effect. On the other hand, in anaphylactic shock resulting from an allergic reaction, corticosteroids may increase or restore cardiovascular responsiveness to adrenergic drugs.

## CONTRAINDICATIONS FOR USE

Corticosteroids are contraindicated in systemic fungal infections and in people who are hypersensitive to drug formulations. They should be used with caution in clients at risk of infections (they may decrease resistance), clients with infections (they may mask signs and symptoms so that infections become more severe before they are recognized and treated), diabetes mellitus (they cause or increase hyperglycemia), peptic ulcer disease, inflammatory bowel disorders, hypertension, congestive heart failure, and renal insufficiency.

## *Nursing Process*

### Assessment related to
### initiation of corticosteroid therapy

- Each client should be thoroughly assessed before long-term, systemic corticosteroid therapy is initiated. Assessment may include diagnostic tests for diabetes mellitus, tuberculosis, and peptic ulcer disease because these conditions may develop from or be exacerbated by administration of corticosteroid drugs. If one of these conditions is present, corticosteroid therapy must be altered and other drugs given concomitantly.
- If acute infection is found on initial assessment, it should be treated with appropriate antibiotics either before corticosteroid drugs are started or concomitantly with corticosteroid therapy. This is necessary because corticosteroids may mask symptoms of infection and impair healing. Thus, even relatively minor infections can become serious if left untreated during corticosteroid therapy. If infection occurs during long-term corticosteroid therapy, appropriate antibiotic therapy (as determined by culture of the causative microorganism and antibiotic sensitivity studies) is again

indicated. Also, increased doses of corticosteroids are usually indicated to cope with the added stress of the infection.

### Assessment related to
### previous or current corticosteroid therapy

Initial assessment of every client should include information about previous or current treatment with systemic corticosteroids. This can usually be determined by questioning the client or reviewing medical records.

- If the nurse determines that the client has taken corticosteroids in the past, additional information is needed about the specific drug and dosage taken, the purpose and length of therapy, and when therapy was stopped. Such information is necessary for planning nursing care. If the client had an acute illness and received an oral or injected corticosteroid for 1 to 2 weeks or received corticosteroids by local injection or application to skin lesions, no special nursing care is likely to be required. If, however, the client took systemic corticosteroids for more than 1 to 2 weeks during the past year (approximately), nursing observations must be especially vigilant. Such a client may be at higher risk for developing acute adrenocortical insufficiency during stressful situations. If the client is having surgery, corticosteroid therapy is restarted either before or on the day of surgery and continued, in decreasing dosage, for a few days after surgery. In addition to anesthesia and surgery, potentially significant sources of stress include hospitalization, various diagnostic tests, concurrent infection or other illnesses, and family problems.
- If the client is currently taking a systemic corticosteroid drug, again the nurse must identify the drug, the dosage and schedule of administration, the purpose for which the drug is being taken, and the length of time involved. Once this basic information is obtained, the nurse can further assess client status and plan nursing care. Some specific factors include the following:
  - If the client will undergo anesthesia and surgery, expect that higher doses of corticosteroids will be given for several days. This may be done by changing the drug, the route of administration, and the dosage. Specific regimens vary according to type of anesthesia, surgical procedure, client condition, physician preference, and other variables. A client having major abdominal surgery may be given 300 to 400 mg of hydrocortisone (or the equivalent dosage of other agents) on the day of surgery and then be tapered back to maintenance dosage within a few days.
  - Note that additional corticosteroids may be given in other situations as well. One extra dose may be adequate for a short-term stress situation, such as an angiogram or other invasive diagnostic test.
  - Using all available data, assess the likelihood of the client's having acute adrenal insufficiency (sometimes called adrenal crisis).
  - Assess for signs and symptoms of adrenocortical excess (hypercorticism, Cushing's disease).
  - Assess for signs and symptoms of the disease for which long-term corticosteroid therapy is being given.

### Nursing diagnoses

- Body Image Disturbance related to cushingoid changes in appearance

- Altered Nutrition: Less than Body Requirements related to protein and potassium losses
- Altered Nutrition: More than Body Requirements related to sodium and water retention and hyperglycemia
- Altered Tissue Perfusion related to atherosclerosis and hypertension
- Excess Fluid Volume related to sodium and water retention
- High Risk for Injury related to adverse drug effects of impaired wound healing; increased susceptibility to infection; weakening of skin and muscles; osteoporosis, gastrointestinal ulceration, diabetes mellitus, hypertension, and acute adrenocortical insufficiency
- Ineffective Individual Coping related to chronic illness and long-term drug therapy
- Ineffective Individual Coping related to drug-induced mood changes, irritability, insomnia
- Knowledge Deficit related to disease process and corticosteroid drug therapy

### Planning/Goals

*The client will:*

- Receive or take the drug correctly
- Receive and practice measures to decrease the need for corticosteroids and minimize adverse effects
- Be monitored regularly for adverse drug effects
- Keep appointments for follow-up care
- Be assisted to cope with body image changes
- Verbalize or demonstrate essential drug information

### Interventions

Use supplementary drugs as ordered and nondrug measures to decrease dosage and side effects of corticosteroid drugs. Some specific measures include the following:

- Help clients to set reasonable goals of drug therapy. For example, partial relief of symptoms may be better than complete relief if the latter requires larger doses or longer periods of treatment with systemic drugs.
- In clients with bronchial asthma and COPD, bronchodilating drugs and other treatment measures should be continued during corticosteroid therapy.
- In clients with rheumatoid arthritis, rest, physical therapy, salicylates or other nonsteroid anti-inflammatory drugs, and local injections of corticosteroid drugs into joints when only one or two are involved are continued during systemic corticosteroid therapy.
- Help clients to identify stressors and to find ways to modify or avoid stressful situations when possible. For example, most clients probably do not think of extreme heat or cold or minor infections as significant stressors. They can be, however, for people taking corticosteroid drugs. This assessment of potential stressors must be individualized because a situation viewed as stressful by one client may not be stressful to another.
- Encourage activity, if not contraindicated, to slow demineralization of bone (osteoporosis). This is especially important in postmenopausal women, who are very susceptible to osteoporosis. Walking is preferred if the client is able. Range-of-motion exercises are indicated in immobilized or bedfast people. Also, bedfast clients taking corticosteroid drugs should have their positions changed frequently because these drugs thin the skin and increase the risk of pressure sores. This risk is further increased if edema also is present.
- Dietary changes may be beneficial in some clients. Salt restriction may help prevent hyponatremia, fluid retention, and edema. Foods high in potassium may help prevent hypokalemia. A diet high in protein, calcium, and vitamin D may help to prevent osteoporosis. Increased intake of vitamin C may help to decrease bleeding in the skin and soft tissues.
- Avoid exposing the client to potential sources of infection by washing hands frequently, using aseptic technique when changing dressings, keeping health-care personnel and visitors with colds or other infections away from the client, and following other appropriate measures. Reverse or protective isolation of the client is sometimes indicated, commonly for those who have had organ transplants and are receiving corticosteroids to help prevent rejection of the transplanted organ.

*Teach clients on long-term systemic corticosteroid therapy to:*

- Wear a special alert bracelet or tag or carry an identification card stating the drug being taken; the dosage; the physician's name, address, and telephone number; and instructions for emergency treatment. If an accident or emergency situation occurs, health-care providers must know about corticosteroid drug therapy to give additional amounts during the stress of the emergency.
- Report to all health-care providers consulted that corticosteroid drugs are being taken or have been taken within the past year. Current or previous corticosteroid therapy can influence treatment measures. Such knowledge increases the ability to provide appropriate treatment.
- Maintain regular medical supervision. This is extremely important so that the physician can detect adverse reactions, evaluate disease status, and evaluate drug response and indications for dosage change, as well as other responsibilities that can be carried out only with personal contact between the physician and the client. Periodic blood tests, x-ray studies, and other tests may be performed during long-term corticosteroid therapy.
- Take no other drugs, prescription or nonprescription, without notifying the physician who is supervising corticosteroid therapy. Corticosteroid drugs influence reactions to many other drugs, and many other drugs interact with corticosteroids to either increase or decrease their effects. Thus, taking other drugs can either cancel or decrease the expected therapeutic benefits or increase the incidence or severity of adverse reactions.
- Ask the physician about the amount and kind of activity or exercise needed. As a general rule, being as active as possible helps to prevent or delay osteoporosis, a common adverse reaction. However, increased activity may not be desirable for everyone. A client with rheumatoid arthritis, for example, may become too active when drug therapy relieves joint pain and increases mobility.
- Follow instructions for other measures used in treatment of the particular condition. For example, other drugs and physical therapy may be prescribed for rheumatoid arthritis. Such measures may allow smaller doses of corticosteroids, which are greatly to the client's advantage in decreasing adverse reactions.

- Recognize stress situations that necessitate increases in drug dosage. Clarify with the physician predictable sources of stress and the amount of drug to be taken if the stress cannot be avoided. This requires commitment and cooperation between the client and health-care personnel. Close supervision is necessary, especially during the first few months of corticosteroid therapy. Common stresses include infections such as the common cold, extremes of heat or cold, surgical procedures, illness, or death of a family member. However, many stress situations are acute and unpredictable and elicit different responses from different clients.
- If diabetes mellitus results from corticosteroid therapy, teach the client as you would any other diabetic: that is, teach about drug therapy, diet, and blood glucose testing, and provide other necessary information.

### Evaluation

- Interview and observe for relief of symptoms for which corticosteroids were prescribed.
- Interview and observe for accurate drug administration.
- Interview and observe for use of nondrug measures indicated for the condition being treated.
- Interview and observe for adverse drug effects on a regular basis.
- Interview regarding drug knowledge and effects to be reported to health-care providers.

## Principles of therapy

### RISK–BENEFIT FACTORS

1. Because corticosteroid drugs can cause serious adverse reactions, indications for their clinical use should be as clear-cut as possible. They are relatively safe for short-term treatment of self-limiting conditions, such as allergic reactions or acute exacerbations of chronic conditions. Long-term use of pharmacologic doses (more than 20 mg of hydrocortisone daily or its equivalent) is almost always accompanied by adverse reactions. For this reason, long-term corticosteroid therapy should be reserved for life-threatening conditions or severe, disabling symptoms that do not respond to treatment with more benign drugs or other measures. Both physician and client should be convinced that the anticipated benefits of long-term therapy are worth the risks.
2. The goal of corticosteroid therapy is usually to reduce symptoms to a tolerable level. Total suppression of symptoms is likely to require excessively large doses and produce excessive adverse effects.

### DRUG SELECTION

Choice of corticosteroid drug is influenced by many factors, including the purpose for use, characteristics of specific drugs, desired route of administration, charac-

teristics of individual clients, and expected side effects. Some guidelines for rational drug choice include the following:

1. *Adrenocortical insufficiency*, whether caused by Addison's disease, adrenalectomy, or inadequate corticotropin, requires replacement of both glucocorticoids and mineralocorticoids. Hydrocortisone and cortisone are usually the drugs of choice because they have greater mineralocorticoid activity compared with other corticosteroids. If additional mineralocorticoid activity is required, fludrocortisone is most convenient because it can be given orally.
2. *Nonendocrine disorders*, in which anti-inflammatory, antiallergic, antistress, and immunosuppressive effects are desired, can be treated by a corticosteroid drug with primarily glucocorticoid activity. Prednisone is often the glucocorticoid of choice. It has less mineralocorticoid activity than hydrocortisone and is less expensive than newer synthetic glucocorticoids.
3. *Respiratory disorders.* Beclomethasone (Vanceril), dexamethasone (Decadron), flunisolide (Aerobid), and triamcinolone (Azmacort) are corticosteroids formulated to be given by oral or nasal inhalation. Their use replaces, prevents, delays, or decreases use of systemic drugs and thereby decreases risks of serious adverse effects. Higher doses may suppress adrenocortical function.
4. *Cerebral edema* associated with brain tumors, craniotomy, or head injury. Dexamethasone (parenterally or orally) is considered the corticosteroid of choice because it is thought to penetrate the blood-brain barrier more readily and achieve higher concentrations in cerebrospinal fluids and tissues. With brain tumors, the drug is more effective in metastatic lesions and glioblastomas than astrocytomas and meningiomas.
5. *Acute, life-threatening situations* require a drug that can be given parenterally, usually IV. This limits the choice of drugs because not all are available in injectable preparations. Hydrocortisone, dexamethasone, and methylprednisolone are among those that may be given parenterally.

### DOSAGE FACTORS

Dosage of corticosteroid drugs is influenced by many factors, such as the specific drug to be given, the desired route of administration, the reason for use, expected adverse effects, and client characteristics. Generally, the smallest effective dose should be given for the shortest effective time. Dosage guidelines include the following:

1. Dosage must be individualized according to the severity of the disorder being treated, whether the disease is acute or chronic, and the client's response to

drug therapy. If life-threatening disease is present, high doses are usually given until acute symptoms are brought under control. Then, dosage is gradually reduced until a maintenance dose is determined or the drug is discontinued. If the disease is not life-threatening, the physician may still choose to prescribe relatively high doses initially and reduce to maintenance doses or may choose to start with low doses and increase to a maintenance level.

2. Physiologic doses (about 20 mg of hydrocortisone or its equivalent daily) are given to replace or substitute for endogenous adrenocortical hormone. Pharmacologic doses (multiples of physiologic doses) are usually required for anti-inflammatory, antiallergic, anti-stress, and immunosuppressive effects.

3. New drugs are compared to hydrocortisone. They are more potent than hydrocortisone on a weight basis but are equipotent in anti-inflammatory effects when given in equivalent doses (see Table 24-1). Statements of equivalency with hydrocortisone are helpful in evaluating new drugs, comparing different drugs, and changing drugs or dosages. However, dosage equivalents generally apply only to drugs given orally or IV. When the drugs are given by other routes, equivalency relationships are likely to be changed.

4. Dosage for children is calculated according to severity of disease rather than weight.

5. Dosage must be reduced if hypoalbuminemia is present. Normally, corticosteroids are highly bound to serum proteins, especially albumin. With hypoalbuminemia, more drug is unbound and pharmacologically active. This increases the incidence and severity of adverse effects if dosage is not reduced.

6. For people receiving chronic corticosteroid therapy, dosage must be increased during periods of stress. Although an event that is stressful for one client may not be stressful for another, some common sources of stress for most people include surgery and anesthesia, infections, anxiety, and extremes of temperature. Some guidelines for corticosteroid dosage during stress include the following:

   a. During *minor or relatively mild illness* (viral upper respiratory infection, any febrile illness, strenuous exercise, gastroenteritis with vomiting and diarrhea, minor surgery), doubling the daily maintenance dose is usually adequate. Once the stress period is over, dosage may be reduced abruptly to the usual maintenance dose.

   b. During *major stress or severe illness*, even larger doses are necessary. For example, a client undergoing abdominal surgery may require 300 to 400 mg of hydrocortisone on the day of surgery. This dose can gradually be reduced to usual maintenance doses within about 5 days if postoperative recovery is uncomplicated. As a general rule, it is better to administer excessive doses temporarily than to risk inadequate doses and adrenal insufficiency. The client also may require sodium chloride and fluid replacement, antibiotic therapy if infection is present, and supportive measures if shock occurs.

   An acute stress situation of short duration, such as traumatic injury or invasive diagnostic tests (angiograms, pneumoencephalograms), can usually be treated with a single dose of about 100 mg of hydrocortisone immediately after the injury or before the diagnostic test.

   c. Many chronic diseases that require long-term corticosteroid therapy are characterized by exacerbations and remissions. Dosage of corticosteroids usually must be increased during acute flare-ups of disease symptoms but can then be decreased gradually to maintenance levels.

## SELECTION OF ROUTE OF ADMINISTRATION

Corticosteroid drugs can be given by several different routes to achieve local or systemic effects. When feasible, they should be given locally rather than systemically to prevent or decrease systemic toxicity. When corticosteroids must be given systemically, the oral route is preferred. Parenteral administration is indicated only for clients who are seriously ill or unable to take oral medications.

## SCHEDULING GUIDELINES

Scheduling of drug administration is more important with corticosteroids than with most other drug classes. Most adverse effects occur with long-term administration of high doses. A major adverse reaction is suppression of the HPA axis and subsequent loss of adrenocortical function. Although opinions differ, the following schedules are often recommended to prevent or minimize HPA suppression:

1. *Short-term use (10 days or less) in acute situations*: Corticosteroids can be given in relatively large, divided doses for about 48 to 72 hours until the acute situation is brought under control. At times, also, continuous IV infusions may be given. After acute symptoms subside or 48 to 72 hours have passed, the dosage is tapered so that a slightly smaller dose is given each day until the drug can be discontinued completely. Such a regimen may be useful in allergic reactions, contact dermatitis, exacerbations of chronic conditions (*e.g.*, rheumatoid arthritis, bronchial asthma), and stressful situations such as surgery.

2. *Replacement therapy in cases of chronic adrenocortical insufficiency*: Daily administration is preferred. The entire daily dose can be taken each morning, between 6 and 9 AM. This schedule simulates normal endogenous corticosteroid secretion.

3. *Other chronic conditions*: Alternate-day therapy (ADT) is usually preferred. ADT involves giving a double dose every other morning. This schedule allows rest periods so that adverse effects are decreased while anti-inflammatory effects continue.

   a. ADT seems to be as effective as more frequent administration in most clients with bronchial asthma, ulcerative colitis, and other conditions for which long-term corticosteroid therapy is prescribed.

   b. ADT is used only for maintenance therapy; that is, clinical signs and symptoms are controlled initially with more frequent drug administration. ADT can be started once symptoms have subsided and stabilized.

   c. ADT does not retard growth in children as do other schedules.

   d. ADT probably decreases susceptibility to infection.

   e. Intermediate-acting glucocorticoids, such as prednisone, prednisolone, and methylprednisolone, are the drugs of choice for ADT.

   f. ADT is not usually indicated in clients who have received long-term corticosteroid therapy. First, these clients already have maximal HPA suppression, so a major advantage of ADT is lost. Second, if they are transferred to ADT, recurrence of symptoms and considerable discomfort may occur on days when drugs are omitted. Clients with severe disease and very painful or disabling symptoms also may experience severe discomfort with ADT.

## USE IN CHILDREN

Corticosteroids are used for the same conditions in children as in adults. With long-term use, corticosteroids may impair growth and development by their effects on protein and bone metabolism. If stunting of growth occurs, most children have a "catch-up" spurt of growth when the drug is discontinued, so permanent stunting is unusual.

Parents and health-care providers can monitor drug effects by taking weekly recordings of height and weight. Alternate-day therapy is less likely to impair normal growth and development than daily administration.

## USE IN OLDER ADULTS

Corticosteroids are used for the same conditions in older adults as in younger ones. Older adults are especially likely to have conditions that are aggravated by the drugs (*e.g.*, congestive heart failure, hypertension, diabetes mellitus, arthritis, and concomitant drug therapy that increases risks of gastrointestinal ulceration and bleeding). Consequently, risk–benefit ratios of corticosteroid therapy should be carefully considered, especially for long-term therapy.

When used, lower doses are usually indicated because of decreased muscle mass, plasma volume, hepatic metabolism, and renal excretion in older adults. In addition, therapeutic and adverse responses should be monitored regularly by a health-care provider (*e.g.*, blood pressure, serum electrolytes, blood glucose levels).

## NURSING ACTIONS: CORTICOSTEROID DRUGS

| *Nursing Actions* | *Rationale/Explanation* |
| --- | --- |
| **1. Administer accurately**<br>**a.** Read the drug label carefully to be certain of having the correct preparation for the intended route of administration. | Many corticosteroid drugs are available in several different preparations. For example, hydrocortisone is available in formulations for intravenous (IV) or intramuscular (IM) administration, for intra-articular injection, and for topical application in creams and ointments of several different strengths. These preparations cannot be used interchangeably without causing potentially serious adverse reactions and decreasing therapeutic effects. Some drugs are available for only one use. For example, several preparations are for topical use only; beclomethasone is prepared only for oral and nasal inhalation. |

(continued)

## Nursing Actions                                    ## Rationale/Explanation

**b.** With oral corticosteroid drugs, give with or after meals.

Opinion seems divided regarding the effectiveness of this scheduling in relation to meals. The rationale is to decrease gastric irritation and prevent development or aggravation of peptic ulcer disease. Corticosteroid drugs have long been considered ulcerogenic, but there is no valid evidence to substantiate this claim. Many physicians prescribe antacids to be given at the same time as the corticosteroid drug.

**c.** For IV or IM administration:

(1) Follow the manufacturer's directions on the drug vial for the type and amount of diluent to add.

Instructions vary with specific preparations.

(2) Give direct IV injection over at least 1 minute.

To increase safety of administration

(3) Follow the manufacturer's directions for diluting and administering by continuous IV infusions.

Instructions vary with specific preparations.

**d.** For oral inhalation of a corticosteroid, check the instruction leaflet that accompanies the inhaler. If the client also is receiving a bronchodilator, administer it first, then wait a few minutes before giving the corticosteroid inhalation.

Giving a bronchodilating drug by inhalation before giving the corticosteroid increases penetration of the corticosteroid into the tracheobronchial tree and increases its therapeutic effectiveness. Waiting a few minutes between the drugs decreases the likelihood of toxicity from the inhaled fluorocarbon propellants of the aerosol drugs.

**2. Observe for therapeutic effects**

The primary objective of corticosteroid therapy is to relieve signs and symptoms, because the drugs are not curative. Therefore, therapeutic effects depend largely on the reason for use.

**a.** With adrenocortical insufficiency, observe for absence or decrease of weakness, weight loss, anorexia, nausea, vomiting, hyperpigmentation, hypotension, hypoglycemia, hyponatremia, and hyperkalemia.

These signs and symptoms of impaired metabolism do not occur with adequate replacement of corticosteroids.

**b.** With rheumatoid arthritis, observe for decreased pain and edema in joints, greater capacity for movement, and increased ability to perform usual activities of daily living.

**c.** With asthma and chronic obstructive pulmonary disease, observe for decrease in respiratory distress and increased tolerance of activity.

**d.** With skin lesions, observe for decreasing inflammation.

**e.** When the drug is given to suppress the immune response to organ transplants, therapeutic effect is the absence of signs and symptoms indicating rejection of the transplanted tissue.

**3. Observe for adverse effects**

These are uncommon with replacement therapy but common with long-term administration of the pharmacologic doses used for many disease processes. Adverse reactions may affect every body tissue and organ.

**a.** Adrenocortical insufficiency—fainting, weakness, anorexia, nausea, vomiting, hypotension, shock, and if untreated, death

This reaction is likely to occur in clients receiving daily corticosteroid drugs who encounter stressful situations. It is caused by drug-induced suppression of the HPA axis, which makes the client unable to respond to stress by increasing adrenocortical hormone secretion.

**b.** Adrenocortical excess (hypercorticism or Cushing's disease)

Most adverse effects result from excessive corticosteroids.

## Nursing Actions

## Rationale/Explanation

(1) "Moon face," "buffalo hump" contour of shoulders, obese trunk, thin extremities

This appearance is caused by abnormal fat deposits in cheeks, shoulders, breasts, abdomen, and buttocks. These changes are more cosmetic than physiologically significant. However, the alterations in self-image can lead to psychological problems. These changes cannot be prevented, but they may be partially reversed if corticosteroid therapy is discontinued or reduced in dosage.

(2) Diabetes mellitus—glycosuria, hyperglycemia, polyuria, polydipsia, polyphagia, impaired healing, and other signs and symptoms

Corticosteroid drugs can cause hyperglycemia and diabetes mellitus or aggravate preexisting diabetes mellitus by their effects on carbohydrate metabolism.

(3) Central nervous system effects—euphoria, psychological dependence, nervousness, insomnia, depression, personality and behavioral changes, aggravation of preexisting psychiatric disorders

Some clients enjoy the drug-induced euphoria so much that they resist attempts to withdraw the drug or decrease its dosage.

(4) Musculoskeletal effects—osteoporosis, pathologic fractures, muscle weakness and atrophy, decreased linear growth in children

Demineralization of bone produces thin, weak bones that fracture easily. Fractures of vertebrae, long bones, and ribs are relatively common, especially in postmenopausal women and immobilized clients. Myopathy results from abnormal protein metabolism. Decreased growth in children results from impaired bone formation and protein metabolism.

(5) Cardiovascular, fluid, and electrolyte effects—fluid retention, edema, hypertension, congestive heart failure, hypernatremia, hypokalemia, metabolic alkalosis

These effects result largely from mineralocorticoid activity, which causes retention of sodium and water. They are more likely to occur with older corticosteroids, such as hydrocortisone and prednisone.

(6) Gastrointestinal effects—nausea, vomiting, possible peptic ulcer disease, increased appetite, obesity

(7) Increased susceptibility to infection and delayed wound healing

Caused by suppression of normal inflammatory and immune processes and impaired protein metabolism

(8) Menstrual irregularities, acne, excessive facial hair

Caused by excessive sex hormones, primarily androgens

(9) Ocular effects—increased intraocular pressure, glaucoma, cataracts

(10) Integumentary effects—skin becomes reddened, thinner, has stretch marks, and is easily injured

4. **Observe for drug interactions**
   a. Drugs that *increase* effects of corticosteroids:

   (1) Adrenergics (*e.g.*, epinephrine), anticholinergics (*e.g.*, atropine), tricyclic antidepressants (*e.g.*, amitriptyline [Elavil]), antihistamines, and meperidine

   Potentiation of increased intraocular pressure. The combinations are hazardous in glaucoma and should be avoided if possible.

   (2) Diuretics

   Excessive potassium depletion may occur because both diuretics and corticosteroids can cause hypokalemia.

   (3) Estrogens

   Potentiate glycosuria and anti-inflammatory effects of hydrocortisone but not those of dexamethasone, methylprednisolone, prednisolone, or prednisone

   (4) Indomethacin

   Increases ulcerogenic effects

   (5) Salicylates

   May potentiate all effects of corticosteroids by displacing the drug from plasma protein binding sites

*(continued)*

| *Nursing Actions* | *Rationale/Explanation* |
|---|---|
| **b.** Drugs that *decrease* effects of corticosteroids: Antihistamines, barbiturates, chloral hydrate, phenytoin, rifampin | These drugs induce microsomal enzymes in the liver and increase the rate at which corticosteroids are metabolized or deactivated. |
| **5. Teach clients** <br> **a.** With long-term systemic corticosteroid therapy: <br><br> (1) Take the drugs as directed. | This is extremely important with these drugs. Missing a dose or two, stopping the drug, changing the amount or time of administration, or taking extra drug (except as specifically directed during stress situations) or any other alterations may result in complications. Some complications are relatively minor; several are serious, even life-threatening. When these drugs are being discontinued, the dosage is gradually reduced over several weeks. They should not be abruptly stopped. |
| (2) Report to the physician if unable to take a dose orally because of vomiting or some other problem. | In some circumstances, the physician may prescribe one or more injections to prevent potentially serious problems. |
| (3) Avoid exposure to infection when possible. Avoid crowds and people known to have an infection. Also, wash hands frequently and thoroughly. | These drugs increase the likelihood of infection, so preventive measures are necessary. Also, if infection does occur, healing is likely to be slow. |
| (4) Practice safety measures to avoid accidents. | To avoid falls and possible fractures due to osteoporosis; to avoid cuts or other injuries because of delayed wound healing; to avoid soft-tissue trauma because of increased tendency to bruise easily |
| (5) Weigh frequently when starting corticosteroid therapy and at least weekly during long-term maintenance. | An initial weight gain is likely to occur and is usually attributed to increased appetite. Later weight gains may be caused by fluid retention. |
| (6) Muscle weakness and fatigue or disease symptoms may occur when drug dosage is reduced, withdrawn, or omitted (*e.g.*, the nondrug day of ADH). | Although these symptoms may cause some discomfort, they should be tolerated if possible rather than increasing corticosteroid dose. If severe, of course, dosage or time of administration may have to be changed. |
| (7) Dietary changes, if indicated. Possible changes include decreasing salt and increasing potassium, calcium, protein, and vitamins D and C. | These changes may not be necessary in all clients. Limiting salt intake may be important if fluid retention or edema is a problem. The simplest way to do this is to avoid adding table salt to foods and avoid obviously salty foods, such as many snack foods and prepared sandwich meats. If more stringent restrictions seem indicated, consult a dietitian or diet manual. When sodium is retained, potassium is lost. It may be desirable for the client to increase intake of high-potassium foods, such as citrus fruits and juices or bananas. Protein, calcium, and vitamin D may help to prevent or delay osteoporosis, and vitamin C may help to prevent excessive bruising. Meat and dairy products are good sources of protein, calcium, and vitamin D; citrus fruits are good sources of vitamin C. <br> Any diet teaching should be specific to the needs of the individual client and should consider food preferences and usual eating habits. |
| (8) Report to a health-care provider: <br> (a) Stress situations <br> (b) Sore throat, fever, or other signs of infection <br> (c) Weight gain of 5 lb or more in a week | As previously indicated, clients experiencing stress situations require larger doses of corticosteroids. It would be helpful if the physician would instruct the client on what kinds of stress situations the client can handle and for which the physician should be notified. All the other symptoms to |

## Nursing Actions

## Rationale/Explanation

      (d) Swelling in ankles or elsewhere in the body

      (e) Persistent backache or chest pain

      (f) Mental depression or other mood changes

      (g) Changes in sleeping patterns

**b.** With local applications of corticosteroids:

    (1) Use the drug preparation only as directed and for the purpose intended.

    (2) Use hand-held inhalers as follows:

      (a) Shake canister thoroughly.

      (b) Place canister between lips (both open and pursed lips have been recommended).

      (c) Exhale completely.

      (d) Activate canister while taking a slow deep breath.

      (e) Hold breath for 10 seconds or as long as possible.

      (f) Wait at least 1 minute before taking additional inhalations.

      (g) Rinse mouth following inhalations to decrease the incidence of oral thrush.

      (h) Rinse mouthpiece at least once per day.

be reported indicate adverse reactions, such as infection, sodium and fluid retention, fractures of vertebrae or ribs, and psychological problems. If these occur, they must be assessed by the physician to see if any changes in corticosteroid therapy are indicated.

To increase therapeutic effects and decrease adverse reactions. As a general rule, not enough drug is absorbed to cause systemic toxicity. However, systemic toxicity can occur if excess corticosteroid is inhaled or if occlusive dressings are used over skin lesions. Local reactions may occur, especially with large doses. Most of the time, different drug preparations are used for specific purposes, such as eye drops or ear drops or application to skin lesions. These preparations must not be used interchangeably.

## Review and Application Exercises

1. What are the main characteristics and functions of cortisol?
2. What is the difference between glucocorticoid and mineralocorticoid components of corticosteroids?
3. How do glucocorticoids affect body metabolism?
4. What is meant by the HPA axis?
5. What are the mechanisms by which exogenous corticosteroids may cause adrenocortical insufficiency and excess?
6. What are adverse effects associated with chronic use of systemic corticosteroids?
7. For a client on long-term systemic corticosteroid therapy, why is it important to taper the dose and gradually discontinue the drug rather than stop it abruptly?
8. Why is alternate-day administration of a systemic corticosteroid preferred when possible?
9. What are the main differences between administering corticosteroids in adrenal insufficiency and in other disorders?
10. When a corticosteroid is given by inhalation to clients with asthma or other bronchoconstrictive disorder, what is the expected effect?

## Selected References

Beare, P. G., & Myers, J. L. (Eds.) (1990). *Principles and practice of adult health nursing*. St. Louis: C.V. Mosby.

Dahl, S. L. (1992). Rheumatic disorders. In M. A. Koda-Kimble & L. Y. Young (Eds.), *Applied therapeutics: The clinical use of drugs* (5th ed.) (pp. 75-1–75-21). Vancouver, WA: Applied Therapeutics.

(1993). *Drug facts and comparisons*. St. Louis: Facts and Comparisons.

Guyton, A. C. (1991). *Textbook of medical physiology* (8th ed.). Philadelphia: W.B. Saunders.

Hurwitz, L. S., & Porth, C. M. (1990). Alterations in endocrine control of growth and metabolism. In C. M. Porth (Ed.), *Pathophysiology: Concepts of altered health states* (3rd ed.) (pp. 775–795). Philadelphia: J.B. Lippincott.

Paré, P. D., & Montaner, J. S. (1992). Asthma. In W. N. Kelley (Ed.), *Textbook of internal medicine* (2nd ed.) (pp. 1707–1714). Philadelphia: J.B. Lippincott.

Petty, T. L. (1992). Chronic obstructive pulmonary disease. In W. N. Kelley (Ed.), *Textbook of internal medicine* (2nd ed.) (pp. 1717–1722). Philadelphia: J.B. Lippincott.

Spruill, W. J., & Wade, W. E. (1992). Other connective tissue disorders and the use of glucocorticoids. In M. A. Koda-Kimble & L. Y. Young (Eds.), *Applied therapeutics: The clinical use of drugs* (5th ed.) (pp. 76-1–76-15). Vancouver, WA: Applied Therapeutics.

Turka, L.A. (1992). Transplantation immunology. In W. N. Kelley (Ed.), *Textbook of internal medicine* (2nd ed.) (pp. 698–702). Philadelphia: J.B. Lippincott.

### CHAPTER 25

# Thyroid and Antithyroid Drugs

## Description and uses

The thyroid gland produces three hormones: thyroxine, triiodothyronine, and calcitonin. Thyroxine contains four atoms of iodine and is also called $T_4$. Triiodothyronine contains three atoms of iodine and is called $T_3$. Compared to thyroxine, triiodothyronine is more potent and has a more rapid but shorter duration of action. Despite these minor differences, the two hormones produce the same physiologic effects and have the same actions and uses. Calcitonin functions in calcium metabolism and is discussed in Chapter 26.

Production of thyroxine and triiodothyronine depends on the presence of iodine and tyrosine in the thyroid gland. Plasma iodide is derived from dietary sources and from the metabolic breakdown of thyroid hormone, which allows some iodine to be reused. The thyroid gland extracts iodide from the circulating blood, concentrates it, and secretes enzymes that change the chemically inactive iodide to free iodine atoms. Tyrosine is an amino acid derived from dietary protein. It forms the basic structure of thyroglobulin. In a series of chemical reactions, iodine atoms become attached to tyrosine to form the thyroid hormones $T_3$ and $T_4$. Once formed, the hormones are stored within the chemically inactive thyroglobulin molecule.

Thyroid hormones are released into the circulation when the thyroid gland is stimulated by thyrotropin from the anterior pituitary gland. Because the thyroglobulin molecule is too large to cross cell membranes, proteolytic enzymes break down the molecule so that the active hormones can be released. After their release from thyroglobulin, the hormones become largely bound to plasma proteins. Only the small amounts left unbound are biologically active. The bound thyroid hormones are released to tissue cells very slowly. Once in the cells, the hormones combine with intracellular proteins so that they are again stored. They are released slowly within the cell and used over a period of days or weeks. Once used by the cells, the thyroid hormones release the iodine atoms. Most of the iodine is reabsorbed and used to produce new thyroid hormones; the remainder is excreted in the urine.

Thyroid hormones control the rate of cellular metabolism and thereby influence the functioning of virtually every cell in the body. The heart, skeletal muscle, liver, and kidneys are especially responsive to the stimulating effects of thyroid hormones. The brain, spleen, and gonads are less responsive. Thyroid hormones are required for normal growth and development and are considered especially critical for brain and skeletal development and maturation. These hormones are thought to act mainly by controlling intracellular protein synthesis. Some specific physiologic effects include:

1. Increased rate of cellular metabolism and oxygen consumption with a resultant increase in heat production
2. Increased heart rate, force of contraction, and cardiac output (increased cardiac workload)
3. Increased carbohydrate metabolism
4. Increased fat metabolism, including increased lipo-

lytic effects of other hormones and metabolism of cholesterol to bile acids

5. Inhibition of pituitary secretion of thyrotropin

# Thyroid disorders

Thyroid disorders requiring drug therapy are goiter, hypothyroidism, and hyperthyroidism. Hypothyroidism and hyperthyroidism produce opposing effects on body tissues, depending on the levels of circulating thyroid hormone. Specific effects and clinical manifestations are listed in Table 25-1.

## SIMPLE GOITER

Simple goiter is an enlargement of the thyroid gland resulting from iodine deficiency. Inadequate iodine decreases thyroid hormone production. To compensate, the anterior pituitary gland secretes more thyrotropin, which causes the thyroid to enlarge and produce more hormone. If the enlarged gland secretes enough hormone, disfigurement, psychological distress, dyspnea, and dysphagia are the main problems. If the gland cannot secrete enough hormone despite enlargement, hypothyroidism results. Simple or endemic goiter is a common condition in some geographic areas. It is uncommon in the United States, largely because of the widespread use of iodized table salt.

Treatment of simple goiter involves giving iodine preparations and thyroid hormones to prevent further enlargement and promote regression in gland size. Large goiters may require surgical excision.

## HYPOTHYROIDISM

Primary hypothyroidism occurs when disease or destruction of thyroid gland tissue causes inadequate production of thyroid hormones. Some causes of primary hypothyroidism include acute viral thyroiditis; chronic (Hashimoto's) thyroiditis, an autoimmune disorder; and overtreatment of hyperthyroidism with antithyroid drugs, radiation therapy, or surgery. Secondary hypothyroidism occurs when there is decreased thyrotropin from the anterior pituitary gland.

Congenital hypothyroidism (cretinism) occurs when a child is born without a thyroid gland or with a poorly functioning gland. Cretinism is uncommon in the United States but may occur with a lack of iodine in the mother's diet. Symptoms are rarely present at birth, but develop gradually during infancy and early childhood and include poor growth and development, lethargy and inactivity, feeding problems, slow pulse, subnormal tem-

## TABLE 25-1. THYROID DISORDERS AND THEIR EFFECTS ON BODY SYSTEMS

| Hypothyroidism | Hyperthyroidism |
|---|---|
| **Cardiovascular Effects** | |
| Increased capillary fragility | Tachycardia |
| Decreased cardiac output | Increased cardiac output |
| Decreased blood pressure | Increased blood volume |
| Decreased heart rate | Increased systolic blood pressure |
| Cardiac enlargement | Cardiac arrhythmias |
| Congestive heart failure | Congestive heart failure |
| Anemia | |
| More rapid development of atherosclerosis and its complications (*e.g.*, coronary artery and peripheral vascular disease) | |
| **Central Nervous System Effects** | |
| Apathy and lethargy | Nervousness |
| Emotional dullness | Emotional instability |
| Slow speech, perhaps slurring and hoarseness as well | Restlessness |
| Hypoactive reflexes | Anxiety |
| Forgetfulness and mental sluggishness | Insomnia |
| Excessive drowsiness and sleeping | Hyperactive reflexes |
| **Metabolic Effects** | |
| Intolerance of cold | Intolerance of heat |
| Subnormal temperature | Low-grade fever |
| Increased serum cholesterol | Weight loss despite increased appetite |
| Weight gain | |
| **Gastrointestinal Effects** | |
| Decreased appetite | Increased appetite |
| Constipation | Abdominal cramps |
| | Diarrhea |
| | Nausea and vomiting |
| **Muscular Effects** | |
| Weakness | Weakness |
| Fatigue | Fatigue |
| Vague aches and pains | Muscle atrophy |
| | Tremors |
| **Integumentary** | |
| Dry, coarse, and thickened skin | Moist, warm, flushed skin owing to vasodilation and increased sweating |
| Puffy appearance of face and eyelids | Hair and nails soft |
| Dry and thinned hair | |
| Thick and hard nails | |
| **Reproductive Effects** | |
| Prolonged menstrual periods | Amenorrhea or oligomenorrhea |
| Infertility or sterility | |
| Decreased libido | |
| **Miscellaneous Effects** | |
| Increased susceptibility to infection | Dyspnea |
| Increased sensitivity to narcotics, barbiturates, and anesthetics owing to slowed metabolism of these drugs | Polyuria |
| | Hoarse, rapid speech |
| | Increased susceptibility to infection |
| | Excessive perspiration |
| | Localized edema around the eyeballs, which produces characteristic eye changes, including exophthalmos |

perature, and constipation. If the disorder is untreated until the child is several months old, permanent mental retardation is likely to result.

Adult hypothyroidism (myxedema) produces variable signs and symptoms, depending on the amount of functioning thyroid tissue and hormone production. Initially, manifestations are mild and vague. They usually increase in incidence and severity over time as the thyroid gland gradually atrophies, and functioning glandular tissue is replaced by nonfunctioning fibrous connective tissue (see Table 25-1).

Regardless of the cause of hypothyroidism and the age at which it occurs, the specific treatment is replacement of thyroid hormone from an exogenous source. Synthetic thyroid hormones have replaced the desiccated thyroid obtained from the thyroid glands of domestic animals. Synthetic preparations are consistent in potency and clinical effects; they differ primarily in onset and duration of action.

The most clear-cut clinical indication for use of thyroid drugs is hypothyroidism manifested by signs and symptoms and confirmed by diagnostic tests of thyroid function. They also may be used to suppress secretion of thyrotropin by the anterior pituitary gland. Thyroid drugs have been used to treat obesity, menstrual disorders, male and female infertility, and fatigue. They should not be given in any of these situations unless hypothyroidism is present.

## HYPERTHYROIDISM

Hyperthyroidism is characterized by excessive secretion of thyroid hormones. It may be associated with Graves' disease, nodular goiter, thyroiditis, overtreatment with thyroid drugs, functioning thyroid carcinoma, and pituitary adenoma that secretes excessive thyrotropin. Hyperthyroidism usually involves an enlarged thyroid gland that has an increased number of cells and an increased rate of secretion. The hyperplastic thyroid gland may secrete five to 15 times the normal amount of thyroid hormone. As a result, body metabolism is greatly increased. Specific physiologic effects and clinical manifestations of hyperthyroidism are listed in Table 25-1. These effects vary, depending on the amount of circulating thyroid hormone, and they usually increase in incidence and severity with time if hyperthyroidism is not treated.

Thyroid storm or thyrotoxic crisis is a rare but severe complication characterized by extreme symptoms of hyperthyroidism, such as severe tachycardia, fever, dehydration, heart failure, and coma. It is most likely to occur in clients with hyperthyroidism that has been inadequately treated, especially when stressful situations occur (*e.g.*, trauma, infection, surgery, emotional upsets).

## Treatment

Hyperthyroidism is treated by antithyroid drugs, radioactive iodine, surgery, or a combination of these therapeutic methods. The drugs act by decreasing production or release of thyroid hormones. Radioactive iodine acts by emitting rays that destroy thyroid gland tissue. Subtotal thyroidectomy involves surgical excision of thyroid tissue. All these methods reduce the amount of thyroid hormones circulating in the bloodstream. No one method is clearly superior, and each has advantages and disadvantages.

Drug therapy is probably the treatment of choice, at least initially, for most clients. The antithyroid drugs include the thioamide derivatives (propylthiouracil and methimazole) and iodine preparations. The thioamide drugs are preferred by many physicians for clients up to age 30 years and possibly up to age 40. These drugs are inexpensive and relatively safe, and they do not damage the thyroid gland.

Although iodine preparations are the oldest antithyroid drugs, they are no longer used in long-term treatment of hyperthyroidism. They are indicated when a rapid clinical response is needed, as in thyroid storm and acute hyperthyroidism. They are also used to prepare a hyperthyroid person for thyroidectomy. A thioamide drug is given to produce a euthyroid state, and an iodine preparation is given to reduce the size and vascularity of the thyroid gland to reduce the risk of excessive bleeding.

Iodine preparations inhibit the release of thyroid hormones and cause them to be stored within the gland. They reduce blood levels of thyroid hormones more quickly than thioamide drugs or radioactive iodine. Maximal effects are reached in about 10 to 15 days of continuous therapy, and this is probably the primary advantage. Several disadvantages, however, include the following:

1. They may produce goiter, hyperthyroidism, or both.
2. They cannot be used alone. Therapeutic benefits are temporary, and symptoms of hyperthyroidism may reappear and even be intensified if other treatment methods are not also used.
3. Radioactive iodine cannot be used effectively for a prolonged period in a client who has received iodine preparations. Even if the iodine preparation is discontinued, the thyroid gland is saturated with iodine and will not attract enough radioactive iodine for treatment to be effective. Also, if radioactive iodine is given later, acute hyperthyroidism is likely to result because the radioactive iodine causes the stored hormones to be released into the circulation.
4. Although giving a thioamide drug followed by an iodine preparation is standard preparation for thyroidectomy, the opposite sequence of administration

is unsafe. If the iodine preparation is given first and followed by propylthiouracil or methimazole, the client is likely to experience acute hyperthyroidism because the thioamide causes release of the stored thyroid hormones.

Propranolol is used as an adjunctive drug in the treatment of hyperthyroidism. It relieves tachycardia, cardiac palpitations, excessive sweating, and other symptoms. Propranolol is especially helpful during the several weeks required for therapeutic results from antithyroid drugs or from radioactive iodine administration.

Radioactive iodine is effective, inexpensive, and convenient. Probably its main disadvantage is eventual hypothyroidism. A second disadvantage is the delay in therapeutic benefits. Results may not be apparent for 3 months or longer, during which time severe hyperthyroidism must be brought under control with one of the thioamide antithyroid drugs.

Subtotal thyroidectomy is also effective in relieving hyperthyroidism, but this treatment method also has several disadvantages. First, preparation for surgery requires several weeks of drug therapy. Second, there are risks involved in anesthesia and surgery and potential postoperative complications. Third, there is a high risk of eventual hypothyroidism.

## Individual drugs

### THYROID AGENTS (DRUGS USED IN HYPOTHYROIDISM)

**Desiccated thyroid tablets** contain iodine, levothyroxine ($T_4$), thyroglobulin, and triiodothyronine ($T_3$), which are normally present in the human thyroid gland. This preparation is obsolete because it is standardized only by its content of organic iodide. As a result, preparations containing similar amounts of iodide may contain markedly different amounts of $T_4$ and $T_3$, and therapeutic benefits may be lacking or unpredictable.

#### Route and dosage ranges

*Adults:* PO 16–32 mg/d initially, increased by 16–32 mg q2 wk until desired response is obtained; usual maintenance dose is 65–195 mg/d in a single dose
*Older adults:* PO 8–16 mg/d initially, doubled q6–8 wk until desired response is obtained
*Children:* PO 32–65 mg/d for infants up to 1 year of age; 65–195 mg/d for older children, depending on clinical response

**Levothyroxine** (Synthroid, Levothroid) is a synthetic preparation of $T_4$. It is more potent than thyroid, contains a uniform amount of hormone, and can be given parenterally. Compared with liothyronine, levothyroxine has a slower onset and longer duration of action. Levothyroxine is usually considered the drug of choice for long-term treatment of hypothyroidism.

#### Routes and dosage ranges

*Adults:* PO 0.05–0.1 mg/d initially, increased q1–3 wk until the desired response is obtained; usual maintenance dose is 0.1–0.2 mg/d
Myxedema coma, IV 0.2–0.5 mg (0.1 mg/ml) in a single dose; 0.1–0.3 mg may be repeated on the second day if necessary
*Older adults, clients with cardiac disorders, and clients with hypothyroidism of long duration:* PO 0.0125–0.025 mg/d for 6 wk, then dose is doubled q6–8 wk until the desired response is obtained
Myxedema coma, same as adult dosage
*Children:* PO no more than 0.05 mg/d initially, then increased by 0.05–0.1 mg q2 wk until the desired response is obtained; usual dosage range is 0.3–0.4 mg/d
Myxedema coma, same as adult dosage

**Liothyronine** (Cytomel, Triostat) is a synthetic preparation of $T_3$. Compared with levothyroxine, liothyronine has a more rapid onset and a shorter duration of action. Consequently, it may be more likely to produce high concentrations in blood and tissues and cause adverse reactions. Also, it requires more frequent administration if used for long-term treatment of hypothyroidism. Only the intravenous formulation (Triostat) is used in treating myxedema coma.

#### Route and dosage ranges

*Adults:* PO 25 µg/d initially, increased by 12.5–25 µg q1–2 wk until desired response is obtained
Myxedema coma, IV 25-50 µg initially, then adjust dosage according to clinical response. Usual dosage, 65–100 µg/d, with doses at least 4 hours apart and no more than 12 hours apart
*Older adults:* PO 2.5–5 µg/d for 3–6 wk, then doubled q6 wk until the desired response is obtained
Myxedema coma, IV 10–20 µg initially, then adjusted according to clinical response
*Children:* PO 5 µg/d initially, increased by 5 µg/d q3–4 d until the desired response is obtained. Doses as high as 20–80 µg may be required in cretinism.
Myxedema coma, dosage, safety and effectiveness have not been established

**Liotrix** (Euthroid, Thyrolar) contains levothyroxine and liothyronine in a 4:1 ratio, resembling the composition of natural thyroid hormone. The mixture has the same indications for use and the same adverse effects as desiccated thyroid tablets. Euthroid and Thyrolar are available in strengths ranging from 15 to 180 mg in thyroid equivalency. Euthroid-1 and Thyrolar-1 are equivalent to 60 mg of desiccated thyroid.

### Route and dosage ranges

*Adults:* PO 15–30 mg/d initially, increased gradually q1–2 wk until response is obtained

*Older adults, clients with cardiac disorders, and clients with hypothyroidism of long duration:* PO one-fourth to one-half the usual adult dose initially, doubled q8 wk if necessary

*Children:* PO same as adult dosage, increased q2 wk if necessary

## ANTITHYROID AGENTS (DRUGS USED IN HYPERTHYROIDISM)

**Propylthiouracil** is the prototype of the thioamide antithyroid drugs. It can be used alone to treat hyperthyroidism, as part of the preoperative preparation for thyroidectomy, before or after radioactive iodine therapy, and in the treatment of thyroid storm or thyrotoxic crisis. Propylthiouracil acts by inhibiting production of thyroid hormones and peripheral conversion of $T_4$ to the more active $T_3$. It does not interfere with release of thyroid hormones previously produced and stored. Thus, therapeutic effects do not occur for several days or weeks until the stored hormones have been used. **Methimazole** (Tapazole) is similar to propylthiouracil in actions, uses, and adverse reactions, except that it lacks peripheral activity.

Propylthiouracil

### Route and dosage ranges

*Adults:* PO 300–400 mg/d in divided doses q8h, until the client is euthyroid; then 100–150 mg/d in three divided doses, given for maintenance

*Children over 10 years:* PO 150–300 mg/d in divided doses q8h; usual maintenance dose, 100–300 mg/d in two divided doses, q12h

*Children 6–10 years:* 50–150 mg/d in divided doses q8h

Neonatal thyrotoxicosis, 10 mg/kg per day in divided doses

Methimazole

### Route and dosage ranges

*Adults:* PO 15–60 mg/d initially, in divided doses q8h until the client is euthyroid; maintenance, 5–15 mg/d in two or three doses

*Children:* PO 0.4 mg/kg per day initially, in divided doses q8h; maintenance dose, one-half initial dose

**Strong iodine solution** (Lugol's solution) and **saturated solution of potassium iodide** (SSKI) are io-

dine preparations that are sometimes used in short-term treatment of hyperthyroidism. The drugs inhibit release of thyroid hormones, causing them to accumulate in the thyroid gland. Lugol's solution is generally used to treat thyrotoxic crisis and to decrease the size and vascularity of the thyroid gland before thyroidectomy. SSKI is more often used as an expectorant but may be given as preparation for thyroidectomy. Iodine preparations should not be followed by propylthiouracil, methimazole, or radioactive iodine because the latter drugs cause release of stored thyroid hormone and may precipitate acute hyperthyroidism.

Strong iodine solution

### Route and dosage ranges

*Adults and children:* PO 2–6 drops three times per day for 10 days before thyroidectomy

Potassium iodide solution

### Route and dosage ranges

*Adults and children:* PO 5 drops three times per day for 10 days before thyroidectomy

**Sodium iodide** $^{131}$**I** (Iodotope) is a radioactive isotope of iodine. The thyroid gland cannot differentiate between regular iodide and radioactive iodide, so it picks up the radioactive iodide from the circulating blood. As a result, small amounts of radioactive iodide can be used as a diagnostic test of thyroid function, and larger doses are used therapeutically to treat hyperthyroidism. Therapeutic doses act by emitting beta and gamma rays, which destroy thyroid tissue and thereby decrease production of thyroid hormones. It is also used to treat thyroid cancer.

Radioactive iodide is usually given in a single dose on an outpatient basis. For most clients, no special radiation precautions are necessary. If a very large dose is given, the client may be isolated for 8 days, which is the half-life of radioactive iodide. Therapeutic effects are delayed for several weeks or up to 6 months. During this time, symptoms may be controlled with thioamide drugs or propranolol. Radioactive iodide is usually given to middle-aged and elderly people; it should not be given during pregnancy and lactation.

### Routes and dosage ranges

*Adults and children:* PO, IV, dosage as calculated by a radiologist trained in nuclear medicine

**Propranolol** (Inderal) is an antiadrenergic, not an antithyroid, drug. It does not affect thyroid function, hormone secretion, or hormone metabolism. It is most often used to treat cardiovascular conditions, such as arrhythmias, angina pectoris, and hypertension. When given to clients with hyperthyroidism, propranolol blocks beta-adrenergic receptors in various organs and thereby controls symptoms of hyperthyroidism resulting from excessive stimulation of the sympathetic nervous system. These symptoms include tachycardia, palpitations, excessive sweating (hyperhidrosis), tremors, and nervousness. Propranolol is useful for controlling symptoms during the delayed response to thioamide drugs and radioactive iodine, before thyroidectomy, and in treating thyrotoxic crisis. When the client becomes euthyroid and hyperthyroid symptoms are controlled by definitive treatment measures, propranolol should be discontinued.

### Route and dosage range

*Adults:* PO 40–160 mg/d in divided doses

## Nursing Process

### Assessment

- Assess for signs and symptoms of thyroid disorders (see Table 25-1). During the course of treatment with thyroid or antithyroid drugs, the client's blood level of thyroid hormone may range from low to normal to high. At either end of the continuum, signs and symptoms may be dramatic and obvious. As blood levels change toward normal as a result of treatment, signs and symptoms become less obvious. If presenting signs and symptoms are treated too aggressively, they may change toward the opposite end of the continuum and indicate adverse drug effects. Thus, each client receiving a drug that alters thyroid function must be assessed for indicators of hypothyroidism, euthyroidism, and hyperthyroidism.
- Check laboratory reports of diagnostic test values. Commonly used tests of thyroid function and their normal values are resin $T_3$ uptake ($RT_3U$), 25% to 45%; serum $T_3$, 0.08 to 0.20 $\mu$g/100 ml; serum $T_4$, 5 to 12 $\mu$g/100 ml; serum thyroid-stimulating hormone (TSH), 0.5 to 5 $\mu$U/ml.

### Nursing diagnoses

- Decreased Cardiac Output related to disease or drug-induced hypothyroidism
- Altered Nutrition: Less than Body Requirements with hyperthyroidism
- Altered Nutrition: More than Body Requirements with hypothyroidism
- Body Image Disturbance related to weight gain with hypothyroidism or weight loss and exophthalmos with hyperthyroidism
- Ineffective Individual Coping related to disease process and long-term drug therapy
- Constipation with hypothyroidism, diarrhea with hyperthyroidism
- Ineffective Thermoregulation related to changes in metabolism rate and body heat production
- Knowledge Deficit: Disease process and drug therapy

### Planning/Goals

*The client will:*

- Achieve normal blood levels of thyroid hormone
- Receive or take drugs accurately
- Experience relief of symptoms of hypothyroidism or hyperthyroidism
- Be assisted to cope with symptoms until therapy becomes effective
- Avoid preventable adverse drug effects
- Be monitored regularly for therapeutic and adverse responses to drug therapy

### Interventions

Use nondrug measures to control symptoms, increase effectiveness of drug therapy, and decrease adverse reactions. Some areas for intervention include the following:

- **Environmental temperature**. Regulate for the client's comfort, when possible. Clients with hypothyroidism are very intolerant of cold owing to their slow metabolism rate. Chilling and shivering should be prevented because of added strain on the heart. Provide blankets and warm clothing as needed. Clients with hyperthyroidism are very intolerant of heat and perspire excessively owing to their rapid metabolism rate. Provide cooling baths and lightweight clothing as needed.
- **Diet**. Despite a poor appetite, *hypothyroid* clients are often overweight. Thus, a low-calorie, weight reduction diet may be indicated. In addition, an increased intake of high-fiber foods is usually needed to prevent constipation as a result of decreased gastrointestinal secretion and motility. Despite a good appetite, *hyperthyroid* clients are often underweight because of rapid metabolism rates. They often need extra calories and nutrients to prevent tissue breakdown. These can be provided by extra meals and snacks. The client may wish to avoid highly seasoned and high-fiber foods because they may increase diarrhea.
- **Fluids**. With *hypothyroidism*, clients need an adequate intake of low-calorie fluids to prevent constipation. With *hyperthyroidism*, clients need large amounts of fluids (3000–4000 ml/d) unless contraindicated by cardiac or renal disease. The fluids are needed to eliminate heat and waste products produced by the hypermetabolic state. Much of the client's fluid loss is visible as excessive perspiration and urine output.
- **Activity**. With *hypothyroidism*, encourage activity to maintain cardiovascular, respiratory, gastrointestinal, and musculoskeletal function. With *hyperthyroidism*, encourage rest and quiet, nonstrenuous activity. Because clients differ in what they find restful, this must be determined with each one. A quiet room, reading, and soft music may be helpful. Mild sedatives are often given. The client is caught in the dilemma of needing rest because of the high metabolic rate but being unable to rest because of nervousness and excitement.
- **Skin care**. *Hypothyroid* clients are likely to have edema and dry skin. When edema is present, inspect pressure points, turn often, and avoid trauma when possible. Edema increases risks of skin breakdown and decubitus ulcer formation. Also, increased capillary fragility increases the likelihood of bruising from seemingly minor trauma. When skin

is dry, use soap sparingly and lotions and other lubricants freely.
- **Eye care**. *Hyperthyroid* clients are likely to have exophthalmos. In mild cases, use measures to protect the eye. For example, dark glasses, local lubricants, and patching of the eyes at night may be needed. Diuretic drugs and elevating the head of the bed may help reduce periorbital edema and eyeball protrusion. If the eyelids cannot close, they are sometimes taped shut to avoid corneal abrasion. In severe exophthalmos, the above measures are taken and large doses of corticosteroids are usually given.

*Teach clients:*
- That the duration of drug therapy for hypothyroidism is usually lifelong and for hyperthyroidism is usually 1 year
- That periodic tests of thyroid function will be needed
- That dosage adjustments will be made according to clinical response and results of thyroid function tests
- To monitor response to drug therapy by weighing themselves at least weekly and recording their pulse rate daily

### Evaluation

- Interview and observe for compliance with instructions for taking medications.
- Observe for relief of symptoms.
- Check laboratory reports for normal blood levels of thyroid hormones.
- Interview and observe for adverse drug effects.
- Check appointment records for compliance with follow-up procedures.

## Principles of therapy

### THYROID DRUGS

### Drug selection

Levothyroxine is considered the drug of choice for thyroid hormone replacement because of uniform potency, once-daily dosing, and low cost.

### Dosage factors

Dosage is influenced by the choice of drug, the client's age, the client's general condition, severity and duration of hypothyroidism, and clinical response to drug therapy. Specific factors include the following:

1. Dosage must be individualized to approximate the amount of thyroid hormone needed to make up the deficit in endogenous hormone production.
2. As a general rule, initial dosage is relatively small. Dosage is gradually increased at about 2-week intervals in most clients until an optimum response is obtained, and symptoms are relieved. Maintenance dosage for long-term therapy is based on the client's

clinical status and periodic laboratory tests, such as measurement of serum $T_3$ and $T_4$.
3. Infants requiring thyroid hormone replacement need relatively large doses. After thyroid drugs are started, the maintenance dosage is determined by periodic radioimmunoassay of serum $T_4$ and by periodic x-ray studies to follow bone development.
4. Clients who are elderly or have cardiovascular disease are given small initial doses. Also, increments are smaller and made at longer intervals, usually about 8 weeks. The primary reason for very cautious thyroid replacement in such clients is the high risk of adverse effects on the cardiovascular system.

### Hypothyroidism and the metabolism of other drugs

Changes in the rate of body metabolism affect the metabolism of various drugs. Most drugs given to a client with hypothyroidism have a prolonged effect because drug metabolism in the liver is delayed, and the glomerular filtration rate of the kidneys is decreased. Also, drug absorption from the gastrointestinal system or a parenteral injection site may be slowed. As a result, dosage of most other drugs should be reduced. For example, people with hypothyroidism are especially sensitive to narcotics, barbiturates and other sedative-type drugs, and anesthetics. If these drugs are necessary, they are given very cautiously and in dosages of about one-third to one-half the usual dose. Even then, clients must be observed very closely for respiratory depression.

Once thyroid replacement therapy is started and stabilized, the client becomes euthyroid, has a normal rate of metabolism, and can tolerate usual doses of most drugs if other influencing factors are not present. On the other hand, excessive doses of thyroid drugs may produce hyperthyroidism and a greatly increased rate of metabolism. In this instance, larger doses of most other drugs are necessary to produce the same effects. Rather than increasing dosage of other drugs, though, dosage of thyroid drugs should be reduced so that the client is euthyroid again.

### Duration of replacement therapy

Thyroid replacement therapy in the client with hypothyroidism is lifelong. Medical supervision is needed frequently during early treatment and at least annually after the client's condition has stabilized and maintenance dosage has been determined.

### Adrenal insufficiency

If adrenal insufficiency is present in a client who needs thyroid drugs, that insufficiency must be corrected by giving corticosteroid drugs before starting thyroid replacement, because thyroid hormones increase tissue metabolism and tissue demands for adrenocortical hormones. If adrenal insufficiency is not treated first, administration of thyroid hormone may cause acute adrenocortical insufficiency.

## ANTITHYROID DRUGS

### Dosage factors

Dosage of the thioamide antithyroid drugs is relatively large until a euthyroid state is reached, in about 6 to 8 weeks. Then a maintenance dose, in the smallest amount that prevents recurrent symptoms of hyperthyroidism, is given for 1 year or longer. Dosage should be decreased if the thyroid gland enlarges or signs and symptoms of hypothyroidism occur.

### Duration of antithyroid therapy

No clear-cut guidelines exist regarding duration of antithyroid drug therapy because exacerbations and remissions occur. It is usually continued until the client is euthyroid for 6 to 12 months. Then diagnostic tests to evaluate thyroid function or a trial withdrawal may be implemented to determine whether the client is likely to remain euthyroid without further drug therapy. If the drug is to be discontinued, this is usually done gradually over weeks or months.

### Use in pregnancy

When iodine preparations and thioamide antithyroid drugs are used during pregnancy, they can cause goiter and hypothyroidism in the fetus or newborn.

### Hyperthyroidism and the metabolism of other drugs

Treatment of hyperthyroidism changes the rate of body metabolism, including the rate of metabolism of many drugs. During the hyperthyroid state, drug metabolism may be very rapid, and higher doses of most drugs may be necessary to achieve therapeutic results. When the client becomes euthyroid, the rate of drug metabolism is decreased. Consequently, doses of all medications should be evaluated and probably reduced to avoid severe adverse reactions.

### Iodine ingestion and hyperthyroidism

Iodine is present in foods (especially seafood), in many medications used to treat pulmonary and other diseases (*e.g.*, Calcidrine, Organidin, Quadrinal), and in many contrast dyes used for gallbladder and other radiologic procedures. Ingestion of large amounts of iodine from these sources may result in goiter and hyperthyroidism. These conditions can develop in clients with no history of thyroid disease, but they are probably more likely in those with underlying thyroid problems.

## USE IN CHILDREN

For *hypothyroidism* in children, levothyroxine or liothyronine is given. For congenital hypothyroidism (cretinism), drug therapy should be started as soon after birth as the condition is diagnosed and continued for life. One of the drugs may be given for hypothyroidism occurring at any age. Adequate replacement of thyroid hormone is necessary for normal growth and development, and dosage needs may change with growth. Recording height and weight at regular intervals and comparing them with growth charts is one way to monitor drug effects on growth. Adverse drug effects are similar to those seen in adults, and children should be monitored closely.

For *hyperthyroidism* in children, a thioamide antithyroid drug (propylthiouracil or methimazole) is used. Potential risks of adverse effects are similar to those in adults. Because radioactive iodine may cause cancer and chromosome damage in children, it should be used only for hyperthyroidism that cannot be controlled by other antithyroid drugs or surgery.

## USE IN OLDER ADULTS

Signs and symptoms of thyroid disorders may mimic those of other disorders that often occur in older adults (*e.g.*, congestive heart failure). Therefore, a thorough physical examination and diagnostic tests of thyroid function are necessary before starting any type of treatment.

For *hypothyroidism*, levothyroxine is usually given. Thyroid replacement hormone increases the workload of the heart and may cause serious adverse effects in older adults, especially those with cardiovascular disease. Cardiac effects also may be increased in clients receiving bronchodilators or other cardiac stimulants. To decrease adverse effects, the drugs should be given in small initial doses and increased gradually, if necessary, at intervals of about 6 to 8 weeks. Blood pressure and pulse should be monitored regularly. As a general rule, do not give the drug if the resting heart rate is more than 100 beats per minute.

For *hyperthyroidism*, propylthiouracil or methimazole may be used, but radioactive iodine is often preferred because it is associated with fewer adverse effects than other antithyroid drugs or surgery. Clients should be monitored closely for hypothyroidism, which usually develops within a few years after receiving treatment for hyperthyroidism.

# NURSING ACTIONS: THYROID AND ANTITHYROID DRUGS

*Nursing Actions* | *Rationale/Explanation*

**1. Administer accurately**
  **a.** With thyroid drugs:

(1) Administer in a single daily dose, usually before breakfast.

This allows peak drug activity during daytime hours and is less likely to interfere with sleep.

(2) Check the pulse rate before giving the drug. If the rate is over 100 per minute or if any changes in cardiac rhythm are noted, consult the physician before giving the dose.

Tachycardia or other cardiac arrhythmias may indicate adverse cardiac effects. Dosage may need to be reduced or the drug stopped temporarily.

(3) Do not switch among various brands or generic forms of the drug.

Differences in bioavailability have been identified among available products. Changes in preparations may alter dosage and therefore symptom control.

  **b.** With antithyroid and iodine drugs:

(1) Administer q8h.

All these drugs have rather short half-lives and must be given frequently and regularly to maintain therapeutic blood levels. In addition, if iodine preparations are not given every 8 hours, symptoms of hyperthyroidism may recur.

(2) Dilute iodine solutions in a full glass of fruit juice or milk, if possible, and have the client drink the medication through a straw.

Dilution of the drug reduces gastric irritation and masks the unpleasant taste. Using a straw prevents staining the teeth.

**2. Observe for therapeutic effects**
  **a.** With thyroid drugs, observe for:

(1) Increased energy and activity level, less lethargy and fatigue

(2) Increased alertness and interest in surroundings

(3) Increased appetite

(4) Increased pulse rate and temperature

(5) Decreased constipation

(6) Reversal of coarseness and other changes in skin and hair

(7) With cretinism, increased growth rate (record height periodically)

(8) With myxedema, diuresis, weight loss, and decreased edema

(9) Increased serum $T_4$

Therapeutic effects result from a return to normal metabolic activities and relief of the symptoms of hypothyroidism. Therapeutic effects may be evident as early as 2 or 3 days after drug therapy is started or delayed up to about 2 weeks. All signs and symptoms of myxedema should disappear in about 3 to 12 weeks.

(10) Decreased serum cholesterol and possibly decreased creatine phosphokinase, lactic dehydrogenase, and aspartate aminotransferase

These tests are often elevated with myxedema and may return to normal when thyroid replacement therapy is begun.

  **b.** With antithyroid and iodine drugs, observe for:

(1) Slower pulse rate

(2) Slower speech

(3) More normal activity level (slowing of hyperactivity)

(4) Decreased nervousness

With propylthiouracil and methimazole, some therapeutic effects are apparent in 1 or 2 weeks, but euthyroidism may not occur for 6 or 8 weeks.
With iodine solutions, therapeutic effects may be apparent within 24 hours. Maximal effects occur in about 10 to 15 days. However, therapeutic effects may not be sustained.

*(continued)*

## Nursing Actions                                 ## Rationale/Explanation

(5) Decreased tremors

(6) Improved ability to sleep and rest

(7) Weight gain

Symptoms may reappear if the drug is given longer than a few weeks, and they may be more severe than initially.

### 3. Observe for adverse effects

**a.** With thyroid drugs, observe for tachycardia and other cardiac arrhythmias, angina pectoris, myocardial infarction, congestive heart failure, nervousness, hyperactivity, insomnia, diarrhea, abdominal cramps, nausea and vomiting, weight loss, fever, intolerance to heat.

Most adverse reactions stem from excessive doses, and signs and symptoms produced are the same as those occurring with hyperthyroidism. Excessive thyroid hormones make the heart work very hard and fast in attempting to meet tissue demands for oxygenated blood and nutrients. Symptoms of myocardial ischemia occur when the myocardium does not get an adequate supply of oxygenated blood. Symptoms of congestive heart failure occur when the increased cardiac workload is prolonged. Cardiovascular problems are more likely to occur in clients who are elderly or who already have heart disease.

**b.** With propylthiouracil and methimazole, observe for:

(1) Hypothyroidism—bradycardia, congestive heart failure, anemia, coronary artery and peripheral vascular disease, slow speech and movements, emotional and mental dullness, excessive sleeping, weight gain, constipation, skin changes, and others

(2) Blood disorders—leukopenia, agranulocytosis, hypoprothrombinemia

Leukopenia may be difficult to evaluate because it may occur with hyperthyroidism and with antithyroid drugs. Agranulocytosis occurs rarely but is the most severe adverse reaction; the earliest symptoms are likely to be sore throat and fever. If these occur, report them to the physician immediately.

(3) Integumentary system—skin rash, pruritus, alopecia

(4) CNS—headache, dizziness, loss of sense of taste, drowsiness, paresthesias

(5) Gastrointestinal system—nausea, vomiting, abdominal discomfort, gastric irritation, cholestatic hepatitis

(6) Other—lymphadenopathy, edema, joint pain, drug fever

**c.** With iodine preparations, observe for:

Adverse effects are uncommon with short-term use.

(1) Iodism—metallic taste, burning in mouth, soreness of gums, excessive salivation, gastric or respiratory irritation, rhinitis, headache, redness of conjunctiva, edema of eyelids

(2) Hypersensitivity—acneiform skin rash, pruritus, fever, jaundice, angioedema, serum sickness

Allergic reactions rarely occur.

(3) Goiter with hypothyroidism

Uncommon but may occur in adults and newborns whose mothers have taken iodides for long periods

(continued)

| *Nursing Actions* | *Rationale/Explanation* |
|---|---|
| **4. Observe for drug interactions** | |
| **a.** Drugs that *increase* effects of the thyroid hormones: | |
| (1) Antidepressants (tricyclic), epinephrine, levarterenol | These drugs primarily increase catecholamines. When combined with thyroid hormones, excessive cardiovascular stimulation may occur and cause myocardial ischemia, cardiac arrhythmias, hypertension, and other adverse cardiovascular effects. |
| (2) Clofibrate, phenobarbital, and phenytoin | Potentiate thyroid drugs by displacement from plasma protein-binding sites or by slowing liver metabolism |
| **b.** Drugs that *decrease* effects of thyroid hormones: | |
| (1) Antihypertensives | These agents decrease the cardiovascular effects of catecholamines (epinephrine and norepinephrine) and thyroid hormone so that angina pectoris is less likely to occur. |
| (2) Cholestyramine resin (Questran) | This drug decreases gastrointestinal absorption of thyroid hormones. Cholestyramine binds $T_4$ and $T_3$ almost irreversibly. If it is necessary to give these drugs concurrently, give the resin at least 4 or 5 hours before or after giving the thyroid drug. |
| (3) Estrogens, including oral contraceptives containing estrogens | Estrogens inhibit thyroid hormones by increasing thyroxine-binding globulin. This increases the amount of bound, inactive thyroid hormones in clients with hypothyroidism. This decreased effect does not occur in clients with adequate thyroid hormone secretion because the increased binding is offset by increased $T_4$ production. Women taking oral contraceptives may need larger doses of thyroid hormone replacement than would otherwise be needed. |
| (4) Propranolol (Inderal) | This drug decreases cardiac effects of thyroid hormones. It is used in hyperthyroidism to reduce tachycardia and other symptoms of excessive cardiovascular stimulation. |
| **c.** Drugs that *increase* effects of antithyroid drugs: | |
| (1) Chlorpromazine, sulfonamides, oral antidiabetic drugs, xanthines | Increased risk of goiter |
| (2) Lithium | Acts synergistically to produce hypothyroidism |
| **5. Teach clients** | |
| **a.** Take thyroid and antithyroid drugs as directed. | Thyroid replacement hormones must be continued throughout life. Thioamide antithyroid drugs must be taken for 1 year or longer. |
| **b.** Report adverse effects (hyperthyroidism, hypothyroidism, iodism, and others). | Drug dosage may need to be reduced or the drug discontinued. |
| **c.** Avoid over-the-counter drugs or consult with physician before taking them. | Many preparations contain iodide, which can increase the likelihood of goiter with thioamides and the risk of adverse reactions from excessive doses of iodide. For example, cough syrups, some asthma medications, and some multivitamins contain iodide. |
| **d.** Ask the physician if it is necessary to avoid or restrict amounts of seafood or iodized salt. | These sources of iodide may need to be reduced or omitted during antithyroid drug therapy. |

## Review and Application Exercises

1. Where is TSH produced and what is its function?
2. What is the role of thyroid hormones in maintaining body functions?
3. What signs and symptoms are associated with hypothyroidism?
4. In primary hypothyroidism, are blood levels of TSH increased or decreased?
5. What is the drug of first choice for treating hypothyroidism?
6. What are adverse effects of drug therapy for hypothyroidism?
7. What signs and symptoms are associated with hyperthyroidism?
8. Which drugs reduce blood levels of thyroid hormone in hyperthyroidism, and how do they act?
9. What are adverse effects of drug therapy for hyperthyroidism?
10. When propranolol is used in the treatment of hyperthyroidism, what are its expected effects?
11. What is the effect of thyroid disorders on metabolism of other drugs?

## Selected References

Beare, P. G., & Myers, J. L. (Eds.) (1990). *Principles and practice of adult health nursing.* St. Louis: C.V. Mosby.

Dong, B. J. (1992). Thyroid disorders. In M. A. Koda-Kimble & L. Y. Young (Eds.), *Applied therapeutics: The clinical use of drugs* (5th ed.) (pp. 71-1–71-30). Vancouver, WA: Applied Therapeutics.

(1993). *Drug facts and comparisons.* St. Louis: Facts and Comparisons.

Guyton, A. C. (1991). *Textbook of medical physiology* (8th ed.). Philadelphia: W.B. Saunders.

Hancock, M. R. (1992). Nursing management of adults with disorders of the thyroid gland. In L. O. Burrell (Ed.), *Adult nursing in hospital and community settings* (pp. 1113–1136). Norwalk, CT: Appleton & Lange.

Hurwitz, L. S., & Porth, C. M. (1990). Alterations in endocrine control of growth and metabolism. In C. M. Porth (Ed.), *Pathophysiology: Concepts of altered health states* (3rd ed.) (pp. 775–795). Philadelphia: J.B. Lippincott.

Utiger, R. D. (1992). Disorders of the thyroid gland. In W. N. Kelley (Ed.), *Textbook of internal medicine* (2nd ed.) (pp. 1992–2001). Philadelphia: J.B. Lippincott.

### CHAPTER 26

# Hormones that Regulate Calcium and Phosphorus Metabolism

## Description

Calcium and phosphorus metabolism is regulated primarily by three hormones: parathyroid hormone, calcitonin, and vitamin D (calciferol). These hormones are interrelated in a complex homeostatic mechanism of which the main goal is to maintain normal serum levels of calcium.

### PARATHYROID HORMONE

Parathyroid hormone is secreted by the parathyroid glands, located immediately behind the thyroid gland. The primary function of parathyroid hormone is to maintain normal calcium levels in the serum or extracellular fluid. Parathyroid hormone secretion is stimulated by low serum calcium levels and inhibited by normal or high levels. Thus, secretion is controlled by a negative feedback system, as are most other hormonal secretions. Because phosphate is closely related to calcium in body functions, parathyroid hormone also regulates phosphate metabolism. As a general rule, when serum calcium levels go up, serum phosphate levels go down, and vice versa. Thus, an inverse relationship between calcium and phosphate is maintained.

When the serum calcium level falls below the normal range, parathyroid hormone raises the level by acting on bone, intestines, and kidneys. The effect of parathyroid hormone on bone is to increase bone breakdown or resorption, thereby causing calcium to move from bone into the serum. The effect on intestines is to increase absorption of calcium ingested in food, and the effect on the kidneys is to increase reabsorption of calcium in the renal tubules (thereby decreasing urinary excretion). The opposite effects occur with phosphate; that is, parathyroid hormone decreases serum phosphate and increases urinary phosphate excretion.

Disorders of parathyroid function are related to deficient production of parathyroid hormone (hypoparathyroidism) or excessive production (hyperparathyroidism). Hypoparathyroidism is most often caused by removal of or damage to the parathyroid glands during thyroidectomy or other neck surgery. There are normally four parathyroid glands. Removal of two causes little, if any, change in normal function. If even a small amount of parathyroid tissue remains, a transient hypoparathyroidism may occur, but the tissue usually enlarges and secretes sufficient parathyroid hormone to meet body requirements. Hyperparathyroidism is most often caused by a tumor or hyperplasia of one of the glands. It also may result from ectopic secretion of parathyroid hormone by malignant tumors (*e.g.*, carcinomas of the lung, pancreas, kidney, ovary, prostate gland, or bladder).

Clinical manifestations and treatment of hypoparathyroidism are the same as those of hypocalcemia, which is discussed later in this chapter. Treatment of

Anne Collins Abrams: CLINICAL DRUG THERAPY, Fourth Edition.
© 1995 J.B. Lippincott Company.

hypocalcemia includes giving a calcium preparation and perhaps vitamin D. Clinical manifestations of hyperparathyroidism are those of hypercalcemia, also discussed later in this chapter. When hypercalcemia is caused by a tumor of parathyroid tissue, the usual treatment of choice is surgical excision. When it is caused by malignant tumor, treatment of the tumor with surgery, irradiation, or chemotherapy may reduce production of parathyroid hormone.

## CALCITONIN

Calcitonin is a hormone secreted by the thyroid gland. Its secretion is controlled by the concentration of ionized calcium in the blood flowing through the thyroid gland. When the serum level of ionized calcium is increased, secretion of calcitonin is increased. Calcitonin lowers serum calcium levels primarily by decreasing movement of calcium from bone to serum. Calcitonin also increases renal excretion of calcium, phosphate, sodium, and chloride, but its primary function is to lower serum calcium in the presence of hypercalcemia. Its action is rapid but of short duration. Thus, it has little effect on long-term calcium metabolism. Synthetic preparations of calcitonin are available for clinical use in the treatment of hypercalcemia and Paget's disease.

## VITAMIN D (CALCIFEROL)

Vitamin D is a fat-soluble vitamin that includes both ergocalciferol (obtained from foods) and cholecalciferol (formed by exposure of skin to sunlight). It functions as a hormone and plays an important role in calcium metabolism. The main action of vitamin D is to raise serum calcium levels by increasing intestinal absorption of dietary calcium and mobilizing calcium from bone. Vitamin D is not physiologically active in the body. It must be converted to an active metabolite (1,25-dihydroxyvitamin D or calcitriol) by a series of reactions in the liver and kidneys. Parathyroid hormone and adequate renal function are required to produce the active metabolite.

The recommended intake of vitamin D is 10 µg (400 units) daily from infancy through 24 years and 5 µg (200 units) for people older than 24 years. Milk that has been fortified with vitamin D is the best food source. Exposure of skin to sunlight is also needed to supply adequate amounts of vitamin D.

Deficiency of vitamin D causes inadequate absorption of calcium and phosphorus. This, in turn, leads to low levels of serum calcium and stimulation of parathyroid hormone secretion, which raises serum calcium levels by moving calcium from bone into serum. In children, this sequence of events produces inadequate mineralization of bone (rickets), a condition now rare in the United States. In adults, vitamin D deficiency causes osteomalacia, a condition characterized by decreased bone density and strength. Osteomalacia is more likely to occur during times of increased need for calcium, such as pregnancy and lactation.

Clinical indications for use of vitamin D supplements include prevention and treatment of rickets and osteomalacia, treatment of hypoparathyroidism, and treatment of chronic hypocalcemia when calcium supplements fail to maintain normal serum calcium levels. The major adverse reaction resulting from high dosage or prolonged administration is hypervitaminosis D. This condition of excessive accumulation of vitamin D produces signs and symptoms of hypercalcemia. The first step in treatment is to stop the administration of vitamin D. Other treatment measures are the same as for hypercalcemia from other causes and are described later in this chapter.

## CALCIUM AND PHOSPHORUS

Calcium and phosphorus are discussed together because they are closely related physiologically. They are both required, as calcium phosphate, in formation and maintenance of bones and teeth. They are also found in many of the same foods, are absorbed together, and are both regulated by parathyroid hormone.

### Calcium

Calcium is the most abundant cation in the body. About 98% of calcium is located in the bones and teeth; the rest is in the extracellular fluid and soft tissues. About half of the total serum calcium is ionized and physiologically active. This seemingly small amount of calcium performs vital functions. Small fluctuations in the amount of ionized calcium have profound effects on body organs. The other half of serum calcium is bound, mostly to serum proteins, and is physiologically inactive. There is constant shifting of calcium among the different forms. This is part of the homeostatic mechanism that acts to maintain serum calcium levels at about 8.5 to 10 mg/100 ml.

Calcium performs vital functions in the body, including the following:

1. Participating in many metabolic processes. Calcium is important in the regulation of:
   a. Cell membrane permeability and function
   b. Nerve cell excitability and transmission of impulses
   c. Muscle cell excitation and coupling, including the electrophysiologic slow calcium channel response in cardiac and smooth muscle
   d. Blood coagulation and platelet adhesion processes
   e. Hormone secretion
   f. Enzyme activity

2. Building and maintaining bones and teeth. Bone calcium is mainly composed of calcium phosphate and calcium carbonate. In addition to these bound forms, a small amount of calcium is available for exchange with serum. This acts as a reserve supply of calcium. Calcium is constantly shifting between bone and serum as bone is formed and broken down. Calcium is taken from the serum and used in the formation of new bone by osteoblast cells; it is transferred from bone to the serum when bone is broken down by osteoclast cells. The latter process is called bone resorption. When serum calcium levels become low, calcium moves into serum at the expense of bone calcium.

The calcium requirement of normal adults is about 1000 mg daily. Increased daily amounts are needed by growing children (1200 mg), pregnant or lactating women (1200 mg), and postmenopausal women who do not take replacement estrogens (1500 mg to prevent osteoporosis).

The best source of calcium is milk or milk products. Three 8-oz glasses of milk daily contain approximately the amount needed by healthy adults. Calcium in milk is readily used by the body because milk also contains lactose and vitamin D, both of which are involved in calcium absorption. Other sources of calcium include vegetables (*e.g.*, broccoli, spinach, kale, mustard greens) and seafood (*e.g.*, clams, oysters).

Only about 30% of dietary calcium is absorbed. Some factors that aid calcium absorption include the presence of vitamin D, increased acidity of gastric secretions, the presence of lactose, moderate amounts of fat, high protein intake, and a physiologic need. Factors that inhibit calcium absorption include the following:

Vitamin D deficiency
High-fat diet, which leads to formation of insoluble calcium salts in the intestine
The presence of oxalic acid (from beet greens, chard), which combines with calcium to form insoluble calcium oxalate in the intestine
Alkalinity of intestinal secretions, which leads to formation of insoluble calcium phosphate
Diarrhea or other conditions of rapid intestinal motility, which do not allow sufficient time for absorption
Immobilization
Mental or emotional stress

Calcium is lost from the body in feces, urine, and sweat. In lactating women, relatively large amounts are lost in breast milk.

## Phosphorus

1. Phosphorus is one of the most important elements in normal body function. Most phosphorus is combined with calcium in bones and teeth as calcium phosphate (about 80%). The remainder is distributed in every body cell and in extracellular fluid. It is combined with carbohydrates, lipids, proteins, and a variety of other compounds.

2. Most phosphorus is located intracellularly (as the phosphate ion), where it performs many metabolic functions:
   a. It is an essential component of deoxyribonucleic acid, ribonucleic acid, and other nucleic acids in body cells. Thus, it is required for cell reproduction and body growth.
   b. It combines with fatty acids to form phospholipids, which are components of all cell membranes in the body. This reaction also prevents excessive amounts of free fatty acids.
   c. It forms a phosphate buffer system, which helps to maintain acid-base balance. When excess hydrogen ions are present in kidney tubules, phosphate combines with them and allows their excretion in urine. At the same time, bicarbonate is retained by the kidneys and contributes to alkalinity of body fluids. Although there are other buffering systems in the body, failure of the phosphate system leads to metabolic acidosis (retained hydrogen ions or acid and lost bicarbonate ions or base).
   d. It is necessary for cell use of glucose and production of energy.
   e. It is necessary for proper function of several B vitamins; that is, the vitamins function as coenzymes in various chemical reactions only when combined with phosphate.

3. Daily requirements for phosphorus are about 800 mg for normal adults and about 1200 mg for growing children and pregnant or lactating women. Phosphorus is widely available in foods. Good sources are milk and dairy products, meat, poultry, fish, eggs, and nuts. There is little risk of phosphorus deficiency with an adequate intake of calcium and protein.

About 70% of dietary phosphorus is absorbed from the gastrointestinal tract. The most efficient absorption occurs when calcium and phosphorus are ingested in approximately equal amounts. Because this equal ratio is present in milk, milk is probably the best source of phosphorus. Generally, factors that increase or decrease calcium absorption act the same way on phosphorus absorption. Vitamin D enhances, but is not essential for, phosphorus absorption. Large amounts of calcium or aluminum in the gastrointestinal tract may combine with phosphate to form insoluble compounds and thereby decrease absorption of phosphorus.

Phosphorus is lost from the body primarily in urine. In people with acute or chronic renal failure, phosphorus intake is restricted because excretion is impaired.

# Hypocalcemia

Hypocalcemia may result from several causes, including inadequate dietary intake of calcium and vitamin D, inadequate absorption of calcium and vitamin D with diarrhea or malabsorption syndromes, hypoparathyroidism, and impaired renal function. Hypocalcemia associated with renal failure is caused by two mechanisms. First, inability to excrete phosphate in urine leads to accumulation of phosphate in the blood (hyperphosphatemia). Because phosphate levels are inversely related to calcium levels, hyperphosphatemia induces hypocalcemia. Second, when kidney function is impaired, vitamin D conversion to its active metabolite is impaired. This results in decreased intestinal absorption of calcium.

Clinical manifestations of hypocalcemia are characterized by increased neuromuscular irritability, which may progress to tetany. Tetany is characterized by numbness and tingling of the lips, fingers, and toes; twitching of facial muscles; spasms of skeletal muscle; carpopedal spasm; laryngospasm; and convulsions. In young children, hypocalcemia may be manifested by convulsions rather than tetany and erroneously diagnosed as epilepsy. This may be a serious error because anticonvulsant drugs used for epilepsy may further decrease serum calcium levels.

## INDIVIDUAL DRUGS USED IN HYPOCALCEMIA

The drugs used to treat hypocalcemia are calcium and vitamin D preparations (Table 26-1). Several calcium salts may be used intravenously for acute hypocalcemia and orally for less severe or chronic hypocalcemia. These preparations differ mainly in the amounts of calcium they contain and the routes by which they may be given. Vitamin D is used in chronic hypocalcemia if calcium preparations alone cannot maintain serum calcium levels within normal range.

## Nursing Process (Hypocalcemia)

### Assessment

- Assess for conditions in which hypocalcemia is likely to occur (*e.g.*, inadequate intake or absorption of calcium and vitamin D).

### TABLE 26-1. DRUGS USED IN HYPOCALCEMIA

| Generic/Trade Name | Routes and Dosage Ranges | |
|---|---|---|
| | *Adults* | *Children* |
| **Calcium Preparations** | | |
| **Calcium carbonate, precipitated** (40% calcium) (Os-Cal 500) | PO 1–1.5 g 3 times daily with meals (maximal daily dose, 8 g) | |
| **Calcium chloride** (27% calcium) | PO 6–8 g daily in 4 divided doses<br>IV 500 mg–1 g (5–10 ml of 10% solution) by slow injection | PO 300 mg/kg per day of a 2% solution in 4 divided doses |
| **Calcium glubionate** (6% calcium) (Neo-Calglucon) | PO 15 ml 3 times daily<br>Pregnancy or lactation, PO 15 ml 4 times daily | PO 10 ml 3 times daily |
| **Calcium gluceptate** (8% calcium) | IV 5–20 ml<br>IM 2–5 ml | IM 2–5 ml |
| **Calcium gluconate** (9% calcium) (Kalcinate) | PO 1–2 g 3 or 4 times daily<br>IV 5–20 ml of 10% solution | PO, IV 500 mg/kg per day in divided doses |
| **Calcium lactate** (13% calcium) | PO 1–3 g 3 times daily with meals | PO 500 mg/kg per day in divided doses |
| **Calcium phosphate dibasic** (30% calcium) (Dical-D) | PO 0.5–1.5 g 2 or 3 times daily with meals | Dosage not established |
| **Vitamin D Preparations** | | |
| **Calcifediol** (Calderol) | PO 50–100 µg daily | Dosage not established |
| **Calcitriol** (Rocaltrol) | PO 0.25 µg daily initially, then adjusted according to serum calcium levels (usual daily maintenance dose, 0.5–1 µg) | |
| **Cholecalciferol** (Delta-D) | PO 400–1000 IU daily | Dosage not established |
| **Dihydrotachysterol** (Hytakerol) | PO 0.8–2.4 mg daily, then decreased for maintenance according to serum calcium levels (usual daily maintenance dose, 0.2–1.0 mg) | |
| **Ergocalciferol (vitamin D)** (Drisdol) | PO 50,000–200,000 units daily initially (average daily maintenance dose, 25,000–100,000 units) | |

- Assess dietary intake of dairy products and other calcium-containing foods.
- Observe for the previously described clinical manifestations.
- Check serum calcium reports for decreased values. Although laboratories differ slightly in normal values, the total serum calcium level is about 8.8 to 10.3 mg/100 ml (SI units 2.2–2.6 mmol/L). About half of the total serum calcium (e.g., 4–5 mg/100 ml) should be free ionized calcium, the physiologically active form. To interpret serum calcium levels accurately, serum albumin levels and acid-base status must be considered. Low serum albumin decreases the total serum level of calcium by decreasing the amount of calcium that is bound to protein. However, the unbound, ionized concentration is normal. Metabolic and respiratory alkalosis increase binding of calcium to serum proteins, thereby maintaining normal total serum calcium but decreasing the ionized values. Conversely, metabolic and respiratory acidosis decrease binding and therefore increase the concentration of ionized calcium.
- Check once daily for *Chvostek's sign*: Tap the facial nerve just below the temple, in front of the ear. If facial muscles twitch, hyperirritability of the nerve and potential tetany are indicated.
- Check for *Trousseau's sign*: Constrict blood circulation in an arm (usually with a blood-pressure cuff) for 3 to 5 minutes. This produces ischemia and increased irritability of peripheral nerves, which causes spasms of the lower arm and hand muscles (carpal spasm) if tetany is present.

### Nursing diagnoses

- Altered Nutrition: Less than Body Requirements with hypocalcemia
- Knowledge Deficit: Recommended daily amounts and dietary sources of calcium and vitamin D
- Knowledge Deficit: Rational use of vitamin and mineral supplements
- High Risk for Injury: Tetany, sedation, seizures from hypocalcemia
- High Risk for Injury: Hypercalcemia related to overuse of supplements
- Constipation with oral calcium supplements

### Planning/Goals

*The client will:*
- Achieve and maintain normal serum levels of calcium
- Increase dietary intake of calcium-containing foods
- Use calcium or vitamin D supplements with the approval and supervision of a health-care provider
- Avoid hypercalcemia from overuse of supplements

### Interventions

Prevent hypocalcemia when possible by assisting clients to maintain an adequate dietary intake of calcium. With an adequate protein and calcium intake, enough phosphorus will also be obtained.
- The best dietary source is milk and other dairy products, including yogurt.
- Unless contraindicated by the client's condition, recommend that adults drink at least two 8-ounce glasses of milk daily. This will furnish about half the daily calcium requirement; the remainder will probably be obtained from other foods.

- Children need about four glasses of milk or an equivalent amount of calcium in milk and other foods to support normal growth and development.
- Pregnant and lactating women also need about four glasses of milk or their equivalents to meet increased needs. Vitamin and mineral supplements are often prescribed during these periods. However, some supplements contain only 250 mg of a calcium salt (equivalent to 8 ounces of milk). This amount does not go very far in meeting a requirement of about 1200 mg.
- Postmenopausal women who take estrogens need the usual adult amount (1000 mg). Those who do not take estrogens need about 1500 mg to prevent or minimize osteoporosis.
- For clients who avoid or minimize their intake of dairy products because of the calories, identify low-calorie sources, such as skim milk and low-fat yogurt.

*Teach clients:*
- Not to take calcium or vitamin D supplements unless recommended by a health-care provider. They are rarely needed if dietary intake is adequate. Taking more than needed to maintain normal body function serves no beneficial purpose. In addition, excessive amounts are potentially more harmful than a minor deficiency.
- If a supplement is recommended, an inexpensive, over-the-counter antacid called Tums contains 200 mg per tablet. Avoid supplements containing bone meal; they may contain lead and other contaminants that are toxic to the human body.
- Exercise, especially if vigorous and weight-bearing, helps to promote and maintain strong bone. Inactivity promotes bone weakening and loss.

### Evaluation

- Check laboratory reports for normal serum calcium levels.
- Interview and observe for relief of symptoms of hypocalcemia
- Interview and observe intake of calcium-containing foods.
- Question about normal calcium requirements and how to meet them.

## Principles of therapy: drugs used in hypocalcemia

1. If hypocalcemia is caused by diarrhea or malabsorption, treatment of the underlying condition will decrease loss of calcium from the body and increase absorption.

2. In severe, acute hypocalcemia, intravenous calcium gluconate or calcium chloride is given. For less acute situations or for long-term treatment of chronic hypocalcemia, oral calcium supplements are preferred. Vitamin D is given also if a calcium preparation alone cannot maintain serum calcium levels within a normal range.

3. When vitamin D is given to treat hypocalcemia, dosage is determined by frequent measurement of serum

calcium levels. Usually, higher doses are given initially, then decreased to smaller doses for maintenance therapy.

## CALCIUM–VITAMIN D COMBINATIONS

Calcium salts and vitamin D are combined in a number of commercial preparations. These are promoted as dietary supplements for children and for women during pregnancy and lactation. There is no evidence that these fixed amounts of calcium and vitamin D meet the dietary needs of most people. Therefore, calcium and vitamin D should be prescribed individually. Also, these mixtures are not indicated for maintenance therapy in chronic hypocalcemia.

## DRUG INTERACTIONS

1. Calcium preparations and digitalis preparations have similar effects on the myocardium. Therefore, if calcium is given to a digitalized client, the risks of digitalis toxicity and cardiac arrhythmias are increased. This combination must be used very cautiously.
2. Oral calcium preparations decrease effects of oral tetracycline drugs by combining with the antibiotic and preventing its absorption. They should not be given at the same time or within 2 to 3 hours of each other.

## USE IN CHILDREN

Hypocalcemia is uncommon in children. If it does develop, principles of using calcium or vitamin D supplements are the same as those in adults. Monitor closely for signs and symptoms of adverse drug effects.

## USE IN OLDER ADULTS

Calcium moves from bone to blood to maintain normal serum levels. In older adults, especially women, demineralization and weakening of bone (osteoporosis) increases risks of fractures. Consequently, older adults need to continue their dietary intake of dairy products and other calcium-containing foods. Calcium supplements are often recommended for postmenopausal women, especially those who do not take estrogen replacement drugs. Overuse of supplements should be avoided because it may cause hypercalcemia.

---

## NURSING ACTIONS: DRUGS USED IN HYPOCALCEMIA

| *Nursing Actions* | *Rationale/Explanation* |
|---|---|
| **1. Administer accurately**<br>**a.** Give oral calcium preparations 30 minutes before meals or at bedtime. | To increase absorption |
| **b.** With IV calcium preparations, inject slowly, over at least 2 minutes, check pulse and blood pressure closely, and preferably monitor the electrocardiogram (ECG). | Arrhythmias and hypotension may occur. Hypercalcemia is indicated on the ECG by a prolonged QT interval associated with an inverted T wave. |
| **c.** Do not mix IV calcium preparations with any other drug in the same syringe. | Calcium reacts with some other drugs and forms a precipitate. |
| **2. Observe for therapeutic effects**<br>**a.** Relief of symptoms of neuromuscular irritability and tetany, such as decreased muscle spasms and decreased paresthesias | |
| **b.** Serum calcium levels within normal range (8.5–10 mg/100 ml) | |
| **c.** Absence of Chvostek's and Trousseau's signs | |
| **3. Observe for adverse effects**<br>**a.** Hypercalcemia:<br><br>(1) Gastrointestinal effects—anorexia, nausea, vomiting, abdominal pain, constipation | |

| *Nursing Actions* | *Rationale/Explanation* |
|---|---|
| (2) Central nervous system (CNS) effects—apathy, poor memory, depression, drowsiness, disorientation, coma | |
| (3) Other effects—weakness and decreased tone in skeletal and smooth muscles, dysphagia, polyuria, polydipsia, cardiac arrhythmias | |
| (4) Increased serum calcium | |
| **b.** Hypervitaminosis D—produces hypercalcemia and the clinical manifestations listed above | This is most likely to occur with chronic ingestion of 50,000 or more units of vitamin D daily. In children, accidental ingestion may lead to acute toxicity. |
| **4. Observe for drug interactions**<br>**a.** Drugs that *increase* effects of calcium: | |
| (1) Vitamin D | Increases intestinal absorption of calcium from both dietary and supplemental drug sources |
| **b.** Drugs that *decrease* effects of calcium: | |
| (1) Adrenocorticosteroids (prednisone, others), calcitonin, mithramycin, and phosphates | These drugs lower serum calcium levels by various mechanisms. They are used in the treatment of hypercalcemia and are discussed further in the next section of this chapter. |
| (2) Antacids | Oral calcium preparations are more soluble and better absorbed in an acid medium. Antacids decrease acidity of gastric secretions and therefore may decrease absorption of calcium. |
| (3) Laxatives | These drugs decrease absorption of calcium from the intestinal tract by increasing motility. This allows less time for calcium absorption. |
| **c.** Drugs that *increase* effects of vitamin D: Thiazide diuretics | Thiazide diuretics administered to hypoparathyroid clients may cause hypercalcemia (potentiate vitamin D effects). |
| **d.** Drugs that *decrease* effects of vitamin D: | |
| (1) Anticonvulsants (*e.g.*, phenytoin [Dilantin], primidone [Mysoline], phenobarbital) | These drugs accelerate and change the metabolism of vitamin D in the liver. As a result, vitamin D deficiency, hypocalcemia, and rickets or osteomalacia are likely to develop in clients receiving anticonvulsant drugs for seizure disorders. These problems can be prevented by increasing intake of vitamin D. |
| (2) Cholestyramine resin (Questran) | May decrease intestinal absorption of calcitriol (Rocaltrol) |
| (3) Mineral oil | Mineral oil is a fat and therefore combines with fat-soluble vitamins, such as vitamin D, and prevents its absorption from the gastrointestinal tract. |
| **5. Teach clients**<br>**a.** If calcium or vitamin D is prescribed, take as directed. | To obtain the greatest therapeutic effect with the least likelihood of adverse effects from overdosage |
| **b.** With chronic hypocalcemia, increase dietary intake of calcium and vitamin D with milk and other dairy products. Note that foods that contain oxalic acid (*e.g.*, spinach, rhubarb) and phytic acid (*e.g.*, bran) may decrease absorption of calcium. | |
| **c.** Report signs and symptoms of hypercalcemia. | See 3(a) above. |

# Hypercalcemia

Hypercalcemia occurs with hyperparathyroidism, excessive ingestion of vitamin D, malignant neoplasms, prolonged immobilization, adrenocortical insufficiency, and ingestion of thiazide diuretics, estrogens, and lithium. In hospitalized clients, cancer is a common cause of hypercalcemia, especially carcinomas (of the breast, lung, head and neck, or kidney) and multiple myeloma. Cancer stimulates bone resorption or breakdown, which increases serum calcium levels. Increased urine output leads to fluid volume deficit. This leads, in turn, to increased reabsorption of calcium in renal tubules and decreased renal excretion of calcium. Decreased renal excretion potentiates hypercalcemia.

Clinical manifestations are caused by the decreased ability of nerves to respond to stimuli and the decreased ability of muscles to contract and relax. Hypercalcemia has a depressant effect on nerve and muscle function.

Gastrointestinal problems with hypercalcemia include anorexia, nausea, vomiting, constipation, and abdominal pain. CNS problems include apathy, depression, poor memory, headache, and drowsiness. Severe hypercalcemia may produce lethargy, syncope, disorientation, hallucinations, coma, and death. Other signs and symptoms include weakness and decreased tone in skeletal and smooth muscle, dysphagia, polyuria, polyphagia, and cardiac arrhythmias. In addition, calcium may be deposited in various tissues, such as the conjunctiva, cornea, and kidneys. Calcium deposits in the kidneys (renal calculi) may lead to irreversible damage and impairment of function.

## INDIVIDUAL DRUGS USED IN HYPERCALCEMIA

The agents used in hypercalcemia belong to several therapeutic classes and act by different mechanisms to lower serum calcium levels.

**Calcitonin-salmon** (Calcimar) is used in the treatment of hypercalcemia, Paget's disease, and postmenopausal osteoporosis. In hypercalcemia, calcitonin lowers serum calcium levels by inhibiting bone resorption (*i.e.* movement of calcium from bone to serum). It is most likely to be effective in hypercalcemia caused by hyperparathyroidism, prolonged immobilization, or certain malignant neoplasms. In acute hypercalcemia, calcitonin may be used along with other measures to lower serum calcium levels rapidly. A single injection of calcitonin decreases serum calcium levels in about 2 hours; effects last about 6 to 8 hours. The amount of the decrease is unpredictable and varies extensively among clients. In chronic hypercalcemia, it may lose its effectiveness after several weeks.

Paget's disease is a disorder characterized by an ab-

normal and rapid rate of bone formation and breakdown. Calcitonin slows the rate of bone turnover, improves bone lesions on radiologic examination, and relieves bone pain. In postmenopausal osteoporosis, calcitonin prevents further bone loss and increases bone mass in the presence of adequate calcium and vitamin D.

**Calcitonin-human** (Cibacalcin) is a synthetic preparation with the same number and sequence of amino acids as human calcitonin. It is approved for use in Paget's disease. Compared to calcitonin-salmon, calcitonin-human is more likely to cause nausea and facial flushing and less likely to cause antibody formation and allergic reactions.

### Calcitonin-salmon

#### *Routes and dosage ranges*

*Adults:* Hypercalcemia, SC, IM 4 IU/kg q12h; can be increased after 1 or 2 days to 8 IU/kg q12h; maximum dose, 8 IU/kg q6h

Paget's disease, SC, IM 50–100 IU/d

Postmenopausal osteoporosis, SC, IM 100 IU/d (along with supplemental calcium [1500 mg] and vitamin D [400 units] daily)

### Calcitonin-human

#### *Route and dosage range*

*Adults:* Paget's disease, SC 0.5 mg/d

**Etidronate** (Didronel) and **pamidronate** (Aredia) are chemically related substances that, like calcitonin, lower serum calcium levels by inhibiting calcium resorption from bone. Oral etidronate is used in the symptomatic treatment of Paget's disease and heterotopic ossification (growth of bone in abnormal locations) associated with spinal cord injury or total hip replacement. Intravenous etidronate and pamidronate are used in the treatment of malignancy-associated hypercalcemia. Etidronate is excreted by the kidneys, and dosage must be reduced in the presence of renal insufficiency.

### Etidronate

#### *Routes and dosage ranges*

*Adults:* Paget's disease, PO 5 mg/kg per day for up to 6 months. The course of therapy may be repeated if symptoms recur.

Heterotopic ossification caused by spinal cord injury, PO 20 mg/kg per day for 2 weeks, then 10 mg/kg per day for 10 weeks

Heterotopic ossification associated with total hip replacement, PO 20 mg/kg per day for 1 month preoperatively and continued for 3 months postoperatively

Hypercalcemia of malignancy, IV 7.5 mg/kg per day, diluted in at least 250 ml of 0.9% sodium chloride solution and infused over at least 2 hours daily for 3 successive days

## Pamidronate

### Route and dosage ranges

*Adults:* Hypercalcemia, IV 60–90 mg, reconstituted according to manufacturer's directions, diluted in 1000 ml of 0.9% or 0.45% sodium chloride solution and infused over 24 hours

**Furosemide** (Lasix) is a potent diuretic that increases calcium excretion in urine by preventing its reabsorption in renal tubules. Furosemide can be given IV for rapid effects in hypercalcemic crises or orally for nonemergency situations. (See Chap. 59 for further discussion of diuretic drug therapy.)

### Route and dosage ranges

*Adults:* IV 80–100 mg q2h until a diuretic response is obtained or other treatment measures are initiated
*Children:* IV 20–40 mg q4h until a diuretic response is obtained or other treatment measures are initiated

**Gallium** (Ganite), like calcitonin, etidronate, and pamidronate, inhibits calcium resorption from bone. It is used to treat hypercalcemia of malignancy that does not respond to hydration. It is excreted mainly by the kidneys and contraindicated in severe renal impairment (serum creatinine above 2.5 mg/100 ml).

### Route and dosage ranges

*Adults:* IV 200 mg/m², diluted in 1000 ml of 0.9% sodium chloride or 5% dextrose injection and infused over 24 hours daily for 5 consecutive days

**Hydrocortisone** (Solu-Cortef and others) and **prednisone** (Deltasone and others) are adrenal corticosteroid drugs that may be used to treat hypercalcemia. Because all the glucocorticoids have similar effects, others may be used. In the treatment of hypercalcemia, corticosteroid drugs antagonize effects of vitamin D and therefore decrease intestinal absorption of calcium. They are probably most useful in treating hypercalcemia resulting from excess vitamin D, sarcoidosis, and renal insufficiency. They also may be useful in treating hypercalcemia due to malignant neoplasms (*e.g.,* multiple myeloma, leukemia, lymphomas) by decreasing bone resorption. High doses or prolonged administration of corticosteroids leads to serious adverse reactions. (See Chap. 24 for further discussion of corticosteroid drug therapy.)

## Hydrocortisone

### Route and dosage range

*Adults:* IM, IV 100–500 mg/d

## Prednisone

### Route and dosage range

*Adults:* PO 40–60 mg/d initially, then gradually reduced

**Plicamycin** (Mithracin) probably lowers serum calcium levels by blocking calcium resorption from bone. It is used to treat malignancy-associated hypercalcemia that does not respond to hydration.

### Route and dosage range

*Adults:* IV 25 µg/kg per day for 3 or 4 days, repeated at intervals of 1 wk or more if necessary

**Phosphate salts** (Neutra-Phos) lower serum calcium levels by increasing tissue uptake of calcium. They are effective in the treatment of hypercalcemia of any etiology. A potential adverse reaction to phosphates is calcification of soft tissues due to deposition of calcium phosphate. This can lead to severe impairment of function in the kidneys and other organs. Phosphates should be given only when hypercalcemia is accompanied by hypophosphatemia. Neutra-Phos is a combination of sodium phosphate and potassium phosphate.

### Route and dosage range

*Adults:* PO 1–2 tablets three or four times daily, or contents of 1 capsule mixed with 75 ml of water four times daily

**0.9% Sodium chloride injection** (normal saline) is an IV solution containing water, sodium, and chloride. It is included here because it is the treatment of choice for hypercalcemia and, along with furosemide, is usually effective. The sodium contained in the solution inhibits the reabsorption of calcium in renal tubules and thereby increases urinary excretion of calcium. The solution also relieves the dehydration caused by vomiting and polyuria, and it dilutes the calcium concentration of serum and urine. Saline, 4 to 6 L/d, is given first to hydrate the client, and then furosemide is given.

## Nursing Process (Hypercalcemia)

### Assessment

- Assess dietary intake of calcium and vitamin D.
- Assess for conditions in which hypercalcemia is likely to occur (*e.g.,* cancer, prolonged immobilization).

- Observe for signs and symptoms of hypercalcemia in clients at risk. Electrocardiogram changes indicative of hypercalcemia include a shortened QT interval and an inverted T wave.
- Assess laboratory reports of serum calcium levels for increases (above 10 mg/100 ml total, above 5 mg/100 ml ionized calcium, approximately). To determine whether an increase is significant, consider serum albumin and acid-base balance as described earlier in this chapter.
- If Paget's disease is suspected, assess for an elevated serum alkaline phosphatase and abnormal bone scan reports.

### Nursing diagnoses

- Altered Thought Processes: Confusion with hypercalcemia
- Altered Nutrition: More than Body Requirements with hypercalcemia
- Knowledge Deficit: Disease process and drug therapy for hypercalcemia
- High Risk for Fluid Volume Excess related to large amounts of 0.9% sodium chloride solution used to lower serum calcium levels
- Anxiety related to disease process and treatment
- High Risk for Injury: Hypocalcemia from aggressive treatment of hypercalcemia

### Planning/Goals

*The client will:*
- Achieve normal serum calcium levels
- Comply with instructions for safe drug usage
- Be monitored closely for therapeutic and adverse effects of drugs used to treat hypercalcemia
- Be assisted in reducing dietary calcium intake
- Comply with procedures for follow-up treatment of chronic hypercalcemia
- Avoid preventable adverse effects of treatment for acute hypercalcemia

### Interventions

Prevent or minimize effects of hypercalcemia by assisting clients to decrease dietary calcium intake and prevent precipitation of calcium in the kidneys (formation of renal calculi).
- The most effective measure to decrease dietary calcium is to avoid milk and milk products.
- Antacids containing calcium (*e.g.,* Tums) also should be avoided.
- Measures to decrease formation of renal calculi include forcing fluids to about 3000 to 4000 ml/d and preventing urinary tract infections.

*Teach clients:*
- Expected results of treatment for hypercalcemia
- Nondrug measures to decrease risk of recurrence
- Correct drug administration, including injection techniques if indicated
- To report signs and symptoms of either hypercalcemia or hypocalcemia to a health-care provider

### Evaluation

- Check laboratory reports of serum calcium levels for normal values.
- Interview and observe for decreased intake of dairy products and other calcium-containing foods.
- Interview and observe for accurate drug usage and compliance with follow-up procedures.
- Interview and observe for therapeutic and adverse drug effects.

## Principles of therapy: drugs used in hypercalcemia

Treatment of hypercalcemia depends largely on its cause and severity.

1. When hypercalcemia is caused by an adenoma of a parathyroid gland, surgical excision is indicated. When it is caused by malignancy, excision or treatment is likely to decrease serum calcium levels. When it is caused by excessive intake of vitamin D, the vitamin D preparation should be stopped immediately.

   Clients at risk for hypercalcemia should be monitored for early signs and symptoms so that treatment can be started before severe hypercalcemia develops.
2. Acute hypercalcemia is a medical emergency and requires immediate treatment. The priority is fluid replacement and rehydration. This need can be met by intravenous (IV) saline infusion (0.9% or 0.45% NaCl), 4000 ml/d or more if kidney function is adequate. At the same time, calcium intake is limited. After rehydration, a diuretic, such as furosemide, is usually given IV to increase renal excretion of calcium and to prevent fluid overload. Because sodium, potassium, and water are also lost in the urine, these must be replaced in the IV fluids.

   With mild hypercalcemia, most clients respond to the above treatment, and further drug therapy is not needed. With moderate to severe hypercalcemia of malignancy, etidronate, gallium, or pamidronate may be given. Phosphates should not be used unless hypophosphatemia is present. They are also contraindicated in clients with persistent urinary tract infections and an alkaline urine because calcium phosphate kidney stones are likely to form in such cases.
3. Chronic hypercalcemia requires treatment of the underlying disease process and measures to control serum calcium levels (*e.g.,* a low-calcium diet, high fluid intake, and mobilization). Oral phosphate administration may help if other measures are ineffective.

4. Serum calcium levels should be measured to monitor effects of therapy. In acute hypercalcemia, measure them frequently.
5. For clients with severely impaired renal function who develop hypercalcemia, hemodialysis or peritoneal dialysis with a calcium-free solution is effective and safe.

## USE IN CHILDREN

Guidelines for treating hypercalcemia in children are essentially the same as those for adults, with drug dosages adjusted. Safety, effectiveness, and dosages of etidronate, gallium, and pamidronate have not been established.

## USE IN OLDER ADULTS

Older adults are likely to have chronic cardiovascular and other disorders that may be aggravated by hypercalcemia and its treatment. During infusion of 0.9% sodium chloride (usually 150–200 ml/hr) for acute hypercalcemia, observe older adults closely for signs of congestive heart failure, pulmonary edema, and hypertension.

# NURSING ACTIONS: DRUGS USED IN HYPERCALCEMIA

| *Nursing Actions* | *Rationale/Explanation* |
|---|---|
| **1. Administer accurately** | |
| a. With calcitonin, give at bedtime. | To decrease nausea and discomfort from flushing |
| b. With oral etidronate, give as a single dose or in divided doses. Avoid administration within 2 hours of ingesting dairy products, antacids, or vitamin or mineral supplements. | If gastrointestinal (GI) symptoms occur with the single dose, divided doses may relieve them. Substances containing calcium or other metals decrease absorption of etidronate. |
| With IV etidronate, gallium, and pamidronate, follow manufacturers' instructions. | The drugs require reconstitution and diluting with IV fluids. |
| c. With furosemide, give IV or orally. | |
| d. With hydrocortisone: | |
| (1) Give intravenously (IV) or intramuscularly (IM). | In acute hypercalcemia, IV administration (by bolus injection or by addition to 5% dextrose in water or NaCl injection, given as an IV infusion over several hours) is preferred. |
| (2) Be sure to have the appropriate drug preparation for the ordered route. | Several commercial preparations of hydrocortisone are available. Some are given IV, some IM, and some by either route. Do not assume that any preparation can be given by both routes of administration. |
| (3) Decrease dosage gradually—do not discontinue abruptly. | Abrupt discontinuation can lead to acute adrenal insufficiency. |
| e. With plicamycin, give IV for a limited number of doses. See package insert for specific instructions. | |
| f. With phosphate salts, mix powder forms with water for oral administration. See package inserts for specific instructions. | |
| **2. Observe for therapeutic effects** | |
| a. Decreased serum calcium level | Calcitonin lowers serum calcium levels in approximately 2 hours after injection, and effects last 6 to 8 hours. Corticosteroids require 10 to 14 days to lower serum calcium. Plicamycin lowers serum calcium levels within 24 to 48 hours, but effects last only 3 to 4 days. |

*(continued)*

| *Nursing Actions* | *Rationale/Explanation* |
|---|---|
| **b.** Decreased signs and symptoms of hypercalcemia | |
| **c.** Decreased signs and symptoms of Paget's disease | Decreased serum alkaline phosphatase and radiologic improvement of bone lesions may require several months. Neurologic improvement may require 1 year or more. |
| **3. Observe for adverse effects**<br>**a.** Hypocalcemia | Hypocalcemia may result from vigorous treatment of hypercalcemia, especially with etidronate, gallium, and pamidronate. This can be minimized by monitoring serum calcium levels frequently and adjusting drug dosages and other treatments. |
| **b.** With calcitonin, observe for nausea, vomiting, tissue irritation at injection sites, and allergic reactions. | Adverse reactions are usually mild and transient. |
| **c.** With etidronate and pamidronate, observe for anorexia, nausea, diarrhea, bone pain, fever, and fluid overload. | Adverse effects are more frequent and more severe at higher doses. |
| **d.** With furosemide, observe for dehydration, hypokalemia, hypomagnesemia, and other fluid and electrolyte imbalances. | As furosemide exerts its therapeutic effect of removing excess calcium from the body by increased urine output, water and other electrolytes are lost as well. Adverse reactions can be prevented by avoiding overdosage of furosemide and by careful replacement of the water and electrolytes lost in the urine. Frequent measurements of serum electrolytes help determine amounts of replacement fluids and electrolytes needed. |
| **e.** With gallium, observe for renal impairment, as indicated by increasing blood urea nitrogen and serum creatinine levels. | Nephrotoxicity reportedly develops in approximately 12% of recipients. |
| **f.** With hydrocortisone and prednisone, see Chapter 24. | Adrenal corticosteroids may cause many adverse reactions, especially with high doses or prolonged administration. |
| **g.** With plicamycin, observe for bone marrow depression, nausea, vomiting, and impaired liver function. | These adverse reactions may occur but are much less likely with the small doses used for hypercalcemia than with the large doses used for malignant neoplasms. |
| **h.** With phosphates, observe for nausea, vomiting, and diarrhea. | |
| **4. Observe for drug interactions**<br>**a.** With calcitonin, testosterone and other androgens *increase* effects; parathyroid hormone *decreases* effects. | Androgens and calcitonin have additive effects on calcium retention and inhibition of bone resorption (movement of calcium from bone to serum). Parathyroid hormone antagonizes or opposes calcitonin. Parathyroid hormone *increases* serum calcium concentration, while calcitonin *decreases* it. |
| **b.** With gallium, aminoglycoside antibiotics (*e.g.*, gentamicin), amphotericin B, and other nephrotoxic drugs increase nephrotoxic effects. | |
| **c.** With hydrocortisone and prednisone, see Chapter 24. | |
| **d.** With plicamycin, antineoplastic drugs that cause bone marrow depression (see Chapter 67) increase effects. | |
| **e.** With phosphate salts, avoid concomitant use of antacids containing aluminum and magnesium. | Aluminum and magnesium may combine with phosphate and thereby prevent its absorption and therapeutic effect. |

| *Nursing Actions* | *Rationale/Explanation* |
|---|---|
| **5. Teach clients**<br>**a.** Maintain a low-calcium diet by limiting intake of dairy products. | One serving of milk, cheese, or other dairy product plus fruits and vegetables furnish a daily calcium intake of about 400 mg. |
| **b.** Drink 3 to 4 quarts of fluid daily if able. | To keep the urine dilute. This helps to prevent formation of kidney stones and urinary tract infections. |
| **c.** Report any signs of cystitis, such as burning or discomfort with urination. | Infections in the urinary tract can increase kidney stone formation. If they occur, early treatment is needed. |

## Review and Application Exercises

1. What are major physiologic functions of calcium?
2. What is the normal serum level of calcium?
3. What are some nursing interventions to prevent hypocalcemia?
4. What signs and symptoms may indicate hypocalcemia?
5. How is hypocalcemia treated?
6. What signs and symptoms may indicate hypercalcemia?
7. How is hypercalcemia treated?

## Selected References

Burrell, L. O. (1992). Fluid, electrolyte, and acid-base balances and imbalances and related nursing management. In L. O. Burrell (Ed.), *Adult nursing in hospital and community settings* (pp. 100–140). Norwalk, CT: Appleton & Lange.

Cuddy, P. G. (1992). Fluid and electrolyte disorders. In M.A. Koda-Kimble & L. Y Young (Eds.), *Applied therapeutics: The clinical use of drugs* (5th ed.) (pp. 28-1–28-21). Vancouver, WA: Applied Therapeutics.

Davis, J. R., & Sherer, K. (1994). *Applied nutrition and diet therapy for nurses* (2nd ed.). Philadelphia: W.B. Saunders.

Eschleman, M. M. (1991). *Introductory nutrition and diet therapy* (2nd ed.). Philadelphia: J.B. Lippincott.

Guyton, A. C. (1991). *Textbook of medical physiology* (8th ed.). Philadelphia: W.B. Saunders.

Juneau, B. (1992). Normal and altered fluid and electrolyte balance. In B. L. Bullock & P. P. Rosendahl (Eds.), *Pathophysiology: Adaptations and alterations in function* (3rd ed.) (pp. 178–194). Philadelphia: J.B. Lippincott.

Lobaugh, B., & Drezner M. K. (1992). Evaluation of hypercalcemia and hypocalcemia. In W. N. Kelley (Ed.), *Textbook of internal medicine* (2nd ed.) (pp. 2115–2121). Philadelphia: J.B. Lippincott.

### CHAPTER 27

# Antidiabetic Drugs

There are two types of antidiabetic drugs: insulin and oral sulfonylurea agents. Because these drugs are used to lower blood glucose, they are also called hypoglycemic agents. Diabetes mellitus is a common, complex disorder. To understand clinical usage of antidiabetic drugs, it is necessary to understand the characteristics of endogenous insulin, diabetes mellitus, and the drugs.

## Endogenous insulin

Insulin is a protein hormone (51 amino acids in two chemically linked chains) secreted by beta cells in the pancreas. The average adult pancreas secretes a basal amount of approximately 0.5 to 1 unit/h and additional amounts after meals or when the blood sugar level exceeds 100 mg/100 ml, with an average daily secretion of about 50 units.

Insulin is secreted into the bloodstream, circulates mainly in an unbound form, has a short plasma half-life of about 6 minutes, is cleared from circulating blood within 10 to 15 minutes, and is transported to most body cells. At the cellular level, insulin binds with receptors on the surface of the cell membrane to produce an insulin-receptor complex, which then alters cellular metabolism by activating some intracellular enzymes and inactivating others. As a result, the cell membrane becomes highly permeable to glucose and allows its rapid entry into the cells. The cell membrane also becomes more permeable to amino acids and electrolytes, such as potassium, magnesium, and phosphate ions. The movement of these substances into and out of the cell produces additional changes in cellular metabolism. The insulin that does not combine with receptors is metabo-lized in the liver (about 50%), kidneys (about 25%), plasma, and muscles.

Physiologically, insulin plays a major role in metabolism of carbohydrate, fat, and protein. These foodstuffs are broken down into molecules of glucose, lipids, and amino acids, respectively. These molecules enter the cells and are converted to energy for cellular activities. The energy can be used immediately or converted to storage forms for later use. When carrying out its metabolic functions, the overall effect of insulin is to lower blood glucose levels, primarily by the following mechanisms:

1. In the liver, insulin acts to *decrease* breakdown of glycogen (glycogenolysis), formation of new glucose from fatty acids and amino acids (gluconeogenesis), and formation of ketone bodies (ketogenesis). At the same time, it acts to *increase* synthesis and storage of glycogen and fatty acids.
2. In adipose tissue, insulin acts to *decrease* breakdown of fat (lipolysis) and to *increase* production of glycerol and fatty acids.
3. In muscle tissue, insulin acts to *decrease* protein breakdown and amino acid output and to *increase* amino acid uptake, protein synthesis, and glycogen synthesis.

### EFFECTS OF INSULIN ON CARBOHYDRATE METABOLISM

Specific effects of insulin on carbohydrate metabolism include the following:

1. It increases glucose transport into most body cells. Complete lack of insulin allows transport of about one fourth the normal amount of glucose. Insulin

Anne Collins Abrams: CLINICAL DRUG THERAPY, Fourth Edition.
© 1995 J.B. Lippincott Company.

facilitates glucose transport into skeletal muscle, adipose tissue, the heart, and some smooth muscle organs, such as the uterus. It does not increase glucose transport into brain cells, red blood cells, intestinal mucosal cells, or tubular epithelial cells of the kidney.
2. It regulates glucose metabolism and homeostasis.

The main goal of glucose metabolism is to produce energy for cellular functions. If excess glucose is present after this need is met, it is converted to glycogen and stored for future energy needs or converted to fat and stored. The excess glucose transported to liver cells is converted to fat only after glycogen stores have been saturated. When insulin is absent or blood glucose levels are low, these stored forms of glucose can be reconverted. The liver is especially important in restoring blood sugar levels by breaking down glycogen or by forming new glucose.

## EFFECTS OF INSULIN ON FAT METABOLISM

Specific effects of insulin on fat metabolism include the following:

1. Insulin promotes transport of glucose into fat cells. Once inside the cell, glucose is broken down. One of the breakdown products is alpha-glycerophosphate, which combines with fatty acids to form triglycerides. This is the mechanism by which insulin promotes fat storage.
2. When insulin is lacking, fat is not stored in the fat cells. Instead, it is released into the bloodstream in the form of free fatty acids. Blood concentrations of other lipids (triglycerides, cholesterol, phospholipids) are also increased. The high blood lipid concentration probably accounts for the atherosclerosis that tends to develop early and progress more rapidly in people with diabetes mellitus. Also, when more fatty acids are released than the body can use as fuel, some fatty acids are converted into ketone bodies. Excessive amounts of ketones produce acidosis and coma.

## EFFECTS OF INSULIN ON PROTEIN METABOLISM

Effects of insulin on protein metabolism and growth include the following:

1. Insulin increases the total amount of body protein by increasing transport of amino acids into cells and synthesis of protein within the cells. The basic mechanism of these effects is unknown.
2. Insulin potentiates the effects of growth hormone.

3. Lack of insulin causes protein depletion and breakdown into amino acids. These amino acids are released into the bloodstream and transported to the liver for energy or gluconeogenesis. These proteins are not replaced by synthesis of new proteins. The overall consequences of protein wasting include abnormal functioning of many body organs, severe weakness, and weight loss.

# Diabetes mellitus

## CHARACTERISTICS

Diabetes mellitus is a chronic systemic disease characterized by metabolic and vascular abnormalities. Metabolic problems occur early in the disease process and are related to changes in the metabolism of carbohydrate, fat, and protein. One of the primary clinical manifestations of disordered metabolism is hyperglycemia. Vascular problems include rapid development and progression of atherosclerosis throughout the body and changes in small blood vessels, which especially affect the retina and kidneys. Clinical manifestations of vascular disorders may include hypertension, myocardial infarction, stroke, retinopathy, blindness, nephropathy, and peripheral vascular disease.

## CLASSIFICATIONS

The two major classifications of diabetes mellitus are type I and type II. Although both types are characterized by hyperglycemia, they differ significantly in onset, course, treatment, and pathologic changes. Secondary diabetes may be induced by certain disease processes, certain drugs, and pregnancy.

### Type I

Type I, or insulin-dependent, diabetes mellitus is thought to be a genetically related autoimmune disorder characterized by the production of antibodies against pancreatic beta cells and the body's own insulin. The anti-beta cell antibodies produce an inflammatory reaction in the beta cell area that gradually destroys the cells and reduces insulin secretion. When 10% or fewer functioning beta cells remain, hyperglycemia and other symptoms of diabetes develop. Eventually, all the beta cells are destroyed, and no insulin is produced. The anti-insulin antibodies destroy or decrease the effectiveness of insulin.

Type I diabetes may occur at any age but usually starts before 20 years of age. It generally has a sudden onset; produces more severe symptoms; is more difficult to control (*i.e.*, it tends to be labile or brittle); produces a high incidence of complications, such as diabetic keto-acidosis (DKA) and renal failure; and requires administration of exogenous insulin. Only 5% of diabetics have type I diabetes.

## Type II

Type II, or non–insulin-dependent, diabetes mellitus (NIDDM) involves insulin resistance rather than an insulin deficiency. In fact, many people have normal or high blood levels of insulin. Their symptoms are thought to result from a defect in insulin receptors (*e.g.*, low numbers or impaired binding capacity) or a defect in insulin-receptor effects on cellular metabolism. When the number of insulin receptors in muscle, adipose, and other target tissues declines, available insulin may not bind with enough cellular receptors to perform its metabolic functions.

Obesity is considered to be a major cause of type II diabetes. With obesity and chronic ingestion of excess calories, more insulin is required. The increased need leads to prolonged stimulation and eventual "fatigue" of pancreatic beta cells. As a result, the cells become less responsive to elevated blood sugar levels and less able to produce enough insulin to meet metabolic needs.

Type II diabetes may occur at any age but usually starts after 40 years of age. It usually has a gradual onset, produces less severe symptoms initially, is easier to control (tends to be more stable), causes less DKA and renal failure but more myocardial infarctions and strokes, and does not necessarily require exogenous insulin, because endogenous insulin is still produced by pancreatic beta cells. Thus, insulin may be present but unable to act effectively to lower blood sugar. Approximately 90% of diabetics have type II diabetes; 20% to 30% of them require exogenous insulin.

## ETIOLOGY

Disease-induced diabetes mellitus can result from any condition that damages or removes pancreatic beta cells. In addition to the autoimmune process described previously, such conditions include cancer, pancreatitis, surgical excision of pancreatic tissue, and viral infections.

Hormone-induced diabetes may result from excessive amounts of some hormones, whether from endogenous oversecretion or from excessive administration of exogenous hormones. These include adrenal corticosteroids, growth hormone, glucagon, and thyroid hormone.

Other diabetogenic drugs, in addition to certain hormones, include diazoxide, epinephrine, thiazide diuretics, phenothiazine antipsychotic drugs, propranolol, and phenytoin.

Gestational diabetes is a type of glucose intolerance that develops during pregnancy in women previously unknown to be diabetic. It occurs in about 2% of pregnancies and requires insulin therapy to decrease risks of birth defects. It usually subsides after delivery, but as many as 30% of these women are estimated to develop type II diabetes within 10 to 15 years.

## SIGNS AND SYMPTOMS

Most signs and symptoms of diabetes mellitus stem from a relative or absolute lack of insulin and the subsequent metabolic abnormalities. The incidence and severity of clinical manifestations are correlated with the amount of effective insulin. In type I diabetes, insulin secretion is absent or severely impaired. Clinical signs and symptoms may be precipitated by infection, rapid growth, pregnancy, or other factors that increase demand for insulin. In type II diabetes, insulin is secreted but is inadequate or ineffective, especially when insulin demand is increased by obesity, pregnancy, aging, or other factors. In many people, signs and symptoms occur with obesity and subside with normal weight.

Most early manifestations result from disordered carbohydrate metabolism, which causes excess glucose to accumulate in the blood (hyperglycemia). Hyperglycemia produces glucosuria, which in turn produces polydipsia, polyuria, dehydration, and polyphagia.

Glucosuria usually appears when the blood glucose level is about twice the normal value and the kidneys receive more glucose than can be reabsorbed. However, renal threshold varies, and the amount of glucose lost in the urine does not accurately reflect blood glucose. In very young people, glucose tends to appear in urine at much lower or even normal blood glucose levels. In older people, the ability of the kidneys to excrete excess glucose from the blood is decreased. Therefore, some older people can have rather high blood glucose levels with little or no glucose appearing in the urine.

When large amounts of glucose are present, water is pulled into the renal tubule. This results in a greatly increased urine output (polyuria). The excessive loss of fluid in urine (osmotic diuresis) leads to increased thirst (polydipsia) and, if fluid intake is inadequate, to fluid volume deficit (dehydration). Dehydration also occurs because high blood glucose levels increase osmotic pressure in the bloodstream, and fluid is pulled out of the cells in the body's attempt to regain homeostasis.

Polyphagia (increased appetite) occurs because the body cannot use ingested foods. Many people with diabetes lose weight because of abnormal metabolism.

## COMPLICATIONS

Complications of diabetes mellitus are common and potentially disabling or life-threatening. They are attributed to insulin deficiency and the resultant metabolic abnormalities. These metabolic abnormalities, especially those associated with hyperglycemia, can cause early, acute complications, such as DKA or nonketotic hyperosmolar coma. Eventually, metabolic abnormalities lead to changes in structure and function of blood vessels and other body tissues.

1. **Ketoacidosis.** This acute, life-threatening complication of diabetes occurs with severe insulin deficiency. In the absence of insulin, glucose cannot be used by body cells for energy, and fat is mobilized from adipose tissue to furnish a fuel source. The mobilized fat circulates in the bloodstream, from which it is extracted by the liver and broken down into glycerol and fatty acids. The fatty acids are further changed in the liver to ketone bodies (acetoacetic acid, acetone, beta-hydroxybutyric acid), which then enter the bloodstream and are circulated to body cells for metabolic conversion to energy, carbon dioxide, and water.

Owing to these metabolic abnormalities, clinical signs and symptoms develop rather rapidly because ketone bodies tend to be produced more rapidly than body cells can use them. Thus, they accumulate and produce acidemia (a drop in blood pH and an increase in blood hydrogen ions). The body attempts to buffer the acidic hydrogen ions by exchanging them for intracellular potassium ions. Thus, hydrogen ions enter body cells, and potassium ions leave the cells to be excreted in the urine. Another attempt to remove excess acid involves the lungs. Deep, labored respirations, called Kussmaul respirations, eliminate more carbon dioxide and prevent formation of carbonic acid. A third attempt to regain homeostasis involves the kidneys, which excrete some of the ketones, thereby producing acetone in the urine.

DKA worsens as the compensatory mechanisms fail. Clinical signs and symptoms vary and become progressively more severe. Early ones include blurred vision, anorexia, nausea and vomiting, thirst, and polyuria. Later ones include drowsiness, which progresses to stupor and coma, Kussmaul breathing, dehydration and other signs of fluid and electrolyte imbalances, and decreased blood pressure, increased pulse, and other signs of shock.

2. **Hyperglycemic hyperosmolar nonketotic coma.** This is another type of diabetic coma that is potentially life threatening. It is relatively rare and carries a high mortality rate. The term *hyperosmolar* refers to an excessive amount of glucose, electrolytes, and other solutes in the blood in relation to the amount of water.

Like DKA, hyperosmolar coma is characterized by hyperglycemia, which leads to osmotic diuresis and resultant thirst, polyuria, dehydration, and electrolyte losses, as well as neurologic signs ranging from drowsiness to stupor to coma. Additional clinical problems may include hypovolemic shock, thrombosis, renal problems, or stroke. Hyperosmolar coma differs from DKA because it occurs in people with previously unknown or mild diabetes; because of the lack of ketosis; because it follows an illness; and because it occurs in hyperglycemic conditions other than diabetes (*e.g.*, severe burns, corticosteroid drug therapy).

3. **Cardiovascular complications.** Diabetics develop generalized atherosclerosis that, compared to nondiabetics, occurs at an earlier age, progresses more rapidly, and becomes more severe. Changes occur in large and small blood vessels. Reasons for vascular changes are unclear, but the sequence of events is thought to involve damage to the endothelial lining, followed by platelet aggregation, lipid deposition, plaque formation, and thrombosis in the damaged area.

Vascular disease is a leading cause of death in diabetics. It is also a leading cause of morbidity, because diabetics are much more likely to have myocardial infarction, peripheral arterial insufficiency, kidney failure, and blindness than nondiabetics. Other vascular complications include angina pectoris, congestive heart failure, hypertension, and cerebral thrombosis (stroke).

4. **Nephropathy.** The several types of kidney lesions in diabetes mellitus are collectively called *diabetic nephropathy*. One such lesion is diffuse glomerulosclerosis, which is found in about 90% of people who have had diabetes for more than 10 years. Another lesion is called *nodular glomerulosclerosis*, or Kimmelstiel-Wilson syndrome. It occurs in 10% to 25% of diabetics. A third lesion is acute or chronic pyelonephritis. Although pyelonephritis also occurs in nondiabetics, it is usually more severe in diabetics. A fourth lesion involves atherosclerosis and arteriosclerosis of renal arteries as a manifestation of generalized atherosclerosis. These disorders all produce abnormal renal function and may cause renal failure.

5. **Retinopathy.** This is the most common and most serious ocular complication of diabetes, although cataract formation and glaucoma may develop at an earlier age in the diabetic. Diabetic retinopathy is related to the duration of diabetes. About 50% of diabetics have some degree of retinopathy after 10 years, about 80% to 90% after 20 years. Retinopathy results from vascular changes, and the severity is correlated with the degree of generalized vascular disease. Hemorrhage, edema, and exudates may be seen through the ophthalmoscope. Retinal detachment may occur.

6. **Neuropathy.** Several nonspecific neurologic disorders are often associated with diabetes mellitus. The degenerative changes in nerves that produce neuropathy are attributed to sorbitol, an alcohol produced by glucose metabolism.

In the extremities, neuropathy causes discomfort

and impairment of sensory and motor functions. Injuries often result, usually in the feet, and even minor injuries may eventually necessitate leg amputation. In the cardiovascular system, silent myocardial infarction, postural hypotension, and impaired response to sympathetic or parasympathetic stimulation may occur. Another autonomic manifestation is the absence of warning signs of hypoglycemia. In the gastrointestinal system, neuropathy may cause disturbances of motility (*e.g.*, gastroparesis) and changes in bowel function. In the genitourinary system, bladder atony may cause urine retention and urinary tract infections. Impotence and retrograde ejaculation may occur in men.

7. *Other complications.* Arthropathy and osteolysis may develop, probably from trauma and decreased ability to perceive pain. Diabetics are more susceptible to infections, especially tuberculosis, pneumonia, and urinary tract and skin infections. When infections occur, they tend to progress more rapidly and become more severe. Formerly, it was thought that infections were caused and perpetuated by hyperglycemia because microorganisms thrive on glucose. More recently, however, infections have been attributed to impairment of phagocytosis and other defense mechanisms. Women with diabetes are more likely to develop toxemia and other complications of pregnancy. Babies born to diabetic mothers are more likely to be premature or stillborn.

## Hypoglycemic drugs

Individual insulins and oral hypoglycemic drugs are listed in Tables 27-1 and 27-2, respectively.

### INSULIN

1. Commercially available insulin preparations are combinations of beef and pork insulins, single-component pork insulin, and human insulin. Early products contained proinsulin and other protein contaminants that caused a relatively high incidence of allergic reactions and insulin antibody formation. Newer products are highly purified and less likely to be antigenic. Beef insulin differs from human insulin by three amino acids and is more antigenic than pork insulin. Pork insulin differs from human insulin by one amino acid. Human insulin is produced in the laboratory with recombinant deoxyribonucleic acid techniques using strains of *Escherichia coli* or yeast or by enzymatically modifying pork insulin to replace the single different amino acid. Thus, human insulin has the same number and sequence of amino acids as

endogenous insulin. It is not derived from the human pancreas.

2. Insulin cannot be given orally because it is a protein that is destroyed by proteolytic enzymes in the gastrointestinal tract. It is given only by the parenteral route.

3. Insulin preparations differ primarily in onset and duration of action. They are usually categorized as short-, intermediate-, or long-acting insulins. Short-acting insulins have a rapid onset and a short duration of action. Intermediate- and long-acting insulins are modified by adding protamine (a large, insoluble protein), zinc, or both to slow absorption and prolong drug action.

4. Insulin preparations are available in two concentrations, U-40 and U-100. These terms refer to the concentration or number of units of insulin per milliliter of fluid. For example, U-100 contains 100 units of insulin per milliliter. Each concentration must be given with a syringe calibrated for that concentration (*e.g.*, U-100 insulin can be accurately measured only in a U-100 syringe). In the United States, U-100 insulin and U-100 insulin syringes are used almost exclusively.

   In addition, a stable mixture of 70% NPH and 30% regular insulin (*e.g.*, Humulin 70/30) is available. The mixture is more convenient and may be more accurately measured when both an intermediate- and a short-acting insulin are needed.

5. Insulin absorption is delayed or decreased when it is injected into subcutaneous tissue with lipodystrophy or other lesions, when circulatory problems (*e.g.*, edema or hypotension) are present, by insulin-binding antibodies (which develop after 2 or 3 months of insulin administration), and by injecting cold (*i.e.*, refrigerated) insulin.

6. Temperature extremes can cause loss of potency. Insulin retains potency up to 36 months under refrigeration and about 18 to 24 months at room temperature. At high temperatures (about 100°F or 37.8°C), insulin loses potency in about 2 months. If frozen, insulin remains potent but tends to clump or precipitate. This prevents withdrawal of an accurate dose, and the vial should be discarded.

### ORAL HYPOGLYCEMIC DRUGS

The oral hypoglycemic drugs, called sulfonylureas, are chemically related to sulfonamide antibacterial drugs; are well absorbed with oral administration; have the same mechanisms of action, indications for use, and contraindications; are more than 90% bound to plasma proteins; produce hypoglycemia as a major adverse effect; are extensively metabolized in the liver; and are excreted primarily by the kidneys (except for glyburide,

## TABLE 27-1. INSULINS

| Generic/Trade Name | Characteristics | Routes and Dosage Ranges | Action (h) | | |
| --- | --- | --- | --- | --- | --- |
| | | | **Onset** | **Peak** | **Duration** |
| **Short-Acting Insulins** | | | | | |
| **Insulin injection** (Insulin, Regular Iletin I Purified preparations: Regular Iletin II [beef or pork], Actrapid [pork], Velosulin [pork] Human Insulin: Humulin R, Novolin R) | 1. A clear liquid solution with the appearance of water 2. The hypoglycemic drug of choice for diabetics experiencing acute or emergency situations, diabetic ketoacidosis, hyperosmolar nonketotic coma, severe infections or other illnesses, major surgery, and pregnancy 3. The only insulin preparation that can be given IV 4. Rarely used alone for long-term maintenance but may be combined with an intermediate-acting insulin (e.g., NPH) for this purpose | SC, dosage individualized according to blood and urine glucose levels. For sliding scale, 5–20 units before meals and bedtime, depending on blood glucose levels or urine levels of glucose and acetone IV, dosage individualized. For ketoacidosis, regular insulin may be given by direct injection, intermittent infusion, or continuous infusion. One regimen involves an initial bolus injection of 10–20 units followed by a continuous low-dose infusion of 2–10 units/h, based on hourly blood and urine glucose levels | 1/2–1 | 2–3 | 5–7 |
| **Prompt insulin zinc suspension** (Semilente Insulin, Semilente Iletin I Purified preparation: Semitard [pork]) | 1. Modified by chemical combination with zinc to produce small crystals, which are rapidly absorbed 2. Rarely used alone; most often used in combination with intermediate (Lente) or long-acting (Ultralente) insulins 3. A suspension that is milky or cloudy when mixed thoroughly in the drug vial 4. Given *only* SC 5. Not recommended in emergencies | SC, dosage individualized. Initially, 10–20 units once or twice daily may be given. | 1/2–1 1/2 | 4–6 | 12–16 |
| **Intermediate Acting Insulins** | | | | | |
| **Isophane insulin suspension** (NPH Iletin I, NPH Insulin Purified preparations: Insulatard NPH, Iletin II [beef or pork], NPH purified pork Human insulin: Humulin N, Novolin N) | 1. Commonly used for long-term administration 2. Modified by addition of protamine (a protein) and zinc 3. A suspension with a cloudy appearance when correctly mixed in the drug vial 4. Given *only* SC 5. Not recommended for use in acute situations 6. Hypoglycemic reactions are more likely to occur during mid-to-late afternoon | SC, dosage individualized. Initially, 7–26 units may be given once or twice daily. | 1–1 1/2 | 8–12 | 18–24 |
| **Insulin zinc suspension** (Lente insulin Lente Iletin I Purified preparations: Lente Iletin II [beef or pork], Lente purified pork Human insulin: Novolin L) | 1. Modified by addition of zinc 2. A mixture of 30% Semilente and 70% Ultralente. The small crystals of Semilente are rapidly absorbed, and the large crystals of Ultralente are slowly absorbed 3. May be used interchangeably with NPH insulin 4. A suspension with a cloudy appearance when correctly mixed in the drug vial 5. Given *only* SC | SC, dosage individualized. Initially, 7–26 units may be given once or twice daily. | 1–2 | 8–12 | 18–24 |
| **Long-Acting Insulin** | | | | | |
| **Extended insulin zinc suspension** (Ultralente Purified preparation: Ultratard [beef]) | 1. Modified by addition of zinc and formation of large crystals, which are slowly absorbed 2. Hypoglycemic reactions are frequent and likely to occur during sleep. 3. Rarely used alone; may be combined with Lente or Semilente | SC, dosage individualized. Initially, 7–26 units may be given once daily | 4–8 | 10–30 | 36 plus |

*(continued)*

**TABLE 27-1. INSULINS** *(Continued)*

| Generic/Trade Name | Characteristics | Routes and Dosage Ranges | Action (h) | | |
|---|---|---|---|---|---|
| | | | **Onset** | **Peak** | **Duration** |
| *Insulin Mixtures* | | | | | |
| **NPH 70%** **Regular 30%** (Humulin 70/30, Novolin 70/30, Mixtard 70/30) | 1. Stable mixture 2. Onset, peak, and duration of action same as individual components | SC, dosage individualized | | | |

which is excreted about 50% in urine and 50% in bile). The drugs vary in duration of action.

The four older agents are called first-generation sulfonylureas. Metabolism of acetohexamide (Dymelor) and chlorpropamide (Diabinese) produces active metabolites that contribute to their duration of action. Metabolism of tolazamide (Tolinase) and tolbutamide (Orinase) produces inactive metabolites.

The two newer agents, glipizide (Glucotrol) and gly-

buride (DiaBeta, Micronase), are called second-generation sulfonylureas. They are similar in therapeutic and adverse effects. Compared to first-generation drugs, they produce similar hypoglycemia but are less likely to cause other adverse effects. They are metabolized to inactive compounds, which may be advantageous in clients with impaired renal function.

In addition to their hypoglycemic actions, oral antidiabetic drugs have other pharmacologic activities. For

**TABLE 27-2. ORAL HYPOGLYCEMIC AGENTS**

| Generic/Trade Name | Characteristics | Route and Dosage Ranges | Duration of Action (h) |
|---|---|---|---|
| *First-Generation Sulfonylureas* | | | |
| **Acetohexamide** (Dymelor) | 1. Intermediate-acting agent 2. Hypoglycemic activity due to the parent drug and an active metabolite 3. Readily absorbed from the gastrointestinal (GI) tract, metabolized in the liver, and excreted in urine 4. Has uricosuric properties; therefore, is probably the preferred oral agent for diabetics with gout | PO, dosage individualized. Usual range, 250 mg–1.5 g; maximal daily dose, 1.5 g. Dosages of 1 g or less daily can be given in a single dose. Dosage of 1.5 g daily should be given in two divided doses, before morning and evening meals. | 12–24 |
| **Chlorpropamide** (Diabinese) | 1. Long-acting agent 2. When chlorpropamide therapy is started, therapeutic effects may not be evident for 1–2 wk. When the drug is discontinued, several weeks are required for complete elimination of the drug from the body. These effects are due to the long half-life of the drug. | PO, dosage individualized. Initially, 100–250 mg daily in a single dose. Dosage may be increased or decreased by 50–125 mg at weekly intervals. Usual maintenance dose is 100–500 mg daily. Avoid doses greater than 750 mg daily. | Up to 60 |
| **Tolazamide** (Tolinase) | Similar to other sulfonylurea hypoglycemic agents except it does not have antidiuretic action. Consequently, tolazamide may be useful in diabetics with congestive heart failure, hepatic cirrhosis, or other conditions characterized by fluid retention and edema. | PO, dosage individualized. Initially, 100–250 mg daily is given in a single dose. Dosage may be adjusted every 4–6 d, as needed. If 500 mg or more is required daily, two divided doses are given. | 10–16 |
| **Tolbutamide** (Orinase) | 1. Short-acting agent 2. One of the most frequently used oral antidiabetic drugs | PO, dosage individualized. Initially, 500 mg is given in divided doses, twice daily Maintenance dose is 250 mg–3 g daily, in divided doses. | 6–12 |
| *Second-Generation Sulfonylureas* | | | |
| **Glipizide** (Glucotrol) | 1. Greater hypoglycemic effect per milligram than first-generation drugs 2. May cause less toxicity than first-generation drugs | PO 5 mg daily in a single dose, 30 minutes before breakfast | 24 |
| **Glyburide** (DiaBeta, Micronase) | See glipizide, above | PO 2.5–5 mg daily in a single dose | 24 |

example, acetohexamide, tolazamide, glyburide, and glipizide have mild diuretic effects; acetohexamide has uricosuric effects; and chlorpropamide may potentiate the action of antidiuretic hormone.

## MECHANISMS OF ACTION

Exogenous insulin has the same mechanism of action as the endogenous hormone. Oral hypoglycemic agents lower blood glucose by increasing secretion of insulin, increasing peripheral use of glucose, decreasing production of glucose in the liver, and increasing the number of insulin receptors or altering postreceptor actions to increase tissue responsiveness to insulin. Because the drugs stimulate pancreatic beta cells to produce and release more insulin, they are effective only when functioning pancreatic beta cells are present.

## INDICATIONS FOR USE

The primary clinical indication for insulin is treatment of diabetes mellitus. Because diabetes is characterized by a relative or absolute lack of the natural pancreatic hormone, insulin from a source outside the body is needed as a substitute or replacement. Insulin is the only effective treatment for type I diabetes, because little, if any, endogenous insulin is produced and metabolism is severely impaired. Insulin is required for 20% to 30% of type II diabetics who cannot control their disease with diet, weight control, and oral hypoglycemic drugs. It may be needed for all diabetics during times of stress, such as infection or surgery. Insulin also is used to control diabetes induced by chronic pancreatitis, surgical excision of pancreatic tissue, hormones and other drugs, and pregnancy (gestational diabetes). In nondiabetics, insulin is used to prevent or treat hyperglycemia induced by intravenous (IV) hyperalimentation solutions and to treat hyperkalemia. In hyperkalemia, an IV infusion of insulin and dextrose solution causes potassium to move from the blood into the cell; it does not eliminate potassium from the body.

Oral hypoglycemic agents are indicated for clients with symptomatic type II diabetes that cannot be controlled by diet or weight loss.

## CONTRAINDICATIONS FOR USE

The only clear-cut contraindication to the use of insulin is hypoglycemia (because of the risk of brain damage). Beef or pork insulin is contraindicated in clients allergic to the animal proteins.

Oral hypoglycemic drugs are contraindicated in clients with hypersensitivity to sulfonylureas, with severe renal or hepatic impairment, and during pregnancy.

They are unlikely to be effective during periods of stress, such as major surgery, severe illness, or infection. Insulin is usually required in these circumstances.

## Nursing Process

### Assessment

Assess the client's knowledge, attitude, and condition in relation to diabetes, the prescribed treatment plan, and complications. Assessment data should include past manifestations of the disease process and the client's response to them, present status, and potential problem areas.

- *Historic data* include age at onset of diabetes, prescribed control measures and their effectiveness, the ease or difficulty of complying with the prescribed treatment, occurrence of complications such as ketoacidosis, and whether other disease processes have interfered with diabetes control.
- *Assess the client's current status*, including subjective and objective information related to the following areas:
  - **Diet**. Ask how many calories are prescribed, how they are calculated (food exchanges, weighing portions, or other), who prepares the food, what factors help in following the diet, what factors interfere with following the diet, what the present weight is, and whether there has been a recent increase or decrease in weight. Also, list specific foods eaten at home during a 1- to 3-day period. This information assists in evaluating the nutritional adequacy of the diet actually taken and the client's adherence to the prescribed diet.
  - **Activity**. Ask the client to describe usual activities of daily living, including those related to work, home, and recreation.
  - **Medication**. If the client takes insulin, ask what kind, how much, who administers it, usual time of administration, sites used for injections, if a hypoglycemic reaction to insulin has ever been experienced, and if so, how it was handled. This information helps to assess knowledge, usual practices, and teaching needs. If the client takes an oral antidiabetic drug, ask the name, the prescribed dosage, and the dosage actually taken.
  - **Monitoring methods**. Blood or urine testing for glucose are the two methods of monitoring disease control and response to treatment. Try to determine the method used, the frequency of testing, and the pattern of results. If possible, observe the client performing and interpreting an actual test to assess accuracy.
  - **Skin and mucous membranes**. Inspect for signs of infection and any other lesions. Infections are relatively common in axillary and groin areas, because these are areas with large numbers of microorganisms. Periodontal disease, also called pyorrhea, is relatively common and may be manifested by inflammation and bleeding of the gums. Women with diabetes are susceptible to monilial vaginitis and infections underneath the breasts. Check the sites of insulin injection for atrophy (dimpling or indentation), hypertrophy (nodules or lumps), and fibrosis (hardened areas). Check the lower leg for brown spots;

these are caused by small hemorrhages into the skin and may indicate widespread changes in the blood vessels.

Problems are especially likely to develop in the feet from infection, trauma, pressure, vascular insufficiency, and neuropathy. Therefore, inspect the feet for calluses, ulcers, and signs of infection. When such problems develop, sensory impairment from neuropathy may delay detection, and impaired circulation may delay healing. Check pedal pulses, color, and temperature in both feet to assist in evaluating the adequacy of arterial blood flow to the feet.

- **Eyes**. Ask if the client has experienced any changes in visual acuity or blurring of vision and if eyes are examined regularly. Diabetics are prone to develop retinopathy, cataracts, and possibly glaucoma.
- **Cardiovascular system**. Because atherosclerosis tends to develop in diabetics, they are susceptible to a number of cardiovascular problems, such as hypertension, angina pectoris, myocardial infarction, and peripheral vascular disease. Therefore, check blood pressure, ask if chest pains ever occur, and ask about pain in the legs with exercise (intermittent claudication).
- **Genitourinary system**. Diabetics are likely to have kidney and bladder problems. Assess for signs of urinary tract infection, such as burning on urination; albumin, white blood cells, or blood in urine; edema; increased urination at night; difficulty voiding; generalized itching; easy bleeding and bruising; fatigue; and muscular weakness. Impotence may develop in male diabetics and is probably caused by neuropathy.
- Assess blood sugar reports for increases or decreases. Two or more fasting blood glucose levels above 140 mg/100 ml are diagnostic of diabetes mellitus. Also, 2-hour postprandial blood sugars above 140 mg/100 ml for people younger than 50 years and above 180 mg for people over 60 are significant. Decreased blood sugar levels are especially dangerous at 40 mg/100 ml or below.
- Assess the glycosylated hemoglobin (also called glycohemoglobin and hemoglobin $A_{1c}$) level when available. This test indicates glucose bound to hemoglobin in red blood cells when the red blood cell is exposed to high levels of blood glucose. The binding is irreversible and lasts for the life span of the red blood cell (about 120 days). Thus, the test reflects the average blood sugar for about 2 to 3 months before the test is done and indicates whether blood sugar is being controlled within desirable ranges.

Test results are not affected by several factors that alter blood sugar levels, such as time of day, food intake, exercise, recently administered antidiabetic drugs, emotional stress, or patient cooperation. The test is especially useful with children, labile diabetics, and those who have abnormal renal thresholds for glucose, who do not test blood glucose regularly, or who change their usual habits before a scheduled appointment with a health-care provider so that their blood sugar control appears better that it actually is.

### Nursing diagnoses

- Altered Tissue Perfusion related to atherosclerosis and vascular impairment
- Sensory-Perceptual Alterations related to impaired vision
- Sensory-Perceptual Alterations related to neuropathy, especially in the legs

- Ineffective Individual Coping related to chronic illness and required treatment
- Anxiety: Managing a chronic illness, finger sticks, insulin injections
- High Risk for Injury: Trauma, infection, hypoglycemia, hyperglycemia
- High Risk for Noncompliance related to inability or unwillingness to manage the disease process and required treatment
- Knowledge Deficit: Disease process and management
- Knowledge Deficit: Administration and effects of antidiabetic drugs
- Knowledge Deficit: Interrelationships among diet, exercise, and antidiabetic drugs
- Knowledge Deficit: Management of hypoglycemia, "sick days," and other complications

### Planning/Goals

*The client will:*
- Learn self-care activities at an individualized pace and style
- Manage drug therapy to prevent or minimize hypoglycemia and other adverse effects
- Develop a consistent pattern of diet and exercise
- Use available resources to learn about the disease process and how to manage it
- Administer antidiabetic drugs accurately
- Self-monitor blood glucose or urine glucose appropriately
- Keep appointments for follow-up and monitoring procedures by a health-care provider

### Interventions

Use nondrug measures to improve control of diabetes and to help prevent complications.
- Assist the client in maintaining the prescribed diet. Specific measures vary but may include teaching the client and family about the importance of diet, referring the client to a dietitian, and helping the client identify and modify factors that decrease compliance with the diet. If the client is obese, assist in developing a program to lose weight and then maintain weight at a more nearly normal level.
- Assist the client to develop and maintain a regular exercise program.
- Perform and interpret blood tests for glucose accurately, and teach clients and family members to do so. Self-monitoring of blood glucose levels allows the client to see the effects of diet, exercise, and hypoglycemic medications on blood glucose levels and may promote compliance.

Several products are available for home glucose monitoring. All involve obtaining a drop of capillary blood from a finger with a sterile lancet. The blood is placed on a semipermeable membrane that contains a reagent. The amount of blood glucose, in milligrams per 100 ml, can be read visually or with various machines (*e.g.*, Accu-Chek Glucometer). The latter method is more accurate but less convenient and more expensive than visual reading.
- Test urine for acetone when the client is sick, when blood glucose levels are above 250 mg/100 ml, and when episodes of nocturnal hypoglycemia are suspected. Also teach clients and family members to test urine when indicated.
- Promote early recognition and treatment of problems by observing for signs and symptoms of urinary tract infection, peripheral vascular disease, vision changes, ketoacidosis,

hypoglycemia, and others. Teach clients and families to observe for these conditions and report their occurrence.

- Discuss the importance of regular visits to the physician, clinic, or other facility for blood sugar measurements, weights, blood pressure measurements, and eye examinations.
- Perform and teach correct foot care. Have the client observe the following safeguards: Avoid going barefoot to prevent trauma to the feet; wear correctly fitted shoes; wash the feet daily with warm water, dry well, inspect for any lesions or pressure areas, and apply lanolin if the skin is dry; wear cotton or wool socks, because they are more absorbent than synthetic materials, such as nylon; cut toenails straight across and only after the feet have been soaked in warm water and washed thoroughly. Teach the client to avoid use of hot-water bottles or electric heating pads, cutting toenails if vision is impaired, use of strong antiseptics on the feet, and cutting corns or calluses. Also teach the client to report any lesions on the feet to the physician.

### Teach clients:

- The nature and characteristics of diabetes mellitus and proposed control measures. Few diseases require as much adaptation in activities of daily living as diabetes mellitus. Thus, the client must be well informed to control the disease, minimize complications, and achieve an optimum quality of life.
- Signs and symptoms of hyperglycemia: increased urine glucose and excessive thirst, hunger, and urine output. Persistent hyperglycemia may indicate a need to change some aspect of the treatment program, such as diet or medication.
- Symptoms of hypoglycemia: sweating, nervousness, hunger, weakness, tremors, and mental confusion. Hypoglycemia may indicate too much medication or exercise or too little food. If it occurs, take about 4 oz of orange juice, two lumps of sugar, or a few bites of candy. Repeat in 10 to 15 minutes if necessary. Avoid taking so much sugar that hyperglycemia occurs.
- The importance of diet, weight control, and exercise in control of diabetes. Maintaining normal weight and avoiding excessive caloric intake decrease the need for medication, decrease the workload of the pancreas, and help the body use insulin more efficiently. Exercise improves use of insulin and helps to promote more normal blood glucose levels.
- Measures to delay, prevent, or decrease severity of complications. These measures are wide ranging and include regular medical supervision, regular vision and glaucoma testing, and special foot care. The goal of such measures is to prevent complications. If they cannot be prevented, early recognition and treatment may minimize their severity.
- Take only drugs prescribed by a physician who knows the client has diabetes. Avoid other prescriptions and over-the-counter drugs unless these are discussed with the physician treating the patient, because adverse reactions and interactions may occur. For example, aspirin and other salicylates increase the likelihood of hypoglycemia. These drugs are often included in over-the-counter preparations for pain.
- Test blood regularly for glucose. A frequently recommended schedule is before meals and at bedtime.

### Evaluation

- Check blood sugar reports regularly for normal or abnormal values.
- Check glycosylated hemoglobin reports when available.
- Interview and observe for therapeutic and adverse responses to antidiabetic drugs.
- Interview and observe for compliance with prescribed treatment.
- Interview clients and family members about the frequency and length of hospitalizations for diabetes mellitus.

## Principles of therapy

### TREATMENT REGIMENS

Once a diagnosis of diabetes mellitus is established, the physician must choose a treatment regimen to control the disease process. The goal of treatment is to maintain blood sugar at normal or near-normal levels. There is increasing evidence that strict control of blood sugar decreases complications of diabetes. Home monitoring of blood glucose and insulin infusion pumps allow frequent adjustments of insulin dosage according to blood sugar levels.

The treatment regimen chosen for a particular diabetic client depends on the type of diabetes, the client's age and general condition, and the client's ability and willingness to comply with the prescribed therapy.

In type I diabetes, the only effective treatment measures are insulin, diet, and exercise. In type II diabetes, the treatment of choice is diet therapy and weight control. If this regimen is ineffective, an oral agent or insulin may be added.

### GUIDELINES FOR INSULIN THERAPY

#### Choice of preparation

When insulin therapy is indicated, the physician may choose from several preparations that vary in composition, onset and duration of action, and other characteristics. Some factors to be considered include the following:

1. Human insulin is preferred for newly diagnosed type I diabetes, gestational diabetes, poorly controlled diabetes, and diabetics undergoing surgery or experiencing illness that requires short-term insulin therapy. Human insulin is less likely to cause allergic reactions and insulin-antibody formation, but it is more expensive than older preparations.
2. Isophane insulin (NPH) or insulin zinc suspension (Lente) is probably the insulin of choice for clients who require long-term insulin therapy.
3. Regular insulin (insulin injection) is the only prepa-

ration that has a rapid onset of action and can be given IV. Therefore, it is the insulin of choice during acute situations, such as diabetic ketoacidosis, severe infection or other illness, and surgical procedures.

4. For some clients, a combination of regular insulin and an intermediate-acting insulin, most often NPH, provides more consistent control of blood glucose levels.

5. For clients with local or systemic manifestations of insulin allergy, the insulin of choice is either human insulin or purified pork insulin.

## Dosage factors

Dosage of insulin must be individualized according to blood glucose levels. An initial dose of approximately 0.5 to 1 unit/kg per day may be started and then adjusted to maintain blood glucose levels (tested before meals and at bedtime) of 80 to 140 mg/100 ml. However, many factors influence blood glucose response to exogenous insulin and therefore influence insulin requirements.

1. Factors that increase insulin requirements include weight gain, increased caloric intake, pregnancy, decreased activity, acute infections, hyperadrenocorticism (Cushing's disease), primary hyperparathyroidism, acromegaly, hypokalemia, and drugs such as adrenocorticosteroids, thyroid, epinephrine, and thiazide diuretics.

2. Factors that decrease insulin requirements include weight reduction; decreased caloric intake; increased physical activity; development of renal insufficiency; stopping administration of adrenocorticosteroids, thyroid, epinephrine, and diuretics; hypothyroidism; hypopituitarism; recovery from hyperthyroidism; recovery from acute infections; and the "honeymoon period," which sometimes occurs with type I diabetes.

   Renal insufficiency decreases dosage requirements because a smaller proportion of a given dose is metabolized than with normal renal function. The honeymoon period, characterized by recovery of islet cell function and temporary production of insulin, may occur after diabetes is first diagnosed. Insulin requirements may decrease rapidly, and if the dosage is not decreased, severe hypoglycemic reactions may result.

3. In acute situations, dosage of regular insulin needs frequent adjustments based on measurements of blood glucose. A sliding scale, in which dosage is specified for various blood sugar levels, is often used. If insulin is given IV in a continuous infusion, about 20% to 30% of the added insulin becomes bound to the container of IV fluids and to the plastic infusion set. It is recommended that 10 to 50 ml of the solution be discarded to saturate binding sites.

4. Dosage of insulin for long-term therapy is usually determined by trial and error. One such method involves an intermediate-acting insulin preparation, such as NPH or Lente, given 30 to 60 minutes before breakfast, in an initial dose of 10 to 26 units daily. This dose may be increased by 2 to 10 units at daily to weekly intervals, depending on blood glucose levels. Once hyperglycemia is relatively well controlled with an insulin dose, additional changes in dosage should generally be small (1 or 2 units at a time) and no more often than every 2 or 3 days. Occasional dosage adjustments may be necessary because of illness or changes in physical activity.

A second method involves initial use of regular insulin. Five to 10 units are given 15 to 30 minutes before meals, and dosage is gradually increased according to blood glucose tests. Once hyperglycemia is relatively well controlled, an intermediate-acting insulin preparation is substituted. This type of insulin is usually given once or twice daily.

A third method involves various combinations of short-acting regular insulin and an intermediate-acting insulin, most often NPH. Many physicians use this method for diabetics who do not achieve satisfactory control with other regimens. Clients or caregivers may mix the insulins, or a commercial preparation containing 70% NPH and 30% regular insulin may be prescribed.

Whichever method is used, regulating insulin dosage to establish and maintain control of hyperglycemia and other manifestations of diabetes may be difficult and time consuming. For example, dosage may be well regulated in a hospital, where diet can be controlled and exercise is limited. When the client leaves the hospital, however, dosage may need to be adjusted. Also, dosage may need to be decreased if the client is being switched from conventional to highly purified or human insulin.

5. Insulin pumps allow continuous subcutaneous administration of regular insulin. A basal amount of insulin is injected (e.g., 1 unit/h or a calculated fraction of the dose used previously) continuously, with bolus injections before meals. This method of insulin administration maintains more normal blood glucose levels and avoids the wide fluctuations that commonly occur with other methods. Candidates for insulin pumps include clients with diabetes that is poorly controlled with more conventional methods and those who are able and willing to care for the devices properly.

## Timing of food intake

Clients receiving insulin need food at the peak action time of the insulin preparation being used and at bedtime. The food is usually taken as a between-meal and a bedtime snack. These snacks help prevent hypoglycemic reactions between meals and at night. When hypoglycemia occurs during sleep, recognition and treatment may be delayed. This delay may allow the reaction to become more severe.

## Diabetic ketoacidosis

Insulin therapy is a major component of any treatment program for DKA. Clients with DKA have a deficiency in the total amount of insulin in the body and a resistance to the action of the insulin that is available, probably owing to acidosis, hyperosmolality, infection, and other factors. To be effective, insulin therapy must be individualized according to frequent measurements of blood glucose. Low doses, given by continuous IV infusion, are preferred in most circumstances.

Other measures that usually must accompany insulin to treat DKA effectively include identification and treatment of conditions that precipitate DKA, administration of IV fluids to correct hyperosmolality and dehydration, administration of potassium supplements to maintain normal serum potassium levels, and administration of sodium bicarbonate to correct metabolic acidosis.

Although other conditions may predispose diabetics to the development of DKA, infection is one of the most common and important. If no obvious source of infection is identified, cultures of blood, urine, and throat swabs are recommended. When infection is identified, antibacterial drug therapy may be indicated.

IV fluids, possibly the most important first step in treating DKA, usually consist of 0.9% sodium chloride, an isotonic solution. Hypotonic solutions are usually avoided because they allow intracellular fluid shifts and may cause cerebral, pulmonary, and peripheral edema.

Although serum potassium levels may be normal at first, they fall rapidly after insulin and IV fluid therapy are begun. Decreased serum potassium levels are caused by expansion of extracellular fluid volume, movement of potassium into cells, and continued loss of potassium in the urine as long as hyperglycemia persists. For these reasons, potassium supplements are usually added to IV fluids. Because both hypokalemia and hyperkalemia can cause serious cardiovascular disturbances, dosage of potassium supplements must be based on frequent measurements of serum potassium levels. Also, continuous or frequent electrocardiogram monitoring is recommended.

Severe acidosis can cause serious cardiovascular disturbances. Specifically, these disturbances usually stem from peripheral vasodilation and decreased cardiac output with hypotension and shock. Acidosis generally can be corrected by giving fluids and insulin.

Sodium bicarbonate may be given if the pH is less than 7.2. If used, sodium bicarbonate should be given slowly and cautiously. Rapid alkalinization can cause potassium to move into body cells faster than it can be replaced IV. The result may be severe hypokalemia and cardiac arrhythmias. Also, giving excessive amounts of sodium bicarbonate can produce alkalosis.

## Treatment of the unconscious client

When a diabetic becomes unconscious and it cannot be determined whether the unconsciousness is caused by DKA or by hypoglycemia from insulin, treat the client for hypoglycemia. If hypoglycemia is the cause of unconsciousness, giving some form of glucose may avert brain damage, which results from severe, prolonged hypoglycemia. If DKA is the cause of unconsciousness, giving glucose will not harm the client. Sudden unconsciousness in the insulin-dependent diabetic is most likely to result from an insulin reaction; DKA usually develops gradually over several days or even weeks.

## Hyperosmolar nonketoacidotic diabetic coma

Treatment of hyperosmolar nonketoacidotic diabetic coma is similar to that of DKA in that insulin, IV fluids, and potassium supplements are major components. Regular insulin is given by continuous IV infusion, and dosage is individualized according to frequent measurements of blood glucose levels. IV fluids are given to correct the profound dehydration and hyperosmolality, and potassium is given IV to replace the large amounts lost in urine during a hyperglycemic state.

## Insulin therapy during the perioperative period

Insulin therapy for diabetics who are having surgery usually consists of regular, short-acting insulin, given IV or subcutaneously. Dosage is determined by frequent measurements of blood glucose. Often these clients are given regular insulin on a sliding scale, in which dosage varies according to blood glucose levels. These tests are performed and insulin is given if indicated at regularly scheduled times, such as before meals and at bedtime or every 6 hours.

This regimen may be used for almost all diabetics having surgery. Even those who have controlled their disease with diet alone or with diet and oral hypoglycemic drugs may need insulin during this period. Those who have been insulin dependent and well controlled with an intermediate-acting insulin need a different regimen during the perioperative period. The changes in insulin therapy are usually necessary because surgery is a stressful situation that tends to increase blood glucose levels and increase the body's need for insulin.

The goal of insulin therapy during the perioperative period is to avoid ketosis from inadequate insulin and hypoglycemia from excessive insulin. The specific actions to reach this goal depend largely on the severity of diabetes and the type of surgical procedure. As a general rule, minor procedures require little change in the usual treatment program. For major operations, diabetes must be well controlled before surgery. For elective procedures, this may mean a delay until the client is in optimum condition to undergo surgery. During and after the operation, the insulin-dependent diabetic may need doses approximating the usual daily requirement; the diabetic receiving oral hypoglycemic drugs will probably need only small doses of insulin.

Along with the insulin, clients need adequate sources of carbohydrate until they can resume oral intake of food and fluids. This is usually supplied by IV solutions of 5% or 10% glucose. It is probably safer for the client to experience a blood glucose level between 150 and 250 mg/100 ml than to risk hypoglycemia.

## ORAL HYPOGLYCEMIC DRUGS

1. Oral antidiabetic drugs are not effective in all clients with type II diabetes mellitus. Even when carefully selected, many clients experience primary or secondary treatment failure. Primary failure involves a lack of initial response to the drugs. Secondary failure means that a therapeutic response occurs when the drugs are first given, but the drugs eventually become ineffective. The reasons for secondary failure are unclear but may include decreased compliance with diet instructions, failure to take the drugs as prescribed, or decreased ability of the pancreatic beta cells to produce more insulin in response to the drugs.
2. All the oral hypoglycemic agents must be used cautiously in clients with impaired renal or hepatic function but especially acetohexamide and chlorpropamide. Tolbutamide, glipizide, or glyburide is preferred in these situations.
3. Dosage of oral hypoglycemic drugs is usually started at lower amounts and increased gradually until the fasting blood glucose level is 110 mg/100 ml or less. The lowest dose that will achieve normal levels of both fasting and postprandial blood sugars is recommended.
4. Oral antidiabetic drugs are not recommended for use during pregnancy because some of these drugs cross the placenta and may cause hypoglycemia and even fetal death. Also, an increased risk of congenital anomalies is possible. A third reason is the risk that women with gestational diabetes will develop overt diabetes because the drugs stimulate an already overstimulated pancreas.

## TREATMENT OF HYPOGLYCEMIA

1. *Orally*. When hypoglycemic reactions occur with insulin or oral agents, treatment consists of the immediate administration of a rapidly absorbed carbohydrate. If the client is awake and can swallow, the carbohydrate is given orally. About 10 g of carbohydrate is usually sufficient and can be furnished by a variety of foods and fluids (*e.g.*, two sugar cubes; 1 to 2 teaspoons of sugar, syrup, honey, or jelly; two or three small pieces of candy; five or six Lifesavers candies; 4 oz of fruit juice, such as orange, apple, or grape; 4 oz of ginger ale; coffee or tea with 2 teaspoons of sugar added). Concentrated glucose products available include gel formulations (*e.g.*, Glutose, Insta-Glucose, Monojel) and chewable tablets (*e.g.*, B-D Glucose). All these products must be swallowed to be effective.
2. *Parenterally*. If the client cannot swallow or is unconscious, carbohydrate cannot be given orally because of the risks of aspiration. Therefore, the treatment choices involve parenteral glucose or glucagon. If the client is in a health-care facility where medical help is readily available, IV glucose in a 50% concentrated solution is the treatment of choice. It acts rapidly to raise blood glucose levels and arouse the client.

   If the client is at home or elsewhere, glucagon may be given if available and there is someone to inject it. A family member may be taught to give glucagon subcutaneously or intramuscularly. It can also be given IV. The usual adult dose is 0.5 to 1 mg. Glucagon is a pancreatic hormone that increases blood sugar by converting liver glycogen to glucose. Thus, it is effective only when liver glycogen is present. Some clients cannot respond to glucagon because glycogen stores are depleted by such conditions as starvation, adrenal insufficiency, or chronic hypoglycemia. The hyperglycemic effect of glucagon occurs more slowly than that of IV glucose and is of relatively brief duration. If the client does not respond to one or two doses of glucagon within 20 minutes, IV glucose is indicated.
3. Once hypoglycemia is relieved, the client should take slowly absorbed carbohydrate and protein foods, such as milk, cheese, and bread. These foods are needed to replace glycogen stores in the liver and to prevent secondary hypoglycemia from rapid use of the carbohydrates given earlier.
4. Although the main goal of treatment is to relieve hypoglycemia and restore the brain's supply of glucose, a secondary goal is to avoid overtreatment and excessive hyperglycemia. Thus, caution is needed in the treatment of hypoglycemia. The client having a hypoglycemic reaction should not use it as an excuse to eat large amounts of food in addition to or instead of the prescribed diet. Health-care personnel caring for the client should avoid giving excessive amounts of glucose. Repeated episodes of hypoglycemia mean that the therapeutic regimen and client compliance must be reevaluated.

## USE IN CHILDREN

Insulin is the only drug indicated for use in type I diabetes. Because children with diabetes cannot produce insulin, insulin is required as replacement therapy. Oral agents are ineffective and should not be given.

## USE IN OLDER ADULTS

General precautions for safe and effective use of antidiabetic drugs apply to older adults, including close monitoring of blood glucose levels. In addition, older adults may have impaired vision or other problems that decrease their ability to perform needed tasks (*e.g.*, self-administration of insulin, monitoring blood glucose levels, managing diet and exercise). They also may have other disorders and take other drugs that complicate management of diabetes. For example, thiazide diuretics, corticosteroids, estrogens, and other drugs may cause hyperglycemia, thereby increasing dosage requirements for antidiabetic drugs.

With oral hypoglycemic drugs, older adults may experience an exaggerated response. This may be averted by starting with a low dose, then increasing or decreasing the dose according to blood glucose levels and clinical response. If hypoglycemic reactions occur, dosage may need to be reduced.

## NURSING ACTIONS: ANTIDIABETIC DRUGS

| *Nursing Actions* | *Rationale/Explanation* |
|---|---|
| **1. Administer accurately**<br>**a.** With insulin: | |
| (1) Store the insulin vial in current use and administer insulin at room temperature. Refrigerate extra vials. | Cold insulin is more likely to cause lipodystrophy, local sensitivity reactions, discomfort, and delayed absorption. Insulin preparations are stable for months at room temperature if temperature extremes are avoided. |
| (2) Avoid freezing temperatures (32°F) or high temperatures (95°F or above). | Extremes of temperature decrease insulin potency and cause clumping of the suspended particles of modified insulins (all except regular insulin). This clumping phenomenon causes inaccurate dosage even if the volume is accurately measured. |
| (3) Use only an insulin syringe calibrated to measure the specific insulin concentration; that is, use only a U-40 insulin syringe to measure U-40 insulin and only a U-100 syringe for U-100 insulin. | For accurate measurement of the prescribed dosage. U-100 insulin and syringes are recommended and are eventually expected to be the only ones available. |
| (4) With modified insulin preparations, which includes all except regular, short-acting insulin, invert and rotate the vial before withdrawing the insulin. Do not shake the vial. | These insulin preparations are suspensions, and the components separate on standing. Unless the particles are resuspended in the solution and distributed evenly, dosage will be inaccurate. Shaking the vial causes air bubbles, which enter the syringe and interfere with accurate measurement of the prescribed dose. |
| (5) When a mixture of two insulins is prescribed, such as regular and NPH, prepare in the following sequence:<br><br>(a) Draw into the insulin syringe the amount of air equal to the total amount of both insulins.<br><br>(b) Draw up the regular insulin first. Inject the equivalent portion of air, and aspirate the ordered dose.<br><br>(c) With the NPH vial, insert the remaining air (avoid injecting regular insulin into the NPH vial), and aspirate the ordered dose. | It is important that the two insulins be drawn up in the same sequence every time. Most authorities recommend that regular insulin *always* be drawn up first. This avoids contamination of the regular insulin with the NPH. Because regular insulin combines with excess protamine in NPH, the concentration of regular insulin is changed when they are mixed. Following the same sequence also leaves the same type of insulin in the needle and syringe (dead space) every time. Although dead space is not usually considered a significant factor with available insulin syringes, it may be with small doses. |

(continued)

*Nursing Actions*                                    *Rationale/Explanation*

(d) Expel air bubbles, if present, and verify that the correct dosage is in the syringe.

(e) Administer the combined insulins *consistently* within 15 minutes of mixing or after a longer period; that is, do not give one dose within 15 minutes of mixing and another 2 hours or days after mixing.

As stated previously, regular insulin combines with excess protamine when combined with NPH insulin. This reaction, which occurs within 15 minutes of mixing, alters the amount of regular insulin present. After about 15 minutes, the mixture is stable for about 1 month at room temperature and 3 months when refrigerated. Thus, to administer the same dose consistently, the mixture must be given at about the same time interval after mixing. NPH and regular insulins are most often combined. The Lente insulins mix well with each other. However, if a Lente insulin is mixed with regular insulin, they interact up to 24 hours. If administered during this time, the dose of each insulin is unknown and variable. After 24 hours, the mixture is stable for 1 month at room temperature and 3 months when refrigerated.

(6) Rotate injection sites systematically, and use all available sites. These include the thighs, abdomen, upper back, upper arms, and buttocks unless some of these locations are contraindicated.

Frequent injection in the same site can cause tissue fibrosis, erratic absorption, and deposits of unabsorbed insulin. Also, if insulin is usually injected into fibrotic tissue where absorption is slow, injection into healthy tissue may result in hypoglycemia because of more rapid absorption. Further, deposits of unabsorbed insulin may initially lead to hyperglycemia. If dosage is increased to control the apparent hyperglycemia, hypoglycemia may occur. In addition, a sudden increase in physical activity is likely to increase subcutaneous blood circulation, causing rapid absorption of insulin.

(7) Rotate sites within the same anatomic area (*e.g.* abdomen) until all sites are used. Avoid random rotation between the abdomen and thigh or arm, for example.

Rates of absorption differ among anatomic sites, and random rotation increases risks of hypoglycemic reactions. Some authorities recommend giving all insulin injections in the abdomen.

(8) Inject insulin at a 90-degree angle into a subcutaneous pocket created by raising subcutaneous tissue away from muscle tissue. Avoid intramuscular injection.

Injection into a subcutaneous pocket is thought to produce less tissue irritation and better absorption than injection into subcutaneous tissue. Intramuscular injection should not be used because of rapid absorption.

2. **Observe for therapeutic effects**

For the most part, therapeutic effects of insulin are associated with decreased hyperglycemia and the signs and symptoms that accompany increases in blood glucose levels.

**a.** Decreased blood glucose levels (normal range [N] = 60–100 mg/100 ml)

The goal of most insulin therapy is normoglycemia, but only if hypoglycemia can be avoided.

**b.** Absent or decreased urine glucose level (N = none)

**c.** Absent or decreased ketones in urine (N = none)

In diabetes, ketonuria indicates insulin deficiency and impending DKA if preventive measures are not taken. Thus, always report the presence of ketones. In addition, when adequate insulin is given, ketonuria decreases. Ketonuria does not often occur with maturity-onset, ketoacidosis-resistant diabetes.

**d.** Absent or decreased pruritus, polyuria, polydipsia, polyphagia, and fatigue

These signs and symptoms occur in the presence of hyperglycemia. When blood sugar levels are lowered with antidiabetic drugs, they tend to subside.

## Nursing Actions                          Rationale/Explanation

**3. Observe for adverse reactions**

**a.** Hypoglycemia—tachycardia, cardiac palpitations, hunger, nausea, blurred vision, weakness and fatigue, confusion, inability to concentrate, muscle tremors and incoordination, sweating, delirium, convulsions, coma

Hypoglycemic reactions are more likely to occur with insulin therapy than with oral antidiabetic drugs. Also, with insulin, they are most likely to occur during the peak activity time of the particular insulin preparation being used. For example, peak activity with regular insulin occurs about 2 to 3 hours after injection. With NPH and Lente insulins, it often occurs 8 to 12 hours after injection but may occur at other times.

**b.** Local allergic reactions—erythema or induration at injection sites

**c.** Systemic allergic reactions—urticaria, edema, nausea and vomiting, diarrhea, dyspnea, occasionally hypotension, shock, and death

**d.** Lipodystrophy—atrophy and "dimpling" at injection site, hypertrophy at injection site

These changes in fatty subcutaneous tissue occur from too-frequent injections into the same site.

**e.** Insulin resistance—requirement of large doses of insulin in the absence of DKA, infection or other factors that serve to increase requirements for insulin

This may be caused by the development of antibodies.

**f.** Somogyi effect—hyperglycemia despite relatively large doses of insulin

This type of hyperglycemia is a rebound phenomenon that may occur following an insulin-induced hypoglycemic reaction. It results from increased secretion of epinephrine, adrenal corticosteroids, and growth hormone in the body's attempt to oppose the excessive insulin.

**4. Observe for drug interactions**

**a.** Drugs that *increase* effects of insulin:

(1) Monoamine oxidase (MAO) inhibitors

These drugs may significantly potentiate and prolong insulin-induced hypoglycemia. Such a combination is hazardous and should be used very cautiously, if at all.

(2) Anabolic steroids, salicylates (*e.g.*, aspirin), sulfinpyrazone (Anturane), sulfonamides, sulfonylureas (*e.g.*, oral antidiabetic drugs)

Increased hypoglycemia

(3) Propranolol (Inderal)

May increase hypoglycemia by inhibiting the normal elevation of blood glucose levels occurring as a homeostatic mechanism in response to hypoglycemia. However, propranolol also may inhibit insulin release. Thus, propranolol may increase or decrease the effects of insulin.

**b.** Drugs that *decrease* effects of insulin:

These drugs are often called *diabetogenic* because of their tendencies to raise blood sugar levels.

(1) Corticosteroids (*e.g.*, hydrocortisone)

Antagonize hypoglycemic effects, produce hyperglycemia

(2) Diuretics (especially thiazide diuretics, such as hydrochlorothiazide)

These drugs antagonize hypoglycemic effects of insulin and may cause hyperglycemia.

(3) Epinephrine

This adrenergic drug tends to raise blood glucose levels and thereby antagonize hypoglycemic effects of insulin.

(4) Glucagon

In small doses, glucagon is used to counteract hypoglycemia induced by insulin. Glucagon raises blood glucose levels by converting liver glycogen to glucose.

(5) Oral contraceptives

Tend to raise blood glucose levels and thereby antagonize insulin effects. Insulin dosage may need to be increased.

(continued)

| *Nursing Actions* | *Rationale/Explanation* |
|---|---|
| (6) Phenytoin (Dilantin) | Inhibits insulin secretion and may cause severe hyperglycemia |
| (7) Propranolol (Inderal) | May inhibit insulin release |
| (8) Thyroid preparations (*e.g.,* levothyroxine [Synthroid]) | May cause hyperglycemia |
| **c.** Drugs that *increase* effects of oral antidiabetics: | |
| (1) Acidifying agents (*e.g.,* ascorbic acid) and probenecid (Benemid) | Increase effects by slowing the rate of urinary excretion |
| (2) Alcohol | Additive hypoglycemia. If alcohol use is chronic and heavy, oral hypoglycemic agents may be metabolized more rapidly and *hyperglycemia* may occur. |
| (3) Allopurinol (Zyloprim), anabolic steroids, chloramphenicol (Chloromycetin), clofibrate (Atromid-S), cyclophosphamide (Cytoxan), guanethidine (Ismelin), MAO inhibitors, sulfinpyrazone (Anturane), tetracyclines | Increase hypoglycemia, mechanisms unclear |
| (4) Anticoagulants, oral | Increase hypoglycemia by slowing metabolism of oral antidiabetic agents and possibly by decreasing their urinary excretion |
| (5) Insulin | Additive hypoglycemia |
| (6) Salicylates (*e.g.,* aspirin) and sulfonamides | Increase hypoglycemia by displacing oral antidiabetic agents from protein-binding sites |
| **d.** Drugs that *decrease* effects of oral antidiabetic agents: | |
| (1) Alcohol | Heavy, chronic intake of alcohol induces metabolizing enzymes in the liver. This increases the rate of metabolism of oral antidiabetic drugs, shortens their half-lives, and may produce hyperglycemia. |
| (2) Beta-blocking agents | Decrease hypoglycemic effects, possibly by decreasing release of insulin in the pancreas |
| (3) Corticosteroids, diuretics, epinephrine, estrogens, and oral contraceptives | These drugs have hyperglycemic effects. |
| (4) Glucagon | Raises blood glucose levels. It is used to treat severe hypoglycemia induced by insulin or oral antidiabetic agents. |
| (5) Nicotinic acid | Large doses have a hyperglycemic effect. |
| (6) Phenytoin (Dilantin) | Inhibits insulin secretion and has hyperglycemic effects |
| (7) Rifampin | Increases the rate of metabolism of oral antidiabetic agents by inducing liver-metabolizing enzymes |
| (8) Thyroid preparations | Antagonize the hypoglycemic effects of oral antidiabetic drugs |
| **5. Teach clients** | |
| **a.** With insulin-dependent diabetics, teach: | |
| (1) Characteristics of the prescribed insulin preparations, including the expected time of peak insulin activity | The client may be able to eat at the time of peak insulin activity and reduce the likelihood of hypoglycemia. If hypoglycemia does occur, it is important that it be recognized as early as possible so that some kind of fast-acting carbohydrate can be taken. |

## Nursing Actions                                    ## Rationale/Explanation

(2) Correct techniques for self-administration of insulin:

    (a) Use sterile technique.

    (b) Draw up insulin in a good light.

    (c) Use appropriate needle and syringe.

    (d) If it is necessary to mix two insulin preparations, draw them up as specified in 1a(5), above.

For accurate dosage

    (e) Inject at a 90-degree angle.

To prevent local reactions

    (f) Rotate injection sites.

To prevent fibrosis, loss, or enlargement of subcutaneous tissue. If these changes occur, unpredictable absorption of the insulin may lead to unstable blood sugar levels and hyperglycemia or hypoglycemia.

    (g) Aspirate.

To avoid inadvertent injection into a blood vessel. Some authorities do not believe aspiration is necessary.

    (h) Change insulin dosage only if instructed to do so and the circumstances are specified.

    (i) Keep several days' supply of insulin, syringes, and needles on hand.

To allow for weather or other conditions that might prevent replacement of insulin or other supplies when needed.

    (j) Carry sugar or candy.

For immediate use if a hypoglycemic reaction occurs

    (k) If illness occurs, take the usual daily dose of insulin; do not omit insulin. Check blood glucose levels frequently. Test urine for ketones if sugar is present; if unable to test own urine, have someone else do it. Rest, keep warm, do not exercise, keep someone with you if possible, and drink some fluids every hour if able—broth and clear soups help.

Diabetics who cannot eat because of nausea, vomiting, or other difficulty commonly omit their insulin. Such a practice increases the likelihood of DKA. Insulin requirements are often increased during illness, probably owing to stress, decreased activity, and other factors. The Joslin Diabetes Foundation recommends keeping a bottle of regular, short-acting insulin on hand even if it is not used ordinarily. The client's physician should be consulted regarding this and the circumstances in which any supplemental insulin should be taken.

    (l) Reduce insulin dosage or eat extra food if you expect to exercise more than usual.

Specific recommendations should be individualized and worked out with the physician in relation to the type of exercise.

**b.** With oral hypoglycemic agents, teach:

    (1) Signs and symptoms of hypoglycemia

Hypoglycemic reactions may occur with oral antidiabetic drugs, although they are less common than with insulin.

    (2) Do not skip meals and snacks.

This increases the risk of hypoglycemic reactions.

    (3) More food may be needed if vigorous exercise is undertaken.

Exercise decreases the need for insulin. Thus, smaller doses of the oral drugs or larger amounts of food are needed. Specific recommendations from the physician will consider the type of exercise.

    (4) Follow the same "sick day rules" as prescribed for clients taking insulin, unless otherwise instructed; that is, take the oral hypoglycemic drug; try to take fluids, such as broths and clear soups, every hour unless vomiting; rest; avoid exercise.

Specific, individualized recommendations should be discussed with the physician before illness occurs. Some clients receiving oral agents need injections of regular, short-acting insulin during episodes of illness.

## Review and Application Exercises

1. What is the function of insulin in normal cellular metabolism?

2. What is the effect of insulin on blood glucose levels?

3. What are the effects of cortisol, epinephrine, glucagon, and growth hormone on blood glucose levels?

4. What are the major differences between type I and type II diabetes?

5. What are sources of exogenous insulin drug preparations?

6. What are advantages and disadvantages of human insulin preparations?

7. What is the rationale for maintaining near-normal blood glucose levels?

8. What is the major risk of maintaining near-normal blood glucose levels?

9. At what blood glucose range is brain damage most likely to occur?

10. Compare regular, NPH, and Lente insulins in terms of onset, peak, and duration of action.

11. In a diabetic client with typical signs and symptoms, distinguish between manifestations of hyperglycemia and hypoglycemia.

12. Contrast insulin and oral hypoglycemic agents in terms of mechanism of action, route of administration, indications for use, contraindications for use, and adverse effects.

13. For an adult client newly diagnosed with type II diabetes, state interventions to assist the client in learning self-care.

14. How could the nurse accurately respond to a child with diabetes mellitus who asks why he cannot take pills like his grandmother does?

15. Prepare a teaching plan for a client starting insulin therapy and for a client starting an oral hypoglycemic drug.

## Selected References

Beare, P. G., & Myers, J. L. (Eds.) (1990). *Principles and practice of adult health nursing*. St. Louis: C.V. Mosby.

Blackshear, P. J. (1992). Type II diabetes. In W. N. Kelley (Ed.), *Textbook of internal medicine* (2nd ed.) (pp. 2022–2029). Philadelphia: J.B. Lippincott.

Campbell, S., & Mooradian, A. D. (1993). Diabetes mellitus. In R. Bressler & M. D. Katz (Eds.), *Geriatric pharmacology* (pp. 409–425). New York: McGraw-Hill.

Cox, D. J., Gonder-Frederick, L. A., Schroeder, D. B., Cryer, P. E., & Clarke, W. L. (1993). Disruptive effects of acute hypoglycemia on speed of cognitive and motor performance. *Diabetes Care, 16*(10), 1391–1393.

Drass, J. (1992). Drugs for diabetes: Insulin injections. *Nursing 92, 22*(11), 40–43.

Dunn, F. L., & McNeill, D. B. (1992). Treatment of endocrine disorders: Diabetes mellitus. In K. L. Melmon, H. F. Morrelli, B. B. Hoffman, & D. W. Nierenberg (Eds.), *Clinical pharmacology: Basic principles in therapeutics* (3rd ed.) (pp. 426–445). New York: McGraw-Hill.

(1993). *Drug facts and comparisons*. St Louis: Facts and Comparisons.

Eisenbarth, G. S. (1992). Type I diabetes. In W. N. Kelley (Ed.), *Textbook of internal medicine* (2nd ed.) (pp. 2029–2034). Philadelphia: J.B. Lippincott.

Guyton, A. C. (1991). *Textbook of medical physiology* (8th ed.). Philadelphia: W.B. Saunders.

Heaman, D. (1992). Normal and altered functions of the pancreas. In B. L. Bullock & P. H. Rosendahl (Eds.), *Pathophysiology: Adaptations and alterations in function* (3rd ed.) (pp. 734–767). Philadelphia: J.B. Lippincott.

Hurwitz, L. S., & Porth, C. M. (1990). Diabetes mellitus. In C. M. Porth (Ed.), *Pathophysiology: Concepts of altered health states* (3rd ed.) (pp. 797–819). Philadelphia: J.B. Lippincott.

King, G. L., & Wolfsdorf, J. I. (1992). Rational use of diet, exercise, oral hypoglycemics, and insulin. In W. N. Kelley (Ed.), *Textbook of internal medicine* (2nd ed.) (pp. 2101–2108). Philadelphia: J.B. Lippincott.

Koda-Kimble, M. A. (1992). Diabetes mellitus. In M. A. Koda-Kimble, & L. Y. Young (Eds.), *Applied therapeutics: The clinical use of drugs* (5th ed.) (pp. 72-1–72-53). Vancouver, WA: Applied Therapeutics.

Melkus, G. D. (1993). Type II non-insulin-dependent diabetes mellitus. *Nursing Clinics of North America, 28*(1), 25–33.

Pandit, M. K., Burke, J., Gustafson, A. B., Minocha, A., & Peiris, A. N. (1993). Drug-induced disorders of glucose tolerance. *Annals of Internal Medicine, 118*, 529–537.

Shlafer, M. (1993). The nurse, pharmacology, and drug therapy: A prototype approach (2nd ed.). Redwood City, CA: Addison-Wesley.

Smith, R. J. (1992). Approach to the patient with hypoglycemia. In W. N. Kelley (Ed.), *Textbook of internal medicine* (2nd ed.) (pp. 2108–2110). Philadelphia: J.B. Lippincott.

Steil, C. F., & Deakins, D. A. (1992). Drugs for diabetes: Oral hypoglycemics. *Nursing 92, 22*(11), 34–39.

Venable, K. M., & Walters, N. G. (1992). Nursing management of adults with disorders of the endocrine pancreas: Diabetes mellitus. In L. O. Burrell (Ed.), *Adult nursing in hospital and community settings* (pp. 1146–1191). Norwalk, CT: Appleton & Lange.

# CHAPTER 28

# Estrogens, Progestins, and Oral Contraceptives

Estrogens and progestins are female sex hormones produced primarily by the ovaries and secondarily by the adrenal cortices in nonpregnant women. In pregnant women, large amounts of estrogens are produced by the placenta.

Like other steroid hormones, estrogens and progestins are synthesized from cholesterol. The ovaries and adrenal glands can manufacture cholesterol or extract it from the blood. Through a series of chemical reactions, cholesterol is converted to progesterone, then to the androgens, testosterone and androstenedione. These male sex hormones are used by the ovaries to produce estrogens. After formation, the hormones are secreted into the bloodstream in response to stimulation by the anterior pituitary gonadotropic hormones, follicle-stimulating hormone (FSH), and luteinizing hormone (LH). In the bloodstream, the hormones combine with serum proteins and are transported to target tissues where they enter body cells. They are thought to cross cell membranes easily, probably because of their steroid molecular structure and lipid solubility. Once inside the cells, they stimulate cellular protein synthesis.

## Estrogens

The main group of female sex hormones is the estrogens. Several estrogens have been identified, but only three are secreted in significant amounts: estradiol, estrone, and estriol. Estradiol is considered the major estrogen because it usually exerts more estrogenic activity than the other two combined. The main function of the estrogens is to promote growth in tissues related to reproduction and sexual characteristics in the female. More specific effects of estrogens on body tissues include the following:

1. **Breasts**. Estrogens stimulate growth of breast tissue at puberty by causing deposition of fat, formation of connective tissue, and construction of ducts. These ducts become part of the milk-producing apparatus after additional stimulation by progesterone.
2. **Sexual organs**. At puberty, estrogen secretion is greatly increased. The increased estrogen produces enlargement and other changes in the sexual organs. The fallopian tubes, uterus, vagina, and external genitalia increase in size. The endometrial lining of the uterus proliferates and develops glands that will later nourish the implanted ovum when pregnancy occurs. The epithelial lining of the vagina becomes more resistant to trauma and infection.
3. **Skeleton**. Estrogen stimulates skeletal growth so that, beginning at puberty, height increases rapidly for several years. Estrogen then causes the epiphyses to unite with the shafts of the long bones, and linear growth is halted. This effect of estrogen is stronger than the similar effect of testosterone in the male. Consequently, females stop growing in height several years earlier than males and on the average are shorter than males. Estrogen also conserves calcium and phosphorus. This action promotes bone formation and decreases bone resorption. An additional skeletal effect of estrogen is to broaden the pelvis in preparation for childbirth.

4. **Skin and subcutaneous tissue.** Estrogen increases vascularity in the skin. This leads to greater skin warmth and likelihood of bleeding in women. Estrogen also causes deposition of fat in subcutaneous tissue, especially in the breasts, thighs, and buttocks, which produces the characteristic female figure.

5. **Anterior pituitary gland.** Estrogens decrease pituitary secretion of FSH and increase secretion of LH when blood levels are sufficiently high. Thus, they control their own secretion, in part, by feedback mechanisms to the anterior pituitary gland.

6. **Metabolism.** In addition to protein anabolism and skeletal effects, estrogen increases sodium and water retention, alters glucose metabolism, increases serum triglycerides, increases high-density lipoproteins (HDL or ''good'' cholesterol because of cardioprotective effects), and decreases low-density lipoproteins (LDL or ''bad'' cholesterol because of cardiotoxic effects).

7. **Blood coagulation.** Estrogen enhances coagulation by increasing blood levels of several clotting factors, including prothrombin and factors VII, IX, and X and probably increases platelet aggregation.

In nonpregnant women, between puberty and menopause, estrogens are secreted in a monthly cycle called the menstrual cycle. During the first half of the cycle, before ovulation, estrogens are secreted in progressively larger amounts. During the second half of the cycle, estrogens and progesterone are secreted in increasing amounts until about 2 days before the onset of menstruation. At that time, secretion of both hormones decreases abruptly. When the endometrial lining of the uterus loses its hormonal stimulation, it is discharged vaginally as menstrual flow.

During pregnancy, the placenta produces large amounts of estrogen, mainly estriol. The increased estrogen causes enlargement of the uterus and breasts, growth of glandular tissue in the breasts, and relaxation of ligaments and joints in the pelvis. All these changes are necessary for growth and birth of the fetus.

Finally, estrogens are inactivated in the liver. They are conjugated with glucuronic acid or sulfuric acid, which makes them water soluble and readily excreted through the kidneys. About 80% of the conjugates are excreted in urine, with the remainder excreted in bile. Impaired liver function increases estrogen activity and may produce signs and symptoms of estrogen excess in males and females.

## Progesterone

Progesterone is a progestin concerned almost entirely with reproduction. In the nonpregnant woman, progesterone is secreted by the corpus luteum during the last half of the menstrual cycle, after ovulation. This hormone continues the changes in the endometrial lining of the uterus begun by estrogens during the first half of the menstrual cycle. These changes provide for implantation and nourishment of a fertilized ovum. When fertilization does not take place, the levels of estrogen and progesterone decrease, and menstruation occurs.

If the ovum is fertilized, progesterone acts to maintain the pregnancy. The corpus luteum produces progesterone during the first few weeks of gestation. Then, the placenta produces the progesterone needed to maintain the endometrial lining of the uterus. In addition to its effects on the uterus, progesterone prepares the breasts for lactation by promoting development of milk-producing cells. Milk is not secreted, however, until the cells are further stimulated by prolactin from the anterior pituitary gland. Progesterone also may help maintain pregnancy by decreasing uterine contractility. This, in turn, decreases the risk of spontaneous abortion.

Progesterone generally has opposite effects on lipid metabolism compared with estrogen. That is, progestins decrease HDL and increase LDL, both of which increase risks of cardiovascular disease. Progesterone also impairs glucose tolerance and makes diabetes mellitus more difficult to control. Like estrogen, progesterone is metabolized in the liver.

## Estrogens and progestins used as drugs

1. When estrogens and progestins are given from exogenous sources as drugs for therapeutic purposes, they produce the same effects as endogenous (naturally occurring) hormones.

2. Several preparations of estrogens and progestins are available for various purposes and routes of administration:

   a. *Naturally occurring, nonconjugated estrogens* (estradiol, estrone) *and natural progesterone* are given intramuscularly because they are rapidly metabolized if given orally. Some crystalline suspensions of estrogens and oil solutions of both estrogens and progesterone prolong drug action by slowing absorption.

   b. *Conjugated estrogens* (Premarin) and some synthetic derivatives of natural estrogens (*e.g.*, ethinyl estradiol) and natural progesterone (*e.g.*, norethindrone) are chemically modified to be effective with oral administration.

   c. *Nonsteroidal, synthetic preparations* are usually given orally or topically. They are chemically altered to slow their metabolism in the liver. They are also less bound to serum proteins than the naturally occurring hormones.

3. Oral contraceptives consist of a synthetic estrogen (*e.g.*, ethinyl estradiol) and a synthetic progestin (*e.g.*, norethindrone). Monophasic contraceptives contain fixed amounts of both components. Biphasics and triphasics contain either fixed amounts of estrogen and varied amounts of progestins or varied amounts of both estrogens and progestins. Biphasic and triphasic preparations mimic normal variations of hormone secretion, decrease the total dosage of hormones, and may decrease adverse effects.

These contraceptives are dispensed in containers with color-coded tablets that must be taken in the correct sequence. Dispensers with 28 tablets contain seven inactive or placebo tablets of a third color. A few contraceptive products contain a progestin only. These are less effective in preventing pregnancy and are more likely to cause vaginal bleeding irregularities, which makes them less acceptable to many women.

## MECHANISM OF ACTION

The precise mechanism by which estrogens and progestins produce their effects is unknown. Estrogens circulate briefly in the bloodstream before reaching target cells, where they enter the cells and combine with receptor proteins in cell cytoplasm. The estrogen-receptor complex then interacts with deoxyribonucleic acid (DNA) to produce ribonucleic acid and new DNA. These substances stimulate cell reproduction and production of various proteins.

Oral contraceptives act by several mechanisms. First, they inhibit hypothalamic secretion of gonadotropin-releasing hormone, which inhibits pituitary secretion of FSH and LH. When these gonadotropic hormones are absent, ovulation and therefore conception cannot occur. Second, the drugs produce cervical mucus that resists penetration of spermatozoa into the upper reproductive tract. Third, the drugs interfere with endometrial maturation and reception of ova that are released and fertilized. These overlapping mechanisms make the drugs highly effective in preventing pregnancy, although they can cause serious adverse reactions as well.

## INDICATIONS FOR USE

### Estrogen

1. *As replacement therapy in deficiency states*. Deficiency states usually result from hypofunction of the pituitary gland or the ovaries and may occur anytime during the life cycle. For example, in the adolescent girl with delayed sexual development, estrogen can be given to produce the changes that normally occur at puberty. In the woman of reproductive age (about age 12 to 45), estrogens are sometimes used in menstrual disorders, including amenorrhea and abnormal uterine bleeding due to estrogen deficiency.

2. *As a component in birth control pills*. Estrogens, usually combined with a progestin, are used widely in the 12- to 45-year age group to control fertility. If pregnancy does occur, estrogens are contraindicated because their use during pregnancy has been associated with the occurrence of vaginal cancer in female offspring and possible harmful effects on male offspring. However, during the postpartum period, estrogen may be given to suppress lactation if the mother is not going to breast-feed.

3. *During menopause*. Estrogens are given to relieve atrophic vaginitis and vasomotor instability, which produces "hot flashes," and to prevent osteoporosis. They also may prevent or delay coronary atherosclerosis and subsequent myocardial infarction. Some authorities have not recommended replacement estrogen therapy during or after menopause because of concern about endometrial cancer, but current opinion is that giving a progestin along with the estrogen negates this risk.

4. *Other clinical uses*. Estrogen is used to treat metastatic breast cancer in women more than 5 years postmenopause, metastatic prostate cancer in men, acne and hirsutism in women with excessive male sex hormone secretion, and excessive height in young girls.

### Progesterone and other progestins

These are probably used most frequently in oral contraceptive pills. They also are used in menstrual disorders, such as amenorrhea, dysmenorrhea, and abnormal uterine bleeding; endometriosis; threatened abortion; infertility; and endometrial cancer. The progestins are used increasingly for conditions formerly treated with estrogens.

The primary clinical indication for the use of oral contraceptives is to control fertility and prevent pregnancy. These preparations also are used to treat various menstrual disorders, such as amenorrhea and dysmenorrhea.

## CONTRAINDICATIONS FOR USE

Because of their widespread effects on body tissues and reported adverse reactions, estrogens, progestins, and oral contraceptives are contraindicated in:

1. Known or suspected pregnancy, because damage to the fetus may result
2. Presence of thromboembolic disorders, such as thrombophlebitis, deep vein thrombosis, or pulmonary embolism

3. Known or suspected cancers of breast or genital tissues, because the drugs may stimulate tumor growth. An exception is use of estrogens for treatment of metastatic breast cancer in women at least 5 years postmenopause.
4. Undiagnosed vaginal or uterine bleeding
5. Fibroid tumors of the uterus
6. Active liver disease or impaired liver function
7. History of cerebrovascular disease, coronary artery disease, thrombophlebitis, hypertension, or conditions predisposing to these disease processes
8. Women older than age 35 who smoke cigarettes. These women have a greater risk of thromboembolic disorders if they take oral contraceptives, possibly because of increased platelet aggregation with estrogen ingestion and cigarette smoking. In addition, estrogen increases hepatic production of blood clotting factors.
9. Family history of breast or reproductive system cancer

## Individual estrogens, progestins, and oral contraceptives

Table 28-1 lists the clinical indications, routes of administration, and dosages of estrogens. Table 28-2 provides the clinical indications, routes of administration, and dosages of progestins. Oral contraceptive agents are listed in Table 28-3.

## *Nursing Process*

### Assessment

Before drug therapy is started, clients need a thorough history and physical examination, including measurements of blood pressure, serum cholesterol, and triglycerides. These parameters must be monitored periodically as long as the drugs are taken.
- Assess for conditions in which estrogens and progestins are used (*e.g.*, menstrual disorders, menopausal symptoms).
- Assess for conditions that increase risks of adverse effects or are contraindications for hormonal therapy (*e.g.*, thromboembolic disorders, pregnancy).
- Record blood pressure with each outpatient contact or regularly with hospitalized clients. Increases are likely because of estrogen-induced increases in angiotensinogen, a precursor to the strong pressor substance, angiotensin. Sodium and water retention also occur.
- Check laboratory reports of cholesterol and triglyceride levels when available.
- Assess diet and presence of cigarette smoking. A high-fat diet increases the risks of gallbladder disease and perhaps other problems; cigarette smoking clearly increases risks

of cardiovascular disease in women over 35 who take oral contraceptives.
- Assess the client's willingness to comply with instructions about drug therapy and follow-up procedures.
- Assess for signs and symptoms of thromboembolic disorders regularly. These are most likely to occur in women over 35 who take oral contraceptives and women or men who take large doses for cancer; they have not been associated with postmenopausal estrogen replacement therapy.

### Nursing diagnoses
- Body Image Disturbance in females, related to effects of hormone deficiency states
- Body Image Disturbance in males, related to feminizing effects and impotence from female hormones
- Altered Tissue Perfusion related to thromboembolic effects of drugs
- High Risk for Fluid Volume Excess related to sodium and water retention
- Knowledge Deficit: Effects of hormonal therapy
- High Risk for Injury related to increased risks of hypertension and gallbladder disease

### Planning/Goals

*The client will:*
- Be assisted to cope with self-concept and body image changes
- Receive or take the drugs accurately
- Experience relief of symptoms for which the drugs are given
- Avoid preventable adverse drug effects
- Keep appointments for monitoring of drug effects

### Interventions
- Assist female clients of childbearing age to choose an appropriate contraceptive method. If the choice is an estrogen-progestin combination, help the client take it accurately.
- Help postmenopausal women plan for adequate calcium and vitamin D in the diet while avoiding excessive amounts.

*Teach clients:*
- Medical supervision, usually every 6 to 12 months, is necessary to check blood pressure, breasts, pelvis, and other areas for possible adverse reactions when these drugs are taken for long periods.
- Women with diabetes should report increased blood glucose levels.
- Women who take oral contraceptives should not smoke cigarettes. Cigarette smoking increases risks of thromboembolic disorders.
- Men who receive estrogens should know that feminizing effects and impotence are temporary and subside when drug therapy is discontinued.

### Evaluation
- Interview and observe for compliance with instructions for taking the drugs.
- Interview and observe for therapeutic and adverse drug effects.

## TABLE 28-1. ESTROGENS

| Generic/Trade Name | Dysfunctional Uterine Bleeding | Menopausal Symptoms | Female Hypogonadism | Postpartum Breast Engorgement* | Prostate Cancer | Other |
|---|---|---|---|---|---|---|
| **Chlorotrianisene** (Tace) | | PO 12–25 mg daily for 21 d, followed by 7 d without the drug | PO 12–25 mg daily for 21 d | PO 72 mg twice daily for 2 d; 12 mg four times daily for 7 d, or 50 mg q6h for 6 doses | PO 12–25 mg daily | |
| **Conjugated estrogens** (Premarin) | IM or IV for emergency use, 25 mg, repeated in 6–12 h if necessary | PO 0.3–1.25 mg daily for 21 d followed by 7 d without the drug | PO 2.5–7.5 mg daily in divided doses, cyclically, 20 d on, 10 d off the drug | PO 1.25 mg q4h for 5 d or 3.75 mg q4h for 5 doses | PO 1.25–2.5 mg three times daily | Breast cancer: PO 10 mg t.i.d. for at least 3 mo. Atrophic vaginitis: topically, 2.4 g of vaginal cream inserted daily. Osteoporosis: PO 1.25 mg daily for 21 d, then 7 d without the drug |
| **Dienestrol** (DV) | | | | | | Atrophic or senile vaginitis: topically, vaginal cream applied two or three times daily for about 2 wk, then reduced to three times weekly |
| **Diethylstilbestrol** (Stilbestrol) | | PO 0.2–0.5 mg daily for 21 d, followed by 7 d without the drug | PO 0.2–0.5 mg daily for 21 d, followed by 7 d without the drug | | PO 1–3 mg daily | Breast cancer: PO 15 mg daily. Postcoital contraception: PO 25 mg twice daily for 5 d |
| **Diethylstilbestrol diphosphate** (Stilphostrol) | | | | | PO 50–200 mg three times daily, IV 0.5 g first day, 1 g daily for next 5 d. Maintenance, 0.25–0.5 g one or two times weekly | |
| **Esterified estrogens** (Estratab) | | PO 0.3–1.25 mg daily for 21 d, then 7 d without the drug | PO 2.5–7.5 mg daily, in divided doses, for 21 d, then 7 d without the drug | | PO 1.25–2.5 mg one to three times daily | Breast cancer: PO 10 mg three times daily for at least 3 mo |
| **Estradiol** (Estrace) | | PO 1–2 mg daily for 3 wk, then 1 wk off or daily Monday through Friday, none on Saturday or Sunday | | | PO 1–2 mg three times daily for at least 3 mo | Breast cancer: PO 10 mg three times daily for at least 3 mo |
| **Estradiol cypionate** (Depo-Estradiol) | | IM 1–5 mg q3–4 wk | IM 1.5–2 mg at monthly intervals | | | |

(continued)

**TABLE 28-1. ESTROGENS** *(Continued)*

| Generic/Trade Name | Routes and Dosage Ranges for Various Indications | | | | | |
|---|---|---|---|---|---|---|
| | Dysfunctional Uterine Bleeding | Menopausal Symptoms | Female Hypogonadism | Postpartum Breast Engorgement* | Prostate Cancer | Other |
| **Estradiol transdermal system** (Estraderm) | | Topically to skin, 1 patch one or two times weekly for 3 wk followed by 1 wk off (cyclically) | Same as for menopause | | | |
| **Estradiol valerate** (Delestrogen) | | IM 10–20 mg q4 wk | IM 10–20 mg q4 wk | IM 10–25 mg at end of first-stage labor | IM 30 mg q1–2 wk | |
| **Estrone** (Theelin) | IM 2–4 mg daily for several days until bleeding is controlled, followed by progestin for 1 wk | IM 0.1–0.5 mg weekly in single or divided doses | IM 0.1–2 mg weekly | | IM 2–4 mg q3–4 d | |
| **Estropipate** (Ogen) | | PO 0.625–5 mg daily, cyclically | PO 1.25–7.5 mg daily for 3 wk, followed by an 8- to 10-day rest period. Repeat as needed. | | | Ovarian failure: same dosage as for female hypogonadism Atrophic vaginitis: topically, 1–2 g vaginal cream daily |
| **Ethinyl estradiol** (Estinyl, Feminone) | | PO 0.02–0.05 mg daily, cyclically | PO 0.05 mg one to three times daily for 2 wk with addition of progestin for last 2 wk of month | PO 0.5–1 mg daily for 3 d reduced to 0.1 mg after 7 d | PO 0.15–2 mg daily | Breast cancer: PO 1 mg three times daily |
| **Polyestradiol phosphate** (Estradurin) | | | | | IM 40–80 mg every 2–4 wk | |
| **Quinestrol** (Estrovis) | | PO 100 μg daily for 7 d, then 100–200 μg once weekly | | | Atrophic vaginitis: PO 100 μg daily for 7 d, then 100–200 μg weekly | |

*When estrogens are given to prevent breast engorgement and lactation, the first dose should be given within 8 hours after delivery.

# Principles of therapy

## NEED FOR CONTINUOUS SUPERVISION

Because estrogens, progestins, and oral contraceptives are usually taken for several months or years and may cause significant adverse reactions, clients taking these drugs need continued medical supervision. Before the drugs are given, a complete medical history; a physical examination, including breast and pelvic examinations and a Pap smear; urinalysis; and weight and blood pressure measurements are recommended. These examina-

tions should be repeated periodically, at least annually, as long as the client is taking these drugs.

## DRUG SELECTION FACTORS

Choice of estrogen preparation depends on the reason for use and desired route of administration. Conjugated estrogens (*e.g.*, Premarin) are commonly used and may be associated with fewer liver problems than other preparations. Diethylstilbestrol is the only estrogen approved for use as a postcoital contraceptive. Such usage is recommended for females who are victims of rape or incest

## TABLE 28-2. PROGESTINS

| Generic/Trade Name | Routes and Dosage Ranges for Various Indications | | | |
| | Menstrual Disorders | Endometriosis | Endometrial Cancer | Other |
|---|---|---|---|---|
| **Hydroxyprogesterone caproate** (Delalutin) | Amenorrhea, dysfunctional uterine bleeding: IM 375 mg. If no bleeding after 21 d, begin cyclic therapy with estradiol and repeat q4 wk for 4 cycles | | | Uterine adenocarcinoma: IM 1 g or more initially; repeat 1 or more times each week (maximum, 7 g/wk). Stop when relapse occurs or after 12 wk with no response. Test for endogenous estrogen production: IM 250 mg, repeated in 4 wk. Bleeding 7–14 d after injection indicates endogenous estrogen. |
| **Medroxyprogesterone acetate** (Depo-Provera, Provera) | Dysfunctional uterine bleeding: PO 5–10 mg daily for 5–10 days beginning on 16th or 21st day of cycle | | IM 400–1000 mg weekly until improvement, then 400 mg monthly | |
| **Megestrol acetate** (Megace) | Amenorrhea: PO 5–10 mg daily for 5–10 d | | PO 40–320 mg daily in four divided doses for at least 2 mo | Breast cancer: PO 160 mg daily in 4 divided doses for at least 2 mo |
| **Norethindrone** (Norlutin) | Amenorrhea, dysfunctional uterine bleeding: PO 5–20 mg daily, starting on 5th day of menstrual cycle and ending on 25th day | PO 10 mg daily for 2 wk, increase by 5 mg daily every 2 wk to dose of 30 mg. Then give 20–30 mg daily for maintenance up to 6–9 mo | | Norethindrone is also used as a contraceptive (see Table 28-3) |
| **Norethindrone acetate** (Norlutate) | Amenorrhea, dysfunctional uterine bleeding: PO 2.5–10 mg daily, starting on 5th day of menstrual cycle and ending on 25th day | PO 5 mg daily for 2 wk, increased by 2.5 mg daily every 2 wk to dose of 15 mg. Then give 10–15 mg daily for maintenance. | | |
| **Norgestrel** (Ovrette) | | | | Contraception: PO 0.075 mg daily |
| **Progesterone** (Femotrone, Progelan) | Amenorrhea, dysfunctional uterine bleeding: IM 5–10 mg for 6–8 consecutive days | | | |

or whose physical or mental health is threatened by pregnancy. To be effective, the drug should be started within 24 hours if possible and no later than 72 hours after exposure.

## DOSAGE FACTORS

Although dosage needs vary with clients and the conditions for which the drugs are prescribed, a general rule is to use the smallest effective dose for the shortest effective time. Approximately equivalent doses of estrogen preparations are estradiol 50 μg, mestranol 80 μg, diethylstilbestrol 1 mg, and conjugated estrogens 5 mg. Estrogens may be given cyclically, alone or with a progestin. In one regimen, the drug is taken for 3 weeks, then omitted for 1 week; in another, it is omitted the first 5 days of each month. These regimens more closely resemble normal secretion of estrogen and avoid prolonged stimulation of body tissues.

## USE IN SPECIFIC SITUATIONS

### Menopause

In treatment of menopause, estrogen replacement therapy relieves vasomotor and vaginal symptoms and prevents osteoporosis. A commonly prescribed regimen is a conjugated estrogen, such as Premarin, 0.625 mg to 1.25 mg daily for 25 days of each month, with a progestin, such as Provera, 10 mg daily for 10 days of each month, on days 15 to 25 of the cycle. The main function of the progestin is to decrease the risk of endometrial cancer;

**TABLE 28-3.   ORAL CONTRACEPTIVES**

| Trade Name | Phase | Estrogen ($\mu$g) | Progestin (mg) |
|---|---|---|---|
| *Monophasics* | | | |
| Brevicon | | Ethinyl estradiol 35 | Norethindrone 0.5 |
| Demulen 1/35 | | Ethinyl estradiol 35 | Ethynodiol diacetate 1 |
| Demulen 1/50 | | Ethinyl estradiol 50 | Ethynodiol diacetate 1 |
| Genora 0.5/35 | | Ethinyl estradiol 35 | Norethindrone 0.5 |
| Genora 1/35 | | Ethinyl estradiol 35 | Norethindrone 1 |
| Genora 1/50 | | Mestranol 50 | Levonorgestrel 0.15 |
| Levlen | | Ethinyl estradiol 30 | Norethindrone acetate 1 |
| Loestrin 21 1/20 | | Ethinyl estradiol 20 | Norethindrone acetate 1.5 |
| Loestrin 21 1.5/30 | | Ethinyl estradiol 30 | Norethindrone acetate 1 |
| Loestrin Fe 1/20 | | Ethinyl estradiol 20 | Norethindrone acetate 1.5 |
| Loestrin Fe 1.5/30 | | Ethinyl estradiol 30 | Norgestrel 0.3 |
| Lo/Ovral | | Ethinyl estradiol 30 | Norethindrone 0.5 |
| Modicon | | Ethinyl estradiol 35 | Norethindrone 1 |
| N.E.E. 1/35 | | Ethinyl estradiol 35 | Norethindrone 0.5 |
| Nelova 0.5/35E | | Ethinyl estradiol 35 | Norethindrone 1 |
| Nelova 1/35E | | Ethinyl estradiol 35 | Norethindrone 1 |
| Nelova 1/50M | | Mestranol 50 | Norethindrone 1 |
| Norcept-E 1/35 | | Ethinyl estradiol 35 | Levonorgestrel 0.15 |
| Nordette | | Ethinyl estradiol 30 | Norethindrone 1 |
| Norethin 1/35E | | Ethinyl estradiol 35 | Norethindrone 1 |
| Norethin 1/50 | | Mestranol 50 | Norethindrone 1 |
| Norinyl 1 + 35 | | Ethinyl estradiol 35 | Norethindrone 1 |
| Norinyl 1 + 50 | | Mestranol 50 | Norethindrone acetate 1 |
| Norlestrin 1/50 | | Ethinyl estradiol 50 | Norethindrone acetate 1 |
| Norlestrin Fe 1/50 | | Ethinyl estradiol 50 | Norethindrone acetate 2.5 |
| Norlestrin 21 2.5/50 | | Ethinyl estradiol 50 | Norethindrone acetate 2.5 |
| Norlestrin Fe 2.5/50 | | Ethinyl estradiol 50 | Norethindrone 1 |
| Ortho-Novum 1/35 | | Ethinyl estradiol 35 | Norethindrone 1 |
| Ortho-Novum 1/50 | | Mestranol 50 | Norethindrone 0.4 |
| Ovcon-35 | | Ethinyl estradiol 35 | Norethindrone 1 |
| Ovcon-50 | | Ethinyl estradiol 50 | Norgestrel 0.5 |
| Ovral | | Ethinyl estradiol 50 | |
| *Biphasics* | | | |
| Nelova 10/11 | I: 10 d | Ethinyl estradiol 35 | Norethindrone 0.5 |
| | II: 11 d | Ethinyl estradiol 35 | Norethindrone 1 |
| Ortho-Novum | I: 10 d | Ethinyl estradiol 35 | Norethindrone 0.5 |
| 10/11-21 | II: 11 d | Ethinyl estradiol 35 | Norethindrone 1 |
| *Triphasics* | | | |
| Ortho-Novum 7/7/7 | I: 7 d | Ethinyl estradiol 35 | Norethindrone 0.5 |
| | II: 7 d | Ethinyl estradiol 35 | Norethindrone 0.75 |
| | III: 7 d | Ethinyl estradiol 35 | Norethindrone 1 |
| Tri-Levlen | I: 6 d | Ethinyl estradiol 30 | Levonorgestrel 0.05 |
| | II: 5 d | Ethinyl estradiol 40 | Levonorgestrel 0.75 |
| | III: 10 d | Ethinyl estradiol 30 | Levonorgestrel 0.125 |
| Tri-Norinyl | I: 7 d | Ethinyl estradiol 35 | Norethindrone 0.5 |
| | II: 9 d | Ethinyl estradiol 35 | Norethindrone 1 |
| | III: 5 d | Ethinyl estradiol 35 | Norethindrone 0.5 |
| Triphasil | I: 6 d | Ethinyl estradiol 30 | Levonorgestrel 0.05 |
| | II: 5 d | Ethinyl estradiol 40 | Levonorgestrel 0.075 |
| | III: 10 d | Ethinyl estradiol 30 | Levonorgestrel 0.125 |
| *Progestin-Only Products* | | | |
| Micronor | | | Norethindrone 0.35 |
| Nor-Q.D. | | | Norethindrone 0.35 |
| Ovrette | | | Norgestrel 0.075 |

thus, some authorities do not prescribe progestin for the hysterectomized woman. Therapy should be continued indefinitely to prevent osteoporosis.

## Cancer

When estrogens and progestins are used in the treatment of cancer, several factors must be considered. First, the goals of treatment are palliation of symptoms and shrinkage of tumor tissue rather than cure. Second, these drugs have limited effectiveness, and careful selection of recipients is essential. Estrogens are recommended only for men with recurrent or metastatic cancer of the prostate gland and for postmenopausal women with recurrent or metastatic breast cancer. Progestins are used for metastatic cancer of the endometrium. Third, relatively large doses are needed for antineoplastic effects, and the drugs are given continuously rather than cyclically. This means that adverse reactions are more likely to occur and that most symptoms result from hormone excess. Recommended dosages may be decreased. Some studies, for example, indicate that diethylstilbestrol 1 mg daily is as effective as 5 mg daily in the treatment of prostatic cancer. Further, fewer deaths from cardiovascular disease occur with the smaller dose.

## Contraception

When estrogens and progestins are used as oral contraceptives, some guidelines include the following:

1. These drugs are nearly 100% effective in preventing pregnancy. Early products contained larger amounts of estrogen and produced a relatively high incidence of potentially serious adverse effects. Currently available products contain smaller amounts of estrogen, and adverse effects are expected to decrease, although their long-term effects are unknown. Despite the decreased estrogen dosage, oral contraceptives may still be safest when given to nonsmoking women under 35 years of age who do not have a history of thromboembolic problems, diabetes mellitus, hypertension, or migraine.
2. Assess each client's need and desire for oral contraceptives, as well as her willingness to comply with the prescribed regimen. Assessment information includes the client's knowledge about oral contraceptives and other methods of birth control. Compliance involves the willingness to take the drugs as prescribed, to have examinations of breasts and pelvis and blood pressure measurements every 6 to 12 months, and to stop the oral contraceptive peri-

odically (other contraceptive methods can be used during these periods). Assessment also includes identifying clients in whom oral contraceptives are contraindicated or who are at increased risk of adverse reactions.
3. The most effective and widely used oral contraceptives are estrogen-progestin combinations (see Table 28-3). Effects of estrogen components are similar when prescribed in equipotent doses, but progestins differ in progestogenic, estrogenic, antiestrogenic, and androgenic activity. Consequently, adverse effects may differ to some extent, and a client may be able to tolerate one oral contraceptive better than another.
4. Oral contraceptives decrease effects of oral anticoagulants, insulin and oral antidiabetic agents, antihypertensive drugs, and drugs used to lower serum cholesterol. If oral contraceptives are used concurrently with these drug groups, dosage of these groups may need to be increased. If oral contraceptives are discontinued, dosage of the other drugs may need to be decreased.

## USE IN CHILDREN

There is little information about effects of estrogens in children, and the drugs are not indicated for use. Because the drugs cause epiphyseal closure, they should be used with caution prior to completion of bone growth and attainment of adult height.

## USE IN OLDER ADULTS

Estrogens alone or estrogens and progestins are commonly used in postmenopausal women, whether menopause is physiologic or surgically induced by excision of both ovaries. Estrogens prevent vasomotor instability ("hot flashes") and other menopausal symptoms resulting from estrogen deficiency. They also decrease osteoporosis, if taken with adequate amounts of calcium. Progestins reduce the risk of endometrial cancer in women who have not had hysterectomies and simulate normal hormonal changes in women who have had hysterectomies. The risks of thromboembolic disorders (deep vein thrombosis, pulmonary embolism, myocardial infarction, stroke) associated with oral contraceptives have not been reported with the use of estrogens in older women.

In men who receive estrogens for metastatic cancer of the prostate gland, feminizing effects may occur in older men as in younger ones.

## NURSING ACTIONS: ESTROGENS, PROGESTINS, AND ORAL CONTRACEPTIVES

| *Nursing Actions* | *Rationale/Explanation* |
|---|---|
| **1. Administer accurately** | |
| **a.** Give oral estrogens, progestins, and contraceptive preparations after meals or at bedtime. | To decrease nausea, a common adverse reaction |
| **b.** With aqueous suspensions to be given IM, roll the vial between the hands several times. | To be sure that drug particles are evenly distributed through the liquid vehicle |
| **c.** Give oil preparations deeply into a large muscle mass, preferably gluteal muscles. | |
| **2. Observe for therapeutic effects** | Therapeutic effects vary, depending on the reason for use. |
| **a.** With estrogens: | |
| (1) When given for menopausal symptoms, observe for decrease in "hot flashes" and vaginal problems. | |
| (2) When given for amenorrhea, observe for menstruation. | |
| (3) When given for female hypogonadism, observe for menstruation, breast enlargement, axillary and pubic hair, and other secondary sexual characteristics. | |
| (4) When given for postpartum breast engorgement, observe for decreased tenderness and pain and absence of milk secretion. | |
| (5) When used in cancer of the breast or prostate gland, observe for relief of symptoms. | |
| **b.** With progestins: | |
| (1) When given for menstrual disorders, such as abnormal uterine bleeding, amenorrhea, dysmenorrhea, premenstrual discomfort, and endometriosis, observe for relief of symptoms. | |
| **3. Observe for adverse reactions** | Most adverse reactions are attributed to estrogens, although many of the same ones are listed for progestins as well. Thus, observe for similar adverse reactions whether the client is receiving estrogen or progestin alone or in combination as an oral contraceptive drug. |
| **a.** Gastrointestinal system—anorexia, nausea, vomiting, diarrhea, gallbladder disease, cholestatic jaundice | Nausea is the most common adverse reaction. It usually subsides within 1 to 2 weeks of continued drug therapy. |
| **b.** Cardiovascular system: | |
| (1) Thromboembolic conditions, such as thrombophlebitis, pulmonary embolism, cerebral thrombosis, and coronary thrombosis | A greater incidence of blood clotting disorders has been well documented in women taking these drugs, especially oral contraceptives. |
| (2) Hypertension | |
| (3) Edema, weight gain | These are caused by drug-induced fluid retention. |
| **c.** Central nervous system—headache, mental depression, insomnia, nervousness, anxiety | |

*(continued)*

## Nursing Actions

## Rationale/Explanation

**d.** Genitourinary system—vaginal bleeding or spotting, breast engorgement, endometrial cancer, vaginitis due to fungus (*Candida albicans*)

With oral contraceptives, breakthrough bleeding early in the cycle indicates an estrogen deficiency, and bleeding after midcycle indicates a progestin deficiency. Treatment involves altering estrogen or progestin dosage.

**e.** Integumentary system—skin rash, pruritus, acne, hirsutism

**f.** When estrogens are given to men, adverse reactions include gynecomastia, feminizing effects, impotence, atrophy of testicles, and thromboembolic complications.

**g.** Decreased glucose tolerance and increased blood and urine sugar levels

**4. Observe for drug interactions**
**a.** Drugs that *decrease* effects of estrogens, progestins, and oral contraceptives:

(1) Anticonvulsants, barbiturates, rifampin

Decrease effects by inducing enzymes that accelerate metabolism of estrogens and progestins

(2) Antimicrobials—ampicillin, chloramphenicol, neomycin, nitrofurantoin, penicillin V, sulfonamides, tetracyclines

By disrupting the normal bacterial flora of the gastrointestinal tract, antimicrobial drugs may decrease or eliminate enterohepatic circulation of estrogens and their conjugates. This action may decrease effectiveness of the contraceptive or cause breakthrough bleeding.

**5. Teach clients**
**a.** Take estrogens, progestins, or oral contraceptives with meals or food or at bedtime.

To decrease nausea, a common adverse reaction

**b.** If cyclic therapy is prescribed, take the drug for 3 weeks and then omit it for 1 week. Explain that menstruation occurs but pregnancy does not because ovulation has been prevented. With oral contraceptives, consult the physician about what to do if one or more daily doses is omitted for any reason. Another method of contraception may be needed temporarily because ovulation may have occurred.

**c.** Teach women receiving vaginal suppositories of estrogen how to insert them correctly.

**d.** Teach women using transdermal estrogen (*e.g.* Estraderm) to apply it to clean, dry skin, preferably the abdomen; to press tightly about 10 seconds to get a good seal; and to rotate sites so that at least 1 week passes between applications to a site.

To maintain placement and therapeutic effects

**e.** When diethylstilbestrol is used as a postcoital contraceptive, teach clients to take the drug despite the nausea that often occurs.

This drug must be taken as prescribed to be effective in preventing pregnancy.

**f.** Clients should weigh themselves at least weekly and report sudden weight gain.

Fluid retention and edema may occur and produce weight gain.

**g.** Clients should report any unusual vaginal bleeding.

This may be caused by excessive amounts of estrogen.

**h.** Clients should observe for and report adverse reactions, such as calf tenderness, redness, or swelling, which are signs of thrombophlebitis.

## Review and Application Exercises

1. What are reproductive and nonreproductive functions of estrogens?
2. What are the functions of progestins?
3. What is considered the major mechanism of action of oral contraceptives?
4. What are adverse effects of oral contraceptives, and how can they be prevented or minimized?
5. What are the advantages and disadvantages of postmenopausal estrogen replacement therapy?

## Selected References

Barbieri, R. L. (1992). Endocrinology of the female. In W. N. Kelley (Ed.), *Textbook of internal medicine* (2nd ed.) (pp. 2011–2013). Philadelphia: J.B. Lippincott.

Beare, P. G., & Myers, J. L. (Eds.) (1990). *Principles and practice of adult health nursing*. St. Louis: C.V. Mosby.

(1993). *Drug facts and comparisons*. St. Louis: Facts and Comparisons.

Guyton, A. C. (1991). *Textbook of medical physiology* (8th ed.). Philadelphia: W.B. Saunders.

Hoffman, A. R., & Marcus, R. (1992).Treatment of endocrine disorders: Estrogens and progestins. In K. L. Melmon, H. F. Morrelli, B. B. Hoffman, & D. W. Nierenberg (Eds.), *Clinical pharmacology: Basic principles in therapeutics* (3rd ed.) (pp. 446–457). New York: McGraw-Hill.

Maddox, M. A. (1992). Women at midlife: Hormone replacement therapy. *Nursing Clinics of North America, 27*(4), 959–969.

Mehring, P. M. (1990). Alterations in structure and function of the female reproductive system. In C. M. Porth (Ed.), *Pathophysiology: Concepts of altered health states* (3rd ed.) (pp. 637–663). Philadelphia: J.B. Lippincott.

Ruggiero, R. J. (1992). Contraception. In M. A. Koda-Kimble & L. Y. Young (Eds.), *Applied therapeutics: The clinical use of drugs* (5th ed.) (pp. 67-1–67-21). Vancouver, WA: Applied Therapeutics.

Sagraves, R., & Letassy, N. A. (1992). Gynecologic disorders. In M. A. Koda-Kimble & L. Y. Young (Eds.), *Applied therapeutics: The clinical use of drugs* (5th ed.) (pp. 70-1–70-32). Vancouver, WA: Applied Therapeutics.

(1993). Three-month contraceptive injection approved. *FDA Medical Bulletin, 23*(1), 6.

### CHAPTER 29

# Androgens and Anabolic Steroids

## Androgens

Androgens are male sex hormones secreted by the testes in men, the ovaries in women, and the adrenal cortices of both sexes. Like the female sex hormones, the naturally occurring male sex hormones are steroids synthesized from cholesterol. The sex organs and adrenal glands can produce cholesterol or remove it from the blood. Cholesterol then undergoes a series of conversions to progesterone, androgenic prehormones, and finally testosterone. The androgens produced by the ovaries have little androgenic activity and are used mainly as precursor substances for the production of naturally occurring estrogens. The adrenal glands produce about five androgens, including androstenedione and dehydroepiandrosterone, but these ordinarily have little masculinizing effect.

## Anabolic steroids

Anabolic steroids are synthetic drugs with increased anabolic activity and decreased androgenic activity when compared with testosterone. They were developed during attempts to modify testosterone so that its tissue-building and growth-stimulating effects could be retained while its masculinizing effects could be eliminated or reduced.

## Testosterone

Testosterone is normally the only important male sex hormone. It is secreted by the Leydig's cells in the testes in response to stimulation by luteinizing hormone (LH) or interstitial cell-stimulating hormone (ICSH) from the anterior pituitary gland. The main functions of testosterone are related to the development of male sexual characteristics, reproduction, and metabolism. Specific effects of testosterone on body tissues include the following:

1. *Fetal development*. Large amounts of chorionic gonadotropin are produced by the placenta during pregnancy. Chorionic gonadotropin is similar to LH from the anterior pituitary gland. It promotes development of the interstitial or Leydig's cells in fetal testes, which then secrete testosterone. Testosterone production begins about the second month of fetal life. When present, testosterone promotes development of male sexual characteristics, such as the penis, scrotum, prostate gland, seminal vesicles, and seminiferous tubules and suppresses development of female sexual characteristics. In the absence of testosterone, the fetus develops female sexual characteristics.

   Testosterone also provides the stimulus for the descent of the testes into the scrotum. This normally occurs after the seventh month of pregnancy, when the fetal testes are secreting relatively large amounts of testosterone. If the testes do not descend before birth, administration of testosterone or gonadotropic

Anne Collins Abrams: CLINICAL DRUG THERAPY, Fourth Edition.
© 1995 J.B. Lippincott Company.

hormone, which stimulates testosterone secretion, will produce descent in most cases.

2. **Adult development**. Little testosterone is secreted in male children until approximately age 11 to 13 years. At the onset of puberty, testosterone secretion increases rapidly and remains at a relatively high level until about 50 years of age, after which it gradually declines.

   a. The testosterone secreted at puberty acts as a growth hormone to produce enlargement of the penis, testes, and scrotum until about 20 years of age. The prostate gland, seminal vesicles, seminiferous tubules, and vas deferens also increase in size and functional ability. Under the combined influence of testosterone and follicle-stimulating hormone (FSH) from the anterior pituitary gland, sperm production is initiated and maintained throughout the man's reproductive life.

   b. **Skin**. Testosterone increases skin thickness and activity of the sebaceous glands. Acne in the adolescent male is attributed to the increased production of testosterone.

   c. **Voice**. The larynx enlarges and deepens the voice of the adult male.

   d. **Hair**. Testosterone produces the distribution of hair growth on the face, limbs, and trunk typical of the adult male. In men with a genetic trait toward baldness, large amounts of testosterone cause alopecia (baldness) of the scalp.

   e. **Skeletal muscles**. Testosterone is largely responsible for the larger, more powerful muscles of men. This characteristic is caused by the effects of testosterone on protein metabolism. Testosterone helps the body retain nitrogen, form new amino acids, and build new muscle protein. At the same time, it slows the loss of nitrogen and amino acids formed by the constant breakdown of body tissues. Overall, testosterone increases protein anabolism (buildup) and decreases protein catabolism (breakdown).

   f. **Bone**. Testosterone makes bones thicker and longer. After puberty, more protein and calcium are deposited and retained in bone matrix. This causes a rapid rate of bone growth. The height of a male adolescent increases rapidly for a time, then stops as epiphyseal closure occurs. This happens when the cartilage at the end of the long bones in the arms and legs becomes bone. Further lengthening of the bones is then prevented.

   g. **Anterior pituitary function**. High blood levels of testosterone decrease secretion of FSH and of LH or ICSH from the anterior pituitary gland. This, in turn, decreases testosterone production.

After testosterone is secreted by the testes, most of it binds reversibly to plasma proteins. It then circulates in the bloodstream for a half hour or less before it becomes attached to tissues or is broken down into inactive products. The portion that is attached to tissues enters the cells and is changed to dihydrotestosterone. The dihydrotestosterone binds with receptors within the cell and stimulates increased production of protein by the cell. The portion that does not become attached to tissues is converted into androsterone and dehydroepiandrosterone by the liver. These are conjugated with glucuronic or sulfuric acid and excreted in the bile or urine.

## Abuse of androgenic and anabolic steroid drugs

These drugs, especially the anabolic steroids, are widely abused in attempts to enhance muscle development, muscle stregth, and athletic performance. Athletes are considered a high-risk group, because some start taking the drugs in their early teen years and continue for years. Abusers usually take massive doses and often take several drugs or combine injectable and oral drugs for maximum effects. The large doses produce potentially serious adverse effects in several body tissues:

- Liver disorders include benign and malignant neoplasms, cholestatic hepatitis and jaundice, and peliosis hepatis, a disorder in which blood-filled cysts develop in the liver and may lead to hemorrhage or liver failure.
- Central nervous system disorders include aggression, hostility, combativeness, and dependence characterized by preoccupation with drug use, inability to stop taking the drugs, and withdrawal symptoms similar to those that occur with alcohol, cocaine, and narcotics.
- Reproductive system disorders include testicular atrophy, low sperm counts, and impotence in men. They include menstrual irregularities, baldness, hirsutism, and deepening of the voice in women.
- Metabolic disorders include increased serum cholesterol, with increased risk of cardiovascular disease and retention of fluids, with edema and other imbalances. Fluid and electrolyte retention contribute to the increased weight associated with drug use.
- Dermatologic disorders include moderate to severe acne in both sexes, depending on drug dosage.

Many of these adverse effects persist several months after the drugs are stopped and may be irreversible.

Because of their abuse potential, the drugs were legally designated as Schedule III controlled substances in 1991. Although nonprescription sales of the drugs are illegal, they are readily available.

# Characteristics of androgenic and anabolic steroid drugs

Individual androgens and anabolic steroids are listed in Table 29-1.

1. When male sex hormones or androgens are given from exogenous sources for therapeutic purposes, they produce the same effects as the naturally occurring hormones.
2. Male sex hormones given to women antagonize or reduce the effects of female sex hormones. Thus, administration of testosterone to women can suppress menstruation and cause atrophy of the endometrial lining of the uterus.
3. Exogenous androgens are given intramuscularly or orally. Naturally occurring androgens are given by injection because they are rapidly metabolized by the liver if given orally. Some esters of testosterone have been modified to slow the rate of metabolism and thus prolong action.
4. All synthetic anabolic steroids are weak androgens. Consequently, giving these drugs for anabolic effects also produces masculinizing effects. This characteristic limits the clinical usefulness of these drugs in women and children. Profound changes in growth and sexual development may occur if these drugs are given to young children.

## MECHANISM OF ACTION

Androgenic and anabolic drugs penetrate the cell membrane and bind to receptor proteins in the cell cytoplasm. The steroid-receptor complex is then transported to the nucleus where it activates ribonucleic and deoxyribonucleic acid production and stimulates cellular synthesis of protein. Production of protein increases in body cells, especially those associated with male sexual characteristics.

## INDICATIONS FOR USE

With male sex hormones, the most clear-cut indication for use is to treat androgen deficiency states (*e.g.*, hypogonadism, cryptorchidism, impotence, oligospermia) in boys and men. Hypogonadism may result from hypothalamic-pituitary or testicular dysfunction. In prepubertal boys, administration of the drugs stimulates the development of masculine characteristics. In postpubertal men who become androgen deficient, the hormones reestablish and maintain masculine characteristics and functions.

In women, male sex hormones are most often used in the palliative treatment of metastatic breast cancer. These women are usually premenopausal or menopausal and have breast tumors in which growth is stimulated by estrogen, the major female sex hormone. The male sex hormones inhibit the stimulating effects of estrogen. In addition, danazol (Danocrine) may be used to treat endometriosis when other treatment measures are ineffective or contraindicated.

Androgens also have been used in several conditions for which they have been largely replaced by other agents. These include postpartum suppression of breast engorgement and lactation, osteoporosis, and some severe anemias in which androgens stimulate the production of red blood cells.

Anabolic steroids are occasionally used to prevent or treat tissue wasting associated with severe illnesses, burns, trauma, and long-term use of adrenal corticosteroids. All these conditions produce catabolism and negative nitrogen balance. The anabolic steroids can promote tissue buildup (anabolism) and a positive nitrogen balance. However, parenteral hyperalimentation and other nutritional supplements are more effective. These drugs are more often abused for body building purposes than used for therapeutic effects.

## CONTRAINDICATIONS FOR USE

Androgens and anabolic steroids are contraindicated during pregnancy (because of possible masculinizing effects on a female fetus), in clients with preexisting liver disease, and in men with prostate gland disorders. Men with enlarged prostates may develop additional enlargement, and men with prostatic cancer may experience tumor growth. Although not contraindicated in children, these drugs must be used very cautiously and with x-rays approximately every 6 months to evaluate bone growth.

## *Nursing Process*

### Assessment

Before drug therapy is started, clients need a thorough history and physical examination. Periodic monitoring of the client's condition is needed throughout drug therapy.

- Assess for conditions in which androgens and anabolic steroids are used (*e.g.*, deficiency states, debilitating illness).
- Assess for conditions that increase risks of adverse effects or are contraindications (*e.g.*, pregnancy, liver disease, prostatic hypertrophy).
- Check laboratory reports of liver function tests (the drugs may cause cholestatic jaundice and liver damage), serum

**TABLE 29-1. ANDROGENS AND ANABOLIC STEROIDS**

| Generic/Trade Name | Routes and Dosage Ranges for Various Indications | | | |
| --- | --- | --- | --- | --- |
| | *Hypogonadism* | *Anabolic Effects* | *Breast Cancer* | *Other* |
| **Androgens** | | | | |
| **Testosterone** (Android-T Testoject Testaqua Oreton) | IM 10–25 mg two to three times weekly PO 10–40 mg daily Buccal tablets, 5–20 mg daily | | IM 100 mg three times weekly PO 200 mg daily Buccal tablets, 100 mg daily | Cryptorchidism: PO 30 mg daily; buccal tablets, 15 mg daily |
| **Testosterone cypionate** (Depo-Testosterone) | IM 200–400 mg every 4 wk | | | Oligospermia: IM 100–200 mg every 4–6 wk |
| **Testosterone enanthate** (Delatestryl) | IM 200–400 mg every 4 wk | | IM 200–400 mg every 2–4 wk | |
| **Testosterone propionate** (Various) | IM 10–25 mg three to four times weekly | | IM 50–100 mg three times weekly | |
| **Fluoxymesterone** (Halotestin) | PO 5–20 mg daily | | PO 10–40 mg daily in divided doses | Delayed puberty: PO 2 mg daily initially. Increase gradually as necessary. Postpartum breast engorgement: 2.5 mg when active labor begins, then 5–10 mg daily in divided doses for 4–5 d |
| **Methyltestosterone** (Oreton methyl) | PO 10–40 mg daily initially, reduced for maintenance Buccal tablets, half the oral dose | | PO 50–200 mg daily in divided doses Buccal tablets, 25–100 mg daily | Cryptorchidism: PO 30 mg daily; buccal tablets, 15 mg daily Postpartum breast engorgement: PO 80 mg daily for 3–5 d; buccal tablets, 40 mg daily for 3–5 d |
| **Danazol** (Danocrine) | | | | Endometriosis: PO 800 mg daily in 2 divided doses for 6–9 mo Fibrocystic breast disease: PO 100–400 mg daily in two divided doses for 3–6 months |
| **Anabolic Steroids** | | | | |
| **Nandrolone decanoate** (Deca-Durabolin) | | | | Erythropoiesis: IM up to 200 mg every 3–4 wk |
| **Nandrolone phenpropionate** (Durabolin) | | | IM 50–100 mg weekly | Erythropoiesis: IM up to 100 mg weekly |
| **Oxandrolone** (Oxandrin) | | Adults: PO 5–10 mg daily in divided doses (up to 20 mg daily) for 2–4 wk Children: PO 0.1 mg/kg per day | | Osteoporosis (adults): PO 5–10 mg daily in divided doses (up to 20 mg daily) |
| **Oxymetholone** (Anadrol-50) | | | | Erythropoiesis: PO 1–4 mg/kg per day (maximal daily dose, 100 mg) |
| **Stanazolol** (Winstrol) | | Adults: PO 6 mg daily in divided doses Children ages 6–12: PO 2–6 mg daily in divided doses Children under 6: PO 2 mg daily in divided doses | | |
| **Testolactone** (Teslac) | | | PO 250 mg four times daily | |

electrolytes (the drugs may cause sodium and water retention), and serum lipids (the drugs may increase levels and aggravate atherosclerosis).

- Assess weight and blood pressure regularly. These may be elevated by retention of sodium and water with resultant edema, especially in clients with congestive heart failure.
- For children, check x-ray reports of bone growth status initially and about every 6 months while the drugs are being taken.
- Assess the client's attitude toward taking male sex hormones.
- Assess the client's willingness to comply with instructions for taking the drugs and follow-up procedures.

### Nursing diagnoses

- Body Image Disturbance in females related to masculinizing effects and menstrual irregularities
- Sexual Dysfunction in males related to impotence and changes in libido
- Ineffective Individual Coping related to use of androgens and anabolic steroids for nonmedical purposes
- Knowledge Deficit: Physiologic and psychological consequences of overuse and abuse of the drugs to enhance athletic performance
- Noncompliance: Overuse
- Excess Fluid Volume related to sodium and water retention
- High Risk for Injury: Liver disease and other serious adverse drug effects
- High Risk for Violence: Directed at Others related to feelings of aggression and hostility in those who take large doses

### Planning/Goals

*The client will:*
- Use the drugs for medical purposes only
- Receive or take the drugs as prescribed
- Avoid overuse and abuse of drugs for "body building"
- Be counseled regarding effects of overuse and abuse if identified as being at risk (*e.g.*, athletes, especially weight lifters and football players)
- Avoid preventable adverse drug effects
- Comply with monitoring and follow-up procedures

### Interventions

- Assist clients to use the drug correctly.
- Assist clients to reduce sodium intake if edema develops.
- Assist clients with severe injuries or burns to increase intake of protein, calories, and other nutrients.
- Record weight and blood pressure at regular intervals.
- Participate in school or community programs to inform children, parents, coaches, athletic trainers, and others of the risks of inappropriate use of androgens and anabolic steroids.

*Teach clients:*
- Take the drugs only if prescribed and as prescribed. Usage by athletes for body building is inappropriate and, if not prescribed by a licensed physician, illegal.
- Continue medical supervision as long as the drugs are being taken.
- Weigh yourself once or twice weekly, and record the amount.

### Evaluation

- Interview and observe for compliance with instructions for taking prescribed drugs.
- Interview and observe for therapeutic and adverse drug effects.
- Question athletes about illegal use of the drugs.
- Observe athletes for increased weight and behavioral changes that may indicate drug abuse.

## Principles of therapy

1. When androgen or anabolic steroids are used in the treatment of metastatic breast cancer or refractory anemia, the required dosage may be two to three times the amount needed for androgen replacement therapy. These high dosages increase the incidence of adverse reactions.
2. When these drugs are given to women and prepubertal males, good skin care is indicated to decrease the incidence and severity of acne.
3. When these drugs are given for anabolic effects, an adequate intake of protein and calories is necessary to achieve maximum benefit. Similarly, if they are given for anemia, an adequate amount of iron must be available.
4. Drug therapy with androgens and anabolic steroids may be short or long term, depending on the condition in question, the client's response to treatment, and the incidence of adverse reactions. If feasible, intermittent rather than continuous therapy is recommended.
5. Androgens generally potentiate oral anticoagulants, oral antidiabetic agents, and insulin. Dosage of these drugs may need to be decreased during concurrent therapy with androgens or anabolic drugs.

### USE IN CHILDREN

The main indication for use of androgens in children is for boys with established deficiency states. Because the drugs cause epiphyseal closure, hands and wrists should be x-rayed every 6 months to detect bone maturation and prevent loss of adult height. Stimulation of skeletal growth continues for about 6 months after drug therapy is stopped. If premature puberty occurs (precocious sexual development, enlarged penis), the drug should be stopped. The drugs may cause or aggravate acne. Scrupulous hygiene and other antiacne treatment may be needed, especially in adolescent boys.

There is probably no reason to use anabolic steroids to stimulate tissue growth in children. Oral and intravenous supplements are more effective for meeting nutritional needs.

## USE IN OLDER ADULTS

The main indication for use of androgens is a deficiency state in men. Older adults often have hypertension and other cardiovascular disorders that may be aggravated by the sodium and water retention associated with androgens and anabolic steroids. In men, the drugs may increase prostate size and interfere with urination, increase risk of prostatic cancer, and cause excessive sexual stimulation and priapism.

The main reason for use of the drugs in older women is treatment of metastatic breast cancer. Masculinizing effects may occur.

## NURSING ACTIONS: ANDROGENS AND ANABOLIC STEROIDS

| *Nursing Actions* | *Rationale/Explanation* |
|---|---|
| **1. Administer accurately** <br> **a.** Give IM preparations of testosterone, other androgens and anabolic steroids deeply, preferably in the gluteal muscle. | |
| **b.** Give oral preparations before or with meals, in divided doses. | To decrease gastrointestinal disturbances |
| **c.** For buccal preparations: | |
| (1) Give in divided doses. | |
| (2) Place the tablet between the cheek and gum. | Buccal preparations must be absorbed through the mucous membranes. |
| (3) Instruct the client not to swallow the tablet and not to drink, chew, or smoke until the tablet is completely absorbed. | |
| (4) Maintain oral hygiene. | To decrease irritation and risk of infection |
| **2. Observe for therapeutic effects** <br> **a.** When the drug is given for hypogonadism, observe for masculinizing effects, such as growth of sexual organs, deepening of voice, growth of body hair, and acne. | |
| **b.** When the drug is given for anabolic effects, observe for increased appetite, euphoria, or statements of feeling better. | |
| **c.** When the drug is given for cancer, observe for decreased pain and increased reports of feeling better. | |
| **d.** When the drug is given for anemia, observe complete blood count reports for increased red blood cells, hematocrit, and hemoglobin. | |
| **3. Observe for adverse reactions** <br> **a.** Virilism or masculinizing effects: | |
| (1) In adult men with adequate secretion of testosterone—priapism, increased sexual desire, reduced sperm count, and prostate enlargement | |
| (2) In prepubertal boys—premature development of sex organs and secondary sexual characteristics, such as enlargement of the penis, priapism, pubic hair | |

## Nursing Actions

## Rationale/Explanation

(3) In women—masculinizing effects include hirsutism, deepening of the voice, menstrual irregularities

**b.** Jaundice—dark urine, yellow skin and sclera, itching

**c.** Edema

More likely in clients who are elderly or who have heart or kidney disease

**d.** Hypercalcemia

More likely in women with advanced breast cancer

**e.** Difficulty voiding due to prostate enlargement

More likely in middle-aged or elderly men

**f.** Inadequate growth in height of children

**4. Observe for drug interactions**

**a.** Drugs that *decrease* effects of androgens and anabolic agents:

(1) Aminopyrine

Increases the rate of metabolism

(2) Antihistamines

Increase enzyme induction

(3) Barbiturates

Increase enzyme induction and rate of metabolism

(4) Calcitonin

Decreases calcium retention and thus antagonizes calcium-retaining effects of androgens

(5) Chlorcyclizine (Perazil)

Increases metabolism

(6) Estrogens

Antagonize the anticancer effects of androgens

**5. Teach clients**

**a.** Correct use of buccal tablets

**b.** Report adverse reactions, such as jaundice, edema, masculinizing effects.

**c.** Weigh weekly, and report gains.

May indicate fluid retention and edema or a therapeutic effect of anabolic drugs

**d.** Practice frequent and thorough skin cleansing.

To decrease acne, which is most likely to occur in women and children

**e.** With anabolic drugs, eat a well-balanced diet.

Adequate protein and calories are necessary for full anabolic effects. Folic acid is necessary when these drugs are given for anemia.

## Review and Application Exercises

1. How does testosterone promote development of male sexual characteristics?
2. What is the major clinical indication for therapeutic use of testosterone and related androgens?
3. What is the difference between androgenic activity and anabolic activity?
4. What are the adverse effects of using large doses of anabolic steroids in body-building efforts?
5. If your 14-year-old brother said some friends were telling him to take drugs to increase muscle development and athletic ability, how would you reply? Justify your answer.

## Selected References

Beare, P. G., & Myers, J. L. (Eds.) (1990). *Principles and practice of adult health nursing.* St. Louis: C.V. Mosby.

(1993). *Drug facts and comparisons.* St. Louis: Facts and Comparisons.

Guyton, A. C. (1991). *Textbook of medical physiology* (8th ed.). Philadelphia: W.B. Saunders.

Dusek, D. E., & Girdano, D. A. (1992). *Drugs: A factual account* (5th ed.). New York: McGraw-Hill.

Su, T. P., Pagliaro, M., Schmidt, P. J., Pickar, D., Wolkowitz, O., & Rubinow, D. R. (1993). Neuropsychiatric effects of anabolic steroids in male normal volunteers. *Journal of the American Medical Association, 269,* 2760–2764.

# Nutrients, Fluids, and Electrolytes

### CHAPTER 30

# Nutritional Products, Anorexiants, and Digestants

## Nutritional products

Water, carbohydrates, proteins, fats, vitamins, and minerals are required for human nutrition, to promote or maintain health, to prevent illness, and to promote recovery from illness. The first four nutrients are discussed in this chapter; vitamins and minerals are discussed in the following chapters.

Water, carbohydrates, proteins, and fats are necessary for life. Water is second only to oxygen in importance, because a person can live only a few days without water intake. Proteins are basic anatomic and physiologic components of all body cells and tissues. Carbohydrates and fats serve primarily as sources of energy for cell metabolism.

Energy is measured in terms of kilocalories per gram of food oxidized in the body. The term *calorie* is often used instead of *kilocalorie*. Carbohydrates are oxidized first and provide an immediate source of energy; fats are used second and provide a long-term or reserve supply of energy; and proteins are used last. Undernutrition, starvation, and death occur within a few weeks when there is no intake of carbohydrates, proteins, and fats. Table 30-1 lists more specific characteristics of water, carbohydrates, proteins, and fats in relation to normal nutrition.

When inadequate or excessive amounts of these nutrients are ingested, nutritional disorders result. These disorders include water deficit (also called dehydration or fluid volume deficit), water excess (also called water intoxication or fluid volume excess), undernutrition, and obesity. Causes and clinical manifestations of water imbalances are listed in Table 30-2; protein-calorie imbalances are described in Table 30-3.

Numerous products are available to supplement or substitute for dietary intake in clients who cannot ingest, digest, absorb, or use nutrients. For example, liquid formulas are available for oral or tube feedings. Many liquid formulas are nutritionally complete, except for water, when given in sufficient quantities. Others are nutritionally incomplete but useful in certain circumstances. Additional water is given to meet fluid needs. A variety of intravenous (IV) fluids is also available. Most IV fluids are nutritionally incomplete and are designed for short-term use when oral or tube feedings are contraindicated. They are most useful in meeting fluid and electrolyte needs.

When nutrients must be provided parenterally for more than a few days, a special nutritional formula can be given. Parenteral nutritional formulas can be designed to meet all nutritional needs or to supplement other feeding methods. Fat emulsions also are administered to supply additional calories and essential fatty acids. For nutritional deficiencies due to malabsorption of carbohydrates, protein, and fat, pancreatic enzymes may be given to aid digestion.

## Anorexiants and digestants

In nutritional excesses or obesity, anorexiant drugs are sometimes given to decrease appetite (Table 30-4). Amphetamines (see Chap. 16) have been used for this purpose, but they have a high potential for abuse and dependence. Other anorexiant drugs are similar to am-

(*Text continues on p. 322*)

Anne Collins Abrams: CLINICAL DRUG THERAPY, Fourth Edition.
© 1995 J.B. Lippincott Company.

## TABLE 30-1. WATER, CARBOHYDRATES, PROTEINS, AND FATS

| Characteristics | Functions | Requirements | Normal Sources | Normal Losses |
|---|---|---|---|---|
| **Water** | | | | |
| 1. Major chemical constituent of the body<br>2. Intracellular fluid includes the water inside body cells.<br>3. Extracellular fluid includes the water or liquid portion of blood, lymph, spinal fluid, saliva, gastrointestinal secretions, bile, sweat, urine, and the tissue fluid that surrounds body cells. | 1. Serves as a solvent or medium in which all cell metabolism occurs<br>2. Maintains blood volume<br>3. Transports nutrients to body cells<br>4. Assists in maintaining electrolyte balance in blood and cells<br>5. Assists in maintaining body temperature | Approximately 2000–3000 ml daily, depending on activity, environmental temperature, and other factors | 1. Drinking water and other beverages (about 1200 ml/d)<br>2. Water in foods (about 1000 ml/d)<br>3. Water produced by oxidation of foods in the body (about 300 ml/d) | 1. Urine (about 1500 ml/d)<br>2. Insensible losses from skin and lungs (about 900 ml/d)<br>3. Feces (about 100 ml/d) |
| **Carbohydrates** | | | | |
| 1. Chemical substances composed of carbon, hydrogen, and oxygen<br>2. The major source of energy for body activities. When oxidized in the body, carbohydrates furnish 4 kcal of energy per gram.<br>3. They must be broken down into glucose, galactose, or fructose before they can be absorbed. The simple sugars can then be used for energy or stored as glycogen. | 1. Provide glucose, which is necessary for normal cellular metabolism<br>2. Conserve body proteins for tissue building and repair by preventing use of proteins for energy<br>3. Promote normal fat metabolism<br>4. Promote normal function of nerve cells. Glucose is the only source of energy that can be used by the brain.<br>5. Promote growth of normal intestinal bacteria by providing lactose. These bacteria synthesize certain vitamins, mainly vitamin K.<br>6. Promote normal bowel elimination by stimulating peristalsis, absorbing water and increasing the bulk of intestinal contents. This function is fulfilled by complex or indigestible carbohydrates. | Approximately 2000 kcal daily for the average adult female (58 kg or 127 lb) and 2700 kcal for the average adult male (70 kg or 154 lb)<br>Requirements vary, depending on age, size, activity, and other factors. They increase in pregnancy and lactation; rapid growth periods of infancy, early childhood, and adolescence; periods of strenuous activity; and disorders such as fever, hyperthyroidism, severe burns, trauma, or surgery. They decrease with sedentary activities and in elderly people. | Grains, fruits, and vegetables are good sources of carbohydrates and other essential nutrients. Candy and carbonated beverages contain kilocalories but lack other nutrients.<br>Glycogen is a reserve supply of glucose that can be mobilized to meet energy needs. The amount available is relatively small—approximately 110 g in the liver and 225 g in muscle. For some people, this amount would not meet requirements for 24 h during a fasting state. | Waste products from carbohydrate metabolism are mainly carbon dioxide and water. Carbon dioxide is mainly excreted through the lungs, and water may be excreted in urine or used for other metabolic processes. |
| **Proteins** | | | | |
| 1. Chemical substances composed of carbon, hydrogen, water, nitrogen, phosphorus, sulfur, and iron<br>2. When broken down in the body, proteins yield 4 kcal of energy per gram. They are used for energy only when intake of carbohydrates and fats is inadequate. | 1. Furnish amino acids for growth of new tissue and repair of damaged or worn-out tissue. Amino acids are the basic constituents or building blocks of all body cells.<br>2. Serve as components of numerous body fluids and secretions, including enzymes, | Approximately 0.8 g/kg of body weight daily<br>This amount maintains normal nitrogen balance and tissue growth and repair. An average adult female (58 kg) requires about 46 g; an average adult male (70 kg) requires about 56 g.<br>Requirements increase during growth periods | Animal foods, such as meat, fish, poultry, milk, eggs, and cheese, provide "complete" proteins, which contain all the essential amino acids. Proteins from beans, breads, and cereals are incomplete, but they can be combined in ways that provide adequate intake. | Nitrogenous waste products, ammonia, urea, and uric acid are excreted in the urine. |

**TABLE 30-1. WATER, CARBOHYDRATES, PROTEINS, AND FATS** (*Continued*)

| Characteristics | Functions | Requirements | Normal Sources | Normal Losses |
|---|---|---|---|---|
| 3. Most proteins are found in muscle tissue; others are found in soft tissues, bones, teeth, and blood and other body fluids. | many hormones, milk, mucus, and sperm. (Sweat, bile, and urine are normally protein free.) <br> 3. Assist in maintaining normal osmotic pressure in the blood. Albumin is especially important in fulfilling this function. <br> 4. Transport various substances in the blood. Lipid-carrying plasma proteins transport fat-soluble vitamins, cholesterol, triglycerides, and phospholipids. Transferrin carries iron, and another protein carries calcium. Albumin transports free fatty acids, bilirubin, and many drugs. <br> 5. Provide immunoglobulins or antibodies, which are important in resistance to disease | of children, pregnancy and lactation, fever, burn injuries, surgery, hyperthyroidism, and stress. Older adults need the same amount of protein (0.8 g/kg) as younger adults. | | |

### Fats (lipids)

| Characteristics | Functions | Requirements | Normal Sources | Normal Losses |
|---|---|---|---|---|
| 1. Several different chemical substances of which the major ones are triglycerides, phospholipids, and cholesterol. More than 98% of natural fats are triglycerides. <br> 2. Second choice as energy source, after carbohydrates. They furnish 9 kcal of energy per gram. <br> 3. Excess dietary fats are stored, excess carbohydrates and proteins are converted to fat and stored in adipose tissue. | 1. Provide energy for body metabolism <br> 2. Conserve proteins for tissue synthesis by preventing use of proteins for energy <br> 3. Protect organs from injury <br> 4. Conserve body heat and help maintain normal body temperature <br> 5. Conserve thiamine, a vitamin that is required for carbohydrate metabolism but not fat metabolism <br> 6. Promote intestinal absorption of fat-soluble vitamins <br> 7. Increase palatability of foods <br> 8. Slow gastric emptying, thereby increasing and prolonging satiety <br> 9. Promote normal growth and development <br> 10. Serve as essential components of cells and cell membranes <br> 11. Protect against entry of foreign substances and loss of water through the skin | Approximately 50–130 g daily (900–1200 kilocalories in a 3000-kcal diet). Requirements depend on weight, size, amount of carbohydrate ingested, physical activity, and other factors | High amounts of fat are contained in meat, egg yolk, cheese, butter, whole milk, salad dressings, cream, and ice cream. <br> In addition to food sources, triglycerides and cholesterol are formed in the liver. Cholesterol in foods is only about 50% absorbed. | Fats are excreted in sweat, bile, and feces or are oxidized to carbon dioxide and water, which are excreted. |

## TABLE 30-2. WATER IMBALANCES

### Water Deficit

| Causes | Signs and Symptoms |
|---|---|
| 1. Inadequate fluid intake, most likely to occur in people who are comatose, unable to swallow, or otherwise incapacitated<br>2. Excessive fluid loss due to vomiting, diarrhea, fever, diuretic drug therapy, high environmental temperatures, strenuous physical activity, or excessive sweating<br>3. A combination of 1 and 2 | 1. Thirst<br>2. Oliguria and concentrated urine<br>3. Weakness<br>4. Dry tongue and oral mucous membranes<br>5. Flushed skin<br>6. Weight loss<br>7. Fever<br>8. Increased hematocrit<br>9. Mental disturbances ranging from mild confusion to delirium, convulsions, and coma<br>10. Hypovolemic shock if the deficiency is severe or develops rapidly |

### Water Excess

| Causes | Signs and Symptoms |
|---|---|
| 1. Excessive intake, most likely to occur with excessive amounts or rapid infusion of IV fluids<br>2. Impaired excretion of fluids due to endocrine, renal, cardiovascular, or central nervous system disorders | 1. Drowsiness<br>2. Weakness and lethargy<br>3. Weight gain<br>4. Edema<br>5. Low serum sodium and hematocrit<br>6. Disorientation<br>7. Circulatory overload and pulmonary edema if water excess is severe or develops rapidly |

phetamines but are promoted for use only in appetite control. These drugs are of limited effectiveness in obesity and lose their appetite-suppressant effects in about 4 to 6 weeks. They are useful only for short-term therapy and as part of a weight-reduction program that also includes calorie restriction, exercise, medical supervision, and psychological support. These drugs may lead to abuse and dependence of the amphetamine type, and their use is regulated by the Controlled Substances Act. Anorexiant drugs are contraindicated in cardiovascular disease, hyperthyroidism, glaucoma, and agitated psychological disturbances.

Phenylpropanolamine is an adrenergic drug commonly used as a nasal decongestant in over-the-counter cold remedies. It is also the active ingredient in over-the-counter appetite suppressants (*e.g.*, Dexatrim, Acutrim). Effectiveness of the drug in weight reduction is limited, and its use has been associated with psychosis, hypertension, stroke, renal failure, cardiac arrhythmias, and death. These adverse effects have occurred with recommended doses but are especially likely with overdoses or concomitant use of other stimulants, such as caffeine.

# Individual nutritional products for oral or tube feeding

## NUTRITIONALLY COMPLETE LIQUID FORMULAS FOR GENERAL USE

**Compleat** (tube feeding [TF] 1600 ml), **Ensure** (orally [PO] or TF 2000 ml), **Isocal** (PO or TF 2000 ml), **Meritene** (PO or TF 1200 ml), **Osmolite** (TF 2000 ml), **Sustacal** (PO or TF 1080 ml), and **Sustagen** (PO or TF 1000 ml) are examples of formulas that provide Recommended Dietary Allowances for protein, vitamins, and minerals. Most of the formulas provide 1 calorie per milliliter.

When given in the designated amounts, these formulas meet basic nutritional needs for adults. However, amounts should be individualized according to nutritional needs and whether the formula is being used to supplement or substitute for other sources of food and fluids. **PediaSure** is a nutritionally complete formula for enteral use in children 1 to 6 years old.

## NUTRITIONAL AGENTS FOR SPECIFIC USES (DEFINED FORMULA OR ELEMENTAL DIETS)

**Lofenalac** is a low-phenylalanine preparation used only in infants and children with phenylketonuria, a metabolic disorder in which phenylalanine cannot be metabolized normally. Lofenalac is inadequate for com-

## TABLE 30-3. CARBOHYDRATE, PROTEIN, AND FAT IMBALANCES

### Protein–Calorie Deficit

| Causes | Signs and Symptoms |
|---|---|
| 1. Inadequate intake of protein, carbohydrate, and fat<br>2. Impaired ability to digest, absorb, or use nutrients<br>3. Excessive losses | 1. Weight loss with eventual loss of subcutaneous fat and muscle mass<br>2. Increased susceptibility to infection<br>3. Weakness and fatigability<br>4. Dry, scaly skin<br>5. Impaired healing<br>6. Impaired growth and development in children<br>7. Edema<br>8. Decreased hemoglobin<br>9. Acidosis<br>10. Disordered brain function<br>11. Coma<br>12. Starvation |

### Protein–Calorie Excess

| Causes | Signs and Symptoms |
|---|---|
| 1. Excessive intake, especially of carbohydrates and fats | 1. Weight gain<br>2. Obesity |

**TABLE 30-4. ANOREXIANTS**

| Generic/ Trade Name | Route and Dosage Range (Adults) | Status Under Controlled Substances Act | Remarks |
|---|---|---|---|
| **Benzphetamine** (Didrex) | PO 25–50 mg one to three times daily | Schedule III | Dosages not established for children under 12 years of age |
| **Diethylpropion** (Tenuate) | PO 25 mg three times daily | Schedule IV | |
| **Fenfluramine** (Pondimin) | PO 20–40 mg three times daily; maximal daily dose, 120 mg | Schedule IV | Fenfluramine generally has the same actions, uses, and characteristics as the other nonamphetamine anorexiant drugs. An important difference, however, is that fenfluramine depresses, rather than stimulates, the central nervous system. |
| **Mazindol** (Sanorex) | PO 1 mg three times daily | Schedule III | |
| **Phendimetrazine** (Plegine) | PO 35 mg two or three times daily or 105 mg once daily | Schedule III | |
| **Phentermine hydrochloride** (Fastin) | PO 8.0 mg three times daily or 15–37 mg daily in the morning | Schedule IV | |
| **Phentermine resin** (Ionamin) | PO 15–30 mg once daily | Schedule IV | |

plete nutrition and growth, although it meets Food & Drug Administration requirements for infant formulas. For growth needs, it is recommended that about 85% of the child's protein needs be supplied with Lofenalac and the remaining 10% to 15% be supplied with foods containing phenylalanine, which is an essential amino acid.

**MBF, Nursoy, ProSobee, Isomil**, and **Soyalac** are hypoallergenic, milk-free formulas. They derive their protein from soybean products rather than milk. They provide 20 calories/oz when mixed or diluted as directed and provide all other essential nutrients for normal growth and development. They are used as milk substitutes for clients who are allergic to milk (most often infants).

**Nutramigen** is a nutritionally complete hypoallergenic formula containing predigested protein. It is used for infants and children who are allergic to ordinary food proteins or who have diarrhea or other gastrointestinal (GI) problems.

**Portagen** is a nutritionally complete formula that contains medium-chain triglycerides, an easily digested form of fat. It is used primarily in clients with fat malabsorption problems. It may be used as the complete diet, as a beverage with meals, or as an addition to various recipes. It may induce coma in clients with severe hepatic cirrhosis.

**Precision diets** are nutritionally complete, low-residue formulas for oral or tube feedings. The **high-nitrogen diet** provides 125 g of protein or 20 g of nitrogen, 3000 kcal, and recommended amounts of essential vitamins and minerals in 10 3-oz servings. The **low-residue** formula contains 45 g of protein or 7.2 g of nitrogen

(a maintenance amount of protein), 1900 kcal, and essential vitamins and minerals in six 3-oz servings. The **isotonic** diet contains the same amounts of protein, vitamins, and minerals as the low-residue formula but is isotonic rather than hypertonic and provides 1500 kcal in six 2-oz servings.

These preparations are ingested or given by tube slowly over 4 hours. The carbohydrate content may produce hyperglycemia; therefore, they should not be used in clients with diabetes mellitus. These formulas can be given to children if the amount is calculated to provide recommended amounts of nutrients for the particular age group.

**Pregestimil** is an infant formula that contains easily digested protein, fat, and carbohydrate. It is used in infants with diarrhea, dietary intolerances, or malabsorption syndromes.

**Pulmocare** was designed for clients with chronic obstructive pulmonary disease. Because of impaired breathing, these clients have difficulty eliminating sufficient quantities of carbon dioxide, a waste product of carbohydrate metabolism. When carbon dioxide accumulates in the body, it may produce respiratory acidosis and eventually respiratory failure. Pulmocare contains more fat and less carbohydrate than most other formulas. Consequently, its metabolism produces less carbon dioxide. It contains 1.5 calories/ml.

**TraumaCal**, a high-protein formula with easily assimilated amino acids and other nutrients, was developed for clients with severe trauma or burn injuries to help meet nutritional needs and promote healing. It contains 1.5 calories/ml.

**Vivonex** is a nutritionally complete diet that contains crystalline amino acids as its protein or nitrogen source. It can be used for oral or tube feedings. It requires virtually no digestion and leaves virtually no fecal residue, so it is especially useful in GI disorders. The amount, concentration, and rate of administration can be adjusted to meet nutritional needs and tolerance in adults and children.

## NUTRITIONALLY INCOMPLETE SUPPLEMENTS

**Amin-Aid** is used as a source of protein for clients with acute and chronic renal insufficiency in whom dietary protein must be restricted. Amin-Aid supplies amino acids, carbohydrate, and a few electrolytes.

**Casec** is an oral protein supplement for use in infants, children, or adults.

**Citrotein** is an oral dietary supplement that provides protein, vitamins, and minerals. It is especially useful when appetite and food intake are decreased or during rapid growth periods when intake does not meet nutritional needs.

**Gevral Protein** is an oral supplement used to increase intake of protein, vitamins, and minerals. The powder can be mixed with water, milk, or other cold liquids, added to cereals, or mixed into desserts.

**Lipomul** (corn oil) and **Microlipid** (safflower oil) are fat supplements containing unsaturated fats.

**Lonalac**, an oral supplement, is used as a milk substitute in sodium-restricted diets or to increase protein intake when sodium must be restricted.

**MCT Oil** is a preparation of medium-chain triglycerides derived from coconut oil. MCT Oil is more easily digested than fats contained in most foods, which are mainly long-chain triglycerides. The medium-chain triglycerides are water soluble, are absorbed into the portal vein rather than lymphatic channels, and do not require the presence of bile salts for absorption. Thus, they are useful in children or adults with fat malabsorption syndromes. Although they are useful as a caloric substitute for dietary fat (1 tablespoon provides 115 kcal), they do not promote absorption of fat-soluble vitamins or provide essential fatty acids as the long-chain triglycerides do. MCT Oil can be mixed with fruit juices, used with salads or vegetables, or used in cooking and baking. Limited amounts of this product should be used in clients with severe hepatic cirrhosis because of the risk of precipitating encephalopathy and coma.

**Polycose** is an oral supplement used to increase caloric intake. Derived from carbohydrate, Polycose may be used by clients on protein-, electrolyte-, or fat-restricted diets. Available in liquid and powder, Polycose may be mixed with water or other beverages and with foods. Amounts taken should be determined by taste, calories needed, and tolerance.

## COMPLETE INFANT FORMULAS

**Enfamil, Similac**, and **SMA** are commonly used complete nutritional formulas for full-term infants or premature infants who can be bottle-fed. Either may be used alone for bottle-fed infants or as a supplement for breast-fed infants. These preparations are quite similar to human breast milk. Their only deficiency is in iron, which may be given separately or in a formula preparation containing iron.

# Intravenous fluids

**Dextrose injection** is available in preparations containing 2.5%, 5%, 10%, 20%, 25%, 30%, 40%, 50%, 60%, and 70% dextrose. The most frequently used concentration is 5% dextrose in water or sodium chloride injection. A concentration of 5% dextrose in water is approximately isotonic with blood. It provides water and 170 kcal/L. The dextrose is rapidly used, leaving "free" water for excreting waste products, maintaining renal function, and maintaining urine output. The 10% dextrose solution provides double the amount of calories in the same volume of fluid but is hypertonic and therefore may cause phlebitis. The 20% to 50% solutions are used primarily to provide calories in parenteral nutrition. They are hypertonic and must be given through a central or subclavian catheter.

**Dextrose and sodium chloride injection** is available in various concentrations. The most frequently used are 5% dextrose in 0.225% or 0.45% sodium chloride (also called $D_5$ 1/4 and $D_5$ 1/2 normal saline, respectively). These provide about 170 kcal/L, water, sodium, and chloride. They are frequently used for maintenance therapy, usually with added potassium chloride, in clients who cannot eat or drink. They also are used for replacement therapy when large amounts of fluid are lost, for keeping IV lines open, and for administering medications.

**Crystalline amino acid solutions** (Aminosyn, Freamine) contain essential and nonessential amino acids. These solutions are most often used with concentrated dextrose injection in parenteral nutrition.

**Fat emulsions** (Intralipid, Liposyn) provide a source of concentrated calories and essential fatty acids. The emulsion is usually given as part of parenteral nutrition. More calories can be supplied with a fat emulsion than with dextrose-protein solutions alone. It is available in 10% and 20% emulsions; 500 ml of 10% emulsion provides 550 calories. Fat emulsions should not provide more than 60% of total caloric intake.

# Pancreatic enzymes

**Pancreatin** is an oral preparation of pancreatic enzymes used to aid digestion and absorption of dietary carbohydrate, protein, and fat in conditions characterized by pancreatic enzyme deficiency. These conditions include cystic fibrosis, chronic pancreatitis, pancreatectomy, and pancreatic obstruction. **Pancrelipase** (Viokase) is essentially the same as pancreatin except that it may be more effective in steatorrhea (excess fat in the feces).

## Pancreatin

### *Route and dosage ranges*

*Adults:* PO 1 or 2 capsules or tablets with meals or snacks

*Children:* PO 1 or 2 capsules or tablets with each meal initially, increased in amount or frequency if necessary and adverse effects do not occur

## Pancrelipase

### *Route and dosage ranges*

*Adults:* PO 1–3 capsules or tablets before or with meals or snacks; or 1 or 2 packets of powder with meals or snacks

# *Nursing Process*

## Assessment

Assess each client for current or potential nutritional disorders. Some specific assessment factors include the following:

- What are usual drinking and eating patterns? Does fluid intake seem adequate? Does food intake seem adequate in terms of normal nutrition? Is the client financially able to purchase sufficient food? What are fluid and food likes and dislikes?
- Does the client know the basic foods for normal nutrition? Does the client view nutrition as important in maintaining health?
- Does the client appear overweight or underweight? How does current weight compare with the ideal weight for age and height?
- Does the client have symptoms, disease processes, treatment measures, medications, or diagnostic tests that are likely to interfere with nutrition? For example, many illnesses and oral medications cause anorexia, nausea, vomiting, and diarrhea.
- Are any conditions present that increase or decrease nutritional requirements?
- Check available reports of laboratory tests, such as serum proteins, complete blood count, and blood glucose. Nutritional disorders, as well as many other disorders, may cause abnormal values.

## Nursing diagnoses

- Altered Nutrition: Less than Body Requirements related to inadequate intake
- Altered Nutrition: Less than Body Requirements related to impaired ability to digest and absorb nutrients
- Altered Nutrition: More than Body Requirements related to excessive intake
- High Risk for Fluid Volume Deficit related to inadequate intake
- High Risk for Fluid Volume Excess related to excessive intake
- Diarrhea related to enteral nutrition
- Altered Growth and Development related to nutrient deficiency
- Altered Protection related to nutrient deficiency
- High Risk for Self-Care Deficit: Feeding
- Body Image Disturbance related to excessive weight loss or weight gain
- Knowledge Deficit: Normal nutrition
- Knowledge Deficit: Nutritional needs during illness
- High Risk for Infection related to microbial contamination of enteral formulas
- High Risk for Infection related to impaired tissue integrity with parenteral therapy

## Planning/Goals

*The client will:*
- Improve nutritional status in relation to body needs
- Maintain fluid and electrolyte balance
- Avoid complications of enteral nutrition, including aspiration, diarrhea, fluid volume deficit or excess, and infection
- Avoid complications of parenteral nutrition, including fluid volume deficit or excess and infection
- Identify the types and amounts of foods to meet nutritional needs
- Avoid overuse and abuse of anorexiant drugs

## Interventions

Implement measures to prevent nutritional disorders by promoting a well-balanced diet for all clients. Depending on the client's condition, diet orders, food preferences, knowledge and attitudes about nutrition, and other factors, specific activities may include the following:

- Provide food and fluid the client is willing and able to take, at preferred times when possible.
- Assist the client to a sitting position, cut meat, open containers, feed the client, and perform other actions if indicated.
- Treat symptoms or disorders that are likely to interfere with nutrition, such as pain, nausea, vomiting, or diarrhea.
- Consult with the physician or dietitian when needed, especially when special diets are ordered. Compliance is improved when the ordered diet differs as little as possible from the usual diet. Also, preferred foods often may be substituted for disliked ones.
- Promote exercise and activity. For the undernourished client, this may increase appetite, improve digestion, and aid bowel elimination. Exercise may distract the overweight or obese client from hunger.
- Minimize the use of sedative-type drugs when appropriate. Although no one should be denied pain relief, strong anal-

gesics and other sedatives may cause drowsiness and decreased desire or ability to eat and drink.

- Weigh clients at regular intervals.

*Teach clients:*

- The importance of nutrition in promoting health and recovery from illness
- The kinds and amounts of food and fluids needed for normal nutrition
- Ways of adapting restricted diets to increase their acceptability
- Benefits to be gained from nutritional agents, whether given orally, intravenously, or by tube feeding
- Benefits and techniques of weight control
- That anorexiants are ineffective unless combined with restricted calorie intake and increased exercise

### Evaluation

- Observe the undernourished client for quantity and quality of nutrient intake, weight gain, and improvement in laboratory tests of nutritional status (*e.g.*, serum proteins, blood sugar, electrolytes).
- Observe the obese client for food intake, weight loss, and appropriate use of exercise or anorexiant drugs.
- Observe children for quantity and quality of food intake and appropriate increases in height and weight.
- Interview and observe for signs and symptoms of complications of enteral and parenteral nutrition.

## Principles of therapy

### MANAGING FLUID DISORDERS

#### Fluid deficiency

Treatment of fluid deficiency is aimed toward increasing intake or decreasing loss, depending on causative factors. The safest and most effective way of replacing body fluids is to give oral fluids when possible. Water is probably best, at least initially. Fluids containing large amounts of carbohydrate, fat, or protein are hypertonic and may increase fluid volume deficit if taken without sufficient water. If the client cannot take oral food or fluids for a few days or can take only limited amounts, IV fluids can be used to provide complete or supplemental amounts of fluids. Frequently used solutions include 5% dextrose in water or sodium chloride.

To meet fluid needs over a longer period, a nasogastric or other GI tube may be used to administer fluids. Fluid needs must be assessed carefully for the client receiving food and fluid only by tube. Additional water is almost always needed after or between administrations of commercial tube-feeding formulas. Most of these formulas are hyperosmolar (hypertonic) and will intensify fluid deficit if an inadequate amount of water accompanies them. Some nurses are reluctant to give additional water or other fluids when tube-feeding formulas are used. They may give only 50 to 100 ml of water to rinse the tube even when obvious signs of fluid deficit are present (*e.g.*, concentrated urine, poor skin turgor, dry mucous membranes).

Another way of meeting long-term fluid needs when the GI tract cannot be used is parenteral nutrition. These IV solutions provide other nutrients as well as fluids.

Optimal amounts of fluid may vary greatly. For most clients, 2000 to 3000 ml daily is adequate. A person with severe heart failure or oliguric kidney disease needs smaller amounts, but someone with extra losses (*e.g.*, vomiting, diarrhea) needs more.

#### Fluid excess

Treatment of fluid excess is aimed toward decreasing intake and increasing loss. In acute circulatory overload or pulmonary edema, the usual treatment is to stop fluid intake (if the client is receiving IV fluids, slow the rate but keep the vein open for medication) and administer diuretics. Because fluid excess may be a life-threatening emergency, prevention is better than treatment.

### MANAGING UNDERNUTRITION

The goal of treatment is to provide an adequate quantity and quality of nutrients to meet tissue needs. Requirements for nutrients vary with age, level of activity, level of health or illness, and other factors that must be considered when designing appropriate therapy.

#### Oral feedings

The safest and most effective way of increasing nutritional intake is by oral feedings when feasible. High-protein, high-calorie foods can be included in many diets and given as between-meal or bedtime snacks. If the client cannot ingest enough food and fluid, many of the commercial nutritional preparations can be given as between-meal supplements to increase intake of protein and calories. These preparations vary in taste and acceptability. Measures to improve taste may include chilling, serving over ice, or mixing with fruit juice or another beverage. Specific methods depend on the client's taste preferences and the available formula. Refer to instructions, usually on the labels, for appropriate diluting and mixing of beverages.

#### Enteral (tube) feedings

When oral feeding is contraindicated but the GI tract is functioning, tube feeding has several advantages over IV fluids, especially for long-term use. First, tube feeding is usually safer, more convenient, and more economical. Second, it helps to prevent GI atrophy, maintain GI function, and maintain immune system function. Third, several tubes and placement sites are available. For example, a nasogastric tube may be used for about 4 weeks. For long-term feedings, a gastrostomy tube may be placed percutaneously (called percutaneous endoscopic gastrostomy tubes) or surgically. Nasoenteric tubes are recommended for clients at high risk of aspiration from gastric feedings or with gastric disorders. Except for gastrostomy tubes, the tubes should be soft and small bore to decrease trauma.

When tube feedings are the client's only source of nutrients, they should be nutritionally complete and given in amounts calculated to provide adequate water, protein, calories, vitamins, and minerals. Although tube-feeding formulas vary in osmolality and volume needed for adequate intake of nutrients, any of the complete formulas can be used effectively. Other guidelines include the following:

1. Once the kind and amount of formula are chosen, the method of feeding is selected. For feedings that enter the stomach, an intermittent schedule of administration every 4 to 6 hours, over 30 to 60 minutes, is usually recommended. For feedings that enter the duodenum or jejunum, a continuous drip method is required because the small bowel cannot tolerate the larger volumes of intermittent feedings. Continuous feedings require an infusion pump for accurate control of the flow rate.
2. A common practice has been to initiate feedings with small amounts of diluted solution (*i.e.*, half strength), then increase to larger amounts and full strength. The rationale is to decrease the diarrhea and dehydration that may ensue when hypertonic solutions are given, and water is drawn into the GI tract. Some authorities question the value of this regimen and prefer starting with small amounts of full-strength formulas. Isocal and Osmolite are isotonic and should be given full strength. Most formulas provide 1 kcal/ml so that caloric intake can be quickly calculated. Water can be given with, after, or between regular feedings and with medications, according to the client's fluid needs.
3. Other than problems resulting from hypertonic solutions and inadequate fluid intake (diarrhea, fluid volume deficit, hypernatremia), a major complication of tube feeding is aspiration of the formula into the lungs. This is more likely to occur with unconscious clients. It can be prevented by correctly positioning clients, verifying tube placement (before every intermittent feeding and about every 4 hours with continuous feedings), and giving feedings slowly.

## Parenteral feedings

Parenteral feedings are indicated when the GI tract is nonfunctioning; when enteral feedings would aggravate conditions such as inflammatory bowel diseases or pancreatitis; and when nutritional needs cannot be met by enteral feedings. For short-term use (about 3–5 days) of IV fluids, the goal is to provide adequate amounts of fluids and electrolytes and enough carbohydrate to minimize oxidation of body protein and fat for energy. Choice of specific solution depends on individual needs but probably should contain at least 5% dextrose. A frequently used solution is 5% dextrose in 0.22% sodium chloride, 2000 to 3000 ml/24 hours. Potassium chloride is often added, and vitamins may be added. These solutions are nutritionally inadequate.

## Parenteral nutrition

For long-term IV feedings (weeks to months), the goal is to provide all nutrients required for normal body functioning, including tissue growth. This goal can be met with parenteral nutrition. Basic nutritional solutions provide water, carbohydrate, protein, vitamins, and minerals. Originally, calories were supplied primarily by 25% to 50% glucose. This resulted in a hypertonic solution that had to be given in a central vein so it could be diluted rapidly. Although effective, central parenteral nutrition requires special techniques to increase safety and decrease complications. For example, a physician must insert the central IV catheter, and placement must be verified by a chest x-ray. Complications include air embolism and pneumothorax. Peripheral parenteral nutrition (PPN) was then developed. PPN, which contains 5% or 10% dextrose, can be given alone or in combination with oral or enteral feedings to increase nutrient intake.

Later, IV fat emulsions were developed to provide additional calories and essential fatty acids (in a small fluid volume). These solutions are isotonic and may be given centrally or peripherally. When given peripherally, they are coinfused with the PPN solution. The fat emulsion is thought to protect the vein and decrease or delay phlebitis.

Home administration of central parenteral nutrition and PPN is increasing. Guidelines for both methods include the following:

1. Administer with an infusion pump to control the flow rate accurately. The solution must be given at a consistent rate so that nutrients can be used and complications prevented. The initial flow rate is usually 50 ml/h; flow rate is then increased as tolerated to meet nutritional requirements (about 1500–3000 ml/d). With home administration, the entire daily amount may be infused overnight.
2. To prevent infection, several measures are indicated. First, the IV catheter must be inserted with aseptic technique. Second, all solutions must be prepared aseptically in the pharmacy under a laminar flow hood. Third, use an 0.45- to 0.22-$\mu$m in-line filter.

Fourth, change solution containers and tubing every 24 hours. Fifth, change the dressing at the venipuncture site at least every 48 hours. Most hospitals and home health agencies have established protocols regarding dressing changes. These usually include cleansing around the catheter with povidone-iodine solution (Betadine), applying povidone-iodine ointment, and reapplying an occlusive dressing. Sterile technique is used throughout.

3. "Piggyback" fat emulsions into the IV line beyond the filter.

## MANAGING OVERWEIGHT OR OBESITY

1. For effective weight loss and continued weight control, the main elements are decreasing caloric intake and increasing exercise (caloric output). This largely depends on the client's motivation and self-discipline in changing eating habits. This is very difficult for most people to do.

2. Many reduction diets and regimens have been proposed. Among the more successful programs are groups that meet regularly and offer psychological support and diet plans. Among the more radical treatments are surgical procedures that limit the amount of food and fluid that can be ingested.

3. Drug therapy has a limited role in weight control. Anorexiant drugs are effective for only a few weeks, so they may be helpful in initiating a weight-reduction program. Many clients regain weight, however, when the drugs are stopped.

4. The role of the nurse may involve counseling about benefits to be gained from weight loss, the undesirability and hazards of "fad" diets, and specific ways of decreasing caloric intake, such as low-calorie snacks, participating in noneating activities, and not buying favorite high-calorie foods. Any program for weight control must be individualized, and continued support must be available.

## NUTRITIONAL SUPPORT FOR CHILDREN

Children generally need increased amounts of water, protein, carbohydrate, and fat in proportion to their size to support growth and increased physical activity. However, reports of childhood obesity and inadequate exercise abound. Therefore, the goal of nutritional support is to meet needs without promoting obesity.

With tube feedings, to prevent nausea and regurgita-tion, the recommended rate of administration is no more than 5 ml every 5 to 10 minutes for premature and small infants and 10 ml/min for older infants and children. Preparation of formulas, positioning of children, and administration are the same as for adults to prevent aspiration, diarrhea, and infection.

Parenteral nutrition may be indicated in infants and children who cannot eat or be fed enterally. With newborns, especially preterm and low–birth-weight infants, parenteral nutrition is needed within about 3 days of birth because they have little nutritional reserve. However, lipid emulsions should be given very cautiously in preterm infants because deaths have been attributed to increased serum levels of lipids and free fatty acids. With other infants and children, parenteral nutrition may be used during medical illnesses or perioperative conditions to improve or maintain nutritional status. Overall, benefits include weight gain, increased height, increased liver synthesis of plasma proteins, and improved healing and recovery.

## NUTRITIONAL SUPPORT FOR OLDER ADULTS

Older adults are at risk of developing deficits and excesses in fluid volume. Inadequate intake is common and may result from numerous causes (*e.g.,* impaired thirst mechanism, impaired ability to obtain and drink fluids, inadequate water with hyperosmolar tube feedings). Increased losses also occur with diuretic drugs, which are commonly prescribed for older adults. Fluid volume excess is most likely to occur with large amounts or rapid administration of IV fluids, especially in older adults with impaired cardiovascular function.

Older adults also are at risk of undernutrition and overnutrition in terms of protein, carbohydrate, and fat intake. Inadequate intake may result from the inability to obtain and prepare food, as well as disease processes that interfere with the ability to digest and use nutrients. When alternative feeding methods (tube feedings, IV fluids) are used, careful assessment of nutritional status is required to avoid deficits or excesses. Excessive intake may result from continuing usual eating patterns while exercising less. Caloric needs are usually decreased in older adults, primarily because of slowed metabolism and decreased physical activity. With the high incidence of atherosclerosis and cardiovascular disease in older adults, it is especially important that fat intake be reduced.

# NURSING ACTIONS: NUTRITIONAL PRODUCTS AND ANOREXIANTS

| *Nursing Actions* | *Rationale/Explanation* |
|---|---|

**1. Administer accurately**

**a.** For oral supplemental feedings:

(1) Give at the preferred time and temperature, when possible.

To increase the likelihood the feeding will be taken. Chilling the formula may increase palatability.

(2) Mix powders or concentrated liquid preparations in preferred beverages if not contraindicated.

Some can be mixed with fruit juice, milk, tea, or coffee, which may improve taste and acceptability.

(3) Provide flavoring packets when available and preferred by the client.

To improve taste and add variety.

**b.** For IV feedings:

(1) Administer fluids at the prescribed flow rate. Use an infusion control device for hyperalimentation solutions.

To administer sufficient fluids without a rapid flow rate. Rapid flow rates or large amounts of IV fluids can cause circulatory overload and pulmonary edema. In addition, hyperglycemia and osmotic diuresis may occur with hyperalimentation solutions.

(2) With IV fat emulsions, connect to the primary IV line beyond the filter; start slowly (0.5–1 ml/min) for about 30 minutes. If no adverse effects occur, increase rate to a maximum of 125 ml/h for the 10% solution or 60 ml/h for a 20% solution.

Lipid emulsions should not be filtered.

(3) Use sterile technique when changing containers, tubings, or dressings.

To prevent infection

(4) When adding drugs, use sterile technique, and add only those drugs known to be compatible with the IV solution.

To avoid physical or chemical incompatibility

(5) Do not administer antibiotics or other drugs through central venous catheters.

To avoid incompatibilities and possible precipitation or inactivation of the drug or fluid components

**c.** For tube feedings:

(1) Have the client sitting, if possible.

To decrease risks of aspirating formula into lungs

(2) Check tube placement before each feeding by aspirating stomach contents or instilling air into the tube while listening over the stomach with a stethoscope.

To prevent aspiration or accidental instillation of feedings into lungs

(3) Give the solution at room temperature.

Cold formulas may cause abdominal cramping.

(4) If giving by intermittent instillation, do not give more than 500 ml per feeding, including water for rinsing the tube.

To avoid gastric distention, possible vomiting, and aspiration into lungs

(5) Give by gravity flow (over 30–60 minutes) or infusion pump.

Rapid administration may cause nausea, vomiting, and other symptoms.

(6) With continuous feedings, change containers and tubing daily. With intermittent bolus feedings, rinse all equipment after each use, and change at least every 24 hours.

Most tube feeding formulas are milk based and provide a good culture medium for bacterial growth. Clean technique, not sterile technique, is required.

(7) Give an adequate amount of water, based on assessment of fluid needs. This may be done by mixing water with the tube feeding formula, giving it after the tube feeding, or giving it between feedings.

To avoid dehydration and promote fluid balance. Most clients receiving 1500 to 2000 ml of tube feeding formula daily will need 1000 ml or more of water daily.

*(continued)*

## Nursing Actions

## Rationale/Explanation

(8) Rinse nasogastric tubes with at least 50 to 100 ml water after each bolus feeding or administration of medications through the tube.

To keep the tube patent and functioning. This water is included in calculation of fluid intake.

(9) When medications are ordered by tube, liquid preparations are preferred over crushed tablets or powders emptied from capsules.

Tablets or powders may stick in the tube lumen. This may mean the full dose of the medication does not reach the stomach. Also, the tube is likely to become obstructed.

**d.** With pancreatic enzymes, give with meals or food.

To obtain therapeutic effects, these agents must be in the small intestine when food is present.

**e.** With anorexiant drugs:

(1) Give single-dose drugs in the early morning.

For maximum appetite-suppressant effects during the day

(2) Give multiple-dose preparations 30 to 60 minutes before meals and the last dose of the day about 6 hours before bedtime.

For maximum appetite-suppressant effects at mealtime and to avoid interference with sleep from the drug's stimulating effects on the central nervous system (CNS)

2. **Observe for therapeutic effects**
   **a.** With water and other fluids, observe for fluid balance (amber-colored urine, about 1500 ml daily; moist mucous membranes in the oral cavity; adequate skin turgor).

   **b.** With nutritional formulas given orally or by tube feeding, observe for weight gain and increased serum albumin. For infants and children receiving milk substitutes, observe for decreased diarrhea and weight gain.

Therapeutic effects depend on the reason for use (that is, prevention or treatment of undernutrition).

   **c.** With parenteral hyperalimentation, observe for weight maintenance or gain and normal serum levels of glucose, electrolytes, and protein.

These are indications of improved metabolism, nitrogen balance, and nutritional status. When parenteral hyperalimentation is used for gastrointestinal malabsorption syndromes, diarrhea and other symptoms are usually relieved when oral feedings are stopped.

   **d.** With pancreatic enzymes, observe for decreased diarrhea and steatorrhea.

The pancreatic enzymes function the same way as endogenous enzymes to aid digestion of carbohydrate, protein, and fat.

   **e.** With anorexiant drugs, observe for decreased caloric intake and weight loss.

The recommended rate of weight loss is about 2 to 3 lb weekly.

3. **Observe for adverse effects**
   **a.** With fluids, observe for peripheral edema, circulatory overload, and pulmonary edema (severe dyspnea, crackles).

Fluid excess is most likely to occur with rapid administration or large amounts of IV fluids, especially in people who are elderly or have congestive heart failure.

   **b.** With commercial nutritional formulas (except Osmolite and Isocal), observe for hypotension, tachycardia, increased urine output, dehydration, nausea, vomiting, or diarrhea.

These adverse reactions are usually attributed to the hyperosmolality or hypertonicity of the preparations. They can be prevented or minimized by starting with small amounts of formula, given slowly.

   **c.** With parenteral hyperalimentation, observe for elevated blood and urine glucose levels, signs of infection (fever, inflammation at the venipuncture site), concentrated urine of high specific gravity (1.035 or above), hypertension, dyspnea.

These signs and symptoms indicate complications of therapy. Except for infection, they are likely to occur when the solution is given in a concentration or at a rate that delivers more glucose than can be used. This produces hyperglycemia, which in turn causes excessive amounts of fluid to be excreted in the urine (osmotic diuresis). Hyperglycemic, hyperosmolar, nonketotic coma also may occur.

   **d.** With IV fat emulsions, observe for signs of fat embolism (dyspnea, fever, chills, pain in the chest and back), phlebitis from vein irritation, and sepsis from contamination. Hyperlipidemia and hepatomegaly also may occur.

Thrombophlebitis and sepsis are the most frequent adverse effects.

| *Nursing Actions* | *Rationale/Explanation* |
|---|---|
| **e.** With anorexiant drugs, observe for: | |
| (1) Nervousness, insomnia, hyperactivity | These adverse effects are caused by excessive stimulation of the CNS. They are more likely to occur with large doses or too frequent administration. |
| (2) Hypertension | Anorexiant drugs stimulate the sympathetic nervous system and may cause or aggravate hypertension. |
| (3) Development of tolerance to appetite-suppressant effects | This usually occurs within 4 to 6 weeks and is an indication for discontinuing drug administration. Continued administration does not maintain appetite-suppressant effects but increases incidence of adverse effects. In addition, taking large doses of the drug does not restore appetite-suppressant effects. |
| (4) Signs of psychological drug dependence | More likely with large doses or long-term use |
| (5) With fenfluramine, observe for drowsiness during use and mental depression when the drug is discontinued. | Fenfluramine causes CNS depression rather than the stimulation that occurs with other anorexiant drugs. |
| **4. Observe for drug interactions with anorexiants** | |
| **a.** Drugs that *increase* effects: | |
| (1) Alkalinizing agents (*e.g.,* sodium bicarbonate) | Potentiate anorexiants by increasing gastrointestinal absorption and decreasing urinary excretion |
| (2) Antidepressants, tricyclic | May increase hypertensive effects of anorexiants |
| (3) Monoamine oxidase (MAO) inhibitors | Increase hypertensive effects. Anorexiants should not be given within 2 weeks of MAO inhibitors because of possible hypertensive crisis. |
| (4) Other CNS stimulants | Additive stimulant effects |
| (5) Other sympathomimetic drugs (*e.g.,* epinephrine, isoproterenol) | Additive hypertensive and other cardiovascular effects |
| **b.** Drugs that *decrease* effects: | |
| (1) Acidifying agents (*e.g.,* ascorbic acid) | Decrease gastrointestinal absorption and increase urinary excretion |
| (2) Antihypertensive drugs | Anorexiants have blood pressure-raising effects that antagonize blood pressure-lowering effects of drugs used for hypertension |
| (3) CNS depressants (*e.g.,* alcohol, chlorpromazine) | Antagonize or decrease effects |
| **5. Teach clients** | |
| **a.** Most intravenous fluids are nutritionally inadequate and useful only for short-term treatment. Thus, return to oral feedings is desirable as soon as tolerated after surgery or illness. | |
| **b.** Take pancreatic enzymes with food. | To obtain the therapeutic benefit of increased digestion and absorption of foods |
| **c.** Take anorexiants in the dosage and for the length of time prescribed. | Excessive dosage will cause potentially serious adverse reactions. These drugs lose their appetite-depressant effects in 4 to 6 weeks. Prolonged use may lead to psychological dependence. |

## Review and Application Exercises

1. How does an adequate fluid balance help to maintain normal body functioning?
2. Differentiate clients who are at high risk of developing fluid imbalances.
3. When assessing a client's fluid balance, what signs and symptoms indicate fluid volume deficit or excess?
4. What are pharmacologic and nonpharmacologic interventions to restore fluid balance when an imbalance occurs?
5. For clients who are unable to ingest food, which nutrients can be provided with IV nutritional formulas?
6. How do peripheral intravenous nutritional formulas differ from those that must be given with a "deep line"?
7. What is the role of lipid emulsions in parenteral nutrition?
8. In an infant receiving parenteral nutrition, what is the best way to assess the adequacy of nutritional status?
9. In an outpatient or home care client with a protein-calorie deficit and various commercial nutritional supplements or replacement formulas:

    Analyze the types and amounts of nutrients provided.

    Choose a supplement to recommend to the client or caregiver.

    Designate the amount to be taken daily for optimum nutritional status.

    Suggest ways to increase palatability and client ingestion of the nutrients.

10. With an obese client who requests anorexiant drugs to assist with weight loss, discuss the advantages and disadvantages of drug therapy versus nonpharmacologic weight loss measures.

## Selected References

Campbell, S. M. (1992). Adult enteral nutrition. In M. A. Koda-Kimble & L. Y. Young (Eds.), *Applied therapeutics: The clinical use of drugs* (5th ed.) (pp. 31-1–31-8). Vancouver, WA: Applied Therapeutics.

Corman, L. C. (1993). The role of nutrition in sickness and in health. *Medical Clinics of North America, 77*(4), 711–724.

Davis, J. R., & Sherer, K. (1994). *Applied nutrition and diet therapy for nurses* (2nd ed.). Philadelphia: W.B. Saunders.

(1993). *Drug facts and comparisons*. St. Louis: Facts and Comparisons.

Ebbert-Sauer, M. L. (1992). Adult parenteral nutrition. In M. A. Koda-Kimble & L. Y. Young (Eds.), *Applied therapeutics: The clinical use of drugs* (5th ed.) (pp. 30-1–30-14). Vancouver, WA: Applied Therapeutics.

Gerlach, M. J., McDermott, M. M., Burrell, L. O., Lukens, L., McCall, C.Y., Walters, N.G., & Lillis, P.P. (1992). Nursing management of adults with common problems of the gastrointestinal system. In L.O. Burrell (Ed.), *Adult nursing in hospital and community settings*, (pp. 1321–1378). Norwalk, CT: Appleton & Lange.

Schwartz, R.S. (1992). Geriatric clinical nutrition. In W.N. Kelley (Ed.), *Textbook of internal medicine* (2nd ed.) (pp. 2391–2395). Philadelphia: J.B. Lippincott.

Thornhill, D. G., & Pleuss, J. (1990). Alterations in nutritional status. In C. M. Porth (Ed.), *Pathophysiology: Concepts of altered health states* (3rd ed.) (pp 743–765). Philadelphia: J.B. Lippincott.

Wesley, J. R. (1992). Efficacy and safety of total parenteral nutrition in pediatric patients. *Mayo Clinic Proceedings, 67*, 671–675.

Williams, L., Davis, J. A., & Lowenthal, D. T. (1993). The influence of food on the absorption and metabolism of drugs. *Medical Clinics of North America, 77*(4), 815–829.

Young, C., & White, S. (1992). Preparing patients for tube feeding at home. *American Journal of Nursing, 92*, 46–53.

# CHAPTER 31

# Vitamins

## Description and uses

Vitamins are a group of substances necessary for normal body metabolism of fat, carbohydrate, and protein. They act mainly as coenzymes to help convert carbohydrate and fat into energy and form bones and tissues. These compounds vary greatly in chemical structure and function. They are effective in small amounts and are normally obtained from foods. Vitamins are usually classified as fat soluble (A, D, E, K) and water soluble (B complex, C). Fat-soluble vitamins are absorbed from the intestine with dietary fat, and absorption requires the presence of bile salts and pancreatic lipase. These vitamins are relatively stable in cooking. Water-soluble vitamins are readily absorbed but are also readily lost by improper cooking and storage. Vitamin D is discussed in Chapter 26 because of its major role in bone metabolism.

Table 31-1 summarizes the characteristics, functions, food sources, and recommended amounts of vitamins. The recommended dietary allowances (RDAs) were established by the Food and Nutrition Board of the National Academy of Sciences for daily intake by healthy adults and children. The RDAs were revised in 1989. When inadequate amounts of vitamins are ingested, vitamin deficiencies result. Deficiency states are uncommon in people who can eat and are generally healthy. They are more likely to occur with disease processes that interfere with absorption or use of vitamins. When excessive amounts of fat-soluble vitamins are taken, excess states may occur because fat-soluble vitamins accumulate in the body. Excess states do not occur with dietary intake of water-soluble vitamins because these vitamins are rapidly excreted in the urine. Causes and clinical manifestations of vitamin disorders are listed in Table 31-2.

### PRESCRIPTION VITAMINS

When vitamins are prescribed by a physician to prevent or treat deficiencies, they exert the same physiologic effects as those obtained from foods. Synthetic vitamins have the same structure and function as natural vitamins derived from plant and animal sources. There is no evidence that natural vitamins are superior to synthetic vitamins. Natural vitamins are usually much more expensive.

### NONPRESCRIPTION VITAMINS

There are many commercially available vitamin preparations; some contain a single vitamin, and some contain multiple vitamins. The only clear-cut indications for use of these products are prevention and treatment of vitamin deficiencies. Because vitamins are essential nutrients, some people believe that large doses (megadoses) promote health and provide other beneficial effects. There is no evidence that amounts beyond those needed for normal body functioning serve any beneficial effects; excessive intake of vitamins causes harmful effects. Thus, "megavitamins" should never be self-prescribed.

Many multivitamin preparations do not require a physician's prescription. These preparations vary widely in number, type, and amount of specific ingredients. Although useful in certain situations, they cannot be used interchangeably or indiscriminately with safety. More specific characteristics include the following:

1. Preparations promoted for use as dietary supplements may contain 50% of the amounts recom-

(*Text continues on p. 336*)

**TABLE 31-1.    VITAMINS AS NUTRIENTS**

| | Characteristics | Functions | Recommended Dietary Allowances (RDAs) | Dietary Sources |
|---|---|---|---|---|
| **Fat-Soluble Vitamins** | | | | |
| Vitamin A (Retinol) | 1. Obtained from animal foods and plant foods that contain carotenoids (precursors of vitamin A) <br> 2. About one third of carotenoids are absorbed, and they become active in body functioning only after conversion to retinol in the wall of the small intestine. <br> 3. Retinol, another name for preformed vitamin A, is the physiologically active form. <br> 4. Vitamin A activity is expressed in retinol equivalents (RE), which include both preformed Vitamin A and carotenoids. 1 RE = 1 μg retinol or 6 μg beta-carotene. | Required for normal vision, growth, bone development, skin, and mucous membrane | Women: 800 RE (4000 IU) <br> Men: 1000 RE (5000 IU) <br> Pregnant women: 1000 RE (5000 IU) <br> Lactating women: 1200 RE (6000 IU) <br> Children 1–10 years: 400–700 RE (2000–3500 IU); 11 years and older: same as adults | Preformed vitamin A— meat, butter and fortified margarine, egg yolk, whole milk, cheese made from whole milk <br> Carotenoids—turnip and collard greens, carrots, sweet potatoes, squash, apricots, peaches, cantaloupe |
| Vitamin E | 1. A group of substances called tocopherols, of which alpha-tocopherol is most biologically active <br> 2. Vitamin E activity is expressed in milligrams of alpha-tocopherol equivalents (alpha TE). | It is thought to act as an antioxidant in preventing destruction of certain fats, including the lipid portion of cell membranes. It also may increase absorption, hepatic storage, and use of vitamin A. | Women: 8 mg alpha TE <br> Men: 10 mg alpha TE <br> Children up to 10 years: 3–7 mg alpha TE; 11 years and older, same as adults | Cereals, green vegetables, egg yolk, milk fat, butter, meat, vegetable oils |
| Vitamin K | 1. Occurs naturally in two forms: phytonadione ($K_1$), found in plant foods, and menaquinone ($K_2$), synthesized in the intestine by bacteria <br> 2. Absorbed mainly from the upper intestine in the presence of bile and dietary fats | Essential for normal blood clotting. Activates precursor proteins, found in the liver, into clotting factors: prothrombin (factor II), proconvertin (factor VII), plasma thromboplastin component (factor IX), and Stuart factor (factor X) | 1 μg/kg | Green leafy vegetables (spinach, kale, cabbage, lettuce), cauliflower, tomatoes, wheat bran, cheese, egg yolk, liver |
| Vitamin D | See Chapter 26. | | | |
| **Water-Soluble Vitamins** | | | | |
| **B-Complex Vitamins** | | | | |
| Biotin | Must be obtained from dietary intake. There is also some synthesis by intestinal bacteria, and a portion is absorbed. | Essential in fat and carbohydrate metabolism | Not established; provisionally set at 30–100 μg | Meat, especially liver, egg yolk, nuts, cereals; most vegetables |
| Cyanocobalamin (vitamin $B_{12}$) | In addition to food sources, some is also obtained from tissue storage in the liver and from recovery of cyanocobalamin secreted in bile and reabsorbed in the small intestine. | Essential for normal metabolism of all body cells (especially those of the bone marrow, nervous tissue, and gastrointestinal tract); normal red blood cells; growth; and metabolism of carbohydrate, protein, and fat | Adults: 2 μg <br> Children: 0.7–1.4 μg <br> Infants: 0.3–0.5 μg | Meat, especially liver, eggs, fish, cheese |

**TABLE 31-1. VITAMINS AS NUTRIENTS** *(Continued)*

| | Characteristics | Functions | Recommended Dietary Allowances (RDAs) | Dietary Sources |
|---|---|---|---|---|
| Folic acid (folate) | 1. Obtained from foods and the enterohepatic cycle. The latter provides an endogenous source, because folate is excreted in bile, reabsorbed in the small bowel, and reused. 2. May be lost from vegetables stored at room temperature or cooked at high temperatures. | Essential for normal metabolism of all body cells, for normal red blood cells, and for growth | Women: 180 $\mu$g<br>Men: 200 $\mu$g<br>Pregnant woman: 400 $\mu$g<br>Lactating women: 260–280 $\mu$g<br>Children, 1–10 years: 50–100 $\mu$g; 11–14 years, 150 $\mu$g; Infants: 25–35 $\mu$g | Liver, kidney beans, fresh green vegetables (spinach, broccoli, asparagus) |
| Niacin (vitamin B$_3$) | 1. Obtained from food and endogenous synthesis from tryptophan. 2. Niacin activity is expressed in niacin equivalents (NE): 1 mg of niacin or 60 mg tryptophan = 1 NE. | Essential for glycolysis, fat synthesis, and tissue respiration. It functions as a coenzyme in many metabolic processes (after conversion to nicotinamide, the physiologically active form). | Women: 15 NE<br>Men: 20 NE<br>Pregnant women: 17 NE<br>Lactating women: 20 NE<br>Children, 1–10 years: 9–13 NE<br>Males, 11–14 years, 17 NE; females, 11–14 years, 15 NE<br>Infants: 5–6 NE | Meat, poultry, fish, peanuts |
| Pantothenic acid (vitamin B$_5$) | | A component of coenzyme A and essential for cellular metabolism (intermediary metabolism of carbohydrate, fat, and protein; release of energy from carbohydrate; fatty acid metabolism; synthesis of cholesterol, steroid hormones, phospholipids, and porphyrin) | Not established. Estimated at 4–7 mg. | Eggs, liver, salmon, yeast, cauliflower, broccoli, lean beef, potatoes, tomatoes |
| Pyridoxine (vitamin B$_6$) | Occurs in three forms (pyridoxal, pyridoxine, and pyridoxamine), all of which are converted in the body to pyridoxal phosphate, the physiologically active form. | 1. Serves as a coenzyme in many metabolic processes 2. Functions in metabolism of carbohydrate, protein, and fat 3. Required for formation of tryptophan and conversion of tryptophan to niacin 4. As part of the enzyme phosphorylase, helps release glycogen from the liver and muscle tissue 5. Functions in metabolism of the central nervous system 6. Helps maintain cellular immunity | Women: 1.6 mg<br>Men: 2 mg<br>Pregnant women: 2.2 mg<br>Lactating women: 2.1 mg<br>Children, 1–10 years: 1–1.4 mg<br>Males, 11–14 years, 1.7 mg; females 11–14 years, 1.4 mg<br>Infants: 0.3–0.6 mg | Yeast, wheat germ, liver and other glandular meats, whole grain cereals, potatoes, legumes |
| Riboflavin (vitamin B$_2$) | | 1. Serves as a coenzyme in metabolism 2. Necessary for growth 3. May function in production of corticosteroids and red blood cells and in gluconeogenesis | Women: 1.3 mg<br>Men: 1.7 mg<br>Pregnant women: 1.6 mg<br>Lactating women: 1.7 mg<br>Children, 1–10 years: 0.8–1.2 mg<br>Males, 11–14 years, 1.5 mg; females, 11–14 years, 1.3 mg<br>Infants: 0.4–0.5 mg | Milk, cheddar and cottage cheese, meat, eggs, green leafy vegetables |

*(continued)*

**TABLE 31-1. VITAMINS AS NUTRIENTS** *(Continued)*

| | Characteristics | Functions | Recommended Dietary Allowances (RDAs) | Dietary Sources |
|---|---|---|---|---|
| Thiamine (vitamin B₁) | | A coenzyme in carbohydrate metabolism and essential for energy production | Women: 1.1 mg<br>Men: 1.5 mg<br>Pregnant women: 1.5 mg<br>Lactating women: 1.6 mg<br>Children, 1–10 years: 0.7–1 mg<br>Males, 11–14 years, 1.3 mg; females, 11–14 years, 1.1 mg<br>Infants: 0.3–0.4 mg | Meat, poultry, fish, egg yolk, dried beans, whole grain cereal products, peanuts |
| *Vitamin C*<br>Vitamin C (ascorbic acid) | 1. Dietary vitamin C is well absorbed from the intestinal tract and distributed widely in body tissues.<br>2. Not stored in body to a significant extent. Once tissues are saturated with about 1500 mg, any excess is excreted in the urine. | 1. Essential for collagen formation (collagen is a fibrous protein in connective tissue throughout the body, including skin, ligaments, cartilage, bone, and teeth)<br>2. Required for wound healing and tissue repair, metabolism of iron and folic acid, synthesis of fats and proteins, preservation of blood vessel integrity, and resistance to infection | Adults: 60 mg<br>Pregnant women: 70 mg<br>Lactating women: 90–95 mg<br>Children, infancy–14 years: 30–50 mg; 15 years and older, 60 mg | Fruits and vegetables, especially citrus fruits and juices |

mended for daily intake. In healthy people who eat a well-balanced diet, nutrient needs may be greatly exceeded.

2. Preparations for therapeutic use may contain 300% to 500% of the amounts recommended for daily intake in normal circumstances. These should not contain more than recommended amounts of vitamin D, folic acid, and vitamin A.

3. Multivitamin preparations often contain minerals as well, usually in amounts much smaller than those recommended for daily intake.

Individual vitamin preparations are listed in Table 31-3.

## Nursing Process

### Assessment

Assess each client for current or potential vitamin disorders during an overall assessment of nutritional status. Specific assessment factors related to vitamins include the following:

- Deficiency states are more common than excess states.
- People with other nutritional deficiencies are likely to have vitamin deficiencies as well.
- Deficiencies of water-soluble vitamins (B complex and C) are more common than those of fat-soluble vitamins.

- Vitamin deficiencies are usually multiple, and signs and symptoms often overlap, especially with B-complex deficiency states.
- Vitamin requirements are generally increased during infancy, pregnancy, lactation, fever, hyperthyroidism, and probably most illnesses. Thus, a vitamin intake that is normally adequate may become inadequate in certain circumstances.
- Vitamin deficiencies are likely to occur in people who are poor, elderly, chronically or severely ill, or alcoholic.
- Vitamin excess states are uncommonly caused by excessive dietary intake but may occur with use of vitamin drug preparations, especially if megadoses are taken.

### Nursing diagnoses

- High Risk for Altered Nutrition: Less than Body Requirements related to vitamin deficiency
- High Risk for Altered Nutrition: More than Body Requirements related to vitamin excess with overuse of supplements
- High Risk for Injury related to vitamin deficiency or overdose
- Knowledge Deficit: Importance of adequate vitamin intake in normal body functioning
- Knowledge Deficit: Dietary sources of various vitamins
- Knowledge Deficit: Adverse effects of self-prescribed megadoses of vitamins

### Planning/Goals

*The client will:*

- Ingest appropriate amounts and sources of dietary vitamins

## TABLE 31-2. VITAMIN IMBALANCES

| | Deficiency States | | Excess States | |
|---|---|---|---|---|
| | *Causes* | *Signs and Symptoms* | *Causes* | *Signs and Symptoms* |
| **Fat-Soluble Vitamins** | | | | |
| Vitamin A | Rarely caused by inadequate dietary intake in the United States; usually occurs with disease processes that interfere with intake, absorption, or use. Absorption is decreased with a lack of dietary fat or bile salts (from biliary tract obstruction), inflammatory gastrointestinal (GI) conditions, and other conditions characterized by malabsorption and diarrhea. Hepatitis or hepatic cirrhosis may prevent liver storage of vitamin A. | Night blindness Xerophthalmia, which may progress to corneal ulceration and blindness Changes in skin and mucous membranes that lead to skin lesions and infections, respiratory tract infections, and urinary calculi | Excessive intake of vitamin A, which is unlikely with dietary intake but can occur with vitamin abuse | Anorexia Vomiting Irritability Headache Skin changes (dryness, itching, desquamation, dermatitis) Later manifestations may include fatigue, pain in muscles, bones, and joints, gingivitis, enlargement of spleen and liver, altered liver function, increased intracranial pressure, and other neurologic signs. Congenital abnormalities may occur in newborns whose mothers took excessive vitamin A during pregnancy. Acute toxicity, with increased intracranial pressure, bulging fontanels, and vomiting, may occur in infants who are given vitamin A. |
| Vitamin E | Deficiency is rare. | | Excessive state not established | |
| Vitamin K | Inadequate intake, absorption, or use. Rarely caused by inadequate intake after infancy. Occurs commonly in newborns owing to lack of dietary intake of vitamin K and lack of intestinal synthesis of the vitamin during the first week of life. After infancy, deficiency usually results from diseases that interfere with absorption (biliary tract and GI disorders) or use (hepatic cirrhosis and hepatitis). In alcoholics, deficiency commonly occurs and probably results from decreased intake and impaired use. Drug-induced deficiency occurs with oral coumarin anticoagulants and some other drugs that act as vitamin K antagonists. Also, antibiotics reduce bacterial synthesis of vitamin K in the intestine, but this is a rare cause of deficiency. | Abnormal bleeding (melena, hematemesis, hematuria, epistaxis, petechiae, ecchymoses, hypovolemic shock) | Unlikely to occur from dietary intake; may occur when vitamin K is given as an antidote for oral anticoagulants | Clinical manifestations rarely occur. However, when vitamin K is given to someone who is receiving warfarin (Coumadin), the client can be made "warfarin-resistant" for 2–3 wk. |
| Vitamin D | See Chapter 26. | | | |

*(continued)*

**TABLE 31-2.   VITAMIN IMBALANCES**  *(Continued)*

| | Deficiency States | | Excess States | |
| --- | --- | --- | --- | --- |
| | *Causes* | *Signs and Symptoms* | *Causes* | *Signs and Symptoms* |
| *Water-Soluble Vitamins* | | | Excess states do not occur with dietary intake of water-soluble vitamins but may occur with megadoses. Megadoses should be avoided. | |
| Biotin | Inadequate intake or impaired absorption. Biotin deficiency is rare. | Anorexia<br>Nausea<br>Depression<br>Muscle pain<br>Dermatitis | | |
| Cyanocobalamin (vitamin $B_{12}$) | Usually impaired absorption from a lack of hydrochloric acid or intrinsic factor in the stomach | Megaloblastic or pernicious anemia:<br>1. Decreased numbers of red blood cells (RBCs)<br>2. Abnormally large, immature RBCs<br>3. Fatigue<br>4. Dyspnea<br>5. With severe deficiency, leukopenia, thrombocytopenia, cardiac arrhythmias, heart failure, or infections may occur.<br>Neurologic signs and symptoms:<br>1. Paresthesias in hands and feet<br>2. Unsteady gait<br>3. Depressed deep-tendon reflexes<br>4. With severe deficiency, loss of memory, confusion, delusions, hallucinations, and psychosis may occur. Nerve damage may be irreversible. | | |
| Folic acid | Inadequate diet<br>Impaired absorption (intestinal disorders)<br>Greatly increased requirements (pregnancy, lactation, hemolytic anemias)<br>Ingestion of folate antagonist drugs (*e.g.*, methotrexate)<br>Alcoholism is a common cause. It interferes with intake and absorption. | Megaloblastic anemia that cannot be distinguished from the anemia produced by $B_{12}$ deficiency<br>Impaired growth in children<br>Glossitis<br>GI problems (folic acid deficiency does not produce neurologic signs and symptoms as $B_{12}$ deficiency does) | | |
| Niacin (vitamin $B_3$) | Inadequate diet or impaired absorption | Pellagra:<br>1. Erythematous skin lesions<br>2. GI problems (stomatitis, glossitis, enteritis, diarrhea)<br>3. CNS problems (headache, dizziness, insomnia, depression, memory loss)<br>4. With severe deficiency, delusions, hallucinations, and impairment of peripheral motor and sensory nerves may occur. | | |
| Pantothenic acid (vitamin $B_5$) | No deficiency state established | | | |

**TABLE 31-2. VITAMIN IMBALANCES** (*Continued*)

| | Deficiency States | | Excess States | |
|---|---|---|---|---|
| | *Causes* | *Signs and Symptoms* | *Causes* | *Signs and Symptoms* |
| *Water-Soluble Vitamins* | | | | |
| Pyridoxine (vitamin B$_6$) | Inadequate intake or impaired absorption | 1. Skin and mucous membrane lesions (seborrheic dermatitis, intertrigo, glossitis, stomatitis) <br> 2. Neurologic problems (convulsions, peripheral neuritis, mental depression) | | |
| Riboflavin (vitamin B$_2$) | Inadequate intake or impaired absorption. Uncommon and usually occurs with deficiencies of other B-complex vitamins | Glossitis and stomatitis <br> Seborrheic dermatitis <br> Eye disorders (burning, itching, lacrimation, photophobia, vascularization of the cornea) | | |
| Thiamine (vitamin B$_1$) | Inadequate diet, especially among pregnant women and infants; impaired absorption due to GI disorders <br> Alcoholism | Mild deficiency—fatigue, anorexia, retarded growth, mental depression, irritability, apathy, lethargy <br> Severe deficiency (beriberi)—peripheral neuritis, personality disturbances, heart failure, edema, Wernicke–Korsakoff syndrome in alcoholics | | |
| Vitamin C (ascorbic acid) | Inadequate dietary intake (most likely in infants, older adults, indigent people, and alcoholics) <br> Increased requirements (people who smoke cigarettes, take oral contraceptives, or have acute or chronic illness) <br> Megadoses that are abruptly discontinued may cause a rebound deficiency. Deficiency also may occur in infants whose mothers took megadoses during pregnancy. | 1. Mild deficiency—irritability, malaise, arthralgia, increased tendency to bleed <br> 2. Severe deficiency—scurvy and adverse effects on most body tissues (gingivitis; bleeding of gums, skin, joints, and other areas; disturbances of bone growth; anemia; and loosening of teeth). If not treated, coma and death may occur. | Megadoses may produce excessive amounts of oxalate in the urine. | Renal calculi |

- Avoid megadoses of vitamin supplements
- Avoid symptoms of vitamin deficiency or overdose

**Interventions**

Implement measures to prevent vitamin disorders; the safest and most effective way to prevent vitamin deficiencies is by increasing dietary intake of vitamins:

- A well-balanced, varied diet that is adequate in proteins and calories is adequate in vitamins for most people. Exceptions are those who have increased requirements or conditions that interfere with absorption or use of vitamins.
- Water-soluble vitamins are often destroyed by cooking or discarded in cooking water. Eating raw fruits and vegetables prevents loss of vitamins during cooking. When fruits

and vegetables are cooked, vitamin losses can be minimized by using small amounts of water, steaming or pressure cooking for the shortest effective time, and keeping cooking utensils covered.

In addition to cooking losses, vitamin C is lost with exposure of foods to air. Consequently, fruits and vegetables, including juices, should be kept covered during storage.

- When vitamin deficiency stems from inadequate dietary intake, correcting the diet is preferred over administering supplemental vitamins when feasible. For vitamin A deficiency, increasing daily intake of plant and animal sources may be sufficient. For vitamin C deficiency, citrus juices can be used therapeutically. Because about 4 oz of orange juice daily meets requirements, larger amounts can relieve defi-

## TABLE 31-3.  VITAMIN DRUG PREPARATIONS

| Generic/Trade Name | Routes and Dosage Ranges |
|---|---|
| *Fat-Soluble Vitamins* | |
| **Vitamin A** (Aquasol A) | Adults with severe deficiency: PO 100,000–500,000 U daily for 3 d, then 50,000 U daily for 2 wk, then 10,000–20,000 U daily for another 2 mo. IM 50,000–100,000 U daily for 3 d, then 50,000 U daily for 2 wk<br>Children over 8 years with severe deficiency: PO, IM, same as adults<br>Infants and children under 8 years: 10,000–15,000 U daily for 10 d |
| **Vitamin E** (Aquasol E) | Adults: PO, IM 60–100 U daily<br>Children: PO, IM 25–60 U daily |
| **Vitamin K** **Menadione sodium diphosphate** (Synkayvite) | Adults and children: PO, IM 5–15 mg daily<br>Adults: PO 5–10 mg daily; SC, IM, IV 5–15 mg daily<br>Children: PO, SC, IM, IV 5–10 mg daily |
| **Phytonadione** (Mephyton Aqua-Mephyton) | Adults and children: PO, SC, IM 2.5–25 mg daily<br>Newborns: IV, IM 0.5–2 mg immediately after birth to *prevent* hemorrhagic disease of neonates; 1–2 mg daily to *treat* hemorrhagic disease |
| *Water-Soluble Vitamins* | |
| *B-Complex Vitamins* | |
| **Calcium pantothenate (B$_5$)** | Adults: PO 10–20 mg daily |
| **Cyanocobalamin (B$_{12}$)** (Rubramin) | Adults and children: PO 10–250 μg daily for 1 mo in an oral therapeutic multivitamin preparation when deficiency is due to increased requirements and gastrointestinal absorption is normal<br>IM, SC, IV 30 μg daily for 5–10 d, then 100–200 μg monthly |
| **Folic acid** (Folvite) | Adults and children: PO, SC, IM, IV up to 1 mg daily until symptoms decrease and blood tests are normal, then maintenance dose of 0.1–0.25 mg daily |
| **Niacin (nicotinic acid), niacinamide (nicotinamide)** | Deficiency, PO, IM, IV 50–100 mg daily<br>Pellagra, 500 mg daily<br>Hyperlipidemia, 2–6 g daily |
| **Pyridoxine (B$_6$)** | Deficiency, PO, IM, IV 10–20 mg daily for 3 wk, then 2–5 mg daily<br>Anemia, peripheral neuritis, 100–200 mg daily<br>Pyridoxine dependency syndrome, up to 600 mg daily |
| **Riboflavin** | PO 5–25 mg daily |
| **Thiamine (B$_1$)** | PO 10–30 mg daily; IM 10–20 mg three times daily for 2 wk, supplemented with 5–10 mg orally; IV 100–200 mg |
| *Vitamin C* | |
| **Vitamin C (ascorbic acid)** | Deficiency, PO, IM, IV 100–500 mg daily<br>Scurvy, 300–1000 mg daily for at least 2 wk<br>Infants receiving formula, 35–50 mg daily for first few weeks of life<br>Urinary acidification, 4–12 g daily in divided doses every 4 h<br>Prophylaxis, 50–100 mg daily |

ciency. When folic acid deficiency anemia stems from dietary lack, one fresh, uncooked fruit or vegetable or one glass of fruit juice added to the daily diet will probably correct the deficiency (except during pregnancy, when folate requirements are increased).

- Even when vitamin supplements are considered necessary, dietary sources should be increased for immediate and long-term benefit.
- Clients receiving only intravenous fluids or a clear liquid diet for more than 2 or 3 days probably need replacement vitamins.

When requirements are increased or absorption is de-

creased, vitamins may be needed as dietary supplements to prevent deficiencies. Vitamin preparations must be chosen carefully because they differ widely in the specific vitamins contained and in the amounts of each. Their use should be based on recommended amounts after assessing eating habits and the usual dietary supply of vitamins.

Some oral multivitamin preparations considered appropriate for supplemental use are Adeflor, Poly-Vi-Flor, Poly-Vi-Sol, Tri-Vi-Flor, Tri-Vi-Sol, and Vi-Daylin for children and Dayalets for adults. These contain less than 150% of the RDA for all ingredients. Preparations containing fluoride require a prescription.

*Teach clients:*

- That the safest and most effective way to obtain needed vitamins is to eat a varied, well-balanced diet
- Which foods are good sources of vitamins, and ways to cook and store them to preserve vitamin content
- To avoid excessive intake of any vitamin preparation. Excessive amounts do not promote health, strength, or youth. Instead, they may cause serious adverse reactions.

With fat-soluble vitamins, the dangers of overdosage have long been known. With water-soluble vitamins, overdosage has been considered wasteful and expensive but not dangerous because these vitamins are rapidly excreted in the urine. However, evidence indicates that prolonged intake of excessive amounts of certain water-soluble vitamins can cause serious adverse effects. For example, large amounts of niacin may cause gastrointestinal problems, flushing, skin rashes, and pruritus and may exacerbate asthma, uricosuria, and gouty arthritis. Long-term ingestion of high doses of pyridoxine has been associated with peripheral neuropathies characterized by decreased sensation in limbs, perioral numbness, and ataxia. These symptoms improved after pyridoxine was withdrawn but were not completely eliminated. Large amounts of vitamin C (1 g or more) may cause diarrhea, uricosuria, and oxalate kidney stones. They also increase estrogen levels, decrease activity of oral anticoagulants, and when taken by pregnant women, have caused scurvy in infants when they no longer received the large amounts to which they were exposed in utero.

### Evaluation

- Interview about and observe the amount and type of food intake.
- Interview about and observe for signs of vitamin deficiency or overdose.

## Principles of therapy

### MANAGING VITAMIN DISORDERS

Vitamin disorders should be recognized as early as possible and appropriate treatment initiated. Early recognition and treatment can prevent a mild deficiency or excess from becoming severe. Some guidelines include the following:

1. *Vitamin deficiency.* For deficiency states, oral vitamin preparations are preferred when possible. They are usually effective (except in malabsorption syndromes), safe, convenient to administer, and relatively inexpensive. If the deficiency involves only a single vitamin, then that vitamin alone is indicated. However, multiple deficiencies are common, and a multivitamin preparation may be needed. Although dosages for deficiencies are generally higher than those for dietary supplements, dosages should be titrated as nearly as possible to the amounts needed by the body.

Multivitamin preparations for treating deficiencies contain more than 150% of the RDA. They should be used only for therapeutic purposes and for limited periods. Some oral preparations considered appropriate for therapeutic use include Abdec, Abdol, Adeflor, Betalin Complex Elixir, Multicebrin, Natalins, Surbex, Tri-Vi-Sol, and Vi-Daylin. Several of these may be used for adults or children. Other preparations are available for use during pregnancy and lactation or for parenteral use.

When fat-soluble vitamins are given to correct deficiency, there is a risk of producing excess states. When water-soluble vitamins are given, excesses are less likely but may occur with large doses. These factors must be considered when determining vitamin dosage.

2. *Vitamin excess.* For excess states, the usual treatment is to stop administration of the vitamin preparation. There are no specific antidotes or antagonists.

### Disorders of fat-soluble vitamins A and K

1. With vitamin A deficiency, increase intake of foods containing vitamin A or carotene when feasible. Use a single, pure form of vitamin A rather than a multivitamin unless multiple deficiencies are present. Give doses no larger than 25,000 U daily unless a severe deficiency is present. Give orally if not contraindicated; give intramuscularly if gastrointestinal absorption is severely impaired or ocular symptoms are severe. With vitamin A excess, immediately stop known sources of the vitamin.

2. With vitamin K deficiency or hypoprothrombinemia, bleeding may occur spontaneously or in response to trauma. Thus, administration of vitamin K and measures to prevent bleeding are indicated. If the deficiency is not severe, oral vitamin K may be given for a few days until serum prothrombin activity returns to a normal range. In obstructive jaundice, bile salts must be given at the same time as oral vitamin K, or vitamin K must be given parenterally. In malabsorption syndromes or diarrhea, parenteral administration is probably necessary. A single dose of vitamin K may be sufficient.

   With severe bleeding, vitamin K may be given intravenously. Intravenous vitamin K must be given very slowly to decrease risks of hypotension and shock. Unfortunately, a therapeutic response does not occur for at least 4 hours. For more rapid control of bleeding, transfusions of plasma or whole blood are needed. When bleeding is caused by oral anticoagulant drugs, avoid overdoses of vitamin K. Oral anticoagulants are usually given for thromboembolic disorders. Giving vitamin K as an antidote to control bleeding reestablishes the risks of thrombi. Measures to prevent bleeding include avoiding trauma, injections, and drugs that may cause bleeding.

## Disorders of B-complex vitamins

1. Most deficiencies of B-complex vitamins are multiple rather than single. Also, many of these vitamins are obtained from the same foods. Treating deficiencies consists of increasing intake of foods containing B-complex vitamins or giving multivitamin preparations. Multivitamin preparations vary greatly in composition and therefore must be carefully chosen. Most preparations contain thiamine, riboflavin, niacin, pyridoxine, and cyanocobalamin. Other vitamins may be included in the formulations.

   If a single deficiency seems predominant, that vitamin may be given alone or in conjunction with a multiple vitamin preparation. For example, thiamine deficiency is common in alcoholic clients, partly because large amounts of thiamine are used to metabolize alcohol.

2. Some relatively rare types of anemia occur with deficiencies of certain B-complex vitamins. One type of anemia occurs with pyridoxine deficiency and is relieved by administration of pyridoxine. Megaloblastic anemias, characterized by abnormally large, immature red blood cells, occur with deficiency of folic acid or vitamin $B_{12}$. If megaloblastic anemia is severe, treatment is usually instituted with folic acid and vitamin $B_{12}$.

   a. In pernicious anemia, vitamin $B_{12}$ must be given by intramuscular or subcutaneous injection because oral forms are not absorbed from the gastrointestinal tract. Vitamin $B_{12}$ injections are specific therapy for pernicious anemia and must be continued for life. Vitamin $B_{12}$ is sometimes given to prevent pernicious anemia in clients who are strict vegetarians, who have had gastrectomy, or who have chronic small bowel disease. Pernicious anemia must be differentiated from other megaloblastic anemias for appropriate therapy. Pernicious anemia and other megaloblastic anemias respond to administration of folic acid. However, if folic acid alone is given to the client with pernicious anemia, hematologic abnormalities disappear but neurologic deterioration continues.

   b. In other types of megaloblastic anemias, vitamin $B_{12}$ or folic acid is indicated. Although both of these are included in many multivitamin preparations, they usually must be given separately for therapeutic purposes. With vitamin $B_{12}$, doses of more than 100 μg are not useful because any excess of that amount is rapidly excreted in urine. It may be given as a single dose of 1000 μg when performing the Schilling test for pernicious anemia. With folic acid, oral administration is indi-

cated for most clients. Daily doses in excess of 1 mg are not useful because any excess is excreted in the urine.

## Disorders of vitamin C

Treatment of vitamin C deficiency involves increased intake of vitamin C from dietary or pharmaceutical sources. Vitamin C (ascorbic acid) is available alone for oral, intramuscular, or intravenous administration. It is also an ingredient in most multiple vitamin preparations for oral or parenteral use.

### USE IN CHILDREN

Children need sufficient amounts of all required vitamins to support growth and normal body functioning. In the healthy child, a varied, well-balanced diet is preferred over vitamin supplements.

If supplements are given, dosages should not exceed recommended amounts. There is a risk of overdosage by children and their parents. Because of manufacturers' marketing strategies, many supplements are available in flavors and shapes (*e.g.*, cartoon characters, animals) designed to appeal to children. Younger children may think of these supplements as "candy" and take more than recommended if they are accessible. Thus, they should be stored out of reach and dispensed by an adult. Parents may lack knowledge of nutrition or be overly concerned about the adequacy of a child's diet. Their wish to promote health may lead them to give supplements when they are not needed or to give more than recommended amounts. Parents may need information about the potential hazards of acute and chronic vitamin overdoses.

### USE IN OLDER ADULTS

Vitamin requirements are the same as for younger adults. However, deficiencies are common in older adults, especially of vitamins A, D, folic acid, riboflavin, and thiamine. Numerous factors may contribute to deficiencies, including limited income, anorexia, lack of teeth or ill-fitting dentures, drugs that decrease absorption of dietary nutrients, and disease processes that interfere with the ability to obtain, prepare, or eat adequate amounts of a variety of foods.

Every older adult should be carefully assessed regarding nutritional status and use of drugs that interact with dietary nutrients. If an older adult cannot eat a varied, well-balanced diet for any reason, a vitamin supplement is probably desirable. In addition, requirements may be increased during illnesses, especially those affecting gastrointestinal function. Overdoses, especially of the fat-soluble vitamins A and D, may cause toxicity and should be avoided.

# NURSING ACTIONS: VITAMINS

| *Nursing Actions* | *Rationale/Explanation* |
|---|---|

**1. Administer accurately**

  **a.** With fat-soluble vitamins:

    (1) Give as directed.

To increase therapeutic effects and avoid adverse reactions

    (2) Do not give oral preparations at the same time as mineral oil.

Mineral oil absorbs the vitamins and thus prevents their systemic absorption.

    (3) For subcutaneous or intramuscular administration of vitamin K, aspirate carefully to avoid intravenous injection, apply gentle pressure to the injection site, and inspect the site frequently. For intravenous injection, vitamin K may be given by direct injection or diluted in intravenous fluids (*e.g.,* 5% dextrose in water or saline).

Vitamin K is given to clients with hypoprothrombinemia, which causes a bleeding tendency. Thus, any injection may cause trauma and bleeding at the injection site.

    (4) Administer intravenous vitamin K slowly, at a rate not to exceed 1 mg/min, whether diluted or undiluted.

Intravenous phytonadione may cause hypotension and shock from an anaphylactic type of reaction.

  **b.** With B-complex vitamins:

    (1) Give parenteral cyanocobalamin (vitamin $B_{12}$) intramuscularly or deep subcutaneously.

    (2) Give oral niacin preparations, except for timed-release forms, with or after meals or at bedtime. Have the client sit or lie down for about ½ hour after administration.

To decrease anorexia, nausea, vomiting, diarrhea, and flatulence. Niacin causes vasodilation, which may result in dizziness, hypotension, and possibly injury from falls. Vasodilation occurs within a few minutes and may last 1 hour.

    (3) Give intramuscular thiamine deeply into a large muscle mass. Avoid the intravenous route.

To decrease pain at the injection site. Hypotension and anaphylactic shock have occurred with rapid intravenous administration and large doses.

**2. Observe for therapeutic effects (mainly decreased signs and symptoms of deficiency)**

  **a.** With vitamin A, observe for improved vision, especially in dim light or at night, less dryness in eyes and conjunctiva (xerophthalmia), improvement in skin lesions.

Night blindness is usually relieved within a few days. Skin lesions may not completely disappear for several weeks.

  **b.** With vitamin K, observe for decreased bleeding and more nearly normal blood coagulation tests (*e.g.,* prothrombin time).

Blood coagulation tests usually improve within 4 to 12 hours.

  **c.** With B-complex vitamins, observe for decreased or absent stomatitis, glossitis, cheilosis, seborrheic dermatitis, neurologic problems (neuritis, convulsions, mental deterioration, psychotic symptoms), cardiovascular problems (edema, heart failure), and eye problems (itching, burning, photophobia).

Deficiencies of B-complex vitamins commonly occur together and produce many similar manifestations.

  **d.** With vitamin $B_{12}$ and folic acid, observe for increased appetite, strength and feeling of well-being, increased reticulocyte counts, and increased numbers of normal red blood cells, hemoglobin, and hematocrit.

Therapeutic effects may be quite rapid and dramatic. The client usually feels better within 24 to 48 hours, and normal red blood cells begin to appear. Anemia is decreased within about 2 weeks, but 4 to 8 weeks may be needed for complete blood count to return to normal.

*(continued)*

| Nursing Actions | Rationale/Explanation |
|---|---|
| **e.** With vitamin C, observe for decreased or absent malaise, irritability, and bleeding tendencies (easy bruising of skin, bleeding gums, nosebleeds, and so on). | |
| **3. Observe for adverse reactions** | |
| **a.** With vitamin A, observe for signs of hypervitaminosis A (anorexia, vomiting, irritability, headache, skin changes [dryness, dermatitis, itching, desquamation], fatigue, pain in muscles, bones, and joints, and other clinical manifestations, and serum levels of vitamin A above 1200 U/100 ml). | Severity of manifestations depends largely on dose and duration of excess vitamin A intake. Very severe states produce additional clinical signs, including enlargement of liver and spleen, altered liver function, increased intracranial pressure, and other neurologic manifestations. |
| **b.** With vitamin K, observe for hypotension and signs of anaphylactic shock with intravenous phytonadione. | Vitamin K rarely produces adverse reactions. Giving intravenous phytonadione slowly may prevent adverse reactions. |
| **c.** With B-complex vitamins, observe for hypotension and anaphylactic shock with parenteral niacin, thiamine, cyanocobalamin, and folic acid; anorexia, nausea, vomiting and diarrhea, and postural hypotension with oral niacin. | Adverse reactions are generally rare. They are unlikely with B-complex multivitamin preparations. They are most likely to occur with large intravenous doses and rapid administration. |
| **d.** With vitamin C megadoses, observe for diarrhea and rebound deficiency if stopped abruptly. | Adverse reactions are rare with usual doses and methods of administration. |
| **4. Observe for drug interactions**<br>**a.** Fat-soluble vitamins: | |
| (1) Bile salts *increase* effects. | Increase intestinal absorption |
| (2) Laxatives, especially mineral oil, *decrease* effects. | Mineral oil combines with fat-soluble vitamins and prevents their absorption if both are taken at the same time. Excessive or chronic laxative use decreases intestinal absorption. |
| (3) Antibiotics may *decrease* effects | With vitamin K, antibiotics decrease production by decreasing intestinal bacteria. With others, antibiotics may cause diarrhea and subsequent malabsorption. |
| **b.** B-complex vitamins: | |
| (1) Cycloserine (antituberculosis drug) *decreases* effects. | By increasing urinary excretion of vitamin B-complex |
| (2) Isoniazid (INH) *decreases* effect. | INH has an antipyridoxine effect. When INH is given for prevention or treatment of tuberculosis, pyridoxine is usually given also. |
| (3) With folic acid: alcohol, methotrexate, oral contraceptives, phenytoin, and triamterene *decrease* effects. | Alcohol alters liver function and leads to poor hepatic storage of folic acid. Methotrexate and phenytoin act as antagonists to folic acid and may cause folic acid deficiency. Oral contraceptives decrease absorption of folic acid. |
| **5. Teach clients**<br>**a.** Avoid large doses of vitamins unless specifically prescribed by the physician. | To avoid adverse effects |
| **b.** If supplementary vitamins are taken, it is probably advisable to consult a physician. | Available preparations differ widely in amounts and types of vitamin content. |
| **c.** Take prescribed vitamins as directed and for the appropriate time. | In pernicious anemia, vitamin $B_{12}$ injections must be taken for the remainder of life. In pregnancy and lactation, vitamins are usually taken only during this period of increased need. |

## Review and Application Exercises

1. What roles do vitamins play in normal body functioning?
2. Identify client populations who are at risk for vitamin deficiencies and excesses.
3. How would you assess a client for vitamin imbalances?
4. What are clinical indications for therapeutic use of specific vitamin drug preparations?
5. Are fat-soluble or water-soluble vitamins more toxic in overdoses and why?
6. For an outpatient or home care client who is likely to have vitamin deficiencies, what information can you provide to increase vitamin intake from food?
7. For a client who asks your advice about taking a multivitamin supplement daily, how would you reply? Justify your answer.

## Selected References

Beare, P. G., & Myers, J. L. (Eds.) (1990). *Principles and practice of adult health nursing*. St. Louis: C.V. Mosby.

Davis, J. R., & Sherer, K. (1994). *Applied nutrition and diet therapy for nurses* (2nd ed.). Philadelphia: W.B. Saunders.

(1993). *Drug facts and comparisons*. St. Louis: Facts and Comparisons.

Eschleman, M. M. (1991). *Introductory nutrition and diet therapy* (2nd ed.). Philadelphia: J.B. Lippincott.

Guyton, A. C. (1991). *Textbook of medical physiology* (8th ed.). Philadelphia: W.B. Saunders.

Shlafer, M. (1993). *The nurse, pharmacology, and drug therapy* (2nd ed.). Redwood City, CA: Addison-Wesley.

Thornhill, D. G., & Pleuss, J. (1990). Alterations in nutritional status. In C. M. Porth (Ed.), *Pathophysiology: Concepts of altered health states* (3rd ed.) (pp 743–765). Philadelphia: J.B. Lippincott.

Williams, L., Davis, J. A., & Lowenthal, D. T. (1993). The influence of food on the absorption and metabolism of drugs. *Medical Clinics of North America, 77*(4), 815–829.

### CHAPTER 32

# Minerals and Electrolytes

## Description and uses

Minerals and electrolytes are essential constituents of bone, teeth, cell membranes, and connective tissue. They are also components of many essential enzymes. In general, they function to maintain fluid, electrolyte, and acid-base balance; maintain osmotic pressure; maintain nerve and muscle function; assist in transfer of essential compounds across cell membranes; and influence the growth process.

Minerals occur in the body and foods mainly in ionic form. Ions are electrically charged particles. Metals (*e.g.*, sodium, potassium, calcium, magnesium) form positive ions or cations; nonmetals (*e.g.*, chlorine, phosphorus, sulfur) form negative ions or anions. These cations and anions combine to form salts or compounds that are physiologically inactive and electrically neutral. When placed in solution, such as a body fluid, the components separate into electrically charged particles called *electrolytes*. For example, sodium and chlorine combine to form sodium chloride (NaCl). (Table salt is composed of NaCl.) In a solution, NaCl separates into $Na^+$ and $Cl^-$ ions. (The plus sign following Na means that Na is a cation. The minus sign following Cl means that Cl is an anion.) At any given time the body must maintain an equal number of positive and negative charges. Therefore, the ions are constantly combining and separating to maintain electrical neutrality or electrolyte balance.

These electrolytes also maintain the acid-base balance of body fluids, which is necessary for normal body functioning. When foods are digested in the body, they produce mineral residues that react chemically as acids or bases. Acids are usually anions, such as chloride, bicarbonate, sulfate, and phosphate. Bases are usually cat- ions, such as sodium, potassium, calcium, and magnesium. If approximately equal amounts of cations and anions are present in the mineral residue, the residue is essentially neutral, and the pH of body fluids does not require adjustment. If there is an excess of cations (base), the body must draw on its anions (acid) to combine with the cations, render them physiologically inactive, and restore the normal pH of the blood. Excess cations are excreted in the urine, mainly in combination with the anion phosphate. If there is an excess of anions (acid), usually sulfate or phosphate, they combine with hydrogen ions or other cations and are excreted in the urine.

### MACRONUTRIENTS

There are 22 minerals thought to be necessary for human nutrition. Some of these (calcium, phosphorus, sodium, potassium, magnesium, chlorine, sulfur) are required in relatively large amounts and thus are sometimes called *macronutrients*. Calcium and phosphorus are discussed in Chapter 26. Sulfur is a component of cellular protein molecules, several amino acids and B vitamins, insulin, and other essential body substances. No recommended dietary allowances (RDAs) have been established; the dietary source is protein foods. The other macronutrients are described here in terms of characteristics, functions, RDAs, and food sources (Table 32-1). Imbalances of macronutrients are classified as deficiency states and excess states. Sodium imbalances (hyponatremia and hypernatremia) are described in Table 32-2, potassium imbalances (hypokalemia and hyperkalemia) in Table 32-3, magnesium imbalances (hypomagnesemia and hypermagnesemia) in Table 32-4, and chloride imbalances (hypochloremic metabolic alkalosis

Anne Collins Abrams: CLINICAL DRUG THERAPY, Fourth Edition.
© 1995 J.B. Lippincott Company.

# TABLE 32-1.  MINERALS AND ELECTROLYTES

| Characteristics | Functions | Recommended Dietary Allowances (RDAs) | Food Sources |
|---|---|---|---|
| **Sodium** | | | |
| 1. Major cation in extracellular body fluids (blood, lymph, tissue fluid)<br>2. Small amount in intracellular fluid<br>3. Large amounts of sodium in saliva, gastric secretions, bile, pancreatic and intestinal secretions | 1. Assists in regulating osmotic pressure, water balance, conduction of electrical impulses in nerves and muscles, electrolyte and acid-base balance<br>2. Influences permeability of cell membranes and assists in movement of substances across cell membranes<br>3. Participates in many intracellular chemical reactions | About 2 g (estimated) | 1. Present in most foods. Proteins contain relatively large amounts, vegetables and cereals contain moderate to small amounts, fruits contain little or no sodium.<br>2. Major source of sodium in the diet is table salt added to food in cooking, processing, or seasoning. One teaspoon contains 2.3 g of sodium.<br>3. Water in some areas may contain significant amounts of sodium. |
| **Potassium** | | | |
| 1. Major cation in intracellular body fluids<br>2. Present in all body fluids<br>3. Eliminated from the body primarily in urine. Normally functioning kidneys excrete excessive amounts of potassium, but they cannot conserve potassium when intake is low or absent. The kidneys excrete 10 mEq or more daily in the absence of intake. Potassium excretion is influenced by acid-base balance and aldosterone secretion.<br>4. A small amount of potassium is normally lost in feces and sweat. | 1. Within cells, helps to maintain osmotic pressure, fluid and electrolyte balance, and acid-base balance<br>2. In extracellular fluid, functions with sodium and calcium to regulate neuromuscular excitability. Potassium is required for conduction of nerve impulses and contraction of skeletal and smooth muscle. It is especially important in activity of the myocardium.<br>3. Participates in carbohydrate and protein metabolism. Helps transport glucose into cells and is required for glycogen formation and storage. Required for synthesis of muscle proteins from amino acids and other components. | About 40 mEq | Present in most foods, including meat, whole-grain breads or cereals, bananas, citrus fruits, tomatoes, and broccoli |
| **Magnesium** | | | |
| 1. A cation occurring primarily in intracellular fluid<br>2. Widely distributed in the body, about half in bone tissue and the remainder in soft tissue and body fluids<br>3. Most dietary magnesium is not absorbed from the gastrointestinal tract and is excreted in feces. | 1. Required for conduction of nerve impulses and contraction of muscle<br>2. Especially important in functions of cardiac and skeletal muscles<br>3. Serves as a component of many enzymes<br>4. Essential for metabolism of carbohydrate and protein | About 300 mg for adults. Increased amounts recommended for pregnant or lactating women and children. | Present in many foods; diet adequate in other respects contains adequate magnesium. Good food sources include nuts, cereal grains, dark green vegetables, and seafoods. |
| **Chloride** | | | |
| 1. Ionized form of element chlorine<br>2. The main anion of extracellular fluid<br>3. Almost all chloride is normally excreted by the kidneys. | 1. Functions with sodium to help maintain osmotic pressure and water balance.<br>2. Forms hydrochloric acid (HCl) in gastric mucosal cells<br>3. Helps regulate electrolyte and acid-base balance by competing with bicarbonate ions for sodium<br>4. Participates in a homeostatic buffering mechanism in which chloride shifts in and out of red blood cells in exchange for bicarbonate | 80–110 mEq | Most dietary chloride is ingested as sodium chloride (NaCl), and foods high in sodium are also high in chloride. |

## TABLE 32-2.   SODIUM IMBALANCES

| Causes | Pathophysiology | Signs and Symptoms |
|---|---|---|
| *Hyponatremia* | | |
| 1. Inadequate intake. Unusual but may occur with sodium-restricted diets and diuretic drug therapy or when water only is ingested after water and sodium are lost (*e.g.*, excessive sweating)<br>2. Excessive losses. More common and occur with vomiting, gastrointestinal (GI) suction, diarrhea, excessive water enemas, excessive perspiration, burn wounds, and adrenal insufficiency states (*e.g.*, Addison's disease).<br>3. Excessive dilution of body fluids with water | 1. Decreased serum sodium<br>2. Decreased plasma volume and cardiac output<br>3. Decreased blood flow to kidneys, decreased glomerular filtration rate, and decreased ability of kidneys to excrete water<br>4. Overhydration and swelling of brain cells (cerebral edema). Leads to impaired neurologic and muscular functions.<br>5. GI changes | 1. Serum sodium <135 mEq/L<br>2. Hypotension and tachycardia<br>3. Oliguria and increased blood urea nitrogen (BUN)<br>4. Headache, dizziness, weakness, lethargy, restlessness, confusion, delirium, muscle tremors, convulsions, ataxia, aphasia<br>5. Anorexia, nausea, and vomiting are common; abdominal cramps and paralytic ileus may develop. |
| *Hypernatremia* | | |
| 1. Deficiency of water in proportion to the amount of sodium present. Water deficiency results from lack of intake or excessive losses (diarrhea, diuretic drugs, excessive sweating).<br>2. Excessive intake of sodium. An uncommon cause of hypernatremia because the thirst mechanism is normally activated, and water intake is increased.<br>3. Sodium retention due to hyperaldosteronism and Cushing's disease | 1. Increased serum sodium<br>2. Hypernatremia due to water deficiency decreases fluid volume in extracellular fluid and intracellular fluid compartments (dehydration).<br>3. Hypernatremia due to sodium gain increases extracellular fluid volume and decreases intracellular fluid volume as water is pulled out of cells. | 1. Serum sodium >145 mEq/L<br>2. Lethargy, disorientation, hyperactive reflexes, muscle rigidity, tremors and spasms, irritability, coma, cerebral hemorrhage, subdural hematoma<br>3. Hypotension<br>4. Fever, dry skin, and dry mucous membranes<br>5. Oliguria, concentrated urine with a high specific gravity, and increased BUN |

and hyperchloremic metabolic acidosis) in Table 32-5. Each imbalance is described in terms of causes, pathophysiology, and clinical signs and symptoms.

## MICRONUTRIENTS

The other 15 minerals are required in small amounts and are often called *micronutrients* or *trace elements*. Eight trace elements (chromium, cobalt, copper, fluoride, iodine, iron, selenium, and zinc) have relatively well-defined roles in human nutrition (Table 32-6). Because of their clinical importance, iron imbalances are discussed separately in Table 32-7. Other trace elements (manganese, molybdenum, nickel, silicon, tin, and vanadium) are present in many body tissues. Some are components of enzymes and may be necessary for normal growth, structure, and function of connective tissue. For most of these, requirements are unknown, and states of deficiency or excess have not been identified in humans.

A variety of pharmacologic agents is used to prevent or treat mineral-electrolyte imbalances. Usually, neutral salts of minerals (*e.g.*, potassium chloride) are used in deficiency states, and nonmineral drug preparations are used in excess states.

# Individual agents used in mineral-electrolyte and acid-base imbalances

## ACIDIFYING AGENT

**Ammonium chloride** ($NH_4Cl$) is a systemic acidifying agent occasionally used in the treatment of hypochloremic metabolic alkalosis. As a general rule, chloride is preferably replaced with sodium chloride or potassium chloride rather than ammonium chloride. However, sodium chloride may be contraindicated in an edematous client, or the alkalosis may be unresponsive to sodium or potassium chloride. Ammonium chloride is also sometimes used as a urinary acidifier to facilitate the action or excretion of other drugs.

### Routes and dosage ranges

*Adults:* PO 1–3 g two or four times daily
   IV 100–500 ml of a 2% solution, infused over a 3-h period; dosage depends on client's status and on serum chloride concentration.

## TABLE 32-3. POTASSIUM IMBALANCES

| Causes | Pathophysiology | Signs and Symptoms |
|---|---|---|
| *Hypokalemia* | | |
| 1. Inadequate intake. Uncommon in clients who can eat; may occur in those unable to eat or receiving only potassium-free IV fluids for several days.<br>2. Excessive losses from the gastrointestinal tract (vomiting, gastric suction, diarrhea, overuse of laxatives and enemas) or urinary tract (polyuria from diuretic drugs, renal disease, excessive aldosterone)<br>3. Movement of potassium out of serum and into cells. This occurs with administration of insulin and glucose in treatment of diabetic ketoacidosis and in metabolic alkalosis. | 1. Decreased serum potassium<br>2. Impaired cardiac conduction<br>3. Decreased strength of myocardial contraction and decreased cardiac output. Decreased response to catecholamines and other substances that normally raise blood pressure.<br>4. Neurologic changes due to impaired conduction of nerve impulses<br>5. Impaired function of skeletal, smooth, and cardiac muscle, most likely with serum potassium <2.5 mEq/L. Electrical impulses are slowed until muscle contraction cannot occur.<br>6. Slowed gastric emptying and decreased intestinal motility, probably caused by muscle weakness<br>7. Decreased ability of kidney to concentrate urine and excrete acid. Decreased glomerular filtration rate with prolonged potassium deficiency.<br>8. Impaired carbohydrate metabolism and decreased secretion of insulin | 1. Serum potassium <3.5 mEq/L<br>2. Arrhythmias and electrocardiogram (ECG) changes (depressed ST segment; flattened or inverted T wave; increased amplitude of P wave; prolonged P-R interval; prolonged QRS complex with normal shape and size). Premature atrial and ventricular beats or atrioventricular block may occur, usually in people taking digitalis. Death from cardiac arrest may occur.<br>3. Postural hypotension<br>4. Confusion, memory impairment, lethargy, apathy, drowsiness, irritability, delirium<br>5. Muscle weakness and possibly paralysis. Weakness of leg muscles usually occurs first. Then weakness ascends to include respiratory muscles and cause respiratory insufficiency.<br>6. Abdominal distention, constipation, paralytic ileus<br>7. Polyuria, polydipsia, nocturia. Prolonged deficiency may increase serum creatinine and BUN.<br>8. Hyperglycemia |
| *Hyperkalemia* | | |
| 1. Excess intake. Uncommon with normal kidney function.<br>2. Impaired excretion due to renal insufficiency, oliguria, potassium-saving diuretics, aldosterone deficiency, or adrenocortical deficiency<br>3. Combination of the above factors. Nonfood sources of potassium include potassium supplements, salt substitutes, transfusions of old blood, and potassium salts of penicillin (penicillin G potassium contains 1.7 mEq potassium per 1 million units).<br>4. Movement of potassium from cells into serum with burns, crushing injuries, and acidosis | 1. Increased serum potassium<br>2. Impaired conduction of nerve impulses and muscle contraction<br>3. Impaired cardiac conduction. Hyperkalemia "anesthetizes" nerve and muscle cells so that electrical current cannot be built up to a sufficient level (repolarization) for an electrical impulse to be initiated and conducted. | 1. Serum potassium >5 mEq/L<br>2. Muscle weakness, possibly paralysis and respiratory insufficiency<br>3. Cardiotoxicity, with arrhythmias or cardiac arrest. Cardiac effects are not usually severe until serum levels are 7 mEq/L or above. ECG changes include a high, peaked T wave, prolonged P-R interval, absence of P waves, and prolonged QRS complex. |

## ALKALINIZING AGENTS

**Sodium bicarbonate** has long been used to treat metabolic acidosis, which occurs with severe renal disease, diabetes mellitus, circulatory impairment due to hypotension, shock or fluid volume deficit, and cardiac arrest. The drug dissociates into sodium and bicarbonate ions; the bicarbonate ions combine with free hydrogen ions to form carbonic acid. This action reduces the number of free hydrogen ions and thereby raises blood pH toward normal (7.35–7.45). However, the drug is not generally recommended now unless the acidosis is severe (*e.g.*, pH < 7.1), or clinical shock is present. Even then, usage must be based on frequent measurements of arterial blood gases and careful titration to avoid inducing alkalosis. Alkalosis sensitizes the myocardium and increases the occurrence of arrhythmias. It also alters the oxyhemoglobin dissociation curve so that less oxygen is released, and hypoxemia becomes even more severe. Thus, drug administration may be more harmful than helpful. In most instances, treating the underlying cause of the acidosis is safer and more effective. For example, in diabetic ketoacidosis, fluid replacement and insulin may be effective. In cardiac arrest, interventions to maintain

**TABLE 32-4.   MAGNESIUM IMBALANCES**

| Causes | Pathophysiology | Signs and Symptoms |
|---|---|---|
| *Hypomagnesemia* | | |
| 1. Inadequate dietary intake or prolonged administration of magnesium-free IV fluids<br>2. Decreased absorption, as occurs with alcoholism<br>3. Excessive losses with diuretic drugs, diarrhea, or diabetic acidosis | 1. Decreased serum magnesium<br>2. Impaired conduction of nerve impulses and muscle contraction | 1. Serum magnesium <1.5 mEq/L<br>2. Confusion, restlessness, irritability, vertigo, ataxia, seizures<br>3. Muscle tremors, carpopedal spasm, nystagmus, generalized spasticity<br>4. Tachycardia, hypotension, premature atrial and ventricular beats |
| *Hypermagnesemia* | | |
| 1. Renal failure<br>2. Impaired renal function accompanied by excessive intake of magnesium salts in antacids or cathartics<br>3. Overtreatment of magnesium deficiency | 1. Increased serum magnesium<br>2. Depressant effects on central nervous and neuromuscular systems, which block transmission of electrical impulses | 1. Serum magnesium >2.5 mEq/L<br>2. Skeletal muscle weakness and paralysis, cardiac arrhythmias, hypotension, respiratory insufficiency, drowsiness, lethargy, coma |

circulation and ventilation are more effective in alleviating acidosis.

Sodium bicarbonate also is used to alkalinize the urine. Alkalinization increases solubility of uric acid and sulfonamide drugs and increases excretion of some acids (*e.g.*, salicylates, phenobarbital) when taken in overdose.

### Routes and dosage ranges

*Adults:* PO 325 mg to 2 g, up to four times per day; maximum daily dose, 16 g for adults under 60 years, 8 g for adults over 60 years

IV Dosage individualized according to arterial blood gases

*Children:* IV dosage individualized according to arterial blood gases

## CATION EXCHANGE RESIN

**Sodium polystyrene sulfonate** (Kayexalate) is a cation exchange resin used clinically only in treatment of hyperkalemia. Given orally or rectally, the resin acts in

**TABLE 32-5.   CHLORIDE IMBALANCES**

| Causes | Pathophysiology | Signs and Symptoms |
|---|---|---|
| *Hypochloremic Metabolic Alkalosis* | | |
| 1. Excessive losses of chloride from vomiting, gastric suctioning, diuretic drug therapy, diabetic ketoacidosis, excessive perspiration, or adrenocortical insufficiency<br>2. Excessive ingestion of bicarbonate or base | 1. Decreased serum chloride<br>2. When chloride is lost, the body retains bicarbonate to maintain electroneutrality in extracellular fluids. The result is metabolic alkalosis, a relative deficiency of acid, and a relative excess of base. Hypokalemia is often present as well.<br>3. Hyperexcitability of the nervous system<br>4. Retention of carbon dioxide (acid) as a compensatory attempt to restore acid-base balance<br>5. Fluid loss and decreased plasma volume | 1. Serum chloride <95 mEq/L; arterial blood pH >7.45<br>2. Paresthesias of face and extremities<br>3. Muscle spasms and tetany, which cannot be distinguished from the tetany produced by hypocalcemia<br>4. Slow, shallow respirations<br>5. Dehydration<br>6. Hypotension |
| *Hyperchloremic Metabolic Acidosis* | | |
| 1. Most often caused by dehydration<br>2. Deficient bicarbonate<br>3. Hyperparathyroidism<br>4. Respiratory alkalosis<br>5. Excessive administration of sodium chloride or ammonium chloride | 1. Increased serum chloride<br>2. In dehydration, the kidneys reabsorb water in an attempt to relieve the fluid deficit. Large amounts of chloride are reabsorbed along with the water. The result is metabolic acidosis, a relative excess of acid, and a relative deficiency of base.<br>3. Central nervous system depression<br>4. Increased exhalation of carbon dioxide as a compensatory attempt to restore acid-base balance | 1. Serum chloride >103 mEq/L; arterial blood pH <7.35<br>2. Lethargy, stupor, disorientation, and coma if acidosis is not treated<br>3. Increased rate and depth of respiration |

## TABLE 32-6. SELECTED TRACE ELEMENTS

| Characteristics | Functions | Recommended Dietary Allowances (RDAs) | Food Sources |
|---|---|---|---|
| **Chromium**<br>1. Deficiency state identified in humans and several animal species<br>2. Deficiency produces impaired glucose tolerance (hyperglycemia, glycosuria), impaired growth and reproduction, and decreased life span. | Aids glucose use by increasing effectiveness of insulin and facilitating transport of glucose across cell membranes | Not established | Brewer's yeast and whole wheat products |
| **Cobalt**<br>1. Most body cobalt is stored in the liver; some is stored in the spleen, kidneys, and pancreas.<br>2. Excreted mainly in urine with smaller amounts excreted in feces and perspiration.<br>3. In humans, deficiency of vitamin $B_{12}$ produces pernicious anemia.<br>4. Excess state not established for humans. In animals, excess cobalt produces polycythemia, bone marrow hyperplasia, and increased blood volume. | A component of vitamin $B_{12}$, which is required for normal function of all body cells and for maturation of red blood cells | About 1 mg in the form of vitamin $B_{12}$ | Animal foods, including liver, muscle meats, and shellfish. Fruits, vegetables, and cereals contain no cobalt as vitamin $B_{12}$. |
| **Copper**<br>1. Found in many body tissues including the brain, liver, heart, kidneys, bone, and muscle<br>2. Eliminated from the body in urine, sweat, feces, and menstrual flow<br>3. Human deficiency occurs with lack of food intake, malabsorption syndromes, and prolonged administration of copper-free IV hyperalimentation solutions<br>4. Signs and symptoms of deficiency include decreased serum levels of copper and ceruloplasmin (a plasma protein that transports copper); decreased iron absorption; anemia from impaired erythropoiesis; leukopenia. Death can occur. In infants, three deficiency syndromes have been identified. One is characterized by anemia, a second by chronic malnutrition and diarrhea, and a third (Menke's syndrome) by retarded growth and progressive mental deterioration.<br>5. Copper excess (hypercupremia) may occur in women who take oral contraceptives or who are pregnant and in clients with infections or liver disease. Wilson's disease is a rare hereditary disorder characterized by accumulation of copper in vital organs (brain, liver, kidneys). Signs and symptoms vary according to affected organs. | 1. A component of many enzymes<br>2. Essential for correct functioning of the central nervous, cardiovascular, and skeletal systems<br>3. Important in formation of red blood cells, apparently by regulating storage and release of iron for hemoglobin | Not established; estimated at about 2 mg | Many foods, including liver, shellfish, nuts, cereals, poultry, dried fruits |
| **Fluoride**<br>1. Present in water, soil, plants, and animals in small amounts. Often added to community supplies of drinking water.<br>2. Accumulates in the body until about 50–60 years of age.<br>3. Fluoride deficiency is indicated by dental caries and possibly a greater incidence of osteoporosis.<br>4. Fluoride excess results in mottling of teeth and osteosclerosis. | 1. A component of tooth enamel<br>2. Strengthens bones, probably by promoting calcium retention in bones<br>3. Adequate intake before ages 50–60 years may decrease osteoporosis and fractures during later years. | Not established; average daily intake estimated at about 4 mg | Beef, canned salmon, eggs. Very little in milk, cereal grains, fruits, and vegetables. Fluoride content of foods depends on fluoride content of soil where they are grown. |

*(continued)*

**TABLE 32-6. SELECTED TRACE ELEMENTS** *(Continued)*

| Characteristics | Functions | Recommended Dietary Allowances (RDAs) | Food Sources |
|---|---|---|---|
| *Iodine* | | | |
| 1. Iodine deficiency causes thyroid gland enlargement and may cause hypothyroidism<br>2. Iodine excess (iodism) produces edema, fever, conjunctivitis, lymphadenopathy, stomatitis, vomiting, and coryza. Iodism is unlikely with dietary intake but may occur with excessive intake of drugs containing iodine. | Essential component of thyroid hormones | 150 mg for adults, larger amounts for children and pregnant or lactating women | Seafood is the best source. In vegetables, iodine content varies with the amount of iodine in soil where grown. In milk and eggs, content depends on the amount present in animal feed. |
| *Iron* | | | |
| 1. Nearly three fourths of body iron is in hemoglobin in red blood cells; about one fourth is stored in the liver, bone marrow, and spleen as ferritin and hemosiderin; the remaining small amount is in myoglobin and enzymes or bound to transferrin in plasma.<br>2. Absorption of iron from foods varies widely and is estimated to be about 10% under normal circumstances. It is influenced by several factors:<br>  A. Factors that *increase* absorption:<br>    (1) Presence of dietary ascorbic acid<br>    (2) Acidity of gastric fluids increases solubility of dietary iron.<br>    (3) Presence of calcium. Calcium combines with phosphate, oxalate, and phytate. If this reaction does not occur, iron combines with these substances and produces nonabsorbable compounds.<br>    (4) Physiologic states that increase iron absorption include periods of increased blood formation, such as pregnancy and growth. Also more iron is absorbed when iron deficiency is present.<br>  B. Factors that *decrease* absorption:<br>    (1) Lack of hydrochloric acid in the stomach or administration of antacids, which produces an alkaline environment<br>    (2) Combination of iron with phosphates, oxalates, or phytates in the intestine. This results in insoluble and nonabsorbable compounds.<br>    (3) Increased motility of the intestines, which decreases absorption of iron by decreasing contact time with the mucosa<br>    (4) Steatorrhea or any malabsorption disorder | 1. Essential component of hemoglobin, myoglobin, and several enzymes<br>2. Hemoglobin is required for transport and use of oxygen by body cells; myoglobin aids oxygen transport and use by muscle cells; enzymes are important for cellular respiration. | 10 mg for men and older women<br>18 mg for women during childbearing years and children during periods of rapid growth | Liver and other organ meats, lean meat, shellfish, dried beans and vegetables, egg yolks, dried fruits, molasses, whole grain and enriched breads. Milk and milk products contain essentially no iron. |
| *Selenium* | | | |
| 1. Has antioxidant properties similar to those of vitamin E<br>2. Deficiency most likely with long-term IV therapy. Signs and symptoms include myocardial abnormalities and other muscle discomfort and weakness.<br>3. Highly toxic in excessive amounts. Signs and symptoms include fatigue, peripheral neuropathy, nausea, diarrhea, and alopecia. | Important for function of myocardium and probably other muscles | 70 μg for men; 55 μg for women, increased to 65 μg during pregnancy and 75 μg during lactation | Fish, meat, breads, and cereals |

**TABLE 32-6. SELECTED TRACE ELEMENTS** (*Continued*)

| Characteristics | Functions | Recommended Dietary Allowances (RDAs) | Food Sources |
|---|---|---|---|
| **Zinc** | | | |
| 1. Deficiency may occur in liver cirrhosis, hepatitis, nephrosis, malabsorption syndromes, chronic infections, malignant diseases, myocardial infarction, hypothyroidism, and prolonged administration of zinc-free IV hyperalimentation solutions. Signs and symptoms are most evident in growing children and include impaired growth, hypogonadism in males, anorexia, and sensory impairment (loss of taste and smell). Also, if the client has had surgery, wound healing may be delayed. <br> 2. Zinc excess is unlikely with dietary intake but may develop with excessive ingestion or inhalation of zinc. Ingestion may cause nausea, vomiting, and diarrhea; inhalation may cause vomiting, headache, and fever. | 1. A component of many enzymes that are essential for normal metabolism (*e.g.*, carbonic anhydrase, lactic dehydrogenase, alkaline phosphatase). <br> 2. Necessary for normal cell growth, synthesis of nucleic acids (RNA and DNA), and synthesis of carbohydrates and proteins <br> 3. May be essential for use of vitamin A | 15 mg for adolescents and adults <br> 10 mg for preadolescents <br> 25–30 mg for pregnant and lactating women | Animal proteins, such as meat, liver, eggs, and seafood. Wheat germ is also a good source. |

the colon to release sodium and combine with potassium. Potassium is then eliminated from the body in the feces. Each gram of resin removes about 1 mEq of potassium. This drug is ineffective in severe, acute hyperkalemia because several hours are required to lower serum potassium levels. Thus, the resin is more likely to be used after other measures (*e.g.*, insulin and glucose infusions) have lowered dangerously high serum potassium levels. Insulin and glucose lower serum potassium levels by driving potassium into the cells. They do not remove potassium from the body.

### Routes and dosage ranges

*Adults:* PO 15 g in 100–200 ml of water and 70% sorbitol, one to four times daily

Rectally (retention enema) 30–50 g in 100–200 ml of water and 70% sorbitol q6h

**TABLE 32-7. IRON IMBALANCES**

| Causes | Pathophysiology | Signs and Symptoms |
|---|---|---|
| **Deficiency State** | | |
| 1. Inadequate intake of iron in the diet <br> 2. Faulty absorption of iron <br> 3. Blood loss in gastrointestinal bleeding, heavy or prolonged menstrual flow, traumatic injury, and other conditions | 1. Impaired erythropoiesis <br> 2. Inadequate hemoglobin to transport sufficient oxygen to body tissues <br> 3. Iron deficiency increases absorption of other minerals (*e.g.*, lead, cobalt, manganese) and may produce signs of excess. | 1. Anemia (decrease in red blood cells, hemoglobin, and hematocrit) <br> 2. With gradual development of anemia, minimal symptoms occur <br> 3. With rapid development of anemia or severe anemia, dyspnea, fatigue, tachycardia, malaise, and drowsiness occur. |
| **Acute Excess State** | | |
| Acute iron poisoning usually occurs in small children who take several tablets of an iron preparation. | Acute toxicity | Vomiting, diarrhea, melena, abdominal pain, shock, convulsions, and metabolic acidosis. Death may occur within 24 h if treatment is not prompt. |
| **Chronic Excess State** | | |
| Chronic iron excess (hemochromatosis) is rare but may be caused by long-term ingestion of excessive iron salts (*e.g.*, ferrous sulfate), large numbers of blood transfusions, or a rare genetic trait that promotes iron absorption. | Excess iron is deposited in the heart, pancreas, kidney, liver, and other organs. It impairs cell function and eventually destroys cells. | Cardiac arrhythmias, heart failure, diabetes mellitus, bronze pigmentation of skin, liver enlargement, arthropathy, and others |

# CHELATING AGENTS (METAL ANTAGONISTS)

**Deferoxamine mesylate** (Desferal) is a chelating agent for iron and is the only drug available for removing excess iron from the body. When given orally within a few hours after oral ingestion of iron preparations, deferoxamine combines with the iron in the bowel lumen and prevents its absorption. When given parenterally, it removes iron from storage sites (*e.g.*, ferrin, hemosiderin, transferrin) and combines with the iron to produce a water-soluble compound that can be excreted by the kidneys. The drug can remove about 10 to 50 mg of iron per day. The urine becomes reddish brown from the iron content.

The major indication for use of deferoxamine is acute iron intoxication. It is also used in hemochromatosis due to blood transfusions or hemosiderosis due to certain hemolytic anemias. In these chronic conditions characterized by accumulation of iron in tissues, phlebotomy may be more effective in removing iron. Deferoxamine is more likely to be used in clients who are too anemic or hypoproteinemic to tolerate the blood loss.

### Routes and dosage ranges

*Adults and children:* PO 4–8 g, given within a few hours of oral ingestion of iron preparations
   IM 1 g initially, then 500 mg q4h for 2 doses, then 500 mg q4–12h if needed; maximum dose, 6 g/24 h
   IV 1 g slowly (not to exceed 15 mg/kg per hour), then 500 mg q4h for 2 doses, then 500 mg q4–12h if necessary; maximum dose, 6 g/24 h. This route is used only in the client in shock.

**Penicillamine** (Cuprimine) is a drug that chelates copper, zinc, mercury, and lead to form soluble complexes that are excreted in the urine. The main therapeutic use of penicillamine is to remove excess copper in clients with Wilson's disease (see Table 32-6). It also can be used prophylactically, before clinical manifestations occur, in clients likely to develop this hereditary condition. Penicillamine may be used to treat cystinuria, a hereditary metabolic disorder characterized by large amounts of cystine in the urine and renal calculi. It may be used in lead poisoning and severe rheumatoid arthritis that does not respond to conventional treatment measures.

### Route and dosage ranges

*Adults and older children:* Wilson's disease, PO 250 mg four times per day, increased gradually if necessary up to 2 g/d
   Lead poisoning, PO 250–500 mg twice a day
   Rheumatoid arthritis, PO 125–250 mg/d for 4 weeks, increased by 125–250 mg/d at 1- to 3-mo intervals if necessary

Usual maintenance dose, 500–750 mg/d; maximum dose, 1000–1500 mg/d
*Infants over 6 months and young children:* Wilson's disease, PO 250 mg/d, dissolved in fruit juice
   Lead poisoning, PO 125 mg three times per day

**Succimer** (Chemet) is a drug that chelates lead to form water-soluble complexes that are excreted in the urine. The main therapeutic use is to treat lead poisoning in children with blood levels above 45 µg/100 ml. The most common adverse effects are gastrointestinal (*e.g.*, anorexia, nausea, vomiting, diarrhea).

### Route and dosage ranges

*Children:* PO 10 mg/kg or 350 mg/m$^2$ every 8 hours for 5 days, then every 12 hours for 14 days (total of 19 days of drug administration). For young children who cannot swallow capsules, the capsule contents can be sprinkled on soft food or given with a spoon.

## IRON PREPARATIONS

**Ferrous gluconate** (Fergon) is an oral iron preparation that is effective in treating iron deficiency anemia. It is claimed to be less irritating to gastrointestinal mucosa and therefore better tolerated than ferrous sulfate. Ferrous gluconate contains about 12% elemental iron, so that each 320-mg tablet contains about 38 mg of iron. Indications for use, adverse reactions, and contraindications are the same as for ferrous sulfate.

### Route and dosage ranges

*Adults:* PO 320–640 mg (40–80 mg elemental iron) three times per day
*Children:* PO 100–300 mg (12.5–37.5 mg elemental iron) three times per day
*Infants:* PO 100 mg or 30 drops of elixir initially, gradually increased to 300 mg or 5 ml of elixir daily (15–37.5 mg elemental iron) in divided doses

**Ferrous sulfate** (Feosol), which contains 20% elemental iron, is the prototype of oral iron preparations and the preparation of choice for prevention or treatment of iron deficiency anemia. It may be used as an iron supplement during periods of increased requirements (*e.g.*, childhood, pregnancy). Nausea and other gastrointestinal symptoms may result from gastric irritation. Ferrous sulfate and other oral iron preparations discolor feces, producing a black-green color that may be mistaken for blood in the stool. Contraindications to oral iron preparations include peptic ulcer disease, inflammatory intestinal disorders, anemias other than iron deficiency anemia, multiple blood transfusions, hemochromatosis, and hemosiderosis.

### Route and dosage ranges

*Adults:* PO 300 mg–1.2 g (60–240 mg elemental iron) daily in three or four divided doses

*Children 6–12 years:* PO 120–600 mg (24–120 mg elemental iron) daily in divided doses

*Infants and children under 6 years:* 300 mg (60 mg elemental iron) daily in divided doses

**Iron dextran injection** (InFeD) is a parenteral form of iron useful in treating confirmed iron deficiency anemia when oral supplements are not feasible. One ml equals 50 mg of elemental iron. Reasons for using iron dextran injection include peptic ulcer or inflammatory bowel disease that is likely to be aggravated by oral iron preparations; the client's inability or unwillingness to take oral preparations; and a shortage of time for correcting the iron deficiency (*e.g.*, late pregnancy or preoperative status). One of the major advantages of parenteral iron is that body iron stores can be replenished rapidly. The drug is contraindicated in anemias not associated with iron deficiency and hypersensitivity to the drug (fatal anaphylactoid reactions have occurred).

See the manufacturer's literature regarding calculation of dosage.

## MAGNESIUM PREPARATION

**Magnesium sulfate** is given parenterally in hypomagnesemia, convulsions associated with pregnancy (eclampsia), and prevention of hypomagnesemia in total parenteral nutrition. Therapeutic effects in these conditions are attributed to the drug's depressant effects on the central nervous system and smooth, skeletal, and cardiac muscle. Therapeutic uses of magnesium salts as antacids and cathartics are discussed in Chapters 63 and 64, respectively. Magnesium preparations are contraindicated in clients who have impaired renal function or who are comatose.

### Routes and dosage ranges

*Adults:* Hypomagnesemia, IM 1–2 g (2–4 ml of 50% solution) once or twice daily based on serum magnesium levels

Eclampsia, IM 1–2 g (2–4 ml of 50% solution) initially, then 1 g q30 min until seizures stop

Convulsive seizures, IM 1 g (2 ml of 50% solution) repeated PRN

IV, do not exceed 150 mg/min (1.5 ml/min of a 10% solution, 3 ml/min of a 5% solution)

*Older children:* IM, same dosage as adults

## POTASSIUM PREPARATIONS

**Potassium chloride** is usually the drug of choice for preventing or treating hypokalemia, because deficiencies of potassium and chloride often occur together. It is often prescribed for clients who are receiving potassium-losing diuretics (*e.g.*, hydrochlorothiazide, furosemide), those who are receiving digitalis preparations (hypokalemia increases risks of digitalis toxicity), and those who are receiving only intravenous fluids because of surgical procedures, gastrointestinal disease, or other conditions. Potassium chloride also may be used to replace chloride in hypochloremic metabolic alkalosis.

Potassium chloride can be given orally or intravenously. Oral preparations are recommended when feasible, but one disadvantage of oral liquid preparations is an unpleasant taste. This has led to production of various flavored powders, liquids, and effervescent tablets (*e.g.*, Kay Ciel Elixir, K-Lor, Klorvess). Tablets containing a wax matrix (*e.g.*, Slow-K) are effective and may be better tolerated by most clients than liquid formulations. Intravenous preparations of potassium chloride must be diluted before administration to prevent hyperkalemia, cardiotoxicity, and severe pain at the injection site.

Potassium chloride is contraindicated in clients with renal failure and in those receiving potassium-saving diuretics, such as triamterene, spironolactone, or amiloride.

**Potassium gluconate** (Kaon) and **potassium bicarbonate and citrate** (K-Lyte) are oral preparations of potassium salts other than chloride. They are supposedly more palatable and therefore more likely to be taken than oral potassium chloride preparations. The major indication for their use is the occasional hypokalemia associated with hyperchloremia. If given to a client with hypokalemia and hypochloremia, these preparations do not replace chloride, and another source of chloride must be given. Adverse reactions and contraindications are the same as for potassium chloride.

### Routes and dosage ranges

*Adults:* PO 15–20 mEq two to four times per day

IV (potassium chloride injection), about 40–100 mEq/24 h. Dosage must be individualized and depends on serum potassium levels and total potassium body stores. Potassium chloride (KCl) must be diluted. A generally safe dosage range is 20–60 mEq, diluted in 1000 ml of dextrose or sodium chloride IV solution and given no faster than 10–15 mEq/h or 60–120 mEq/24 h.

## SODIUM PREPARATIONS

**Sodium chloride injection** is available in several concentrations and sizes for intravenous use. Concentrations are 0.45% (hypotonic solution), 0.9% (isotonic), and 3% (hypertonic). Sodium chloride is also available in combination with dextrose. Five percent dextrose in 0.22% sodium chloride and 5% dextrose in 0.45% sodium chloride are among the most frequently used solutions for intravenous fluid therapy. They contain 38.5

and 77 mEq/L, respectively, of sodium and chloride. Isotonic or 0.9% sodium chloride contains 154 mEq of both sodium and chloride. This solution may be used to treat hyponatremia. The 3% solution contains 513 mEq of sodium and chloride per liter. It may be used in severe hyponatremia but is rarely necessary. Because of the high risk of circulatory overload and pulmonary edema, it must be given in small amounts (200–400 ml) and administered slowly (no faster than 100 ml/h).

### Route and dosage range

*Adults:* IV 1500–3000 ml of 0.22%, 0.45% solution/24 h depending on client's fluid needs; about 50 ml/h to keep IV lines open

## ZINC PREPARATION

**Zinc sulfate** is available in tablets containing 110, 200, or 220 mg of zinc sulfate (equivalent to 25, 47, and 50 mg of elemental zinc, respectively) and in capsules containing 220 mg of zinc sulfate (equivalent to 50 mg of elemental zinc). It is also an ingredient in several vitamin-mineral combination products. Zinc sulfate is given orally as a dietary supplement to prevent or treat zinc deficiency. In malnourished clients, it may be used to promote wound healing after surgery. There is no evidence, though, that zinc promotes wound healing or has any other beneficial effect in the absence of zinc deficiency.

### Route and dosage range

*Adults:* PO 25–50 mg elemental zinc daily

## MULTIPLE MINERAL-ELECTROLYTE PREPARATIONS

There are numerous commercially prepared electrolyte solutions for intravenous use. One group provides *maintenance* amounts of fluids and electrolytes when oral intake of food and fluids is restricted or contraindicated. These solutions differ slightly in the number and amount of particular electrolytes. A second group provides *replacement* amounts of electrolytes (mainly sodium and chloride) when electrolytes are lost from the body in abnormal amounts. This group includes Normosol-R (Abbott), and Plasma-Lyte 148 (Travenol). These electrolyte preparations are available with dextrose 2.5% to 10%. Ringer's solution is another replacement fluid that is used fairly often. It is manufactured by several different companies; health-care agencies use one manufacturer's products for the most part.

Several oral electrolyte solutions (*e.g.,* Lytren, Pedialyte) contain sodium, chloride, potassium, calcium, magnesium, and other electrolytes along with a small amount of dextrose. They are used to supply maintenance amounts of fluids and electrolytes when oral intake is restricted. They are especially useful in children for treatment of diarrhea and may prevent severe fluid and electrolyte depletion. The amount given must be carefully prescribed and calculated to avoid excessive intake. They should not be used in severe circumstances in which intravenous fluid and electrolyte therapy are indicated. They must be cautiously used with impaired renal function. They should not be mixed with other electrolyte-containing fluids, such as milk or fruit juices.

### Routes and dosage ranges

*Adults:* IV 2000–3000 ml/24 h, depending on individual fluid and electrolyte needs
*Children:* IV, PO, amount individualized according to fluid and electrolyte needs

## *Nursing Process*

### Assessment

Assess each client for current or potential mineral-electrolyte or acid-base disorders. This is usually done in an overall assessment of nutritional status. Specific assessment factors related to minerals and electrolytes include the following:

- Deficiency states are probably more common than excess states unless a mineral-electrolyte supplement is being taken. However, deficiencies and excesses may be equally harmful, and both must be assessed.
- Clients with other nutritional deficiencies are likely to have mineral-electrolyte deficiencies as well. Moreover, deficiencies are likely to be multiple, with overlapping signs and symptoms.
- Many drugs influence gains and losses of minerals and electrolytes, including diuretics and laxatives.
- Minerals and electrolytes are lost with gastric suction, polyuria, diarrhea, excessive perspiration, and other conditions.
- Assess laboratory reports when available.
  - Check the complete blood count for decreased red blood cells, hemoglobin, and hematocrit. Reduced values may indicate iron deficiency anemia, and further assessment is needed.
  - Check serum electrolyte reports for increases or decreases. All major minerals can be measured in clinical laboratories. The ones usually measured are sodium, chloride, and potassium; carbon dioxide content, a measure of bicarbonate, is also assessed. Normal values vary to some extent with the laboratory and the method of measurement, but a general range of normal values is sodium, 135 to 145 mEq/L; chloride, 95 to 105 mEq/L; potassium, 3.5 to 5 mEq/L; and carbon dioxide, 22 to 26 mEq/L. Minor differences in these values are insignificant.

### Nursing diagnoses

- High Risk for Altered Nutrition: Less than Body Requirements related to mineral-electrolyte deficiency
- High Risk for Altered Nutrition: More than Body Requirements related to excessive intake of drug preparations

- High Risk for Injury related to mineral-electrolyte deficiency or overdose
- Knowledge Deficit: Importance of adequate mineral-electrolyte intake in normal body functioning
- Knowledge Deficit: Dietary sources of various mineral-electrolyte nutrients

## Planning/Goals

*The client will:*
- Have an adequate dietary intake of minerals and electrolytes
- Avoid mineral-electrolyte supplements unless recommended by a health-care provider
- Participate in follow-up procedures and laboratory tests as requested when mineral-electrolyte drugs are prescribed
- Take mineral-electrolyte drugs as prescribed
- Avoid adverse effects of drug preparations

## Interventions

Implement measures to prevent mineral-electrolyte disorders:
- Promote a varied diet. A diet adequate in protein and calories generally provides adequate minerals and electrolytes.
- If assessment data reveal potential development of a disorder, start preventive measures as soon as possible. For clients able to eat, foods high in iron may at least delay onset of iron deficiency anemia, foods high in potassium may prevent hypokalemia with diuretic therapy, and salty foods along with water help to prevent problems associated with excessive perspiration. For people unable to eat, intravenous fluids and electrolytes are usually given. Generally, oral food intake or tube feeding is preferable to intravenous therapy.
- Treat underlying disorders that contribute to the mineral-electrolyte deficiency or excess. Measures to relieve anorexia, nausea, vomiting, diarrhea, pain, and other symptoms help to increase intake or decrease output of certain minerals. Measures to increase urine output, such as forcing fluids, help to increase output of some minerals in the urine and therefore prevent excess states from developing.
- Mineral supplements are recommended only for current or potential deficiencies. They provide no beneficial effects in the absence of deficiency, and all are toxic if taken in excessive amounts. When deficiencies are identified, treat with foods when possible. Next, use oral mineral supplements. Use parenteral supplements only for clear-cut indications, because they are potentially the most hazardous.
- For clients who have nasogastric tubes to suction, irrigate the tubes with isotonic sodium chloride solution. The use of tap water is contraindicated because it is hypotonic and would pull electrolytes into the stomach. Electrolytes are then lost in the aspirated and discarded stomach contents. For the same reason, only 2 to 3 teaspoons of ice chips or water are allowed per hour. Clients often request ice chips or water frequently and in larger amounts than desirable; the nurse must explain the reason for the restrictions.
- If tap-water enemas are ordered to be given until clear of feces, give no more than three. Isotonic sodium chloride is preferred to tap water. Still, no more than three enemas should be given consecutively.

*Teach clients:*
- The best source of minerals and electrolytes is a well-balanced diet with a variety of foods. A well-balanced diet contains all the minerals needed for health in most people. An exception is iron, which is often needed as a dietary supplement in women and children.
- The safest course of action is to take drug preparations only on a health-care provider's advice, in the amounts and for the length of time prescribed. All minerals are toxic when taken in excess. Also, there is no benefit to taking more than the body needs.
- To keep all mineral-electrolyte substances out of reach of children to prevent accidental overdose. Acute iron intoxication is a relatively common problem among small children.
- To keep appointments with health-care providers for periodic blood tests and other follow-up procedures when mineral-electrolyte supplements are prescribed. This will help prevent ingestion of excessive amounts.

## Evaluation

- Interview about and observe the amount and type of food intake in relation to required minerals and electrolytes.
- Interview and observe for signs of mineral-electrolyte deficiency or excess.

# Principles of therapy

### DIET SUPPLEMENTS

Some people take mineral preparations as dietary supplements in an effort to promote health and prevent deficiencies. They are rarely needed for this purpose by people who eat a balanced and varied diet; who have no increased need for nutrients, such as growth or pregnancy; and who have no abnormal losses of nutrients, such as those caused by gastrointestinal diseases. In fact, dietary supplements in a person who eats adequately could exceed nutrient needs by more than 100%. No known benefit to health results from ingesting more mineral nutrients than the body needs, and harm may result because all minerals are toxic at high doses.

### PREVENTION OF AN EXCESS STATE

When a mineral is given to correct a deficiency state, there is a risk of producing an excess state. Because both deficiency and excess states may be harmful, the amount of mineral supplement should be titrated as closely as possible to the amount needed by the body. Larger doses are needed to treat deficiency states than are needed to prevent deficiencies from developing. In addition to producing potential toxicity, large doses of one mineral may cause a relative deficiency of another mineral or nutrient.

### DRUG SELECTION

Oral drug preparations are preferred, when feasible, for preventing or treating mineral disorders. They are generally safer, less likely to produce toxicity, more convenient to administer, and less expensive than parenteral preparations.

## PRINCIPLES OF TREATING SODIUM DISORDERS

### Hyponatremia

Treatment of hyponatremia is aimed at restoring normal levels of serum sodium. This can be done with isotonic sodium chloride solution when hyponatremia is caused by sodium depletion and with restriction of water when hyponatremia is caused by fluid volume excess (water intoxication).

### Hypernatremia

Treatment of hypernatremia requires administration of sodium-free fluids, either orally or intravenously, until serum sodium levels return to normal. Milder states usually respond to increased water intake through the gastrointestinal tract; more severe hypernatremia is likely to require intravenous administration of 5% dextrose in water.

## PRINCIPLES OF TREATING POTASSIUM DISORDERS

### Hypokalemia

1. Assess for conditions contributing to hypokalemia, and attempt to eliminate them or reduce their impact. Such conditions are generally inadequate intake, excessive loss, or some combination of the two.
2. Assess the severity of the hypokalemia. This is best done on the basis of serum potassium levels and clinical manifestations. Serum potassium levels alone are inadequate because they may not accurately reflect depletion of body potassium.
3. Potassium supplements are indicated in the following circumstances:
   a. When serum potassium level is below 3 mEq/L on repeated measurements, even if the client is asymptomatic
   b. When serum potassium is 3 to 3.5 mEq/L and clear-cut symptoms or electrocardiogram (ECG) changes indicate hypokalemia. Some clinicians advocate treatment in the absence of symptoms.
   c. In clients receiving digitalis preparations, if necessary to maintain serum potassium levels above 3.5 mEq/L. Such usage is indicated because hypokalemia increases digitalis toxicity.

4. Although opinions differ, potassium supplements are probably not indicated for prevention of hypokalemia except in clients with hypokalemic periodic paralysis, a rare disorder. Thus, use of potassium supplements with diuretic therapy is not indicated unless hypokalemia develops or digitalis preparations are being given.
5. When potassium supplements are necessary, oral administration is preferred. Oral preparations are usually effective and less likely to cause hyperkalemia than intravenous preparations.
6. Potassium chloride is the drug of choice in most instances because it replaces potassium and chloride. Liquids, powders, and effervescent tablets for oral use must be diluted in at least 4 oz of water or juice to improve taste and decrease gastric irritation. Controlled-release tablets or capsules with KCl in a wax matrix or microencapsulated form are preferred by most clients.
7. Intravenous KCl is indicated when a client cannot take an oral preparation or has severe hypokalemia. The serum potassium level should be measured, total body deficit estimated, and adequate urine output established before intravenous potassium therapy begins.
   a. Intravenous KCl must be well diluted to prevent sudden hyperkalemia, cardiotoxic effects, and phlebitis at the venipuncture site. The usual dilution is KCl 20 to 60 mEq/1000 ml of intravenous fluid.
   b. Dosage must be individualized. Clients receiving intravenous fluids only are usually given 40 to 60 mEq of KCl daily. This can be given safely with 20 mEq KCl/L of fluids and a flow rate of 100 to 125 ml/h. In severe deficits, a higher concentration and a higher flow rate may be necessary. In these situations, an infusion pump to control flow rate accurately and continuous cardiac monitoring for detection of hyperkalemia are necessary. Also, serum potassium levels must be checked frequently and dosage adjusted if indicated. No more than 100 to 200 mEq KCl should be given within 24 hours, even if several days are required to replace the estimated deficit.
   c. Do not administer potassium-containing intravenous solutions into a central venous catheter. There is a risk of hyperkalemia and cardiac arrhythmias or arrest because there is limited time for the solution to be diluted in the blood returning to the heart.
   d. In critical situations, KCl usually should be given in sodium chloride solutions rather than dextrose solutions. Administering dextrose solutions may increase hypokalemia by causing some potassium to leave the serum and enter cells.

## Hyperkalemia

1. Eliminate any exogenous sources of potassium, such as potassium supplements, penicillin G potassium, salt substitutes, and blood transfusion with old blood.
2. Treat acidosis if present, because potassium leaves cells and enters the serum with acidosis.
3. Use measures that antagonize the effects of potassium, that cause potassium to leave the serum and reenter cells, and that remove potassium from the body. Appropriate measures are determined mainly by serum potassium levels and ECG changes. Continuous cardiac monitoring is required.

   Severe hyperkalemia (serum potassium above 7 mEq/L and ECG changes indicating hyperkalemia) requires urgent treatment. Immediate intravenous administration of sodium bicarbonate 45 mEq, over a 5-minute period, causes rapid movement of potassium into cells. This can be repeated in a few minutes if ECG changes persist.

   Calcium gluconate 10%, 5 to 10 ml intravenously, is also given early in treatment. It acts to decrease the cardiotoxic effects of hyperkalemia. It is contraindicated if the client is receiving digitalis, and it cannot be added to fluids containing sodium bicarbonate because insoluble precipitates are formed.

   The next step is intravenous infusion of glucose and insulin. This also causes potassium to move into cells, although not as quickly as sodium bicarbonate.
4. When hyperkalemia is less severe or when it has been reduced by the above measures, sodium polystyrene sulfonate, a cation exchange resin, can be given orally or rectally to remove potassium from the body. Each gram of the resin combines with 1 mEq potassium, and both are excreted in feces. The resin is usually mixed with water and sorbitol, a poorly absorbed, osmotically active alcohol that has a laxative effect. The sorbitol offsets the constipating effect of the resin and aids in its expulsion. Oral administration is preferred, and several doses daily may be given until serum potassium is normal. When given as an enema, the solution must be retained from one to several hours, or repeated enemas must be given for therapeutic effect.
5. If the above measures fail to reduce hyperkalemia, peritoneal dialysis or hemodialysis may be used.

## PRINCIPLES OF TREATING MAGNESIUM DISORDERS

### Hypomagnesemia

1. Prevent, when possible, by giving parenteral fluids with magnesium when the fluids are the only source of nutrients. Multiple electrolyte intravenous solutions contain magnesium chloride or acetate, and magnesium can be added to solutions for total parenteral nutrition.
2. Magnesium sulfate, intravenously or intramuscularly, can be given daily as long as hypomagnesemia persists or continuing losses occur. Initial dosage may be larger, but the usual maintenance dose is about 8 mEq daily. A 10% solution is available in 10-ml vials that contain 8 mEq of magnesium sulfate for adding to intravenous solutions. A 50% solution is available in 2-ml vials (8 mEq) for intramuscular administration.
3. Check serum magnesium levels daily.

### Hypermagnesemia

1. Stop any source of exogenous magnesium, such as magnesium sulfate or magnesium-containing antacids, cathartics, or enemas.
2. Have calcium gluconate available for intravenous administration. It is an antidote for the sedative effects of magnesium excess.
3. Increase urine output by increasing fluid intake, if feasible. This increases removal of magnesium from the body in urine.
4. Clients with chronic renal failure are the most likely to develop hypermagnesemia. They are likely to require peritoneal dialysis or hemodialysis to lower serum magnesium levels.

## PRINCIPLES OF TREATING IRON DEFICIENCY AND EXCESS

### Iron deficiency anemia

1. Anemia is a symptom, not a disease. Therefore, the underlying cause must be identified and eliminated, if possible.
2. Assess the client's intake of and attitude toward foods with high iron content. Encourage increased dietary intake of these foods.
3. Use oral iron preparations when possible. They are generally safe, effective, convenient to administer, and relatively inexpensive. Ferrous preparations (sulfate, gluconate, fumarate) are better absorbed than ferric preparations. Other iron salts do not differ significantly from ferrous sulfate. Ferrous sulfate is usually the drug of choice for oral iron therapy. Slow-release or enteric-coated products tend to decrease absorption of iron.
4. Dosage is calculated in terms of elemental iron. Iron preparations vary greatly in the amount of elemental iron they contain. Ferrous sulfate, for example, contains 20% iron; thus, each 300-mg tablet furnishes

about 60 mg of elemental iron. With the usual regimen of one tablet three times daily, a daily dose of 180 mg of elemental iron is given. For most clients, probably half that amount (30 mg three times daily) would correct the deficiency. However, tablets are not manufactured in sizes to allow this regimen, and liquid preparations are not very popular with clients. Thus, relatively large doses are usually given, but smaller doses may be just as effective, especially if gastrointestinal symptoms become a problem with higher dosages. Whatever the dose, only about 10% to 15% of the iron is absorbed. Most of the remainder is excreted in feces, which turn dark green or black.

5. Oral iron preparations are better absorbed if taken on an empty stomach. However, because gastric irritation is a common adverse reaction, they are more often given with or immediately after meals.

6. Although normal hemoglobin levels return after about 2 months of oral iron therapy, an additional 6-month period of drug therapy is recommended to replenish the body's iron stores.

7. Reasons for failure to respond to iron therapy include continued blood loss, failure to take the drug as prescribed, or defective iron absorption. These factors must be reevaluated if no therapeutic response is evident within 3 to 4 weeks after drug therapy is begun.

8. Parenteral iron is indicated when oral preparations may further irritate a diseased gastrointestinal tract, when the client is unable or unwilling to take the oral drugs, or when the anemia must be corrected relatively rapidly.

9. For severe iron deficiency anemia, blood transfusions may be most effective.

### Iron excess

1. Acute iron overdosage requires treatment as soon as possible, even if overdosage is only suspected, and the amount taken is unknown. It is unnecessary to wait until serum iron level is measured.

   If treatment is begun shortly after oral ingestion of iron, induced vomiting or aspiration of stomach contents by nasogastric tube is helpful. This can be followed by lavage with 1% sodium bicarbonate solution to form insoluble iron carbonate compounds. The next step is to instill in the stomach 5 to 8 g of deferoxamine dissolved in 50 ml of distilled water to bind the iron remaining in the gastrointestinal tract and prevent its absorption. Finally, deferoxamine is given intramuscularly or intravenously to bind with iron in tissues and allow its excretion in the urine. Throughout the treatment period, supportive measures may be needed for gastrointestinal hemorrhage, acidosis, and shock.

2. For chronic iron overload or hemochromatosis, the first step in treatment is to stop the source of iron, if possible. Phlebotomy is the treatment of choice for most clients because withdrawal of 500 ml of blood removes about 250 mg of iron. Phlebotomy may be needed as often as weekly and for as long as 2 to 3 years. For clients resistant to or intolerant of phlebotomy, deferoxamine can be given. About 10 to 50 mg of iron is excreted daily in the urine with deferoxamine administration.

### PRINCIPLES OF TREATING ACID-BASE DISORDERS

#### Metabolic acidosis

1. Assess the presence and severity of acidosis by measuring arterial blood gases. Results reflecting acidosis are decreased pH (less than 7.35) and decreased bicarbonate (less than 22 mEq/L).

2. Assess and treat the underlying condition, such as diabetic ketoacidosis.

3. If this does not relieve acidosis, or if acidosis is severe (arterial blood pH less than 7.2), sodium bicarbonate may be given parenterally to alkalinize the blood. It can be given by direct injection into a vein or as a continuous intravenous infusion. Ampules and prefilled syringes are available in 8.4% solution (50 ml contains 50 mEq) or 7.5% solution (50 ml contains 44.6 mEq). Intravenous solutions of 5% and 1.4% sodium bicarbonate are also available in 500-ml bottles.

4. Monitor arterial blood gases and serum potassium levels frequently. Overtreatment of acidosis with sodium bicarbonate will produce alkalosis. Serum potassium levels may change from high to normal levels initially (because acidosis causes potassium to be drawn into the bloodstream) to severely low levels as potassium reenters cells with treatment of acidosis. Thus, potassium replacement is likely to be needed during treatment of acidosis.

5. During severe acidosis, effective ventilation measures are needed along with sodium bicarbonate to remove carbon dioxide from the blood.

6. In lactic acidosis, larger doses of sodium bicarbonate may be required than in other types of acidosis. This is because of continued production of large amounts of lactic acid by body metabolism.

7. Chronic metabolic acidosis may occur with chronic renal failure. Sodium bicarbonate or citrate (which is converted to bicarbonate in the body) can be given orally in a dose sufficient to maintain a normal serum bicarbonate level.

## Metabolic alkalosis

1. Assess the presence and severity of the alkalosis by measuring arterial blood gases. Values indicating alkalosis are increased pH (above 7.45) and increased bicarbonate (above 26 mEq/L).
2. Assess and treat the underlying condition. Often, volume depletion and hypochloremia are present and can be corrected with isotonic 0.9% sodium chloride solution. If hypokalemia and hypochloremia are present, potassium chloride will likely replace both deficits.
3. In severe alkalosis that does not respond to the above therapy, ammonium chloride can be given, but it must be given cautiously to avoid inducing acidosis.

## USE IN CHILDREN

Children need sufficient amounts of minerals and electrolytes to support growth and normal body functioning. In the healthy child, a varied, well-balanced diet is generally preferred over supplements. However, iron deficiency is common in young children and teenage girls, and an iron supplement is often needed.

If supplements are given, dosages should not exceed recommended amounts. All minerals and electrolytes are toxic in overdose and may cause life-threatening adverse effects. All such drugs should be kept out of reach of young children and should never be referred to as "candy."

## USE IN OLDER ADULTS

Mineral-electrolyte requirements are the same as for younger adults, but deficiencies of calcium and iron are common in older adults. Numerous factors may contribute to deficiencies, including limited income, anorexia, lack of teeth or ill-fitting dentures, drugs that decrease absorption of dietary nutrients, and disease processes that interfere with the ability to obtain, prepare, or eat adequate amounts of a variety of foods. Diuretic drugs, frequently prescribed for cardiovascular disorders in older adults, may cause potassium deficiency unless serum levels are carefully monitored and preventive measures taken.

Excess states also may occur in older adults. For example, decreased renal function promotes retention of magnesium and potassium. Hyperkalemia also may occur with the use of potassium supplements or salt substitutes. All minerals and electrolytes are toxic in overdose.

Every older adult should be assessed carefully regarding nutritional status and use of drugs that interact with dietary nutrients. Serum levels of minerals and electrolytes should be monitored carefully during illness and measures taken to prevent either deficiency or excess states.

# NURSING ACTIONS: MINERAL–ELECTROLYTE PREPARATIONS

| *Nursing Actions* | *Rationale/Explanation* |
| --- | --- |
| **1. Administer accurately**<br>**a.** Give oral mineral–electrolyte preparations with food or immediately after meals. | To decrease gastric irritation. Iron and possibly some other agents are better absorbed when taken on an empty stomach. However, they are better tolerated when taken with food. |
| **b.** Give IV preparations slowly, as a general rule. | The primary danger of rapid IV injection or infusion is a transient excess in serum, which may cause cardiac arrhythmias or other serious problems. |
| **c.** Do not mix minerals and electrolytes with any other drug in a syringe. | High risk of physical incompatibility and precipitation of drugs |
| **d.** For IV infusion, most minerals and electrolytes are compatible with solutions of dextrose or sodium chloride. Do not mix with other solutions until compatibility is determined. | To avoid physical incompatibility and precipitation of contents |

*(continued)*

## Nursing Actions

## Rationale/Explanation

**e.** For IV sodium chloride (NaCl) solutions:

(1) Give fluids at the prescribed flow rate.

Flow rates depend largely on reasons for use. For example, if a client is receiving no oral fluids (NPO) or only small amounts, the flow rate is often 100 to 125 ml/h or 2400 to 3000 ml/24 hours. If used as a vehicle for IV antibiotics, the rate is often 50 ml/h or keep open rate (KOR). If the client is dehydrated, 150 to 200 ml/h may be given for a few hours or until a certain amount has been given. (Restrictions in time or amount are necessary to avoid circulatory overload or pulmonary edema.)

(2) Give hypertonic saline solution (3% sodium chloride injection) slowly. Also, give no more than 200 to 400 ml at one time.

To avoid circulatory overload and sclerosing the veins

**f.** For potassium supplements:

(1) Mix liquids, powders, and effervescent tablets in at least 4 oz of juice, water, or carbonated beverage.

To dilute, disguise the unpleasant taste, and decrease gastric irritation

(2) Give oral preparations with or after meals.

To decrease gastric irritation

(3) Never give undiluted potassium chloride (KCl) IV.

Transient hyperkalemia may cause life-threatening cardiotoxicity. Severe pain and vein sclerosis also may result.

(4) Dilute IV KCl 20 to 60 mEq in 1000 ml of IV solution, such as dextrose in water. Be sure that KCl is mixed well with the IV solution.

Dilution decreases risks of hyperkalemia and cardiotoxicity. It also prevents or decreases pain at the infusion site.

(5) Generally, give potassium-containing IV solutions at a rate that administers about 10 mEq/h or less.

This is the safest amount and rate of potassium administration. It is also usually effective.

(6) For life-threatening arrhythmias caused by hypokalemia, potassium can be replaced with 20 to 40 mEq/h with appropriate cardiac monitoring.

Risks of hyperkalemia and life-threatening cardiotoxicity are greatly increased with high concentrations or rapid flow rates. Constant electrocardiogram monitoring is the best way to detect hyperkalemia.

**g.** For magnesium sulfate ($MgSO_4$):

(1) Read the drug label carefully to be sure you have the correct preparation for the intended use.

$MgSO_4$ is available in concentrations of 10%, 25%, and 50% and in sizes of 2-, 10-, and 20-ml ampules, as well as a 30-ml multidose vial.

(2) For IM administration, small amounts of 50% solution are usually used (1 g $MgSO_4$ = 2 ml of 50% solution).

(3) For IV use, a 5% or 10% solution is used for direct injection, intermittent infusion, or continuous infusion. Whatever concentration is used, administer no more than 150 mg/min (1.5 ml/min of 10% solution; 3 ml/min of 5% solution).

**h.** For sodium bicarbonate ($NaHCO_3$):

(1) Read the label carefully to be sure you have the correct solution.

$NaHCO_3$ is available in several concentrations and sizes, such as 50-ml ampules or prefilled syringes with 50 mEq drug (8.4% solution) or 44.6 mEq drug (7.5% solution), 500-ml bottles with 297.7 mEq drug (5% solution) or 83 mEq drug (1.4% solution).

(2) Inject directly into the vein or into the tubing of a flowing IV infusion solution in emergencies, such as cardiac arrest.

## Nursing Actions

## Rationale/Explanation

(3) In nonemergency situations, titrate flow rate of infusions according to arterial blood gases.

To avoid iatrogenic alkalosis

(4) Flush IV lines before and after injecting and do not add any other medications to an IV containing $NaHCO_3$

$NaHCO_3$ is highly alkaline and may cause precipitation of other drugs.

(5) Monitor arterial blood gases for increased pH after each 50 to 100 mEq of $NaHCO_3$.

To avoid overtreatment and metabolic alkalosis

**i.** For iron preparations:

(1) Dilute liquid iron preparations, give with a straw, and have the client rinse the mouth afterward

To prevent temporary staining of teeth

(2) To give iron dextran intramuscularly, use a 2- to 3-inch needle and Z-track technique to inject the drug into the upper outer quandrant of the buttock.

To prevent discomfort and staining of subcutaneous tissue and skin

(3) To give iron dextran IV (either directly or diluted in sodium chloride solution and given over several hours), do not use the multidose vial.

The multidose vial contains phenol as a preservative and is not suitable for IV use. Ampules of 2 ml or 5 ml are available without preservative.

**j.** Refer to the individual drugs or package literature for instructions regarding administration of ammonium chloride, deferoxamine, penicillamine, tromethamine, and multiple electrolyte solutions.

**2. Observe for therapeutic effects**
**a.** With NaCl, observe for decreased symptoms of hyponatremia and increased serum sodium level.

Therapeutic effects should be evident within a few hours.

**b.** With KCl or other potassium preparations, observe for decreased signs of hypokalemia and increased serum potassium levels.

**c.** With $MgSO_4$, observe for decreased signs of hypomagnesemia, increased serum magnesium levels, or control of convulsions.

**d.** With zinc sulfate ($ZnSO_4$), observe for improved wound healing.

**e.** With sodium bicarbonate ($NaHCO_3$), observe for decreased manifestations of acidosis and a rise in blood pH and bicarbonate levels.

**f.** With iron preparations, observe for:

Therapeutic effects are usually evident within a month unless other problems are also present (*e.g.*, vitamin deficiency, achlorhydria, infection, malabsorption).

(1) Increased vigor and feeling of well-being

(2) Improved appetite

(3) Less fatigue

(4) Increased RBC, hemoglobin, and hematocrit

(5) With parenteral iron, observe for an average increase in hemoglobin of 1 g/week.

(continued)

| *Nursing Actions* | *Rationale/Explanation* |
|---|---|
| **3. Observe for adverse effects** | |
| **a.** Mineral–electrolyte excess states: | These are likely to occur with excessive dosages of supplements. They can usually be prevented by using relatively low doses in nonemergency situations and by frequent monitoring of serum levels of electrolytes and iron. |
| (1) With NaCl injection, observe for hypernatremia and circulatory overload. | These are most likely to occur with rapid infusion of large amounts or with heart or kidney disease, which decreases water excretion and urine output. They also may occur with hypertonic solutions (*e.g.*, 3% NaCl), but these are infrequently used. |
| (2) With potassium preparations, observe for hyperkalemia. | This is most likely to occur with rapid IV administration, high dosages or concentrations, or in the presence of renal insufficiency and decreased urine output. |
| (3) With magnesium preparations, observe for hypermagnesemia. | See potassium preparations, above. |
| (4) With NaHCO$_3$ observe for metabolic alkalosis. | This is most likely to occur when large amounts of NaHCO$_3$ are given IV. |
| **b.** Gastrointestinal (GI) symptoms—anorexia, nausea, vomiting, diarrhea, and abdominal discomfort from gastric irritation | Most oral preparations of minerals and electrolytes are likely to cause gastric irritation. Taking the drugs with food or 8 oz of fluid may decrease symptoms. |
| **c.** Cardiovascular symptoms: | |
| (1) Cardiac arrhythmias | Potentially fatal arrhythmias may occur with hyperkalemia or hypermagnesemia. |
| (2) Hypotension, tachycardia, other symptoms of shock | May occur with deferoxamine and iron dextran injections |
| (3) Circulatory overload and possible pulmonary edema | Most likely to occur with large amounts of NaCl or NaHCO$_3$ |
| **d.** With Kayexalate, observe for hypokalemia, hypocalcemia, hypomagnesemia, and edema. | Although this drug is used to treat hyperkalemia, it removes calcium and magnesium ions as well as potassium ions. Because it acts by trading sodium for potassium, the sodium retention may lead to edema. |
| **4. Observe for drug interactions** | |
| **a.** Drugs that *increase* effects of minerals and electrolytes and related drugs: | |
| (1) Acidifying agents (ammonium chloride): effects are increased by sodium chloride, potassium chloride, and ascorbic acid. | Systemic acidification by increased serum chloride; also increased urine acidity |
| (2) Alkalinizing agents (sodium bicarbonate): effects are increased by antacids, such as magnesium hydroxide, calcium carbonate, and aluminum hydroxide. | Small amounts of antacids may be absorbed to produce additive effects. |
| (3) Cation exchange resin (Kayexalate): diuretics increase potassium loss; other sources of sodium increase the likelihood of edema. | Additive effects |
| (4) Iron salts: | |
| (a) Allopurinol (Zyloprim) | This drug may increase the concentration of iron in the liver. It should not be given concurrently with any iron preparation. |
| (b) Ascorbic acid (vitamin C) | In large doses of 1 g or more, ascorbic acid increases absorption of iron by acidifying secretions. |

## *Nursing Actions*

## *Rationale/Explanation*

(5) Potassium salts:

    (a) Spironolactone, triamterene, amiloride

These drugs are potassium-saving diuretics. They should *not* be given with a potassium supplement because of additive risks of producing life-threatening hyperkalemia.

    (b) Salt substitutes (*e.g.*, Neo-Curtasol)

These contain potassium rather than sodium and may cause hyperkalemia if given with potassium supplements.

    (c) Penicillin G potassium

This potassium salt of penicillin contains 1.7 mEq of potassium per 1 million units. It may produce hyperkalemia if given in combination with potassium supplements.

**b.** Drugs that *decrease* effects of minerals and electrolytes and related drugs:

(1) Acidifying agents: effects are decreased by alkalinizing agents.

Alkalinizing agents neutralize the effects of acidifying agents.

(2) Alkalinizing agents: effects are decreased by acidifying drugs.

Acidifying drugs neutralize effects of alkalinizing agents.

(3) Oral iron salts:

    (a) Antacids containing carbonate

The antacids decrease iron absorption by forming an insoluble, nonabsorbable compound of iron carbonate.

    (b) Magnesium trisilicate

This antacid decreases absorption of iron.

    (c) Pancreatic extracts

These inhibit iron absorption by increasing alkalinity of GI fluids.

(4) Potassium salts:

    (a) Calcium gluconate

Decreases cardiotoxic effects of hyperkalemia and is therefore useful in the treatment of hyperkalemia

    (b) Sodium polystyrene sulfonate (Kayexalate)

Used in treatment of hyperkalemia because it removes potassium from the body

## 5. Teach clients

**a.** With iron preparations, teach:

(1) To take with or after meals, at least initially

To decrease gastric irritation. If no anorexia, nausea, vomiting, or other problems occur, the drug can be tried before meals because it is better absorbed from an empty stomach.

(2) To dilute and take liquid iron preparations through a straw

To avoid staining the teeth

(3) That the drug turns stools dark green or black

**b.** Potassium preparations *must* be taken as directed.

The unpleasant taste of oral solutions apparently reduces compliance with physician's orders.

(1) Mix oral solutions or effervescent tablets with at least 4 oz of water or juice.

To improve the taste

(2) Take after meals

To further dilute the drug and decrease gastric irritation

(3) Do *not* stop taking the drug without notifying the physician who prescribed it, especially if also taking digitalis or diuretics.

Serious problems may develop from low levels of potassium in the blood.

## Review and Application Exercises

1. What are the major roles of minerals and electrolytes in normal body functioning?
2. How would you assess a client for hypokalemia?
3. When a client is given potassium supplements for hypokalemia, how do you monitor for therapeutic and adverse drug effects?
4. Identify client populations at risk of developing hyperkalemia.
5. List interventions to decrease risks of developing hyperkalemia.
6. If severe hyperkalemia develops, how is it treated?
7. What are some causes of iron deficiency anemia?
8. In a client with iron deficiency anemia, what information could you provide about good food sources of iron?
9. What are advantages and disadvantages of iron supplements?

## Selected References

Beare, P. G., & Myers, J. L. (Eds.) (1990). *Principles and practice of adult health nursing.* St. Louis: C.V. Mosby.

Bolinger, A. M. (1992). Anemias. In M. A. Koda-Kimble & L. Y. Young (Eds.), *Applied therapeutics: The clinical use of drugs* (5th ed.) (pp. 50-1–50-14). Vancouver, WA: Applied Therapeutics.

Cuddy, P. G. (1992). Fluid and electrolyte disorders. In M. A. Koda-Kimble & L. Y. Young (Eds.), *Applied therapeutics: The clinical use of drugs* (5th ed.) (pp. 28-1–28-21). Vancouver, WA: Applied Therapeutics.

Davis, J. R., & Sherer, K. (1994). *Applied nutrition and diet therapy for nurses* (2nd ed.). Philadelphia: W.B. Saunders.

(1993). *Drug facts and comparisons.* St. Louis: Facts and Comparisons.

Eschleman, M. M. (1991). *Introductory nutrition and diet therapy* (2nd ed.). Philadelphia: J.B. Lippincott.

Guyton, A. C. (1991). *Textbook of medical physiology* (8th ed.). Philadelphia: W.B. Saunders.

Thornhill, D. G., & Pleuss, J. (1990). Alterations in nutritional status. In C. M. Porth (Ed.), *Pathophysiology: Concepts of altered health states* (3rd ed.) (pp. 743–765). Philadelphia: J.B. Lippincott.

# Drugs Used to Treat Infections

### CHAPTER 33

# General Characteristics of Antimicrobial Drugs

Antimicrobial drugs are used to prevent or treat infections caused by pathogenic (disease-producing) microorganisms. People are surrounded by microorganisms, few of which cause disease in normal circumstances. Infections are usually prevented by the body's defense mechanisms against pathogenic invasion of tissues. If infections do occur, these mechanisms help eliminate them. Conditions that impair the defense mechanisms increase the incidence and severity of infections. The type, number, and virulence of the infective microorganism also are influential factors. To participate effectively in antimicrobial drug therapy, the nurse must be knowledgeable about the host, the microorganism, and antimicrobial drugs.

## Host defense mechanisms

The major defense mechanisms of the human body are intact skin and mucous membranes, various anti-infective secretions, mechanical movements, phagocytic cells, and the immune and inflammatory processes. The skin prevents penetration of foreign particles, and its secretions and indigenous bacterial flora inhibit growth of pathogenic microorganisms. Secretions of the gastrointestinal, respiratory, and genitourinary tracts (*e.g.*, gastric acid, mucus) kill, trap, or inhibit growth of microorganisms. Coughing, swallowing, and peristalsis help to remove foreign particles and pathogens trapped in mucus, as does the movement of cilia. Phagocytic cells in various organs and tissues engulf and digest pathogens and cellular debris. The immune system produces lymphocytes and antibodies. The inflammatory process (see Chap. 1) is the body's response to injury by microorganisms, foreign particles, chemical agents, or physical irritation of tissues. Inflammation localizes, destroys, neutralizes, dilutes, or removes the injurious agent so that tissue healing can occur.

Many factors impair host defense mechanisms and predispose to infection by disease-producing microorganisms:

1. Breaks in the skin and mucous membranes related to trauma, inflammation, open lesions, or insertion of prosthetic devices, tubes, and catheters for diagnostic or therapeutic purposes
2. Impaired blood supply
3. Neutropenia and other blood disorders
4. Malnutrition
5. Poor personal hygiene
6. Suppression of indigenous bacterial flora by antimicrobial drugs
7. Suppression of the immune system and the inflammatory response by immunosuppressive drugs, cytotoxic antineoplastic drugs, and adrenal corticosteroids
8. Diabetes mellitus and other chronic diseases
9. Advanced age

## Microorganisms and infections

Microorganisms are everywhere in the environment, including air, food, water, and soil. They also are present in the human body, especially on the skin and in the mouth, upper respiratory tract, genitals, and colon.

Anne Collins Abrams: CLINICAL DRUG THERAPY, Fourth Edition.
© 1995 J.B. Lippincott Company.

These microorganisms (bacteria, viruses, fungi, and others) usually live in a state of balance with the human host and do not cause disease. Infection results when the balance is upset by decreased host resistance or increased numbers and virulence of microorganisms. In an infection, microorganisms initially attach to host cell receptors (*i.e.*, proteins, carbohydrates, lipids, or combinations of these structures) much as drug molecules bind with cell receptors. For example, some bacteria have hair-like structures that attach them to skin and mucous membranes. Most microorganisms preferentially attach themselves to particular body tissues. The microorganisms may then invade tissues, multiply, and produce infection. Some microorganisms become embedded in a layer of mucus, which protects them from normal body defense mechanisms.

1. Microorganisms are classified according to groups or species.
   a. *Bacteria* are subclassified according to whether they are aerobic (require oxygen) or anaerobic (cannot live in the presence of oxygen), their reaction to Gram's stains (gram-positive or gram-negative), and their shape (cocci [oval], bacilli [rod-shaped], spirilla [spiral]). In addition, various strains develop as an organism adapts to its environment. Many bacteria can survive in living (humans, animals) or nonliving (objects, air, food, soil, water) environments.
   b. *Viruses* are intracellular parasites that survive only in living tissues. They are classified in several different ways according to host, origin, and other characteristics. Like bacteria, viruses produce many strains.
   c. *Fungi* are plant-like organisms that live as parasites on living tissue or as saprophytes on decaying organic matter. About 50 species are pathogenic in humans.
2. The human body normally has areas that are sterile and areas that contain microorganisms.
   a. *Sterile areas* are the lower respiratory tract (trachea, bronchi, lungs), much of the gastrointestinal and genitourinary tracts, the musculoskeletal system, and the body cavities. Body fluids also are sterile.
   b. *Indigenous skin flora* includes staphylococci, streptococci, diphtheroids, and transient environmental organisms. The upper respiratory tract contains staphylococci, streptococci, pneumococci, diphtheroids, and *Haemophilus influenzae*. The external genitalia contain skin organisms; the vagina contains lactobacilli, *Candida*, and *Bacteroides*. The colon contains *Escherichia coli*, *Klebsiella*, *Enterobacter*, *Proteus*, *Pseudomonas*, *Bacteroides*, *Clostridia*, lactobacilli, streptococci, and staphylococci. Microorganisms that are part of the in-

digenous flora and are nonpathogenic in one area of the body may become pathogenic in other parts of the body. For example, *E. coli* often causes urinary tract infections.

3. *Common human pathogens* are viruses, gram-positive streptococci and staphylococci, and gram-negative intestinal organisms (*E. coli*, *Bacteroides*, *Klebsiella*, *Proteus*, and *Pseudomonas* species and others; Table 33-1). These microorganisms are usually spread by air, direct contact with an infected person, or contaminated hands, food, water, and objects. Some also may be spread by a carrier (a person who transmits a pathogenic organism but does not have an active infection). For example, some people "carry" pathogenic strains of staphylococci in their upper respiratory tracts (*e.g.*, anterior nares).

4. *"Opportunistic" microorganisms* may be part of the indigenous flora and are usually nonpathogenic. They become pathogens, however, in hosts whose defense mechanisms are impaired. Opportunistic infections are likely to occur in people with severe burns, cancer, prolonged intravenous fluid therapy, indwelling urinary catheters, and antibiotic or corticosteroid drug therapy.
   a. Opportunistic bacterial infections may involve drug-resistant gram-negative microorganisms. These infections are serious and may be life threatening.
   b. Fungi of the *Candida* genus, especially *Candida albicans*, may cause life-threatening bloodstream or deep tissue infections, such as brain abscesses.
   c. Viral infections may cause fatal pneumonia in renal, cardiac, and bone marrow transplant recipients.

5. Microorganisms may develop resistance to antimicrobial drugs by producing enzymes that destroy or inactivate the drug, reducing their permeability to the drug, changing their metabolic pathways, genetically mutating, and transferring genetic material (deoxyribonucleic acid or plasmids) between microorganisms. Resistant organisms grow and multiply when susceptible organisms (*e.g.*, indigenous flora) are suppressed by antimicrobial drugs or when normal body defenses are impaired by immunosuppressive disorders or drugs. **The development of drug-resistant microorganisms is increased by widespread use of antimicrobial drugs, especially broad-spectrum agents, and by interrupted or inadequate antimicrobial treatment of infections.**

6. Infections are often categorized as community-acquired or hospital-acquired (nosocomial). Because the microbial environments differ, the two types of infections usually have different etiologies and require different antimicrobial drugs. As a general rule, community-acquired infections are less severe and easier to treat. Nosocomial infections may be more

**TABLE 33-1. COMMON BACTERIAL PATHOGENS**

### Gram-Positive Bacteria

#### Staphylococci

Some species of staphylococci are pathogenic. They may produce endotoxins that destroy tissue cells. Some produce enterotoxins and cause a common type of food poisoning. *Staphylococcus aureus* and *Staphylococcus epidermidis* are widespread human pathogens, commonly present on skin and mucous membranes of the nose and mouth. They are spread by direct and indirect contact with people who are carriers, people with staphylococcal infections, animals, and nonliving environments, such as mop water and the cooling coils of air-conditioning systems. *S. aureus* causes boils, carbuncles, surgical wound infections, and internal abscesses. *S. epidermidis* causes endocarditis, bacteremia, and other serious infections.

#### Streptococci

*Streptococcus viridans, Streptococcus pneumoniae,* and *Streptococcus pyogenes* are three strains that are pathogenic to humans. *S. viridans* (alpha-hemolytic streptococcus) is part of the indigenous bacterial flora of the upper respiratory tract. It does not cause disease unless the mucosal barrier is damaged by trauma, previous infection, or surgical manipulation. Such damage allows the organisms to enter the bloodstream and gain access to other parts of the body. For example, the organisms may cause subacute bacterial endocarditis if they reach damaged heart valves. *S. pneumoniae* causes about three fourths of all bacterial pneumonias. *S. pyogenes* (beta-hemolytic streptococcus) causes severe pharyngitis ("strep throat"), scarlet fever, rheumatic fever, and acute bacterial endocarditis. These infections are usually spread by inhalation of droplets from the upper respiratory tracts of carriers or people with infections. The organism also grows in milk.

### Gram-negative Bacteria

#### Bacteroides

*Bacteroides* are anaerobic bacteria normally found in the digestive, respiratory, and genital tracts. They also may be found in the bloodstream and necrotic tissue. The most common bacteria in the colon, they greatly outnumber *Escherichia coli. Bacteroides fragilis* is the species most often seen.

#### Escherichia coli

*E. coli* inhabits the intestinal tract of humans and animals and is normally nonpathogenic in the intestinal tract. The organism may be beneficial by synthesizing vitamins and by competitively discouraging growth of possible pathogens. It may cause infection when allowed access to other parts of the body. For example, *E. coli* causes most urinary tract infections. The presence of *E. coli* in milk or water indicates fecal contamination.

#### Klebsiella

*Klebsiella* organisms are often associated with respiratory infections and may infect the urinary tract, bloodstream, and meninges. *Klebsiella pneumoniae* is a relatively common cause of pneumonia, especially in people with bronchitis or other pulmonary disease.

#### Proteus

*Proteus* organisms are normally found in the intestinal tract and in decaying matter. They most often cause urinary tract and wound infections but may infect any tissue. Infection usually occurs with antibiotic therapy, which decreases drug-sensitive bacteria and allows drug-resistant bacteria to proliferate.

#### Pseudomonas

These organisms are found in water, soil, and normal skin and intestines. *Pseudomonas aeruginosa* is the species most often associated with human disease. It can cause infections of wounds, burns, eyes, and ears, as well as pneumonia. Infection is more likely to occur in hosts who are very young or very old or who have impaired immune systems.

#### Serratia

*Serratia marcescens* is found in infected people, water, soil, milk, and feces. Formerly believed nonpathogenic to humans, the organism is now known to cause septicemia and infections of the urinary tract, respiratory tract, skin, and burn wounds. It also may cause hospital epidemics and produce drug-resistant strains.

#### Salmonella

About 1400 species of *Salmonella* have been identified; several are pathogenic to humans. The organisms cause gastroenteritis, typhoid fever, septicemia, and a severe, sometimes fatal type of food poisoning.

#### Shigella

*Shigella* contains several species that cause gastrointestinal problems ranging from mild diarrhea to severe and often fatal dysentery.

severe and difficult to manage because they often result from drug-resistant microorganisms and occur in people whose resistance to disease is impaired. Drug-resistant strains of staphylococci, *Pseudomonas*, and *Proteus* are common causes of nosocomial infections. The microorganisms that cause nosocomial infections often vary among health-care agencies, depending primarily on the antimicrobial drugs used to treat infections in that environment.

# Characteristics of anti-infective drugs

## TERMINOLOGY

Several terms are used to describe these drugs. *Antiinfective* and *antimicrobial* include antibacterial, antiviral, and antifungal drugs; *antibacterial* and *antibiotic* usually refer only to drugs used in bacterial infections. Most of the drugs in this section are antibacterials. Antiviral and antifungal drugs are discussed in Chapters 42 and 43, respectively.

Additional terms for antibacterial drugs include *broad spectrum*, for those effective against several groups of microorganisms, and *narrow spectrum* for those effective against a few groups. The action of an antibacterial drug is usually described as *bactericidal* (kills the microorganism) or *bacteriostatic* (inhibits growth of the microorganism). Whether a drug is bactericidal or bacteriostatic often depends on its concentration at the infection site and the susceptibility of the microorganism to the drug.

## MECHANISMS OF ACTION

Anti-infectives act against microorganisms by several mechanisms, including the following:

1. Inhibition of bacterial cell wall synthesis or activation of enzymes that disrupt bacterial cell walls (*e.g.*, penicillins, cephalosporins, cycloserine, vancomycin, bacitracin)
2. Inhibition of protein synthesis by bacteria or production of abnormal bacterial proteins (*e.g.*, chloramphenicol, tetracyclines, erythromycin, clindamycin, aminoglycosides). These drugs bind irreversibly to bacterial ribosomes, intracellular structures that synthesize proteins. When antimicrobial drugs are bound to the ribosomes, bacteria cannot synthesize the proteins necessary for cell walls and other structures.
3. Disruption of bacterial cell membranes (*e.g.*, polymyxins, colistimethate, antifungals)
4. Inhibition of organism reproduction by interfering with nucleic acid synthesis (*e.g.*, rifampin, anti–acquired immunodeficiency syndrome [AIDS] antivirals)
5. Inhibition of cell metabolism and growth (*e.g.*, sulfonamides, trimethoprim)

## INDICATIONS FOR USE

The clinical indications for use of anti-infectives are prevention and treatment of infections. Treatment may be directed therapy (against a specific organism identified by culture) or empiric (against the most likely pathogens until a specific organism is identified). Generally accepted prophylactic uses include the following:

1. Penicillin in group A streptococcal infections to prevent rheumatic fever, rheumatic heart disease, and glomerulonephritis
2. Antibiotics to prevent bacterial endocarditis in clients with cardiac valvular disease

3. Isoniazid to prevent tuberculosis (see Chap. 41)
4. Antibiotics during the perioperative period for selected high-risk clients (those whose resistance to infection is lowered due to age, poor nutrition, disease, or drugs) and for selected high-risk surgical procedures (cardiac surgery, gastrointestinal surgery, certain orthopedic procedures, organ transplants)
5. Antibiotics to prevent gonorrhea and syphilis after exposure has occurred

## Nursing Process

### Assessment

Assess for current or potential infection:

- General signs and symptoms of infection are the same as those of inflammation, although the terms are not synonymous. Inflammation is the normal response to any injury; infection requires the presence of a microorganism. The two often occur together. Inflammation may weaken tissue, allowing microorganisms to invade and cause infection. Infection (tissue injury by microorganisms) arouses inflammation. Local signs include redness, heat, edema, and pain; systemic signs include fever and leukocytosis. Specific manifestations depend on the site of infection. Common sites are the respiratory tract, surgical or other wounds, and the genitourinary tract.
- Assess culture reports for causative organisms and susceptibility reports for appropriate antibacterial drug therapy.
- Assess clients for drug allergies. If present, ask about specific signs and symptoms.
- Assess each client for the presence of factors that increase risks of infection (see the section Host Defense Mechanisms above).

### Nursing diagnoses

- Fatigue related to infection
- Self-Care Deficit related to infection
- Activity Intolerance related to fatigue
- Diarrhea related to antimicrobial therapy
- Altered Nutrition: Less than Body Requirements related to anorexia, nausea, and vomiting associated with antimicrobial therapy
- High Risk for Injury related to infection or adverse drug effects
- High Risk for Infection related to mutant strains of drug-resistant microorganisms
- Knowledge Deficit: Methods of preventing infections
- Knowledge Deficit: Appropriate use of anti-infective drugs

### Planning/Goals

*The client will:*

- Receive antimicrobial drugs accurately when given by health-care providers
- Take drugs as prescribed and for the length of time prescribed when self-administered as an outpatient

- Experience decreased fever, white blood cell (WBC) count, and other signs and symptoms of infection
- Be monitored regularly for therapeutic and adverse drug effects
- Verbalize and practice measures to prevent future infections
- Be safeguarded against nosocomial infections by health-care providers

## Interventions

- Use measures to prevent and minimize the spread of infection.
  - Wash hands thoroughly and often. This is probably the most effective method of preventing infections.
  - Support natural defense mechanisms by promoting general health measures, such as nutrition, fluid and electrolyte balance, rest, and exercise.
  - Keep the client's skin clean and dry, especially the hands, underarms, groin, and perineum, because these areas harbor large numbers of microorganisms. Also, take care to prevent trauma to the skin and mucous membrane. Damaged tissues are susceptible to infection.
  - Treat all body fluids (e.g., blood, aspirates from abdomen or chest) and body substances (e.g., sputum, feces, urine, wound drainage) as infectious. Major elements of "universal precautions" to prevent transmission of hepatitis B, human immunodeficiency virus, and other pathogens include wearing gloves when likely to be exposed to any of the above materials and thorough handwashing when the gloves are removed. Rigorous and consistent use of the recommended precautions helps to protect health-care providers and clients.
  - Implement isolation procedures appropriately.
  - To prevent spread of respiratory infections, have client wash hands after coughing, sneezing, or contact with infected people; cover mouth and nose with tissues when sneezing or coughing and dispose of tissues by placing them in a paper bag and burning it; expectorate sputum (swallowing may cause reinfection); avoid crowds when possible, especially during influenza season (approximately November through February); recommend annual influenza vaccine to high-risk populations (e.g., people with chronic diseases, such as diabetes, heart, lung, or renal problems; older adults; and health-care personnel who are likely to be exposed).
  - Assist or instruct clients at risk about pulmonary hygiene measures to prevent accumulation or promote removal of respiratory secretions. Such secretions promote bacterial growth. These measures include ambulating, turning, coughing and deep-breathing exercises, and incentive spirometry.
  - Use sterile technique when changing any dressing. If a wound is not infected, sterile technique helps prevent infection; if the wound is already infected, sterile technique avoids introducing new bacteria. For all but the smallest of dressings without drainage, remove the dressing with clean gloves, discard it in a plastic or foil-lined moisture-proof bag, and wash hands before putting on sterile gloves to apply the new dressing.

- To minimize spread of staphylococcal infections, infected personnel with skin lesions should not work until lesions are healed; infected patients should be isolated. Personnel with skin lesions probably spread more staphylococci than clients because personnel are more mobile.
- For clients with infections, monitor temperature for fever increase or decrease, and monitor WBC count for decrease.
- For clients receiving antimicrobial therapy, maintain a total fluid intake of about 3000 ml/24 hours, if not contraindicated by the client's condition. An adequate intake and avoidance of fluid volume deficit may help to decrease drug toxicity, especially with aminoglycoside antibiotics. On the other hand, a client receiving intravenous antibiotics, with 50 to 100 ml of fluid per dose, may be at risk of developing fluid volume overload.

*Teach clients:*

- The importance of handwashing, maintaining nutrition and fluid balance, getting adequate rest, and handling secretions correctly. These measures help the body to fight the infection, prevent further infection, and enhance the effectiveness of anti-infective drugs.
- The importance of taking all prescribed doses of an antimicrobial and not stopping when symptoms subside. Reasons include adequate treatment of the current infection and prevention of new infections that may be harder to treat (e.g., infections caused by drug-resistant organisms are usually more serious and often require more expensive and more toxic drugs). If problems occur with taking the drug, report them to the prescribing physician rather than stopping the drug.
- Not to take antimicrobials left over from a previous illness or prescribed for someone else. Even if infection is present and anti-infective treatment appears needed, the likelihood of having the appropriate drug on hand, and in adequate amounts, is extremely small. Thus, taking drugs not prescribed for the particular illness tends to maximize risks and minimize benefits. Also, if the infection is viral, most antimicrobials are ineffective unless a bacterial superinfection develops.
- To report any other drugs being taken to the prescribing physician. Drug interactions may occur, and changes in drug therapy may be indicated.
- To report any drug allergies to all health-care providers and wear a medical identification emblem that lists allergens.
- That some antibiotics (e.g., ampicillin, nitrofurantoin, penicillin V, sulfonamides, tetracyclines) decrease the effectiveness of estrogens and oral contraceptives. Women taking these drugs should use another method of contraception. Inadequate blood levels of estrogen may be indicated by breakthrough bleeding and are thought to result from reduced enterohepatic recirculation of estrogens. This, in turn, probably results from drug-induced decreases in intestinal bacterial flora.

## Evaluation

- Interview and observe for compliance with instructions for using anti-infective drugs.
- Interview and observe for practices to prevent infection.
- Observe for adverse drug effects.

# Principles of therapy

## RATIONAL USE OF ANTIMICROBIAL DRUGS

Antimicrobials are among the most frequently used drugs worldwide. Although benefits of the drugs can be great when they are used rationally, much usage is considered inappropriate and excessive. Many authorities are alarmed about the increasing prevalence of drug-resistant microorganisms that such misuse engenders. Some guidelines for rational use include:

1. Stop the long-term pattern of use in which a powerful new antimicrobial drug is developed and widely used, then becomes ineffective in some infections because of microbial resistance. Such a pattern began with the penicillins and is evident with currently available antibacterial drugs. Thus, indiscriminant, "routine" use of the most powerful, broadest spectrum drugs when others may be just as effective leaves no drugs in reserve for serious infections or infections caused by resistant organisms.
2. Give the most narrow-spectrum drug likely to be effective in a given infection. Use of broad-spectrum drugs alters the normal body flora more extensively and increases adverse drug effects and the emergence of drug-resistant microorganisms.
3. Give antibacterial drugs only when a significant bacterial infection is diagnosed or strongly suspected or when there is an established indication for prophylaxis. These drugs should not be used for viral or trivial infections. They are ineffective in viral infections; they may allow the growth of drug-resistant organisms in trivial infections.
4. Minimize antimicrobial drug therapy for fever unless other clinical manifestations or laboratory data indicate infection.
5. Use the drugs along with other interventions to decrease microbial proliferation, such as frequent and thorough handwashing, preoperative skin and bowel cleansing, and drainage of abscesses.

## COLLECTION OF SPECIMENS

Collect specimens for culture and Gram's stain before giving the first dose of an anti-infective. For best results, specimens must be collected accurately and taken directly to the laboratory. If delayed, contaminants may overgrow pathogenic microorganisms.

## DRUG SELECTION

Choosing an antimicrobial drug for treating an infection should be based on several factors. One factor is culture and susceptibility studies. Culture identifies the causative organism; susceptibility tests determine which drugs are likely to be effective against the organism. Culture and susceptibility studies are especially important with suspected gram-negative infections because of the high incidence of drug-resistant microorganisms. Because these tests require 48 to 72 hours, the physician usually prescribes for immediate administration a drug that is likely to be effective. A second factor is knowledge of the organisms most likely to infect particular body tissues. For example, urinary tract infections are often caused by *E. coli*, and a drug effective against this organism is indicated. A third factor is a drug's ability to penetrate infected tissues. Several antimicrobials are effective in urinary infections because they are excreted in the urine. However, the choice of an effective antimicrobial drug may be limited in infections of the brain, eyes, gallbladder, or prostate gland because many drugs are unable to reach therapeutic concentrations in those tissues. A fourth factor involves a drug's toxicity and the risk-to-benefit ratio. That is, a less toxic drug should generally be used for mild infections, and the more toxic drugs should be reserved for serious infections. A fifth factor is drug cost. If an older, less expensive drug meets the criteria for rational drug selection and is likely to be effective in a given infection, it should be used in preference to more expensive agents.

## ANTIBIOTIC COMBINATION THERAPY

Antimicrobial drugs are often used in combination. One indication for combination therapy is an infection known or thought to be caused by multiple microorganisms (*e.g.*, abdominal and pelvic infections). A second indication is a serious infection in which a combination is synergistic (*e.g.*, an aminoglycoside and an antipseudomonal penicillin for pseudomonal infections). A third indication is the likely emergence of drug-resistant organisms (*e.g.*, tuberculosis is routinely treated with three or more drugs). A fourth indication is fever or other signs of infection in a client whose immune system is suppressed (*e.g.*, a client with cancer and chemotherapy-induced neutropenia, a client with AIDS, or a client with a bone marrow or solid organ transplant). Staphylococci and the gram-negative organisms *E. coli*, *Klebsiella pneumoniae*, and *Pseudomonas aeruginosa* often cause infections in neutropenic cancer patients. Transplant and AIDS patients may develop a variety of bacterial, viral, or fungal infections.

## DOSAGE

Dosage (amount and frequency of administration) should be individualized according to characteristics of the chosen drug and the client's condition. For example, dosage may need to be increased for serious infections or reduced if the client has renal impairment or other disorders that delay drug elimination. Reports of susceptibility tests usually state the minimum inhibitory concentration (MIC) of drug that is effective against a microorganism. The MIC may be used as a guideline for achieving therapeutic blood levels of the antimicrobial agent.

## ROUTE OF ADMINISTRATION

Most antimicrobial drugs are given orally or intravenously for systemic infections. The route of administration depends on the client's condition (*e.g.*, location and severity of the infection, ability to take oral drugs) and the available drug dosage forms. In serious infections, the intravenous route is usually preferred.

## DURATION OF THERAPY

Duration of therapy varies from a single dose to years, depending on the reason for use. For most acute infections, the average duration is about 7 to 10 days or until the recipient has been afebrile and asymptomatic for 48 to 72 hours.

## PERIOPERATIVE USE

When used to prevent infections associated with surgery, antimicrobials should be given shortly before the scheduled operation. This provides effective tissue concentration during the procedure, when contamination occurs. The choice of drug depends on the pathogens most likely to enter the operative area. A first-generation cephalosporin, such as cefazolin (Kefzol), is often used, usually in a single preoperative dose. Postoperative antimicrobials are indicated with dirty, traumatic wounds or ruptured viscera.

## USE IN RENAL INSUFFICIENCY

In renal insufficiency or failure, antimicrobial drug therapy requires extreme caution. Many drugs are excreted primarily by the kidneys; some are nephrotoxic and may further damage the kidneys. In the presence of renal failure, they are likely to accumulate and produce toxic effects. Thus, dosage reductions are necessary for some drugs. Methods of calculating dosage are usually based on rates of creatinine clearance.

The following formula may be used to estimate creatinine clearance:

Males: Weight in kg × (140 minus age), divided by
72 × serum creatinine (mg/100 ml)
Females: 0.85 × above value

Dosage may be reduced by giving smaller individual doses, by increasing the time interval between doses, or both. Anti-infective drugs can be categorized as follows in relation to renal disease:

1. Drugs that should not be given in the presence of renal disease (*i.e.*, creatinine clearance of less than 30 ml/min) unless the infecting organism is sensitive only to a particular drug. This group includes all tetracyclines except doxycycline (Vibramycin).
2. Drugs that are not used in renal disease unless the infection is caused by organisms resistant to safer drugs. If used, dosage must be carefully adjusted, renal function must be closely monitored, and the recipient must be closely observed for adverse effects. These drugs include all the aminoglycosides, carbenicillin, cephalexin, colistin, amphotericin B, ethambutol, and flucytosine. Serum drug levels are recommended for monitoring aminoglycoside antibiotics.
3. Drugs that require dosage reduction in severe renal failure. These include penicillin G, ampicillin, methicillin, oxacillin, trimethoprim-sulfamethoxazole, and most cephalosporins.
4. Drugs that require little or no dosage adjustment. These include cloxacillin, dicloxacillin, nafcillin, erythromycin, doxycycline, clindamycin, chloramphenicol, rifampin, and isoniazid.

An additional factor is important in clients with acute or chronic renal failure who are receiving hemodialysis or peritoneal dialysis: some drugs are removed by dialysis, and an extra dose may be needed during or after dialysis.

## USE IN LIVER DISEASE

In severe liver disease, antimicrobial drugs that are excreted by the liver must be reduced in dosage. These include erythromycin, clindamycin, and chloramphenicol. The antitubercular drugs rifampin and isoniazid have longer half-lives in clients with cirrhosis. Dosing in liver disease is not well defined.

## USE IN CHILDREN

Antimicrobial drugs are commonly used in hospitals and ambulatory settings for respiratory infections, otitis media, and other infections. General principles of pediatric (see Chap. 3) and antimicrobial drug therapy apply. Other guidelines include the following:

1. *Penicillins and cephalosporins* are considered safe for most age groups. However, they are eliminated more slowly in neonates because of immature renal function and must be used cautiously. Aztreonam (Azac-

tam) and imipenem-cilastatin (Primaxin) have not been established as safe and effective in children under 12 years old.

2. *Erythromycin* is generally considered safe. The newer macrolides, azithromycin (Zithromax) and clarithromycin (Biaxin) have not been established as safe and effective in children but are expected to be approved for pediatric use.

3. *Aminoglycosides* (*e.g.*, gentamicin and others) may cause nephrotoxicity and ototoxicity in any client population. Neonates are at high risk because of immature renal function.

4. *Tetracyclines* are contraindicated in children under 8 years old because of drug effects on teeth and bone (see Chap. 37).

5. When *clindamycin* (Cleocin) is given to neonates and infants, liver and kidney function should be monitored.

6. Quinolones such as *ciprofloxacin* (Cipro), *norfloxacin* (Noroxin), and others are not recommended for use in children (younger than 18 years of age) because safety and effectiveness have not been established. In addition, cartilage and function of weight-bearing joints have been impaired in young animals given the drugs.

7. *Isoniazid* (INH) is used to prevent tuberculosis, and isoniazid and rifampin (Rifadin) are used to treat tuberculosis in children as in adults. Ethambutol (Myambutol) is not recommended for children under 13 years old.

8. *Trimethoprim* (often given in combination with sulfamethoxazole as Bactrim or Septra) has not been proven safe for children under 12 years of age.

## USE IN OLDER ADULTS

Antimicrobial drugs are commonly used in hospitals and ambulatory settings for infections in older adults as in younger adults. General principles of geriatric (see Chap. 3) and antimicrobial drug therapy apply. Other guidelines include the following:

1. *Penicillins* are generally safe. However, hyperkalemia may occur with large intravenous doses of penicillin G potassium (1.7 mEq potassium per 1 million units), and hypernatremia may occur with ticarcillin (Ticar), which contains 5.6 mEq sodium per gram. Hyperkalemia and hypernatremia are more likely to occur with impaired renal function, a common condition in older adults.

2. *Cephalosporins* (cefazolin and others) are generally considered safe but may cause or aggravate renal impairment, especially when other nephrotoxic drugs are used concurrently. Dosage of several cephalosporins needs to be reduced in the presence of renal impairment (see Chap. 35).

3. *Erythromycin* is generally safe. Two related drugs, azithromycin and clarithromycin, have not been used extensively in older adults but seem to be relatively safe. Dosage of clarithromycin should be reduced with severe renal impairment.

4. *Aminoglycosides* (*e.g.*, gentamicin and others) are contraindicated in the presence of impaired renal function if less toxic drugs are effective against causative microorganisms. Older adults are at high risk of nephrotoxicity and ototoxicity from these drugs. Several specific interventions to decrease adverse drug effects are described in Chapter 36.

5. *Clindamycin* may cause diarrhea and should be used with caution in the presence of gastrointestinal disease, especially colitis.

6. *Trimethoprim-sulfamethoxazole* (Bactrim, Septra) may cause an increased risk of severe adverse effects in older adults, especially those with impaired liver or kidney function. Severe skin reactions and bone marrow depression are the most frequently reported severe reactions.

7. *Tetracyclines* (except doxycycline) and nitrofurantoin (Macrodantin) are contraindicated in the presence of impaired renal function if less toxic drugs are effective against causative organisms.

## GENERAL NURSING ACTIONS: ANTIMICROBIAL DRUGS

| *Nursing Actions* | *Rationale/Explanation* |
| --- | --- |
| **1. Administer accurately**<br>  **a.** Schedule at evenly spaced intervals around the clock. | To maintain therapeutic blood levels |
|   **b.** Give most oral anti-infective drugs on an empty stomach (1 hour before or 2 hours after meals). Notable exceptions are amoxicillin and bacampicillin, which can be scheduled without regard to meals. | To prevent drug inactivation by gastric acid and to promote absorption |

## Nursing Actions

## Rationale/Explanation

**c.** For oral and parenteral solutions from powder forms, follow label instructions for mixing and storing. Check expiration dates.

Several antimicrobial drugs are marketed in powder forms because they are unstable in solution. When mixed, measured amounts of diluent must be added for drug dissolution and the appropriate concentration, usually expressed in milligrams per milliliter (mg/ml). Parenteral solutions are often prepared in the pharmacy. Most solutions require refrigeration for longer periods of stability. None of the solutions should be used after the expiration date because drug decomposition is likely.

**d.** Give parenteral anti-infective solutions *alone*; do not mix with any other drug in a syringe or IV solution.

To avoid chemical and physical incompatibilities that may cause drug precipitation or inactivation

**e.** Give IM anti-infective drugs deeply into large muscle masses (preferably gluteal muscles), and rotate injection sites.

Most parenteral solutions are irritating to tissues. IM injection is not the preferred route for most anti-infective drugs.

**f.** For IV administration, use dilute solutions, give slowly, and flush tubing with at least 10 ml of IV solution.

Most anti-infective drugs that are given IV can be given by intermittent infusion. Although instructions vary with specific drugs, most reconstituted drugs can be further diluted with 50 to 100 ml of IV fluid ($D_5W$, NS, $D_5$–1/4% or $D_5$–1/2% NaCl) and infused over 20 to 60 minutes. This method causes less vein irritation and thrombophlebitis, avoids drug deactivation, and provides therapeutic serum levels. Flushing is necessary for two reasons. First, most tubing holds about 10 ml. If not rinsed, as much as 10% of a dose mixed in 100 ml may remain in the tubing. Even more remains when the dose is mixed in smaller amounts of fluid. Second, rinsing reduces the risk of contact between incompatible drugs in the tubing.

**2. Observe for therapeutic effects**

**a.** With local infections, observe for decreased redness, edema, heat, and pain.

Signs and symptoms of inflammation and infection usually subside within about 48 hours after anti-infective therapy is begun. Although systemic manifestations of infection are similar regardless of the cause, specific manifestations vary with the type or location of the infection.

**b.** With systemic infections, observe for decreased fever and white blood cell count, increased appetite, and reports of feeling better.

**c.** With wound infections, observe for decreased signs of local inflammation and decreased drainage. Drainage also may change from purulent to serous.

**d.** With respiratory infections, observe for decreased dyspnea, coughing, and secretions. Secretions may change from thick and colored to thin and white.

**e.** With urinary tract infections, observe for decreased urgency, frequency, and dysuria. If urinalysis is done, check the laboratory report for decreased bacteria and white blood cells.

**3. Observe for adverse effects**

**a.** Hypersensitivity

Hypersensitivity may occur with most anti-infectives but is more common with penicillins.

  (1) Anaphylaxis–hypotension, respiratory distress, urticaria, angioedema, vomiting, diarrhea

Anaphylaxis usually occurs within minutes after taking the drug. Hypotension results from vasodilation and circulatory collapse. Respiratory distress results from bronchospasm or laryngeal edema.

| *Nursing Actions* | *Rationale/Explanation* |
|---|---|
| (2) Serum sickness—fever, vasculitis, generalized lymphadenopathy, edema of joints, bronchospasm, urticaria | This is a delayed allergic reaction, occurring 1 week or more after the drug is started. Signs and symptoms are caused by inflammation. |
| **b.** Superinfection | Superinfection is a new or secondary infection that occurs during anti-infective therapy of a primary infection. Superinfections are relatively common and potentially serious because responsible microorganisms are often drug-resistant staphylococci, gram-negative organisms (*Proteus* or *Pseudomonas*) or fungi (*Candida*). Infections with these organisms are often difficult to treat. |
| (1) Stomatitis—sore mouth, white patches on oral mucosa, black furry tongue | |
| (2) Diarrhea | |
| (3) Monilial vaginitis—rash in perineal area, itching, vaginal discharge | |
| (4) New localized signs and symptoms—redness, heat, edema, pain, drainage, cough | |
| (5) Recurrence of systemic signs and symptoms—fever, malaise | |
| **c.** Phlebitis at venipuncture sites; pain at IM injection sites | Parenteral solutions of many anti-infective drugs are irritating to tissues. |
| **d.** Gastrointestinal symptoms—nausea, vomiting, diarrhea | These are common with oral anti-infective agents and probably result from irritation of gastrointestinal mucosa and changes in gastrointestinal flora. |
| **4. Observe for drug interactions** | See following chapters. The most significant interactions are those that alter anti-infective effectiveness or increase drug toxicity. |
| **5. Teach clients**<br>**a.** Take oral drugs at evenly spaced intervals, around the clock. | To maintain effective blood levels |
| **b.** Take oral drugs on an empty stomach, 1 hour before or 2 hours after a meal unless instructed otherwise. | Food decreases absorption of most oral anti-infectives. If the drug causes intolerable nausea or vomiting, a few bites of food (*e.g.*, crackers) may be taken. |
| **c.** Take drugs with a full glass of water. | To decrease gastric irritation and increase rates of dissolution and absorption (tablets and capsules) |
| **d.** Report nausea, vomiting, diarrhea, skin rash, recurrence of symptoms for which the anti-infective drug was prescribed, or signs of new infection (*e.g.*, fever, cough, sore mouth, drainage). | These problems may indicate adverse effects of the drug, lack of therapeutic response to the drug, or a superinfection. Any of these requires evaluation and may indicate changes in drug therapy. |

## Review and Application Exercises

1. How does the body defend itself against infection?
2. When assessing a client, what signs and symptoms may indicate an infectious process?
3. Do all infections require antimicrobial drug therapy? Why or why not?
4. With antimicrobial drug therapy, what is meant by the terms bacteriostatic, bactericidal, antimicrobial spectrum of activity, and minimum inhibitory concentration?
5. Why is it important to identify the organism causing an infection?
6. Why are infections of the brain, eye, and prostate

gland more difficult to treat than infections of the gastrointestinal, respiratory, and urinary tracts?

**7.** What factors promote the development of drug-resistant microorganisms, and how can they be prevented or minimized?

**8.** What are common adverse effects associated with antimicrobial drug therapy?

**9.** When teaching a client about a prescribed antibiotic, a common instruction is to take all the medicine and not to stop prematurely. Why is this information important?

**10.** When a dose of an antibiotic is prescribed to prevent postoperative infection, should it be given before, during, or after surgery? Why?

## Selected References

(1993). Antimicrobial prophylaxis in surgery. *The Medical Letter on Drugs and Therapeutics, 35,* 91–93.

Beare, P. G., & Myers, J. L. (Eds.) (1990). *Principles and practice of adult health nursing.* St. Louis: C.V. Mosby.

Breitenbucher, R. B., & Peterson, P. K. (1990). Infections in the elderly. In G. L. Mandell, R. G. Douglas Jr, & J. E. Bennett (Eds.), *Principles and practice of infectious diseases* (3rd ed.) (pp. 2315–2320). New York: Churchill Livingstone.

(1994). *Drug facts and comparisons.* St. Louis: Facts and Comparisons.

Dunne, W. M. (1990). Mechanisms of infectious disease. In C. M. Porth (Ed.), *Pathophysiology: Concepts of altered health states* (3rd ed.) (pp. 145–163). Philadelphia: J.B. Lippincott.

Ericsson, C. D. (1992). Approach to surgical infections, including burns and postoperative infections. In W. N. Kelley (Ed.), *Textbook of internal medicine* (2nd ed.) (pp. 1641–1644). Philadelphia: J.B. Lippincott.

Guglielmo, B. J. (1992). Principles of antimicrobial therapy. In M. A. Koda-Kimble & L. Y. Young (Eds.), *Applied therapeutics: The clinical use of drugs* (5th ed.) (pp. 33-1–33-12). Vancouver, WA: Applied Therapeutics.

Hammerschlag, M. R. (1993). Azithromycin and clarithromycin. *Pediatric Annals, 22*(3), 160–166.

Kunin, C. M. (1993). Resistance to antimicrobial drugs—A worldwide calamity. *Annals of Internal Medicine, 118,* 557–561.

Levy, S. B. (1993). Confronting multidrug resistance. *Journal of the American Medical Association, 269,* 1840–1842.

Moellering Jr., R. C. (1990). Principles of anti-infective therapy. In G. L. Mandell, R. G. Douglas Jr., & J. E. Bennett (Eds.), *Principles and practice of infectious diseases* (3rd ed.) (pp 206–218). New York: Churchill Livingstone.

Murray, B. E. (1992). Antimicrobial therapeutic agents. In W. N. Kelley (Ed.), *Textbook of internal medicine* (2nd ed.) (pp. 1564–1575). Philadelphia: J.B. Lippincott.

O'Hanley, P. D., Tam, J. Y., & Holodniy, M. (1992). Infectious disorders. In K. L. Melmon, H. F. Morrelli, B. B. Hoffman, & D. W. Nierenberg (Eds.), *Clinical pharmacology: Basic principles in therapeutics* (3rd ed.) (pp. 642–720). New York: McGraw-Hill.

Streit, L. A. (1992). Nursing management of adults with infections. In L. O. Burrell (Ed.), *Adult nursing in hospital and community settings* (pp. 79–99). Norwalk, CT: Appleton & Lange.

Van Scoy, R. E., & Wilkowske, C. J. (1992). Prophylactic use of antimicrobial agents in adult patients. *Mayo Clinic Proceedings, 67,* 288–292.

# CHAPTER 34

# Penicillins

## Penicillins

The penicillins are effective, safe, and widely used antimicrobial agents. The group includes natural extracts from the *Penicillium* mold and several semisynthetic derivatives. When penicillin G, the prototype, was introduced, it was effective against streptococci, staphylococci, gonococci, meningococci, *Treponema pallidum*, and other organisms. It had to be given parenterally because it was destroyed by gastric acid, and injections were very painful. With extensive use, strains of drug-resistant staphylococci appeared. Later penicillins were developed to increase gastric acid stability, beta-lactamase stability, and antimicrobial spectrum of activity, especially against gram-negative microorganisms.

The basic chemical structure of penicillin is 6-aminopenicillanic acid, which contains a beta-lactam ring and side chains. The beta-lactam ring is essential for antibacterial activity, and penicillins are often called beta-lactam antibiotics. Most penicillins are susceptible to destruction by beta-lactamases, a group of enzymes produced by some bacteria that open the beta-lactam ring and inactivate the drug. Penicillinase is a beta-lactamase enzyme that acts specifically on penicillins. This is a major mechanism by which microorganisms develop resistance to beta-lactam antibiotics (penicillins, cephalosporins, and others). Semisynthetic derivatives are formed by adding side chains to the penicillin nucleus.

After absorption, penicillins are widely distributed and achieve therapeutic concentrations in most body fluids, including joint, pleural, and pericardial fluids and bile. Therapeutic levels are not usually obtained in intra-ocular and cerebrospinal fluids unless inflammation is present because normal cell membranes act as barriers to drug penetration. Penicillins are rapidly excreted by the kidneys and produce high drug concentrations in the urine (an exception is nafcillin, which is excreted by the liver).

## MECHANISM OF ACTION

Penicillins kill bacteria by inhibiting synthesis of the bacterial cell wall. The mechanism of their antibacterial action involves binding of drug molecules to protein molecules (called penicillin-binding proteins) in bacterial cell membranes. This binding produces a defective cell wall that allows intracellular contents to leak out, destroying the microorganism. In sub-bactericidal concentrations, penicillins may inhibit growth, decrease viability, and alter the shape and structure of organisms. The latter characteristic may help to explain the development of mutant strains of microorganisms exposed to the drugs. Penicillins are most effective when bacterial cells are dividing.

## INDICATIONS FOR USE

Clinical indications for use of penicillins include bacterial infections caused by susceptible microorganisms. They are often the drugs of choice for treatment of streptococcal pharyngitis, pneumococcal pneumonia, gonorrhea, and syphilis and for prevention of bacterial endocarditis in clients with valvular heart disease who must undergo dental or surgical procedures. They are often useful in respiratory infections, cholecystitis, and cellulitis.

Anne Collins Abrams: CLINICAL DRUG THERAPY, Fourth Edition.
© 1995 J.B. Lippincott Company.

## CONTRAINDICATIONS FOR USE

Contraindications include hypersensitivity or allergic reactions to any penicillin preparation.

# Subgroups and individual penicillins

Individual penicillins are listed, with routes of administration and dosage ranges, in Table 34-1.

## PENICILLINS G AND V

**Penicillin G**, the prototype of the penicillins, is widely used. Because of its effectiveness and minimal toxicity, it is recommended for treatment of infections caused by susceptible microorganisms. Although most staphylococci and some gonococci have developed resistance to penicillin G, the drug is still effective in most streptococcal infections. Thus, it is the drug of choice to treat streptococcal pharyngitis and to prevent rheumatic fever, a complication of streptococcal pharyngitis.

Numerous preparations of penicillin G are available for various purposes and routes of administration. They cannot be used interchangeably. Only aqueous preparations can be given intravenously. Preparations containing benzathine or procaine can be given only intramuscularly. Long-acting repository forms have additives that decrease their solubility in tissue fluids and delay their absorption. When penicillin G is given orally, large doses must be given to offset the portion destroyed by gastric acid.

**Penicillin V** is derived from penicillin G and has the same antibacterial spectrum. It is not destroyed by gastric acid and is given only orally. It is better absorbed and produces higher blood levels than penicillin G. The potassium salt is preferred because it is better absorbed than plain penicillin V.

## PENICILLINASE-RESISTANT (ANTISTAPHYLOCOCCAL) PENICILLINS

This group includes five drugs (**cloxacillin, dicloxacillin, methicillin, nafcillin**, and **oxacillin**) that are effective in treating infections caused by staphylococci resistant to penicillin G. They are specifically formulated to resist the action of beta-lactamase (penicillinase) enzymes that inactivate other penicillins. These drugs are recommended for use only in known or suspected staphylococcal infections. Methicillin-resistant *Staphylococcus aureus* infections are increasing. Although called methicillin resistant, these staphylococcal microorganisms are resistant to the other antistaphylococcal drugs as well.

## AMPICILLINS

**Ampicillin** is a broad-spectrum, semisynthetic penicillin that is bactericidal for several types of gram-positive and gram-negative bacteria. It has been effective against *Proteus mirabilis, Salmonella, Shigella*, and most strains of *Escherichia coli*, but many resistant forms of *Shigella* and *E. coli* are being encountered. Ampicillin is not used against gram-positive cocci because penicillin G or V is less expensive and more effective. It is ineffective against penicillinase-producing staphylococci and gonococci. It is excreted mainly by the kidneys; thus, it is useful in urinary tract infections. Because some is excreted in bile, it is useful in biliary tract infections not caused by biliary obstruction. It is used widely to treat respiratory infections, such as bronchitis and sinusitis, and otitis media.

**Amoxicillin** is similar to ampicillin but is better absorbed and produces more rapid and higher blood levels. It also causes less gastrointestinal distress. **Bacampicillin** is a "pro-drug" that is converted to ampicillin in the body. It has a long duration of action and can be given twice daily. Dosage should be reduced in the presence of renal insufficiency.

## EXTENDED-SPECTRUM (ANTIPSEUDOMONAL) PENICILLINS

The drugs in this group (**carbenicillin, ticarcillin, mezlocillin**, and **piperacillin**) have a broad spectrum of antimicrobial activity. They are especially effective against gram-negative organisms, such as *Pseudomonas, Proteus*, and *E. coli*. They are drugs of choice for pseudomonal infections and are usually given concomitantly with aminoglycoside antibiotics.

Carbenicillin, the first of this group to be developed, is no longer given parenterally for systemic infections. Carbenicillin indanyl sodium, an ester of carbenicillin, is acid stable and therefore can be given orally. Relatively low plasma levels are obtained with the oral drug, but therapeutic levels are obtained in urine. Consequently, oral carbenicillin is used only for treating urinary tract infections caused by susceptible pathogens. Carbenicillin delivers a relatively high amount of sodium to recipients.

Ticarcillin is similar to carbenicillin except that it is more potent on a weight basis and delivers less sodium because the dosage is lower. The other drugs in this group deliver even less sodium, may be more effective against *Pseudomonas* organisms, and are preferred in clients with cardiovascular or other disorders in which sodium intake should be limited. Dosage of these drugs should be reduced in renal failure.

## TABLE 34-1. PENICILLINS

| Generic/Trade Name | Routes and Dosage Ranges | |
| --- | --- | --- |
| | **Adults** | **Children** |
| ***Penicillins G and V*** | | |
| **Penicillin G sodium** | PO 600,000–3 million U daily | PO 25,000–90,000 U/kg per day in divided doses q6–8h |
| **Penicillin G potassium** | IM 300,000–8 million U daily | |
| (Pfizerpen, Pentids, others) | IV 6–20 million U daily by continuous or intermittent infusion q2–4h. Up to 60 million U daily have been given in certain serious infections. | IM, IV 50,000–250,000 U/kg per day in divided doses q4h |
| **Penicillin G benzathine** | PO 400,000–600,000 U q4–6h | PO 25,000–90,000 U/kg per day in three to six divided doses |
| (Bicillin) | IM 1.2–2.4 million U in a single dose | |
| | Prophylaxis of rheumatic fever, IM 1.2 million U monthly or 600,000 U every 2 wk | IM 50,000 U/kg in one dose |
| | Treatment of syphilis, IM 2.4 million U (1.2 million U in each buttock) in a single dose | Prophylaxis of rheumatic fever, IM 1.2 million U monthly or 600,000 U every 1–2 wk |
| **Penicillin G procaine** | IM 600,000–1.2 million U daily in 1 or 2 doses | IM 25,000–50,000 U/kg per day in divided doses q12h |
| (Wycillin, others) | Prevention or treatment of uncomplicated gonorrhea, IM 4.8 million U in a single dose, divided into two or more injections and given at different sites. Probenecid 1 g is given 30 min before the penicillin. | |
| **Penicillin V** | PO 125–500 mg four to six times daily | Same as adults |
| (V-Cillin K, PenVee K, others) | | Infants: PO 15–50 mg/kg per day in three to six divided doses |
| ***Penicillinase-Resistant (Antistaphylococcal) Penicillins*** | | |
| **Cloxacillin** | PO 250–500 mg q6h | Weight 20 kg or more: Same as adults |
| (Tegopen) | | Weight under 20 kg: PO 50–100 mg/kg per day in four divided doses q6h |
| **Dicloxacillin** | PO, IM 125–250 mg q6h | Weight 40 kg or more: Same as adults |
| (Dynapen) | | Weight under 40 kg: 12.5–25 mg/kg per day in four divided doses q6h |
| **Methicillin** | IM 1 g q4–6h | IM 100–200 mg/kg per day in four divided doses q6h |
| (Staphcillin) | IV 1–2 g in 50 ml sodium chloride injection, infused at 10 ml/min q4–6h | |
| **Nafcillin** | IM 500 mg q4–6h | IM, IV 50–100 mg/kg per day in four to six divided doses q4–6h |
| (Unipen) | IV 500 mg–2 g in 15–30 ml sodium chloride injection, infused over 5–10 min, q4h; maximal daily dose, 12 g for serious infections | |
| **Oxacillin** | PO, IM, IV 500 mg–1 g q4–6h. For direct IV injection, the dose should be well diluted and given over 10–15 min. | Weight over 40 kg: Same as adults |
| (Prostaphlin) | | Weight 40 kg or less: PO, IM, IV 50–100 mg/kg per day in four divided doses q6h |
| ***Ampicillins*** | | |
| **Ampicillin** | PO, IM, IV 250–500 mg q6h. In severe infections, doses up to 2 g q4h may be given IV. | Weight over 20 kg: Same as adults |
| (Omnipen, Penbriten, others) | | Weight 20 kg or less: PO, IM, IV 50–100 mg/kg per day in divided doses q6h |
| **Amoxicillin** | PO 250–500 mg q8h | Weight over 20 kg: Same as adults |
| (Amoxil, Larotid, others) | | Weight 20 kg or less: 20–40 mg/kg per day in divided doses q8h |
| **Bacampicillin** | PO 400–800 mg q12h | Weight over 25 kg: Same as adults |
| (Spectrobid) | | |
| ***Extended-Spectrum (Antipseudomonal) Penicillins*** | | |
| **Carbenicillin indanyl sodium** | PO 1–2 tablets (382 mg carbenicillin/tablet) four times daily | PO 30–50 mg/kg per day in divided doses q8h |
| (Geocillin) | | |
| **Ticarcillin** | IM, IV 1–3 g q6h. IM injections should not exceed 2 g/injection. | Weight under 40 kg: 100–300 mg/kg per day q6–8h |
| (Ticar) | | |

*(continued)*

**TABLE 34-1. PENICILLINS** (*Continued*)

| Generic/Trade Name | Routes and Dosage Ranges | |
| --- | --- | --- |
| | *Adults* | *Children* |
| **Mezlocillin** (Mezlin) | IM, IV 200–300 mg/kg per day in four to six divided doses. Usual adult dosage, 3 g q4h or 4 g q6h | Age 1 month–12 years: 300 mg/kg per day in six divided doses, q4h |
| **Piperacillin** (Pipracil) | IV, IM 200–300 mg/kg per day in divided doses q4–6h. Usual adult dosage, 3–4 g q4–6h; maximal daily dose, 24 g | Age under 12 years: Dosage not established |
| *Penicillin/Beta-Lactamase Inhibitor Combinations* | | |
| **Ampicillin/sulbactam** (Unasyn) | IM, IV 1.5–3 g q6h | Age over 12 years, same as adults Age under 12 years, dosage not established |
| **Amoxicillin/potassium clavulanate** (Augmentin) | PO 250–500 mg q8h | Weight under 40 kg: 20–40 mg/kg per day in divided doses q8h |
| **Piperacillin/tazobactam** (Zosyn) | IV 3.375 g q6h | Dosage not established |
| **Ticarcillin/clavulanate** (Timentin) | IV 3.1 g q4–6h | Weight under 60 kg: 200–300 mg/kg per day in divided doses q4–6h |

## PENICILLIN–BETA-LACTAMASE INHIBITOR COMBINATIONS

Beta-lactamase inhibitors are drugs with a beta-lactam structure but little antibacterial activity. They bind irreversibly with beta-lactamase enzymes produced by many bacteria and inactivate the enzymes. Because of this activity, the drugs are combined with several penicillins. In combination, the beta-lactamase inhibitor protects the penicillin from destruction by beta-lactamase enzymes and extends the penicillin's spectrum of antimicrobial activity. Potassium clavulanate, sulbactam, and tazobactam are available in combinations with penicillins.

**Unasyn** is a combination of ampicillin and sulbactam with increased antibacterial activity of ampicillin against beta-lactamase-producing microorganisms, such as *E. coli, Klebsiella, Enterobacter, Bacteroides*, and *S. aureus*. Unasyn is available in vials containing 1 g of ampicillin and 0.5 g of sulbactam or 2 g of ampicillin and 1 g of sulbactam. **Augmentin** contains amoxicillin and potassium clavulanate and may be effective in infections caused by bacteria that are normally resistant to amoxicillin and other beta-lactam antibiotics. Augmentin is available in 250- and 500-mg tablets, each of which contains 125 mg of potassium clavulanate. Thus, two 250-mg tablets are not equivalent to one 500-mg tablet. **Timentin** is a combination of ticarcillin and clavulanate. It is available in an intravenous formulation containing 3 g ticarcillin and 100 mg clavulanate. **Zosyn** is a combination of piperacillin and tazobactam available in an intravenous formulation containing 3 g piperacillin to .375 g tazobactam. Dosage of Zosyn should be reduced for clients with creatinine clearance below 40 ml/minute and those undergoing hemodialysis.

## Nursing Process

General aspects of the nursing process in antimicrobial drug therapy, as described in Chapter 33, apply to the client receiving penicillins. In this chapter, only aspects related specifically to penicillin therapy are included.

### Assessment

Ask clients specifically whether they have ever taken a penicillin and if so, whether they ever had a skin rash, hives, swelling, or difficulty breathing associated with the drug.

### Nursing diagnoses

- High Risk for Injury: Anaphylactic shock
- Knowledge Deficit: Correct administration and usage of penicillins

### Planning/Goals

*The client will:*
- Take penicillins as directed
- Receive prompt and appropriate treatment if anaphylaxis occurs

### Interventions

- After giving a penicillin parenterally in an outpatient setting, keep the client in the area for at least 30 minutes. Anaphylactic reactions are more likely to occur with parenteral than oral use and within a few minutes after injection.
- In any client care setting, keep emergency equipment and supplies readily available.

**Evaluation**

- Observe for improvement in signs of infection.
- Interview and observe for adverse drug effects.

# Principles of therapy

## GUIDELINES RELATED TO HYPERSENSITIVITY TO PENICILLINS

1. Before giving the initial dose of any penicillin preparation, ask the client specifically if he or she has ever taken penicillin and if so, whether an allergic reaction occurred. Penicillin is the most common cause of drug-induced anaphylaxis, a life-threatening hypersensitivity reaction, and a person known to be hypersensitive should generally be given another type of antibiotic.

2. In the rare instance in which penicillin is considered essential, a skin test may be helpful to assess hypersensitivity. Benzylpenicilloyl polylysine (Pre-Pen) or a dilute solution of the penicillin to be administered (10,000 U/ml) may be applied topically to a skin scratch made with a sterile needle. If the scratch test is negative (no urticaria, erythema, or pruritus), the preparation may be injected intradermally. Allergic reactions, including fatal anaphylactic shock, have occurred with skin tests and following negative skin tests.

3. Because anaphylactic shock may occur with administration of the penicillins, especially by parenteral routes, emergency drugs and equipment must be readily available. Treatment may require parenteral epinephrine, oxygen, and insertion of an endotracheal or tracheostomy tube if laryngeal edema occurs.

## DRUG SELECTION, ROUTE, AND DOSAGE

1. Choice of penicillin preparation depends primarily on the organism causing the infection. In many infections, penicillin G is the drug of choice. In many gram-negative infections, ampicillin is useful. In most *Pseudomonas* and *Proteus* infections, an antipseudomonal penicillin is preferred. Most staphylococcal infections are caused by organisms that produce penicillinase, an enzyme that inactivates the above drugs. Thus, in those infections, penicillinase-resistant penicillins are required. Nafcillin is the intravenous agent of choice, and dicloxacillin is the oral agent of choice.

2. Choice of route and dosage depends largely on the seriousness of the infection being treated. For serious infections, penicillins are given intravenously in large

doses. Most penicillins must be given every 4 to 6 hours to maintain therapeutic blood levels. The intramuscular route is rarely used in hospitalized clients but is used more often in ambulatory settings. The oral route is often used, especially for less serious infections and for long-term prophylaxis of rheumatic fever.

## USE IN SPECIFIC SITUATIONS

### Streptococcal infections

When used for streptococcal infections, penicillins should be given for the full prescribed course to prevent complications, such as rheumatic fever, endocarditis, and glomerulonephritis.

### Sexually transmitted diseases

When used for sexually transmitted diseases, it is advisable to refer to the guidelines established by the Centers for Disease Control and Prevention. Recommendations vary according to patterns of bacterial resistance. For example, penicillin-resistant strains of *Neisseria gonorrhoeae* are encountered with increasing frequency.

### With probenecid

Probenecid (Benemid) can be given concurrently with penicillins to increase serum drug levels. Probenecid acts by blocking renal excretion of the penicillins. This action may be useful when high serum levels are needed with oral penicillin preparations or when a single large dose is given for prevention or treatment of gonorrhea or syphilis.

### With an aminoglycoside

A penicillin is often given concomitantly with an aminoglycoside antibiotic for serious infections, such as those caused by *Pseudomonas aeruginosa*. In this instance, the drugs should not be mixed in a syringe or an intravenous solution because that inactivates the aminoglycoside.

## POTENTIAL ELECTROLYTE DISTURBANCES

Excessive amounts of potassium or sodium may be ingested during penicillin therapy. Potassium excess may occur with large intravenous doses of penicillin G potassium, which contains 1.7 mEq of potassium per 1 million U. Hyperkalemia is unlikely with normal renal function but may occur in clients with impaired renal function. Sodium excess may occur when ticarcillin (5.6

mEq sodium/g) is given to clients with renal impairment or congestive heart failure. Hypokalemic metabolic acidosis may occur with ticarcillin in clients with impaired renal function. This occurs because potassium loss is enhanced by high sodium intake.

## USE IN CHILDREN

Penicillins are widely used to treat infections in children and are generally safe. They should be used cautiously in neonates because immature kidney function slows their elimination. Dosages should be based on age, weight, and severity of the infection being treated.

## USE IN OLDER ADULTS

Penicillins are generally safe. With impaired renal function, which often occurs in older adults, hyperkalemia may occur with large intravenous doses of penicillin G potassium, and hypernatremia may occur with ticarcillin. Hypernatremia is less likely with other antipseudomonal penicillins, such as mezlocillin and piperacillin.

Penicillin therapy in debilitated older adults may cause superinfections with *Proteus*, *Pseudomonas*, or *Candida* organisms. In addition to decreased renal function, other disease processes and concurrent drug therapies increase the risks of adverse effects in older adults.

## NURSING ACTIONS: PENICILLINS

| *Nursing Actions* | *Rationale/Explanation* |
|---|---|
| **1. Administer accurately** | |
| **a.** Give most oral penicillins on an empty stomach, about 1 hour before or 2 hours after a meal. Penicillin V, amoxicillin, amoxicillin/clavulanate, and bacampicillin may be given without regard to meals. | To decrease binding to foods and inactivation by gastric acid. The latter four drugs are not significantly affected by food. |
| **b.** Give oral drugs with a full glass of water, preferably; do not give with orange juice or other acidic fluids. | To promote absorption and decrease inactivation, which may occur in an acidic environment |
| **c.** Give IM penicillins deeply into a large muscle mass. | To decrease tissue irritation. |
| **d.** For IV administration, generally dilute reconstituted penicillins in 50 to 100 ml of 5% dextrose or 0.9% sodium chloride injection and infuse over 30 to 60 minutes. | To minimize vascular irritation and phlebitis. Amounts and types of IV solutions may vary. Check manufacturers' literature for specific drugs to ensure compatibility and safety. |
| **e.** Prepare crystalline penicillin G for IV use just before giving. | The drug in crystalline (powder) form is stable for a long time. When diluent is added to form a solution, the drug loses activity rapidly. |
| **f.** Give reconstituted ampicillin IV or IM within 1 hour. | The drug is stable for a limited time in solution. |
| **g.** Do not give methicillin as a continuous IV infusion. | Methicillin is unstable at acid pH, and most solutions used for IV infusions are acidic enough to start breakdown of methicillin in about 20 minutes. |
| **2. Observe for therapeutic effects** | Depend on type of infection. See Chapter 33. |
| **a.** Decreased signs and symptoms of infection for which given | |
| **b.** Absence of signs and symptoms of infection when given prophylactically | |
| **3. Observe for adverse effects**<br>**a.** Hypersensitivity–anaphylaxis, serum sickness | Hypersensitivity is more likely to occur with penicillins than with other anti-infectives. Anaphylaxis may occur within 5 to 30 minutes of penicillin administration. See "Nursing Actions," in Chapter 33 for signs and symptoms of hypersensitivity. |

*(continued)*

## Nursing Actions

## Rationale/Explanation

**b.** Superinfection

See Chapter 33 for signs and symptoms.

**c.** Nausea, vomiting, diarrhea

These gastrointestinal disturbances are more likely to occur with high doses of oral drugs and are probably caused by local irritation of mucosa and changes in gastrointestinal flora.

**d.** Thrombophlebitis at venipuncture sites and pain at intramuscular injection sites

**e.** With carbenicllin and ticarcillin, observe for congestive heart failure (dyspnea, edema, fatigue) and bleeding.

These drugs contain relatively large amounts of sodium. Congestive heart failure is more likely to occur in clients with heart or kidney disease. Bleeding tendencies result from decreased platelet aggregation.

**4. Observe for drug interactions**
   **a.** Drugs that *increase* effects of penicillins:

     (1) Gentamicin and other aminoglycosides

Synergistic activity against *Pseudomonas* organisms when given concomitantly with extended-spectrum (antipseudomonal) penicillins
Synergistic activity against enterococci that cause subacute bacterial endocarditis, brain abscess, meningitis, or urinary tract infection
Synergistic activity against *Staphylococcus aureus* when used with nafcillin or methicillin

     (2) Probenecid (Benemid)

Decreases renal excretion of penicillins, thus elevates and prolongs penicillin blood levels

   **b.** Drugs that *decrease* effects of penicillins:

     (1) Acidifying agents (ammonium chloride, ascorbic acid, cranberry juice, methenamine, methionine, orange juice)

Most oral penicillins are destroyed by acids, including gastric acid. Amoxicillin and penicillin V are acid stable.

     (2) Erythromycin

Erythromycin inhibits the bactericidal activity of penicillins against most organisms but potentiates activity against resistant strains of *S. aureus*.

     (3) Tetracyclines

These bacteriostatic antibiotics slow multiplication of bacteria and thereby inhibit the penicillins, which act against rapidly multiplying bacteria.

**5. Teach clients**
   **a.** Take penicillins (except amoxicillin, amoxicillin/clavulanate, bacampicillin, and penicillin V) on an empty stomach, with at least 8 oz of water, at regular intervals around the clock.

To increase therapeutic effects and decrease adverse effects

   **b.** Report skin rash, hives, itching, severe diarrhea, shortness of breath, fever, sore throat, black tongue, or any unusual bleeding.

These symptoms may indicate a need to discontinue the drug.

   **c.** Discard liquid forms of penicillins after 7 days at room temperature and 14 days when refrigerated.

Liquid forms deteriorate and should not be taken.

## Review and Application Exercises

1. What is the mechanism of penicillin's action against bacteria?
2. What are beta-lactamase enzymes, and what do they do to penicillins?
3. How are penicillins excreted?
4. What are the main differences between penicillin G or V and antistaphylococcal and antipseudomonal penicillins?
5. What is the reason for combining clavulanate, sulbactam or tazobactam with a penicillin?
6. When giving injections of penicillin in an outpatient setting, it is recommended to keep clients in the area and observe them for at least 30 minutes. Why?
7. When probenecid is given concurrently with a penicillin, what is its purpose?
8. What are the signs and symptoms of anaphylaxis?

## Selected References

Beare, P. G., & Myers, J. L. (Eds.) (1990). *Principles and practice of adult health nursing*. St. Louis: C.V. Mosby.

Breitenbucher, R. B., & Peterson, P. K. (1990). Infections in the elderly. In G. L. Mandell, R. G. Douglas Jr, & J. E. Bennett (Eds.), *Principles and practice of infectious diseases* (3rd ed.) (pp. 2315–2320). New York: Churchill Livingstone.

(1993). *Drug facts and comparisons*. St. Louis: Facts and Comparisons.

Dunne, W. M. (1990). Mechanisms of infectious disease. In C. M. Porth (Ed.), *Pathophysiology: Concepts of altered health states* (3rd ed.) (pp. 145–163). Philadelphia: J.B. Lippincott.

Guglielmo, B. J. (1992). Principles of antimicrobial therapy. In M. A. Koda-Kimble & L. Y.Young (Eds.), *Applied therapeutics: The clinical use of drugs* (5th ed.) (pp. 33-1–33-12). Vancouver, WA: Applied Therapeutics.

Kunin, C. M. (1993). Resistance to antimicrobial drugs—A worldwide calamity. *Annals of Internal Medicine, 118*, 557–561.

Moellering, R. C. Jr. (1990). Principles of anti-infective therapy. In G. L. Mandell, R. G. Douglas Jr., & J. E. Bennett (Eds.), *Principles and practice of infectious diseases* (3rd ed.) (pp. 206–218). New York: Churchill Livingstone.

Murray, B. E. (1992). Antimicrobial therapeutic agents. In W. N. Kelley (Ed.), *Textbook of internal medicine* (2nd ed.) (pp. 1564–1575). Philadelphia: J.B. Lippincott.

Neu, H. C. (1990). Penicillins. In G. L. Mandell, R. G. Douglas Jr & J. E. Bennett (Eds.), *Principles and practice of infectious diseases* (3rd ed.) (pp 230–246). New York: Churchill Livingstone.

O'Hanley, P. D., Tam, J. Y., & Holodniy, M. (1992). Infectious disorders. In K. L. Melmon, H. F. Morrelli, B. B. Hoffman, & D. W. Nierenberg (Eds.), *Clinical pharmacology: Basic principles in therapeutics* (3rd ed.). New York: McGraw-Hill.

Streit, L. A. (1992). Nursing management of adults with infections. In L. O. Burrell (Ed.), *Adult nursing in hospital and community settings* (pp. 79–99). Norwalk, CT: Appleton & Lange.

# CHAPTER 35

# Cephalosporins

## Cephalosporins

Cephalosporins are a widely used group of antimicrobial drugs that are derived from a fungus. Although technically cefoxitin (Mefoxin) and cefotetan (cephamycins derived from a different fungus) and loracarbef and moxalactam (synthetic drugs) are not cephalosporins, they are categorized with the cephalosporins because of their similarities to the group. Cephalosporins are also called beta-lactam antibiotics because their chemical structure contains a beta-lactam ring (like the penicillins). They have the same mechanism of action as the penicillins; that is, they inhibit formation of bacterial cell walls. They are broad-spectrum antimicrobial agents with a wide range of activity against gram-positive and gram-negative bacteria. Compared with penicillins, they are generally less active against gram-positive organisms but more active against gram-negative ones.

Once absorbed, cephalosporins are widely distributed into most body fluids and tissues, with maximum concentrations in the liver and kidneys. Many cephalosporins do not reach therapeutic levels in cerebrospinal fluid; exceptions are cefuroxime, a second-generation drug, and the third-generation agents. These drugs reach therapeutic levels when meninges are inflamed. Cephalosporins are excreted through the kidneys (except for cefoperazone, which is excreted in bile).

First-generation cephalosporins have essentially the same spectrum of antimicrobial activity and can be described as a group, with cephalothin (Keflin) as the prototype. They are effective against streptococci (except *Streptococcus faecalis*), staphylococci (except methicillin-resistant *Staphylococcus aureus*), *Neisseria, Salmonella, Shigella, Escherichia, Klebsiella, Bacillus, Corynebacterium*

*diphtheriae, Proteus mirabilis,* and *Bacteroides* (except *Bacteroides fragilis*). They are not effective against *Enterobacter, Pseudomonas,* and *Serratia*.

Second-generation cephalosporins differ from first-generation drugs but are similar to each other. They are more active against some gram-negative organisms than older drugs. Thus, they may be effective in infections resistant to other antibiotics, including those caused by *Haemophilus influenzae, Enterobacter, Klebsiella, Escherichia coli,* and some strains of *Proteus*. Because each of these drugs has a somewhat different antimicrobial spectrum, susceptibility tests must be performed for each drug rather than for the entire group, as was feasible with first-generation drugs. Cefoxitin, for example, is active against *B. fragilis,* an anaerobic organism resistant to most drugs.

Third-generation cephalosporins further extend the spectrum of activity against gram-negative organisms. In addition to activity against the usual enteric pathogens (*e.g., E. coli, Proteus, Klebsiella*), they also are active against several strains resistant to other antibiotics and to first- and second-generation cephalosporins. Thus, they may be useful in infections caused by unusual strains of enteric organisms, such as *Citrobacter, Serratia, Providencia,* and *Enterobacter*. Another difference is that third-generation cephalosporins penetrate inflamed meninges to reach therapeutic concentrations in cerebrospinal fluid. Thus, they may be useful against meningeal infections caused by many common pathogens, including *H. influenzae, Neisseria meningitidis,* and *Streptococcus pneumoniae*. Although some of the drugs are active against *Pseudomonas* organisms, drug-resistant strains emerge when a cephalosporin is used alone for treatment of pseudomonal infection.

Overall, cephalosporins gain gram-negative activity

Anne Collins Abrams: CLINICAL DRUG THERAPY, Fourth Edition.

and lose gram-positive activity as they move from the first to the third generation. The second- and third-generation drugs are more active against gram-negative organisms because they are more resistant to the beta-lactamase enzymes (cephalosporinases) produced by some bacteria to inactivate cephalosporins.

## MECHANISM OF ACTION

Like the penicillins, cephalosporins act by inhibiting bacterial synthesis of cell walls and are more active against bacteria that are rapidly dividing and reproducing.

## INDICATIONS FOR USE

Clinical indications include surgical prophylaxis and treatment of infections of the respiratory tract, skin and soft tissues, bones and joints, urinary tract, and bloodstream (septicemia). Cephalosporins often are used as alternative drugs in infections caused by organisms resistant to other drugs. They are most important clinically for gram-negative infections. In most infections with streptococci and staphylococci, penicillins are more effective and less expensive. In infections caused by methicillin-resistant *S. aureus*, cephalosporins are not clinically effective even if in vitro testing indicates susceptibility.

## CONTRAINDICATIONS FOR USE

A major contraindication for the use of cephalosporins is a previous anaphylactic reaction to penicillin. The chemical structure of cephalosporins is similar to that of penicillins (both groups are beta-lactam antibiotics), and there is a risk of cross-sensitivity between the two groups. However, incidence of cross-sensitivity is thought to be low, especially in clients who have had delayed reactions (*e.g.*, skin rash) to penicillins. Another contraindication is cephalosporin allergy. Immediate allergic reactions with anaphylaxis, bronchospasm, and urticaria occur less often than delayed reactions with skin rash, drug fever, and eosinophilia.

## Individual cephalosporins

Oral drugs are listed in Table 35-1, and parenteral agents are in Table 35-2.

## Nursing Process

General aspects of the nursing process, as described in Chapter 33, apply to the client receiving cephalosporins. In this chapter, only aspects related specifically to cephalosporins are included.

### Assessment

Ask clients specifically if they have ever taken one of the drugs, as far as they know, and whether they ever had a severe reaction (with difficulty breathing and so forth) to penicillin.

### Nursing diagnoses

- High Risk for Injury: Renal impairment
- Knowledge Deficit: Correct administration and usage of cephalosporins

### Planning/Goals

The client will:
- Take oral cephalosporins as directed
- Receive parenteral cephalosporins by appropriate techniques to minimize tissue irritation

### Interventions

- Monitor client response to cephalosporins.
- Monitor dosages for clients with impaired renal function.

### Evaluation

- Observe for improvement in signs of infection.
- Interview and observe for adverse drug effects.

## Principles of therapy

### DRUG SELECTION

The choice of cephalosporin depends on causative organisms, severity of infection, and other factors. Guidelines include the following:

1. When choosing an antimicrobial agent, a cephalosporin may be a good choice when it can be used alone for prophylaxis or treatment. If the cephalosporin must be combined with another antimicrobial agent, a noncephalosporin is preferred. For example, cephalosporins cannot be used alone in the treatment of *Pseudomonas* infections because first- and second-generation drugs are not effective, and third-generation drugs allow emergence of drug-resistant organisms. A cephalosporin could be given concomitantly with an aminoglycoside, but an antipseudomonal penicillin is preferred. Penicillins are less nephrotoxic and less expensive than third-generation cephalosporins.
2. First-generation cephalosporins are often used for surgical prophylaxis, especially with prosthetic implants, because most postimplant infections are caused by gram-positive organisms, such as staphylococci. They also may be used alone for treatment of infections caused by any susceptible organisms in body sites where drug penetration and host defenses

**TABLE 35-1. ORAL CEPHALOSPORINS**

| Generic/Trade Name | Characteristics | Routes and Dosage Ranges | |
| --- | --- | --- | --- |
| | | **Adults** | **Children** |
| *First Generation* | | | |
| **Cefadroxil** (Duricef, Ultracef) | A derivative of cephalexin with no apparent advantage over the parent drug except that it has a longer half-life and can be given less often | PO 1–2 g twice daily | 30 mg/kg per day in two doses q12h |
| **Cephalexin** (Keflex) | 1. Somewhat less active against penicillinase-producing staphylococci than cephalothin 2. First oral cephalosporin; still used extensively | PO 250–500 mg q6h, increased to 4 g q6h if necessary in severe infections | PO 25–50 mg/kg per day in divided doses q6h |
| **Cephradine** (Anspor, Velosef) | Essentially the same as cephalexin, except it also can be given parenterally | PO 250–500 mg q6h, up to 4 g daily in severe infections | PO 25–50 mg/kg per day in divided doses q6h. In severe infections, up to 100 mg/kg per day may be given. |
| *Second Generation* | | | |
| **Cefaclor** (Ceclor) | May be more active against *Haemophilus influenzae* and *Escherichia coli* than cephalothin | PO 250–500 mg q8h | PO 20–40 mg/kg per day in three divided doses q8h |
| **Cefuroxime** (Ceftin) | 1. Can also be given parenterally 2. Available only in tablet form 3. The tablet may be crushed and added to a food (*e.g.*, applesauce), but the crushed tablet leaves a strong, bitter, persistent aftertaste. | PO 250 mg q12h; severe infections, 500 mg q12h; UTI, 125 mg q12h | >12 years, same as adults; <12 years, 125 mg q12h Otitis media, >2 years, 250 mg q12h, <2 years, 125 mg q12h |
| **Cefprozil** (Cefzil) | Similar to cefaclor and cefuroxime | PO 250–500 mg q12–24h | PO 15 mg/kg q12h |
| **Loracarbef** (Lorabid) | A synthetic drug similar to cefaclor | PO 200–400 mg q12h | PO 15–30 mg/kg per day in divided doses q12h |
| *Third Generation* | | | |
| **Cefixime** (Suprax) | First oral third-generation drug | PO 200 mg q12h or 400 mg q24h | PO 4 mg/kg q12h or 8 mg/kg q24h; give adult dose to children 50 kg of weight or 12 years of age or older |
| **Cefpodoxime** (Vantin) | Similar to cefixime except has some activity against staphylococci (except methicillin-resistant *Staphylococcus aureus*) | PO 200–400 mg q12h | PO 5 mg/kg q12h Give 10 mg/kg (400 mg or adult dose) to children 13 years or older with skin and soft-tissue infections |

are not a problem. Cefazolin (Kefzol) and cephapirin (Cefadyl) are frequently used parenteral agents. Cefazolin reportedly reaches a higher serum concentration, is more protein-bound, and has a slower rate of elimination than other first-generation drugs. These factors prolong serum half-life, so cefazolin can be given in smaller doses or less frequently. Cefazolin is also preferred for intramuscular administration because it is less irritating to body tissues.

3. Second-generation cephalosporins also are often used for surgical prophylaxis, especially for gynecologic and colorectal surgery. They are used for treatment of intra-abdominal infections, such as pelvic inflammatory disease, diverticulitis, penetrating wounds of the abdomen, and other infections caused by organisms inhabiting pelvic and colorectal areas.

4. Third-generation cephalosporins are recommended for serious infections caused by susceptible organisms that are resistant to first- and second-generation cephalosporins. They are often used in the treatment of infections caused by *E. coli, Proteus, Klebsiella, Serratia*, and other Enterobacteriaceae, especially when the infections occur in body sites not readily reached by other drugs (*e.g.*, cerebrospinal fluid and bone) and in clients with immunosuppression. Although these drugs are effective against 50% to 75% of *Pseudomonas* strains, they should not be used alone to treat pseudomonal infections because drug resistance develops.

5. Moxalactam is not recommended for use because of bleeding problems from hypoprothrombinemia and platelet dysfunction.

## TABLE 35-2. PARENTERAL CEPHALOSPORINS

| Generic/Trade Name | Characteristics | Routes and Dosage Ranges | |
| --- | --- | --- | --- |
| | | *Adults* | *Children* |
| **First Generation** | | | |
| **Cephalothin** (Keflin) | 1. The first cephalosporin<br>2. Active against streptococci, staphylococci, *Neisseria, Salmonella, Shigella, Escherichia, Klebsiella, Listeria, Bacillus, Haemophilus influenzae, Corynebacterium diphtheriae, Proteus mirabilis*, and *Bacteroides* (except *Bacteroides fragilis*)<br>3. Inactive against enterococci, *Enterobacter, Pseudomonas*, and *Serratia* | IV, IM 1–2 g q4–6h, depending on severity of infection | IV, IM 75–160 mg/kg per day in divided doses q4–6h |
| **Cefazolin** (Kefzol, Ancef) | More active against *Escherichia coli* and *Klebsiella* species than cephalothin | IM, IV 250 mg–1 g q6–8h | IM, IV 50–100 mg/kg per day in three to four divided doses |
| **Cephapirin** (Cefadyl) | No significant differences from cephalothin | IV, IM 500 mg–1 g q4–6h, up to 12 g daily, IV, in serious infections | IV, IM 40–80 mg/kg per day in four divided doses (q6h) |
| **Cephradine** (Anspor, Velosef) | No significant differences from cephalothin except it also can be given orally | IV, IM 500 mg–1 g two to four times daily, depending on severity of infection | IV, IM 75–125 mg/kg per day in divided doses q6h |
| **Second Generation** | | | |
| **Cefamandole** (Mandol) | 1. More active against some gram-negative organisms than cephalothin and other first-generation cephalosporins, especially *H. influenzae, Enterobacter* and *Klebsiella* species, indole-positive strains of *Proteus*, and *E. coli*<br>2. Major clinical usefulness is treatment of gram-negative infections caused by organisms resistant to other cephalosporins | IV, IM 0.5–2 g q4–6h, up to 12 g daily in life-threatening infections | IV, IM 50–150 mg/kg per day in four to six divided doses q4–6h |
| **Cefmetazole** (Zefazone) | Similar to cefoxitin in antibacterial spectrum and clinical use | IV 2 g q6–12h for 5–14 d Surgical prophylaxis, IV 1 or 2 g 30–90 min before surgery, repeated 8 and 16 h later (total of three doses) | |
| **Cefonocid** (Monocid) | 1. Antimicrobial spectrum similar to other second-generation cephalosporins<br>2. Has a long half-life and can therefore be given once daily<br>3. Not approved for use in children | IV, IM 1 g daily (q24h) Surgical prophylaxis, IV, IM 1 g 1 h before procedure | |
| **Ceforanide** (Precef) | 1. Similar to other second-generation cephalosporins<br>2. Has a relatively long half-life and can therefore be given twice daily | IV, IM 0.5–1 g q12h Surgical prophylaxis, IV, IM 0.5–1g 1 h before the procedure | 20–40 mg/kg per day in divided doses q12h |
| **Cefotetan** (Cefotan) | 1. Effective against most organisms except *Pseudomonas*<br>2. Highly resistant to beta-lactamase enzymes<br>3. Dosage must be reduced with renal failure, according to creatinine clearance. | IV, IM 1–2 g q12h for 5–10 d; maximum dose, 3 g q12h in life-threatening infections Perioperative prophylaxis, IV 1–2 g 30–60 min before surgery | |
| **Cefoxitin** (Mefoxin) | 1. The first cephamycin (derived from a different fungus than cephalosporins)<br>2. Compared with cephalothin, cefoxitin is more active against gram-negative bacteria and less active against gram-positive bacteria<br>3. Compared with cefamandole, cefoxitin is more active against indole-positive *Proteus* and *Serratia* but less active against gram-positive bacteria and gram-negative *Enterobacter* and *H. influenzae*.<br>4. A major clinical use may stem from increased activity against *B. fragilis*, an organism resistant to most other antimicrobial drugs. | IV, IM 1–2 q q4–6h | IV, IM 80–160 mg/kg per day in divided doses q4–6h. Do not exceed 12 g/d. |

*(continued)*

## TABLE 35-2. PARENTERAL CEPHALOSPORINS (*Continued*)

| Generic/Trade Name | Characteristics | Routes and Dosage Ranges | |
|---|---|---|---|
| | | *Adults* | *Children* |
| ***Second Generation*** | | | |
| **Cefuroxime** (Ceftin, Kefurox, Zinacef) | 1. Similar to other second-generation cephalosporins<br>2. Penetrates cerebrospinal fluid in presence of inflamed meninges | IV, IM, 750 mg–1.5 g q8h Surgical prophylaxis, IV 1.5 g 30–60 min before initial skin incision, then 750 mg IV or IM q8h if procedure is prolonged | Over 3 mo of age: IV, IM 50–100 mg/kg per day in divided doses q6–8h Bacterial meningitis, IV 200–240 mg/kg per day in divided doses q6–8h, reduced to 100 mg/kg per day on clinical improvement |
| ***Third Generation*** | | | |
| **Cefoperazone** (Cefobid) | 1. Active against gram-negative and gram-positive organisms, including gram-negative organisms resistant to earlier cephalosporins<br>2. Has increased activity against *Pseudomonas* organisms but cannot be used for single-agent treatment of systemic pseudomonal infections<br>3. Excreted primarily in bile; half-life prolonged in hepatic failure | IV, IM 2–4 g/d in divided doses q8–12h | Dosage not established |
| **Cefotaxime** (Claforan) | 1. Antibacterial activity against most gram-positive and gram-negative bacteria, including several strains resistant to other antibiotics. It has activity against some strains of *Pseudomonas aeruginosa* resistant to first- and second-generation cephalosporins.<br>2. Recommended for serious infections caused by susceptible microorganisms | IV, IM 1g q6–8h; maximum dose, 12 g/24h | Weight >50 kg: same as adults Weight <50 kg and age over 1 mo: IV, IM 50–180 mg/kg per day, in divided doses q4–6h Neonates: up to 1 wk of age, IV 50 mg/kg q12h; 1–4 wk, IV 50 mg/kg q8h |
| **Ceftazidime** (Fortaz) | 1. Active against gram-positive and gram-negative organisms<br>2. Especially effective against gram-negative organisms, including *P. aeruginosa* and other bacterial strains resistant to aminoglycosides<br>3. Indicated for serious infections caused by susceptible organisms | IV, IM 1 g q8–12h | 1 month to 12 years: IV 30–50 mg/kg q8h, not to exceed 6 g/d Under 1 mo of age: IV 30 mg/kg q12h |
| **Ceftizoxime** (Cefizox) | 1. Broader gram-negative and anaerobic activity, especially against *B. fragilis*<br>2. More active against gram-positive organisms than moxalactam and more active against *Enterobacteriaceae* than cefoperazone<br>3. Dosage must be reduced with even mild renal insufficiency (creatinine clearance <80 ml/min) | IV, IM 1–2 g q8–12h Gonorrhea, uncomplicated, IM 1 g as a single dose | Over 6 mo of age: IV, IM 5 mg/kg q6–8h, increased to a total daily dose of 200 mg/kg if necessary |
| **Ceftriaxone** (Rocephin) | First third-generation cephalosporin approved for once-daily dosing | IV, IM 1–2 g once daily (q24h) Surgical prophylaxis, IV, IM 1 g ½–2 h before the procedure | IV, IM 50–75 mg/kg per day, not to exceed 2 g daily, in divided doses q12h Meningitis, IV, IM 100 mg/kg per day, not to exceed 4 g daily, in divided doses q12h |
| **Moxalactam** (Moxam) | Antibacterial spectrum is similar to that of cefotaxime, but moxalactam has better activity against anaerobic bacteria and better penetration into cerebrospinal fluid. | IM, IV 1–2 g q8h | Age 1 mo to 12 y: IV, IM 50 mg/kg q6–8h Neonates: up to 1 wk of age, IV 50 mg/kg q12h; 1–4 wk, IV 50 mg/kg q8h |

## ADMINISTRATION AND DOSAGE

Route of administration and dosage depend on several factors. A few cephalosporins are sufficiently well absorbed for oral administration; these are most often used in mild infections and urinary tract infections. Although some cephalosporins can be given intramuscularly, the injections cause considerable pain and induration. Cefazolin is preferred for intramuscular administration because it is less irritating to tissues. The intravenous route is often used, especially with severe infections. Dosages are higher with severe infections and lower with renal failure (except with cefoperazone, which is excreted through the biliary tract).

## PERIOPERATIVE USE

Many of the cephalosporins are used in surgical prophylaxis. The particular drug depends largely on the type of organism likely to be encountered in the operative area. First-generation drugs are often used for procedures associated with gram-positive postoperative infections, such as prosthetic implant surgery. Second-generation cephalosporins are often used for abdominal procedures, especially gynecologic and colorectal surgery, in which enteric gram-negative infections may occur postoperatively. Third-generation drugs should not be used for surgical prophylaxis because they are usually less active against staphylococci than cefazolin; the gram-negative organisms against which they are most useful are rarely encountered in elective surgery; widespread usage for prophylaxis promotes emergence of drug resistant organisms; and they are very expensive.

When used perioperatively, a cephalosporin should be given about 30 to 60 minutes before the first skin incision is made. To be effective, the drug must be present in therapeutic serum and tissue concentrations at the time of surgery. A single dose is usually sufficient. In prosthetic implants, such as arthroplasty and open-heart surgery, the drug may be continued for 3 to 5 days.

## USE IN RENAL FAILURE OR IMPAIRMENT

In renal failure (creatinine clearance <20–30 ml/min), dosage of all cephalosporins except cefoperazone should be reduced by 50%. Cefoperazone is excreted primarily through the bile and therefore does not accumulate with renal failure. Dosage of ceftizoxime should be reduced even with moderate renal impairment (creatinine clearance <80 ml/min).

## USE IN CHILDREN

Cephalosporins are used empirically in children, but few controlled studies have been done. They are generally considered safe. They should be used cautiously in neonates because immature kidney function slows their elimination and increases risks of toxicity. Dosage should be based on age, weight, severity of the infection being treated, and renal function.

## USE IN OLDER ADULTS

Cephalosporins are generally considered safe. They may cause or aggravate renal impairment, especially when other nephrotoxic drugs are used concurrently. Dosage of several cephalosporins must be reduced in the presence of renal impairment, depending on creatinine clearance. Other adverse effects also may be more likely in older adults because of disease processes and concurrent drug therapies.

## NURSING ACTIONS: CEPHALOSPORINS

| Nursing Actions | Rationale/Explanation |
|---|---|
| **1. Administer accurately**<br>**a.** Give oral cephalosporins with food or milk. | To decrease nausea and vomiting. Food delays absorption but does not affect amount of drug absorbed. |
| **b.** Give intramuscular cephalosporins deeply into a large muscle mass. | These drugs are irritating to tissues and cause pain, induration, and possibly sterile abscess. The intramuscular route is infrequently used except for cefazolin. |
| **c.** For intravenous administration, dilute cephalosporins in 50 to 100 ml of 5% dextrose or 0.9% sodium chloride injection and infuse over 30 minutes. | These drugs are irritating to veins and cause phlebitis. This problem can be minimized by adequate dilution of the drug and relatively slow injection rates. Also, changing venipuncture sites helps avoid prolonged irritation of the same vein. Thrombophlebitis is more likely to occur with doses of more than 6 g/d for longer than 3 days. |

*(continued)*

*Nursing Actions*                                    *Rationale/Explanation*

**2. Observe for therapeutic effects**                See Chapter 33.

**a.** Decreased signs of local and systemic inflammation

**b.** Decreased signs of infection for which given

**3. Observe for adverse effects**

**a.** Hypersensitivity—anaphylaxis, serum sickness        Hypersensitivity reactions are similar to those with penicillins but are uncommon.

**b.** Superinfection                                 See Chapter 33 for signs and symptoms.

**c.** Thrombophlebitis at venipuncture sites and pain at intramuscular injection sites        See 1b and c, above.

**d.** Nephrotoxicity—increased blood urea nitrogen and serum creatinine and casts in urine        Renal toxicity is uncommon with cephalosporins but may occur.

**e.** Nausea, vomiting, diarrhea                     May occur with cephalosporins. If diarrhea is severe or contains blood, pus, or mucus, it may indicate pseudomembranous colitis and the need to discontinue the cephalosporin.

**f.** Bleeding                                       Bleeding may occur with cefamandole, cefoperazone, and moxalactam. These drugs may cause hypoprothrombinemia (by killing intestinal bacteria that normally produce vitamin K or a chemical structure that prevents activation of prothrombin) and platelet dysfunction. Hypoprothrombinemia can be treated by administering vitamin K. Vitamin K does not restore normal platelet function or normal bacterial flora in the intestines. Most severe bleeding has been reported with moxalactam; as a result, moxalactam is no longer recommended for use.

**4. Observe for drug interaction**

**a.** Drugs that *increase* effects of cephalosporins:

(1) Loop diuretics (furosemide, ethacrynic acid)        Increased renal toxicity

(2) Gentamicin and other aminoglycoside antibiotics        Additive renal toxicity, especially in older clients, those with renal impairment, those receiving high dosages, and those receiving probenecid

(3) Probenecid                                        Increases blood levels by decreasing renal excretion of the cephalosporins. This may be a desirable interaction to increase blood levels and therapeutic effectiveness or allow smaller doses.

**b.** Drugs that *decrease* effects of cephalosporins
Tetracyclines                                         Tetracyclines are bacteriostatic and slow the rate of bacterial reproduction. Cephalosporins are bactericidal and are most effective against rapidly multiplying bacteria. Thus, tetracyclines should not be given concurrently with cephalosporins.

**5. Teach clients**

**a.** Take oral cephalosporins with food or milk.        To decrease gastrointestinal upset

**b.** Report the occurrence of diarrhea, especially if it is severe or contains blood, pus, or mucus.        The drug may need to be stopped.

## Review and Application Exercises

1. How do cephalosporins perform their bactericidal action?
2. Do the cephalosporins have a narrow or broad spectrum of antimicrobial activity?
3. Why is a cephalosporin the usual drug of first choice for prevention of infections associated with surgical procedures?
4. What is a major mechanism by which microorganisms develop resistance to cephalosporins?
5. Which cephalosporins should be reduced in dosage for clients with renal insufficiency?
6. How do you assess for adequate renal function?
7. What are adverse effects associated with cephalosporins, and how may they be prevented or minimized?

## Selected References

(1993). Antimicrobial prophylaxis in surgery. *Medical Letter on Drugs and Therapeutics, 35,* 91–93.

Beare, P. G., & Myers, J. L. (Eds.) (1990). *Principles and practice of adult health nursing.* St. Louis: C.V. Mosby.

Breitenbucher, R. B., & Peterson, P. K. (1990). Infections in the elderly. In G. L. Mandell, R. G. Douglas Jr, & J. E. Bennett (Eds.), *Principles and practice of infectious diseases* (3rd ed.) (pp. 2315–2320). New York: Churchill Livingstone.

Donowitz, G. R., & Mandell, G. L. (1990). Cephalosporins. In G. L. Mandell, R. G. Douglas Jr, & J. E. Bennett (Eds.), *Principles and practice of infectious diseases* (3rd ed.) (pp. 246–257). New York: Churchill Livingstone.

(1993). *Drug facts and comparisons.* St. Louis: Facts and Comparisons.

Dunne, W. M. (1990). Mechanisms of infectious disease. In C. M. Porth (Ed.), *Pathophysiology: Concepts of altered health states* (3rd ed.) (pp. 145–163). Philadelphia: J.B. Lippincott.

Ericsson, C. D. (1992). Approach to surgical infections, including burns and postoperative infections. In W. N. Kelley (Ed.), *Textbook of internal medicine* (2nd ed.) (pp. 1641–1644). Philadelphia: J.B. Lippincott.

Guglielmo, B. J. (1992). Principles of antimicrobial therapy. In M. A. Koda-Kimble & L. Y. Young (Eds.), *Applied therapeutics: The clinical use of drugs* (5th ed.) (pp. 33-1–33-12). Vancouver, WA: Applied Therapeutics.

Kunin, C. M. (1993). Resistance to antimicrobial drugs—A worldwide calamity. *Annals of Internal Medicine, 118,* 557–561.

(1992). Loracarbef. *Medical Letter on Drugs and Therapeutics, 34,* 87–88.

Moellering, R. C. Jr. (1990). Principles of anti-infective therapy. In G. L. Mandell, R. G. Douglas Jr., & J. E. Bennett (Eds.), *Principles and practice of infectious diseases* (3rd ed.) (pp. 206–218). New York: Churchill Livingstone.

Murray, B. E. (1992). Antimicrobial therapeutic agents. In W. N. Kelley (Ed.), *Textbook of internal medicine* (2nd ed.) (pp. 1564–1575). Philadelphia: J.B. Lippincott.

O'Hanley, P. D., Tam, J. Y., & Holodniy, M. (1992). Infectious disorders. In K. L. Melmon, H. F. Morrelli, B. B. Hoffman, & D. W. Nierenberg (Eds.), *Clinical pharmacology: Basic principles in therapeutics* (3rd ed.) (pp. 642–720). New York: McGraw-Hill.

Rhodes, K. H. (1992). Antibiotic therapy for severe infections in infants and children. *Mayo Clinic Proceedings, 67,* 59–68.

Streit, L. A. (1992). Nursing management of adults with infections. In L. O. Burrell (Ed.), *Adult nursing in hospital and community settings* (pp. 79–99). Norwalk, CT: Appleton & Lange.

Stutman, H. R. (1993). Cefprozil. *Pediatric Annals, 22,* 167–174.

### CHAPTER 36

# Aminoglycosides

## Aminoglycosides

The aminoglycoside antibiotics are bactericidal agents with similar pharmacologic, antimicrobial, and toxicologic characteristics. They are used to treat infections caused by gram-negative microorganisms, such as *Pseudomonas*, *Proteus*, *Escherichia coli*, *Klebsiella*, *Enterobacter*, and *Serratia* species.

These drugs are poorly absorbed (5% or less) from the gastrointestinal (GI) tract. Thus, when given orally, they exert local effects in the GI tract. They are well absorbed from intramuscular injection sites and reach peak effects in 30 to 90 minutes if circulatory status is good. After intravenous administration, peak effects occur within 30 to 60 minutes. Plasma half-life is 2 to 4 hours with normal renal function.

Following systemic administration, aminoglycosides are widely distributed in extracellular fluid and reach therapeutic levels in blood, urine, bone, inflamed joints, and pleural and ascitic fluids. They accumulate in high concentrations in the kidney and inner ear. They are poorly distributed to the central nervous system, intraocular fluids, and respiratory tract secretions.

Systemic drugs are not metabolized; they are excreted unchanged in the urine, primarily by glomerular filtration. Oral drugs are excreted in feces.

### MECHANISM OF ACTION

Aminoglycosides penetrate the cell walls of susceptible bacteria and bind irreversibly to 30S ribosomes, intracellular structures that synthesize proteins. As a result, the bacteria cannot synthesize the proteins necessary for their function and replication.

### INDICATIONS FOR USE

The major clinical use of parenteral aminoglycosides is to treat serious, systemic infections caused by susceptible aerobic, gram-negative organisms. Many hospital-acquired infections are caused by gram-negative organisms. These infections have become more common with control of other types of infections, widespread use of antimicrobial drugs, and diseases (*e.g.*, acquired immunodeficiency syndrome) or treatment measures that lower host resistance (*e.g.*, radical surgery and therapy with antineoplastic or immunosuppressive drugs). The infections occur in the respiratory and genitourinary tracts, skin, wounds, bowel, and bloodstream. Any infection with gram-negative organisms may be serious and potentially life threatening. Management is difficult because the organisms are generally less susceptible to antibacterial drugs, and drug-resistant strains develop rapidly. The few drugs that are effective against them are relatively toxic. In pseudomonal infections, an aminoglycoside is often given concurrently with an antipseudomonal penicillin (*e.g.*, ticarcillin [Ticar]) for synergistic therapeutic effects. The penicillin-induced breakdown of the bacterial cell wall makes it easier for the aminoglycoside to reach its site of action inside the bacterial cell. However, the drugs are chemically and physically incompatible. Therefore, they should not be mixed in a syringe or an intravenous fluid because the aminoglycoside will be deactivated.

A second clinical use is for treatment of tuberculosis.

Anne Collins Abrams: CLINICAL DRUG THERAPY, Fourth Edition.
© 1995 J.B. Lippincott Company.

Streptomycin was often used before the development of other effective and less toxic antitubercular drugs, such as isoniazid and rifampin. Now, streptomycin is no longer marketed and is available only from the Centers for Disease Control and Prevention for treatment of tuberculosis resistant to other antitubercular drugs. Currently, multidrug-resistant strains of the tuberculosis organism, including strains resistant to both isoniazid and rifampin, are being identified with increasing frequency. This development is leading some authorities to recommend an aminoglycoside as part of a three- or four-drug regimen, at least during the first 2 months until culture and susceptibility reports are available.

A third clinical use of aminoglycosides is oral administration to suppress intestinal bacteria. Neomycin and kanamycin may be given before colonoscopy or bowel surgery and to treat hepatic coma. In hepatic coma, intestinal bacteria produce ammonia, which enters the bloodstream and causes encephalopathy. Drug therapy to suppress intestinal bacteria decreases ammonia production. Paromomycin is used mainly in the treatment of intestinal amebiasis.

A few aminoglycosides are administered topically to the eye or to the skin. These are discussed in Chapters 68 and 69, respectively.

## CONTRAINDICATIONS FOR USE

Aminoglycosides are contraindicated in infections for which less toxic drugs are effective. The drugs are nephrotoxic and ototoxic and must be used cautiously in the presence of renal impairment. Dosages are adjusted according to serum drug levels and creatinine clearance. The drugs also must be used cautiously in clients with myasthenia gravis and other neuromuscular disorders because muscle weakness may be increased.

# Individual aminoglycosides

**Amikacin** (Amikin) is a semisynthetic derivative of kanamycin. It has a broader spectrum of antibacterial activity than other aminoglycosides because it resists degradation by most enzymes that inactivate gentamicin and tobramycin. Consequently, its major clinical use is in infections caused by organisms resistant to other aminoglycosides (*e.g., Pseudomonas, Proteus, E. coli, Klebsiella, Enterobacter, Serratia*), whether community or hospital acquired.

### Routes and dosage ranges

*Adults, children, and older infants:* IM, IV 15 mg/kg per day in two or three divided doses, q8–12h

*Neonates:* IM, IV 10 mg/kg initially, then 7.5 mg/kg q12h

**Gentamicin** (Garamycin), a frequently prescribed aminoglycoside, is effective against a number of gram-negative organisms, although resistance of *Pseudomonas* is increasing. Gentamicin acts synergistically with ticarcillin and related penicillins against *Pseudomonas* infections. The combination also inhibits the emergence of resistant bacteria that may occur when either drug is used alone.

### Routes and dosage ranges

*Adults:* IV, IM 3–5 mg/kg per day in three divided doses, q8h (dosage adjusted according to renal function)
*Children:* IV, IM 6–7.5 mg/kg per day in three divided doses, q8h
*Infants and neonates:* IV, IM 7.5 mg/kg per day in three divided doses, q8h
*Premature infants and neonates less than 1 week of age:* IV, IM 5 mg/kg per day in two divided doses, q12h

**Kanamycin** (Kantrex) is occasionally used to decrease bowel bacteria before diagnostic procedures (*e.g.,* colonoscopy) or surgery and in hepatic coma.

### Routes and dosage ranges

*Adults:* IM 15 mg/kg per day in two or three divided doses, q8–12h; maximum dose, 1.5 g/d
Hepatic coma, PO 8–12 g/d in divided doses
Bowel sterilization, PO 1 g q1h for 4 h followed by 1 g q6h for 36–72 h
*Children:* PO 50 mg/kg per day in four divided doses, q6h
IM up to 15 mg/kg per day in two to four divided doses, q6–12h
*Infants and neonates:* IV, IM 5–15 mg/kg per day in two to four divided doses, q6–12h

**Neomycin** (Mycifradin, Otobiotic) is the most toxic aminoglycoside and is recommended for oral or topical use only. It is given orally to decrease bacterial flora in the colon before colonoscopy or bowel surgery and in hepatic coma. Although the drug is poorly absorbed from the GI tract, toxic levels may accumulate when renal disease is present. It is used topically, often in combination with other drugs, for infections of the eye, ear, and skin (burns, wounds, ulcers, dermatoses). When it is used for wound or bladder irrigations, systemic absorption may occur if the area is large or if drug concentration exceeds 0.1%.

### Routes and dosage ranges

*Adults:* Before bowel surgery, PO 4–8 g/d in four divided doses for 1–3 d

Hepatic coma, PO 4–8 g/d in four divided doses for 5–6 d

Infectious diarrhea, PO 50 mg/kg per day in four divided doses

External otitis, topically to ear 2 drops of otic solution three or four times daily

Skin lesions, topically to skin, application of topical ointment or cream two to four times per day

Continuous bladder irrigation, 1 ml Neosporin GU Irrigant (neomycin 40 mg and polymyxin B 200,000 U/ml) in 1000 ml 0.9% sodium chloride irrigating solution over 24 h

*Infants and children:* Infectious diarrhea, PO 50–100 mg/kg per day in four divided doses

External otitis and skin lesions, same as for adults

*Neonates and premature infants:* Infectious diarrhea, PO 10–50 mg/kg per day in four divided doses

**Netilmicin** (Netromycin) is similar to gentamicin in its antimicrobial spectrum but is reportedly less active against *Pseudomonas aeruginosa*. It also may be less nephrotoxic and ototoxic than other aminoglycosides.

### Routes and dosage ranges

*Adults:* IM, IV 4–6.5 mg/kg per day in two or three divided doses, q8–12h

*Infants and children (6 weeks to 12 years):* 5.5–8 mg/kg per day in two to three divided doses, q8–12h

*Neonates (under 6 weeks):* 4–6.5 mg/kg per day, in divided doses, q12h

**Paromomycin sulfate** (Humatin) is an oral aminoglycoside that acts against bacteria and amebae in the intestinal lumen. It is used in the treatment of hepatic coma and intestinal amebiasis. It is ineffective in extraintestinal sites of amebic infection. Paromomycin is not absorbed from the GI tract and is therefore unlikely to cause the ototoxicity and nephrotoxicity associated with systemically absorbed aminoglycosides. However, systemic absorption may occur in the presence of inflammatory or ulcerative bowel disease.

### Route and dosage ranges

*Adults:* Intestinal amebiasis PO 25–35 mg/kg per day, in three divided doses, with meals, for 5–10 d. The course of therapy may be repeated after 2 wk, if necessary.

Hepatic coma, PO 4 g/d in divided doses for 5–6 days

*Children:* Intestinal amebiasis, same as adults

**Tobramycin** (Nebcin) is similar to gentamicin in its antibacterial spectrum, although it may be more active

against *Pseudomonas* organisms, especially when ticarcillin is given concurrently. Tobramycin also may be indicated in serious staphylococcal infections when penicillins or other less toxic drugs are contraindicated or ineffective. It is often used with other antibiotics for septicemia and infections of burn wounds, other soft tissues, bone, the urinary tract, and the central nervous system. Dosage must be reduced with impaired renal function.

### Routes and dosage ranges

*Adults and children:* IM, IV 3–5 mg/kg per day in three or four divided doses, q6–8h

*Neonates (1 week or less):* IM, IV up to 4 mg/kg per day in two divided doses, q12h

## Nursing Process

General aspects of the nursing process as described in Chapter 33 apply to the client receiving aminoglycosides. In this chapter, only aspects related specifically to aminoglycosides are included.

### Assessment

Assess for the presence of factors that predispose to nephrotoxicity or ototoxicity:

- Check laboratory reports of renal function (*e.g.*, serum creatinine, creatinine clearance, and blood urea nitrogen [BUN]) for abnormal values.
- Assess for impairment of balance or hearing, including audiometry reports if available.
- Analyze current medications for drugs that interact with aminoglycosides to increase risks of nephrotoxicity or ototoxicity.

### Planning/Goals

*The client will:*
- Receive dosages individualized by age, weight, renal function, and serum drug levels
- Have serum drug levels monitored regularly and accurately
- Have renal function tests performed regularly
- Be well hydrated during aminoglycoside therapy
- Be observed daily for adverse drug effects

### Interventions

- Monitor laboratory reports of BUN, serum creatinine, creatinine clearance, serum drug levels, and urinalysis as available.
- Force fluids to at least 2000 to 3000 ml daily if not contraindicated. Keeping the client well hydrated reduces nephrotoxicity.
- Avoid concurrent use of other nephrotoxic drugs when possible.
- Weigh clients accurately. The dosage of aminoglycosides is based on weight in kilograms.

### Evaluation

- Interview and observe for improvement in the infection being treated.
- Interview and observe for adverse drug effects.

# Principles of therapy

## LIMITATIONS ON USE

Because of a high incidence of toxicity, aminoglycoside antibiotics should be used only in serious infections caused by susceptible microorganisms and for which less toxic drugs are unavailable.

## CHOICE OF DRUG

Gentamicin is probably the aminoglycoside of choice for systemic infections if resistant microorganisms have not developed in the clinical setting. If gentamicin-resistant organisms have developed, amikacin or tobramycin may be given because they are less susceptible to drug-destroying enzymes. In terms of toxicity, the drugs cause similar effects, except that tobramycin may cause less nephrotoxicity and netilmicin may cause less ototoxicity.

## DRUG DOSAGE

Dosage of aminoglycosides must be carefully regulated because therapeutic doses are close to toxic doses. Some guidelines include the following:

1. An *initial loading dose* is given to achieve therapeutic serum levels rapidly. The amount is based on weight and desired peak serum level. If the client is obese, ideal body weight should be used because aminoglycosides are not significantly distributed in body fat. In clients with normal renal function, the recommended loading dose for gentamicin, tobramycin, and netilmicin is 1.5 to 2 mg/kg of body weight; for amikacin, the loading dose is 5 to 7.5 mg/kg.
2. *Maintenance doses* should be based on serum drug levels. Peak serum levels should be assessed 30 to 60 minutes after drug administration (5–8 µg/ml for gentamicin and tobramycin, 20–30 µg/ml for amikacin, and 4–12 µg/ml for netilmicin). Measurement of peak and trough levels is needed to establish and maintain therapeutic serum levels without excessive toxicity. For gentamicin and tobramycin, peak levels above 10 to 12 µg/ml and trough levels above 2 µg/ml for prolonged periods have been associated with nephrotoxicity. For accuracy, blood samples must be drawn at the correct times.
3. *With impaired renal function*, the dosage of aminoglycoside antibiotics must be reduced. Methods of adjusting drug dosage include measuring serum drug levels or lengthening the time between doses according to creatinine clearance levels. For specific instructions, consult the manufacturer's literature on gentamicin, tobramycin, amikacin, and netilmicin.
4. *In urinary tract infections*, smaller doses can be used than in systemic infections because the aminoglycosides reach high concentrations in the urine. Also, alkalinizing the urine increases the effectiveness of drug therapy. The drugs are much more active in an alkaline environment than in an acidic one.

## GUIDELINES FOR REDUCING TOXICITY

In addition to the previous recommendations, guidelines to decrease the incidence and severity of adverse effects include the following:

1. Identify clients at high risk of adverse effects (*e.g.*, neonates, older adults, clients with renal impairment, and clients with concurrent disease processes or drug therapies that impair blood circulation and renal function).
2. Keep clients well hydrated to decrease drug concentration in serum and body tissues.
3. Avoid concurrent administration of diuretics. Diuretics may increase nephrotoxicity by decreasing fluid volume, thereby increasing drug concentration in serum and tissues. Dehydration is most likely to occur with loop diuretics, such as furosemide (Lasix).
4. Give the drug for no longer than 10 days. Clients are most at risk when high doses are given for prolonged periods.
5. Detect adverse effects early, and reduce dosage or discontinue the drug. Changes in renal function tests that indicate nephrotoxicity may not occur until the client has received an aminoglycoside for about 5 days. If nephrotoxicity occurs, it is usually reversible if the drug is stopped. Early ototoxicity is detectable only with audiometric tests.

## USE IN CHILDREN

Aminoglycosides must be used cautiously in children as with adults. Dosage must be calculated accurately according to weight and renal function. Serum drug levels must be monitored and dosage adjusted as indicated to avoid toxicity. Neonates may have increased risk of nephrotoxicity and ototoxicity because of their immature renal function. Neomycin is not recommended for use in infants and children.

## USE IN OLDER ADULTS

Aminoglycosides should not be used in the presence of impaired renal function if less toxic drugs are effective against causative organisms. When the drugs are given to older adults, extreme caution is required. Because of impaired renal function, other disease processes, and multiple drug therapy, older adults are at high risk of developing nephrotoxicity and ototoxicity. Interventions to decrease the incidence and severity of adverse drug effects are listed above. These interventions are important with any client receiving an aminoglycoside but are especially important with older adults.

# NURSING ACTIONS: AMINOGLYCOSIDES

| *Nursing Actions* | *Rationale/Explanation* |
|---|---|
| **1. Administer accurately** | |
| **a.** For intravenous administration, dilute gentamicin, tobramycin, amikacin, or netilmicin in 50 to 100 ml of 5% dextrose or 0.9% sodium chloride injection and infuse over 30 to 60 minutes. Concentration of gentamicin should not exceed 1 mg/ml. | To achieve therapeutic blood levels |
| **b.** Give intramuscular aminoglycosides in a large muscle mass, and rotate sites. | To avoid local tissue irritation. This is less likely to occur with aminoglycosides than with most other antibiotics. |
| **2. Observe for therapeutic effects** | |
| **a.** Decreased local and systemic signs of infection | See Chapter 33. |
| **b.** Decreased signs and symptoms of the specific infection for which the drug is being given | |
| **3. Observe for adverse effects** | Adverse effects are more likely to occur with parenteral administration of large doses for prolonged periods. However, they may occur with oral administration in the presence of renal impairment and with usual therapeutic doses. |
| **a.** Nephrotoxicity—casts, albumin, red or white blood cells in urine, decreased creatinine clearance, increased serum creatinine, increased blood urea nitrogen. | Renal damage is most likely to occur in clients who are elderly, receive high doses or prolonged therapy, have prior renal damage, or receive other nephrotoxic drugs. This is the most serious adverse reaction. Risks of kidney damage can be minimized by using the drugs appropriately, detecting early signs of renal impairment, and keeping clients well hydrated. |
| **b.** Ototoxicity—deafness or decreased hearing, tinnitus, dizziness, ataxia | This results from damage to the eighth cranial nerve. Incidence of ototoxicity is increased in older clients and those with previous auditory damage, high doses or prolonged duration, and concurrent use of other ototoxic drugs. |
| **c.** Neurotoxicity—respiratory paralysis and apnea | This is caused by neuromuscular blockade and is more likely to occur after rapid intravenous injection, administration to a client with myasthenia gravis, or concomitant administration of general anesthetics or neuromuscular blocking agents (*e.g.*, succinylcholine, tubocurarine). This effect also may occur if an aminoglycoside is administered shortly after surgery, owing to the residual effects of anesthetics or neuromuscular blockers. Neostigmine or calcium may be given to counteract apnea. |
| **d.** Hypersensitivity—skin rash, urticaria | This is an uncommon reaction except with topical neomycin, which may cause sensitization in as many as 10% of recipients. |
| **e.** Nausea, vomiting, diarrhea, peripheral neuritis, paresthesias | Uncommon with parenteral aminoglycosides. Diarrhea often occurs with oral administration. |
| **4. Observe for drug interactions.** | |
| **a.** Drugs that *increase* effects of aminoglycosides: | The listed drugs increase toxicity. |
| (1) Loop diuretics (furosemide, ethacrynic acid, bumetanide) | Increased nephrotoxicity apparently caused by increased drug concentration in serum and tissues when the client is relatively "dehydrated" by potent diuretics |

## Nursing Actions

## Rationale/Explanation

(2) Methoxyflurane (Penthrane) and nephrotoxic anti-microbial agents (amphotericin B, cephalosporins, colistimethate, polymyxin)

Increased nephrotoxicity

(3) Drugs with neuromuscular blocking activity (methoxyflurane, procainamide, promethazine, quinidine, sodium citrate, succinylcholine, tubocurarine)

Increased neuromuscular blockade with possible paralysis of respiratory muscles and apnea. This is most likely to occur with succinylcholine and tubocurarine (see 3c).

**5. Teach clients**

**a.** Report ringing in the ears, loss of hearing, dizziness, or unsteady gait.

These are symptoms of ototoxicity.

**b.** Drink 2000 to 3000 ml of fluid per day if not contraindicated or received by intravenous infusion.

To reduce damage to the kidneys.

**c.** Wash hands thoroughly and often, especially after contact with any secretions or urine.

To help prevent spread of infection and development of drug-resistant organisms

## Review and Application Exercises

1. How do aminoglycosides exert bactericidal effects?
2. Why must aminoglycosides be given parenterally for systemic infections?
3. How are aminoglycosides excreted?
4. What are risk factors for aminoglycoside-induced nephrotoxicity and ototoxicity?
5. How would you assess a client for nephrotoxicity or ototoxicity?
6. What is the reason for giving an aminoglycoside and an antipseudomonal penicillin in the treatment of serious infections caused by *P. aeruginosa?*
7. Why should an aminoglycoside and an antipseudomonal penicillin *not* be combined in a syringe or intravenous fluid for administration?

8. Which laboratory tests need to be monitored regularly for a client receiving a systemic aminoglycoside?
9. When neomycin is given orally, what is the desired effect?
10. What is the rationale for giving an oral aminoglycoside to treat hepatic coma?

## Selected References

(1993). *Drug facts and comparisons.* St. Louis: Facts and Comparisons.

Lietman, P. S. (1990). Aminoglycosides and spectinomycin: Aminocyclitols. In G. L. Mandell, R. G. Douglas Jr., & J. E. Bennett (Eds.), *Principles and practice of infectious diseases* (3rd ed.) (pp. 269–284). New York: Churchill Livingstone.

Rhodes, K. H. (1992). Antibiotic therapy for severe infections in infants and children. *Mayo Clinic Proceedings, 67,* 59–68.

### CHAPTER 37

# Tetracyclines

## Tetracyclines

The tetracyclines are broad-spectrum, bacteriostatic antimicrobial drugs that are similar in chemical structure, pharmacologic properties, and antimicrobial activity. They are effective against a wide range of gram-positive and gram-negative organisms, as well as rickettsiae, mycoplasmas, some protozoa, spirochetes, and others. Most can be given orally or parenterally, and they are widely distributed into most body tissues and fluids. They are excreted in urine and feces. The older tetracyclines are excreted mainly in urine and the newer ones (doxycycline and minocycline) mainly in feces. All tetracyclines are excreted in bile, enter the intestine, and are partially reabsorbed (enterohepatic recirculation).

Tetracyclines decrease the effectiveness of penicillins and cephalosporins and should not be given concurrently with them. Tetracyclines are bacteriostatic and slow the rate of bacterial multiplication; penicillins and cephalosporins are bactericidal agents that are most effective against rapidly multiplying bacteria.

### MECHANISM OF ACTION

Tetracyclines penetrate microbial cells by passive diffusion and an active transport system. Intracellularly, they bind to 30S ribosomes, like the aminoglycosides, and inhibit microbial protein synthesis.

### INDICATIONS FOR USE

Despite a broad spectrum of antimicrobial activity, a tetracycline is the first drug of choice in only a few infections (*e.g.*, cholera, granuloma inguinale, chancroid, Rocky Mountain spotted fever, psittacosis, typhus, trachoma). Other drugs (*e.g.*, penicillin) are usually prefer-

red in gram-positive infections, and most gram-negative organisms are resistant to tetracyclines. However, a tetracycline may be used if bacterial susceptibility is confirmed. Specific clinical indications for tetracyclines include:

1. Treatment of uncomplicated urethral, endocervical, or rectal infections caused by *Chlamydia* organisms
2. Adjunctive treatment, with other antimicrobials, in the treatment of pelvic inflammatory disease and sexually transmitted diseases
3. Long-term treatment of acne. They interfere with the production of free fatty acids and decrease *Corynebacterium* in sebum. These actions decrease the inflammatory, pustular lesions associated with severe acne.
4. Sometimes, as a substitute for penicillin in penicillin-allergic clients. They are effective in treating gonorrhea and syphilis when penicillin cannot be given. They should not be substituted for penicillin for treating streptococcal pharyngitis because microbial resistance is common, and tetracyclines do not prevent rheumatic fever. In addition, they should not be substituted for penicillin in any serious staphylococcal infection because microbial resistance commonly occurs.
5. Doxycycline may be used to prevent traveler's diarrhea due to enterotoxic strains of *Escherichia coli*.
6. Demeclocycline may be used to inhibit antidiuretic hormone in the management of chronic inappropriate antidiuretic hormone secretion.

### CONTRAINDICATIONS FOR USE

The major contraindication for the use of tetracyclines is renal failure. High concentrations of tetracyclines inhibit protein synthesis in human cells. This antianabolic effect increases tissue breakdown (catabolism) and the

Anne Collins Abrams: CLINICAL DRUG THERAPY, Fourth Edition.
© 1995 J.B. Lippincott Company.

amount of waste products to be excreted by the kidneys. The increased workload can be handled by normally functioning kidneys, but waste products are retained when renal function is impaired. This leads to azotemia, increased blood urea nitrogen, hyperphosphatemia, hyperkalemia, and acidosis. If a tetracycline is necessary because of an organism's sensitivity or the host's inability to take other antimicrobial drugs, doxycycline or minocycline should be given.

Nephrotoxicity has occurred from the use of outdated tetracyclines. Expiration dates should be monitored and outdated drugs discarded.

Tetracyclines also are contraindicated in pregnant women and in children up to 8 years of age. During pregnancy, tetracyclines may cause fatal hepatic necrosis in the mother. In the fetus and young child, tetracyclines are deposited in bones and teeth along with calcium. If given during active mineralization of these tissues, tetracyclines can cause permanent brown coloring (mottling) of tooth enamel and can depress bone growth. Tetracyclines should not be used in children unless other drugs are ineffective or contraindicated.

Individual tetracyclines are listed in Table 37-1.

## TABLE 37-1.  TETRACYCLINES

| Generic/Trade Name | Characteristics | Routes and Dosages | |
|---|---|---|---|
| | | **Adults** | **Children** |
| **Tetracycline hydrochloride** (Achromycin, others) | 1. Prototype drug<br>2. Marketed under generic and numerous trade names<br>3. Probably the most frequently used tetracycline<br>4. Parenteral formulation withdrawn from market | PO 250–500 mg q6h | PO 22–44 mg/kg per day in four divided doses |
| **Demeclocycline** (Declomycin) | 1. Has a longer half-life than tetracycline, and smaller doses produce therapeutic serum levels<br>2. The tetracycline most likely to cause photosensitivity<br>3. May be used to promote diuresis when fluid retention is caused by inappropriate secretion of antidiuretic hormone | PO 150 mg q6h or 300 mg q12h<br>Gonorrhea in penicillin-sensitive clients, PO 600 mg initially, followed by 300 mg q12h for 4 days | Age over 8 years, PO 3–6 mg/kg per day in two to four divided doses |
| **Doxycycline** (Vibramycin) | 1. A newer tetracycline that is better absorbed from the gastrointestinal tract than older preparations. Oral administration yields serum drug levels equivalent to those obtained by parenteral administration.<br>2. Highly lipid-soluble; therefore, reaches therapeutic levels in cerebrospinal fluid (CSF), the eye, and the prostate gland<br>3. Can be given in smaller doses and less frequently than other tetracyclines because of long serum half-life (about 18 h)<br>4. Excreted by kidneys to a lesser extent than other tetracyclines and is the only tetracycline considered safe for clients with impaired renal function | PO 100 mg q12h for 2 doses, then once daily or in divided doses; severe infections, 100 mg q12h<br>IV 200 mg the first day, then 100–200 mg daily in one or two doses | PO, IV same as adults for children weighing at least 45 kg<br>Those weighing less than 45 kg:<br>PO 4.4 mg/kg (2 mg/lb) q12h for 2 doses, then 1 mg/kg per day in a single dose; severe infections, 2 mg/kg q12h<br>IV 4.4 mg/kg per day in one or two doses, then 1–2 mg/kg per day, depending on severity of infection |
| **Minocycline** (Minocin) | 1. A relatively new tetracycline that is well absorbed after oral administration<br>2. Like doxycycline, readily penetrates CSF, the eye, and the prostate<br>3. Metabolized more than other tetracyclines, and smaller amounts are excreted in urine and feces | PO, IV 200 mg initially, then 100 mg q12h | Over 12 years old, PO, IV same as adults<br>Under 12 years old, PO, IV 4 mg/kg initially, then 2 mg/kg q12h |
| **Oxytetracycline** (Terramycin) | One of the first tetracyclines developed | PO 250–500 mg q6h, up to 4 g daily in severe infections<br>IM 250 mg daily in a single dose or 200–400 mg daily in two or three divided doses<br>IV 500 mg–1 g daily in two doses; maximal daily dose, 2 g | PO 22–44 mg/kg q6h<br>IM 15–25 mg/kg per day in two or three divided doses<br>IV 10–20 mg/kg per day in two divided doses |

## Nursing Process

See Chapter 33.

## Principles of therapy

1. Culture and sensitivity studies are needed before tetracycline therapy is started because many strains of organisms are either resistant or vary greatly in drug susceptibility. Cross-sensitivity and cross-resistance are common among tetracyclines.
2. The oral route of administration is usually effective and preferred. Parenteral therapy is used when oral administration is contraindicated or for initial treatment of severe infections. Intramuscular injections cause pain, and intravenous infusions cause thrombophlebitis.
3. Tetracyclines decompose with age, exposure to light, and extreme heat and humidity. Because the breakdown products may be toxic, it is important to store

these drugs correctly. Also, the manufacturer's expiration dates on containers should be noted and outdated drugs discarded.

### USE IN CHILDREN

Tetracyclines should not be used in children under 8 years old because of their effects on teeth and bones. In teeth, the drugs interfere with enamel development and may cause a permanent yellow, gray, or brown discoloration. In bone, the drugs form a stable compound in bone-forming tissue and may interfere with bone growth.

### USE IN OLDER ADULTS

Impaired renal function is common among older adults and, with the exceptions of doxycycline (Vibramycin) and minocycline (Minocin), tetracyclines are contraindicated with impaired renal function. Therefore, if a tetracycline is deemed necessary, doxycycline is the drug of choice for older adults.

## NURSING ACTIONS: TETRACYCLINES

| Nursing Actions | Rationale/Explanation |
| --- | --- |
| **1. Administer accurately**<br>**a.** Give most oral tetracycline preparations 1 hour before or 2 hours after meals; give doxycycline and minocycline with food. | Food interferes with absorption of tetracyclines other than doxycycline and minocycline. |
| **b.** Give oral tetracyclines at least 1 hour before or 2 hours after antacids or milk products. | Substances containing aluminum, magnesium, or calcium combine with the drug to form poorly absorbed compounds. |
| **c.** If an oral tetracycline and an iron preparation are ordered, give them as far apart as possible (*e.g.*, tetracycline 3 hours before or 2 hours after the iron supplement). | Iron combines with tetracyclines as do other metallic ions to inhibit absorption. Tetracyclines reach only 10% to 50% of expected serum levels if given with iron. |
| **d.** For parenteral tetracyclines, consult the manufacturer's instructions. | The drugs vary in their routes of administration, methods of preparation, duration of intravenous infusions, and other characteristics. |
| **2. Observe for therapeutic effects**<br>**a.** Decreased local and systemic signs of infection | See Chapter 33. |
| **b.** Decreased signs and symptoms of the specific infection for which the drug is being given | |
| **3. Observe for adverse effects**<br>**a.** Nausea, vomiting, diarrhea | These are the most common adverse reactions and are probably caused by local irritation of gastrointestinal mucosa. After several days of tetracycline therapy, diarrhea may be caused by superinfection. |

## Nursing Actions

## Rationale/Explanation

**b.** Superinfection—sore mouth, white patches on oral mucosa, black furry tongue, diarrhea, skin rash, itching in the perineal area

These signs usually indicate monilial infection. Meticulous oral and perineal hygiene helps prevent these problems. A potentially serious but less common superinfection is colitis, caused by tetracycline-resistant staphylococci. Superinfection is more likely to occur with tetracyclines than with other antibiotics.

**c.** Photosensitivity

This may occur with any tetracycline, but it occurs most often with demeclocycline. It may be prevented by avoiding exposure to sunlight or other sources of ultraviolet light, wearing protective clothing, and using sunscreen lotions.

**d.** Pain and induration with IM injections

This can be minimized by injecting the drug deep into a large muscle mass (*e.g.*, gluteal) and rotating injection sites.

**e.** Thrombophlebitis at the venipuncture site

These drugs are irritating to tissues and cause phlebitis if injected into the same vein for more than 48 to 72 hours.

**f.** Increased blood urea nitrogen and serum creatinine in clients with renal impairment

**g.** Hepatotoxicity—elevated aspartate aminotransferase and other enzymes

Liver toxicity is most likely to occur when renal insufficiency allows accumulation of drug in the blood. It also may occur in pregnant women.

**h.** Blood disorders (neutropenia, thrombocytopenia, anemia) and allergic reactions (skin rash, urticaria, angioedema, anaphylaxis)

These effects rarely occur.

**4. Observe for drug interactions**
   **a.** Drugs that *increase* effects of tetracycline:

   (1) Methoxyflurane (Penthrane)

This anesthetic plus parenteral tetracycline may cause severe nephrotoxicity and death.

   (2) Sulfonamides

The combination is synergistic in certain infections, such as *Nocardia* in brain abscesses, pulmonary or other lesions, lymphogranuloma venereum, and trachoma.

   **b.** Drugs that *decrease* effects of tetracycline:

   (1) Aluminum, calcium, iron, or magnesium preparations (*e.g.*, antacids, ferrous sulfate)

These metals combine with oral tetracyclines to produce insoluble, nonabsorbable compounds that are excreted in feces.

   (2) Cathartics

Decrease absorption

   (3) Sodium bicarbonate

Decreases absorption of tetracyclines about 50%

   (4) Enzyme inducers (*e.g.*, barbiturates, other sedative–hypnotics, phenytoin, carbamazepine)

May increase metabolism of doxycycline

**5. Teach clients**
   **a.** Store tetracyclines in a cool, dry, dark place

The drugs decompose with age and exposure to light, heat, and humidity

   **b.** Take most oral tetracyclines on an empty stomach 1 hour before or 2 hours after meals; take doxycycline and minocycline with food.

Food decreases drug absorption of tetracyclines, except doxycycline and minocycline.

(*continued*)

| *Nursing Actions* | *Rationale/Explanation* |
|---|---|
| **c.** If antacids, iron supplements, or vitamin preparations containing iron must be taken while tetracyclines are also taken, take them as far apart from the tetracyclines as possible (*e.g.*, 3 hours before or 2 hours after the tetracycline). | These drugs combine with tetracyclines with the result that little tetracycline is absorbed. |
| **d.** Do not take milk or milk products with tetracyclines. | Calcium in milk products combines with oral tetracyclines to produce nonabsorbable compounds. |
| **e.** Report severe nausea, vomiting, diarrhea, skin rash, or perineal itching to the physician. | These symptoms may indicate a need for changing or discontinuing tetracycline therapy. |
| **f.** Avoid intense or prolonged exposure to sunlight or to artificial ultraviolet light. If exposure is unavoidable, wear protective clothing, and use a sunscreen lotion. | Tetracyclines, especially demeclocycline, may cause a sunburn or rash reaction. |
| **g.** If the entire prescription of oral tetracycline is not taken, discard the remaining amount. | To avoid having anyone take decomposed tetracyclines, which may have serious results. |

## Review and Application Exercises

1. What is the mechanism of action for tetracyclines?
2. What foods and drugs interfere with the absorption of oral tetracyclines? How can interference be prevented or minimized?
3. What are potentially serious adverse effects of tetracyclines?
4. What is the rationale for long-term, low-dose administration of a tetracycline for acne?
5. Which tetracyclines are contraindicated with renal insufficiency?

## Selected References

(1994). *Drug facts and comparisons.* St. Louis: Facts and Comparisons.
Mandell, G. L., Douglas, R. G. Jr., & Bennett, J. E. (Eds.), *Principles and practice of infectious diseases* (3rd ed.). New York: Churchill Livingstone.
Shlafer, M. (1993). *The nurse, pharmacology, and drug therapy* (2nd ed.). Redwood City, CA: Addison-Wesley.

# CHAPTER 38

# Macrolides

## Macrolides

The macrolide antibiotics include erythromycin, azithromycin (Zithromax), and clarithromycin (Biaxin). Although the drugs differ somewhat in chemical structure, they have the same mechanism of action and similar antimicrobial activity. They may be bacteriostatic or bactericidal, depending largely on drug concentration in infected tissues. They are effective against gram-positive cocci, including group A streptococci, pneumococci, and most staphylococci. They are also effective against species of *Corynebacterium, Treponema, Neisseria*, and *Mycoplasma* and against some anaerobic organisms, such as *Bacteroides* and *Clostridia*. Compared with erythromycin, azithromycin is less active and clarithromycin is more active against most streptococci and staphylycocci. However, streptococci and staphylococci that are resistant to erythromycin also are resistant to azithromycin and clarithromycin. In addition, azithromycin and clarithromycin require less frequent administration and reportedly cause less nausea, vomiting, and diarrhea than erythromycin.

The macrolides are widely distributed in body tissues and fluids, including pleural fluid and sputum, ascitic fluid, and middle-ear exudates. The drugs may enter cerebrospinal fluid when meninges are inflamed. Erythromycin is metabolized primarily in the liver and excreted in bile, with some reabsorption from the gastrointestinal tract. About 20% is excreted in urine. Azithromycin is mainly excreted unchanged in bile, and clarithromycin is metabolized to an active metabolite in the liver and excreted in urine.

## MECHANISM OF ACTION

The macrolides enter microbial cells and attach to 50S ribosomes, thereby inhibiting microbial protein synthesis.

## INDICATIONS FOR USE

Erythromycin is considered one of the safest antibiotics available. It is often used as a penicillin substitute in clients who are allergic to penicillin. Specific clinical indications include:

1. Suppression of intestinal bacteria before colonoscopy or bowel surgery. It is used with neomycin for this purpose.
2. Legionnaires' disease. Erythromycin is the drug of choice for this pneumonia-like disease caused by the gram-negative bacillus *Legionella pneumophila*.
3. Infections caused by *Mycoplasma pneumoniae*
4. Prevention of whooping cough in household contacts
5. Elimination of the diphtheria carrier state as an adjunct to diphtheria antitoxin
6. Substitute for penicillin in prophylaxis of rheumatic fever, gonorrhea, and syphilis and in treatment of pneumococcal pneumonia, streptococcal pharyngitis, and syphilis

Azithromycin and clarithromycin are indicated for the treatment of respiratory tract infections caused by susceptible organisms (*e.g., Streptococcus pyogenes* or *Streptococcus pneumoniae*) and skin or soft tissue infections caused by *Staphylococcus aureus* or *Streptococcus pyogenes*.

Anne Collins Abrams: CLINICAL DRUG THERAPY, Fourth Edition.
© 1995 J.B. Lippincott Company.

**407**

## CONTRAINDICATIONS FOR USE

The drugs are contraindicated in people who have hypersensitivity reactions to macrolides. They also are contraindicated or must be used with caution in clients with preexisting liver disease.

## Individual macrolides

**Erythromycin** is available in numerous preparations, none of which is more effective than erythromycin base or erythromycin stearate. Oral forms, except the estolate salt, are coated or buffered to prevent destruction by gastric acid. The estolate salt is stable in gastric acid. Topical and ophthalmic preparations are discussed in other chapters. For trade names, routes of administration, and dosage ranges, see Table 38-1.

### Azithromycin

#### Route and dosage ranges

*Adults:* PO 500 mg as a single dose on the first day, then 250 mg once daily for 4 days for most infections. For nongonococcal urethritis and cervicitis caused by *Chlamydia trachomatis*, give 1 g as a single dose.

### Clarithromycin

#### Route and dosage ranges

*Adults:* PO 250–500 mg q12h for 7 to 14 days

## Nursing Process

See Chapter 33.

## Principles of therapy

1. Specimens for culture and sensitivity studies should be obtained before the first drug dose because these drugs have a narrow spectrum of antibacterial activity. They are mainly effective against gram-positive organisms, and a number of organisms are resistant. Drug therapy is often started before results are available, especially with serious infections.
2. Erythromycin interferes with the elimination of several drugs, especially those metabolized by the cytochrome P-450 enzymes in the liver. As a result, the affected drugs are eliminated more slowly, their serum levels are increased, and they are more likely to cause adverse effects and toxicity unless dosage is reduced. Interacting drugs include alfentanil (Alfenta), astemizole (Hismanal), bromocriptine (Parlodel), carbamazepine (Tegretol), cyclosporine (Sandimmune), digoxin (Lanoxin), disopyramide (Norpace), methylprednisolone (Medrol), terfenadine (Seldane), theophylline (Theo-Dur), triazolam (Halcion), and warfarin (Coumadin). These drugs represent a variety of drug classes. When erythromycin has been given concurrently with the nonsedating antihistamines astemizole or terfenadine, serious ventricular arrhythmias and fatalities have been reported. Although these interactions have not been reported with azithromycin or clarithromycin, their

### TABLE 38-1. ERYTHROMYCIN PREPARATIONS

| Generic/ Trade Name | Usual Routes and Dosage Ranges | | Remarks |
| --- | --- | --- | --- |
| | *Adults* | *Children* | |
| **Erythromycin base** (E-mycin) | PO 250–500 mg q6h; severe infections, up to 4 g or more daily in divided doses | PO 30–50 mg/kg per day in divided doses q6–12h, severe infections, 100 mg/kg per day in divided doses | |
| **Erythromycin estolate** (Ilosone) | PO 250 mg q6h; maximal daily dose, 4 g | Weight over 25 kg, PO same as adults Weight 10–25 kg, PO 30–50 mg/kg per day in divided doses Weight under 10 kg, PO 10 mg/kg per day in divided doses q6–12h Dosages may be doubled in severe infections. | This preparation may cause cholestatic jaundice and hepatotoxicity. It should not be used with known or suspected hepatic insufficiency. |
| **Erythromycin ethylsuccinate** (E.E.S.) | PO 400 mg four times daily; severe infections, up to 4 g or more daily in divided doses | PO 30–50 mg/kg/day in 4 divided doses q6h. Severe infections, 60–100 mg/kg/day in divided doses | |
| **Erythromycin lactobionate** | IV 15–20 mg/kg per day in divided doses; severe infections, up to 4 g daily | IV same as adults | |
| **Erythromycin stearate** (Erythrocin stearate) | PO 250 mg q6h or 500 mg q12h; severe infections, up to 4 g daily | PO 30–50 mg/kg per day in four divided doses q6h; severe infections, 60–100 mg/kg per day | |

potential occurrence needs to be considered for clients receiving the listed or similar drugs.

3. When erythromycin is used for preoperative bowel preparation, erythromycin base, rather than estolate or stearate, is routinely used. Neomycin and erythromycin base is a useful combination because it suppresses the entire bacterial flora of the colon. However, antibiotic bowel preparation is adjunctive to mechanical bowel cleansing (*e.g.*, liquid diet, laxatives, enemas).

4. In renal failure, the dosage of erythromycin does not need reduction because the drug is excreted primarily by the liver. With clarithromycin, dosage should be reduced; no data are available about azithromycin dosage in renal failure.

5. In liver disease, macrolide antibiotics should be used cautiously, if at all. Because these drugs are eliminated through the liver, they may accumulate and cause toxic effects in the presence of liver disease. In most conditons, other drugs should be substituted.

## USE IN CHILDREN

Erythromycin is commonly used for streptococcal and other infections in children. It is generally considered safe. Azithromycin and clarithromycin have not been approved for use in children.

## USE IN OLDER ADULTS

Erythromycin is generally considered safe. Because it is metabolized in the liver and excreted in bile, it may be useful in clients with impaired renal function. Little information is available about the use of azithromycin and clarithromycin in older adults. A small group given high doses of clarithromycin (1000 mg q12h) for chronic mycobacterial (*Mycobacterium avium* complex or *Mycobacterium abscessus*) lung disease experienced a high incidence of adverse effects, including elevated liver enzymes. The group tolerated smaller doses of 500 mg q12h.

## NURSING ACTIONS: MACROLIDES

| *Nursing Actions* | *Rationale/Explanation* |
| --- | --- |
| **1. Administer accurately**<br>**a.** Give oral erythromycin and azithromycin on an empty stomach, 1 hour before or 2 hours after a meal. Give clarithromycin without regard to food intake. | To aid absorption and maintenance of therapeutic serum drug levels. Food in the gastrointestinal tract decreases absorption of erythromycin and azithromycin but does not interfere with absorption of clarithromycin. |
| **b.** For IV erythromycin, consult the manufacturer's instructions for dissolving, diluting, and administering the drug. Infuse continuously or intermittently (*e.g.*, q6h over 30–60 minutes). | The IV formulation has limited stability in solution, and instructions must be followed carefully to achieve therapeutic effects. Also, instructions differ for intermittent and continuous infusions. IV erythromycin is the treatment of choice for Legionnaires' disease. Otherwise, it is rarely used. |
| **2. Observe for therapeutic effects**<br>**a.** Decreased local and systemic signs of infection | See Chapter 33. |
| **b.** Decreased signs and symptoms of the specific infection for which the drug is being given. | |
| **3. Observe for adverse effects**<br>**a.** Nausea, vomiting, diarrhea | These are the most frequent adverse reactions, reportedly less common with azithromycin and clarithromycin than with erythromycin. |
| **b.** With IV erythromycin, phlebitis at the IV infusion site | The drug is very irritating to body tissues. Phlebitis can be minimized by diluting the drug well, infusing it slowly, and not using the same vein for more than 48 to 72 hours, if possible. |

(*continued*)

## Nursing Actions

## Rationale/Explanation

**c.** Hepatotoxicity—nausea, vomiting, abdominal cramps, fever, leukocytosis, abnormal liver function, and possibly jaundice

More likely to occur with the estolate formulation but has been reported with other preparations as well

**d.** Allergic reactions (anaphylaxis, skin rash, urticaria)

Potentially serious but infrequent

**4. Observe for drug interactions**
  **a.** Drugs that *increase* effects of erythromycin:

  (1) Chloramphenicol (Chloromycetin)

The combination is effective against some strains of resistant *Staphylococcus aureus*.

  (2) Streptomycin

The combination is effective against the enterococcus in bacteremia, brain abscess, endocarditis, meningitis, and urinary tract infections.

  **b.** Drugs that *decrease* effects of macrolides:

  (1) Antacids

Decrease absorption

**5. Teach clients**
  **a.** Take oral erythromycin and azithromycin with water, and minimize food intake just before or after taking the drug.

See Chapter 33.
To increase drug absorption and therapeutic benefits

  **b.** Report severe nausea, vomiting, diarrhea, skin rash, or hives.

These are adverse reactions, and their occurrence may require discontinuation of the drug, decrease in dosage, or other alterations in therapy.

## Review and Application Exercises

1. Why is erythromycin called a penicillin substitute?
2. What are adverse effects with erythromycin, and how may they be prevented or minimized?
3. Why is erythromycin seldom given parenterally?
4. How are the macrolides excreted? What difference does this make in client care?
5. How do azithromycin and clarithromycin differ from erythromycin?

## Selected References

(1993). *Drug facts and comparisons*. St. Louis: Facts and Comparisons.

Hammerschlag, M. R. (1993). Azithromycin and clarithromycin. *Pediatric Annals, 22,* 161–166.

Mandell, G. L., Douglas, R. G. Jr., & Bennett, J. E. (Eds.) (1990). *Principles and practice of infectious diseases* (3rd ed.). New York: Churchill Livingstone.

Wallace, R. J. Jr., Brown, B. A., & Griffith, D. E. (1993). Drug intolerance to high-dose clarithromycin among elderly patients. *Diagnostic Microbiology and Infectious Disease, 16,* 215–221.

### CHAPTER 39

# Miscellaneous Anti-infectives

The drugs described in this chapter are heterogeneous in their characteristics and uses. The nonpenicillin, noncephalosporin beta-lactams and the quinolones (also called fluoroquinolones) are relatively new drugs that are considered significant advances in antimicrobial drug therapy. Most of the other drugs are older and have limited clinical usefulness, mainly because they are more toxic than alternative agents.

## Beta-lactams

**Aztreonam** (Azactam) is a monobactam with activity against a wide spectrum of gram-negative bacteria, including *Enterobacteriaceae*, *Pseudomonas aeruginosa*, and many strains that are resistant to multiple antibiotics. Activity against gram-negative bacteria is similar to that of the aminoglycosides, but the drug does not appear to cause kidney damage or hearing loss. Aztreonam is stable in the presence of beta-lactamase enzymes.

Indications for use include urinary tract infections (UTIs), lower respiratory tract infections, septicemia, and abdominal and gynecologic infections caused by susceptible organisms. Gram-positive and anaerobic bacteria are resistant. Consequently, its ability to preserve normal gram-positive and anaerobic flora may be an advantage over most other antimicrobial agents.

Adverse effects are similar to those for penicillin. Dosage should be reduced in renal impairment.

### Routes and dosage ranges

*Adults:* UTIs, IM, IV 0.5–1.0 g q8–12h
  Systemic infections, 1–2 g q6–12h
*Children:* Dosage not established

**Imipenem/cilastatin** (Primaxin) is a carbapenem bactericidal agent that is distributed in most body fluids. Imipenem is rapidly broken down by an enzyme (dehydropeptidase) in renal tubules and therefore reaches only low concentrations in urine. Cilastatin was synthesized to inhibit the enzyme and increase urine levels of the antibacterial agent. Primaxin contains equal parts of imipenem and cilastatin.

The drug is reportedly effective in infections caused by a wide range of bacteria, including penicillinase-producing staphylococci, *Escherichia coli*, *Proteus* species, *Enterobacter*, *Klebsiella*, *Serratia*, and *P. aeruginosa*. It is effective against *Streptococcus faecalis* (enterococcus) but is not effective against other streptococci. Its main indication for use is treatment of infections caused by organisms resistant to other drugs. Adverse effects are the same as those occurring with other beta-lactam antibiotics. Dosage should be reduced in a client with renal impairment.

### Route and dosage ranges

*Adults:* IV 2–4 g/d, in three to four divided doses
*Children:* IV up to 25 mg/kg q6h

## Quinolones

Quinolones are synthetic, bactericidal, broad-spectrum drugs with activity against gram-negative and gram-positive organisms. The drugs act by interfering with deoxyribonucleic acid gyrase, an enzyme required for bacterial growth and replication. They are indicated for UTIs and some respiratory and sexually transmitted diseases. Indications for use vary with individual agents.

Anne Collins Abrams: CLINICAL DRUG THERAPY, Fourth Edition.
© 1995 J.B. Lippincott Company.

**Cinoxacin** (Cinobac) is used only for UTIs (see Chap. 40). **Enoxacin** (Penetrex) and **norfloxacin** (Noroxin) are used only for UTIs and uncomplicated gonorrhea. **Ciprofloxacin** (Cipro), **lomefloxacin** (Maxaquin), and **ofloxacin** (Floxin) are effective in respiratory, urinary tract, and skin and soft-tissue infections, as well as sexually transmitted diseases caused by chlamydiae and gonorrhea organisms. Lomefloxacin also is approved for prophylactic therapy before transurethral surgical procedures. In some infections, the quinolones allow oral, outpatient treatment that would require parenteral administration and hospitalization with other anti-infective drugs.

The drugs are contraindicated in children under 16 years of age, in pregnant or lactating women, and in those who have experienced a hypersensitivity reaction.

Oral quinolones are generally well absorbed, achieve therapeutic concentrations in most body fluids, and are metabolized to some extent in the liver. The kidneys are the main route of elimination, with about 30% to 60% of an oral dose being excreted unchanged in the urine. Dosage should be reduced in renal impairment.

Ciprofloxacin

### Route and dosage range

*Adults:* UTIs, PO 250 mg q12h
Systemic infections, PO 500–750 mg q12h

Enoxacin

### Route and dosage range

*Adults:* UTIs, PO 200–400 mg q12h for 7–14 d
Gonorrhea, PO 400 mg as a single dose

Lomefloxacin

### Route and dosage range

*Adults:* PO 400 mg once daily
Preoperatively, PO 400 mg as a single dose, 2–6 h before surgery

Norfloxacin

### Route and dosage range

*Adults:* PO 400 mg twice daily

Ofloxacin

### Route and dosage range

*Adults:* PO, IV 200–400 mg q12h for 3 to 10 d
Gonorrhea, PO 400 mg as a single dose

**Chloramphenicol** (Chloromycetin) is a broad-spectrum, bacteriostatic antibiotic that is active against most gram-positive bacteria, most gram-negative bacteria, rickettsiae, chlamydiae, and treponemes. Chloramphen-

icol acts by interfering with microbial protein synthesis. It is well absorbed and diffuses well into body tissues and fluids, including cerebrospinal fluid, but low drug levels are obtained in urine. It is metabolized in the liver and excreted in the urine.

Chloramphenicol is rarely used in infections caused by gram-positive organisms because of the effectiveness and low toxicity of penicillins, cephalosporins, and erythromycin. It is the first drug of choice only in typhoid fever. Otherwise, it is indicated for use in serious infections for which no adequate substitute drug is available. Specific infections include meningococcal, pneumococcal, or *Haemophilus* meningitis in penicillin-allergic clients; anaerobic brain abscess; *Bacteroides fragilis* infections; rickettsial infections and brucellosis when tetracyclines are contraindicated; and *Klebsiella* and *Haemophilus* infections that are resistant to other drugs.

### Routes and dosage ranges

*Adults:* PO, IV 50–100 mg/kg per day, in four divided doses, q6h
*Children and full-term infants over 2 weeks:* PO 50 mg/kg per day, in three or four divided doses, q6–8h

## Polymyxins

**Polymyxin B** (Aerosporin) and **colistin** (Coly-Mycin S) are bactericidal against *Pseudomonas* and other gram-negative organisms except *Proteus*. Because of their toxicity, they are not given parenterally for systemic infections. Polymyxin B may be given intrathecally for meningitis caused by *P. aeruginosa*; colistin may be given orally for bacterial diarrhea caused by *Shigella* or other gram-negative organisms; and both drugs may be given topically for ear infections. When given orally, colistin acts within the bowel lumen because it is poorly absorbed from the gastrointestinal tract. When given topically, the drugs are often combined with others, such as neomycin or bacitracin. A commonly used topical combination preparation is Neosporin.

Polymyxin B sulfate

### Routes and dosage ranges

*Adults:* Intrathecal 50,000 U once daily for 3–4 d, then 50,000 U every other day
Otic solution, 3–4 drops, three or four times daily
*Children over 2 years:* Intrathecal, same as adults
*Children under 2 years:* Intrathecal 20,000 U once daily for 3–4 days or 25,000 U once every other day. Continue with a dosage of 25,000 U once every other day.

Colistin sulfate

### Routes and dosage ranges

*Adults:* PO 5–15 mg/kg per day in three divided doses
Otic suspension, 3–4 drops into ear canal three or
four times daily

*Children:* PO 3–5 mg/kg per day in three divided
doses q8h

**Clindamycin** (Cleocin) is similar to erythromycin
and other macrolides in its mechanism of action and
antimicrobial spectra. It is bacteriostatic in usual doses. It
is effective against gram-positive cocci, including group
A streptococci, pneumococci, and most staphylococci. It
also is effective against species of *Corynebacterium, Treponema, Neisseria,* and *Mycoplasma* and against some anaerobic organisms, such as *Bacteroides* and *Clostridia.*
Clindamycin enters microbial cells and attaches to 50S ribosomes, thereby inhibiting microbial protein synthesis.

Clindamycin is the drug of choice in infections caused
by *B. fragilis.* Because these bacteria are usually mixed
with gram-negative organisms from the gynecologic or
gastrointestinal tracts, clindamycin is usually given with
another drug, such as gentamicin, to treat mixed infections adequately. The drug may be useful as a penicillin
substitute in clients who are allergic to penicillin and
who have streptococcal, staphylococcal, or pneumococcal infections in which the causative organism is sensitive to clindamycin. A topical solution is used in the
treatment of acne.

Clindamycin should not be used for trivial infections
or for treating meningitis. (The drug does not reach
therapeutic concentrations in the central nervous system.) The drug must be used with caution in clients with
renal, hepatic, or gastrointestinal disorders (*e.g.,* colitis).
Clindamycin is widely distributed in body tissues and
fluids, except cerebrospinal fluid. It is metabolized primarily in the liver and excreted in bile.

Clindamycin hydrochloride

### Route and dosage ranges

*Adults:* PO 150–300 mg q6h; up to 450 mg q6h for
severe infections

*Children:* PO 8–16 mg/kg per day in three or four
divided doses q6–8h; up to 20 mg/kg per day in
severe infections

Clindamycin phosphate

### Routes and dosage ranges

*Adults:* IM 600 mg–2.7 g/d in two to four divided
doses q6–8h
IV 600 mg–2.7 g/d in two to four divided doses; up
to 4.8 g/d in life-threatening infections

*Children:* IM, IV 15–40 mg/kg per day in three or four
divided doses q6–8h; up to 40 mg/kg per day in
severe infections

Clindamycin palmitate hydrochloride
(Cleocin Pediatric [75 mg/ml])

### Route and dosage ranges

*Children:* PO 8–12 mg/kg per day in three or four
divided doses; up to 25 mg/kg per day in very severe
infections. For children weighing 10 kg or less, the
minimum dose is 37.5 mg, three times per day.

**Metronidazole** (Flagyl) is effective against anaerobic bacteria, including gram-negative bacilli such as
*Bacteroides;* gram-positive bacilli such as *Clostridia;* and
gram-positive cocci such as *Peptococcus* and *Peptostrep-
tococcus.* It is also effective against protozoa that cause
amebiasis, giardiasis, and trichomoniasis (see Chap. 44).

The main clinical uses of metronidazole are to treat
anaerobic infections, especially intra-abdominal infections, and to prevent infection, especially in colorectal
surgery. It is generally contraindicated during the first
trimester of pregnancy and must be used with caution in
clients with central nervous system or blood disorders.
Because the drug is carcinogenic in rodents and mutagenic in bacteria, it should be used only when necessary.
Metronidazole is widely distributed in body fluids and
tissues, metabolized in the liver, and excreted mostly
(60%–80%) in urine, with a small amount excreted in
feces.

### Routes and dosage ranges

*Adults:* Anaerobic bacterial infection, IV 15 mg/kg as
a loading dose, infused over 1 h, followed by 7.5
mg/kg q6h as a maintenance dose, infused over 1 h;
duration usually 7–10 days; maximum dose 4 g/24 h
Surgical prophylaxis, colorectal surgery, IV 15 mg/
kg, infused over 30–60 min, infusion to be completed about 1 h before surgery, followed by 7.5
mg/kg, infused over 30–60 min at 6 hours and 12
hours after the initial dose

**Spectinomycin** (Trobicin) is used for treatment of
gonococcal infections in people who are allergic to penicillin or whose infection is caused by penicillin-resistant
organisms. Safety for use in pregnant or lactating women
or children has not been established.

### Route and dosage range

*Adults:* IM 2 g in a single dose or 4 g divided into two
equal parts and administered in two gluteal injection sites

**Vancomycin** (Vancocin) is active only against gram-
positive microorganisms. It acts by inhibiting cell-wall

synthesis. It is not absorbed from the gastrointestinal tract after oral administration and is usually given intravenously in systemic infections. Intramuscular injections cause pain and necrosis. When given orally, it acts within the bowel lumen. Vancomycin is mainly used in severe infections caused by penicillin-resistant staphylococci. It also is used in pseudomembranous colitis induced by antibiotics, for reduction of bacterial flora in the bowel, and in staphylococcal enterocolitis. Vancomycin is nephrotoxic and ototoxic.

### Routes and dosage ranges

*Adults:* PO 500 mg q6h or 1 g q12h; maximum dose, 4 g/d

IV 2 g/d in two to four divided doses q6–12h

*Children:* PO, IV 40 mg/kg per day in divided doses

## Nursing Process

See Chapter 33.

## Principles of therapy

1. In the presence of renal impairment, dosage of aztreonam, imipenem/cilastatin, vancomycin, and the quinolones should be reduced.
2. Quinolones are not recommended for use in children because they have been associated with permanent damage in cartilage and joints of young animals of several species. In adults with normal renal function, the drugs should be accompanied by an adequate fluid intake and urine output to prevent drug crystals from forming in the urinary tract. In addition, urinary alkalinizing agents, such as calcium-containing antacids, should be avoided because drug crystals form more readily in alkaline urine. In older adults or others with impaired renal function, the drugs should be used cautiously and in reduced dosages.

3. With chloramphenicol, clients need a complete blood count, platelet count, reticulocyte count, and serum iron every 3 days. These tests are necessary for monitoring drug toxicity, because chloramphenicol may cause bone marrow depression and blood disorders. In addition, the dosage of chloramphenicol must be reduced in clients with impaired liver function, in premature infants, and in full-term infants less than 2 weeks old. In these circumstances, impaired metabolism leads to accumulation and adverse effects. If available, frequent measurements of serum drug levels are probably the most reliable guides for dosage. Therapeutic levels are 10 to 20 μg/ml.
4. With clindamycin, specimens for culture and sensitivity studies should be obtained before the first drug dose. If a client receiving clindamycin develops diarrhea, stools should be checked for white blood cells, blood, and mucus, and a proctoscopy should be done to determine whether the client has pseudomembranous colitis, a potentially fatal adverse reaction. If lesions are seen on proctoscopy, the drug should be stopped immediately. In renal failure, the dosage of clindamycin does not need reduction because it is excreted primarily by the liver. In liver disease, other drugs should be substituted or the dosage should be reduced to prevent accumulation and toxic effects. In children, clindamycin should be given to neonates and infants only if clearly indicated, and then liver and kidney function must be monitored. Diarrhea and pseudomembranous colitis may occur with topical clindamycin for treatment of acne. In older adults, clindamycin should be used cautiously with preexisting inflammatory gastrointestinal disorders (*e.g.*, colitis) or other severe illness. These clients may not tolerate drug-induced diarrhea very well. They should be monitored closely for changes in bowel frequency.
5. With vancomycin, serum levels should be monitored. Therapeutic levels are 10 to 25 μg/ml.

## NURSING ACTIONS: MISCELLANEOUS ANTI-INFECTIVES

| Nursing Actions | Rationale/Explanation |
| --- | --- |
| **1. Administer accurately** <br>   **a.** With *aztreonam*: <br><br>     (1) For IM administration, add 3 ml diluent per gram of drug, and inject into large muscle mass. <br><br>     (2) For IV injection, add 6 to 10 ml sterile water, and inject into vein or IV tubing over 3 to 5 minutes. | |

## *Nursing Actions*

## *Rationale/Explanation*

(3)  For IV infusion, mix in at least 50 ml of 0.9% NaCl or 5% dextrose injection per gram of drug and give over 20 to 60 minutes.

**b.** With *imipenem/cilastatin*, mix reconstituted solution in 100 ml of 0.9% NaCl or 5% dextrose injection. Administer 250- to 500-mg doses over 20 to 30 minutes; give 1-g doses over 40 to 60 minutes.

**c.** With *quinolones*:

(1)  Give oral drugs on an empty stomach, 1 hour before or 2 hours after a meal, except lomefloxacin, which may be given without regard to food intake.

(2)  Give IV infusions over 60 minutes

(3)  When giving ciprofloxacin IV into a primary IV line (*e.g.,* using piggyback or Y connector), stop the primary solution until ciprofloxacin is infused.

**d.** With *chloramphenicol*:

(1)  Give oral drug 1 hour before or 2 hours after meals, q6h around the clock. If GI upset occurs, give with food.

(2)  Mix IV chloramphenicol in 50 to 100 ml of 5% dextrose in water and infuse over 15 to 30 minutes.

**e.** With *clindamycin*:

(1)  Give capsules with a full glass of water.

(2)  Do not refrigerate reconstituted oral solution.

(3)  Give IM injections deeply, and rotate sites. Do not give more than 600 mg in a single injection.

(4)  For IV administration, dilute 300 mg in at least 50 ml of any fluid and give over 10 minutes, *or* dilute 600 mg in 100 ml and give over 20 minutes. *Do not* give clindamycin undiluted or by direct injection.

**f.** With IV *metronidazole*, check the manufacturer's instructions.

**g.** With *vancomycin*, dilute 500-mg doses in 100 ml and 1-g doses in 200 ml of 0.9% NaCl or 5% dextrose injection and infuse over at least 60 minutes.

**2. Observe for therapeutic effects**

**a.** Decreased local and systemic signs of infection

**b.** Decreased signs of the specific infection for which the drug is being given

**3. Observe for adverse effects**
**a.** With aztreonam and imipenem/cilastatin, observe for:

(1)  Phlebitis/thrombophlebitis at venipuncture sites

(2)  Nausea, vomiting, diarrhea

(3)  Skin rash

To promote therapeutic plasma drug levels. Food in the gastrointestinal (GI) tract interferes with absorption of most oral quinolones.

To decrease vein irritation and phlebitis

Manufacturer's recommendation, probably to avoid physical or chemical incompatibilities

To increase absorption and maintain therapeutic blood levels

To avoid esophageal irritation

Refrigeration may thicken the solution and make it difficult to pour.

To decrease pain, induration, and abscess formation

Dilution decreases risks of phlebitis. Cardiac arrest has been reported with bolus injections of undiluted clindamycin.

The drug requires specific techniques for preparation and administration.

To decrease pain and phlebitis at injection sites. Hypotension and flushing of upper extremities may occur with rapid IV administration.

See Chapter 33.

These are the most common adverse drug reactions. Occurrence of others is <0.5.%.

*(continued)*

| *Nursing Actions* | *Rationale/Explanation* |
|---|---|
| **b.** With quinolones, observe for: | The drugs are generally well tolerated and produce relatively few adverse effects. |
| (1) Allergic reactions (anaphylaxis, urticaria) | Uncommon but some fatalities have been reported. |
| (2) Nausea, vomiting, diarrhea, pseudomembranous colitis | Nausea is the most common GI symptom. |
| (3) Headache, dizziness | |
| (4) Crystalluria | Uncommon but may occur with an inadequate fluid intake |
| (5) Other | Adverse effects involving most body systems have been reported with one or more of the quinolones. Most have a low incidence (<1%) of occurrence. |
| **c.** With chloramphenicol, observe for: | |
| (1) Anemia, leukopenia, thrombocytopenia | Blood dyscrasias are the most serious adverse reaction to chloramphenicol. They are caused by bone marrow depression. |
| (2) Clinical signs of infection, bleeding | |
| **d.** With clindamycin, observe for: | |
| (1) Nausea, vomiting, diarrhea | These are the most frequent adverse effects and may be severe enough to require stopping the drug. |
| (2) Pseudomembranous colitis—severe diarrhea, fever, stools containing neutrophils and shreds of mucous membrane | May occur with most antibiotics but is more common with oral clindamycin. It is caused by *Clostridium difficile*. The organism produces a toxin that kills mucosal cells and produces superficial ulcerations that are visible with sigmoidoscopy. Discontinuing the drug and giving oral vancomycin are curative measures. |
| **e.** With metronidazole, observe for central nervous system effects (convulsive seizures, peripheral paresthesias, ataxia, confusion, dizziness, headache), GI effects (nausea, vomiting, diarrhea), and dermatologic effects (skin rash and pruritus, thrombophlebitis at infusion site) | Convulsions and peripheral neuropathy may be serious effects; GI effects are most common |
| **f.** With vancomycin, observe for: | |
| (1) Nephrotoxicity–oliguria, increased blood urea nitrogen and serum creatinine | |
| (2) Ototoxicity—hearing loss, tinnitus | |
| **4. Observe for drug interactions** | |
| **a.** Drugs that *increase* or *decrease* effects of aztreonam and imipenem/cilastatin | See Chapters 34 and 35. Although few interactions have been reported with these drugs, potential interactions are those that occur with other beta-lactam antibiotics. |
| **b.** Drugs that alter effects of quinolones: | |
| (1) Cimetidine, probenecid | These drugs inhibit elimination of quinolones and may increase serum drug levels |
| (2) Antacids, antineoplastic drugs, iron preparations, sucralfate, zinc preparations | Most of these drugs decrease absorption of oral quinolones. |
| **c.** Drugs that *increase* effects of vancomycin: | |
| (1) Aminoglycoside antibiotics | Additive nephrotoxicity and ototoxicity |
| (2) Amphotericin B | Additive nephrotoxicity |
| (3) Cisplatin | Additive nephrotoxicity |

| *Nursing Actions* | *Rationale/Explanation* |
|---|---|
| **d.** Drugs that alter effects of metronidazole | |
| (1) Phenobarbital, phenytoin | These drugs induce hepatic enzymes and decrease effects of metronidazole by accelerating its rate of hepatic metabolism. |
| (2) Cimetidine | May increase effects by inhibiting hepatic metabolism of metronidazole |
| **5. Teach clients** | |
| **a.** Report bleeding (in skin, urine, stool), fever, sore throat, decreased urine output, dizziness, severe diarrhea. | These reactions may indicate that the drug should be discontinued or reduced in dosage. |
| **b.** With quinolones, drink 2 to 3 quarts of fluid daily, if not contraindicated | To prevent drug crystals from developing and damaging urinary tract |

## Review and Application Exercises

1. How do aztreonam and imipenem/cilastatin differ from penicillins and cephalosporins?
2. How do the quinolones exert their antibacterial effects?
3. What are the main clinical uses of the quinolones?
4. What are adverse effects of quinolones, and how may they be prevented or minimized?
5. Why is it important to maintain an adequate fluid intake and urine output with the quinolones?
6. Why are quinolones not given to children?
7. Why is the use of chloramphenicol limited?
8. Which drugs from this chapter may cause pseudomembranous colitis, and why may this condition be life-threatening?

## Selected References

(1993). *Drug facts and comparisons*. St. Louis: Facts and Comparisons.

Guglielmo, J. (1992). Principles of antimicrobial therapy. In M. A. Koda-Kimble & L. Y. Young, (Eds.), *Applied therapeutics: The clinical use of drugs* (5th ed.) (pp. 33-1–33-12). Vancouver, WA: Applied Therapeutics.

Mandell, G. L., Douglas, R. G., Jr., & Bennett, J. E. (Eds.) (1990). *Principles and practice of infectious diseases* (3rd ed.). New York: Churchill Livingstone.

Morita, M. M. (1993). Methicillin-resistant *Staphylococcus aureus*: Past, present and future. *Nursing Clinics of North America, 28*(3), 625–637.

Murray, B. E. (1992). Antimicrobial therapeutic agents. In W. N. Kelley (Ed.), *Textbook of internal medicine* (2nd ed.) (pp. 1564–1575).

Neu, H. C. (1990). Other beta-lactam antibiotics. In G. L. Mandell, R. D. Douglas, Jr., & J. E. Bennett (Eds.), *Principles and practice of infectious diseases* (3rd ed.) (pp. 257–263). New York: Churchill Livingstone.

### CHAPTER 40

# Sulfonamides and Urinary Antiseptics

## Sulfonamides

Sulfonamides were the first synthetic antibacterial agents to be developed. They are bacteriostatic against a wide range of bacteria, including pneumococci, *Neisseria, Escherichia coli, Klebsiella, Proteus, Enterobacter*, and *Haemophilus influenzae*.

Individual drugs vary in extent of systemic absorption and clinical indications. Some are well absorbed and can be used in systemic infections; others are poorly absorbed and exert more local effects. In systemic infections, sulfonamides have largely been replaced by newer, more effective antibacterial agents.

## Urinary antiseptics

Urinary antiseptics are drugs used only to prevent or treat urinary tract infections (UTIs). They are not used in systemic infections because they do not attain therapeutic plasma levels. They are potentially bactericidal for sensitive organisms in the kidneys and bladder because the drugs are concentrated in renal tubules and produce high levels in urine.

### MECHANISM OF ACTION

Sulfonamides act as antimetabolites of para-aminobenzoic acid (PABA), which microorganisms require to produce folic acid; folic acid, in turn, is required for the production of bacterial intracellular proteins. Sulfonamides enter into the reaction instead of PABA, compete for the enzyme involved, and cause formation of nonfunctional derivatives of folic acid. Thus, sulfonamides halt multiplication of new bacteria but do not kill mature, fully formed bacteria. With the exception of the topical sulfonamides used in burn therapy, the presence of pus, serum, or necrotic tissue interferes with sulfonamide action because these materials contain PABA. Some bacteria can change their metabolic pathways to use precursors or other forms of folic acid and thereby develop resistance to the antibacterial action of sulfonamides. Once resistance to one sulfonamide develops, cross-resistance to others is common.

### INDICATIONS FOR USE

A major clinical use of sulfonamides is in UTIs caused by *E. coli, Proteus*, or *Klebsiella* organisms. These drugs are most useful in the treatment of acute and chronic cystitis. They also are used in asymptomatic bacteriuria. In acute pyelonephritis, other agents are usually preferred. Additional uses include ulcerative colitis and uncommon infections, such as chancroid, lymphogranuloma venereum, nocardiosis, toxoplasmosis, and trachoma. Topical sulfonamides are used in the prevention of burn wound infections and treatment of ocular, vaginal, and other soft-tissue infections. For specific clinical indications of individual drugs, see Table 40-1.

Urinary antiseptics are used only for UTIs.

## TABLE 40-1. SULFONAMIDE PREPARATIONS

| Generic/ Trade Name | Characteristics | Clinical Indications | Usual Routes and Dosage Ranges | |
|---|---|---|---|---|
| | | | *Adults* | *Children* |
| **Single Agents** | | | | |
| **Sulfacytine** (Renoquid) | A short-acting agent that is rapidly absorbed and rapidly excreted | Urinary tract infections | PO 500 mg initially, then 250 mg four times daily | |
| **Sulfadiazine** (Microsulfon) | 1. A short-acting, rapidly absorbed, rapidly excreted agent for systemic infections 2. Low solubility 3. Therapeutic blood levels are 10–15 mg/100 ml. | 1. Urinary tract infections 2. Prophylaxis of rheumatic fever in clients allergic to penicillin 3. Nocardiosis 4. Meningococcal meningitis | PO 2–4 g initially, then 2–4 g daily in three to six divided doses | Over 2 mo of age: PO 75 mg/kg initially, then 150 mg/kg per day in four to six divided doses; maximal daily dose, 6 g Prophylaxis of rheumatic fever, PO 500 mg once daily for children weighing less than 30 kg, 1 g daily for children weighing over 30 kg |
| **Sulfamethizole** (Thiosulfil) | A highly soluble, rapidly absorbed, and rapidly excreted agent that is similar to sulfisoxazole in actions and uses | Urinary tract infections | PO 500 mg–1 g three or four times daily | Over 2 mo of age: PO 30–45 mg/kg per day in four divided doses |
| **Sulfamethoxazole** (Gantanol) | 1. Similar to sulfisoxazole in therapeutic effects but absorbed and excreted more slowly. More likely to produce excessive blood levels and crystalluria than sulfisoxazole. 2. An ingredient in mixtures with trimethoprim and phenazopyridine (see Combination Agents, below) | 1. Systemic infections 2. Urinary tract infections | PO 2 g initially, then 1–2 g two or three times daily | Over 2 mo of age: PO 50–60 mg/kg initially, then 30 mg/kg q12h; maximal daily dose, 75 mg/kg |
| **Sulfasalazine** (Azulfidine) | 1. Poorly absorbed, acts within the bowel lumen 2. Does not alter normal bacterial flora in the intestine. Effectiveness in ulcerative colitis may be due to antibacterial (sulfapyridine) and anti-inflammatory (aminosalicylic acid) metabolites. | 1. Ulcerative colitis 2. Regional enteritis (Crohn's disease) | PO 3–4 g daily in divided doses initially; 2 g daily in four doses for maintenance; maximal daily dose, 8 g | PO 40–60 mg/kg per day in three to six divided doses initially, followed by 30 mg/kg per day in four divided doses |
| **Sulfisoxazole** (Gantrisin) | 1. A rapidly absorbed, rapidly excreted sulfonamide that is widely used 2. Highly soluble and less likely to cause crystalluria than most other sulfonamides 3. Available in tablets, parenteral solution, oral suspension and syrup, vaginal cream, and ophthalmic solution and ointment | 1. Urinary tract infections 2. Systemic infections 3. Vaginitis 4. Ocular infections 5. Nocardiosis | PO, IV, SC 2–4 g initially, then 4–8 g daily in three to six divided doses Intravaginally, 2.5–5 g of vaginal cream (10%) twice daily | Over 2 mo of age: PO 75 mg/kg of body weight initially, then 150 mg/kg per day in four to six divided doses; maximal daily dose, 6 g |
| **Combination Agents** | | | | |
| **Sulfamethoxazole–trimethoprim** (Bactrim, Septra, others) | 1. Synergistic effectiveness against many gram-positive and gram-negative organisms, including streptococci (*Streptococcus pneumoniae, Streptococcus viridans, Streptococcus faecalis*); staphylococci (*Staphylococcus epidermidis, Staphylococcus aureus*); *Escherichia coli; Proteus; Enterobacter; Salmonella; Shigella; Serratia; Klebsiella; Nocardia;* and | 1. Acute and chronic urinary tract infections 2. Acute exacerbations of chronic bronchitis 3. Acute otitis media (in children) and acute maxillary sinusitis (in adults) caused by susceptible strains of | Urinary tract infections, trimethoprim 160 mg and sulfamethoxazole 800 mg PO q12h for 10–14 d Shigellosis, same dose as above for 5 d Severe urinary tract infections, PO 8–10 mg (trimethoprim component) per kg/d in two to four divided | Urinary tract infections, otitis media, and shigellosis, PO 8 mg/kg trimethoprim and 40 mg/kg sulfamethoxazole in two divided doses q12h for 10 d Severe urinary tract infections, IV 8–10 mg (trimethoprim component)/kg in two to four divided doses |

*(continued)*

**TABLE 40-1.   SULFONAMIDE PREPARATIONS   (*Continued*)**

| Generic/ Trade Name | Characteristics | Clinical Indications | Usual Routes and Dosage Ranges | |
|---|---|---|---|---|
| | | | *Adults* | *Children* |
| | others. Most strains of *Pseudomonas* are resistant.<br>2. The two drugs have additive antibacterial effects because they interfere with different steps in bacterial synthesis and activation of folic acid, an essential nutrient.<br>3. The combination is less likely to produce resistant bacteria than either agent alone.<br>4. Oral preparations contain different amounts of the two drugs, as follows:<br>  a. "Regular" tablets contain trimethoprim 80 mg and sulfamethoxazole 400 mg.<br>  b. Double-strength tablets (*e.g.,* Bactrim D.S., Septra D.S.) contain trimethoprim 160 mg and sulfamethoxazole 800 mg.<br>  c. The oral suspension contains trimethoprim 40 mg and sulfamethoxazole 200 mg in each 5 ml.<br>5. The intravenous preparation contains trimethoprim 80 mg and sulfamethoxazole 400 mg in 5 ml.<br>6. Dosage must be reduced in renal insufficiency.<br>7. The preparation is contraindicated if creatinine clearance is less than 15 ml/min. | *Haemophilus influenzae* and *S. pneumoniae*<br>4. Shigellosis<br>5. Typhoid fever<br>6. Salmonella infections<br>7. Infection by *Pneumocystis carinii* (prevention and treatment)<br>8. Acute gonococcal urethritis<br>9. Intravenous preparation indicated for *P. carinii* pneumonia, severe urinary tract infections, and shigellosis | doses, up to 14 d<br>*P. carinii* pneumonia, 15–20 mg (trimethoprim component) per kg/d in three to four divided doses, q6–8h, up to 14 d | q6–8h or q12h up to 14 d<br>*P. carinii* pneumonia, IV 15–20 mg (trimethoprim component) per kg/d in three or four divided doses q6–8h up to 14 d |
| **Sulfamethoxazole–phenazopyridine** (Azo Gantanol) | No added benefit beyond that of the drugs given separately | Urinary tract infections with dysuria, frequency, and urgency | PO 4 tablets initially, then 2 tablets twice daily for 2–3 d | |
| **Sulfisoxazole-phenazopyridine** (Azo Gantrisin) | Same as sulfamethoxazole-phenazopyridine | Same as sulfamethoxazole-phenazopyridine | PO 4–6 tablets initially, then 2 tablets four times daily for 2–3 d | |

**Topical Sulfonamides**

| Generic/ Trade Name | Characteristics | Clinical Indications | Adults | Children |
|---|---|---|---|---|
| **Mafenide** (Sulfamylon) | 1. Effective against most gram-negative and gram-positive organisms, especially *Pseudomonas*<br>2. Application causes pain and burning.<br>3. Mafenide is absorbed systemically and may produce metabolic acidosis. | Prevention of bacterial colonization and infection of severe burn wounds | Topical application to burned area, once or twice daily, in a thin layer | Same as adults |
| **Silver sulfadiazine** (Silvadene) | 1. Effective against most *Pseudomonas* species, the most common pathogen in severe burn sepsis, *E. coli, Klebsiella, Proteus*, staphylococci, and streptococci<br>2. Application is painless.<br>3. Does not cause electrolyte or acid-base imbalances<br>4. Significant amounts may be absorbed systemically with large burned areas and prolonged use. | Same as mafenide. Usually the preferred drug. | Same as mafenide | Same as mafenide |

## CONTRAINDICATIONS FOR USE

Sulfonamides are contraindicated in people who have had hypersensitivity reactions to them or to chemically related drugs, such as thiazide diuretics or antidiabetic sulfonylureas. They are also contraindicated in renal failure, late pregnancy, lactation, and children under 2 months of age (except for treatment of congenital toxoplasmosis). Sulfasalazine (Azulfidine) is contraindicated in people who are allergic to salicylates, children under 2 years old, and people with intestinal or urinary tract obstruction. The drugs must be used cautiously in the presence of liver or kidney impairment or blood dyscrasias.

# Individual drugs

Sulfonamides are listed in Table 40-1.

## URINARY ANTISEPTICS

**Cinoxacin** (Cinobac) is a synthetic antibacterial agent used for treatment of initial and recurrent UTIs in adults. It is effective against most gram-negative bacteria that commonly cause UTIs (*E. coli*, *Klebsiella*, *Enterobacter*, and *Proteus* organisms). It exerts bactericidal effects by inhibiting bacterial replication of deoxyribonucleic acid.

### Route and dosage range

*Adults:* PO 1 g daily in two to four divided doses for 7–14 d

**Methenamine mandelate** (Mandelamine) and **methenamine hippurate** (Hiprex) are salts of methenamine that have antibacterial activity only when urine pH is acidic. At a urine pH below 5.5, the drugs are degraded to form formaldehyde, which is the antibacterial component. Acidification of urine is a prerequisite to methenamine effectiveness. Supplemental drug therapy with ascorbic acid or other urinary acidifiers is usually needed. Formaldehyde is active against several gram-positive and gram-negative organisms, including *E. coli*. It is most useful for long-term suppression of bacteria in chronic, recurrent infections. It should generally not be used in acute infections because other anti-infective drugs are more effective. It also should not be used to prevent UTIs in clients with indwelling urinary catheters. Several hours are required for methenamine to be hydrolyzed into formaldehyde and become bacteriostatic. Because catheters continuously empty the bladder, methenamine hydrolyzes in the urine drainage bag rather than the bladder. Methenamine is contraindicated in clients with renal failure.

Methenamine mandelate

### Route and dosage range

*Adults:* PO 1 g four times daily
*Children ages 6–12:* PO 500 mg four times daily
*Children under age 6:* PO 50 mg/kg per day, in three divided doses

Methenamine hippurate

### Route and dosage range

*Adults:* PO 1 g twice daily
*Children:* PO 500 mg–1 g twice daily

**Nalidixic acid** (NegGram) is effective against most gram-negative organisms that cause UTIs, including *E. coli*, *Proteus*, *Klebsiella*, and *Enterobacter* organisms. Bacterial resistance to this drug may develop rapidly (within 48–72 hours).

### Route and dosage range

*Adults:* PO 4 g daily in four divided doses for 1–2 wk, then 2 g/d if long-term treatment is required
*Children:* PO 55 mg/kg per day in four divided doses, reduced to 33 mg/kg per day for long-term use in children under 12 years of age. Contraindicated in infants under 3 months of age.

**Nitrofurantoin** (Furadantin, Macrodantin) has a wide spectrum of antibacterial activity against most gram-positive and gram-negative organisms, including *E. coli*, streptococci, staphylococci, and *Klebsiella*, *Enterobacter*, *Salmonella*, *Shigella*, and some *Proteus* species. It is ineffective against *Pseudomonas* and *Proteus mirabilis*. Despite its broad spectrum, nitrofurantoin generally is not used in systemic infections. It is used primarily for short-term treatment of UTIs or long-term suppression of bacteria in chronic, recurrent UTIs.

An advantage of nitrofurantoin is that bacterial resistance develops slowly and to a limited degree. In contrast to most anti-infective drugs, nitrofurantoin's effectiveness is increased when given with or just after food intake. Macrodantin, a macrocrystalline form of the drug, reportedly causes fewer gastrointestinal adverse effects than Furadantin, a microcrystalline form. Nitrofurantoin is contraindicated in people with severe renal disease.

### Route and dosage range

*Adults:* PO 50–100 mg four times daily
Prophylaxis of recurrent UTIs in women, 50–100 mg at bedtime
*Children over 3 months:* PO 5–7 mg/kg per day, in four divided doses

## OTHER DRUGS USED IN URINARY TRACT INFECTIONS

**Phenazopyridine** (Pyridium) is an azo dye that acts as a urinary tract analgesic. It relieves symptoms of dysuria, burning, and frequency and urgency of urination, which occur with cystitis or urethritis. It has no anti-infective action. It turns urine orange-red, which may be mistaken for blood. It is contraindicated in people with renal insufficiency and severe hepatitis. It is available alone or in fixed-dose combinations with sulfamethoxazole and sulfisoxazole. When indicated, phenazopyridine is better given alone. It can usually be discontinued after 2 to 3 days, whereas the sulfonamide component is given longer.

### Route and dosage range

*Adults:* PO 200 mg three times daily after meals
*Children 6–12 years of age:* PO 12 mg/kg per day, in three divided doses

**Trimethoprim** (Proloprim, Trimpex) is a folate antagonist drug with antibacterial effects. It is available as a single agent for treatment of UTIs caused by susceptible strains of *E. coli, Proteus, Klebsiella,* and *Enterobacter* or in a fixed-dose combination with sulfamethoxazole (see Table 40-1). It is contraindicated in clients with hypersensitivity to trimethoprim or with megaloblastic anemia due to folate deficiency. Rash and pruritus are the most common adverse effects. Nausea, vomiting, glossitis, thrombocytopenia, leukopenia, anemia, and methemoglobinemia occasionally occur.

### Route and dosage range

*Adults:* PO 100 mg q12h for 10 d

## Nursing Process

General aspects of the nursing process in antimicrobial drug therapy, as described in Chapter 33, apply to the client receiving sulfonamides. In this chapter, only aspects related specifically to sulfonamide therapy are included.

### Assessment

Assess clients for signs and symptoms of disorders for which sulfonamides and urinary antiseptics are used:
- For *UTIs*, assess urinalysis reports for white blood cells and bacteria, urine culture reports for type of bacteria, and symptoms of dysuria, frequency, and urgency of urination.
- For *burns*, assess the size of the wound, amount and type of drainage, presence of edema, and amount of eschar.

Ask clients specifically if they have ever taken a sulfonamide and if so, whether they had an allergic reaction.

### Nursing diagnoses
- High Risk for Injury: Hypersensitivity reaction and kidney, liver, or blood disorders
- Knowledge Deficit: Correct administration and usage of sulfonamides

### Planning/Goals

The client will:
- Take sulfonamides as directed
- Receive prompt and appropriate treatment if hypersensitivity occurs

### Interventions
- During sulfonamide therapy, encourage sufficient fluids to produce a urine output of at least 1200 to 1500 ml daily. A high fluid intake decreases the risk of crystalluria (precipitation of crystals in the urine).
- Avoid urinary catheterization when possible. If catheterization is necessary, use sterile technique. The urinary tract is normally sterile except for the lower third of the urethra. Introduction of any bacteria into the bladder may cause infection.
  - A single catheterization has about a 6% chance of introducing infection. With indwelling catheters, bacteria colonize the bladder and produce infection within 2 to 3 weeks, even with meticulous care.
  - When indwelling catheters must be used, measures to decrease the incidence and severity of UTIs include the following: Use a closed drainage system; keep the perineal area clean; force fluids, if not contraindicated, to maintain a dilute urine; and remove the catheter as soon as possible, because infection occurs if the catheter is in place more than a few days. Do not disconnect the system and irrigate the catheter unless obstruction is suspected. *Never* raise the urinary drainage bag above bladder level.
- Force fluids in anyone with a UTI unless contraindicated. Bacteria do not multiply as rapidly in dilute urine. In addition, emptying the bladder frequently allows it to refill with uninfected urine. This decreases the bacterial population of the bladder.
- Teach women to cleanse themselves from the urethral area toward the rectum after voiding or defecating to avoid contamination of the urethral area with bacteria from the vagina and rectum. Also, voiding after sexual intercourse probably helps cleanse the lower urethra and prevent UTI.

### Evaluation
- Observe for improvement in signs of the infection for which a sulfonamide was given.
- Interview and observe for adverse drug effects.

## Principles of therapy

1. With systemically absorbed sulfonamides, an initial loading dose may be given to produce therapeutic blood levels (12 to 15 mg/100 ml) more rapidly. The amount is usually twice the maintenance dose.

2. Urine pH is important in drug therapy with sulfonamides and urinary antiseptics.
   a. With sulfonamide therapy, alkaline urine increases drug solubility and helps prevent crystalluria. It also increases the rate of sulfonamide excretion and the concentration of sulfonamide in the urine. The urine can be alkalinized by giving sodium bicarbonate. Alkalinization is less likely to be needed with sulfisoxazole (because the drug is highly soluble), with the sulfonamides used to treat intestinal infections (because they are not absorbed systemically to any significant extent), or with topical agents used for burn wounds (because there is little systemic absorption).
   b. With mandelamine therapy, urine pH must be acidic (below 5.5) for the drug to be effective. At a higher pH, mandelamine does not hydrolyze to formaldehyde, the antibacterial component. Urine can be acidified by concomitant administration of ascorbic acid.
3. Urine cultures and sensitivity tests are indicated in suspected UTIs because of the great variability in possible pathogens and in their susceptibility to antibacterial drugs, even within the same species or organism. Best results are obtained by using drug therapy indicated by the microorganisms isolated from each client.

## USE IN CHILDREN

Sulfonamides are contraindicated during late pregnancy and lactation and in children under 2 months old (except for treatment of congenital toxoplasmosis). If a fetus or young infant receives a sulfonamide by placental transfer, in breast milk, or by direct administration, the drug displaces bilirubin from binding sites on albumin. As a result, bilirubin may accumulate in the bloodstream (hyperbilirubinemia) and central nervous system (kernicterus) and cause life-threatening toxicity.

Sulfonamides are often used to treat UTIs and acute otitis media in children older than 2 months. Few data are available regarding the effects of long-term or recurrent use of sulfamethoxazole (Gantanol) in children under 6 years old with chronic renal disease. Sulfamethoxazole is often given in combination with trimethoprim (Bactrim, Septra), although trimethoprim has not been established as safe and effective in children under 12 years old. Sulfacytine (Renoquid) is not recommended for use in children under 14 years of age.

## USE IN OLDER ADULTS

Renal function is often impaired in older adults, and a major concern is that sulfonamides may cause further damage. As with younger adults, a fluid intake of about 2 L daily is needed to reduce formation of crystals and stones in the urinary tract.

With the combination of sulfamethoxazole and trimethoprim, older adults are at increased risk of severe adverse effects. Severe skin reactions and bone marrow depression are most often reported. Folic acid deficiency also may occur because both of the drugs interfere with folic acid metabolism.

## NURSING ACTIONS: SULFONAMIDES AND URINARY ANTISEPTICS

| *Nursing Actions* | *Rationale/Explanation* |
|---|---|
| **1. Administer accurately**<br>**a.** Give oral sulfonamide preparations before or after meals, with a full glass of water. | Food in the stomach may delay but does not prevent drug absorption. Giving the drugs before meals probably improves absorption. However, giving with food decreases gastric irritation, anorexia, nausea, and vomiting. Therefore, time of administration in relation to meals can be altered according to the client's tolerance. |
| **b.** For IV trimethoprim-sulfamethoxazole, 5-ml ampule:<br><br>(1) Dilute in 125 ml of 5% dextrose in water, and use within 6 hours.<br><br>(2) Administer over 60 to 90 minutes.<br><br>(3) Flush all IV lines used to remove any residual drug.<br><br>(4) Do not mix with other drugs or solutions. | Manufacturer's recommendations |

*(continued)*

## Nursing Actions

## Rationale/Explanation

**c.** Give nitrofurantoin with or after meals.

Food decreases nausea, vomiting, and diarrhea.

**d.** Apply a thin layer of topical sulfonamides to burn wounds with a sterile gloved hand after the surface has been cleansed of previously applied medication.

Burn wounds can be cleansed in several ways, including immersion in Hubbard tank or whirlpool, shower or tub bath, and spot cleansing with sterile saline, 4″ × 4″ gauze pads, and gloves.

**2. Observe for therapeutic effects**

**a.** Decreased symptoms of urinary tract infection (UTI)—less burning on urination, decreased frequency and urgency of voiding, less fever, sterile urinalysis report

**b.** Less diarrhea with ulcerative colitis or bacillary dysentery

**c.** Lack of fever and wound drainage in burn wounds, evidence of wound healing

Topical sulfonamides for burn therapy are used to prevent rather than treat infection.

**3. Observe for adverse effects**

**a.** Anorexia, nausea, vomiting

These gastrointestinal (GI) symptoms commonly occur with sulfonamides and urinary tract antiseptics, owing to gastric irritation or stimulation of the vomiting center in the medulla.

**b.** Hypersensitivity—skin rash, fever, urticaria, pruritus, serum sickness, occasional anaphylaxis

This is more likely to occur with sulfonamides than urinary tract antiseptics. Sensitization may occur with exposure to a sulfonamide drug or to sulfonamide derivatives, such as thiazide diuretics and oral antidiabetic drugs. The drug should be discontinued if a skin rash appears.

**c.** Nephrotoxicity—oliguria, crystalluria, hematuria

This occurred more often with older, less soluble sulfonamides when drug crystals would form and damage tissues in the urinary tract. Most sulfonamides currently used are relatively soluble. However, adequate fluid intake to produce at least 1200 to 1500 ml of urine daily may prevent crystalluria. Also, alkalinizing urine increases drug solubility and prevents crystals from forming. Nephrotoxicity with urinary antiseptics is uncommon.

**d.** Blood dyscrasias—hemolytic anemia, agranulocytosis, aplastic anemia, others

These are uncommon but potentially life-threatening.

**e.** Central nervous system effects—headache, dizziness, lethargy, mental depression

May occur with sulfonamides

**f.** Phlebitis at the IV site with trimethoprim-sulfamethoxazole

The drug is irritating to tissues. Tissue damage may occur if the drug is allowed to extravasate.

**4. Observe for drug interactions**

**a.** Drugs that *increase* effects of sulfonamides:

(1) Alkalinizing agents (*e.g.*, sodium bicarbonate)

Increase rate of urinary excretion, thereby raising levels of sulfonamides in the urinary tract and increasing effectiveness in UTIs.

(2) Methenamine compounds, urinary acidifiers, paraldehyde

These drugs increase the risk of nephrotoxicity. They should *not* be used with sulfonamides. They may cause precipitation of sulfonamide with resultant blockage of renal tubules.

(3) Tetracyclines

The combination of a tetracycline plus a sulfonamide is preferred treatment of *Nocardia* in brain abscess and lesions of the lungs and other organs, against organisms causing lymphogranuloma venereum, and against organisms causing trachoma. These infections are rare.

## Nursing Actions

## Rationale/Explanation

(4) Salicylates (*e.g.,* aspirin), nonsteroidal anti-inflammatory agents (*e.g.,* ibuprofen, indomethacin), oral anticoagulants, phenytoin, methotrexate

Increase toxicity of sulfonamides by displacing sulfonamides from plasma protein-binding sites, thereby increasing plasma levels of free drug

**b.** Drugs that *decrease* effects of sulfonamides:

(1) Alkalinizing agents (*e.g.,* sodium bicarbonate)

Alkalinizing agents decrease GI absorption of sulfonamides. This results in decreased therapeutic effectiveness in systemic illness. The agents also decrease crystalluria, an adverse effect, by alkalinizing the urine and increasing sulfonamide solubility.

(2) Local anesthetics containing PABA (*e.g.,* procaine, benzocaine)

Increasing the concentration of PABA decreases activity of sulfonamides.

**c.** Drugs that alter effects of nitrofurantoin:

(1) Antacids, alkalinizing agents

May reduce the effectiveness of nitrofurantoin; antacids may impair GI absorption of nitrofurantoin

(2) Acidifying agents

Increase antibacterial activity of nitrofurantoin by decreasing renal excretion. Nitrofurantoin is most active against organisms causing urinary tract infection when urine pH is 5.5 or less.

(3) Probenecid

Decreases renal clearance of nitrofurantoin and may thereby increase its toxicity

**d.** Drugs that alter effects of methenamine:

(1) Acetazolamide (Diamox)

Decreases effect by making urine alkaline. Methenamine requires an acidic pH (5.5 or less) for releasing formaldehyde, the antibacterial product of methenamine breakdown.

(2) Acidifying agents

Increase effects by increasing the rate of liberation of formaldehyde

(3) Alkalinizing agents

Decrease effect by decreasing conversion to formaldehyde

(4) Sulfonamides

See 4a(2), above.

**5. Teach clients**

**a.** Take medication for the full time prescribed.

Sulfonamides and urinary antiseptics are bacteriostatic, and bacterial resistance develops rather readily. Therefore, to be most effective and decrease resistance, these drugs should not be stopped when symptoms subside.

**b.** Take medications before meals; if nausea and vomiting occur, take them with meals.

Absorption from the GI tract is probably better if the drugs are taken on an empty stomach. However, symptoms of GI distress often occur and can be prevented or minimized by taking the medications with food.

**c.** Drink at least 3 quarts of fluid daily, if not contraindicated.

With sulfonamides, an adequate fluid intake and a urine output of at least 1500 ml/d reduce or prevent crystals from forming and damaging the urinary tract. With UTIs, fluids decrease the bacterial population of the urinary tract.

**d.** Report skin rash, fever, sore throat, abnormal bleeding (blood in urine, nose bleed, bruises)

These symptoms may indicate adverse drug effects and the need to discontinue or reduce dosage of the drugs.

**e.** With phenazopyridine, inform the client that the drug turns urine orange-red.

To prevent the client from mistaking the discolored urine for blood from the urinary tract

## Review and Application Exercises

1. How do sulfonamides exert their bacteriostatic effects?
2. Why are sulfonamides often effective in UTIs?
3. What are major adverse effects of sulfonamides, and how may they be prevented or minimized?
4. What is the rationale for combining sulfamethoxazole and trimethoprim?
5. What are important characteristics of urinary antiseptics?

## Selected References

(1993). *Drug facts and comparisons*. St. Louis: Facts and Comparisons.

Mandell, G. L., Douglas, R. G. Jr., & Bennett, J. E. (Eds.) (1990). *Principles and practice of infectious diseases* (3rd ed.). New York: Churchill Livingstone.

Sahai, J. V., & Fendler, K. J. (1992). Urinary tract infections. In M. A. Koda-Kimble & L. Y. Young (Eds.), *Applied therapeutics: The clinical use of drugs* (5th ed.) (pp. 43-1–43-23). Vancouver, WA: Applied Therapeutics.

# CHAPTER 41

# Antitubercular Drugs

## Tuberculosis

Tuberculosis is an infectious disease that usually affects the respiratory system but may involve the kidneys, meninges, bone, adrenal glands, and gastrointestinal tract. It is caused by *Mycobacterium tuberculosis*, the tubercle bacillus. These organisms have unique characteristics that influence the disease process and drug therapy. They multiply slowly; they may lie dormant within the body for many years, encapsulated in calcified tubercles; they resist phagocytosis and survive within phagocytic cells; they rapidly develop resistance to single-drug therapies; and they develop resistance to multiple drugs when treatment is inadequate or incomplete. Drug resistance develops when clients do not take the drugs and doses prescribed for the length of time prescribed. Taking a few doses for a short time inhibits the microorganisms that are most susceptible to the drugs but does not effectively inhibit resistant strains, which grow and flourish.

Tuberculosis has increased during recent years. This increase is largely attributed to a high incidence in people with acquired immunodeficiency syndrome (AIDS) and in immigrants from Southeast Asia, where the disease is endemic. In addition to the increase in number of cases, a major concern is the increase in multidrug-resistant tuberculosis (MDRTB). MDRTB develops in people who receive inadequate drug therapy, and it spreads to previously uninfected contacts. Several outbreaks have occurred in prisons and hospitals, mostly in large urban areas.

## Treatment regimens for tuberculosis

The only effective treatment for tuberculosis is drug therapy. In an effort to provide adequate treatment and promote client compliance, several regimens have been tried and found effective. For several years, recommended treatment involved isoniazid (INH), rifampin (Rifadin), and pyrazinamide for 2 months, followed by INH and rifampin for 4 additional months or for clients unable to tolerate pyrazinamide, INH and rifampin for 9 months. These drugs have been given daily or two or three times weekly. In the intermittent schedule, healthcare providers either administer the drugs or observe the client taking them. This schedule was developed for clients unable or unwilling to self-administer the drugs independently.

With the increasing prevalence of MDRTB, several treatment changes have been recommended by the Centers for Disease Control and Prevention. One recommendation is to perform culture and susceptibility tests with all cases (*i.e.,* do not assume susceptibility to INH and rifampin). A second recommendation is to prescribe four antitubercular drugs (INH, rifampin, pyrazinamide, and either ethambutol or streptomycin) until susceptibility reports become available, then change the regimen if indicated. A third recommendation is directly observed therapy to ensure that the client actually takes the drugs. A fourth recommendation is to continue treatment at least 6 months or 3 months following negative cultures.

Anne Collins Abrams: CLINICAL DRUG THERAPY, Fourth Edition.
© 1995 J.B. Lippincott Company.

**427**

If the client is symptomatic or the culture is positive after 3 months, noncompliance or drug resistance must be considered.

# Characteristics of antitubercular drugs

Antitubercular drugs are divided into primary and secondary agents. Primary drugs (INH, rifampin, pyrazinamide, ethambutol) are used in the initial treatment of tuberculosis. Secondary drugs, used when organisms develop resistance to primary drugs, are less effective, more toxic, or both.

## MECHANISMS OF ACTION

INH inhibits formation of cell walls in mycobacteria. The drug is actively transported into the bacterium, where it kills actively growing organisms and inhibits the growth of dormant organisms in macrophages and tuberculous lesions. Rifampin causes defective, nonfunctional proteins to be produced by the bacterial cell. It also penetrates intact cells and kills intracellular bacteria. This unique ability contributes to its effectiveness in treating tuberculosis because mycobacteria are harbored within host cells. Thus, it acts synergistically with INH. Pyrazinamide is bactericidal against actively growing mycobacteria within macrophages, but its exact mechanism of action is unknown. Ethambutol probably inhibits bacterial synthesis of ribonucleic acid (RNA). Streptomycin acts only against extracellular organisms; it does not penetrate macrophages and tuberculous lesions.

## INDICATIONS FOR USE

INH is used to prevent and treat tuberculosis. Because the drug may cause hepatotoxicity, there is some controversy about who should receive prophylaxis. Generally, though, candidates include the following groups who are at high risk for developing active disease:

1. Household and other close contacts of clients with recently diagnosed tuberculosis. These people should receive INH for 3 months. Then, if a skin test and chest x-ray are negative, the drug may be stopped. If the tests are positive, INH should be continued for 9 additional months.
2. People who are considered newly infected (recent converters from negative to positive skin tests)
3. People with positive skin tests and additional risk factors (lung lesions on chest x-ray; diseases such as diabetes mellitus, silicosis, AIDS, leukemia, or lymphoma; alcoholism; postgastrectomy status; on

chronic hemodialysis; on corticosteroid or other immunosuppressive drugs; immigrants from Southeast Asia)
4. Children and adults under 35 years of age with positive skin tests

In chemotherapy of active tuberculosis, INH should be part of any drug regimen. It is always used in conjunction with one or two other primary antitubercular drugs to inhibit emergence of drug-resistant organisms. Rifampin, pyrazinamide, ethambutol, and streptomycin are used in the treatment of active tuberculosis.

Rifampin also is a drug of choice for prophylaxis of meningitis in close contacts of clients with meningitis. It is being investigated for use in other infections as well, including those caused by some staphylococci, atypical mycobacteria, viruses, and fungi.

## CONTRAINDICATIONS FOR USE

Chemoprophylaxis with INH is contraindicated in clients with hepatic disease, in those who have had reactions to the drug, and in pregnant women. Rifampin is contraindicated in people who have had hypersensitivity reactions and must be used with caution in the presence of liver disease.

# Individual antitubercular drugs

## PRIMARY DRUGS

**INH** (Laniazid, Nydrazid) is the most important antitubercular drug. It is well absorbed from the gastrointestinal tract and widely distributed in body tissues and fluids, including cerebrospinal fluid.

INH is acetylated in the liver to acetylisoniazid, which is more efficiently excreted by the kidneys. Metabolism of INH is genetically determined; some people are "slow acetylators" and others are "rapid acetylators." A person's rate of acetylation may be significant in determining response to INH. Slow acetylators have less $N$-acetyltransferase, the acetylating enzyme, in their livers. In these clients, INH is more likely to accumulate to toxic concentrations, and the development of peripheral neuropathy is more likely. However, there is no significant difference in the clinical effectiveness of INH. Rapid acetylators may require unusually high doses of INH. They also may be more susceptible to serious liver injury related to the formation of hepatotoxic metabolites.

### Route and dosage range

*Adults:* Treatment of active disease, PO, IM 4–5 mg/ kg per day in a single dose (maximum dose, 300 mg/ d), for at least 6 mo

Chemoprophylaxis, PO, IM 300 mg/d in a single dose for 3–12 mo

Disseminated tuberculosis or pulmonary disease resulting from atypical mycobacteria, PO, IM 10–20 mg/kg per day, perhaps for years

*Children:* Treatment of active disease, PO, IM 10–20 mg/kg per day; maximum dose, 300 mg/d for at least 6 mo

Chemoprophylaxis, 10 mg/kg per day in a single dose (maximum dose, 300 mg/d), for 3–12 mo

**Rifampin** is a semisynthetic antibacterial drug that inhibits growth of many gram-positive and gram-negative bacteria, including *Escherichia coli, Pseudomonas, Proteus, Klebsiella, Staphylococcus aureus,* and meningococci, as well as mycobacteria causing tuberculosis. Rifampin is well absorbed following oral administration and diffuses well into body tissues and fluids, with highest concentrations in the liver, lungs, gallbladder, and kidneys. It is metabolized in the liver and excreted primarily in bile; a small amount is excreted in urine. The drug causes a harmless red-orange discoloration of body secretions, including urine, tears, saliva, sputum, perspiration, and feces.

Rifampin is always used with other drugs to prevent the occurrence of drug-resistant organisms. Rifampin and INH in combination eliminate tuberculosis bacilli from sputum and produce clinical improvement faster than any other drug regimen, unless organisms resistant to one or both drugs are causing the disease.

### Route and dosage range

*Adults:* Treatment of active disease, PO 600 mg or 10–20 mg/kg per day in a single dose for at least 6 mo

*Children:* Treatment of active disease, PO 10–20 mg/kg once daily; maximum dose, 600 mg/d for at least 6 mo

**Ethambutol** (Myambutol) is a tuberculostatic drug that inhibits synthesis of ribonucleic acid and thus interferes with mycobacterial protein metabolism. It is well absorbed from the gastrointestinal tract, even when given with food. The extent of tissue distribution is unclear except that diffusion into cerebrospinal fluid is limited. It is excreted primarily by the kidneys, either unchanged or as metabolites. Mycobacterial resistance to ethambutol develops slowly. Ethambutol may be a component in a four-drug regimen for initial treatment of tuberculosis that may be caused by multidrug resistant organisms.

Dosage is determined by body weight because no practical method of measuring serum drug levels is available. Also, dosage is changed during treatment if significant changes in body weight occur. Dosage must be reduced with impaired renal function. To obtain therapeutic serum levels, the total daily dose is given at one time. Ethambutol generally is not recommended for young children whose visual acuity cannot be monitored but may be considered for children of any age when organisms are susceptible to ethambutol and resistant to other drugs.

### Route and dosage range

*Adults and children Over 13 years:* Initial treatment, PO 15 mg/kg per day in a single dose
Retreatment, 25 mg/kg per day for 2 months, then 15 mg/kg per day

*Children Under 13 years:* PO 15–25 mg/kg daily or 50 mg/kg twice weekly; maximum single dose, 2.5 g

**Pyrazinamide** is recommended in initial treatment of tuberculosis, along with INH and rifampin. It was formerly considered a secondary drug, mainly because of hepatotoxicity associated with the high doses (3 g or more daily) commonly used. Recently, smaller doses have been found effective and less toxic, although hepatotoxicity may still occur. Dosage should be reduced for clients with liver disease.

### Route and dosage range

*Adults:* PO 15–30 mg/kg per day, in three or four divided doses to a maximum dose of 2 g/d or 50–70 mg/kg twice weekly to a maximum dose of 4 g

*Children:* Same as for adults

**Streptomycin,** an aminoglycoside formerly used in the treatment of tuberculosis, has been removed from the market. It is available from the Centers for Disease Control and Prevention for treatment of tuberculosis resistant to other antitubercular drugs.

## SECONDARY DRUGS

**Para-aminosalicylic acid** (PAS), **capreomycin** (Capastat), **cycloserine** (Seromycin), and **ethionamide** (Trecator SC) are diverse drugs that share tuberculostatic properties. These drugs are generally less effective or more toxic than primary drugs. They are indicated for use only when other agents are contraindicated or in disease caused by drug-resistant organisms. They must be given concurrently with other tuberculostatic drugs to inhibit emergence of resistant mycobacteria.

*Para-aminosalicylic acid, sodium aminosalicylate*

### Route and dosage range

*Adults:* PO 14–16 g/d in two or three divided doses

*Children:* PO 275–420 mg/kg per day in three or four divided doses

Capreomycin

### Route and dosage range

*Adults:* IM (deep) 20 mg/kg (about 1 g) daily for 2–4 wk, then 1 g two or three times weekly for 6–12 mo or longer
*Children:* No dosage established

Cycloserine

### Route and dosage range

*Adults:* PO 10 mg/kg per day in two divided doses
*Children:* No dosage established

Ethionamide

### Route and dosage range

*Adults:* PO 0.5–1 g/d in three divided doses
*Children:* PO 12–15 mg/kg per day, in three divided doses; maximum dose, 750 mg/d

## Nursing Process

### Assessment

Assess for current or potential tuberculosis:
- For current disease, clinical manifestations include fatigue, weight loss, anorexia, malaise, fever, and a productive cough. In early phases, however, there may be no symptoms. If available, check diagnostic test reports for indications of tuberculosis (chest x-ray, tuberculin skin test, and sputum smear and culture).
- For potential tuberculosis, identify high-risk clients: those who are close contacts of someone with active tuberculosis; those who are elderly or undernourished; those who have diabetes mellitus, silicosis, Hodgkin's disease, leukemia, or AIDS; those who are alcoholics; and those who are receiving immunosuppressive drugs. Most new cases of tuberculosis develop in people previously infected, including immigrants from Southeast Asia and other parts of the world where the disease is endemic. However, the number of new cases with primary infection by multidrug-resistant organisms and rapid progression to active disease is increasing.

### Nursing diagnoses

- Knowledge Deficit: Disease process and need for treatment
- High Risk for Noncompliance related to adverse drug effects and need for long-term treatment
- Knowledge Deficit: Consequences of noncompliance with the drug therapy regimen
- High Risk for Injury: Adverse drug effects

### Planning/goals

*The client will:*
- Take drugs as prescribed
- Keep appointments for follow-up care
- Report adverse drug effects
- Act to prevent spread of the disease

### Interventions

Use measures to prevent the spread of tuberculosis:
- Isolate suspected or newly diagnosed hospitalized clients in a private room for 2 or 3 weeks, until drug therapy has rendered them noninfectious.
- Wear masks with close contact, and wash hands thoroughly afterward.
- Have clients wear masks when out of the room for diagnostic tests.

*Teach clients:*
- About the disease process and the necessity for long-term treatment and follow-up. This is extremely important for the client and the community, because lack of knowledge and failure to comply with the therapeutic regimen lead to disease progression and spread. The American Lung Association publishes many helpful pamphlets, written for the general public, that can be obtained from a local chapter and given to clients and their families. Do not use these as a substitute for personal contact, however.
- Measures to prevent spread of tuberculosis:
  - Cover mouth and nose when coughing or sneezing. This prevents the expulsion of droplet nuclei containing the tubercle bacillus into the surrounding air, where they can be inhaled by and infect others.
  - Cough and expectorate sputum into at least two layers of tissue. Place the used tissues in a waterproof bag, and dispose of the bag, preferably by burning.
  - Wash hands after coughing or sneezing.
- The importance of nutrition and rest in promoting healing

### Evaluation

- Observe for improvement in signs and symptoms of tuberculosis.
- Interview and observe for adverse drug effects.
- Question regarding compliance with instructions for taking antitubercular drugs.

## Principles of therapy

### DRUG REGIMENS

Drug therapy for tuberculosis differs in several respects from drug therapy for other bacterial infections. Some guidelines include the following:

1. Sputum culture and susceptibility reports require 6 to 8 weeks because the tubercle bacillus multiplies slowly. Consequently, initial drug therapy is based on other factors, such as the extent of disease, whether the client has previously received antitubercular drugs, and whether multidrug-resistant strains are being isolated in the particular community. Multidrug-resistant strains may occur anywhere. However, in the United States, they have been most evident in populations with AIDS or in closed environments (*e.g.,* hospitals, prisons).

2. Multiple drugs are required to inhibit emergence of drug-resistant organisms.

3. Duration of drug therapy varies with the purpose, extent of disease, and clinical response. INH for positive tuberculin reactors is given for 12 months. Treatment of active disease with multiple drugs ranges from 6 months to 1 year or more, depending on clinical response and culture reports.

4. Whatever the drug therapy regimen, close supervision is needed during treatment to monitor response and compliance and during the year after completion of drug therapy, because most relapses occur during that time.

## USE IN CHILDREN

INH is used in prevention and treatment of tuberculosis in children as in adults. Hepatotoxicity rarely occurs in children. Rifampin is used in the treatment of tuberculosis. Ethambutol is recommended for children only when the causative organism is resistant to other drugs but susceptible to ethambutol. Pyrazinamide has not been established as safe and effective for use in children and is not recommended because of potential toxicity.

## USE IN OLDER ADULTS

Potentially fatal hepatitis may occur with INH, especially in people who drink alcoholic beverages daily. Liver function tests should be monitored regularly, and the drug should be discontinued if signs and symptoms of hepatotoxicity occur. Pyrazinamide and rifampin also may cause hepatotoxicity. Because these are the drugs of first choice for the first 2 months of tuberculosis therapy, clients must be observed closely for signs of liver dysfunction.

## NURSING ACTIONS: ANTITUBERCULAR DRUGS

| *Nursing Actions* | *Rationale/Explanation* |
|---|---|
| **1. Administer accurately** | |
| **a.** Give INH, ethambutol, and rifampin in a single dose, once daily. | A single dose with the resulting higher blood levels is more effective. Also, fewer doses may increase client compliance with drug therapy. |
| **b.** Give PAS and ethionamide with food. | To minimize nausea, vomiting, and diarrhea |
| **c.** Give rifampin 1 hour before or 2 hours after a meal. | Food delays absorption. |
| **d.** Give capreomycin and parenteral INH by deep intramuscular injection into a large muscle mass, and rotate injection sites. | To decrease local pain and tissue irritation |
| **2. Observe for therapeutic effects** | Therapeutic effects are usually apparent within the first 2 or 3 weeks of drug therapy. |
| **a.** Clinical improvement | |
| (1) Decreased cough, sputum, fever, night sweats, and fatigue | |
| (2) Increased appetite, weight, and feeling of well-being | |
| **b.** Negative sputum smear and culture | |
| **c.** Improvement in chest x-ray studies | |
| **3. Observe for adverse effects** | |
| **a.** Nausea, vomiting, diarrhea | These symptoms are likely to occur with any of the oral antitubercular drugs and are usually most severe with PAS. |
| **b.** Neurotoxicity: | |
| (1) Eighth cranial nerve damage—vertigo, tinnitus, hearing loss | A major adverse reaction to aminoglycoside antibiotics |

*(continued)*

| *Nursing Actions* | *Rationale/Explanation* |
|---|---|
| (2) Optic nerve damage—decreased vision and color discrimination | The major adverse reaction to ethambutol |
| (3) Peripheral neuritis—tingling, numbness, paresthesias | Often occurs with INH but can be prevented by administering pyridoxine (vitamin $B_6$). Also may occur with ethambutol. |
| (4) CNS changes—confusion, convulsions, depression | More often associated with INH but similar changes may occur with ethambutol |
| c. Hepatotoxicity—increased serum aspartate aminotransferase (AST), alanine aminotransferase (ALT), and serum bilirubin; jaundice; and other symptoms of hepatitis | May occur with INH, rifampin, and pyrazinamide, especially if the client already has liver damage |
| d. Nephrotoxicity—increased blood urea nitrogen and serum creatinine, cells in urine, oliguria | A major adverse reaction to aminoglycosides |
| e. Hypersensitivity—fever, tachycardia, anorexia, and malaise are early symptoms. If the drug is not discontinued, exfoliative dermatitis, hepatitis, renal abnormalities, and blood dyscrasias may occur. | Hypersensitivity reactions are more likely to occur between the third and eighth weeks of drug therapy. Early detection and drug discontinuation are necessary to prevent progressive worsening of the client's condition. Severe reactions can be fatal. |
| **4. Observe for drug interactions** | |
| **a.** Drugs that *increase* effects of antitubercular drugs: Other antitubercular drugs | Potentiate antitubercular effects. These drugs are always used in combination of two or more for treatment of tuberculosis. For chemoprophylaxis, INH is used alone. |
| **b.** Drugs that *alter* the effects of INH: | |
| (1) Alcohol and oral antacids decrease effects. | Alcohol induces hepatic enzymes, which accelerate the rate of isoniazid metabolism and may increase the likelihood of toxicity. Oral antacids may decrease absorption of oral INH. |
| (2) Disulfiram | May cause behavioral changes and impairments in coordination |
| (3) Pyridoxine (vitamin $B_6$) | Pyridoxine decreases peripheral neuritis, a common adverse effect of INH, and is usually combined with INH for this purpose. |
| (4) Sympathomimetics | May result in increased blood pressure owing to the MAO inhibitory activity of INH |
| **c.** Drugs that *alter* effects of rifampin: Halothane and INH *increase* effects. | Additive risk of hepatotoxicity |
| **d.** Drugs that *alter* effects of aminoglycosides | See Chapter 36. |
| **5. Teach clients** | |
| **a.** Report adverse reactions to drug therapy: | |
| (1) Severe gastrointestinal problems | |
| (2) Yellowing of sclera, dark urine, clay-colored stools | Characteristics of jaundice and possible liver damage |
| (3) Any changes in vision or hearing | May indicate need to change dosage or discontinue drugs |
| (4) Numbness or tingling of hands or feet | May indicate peripheral neuritis, which can usually be controlled by taking pyridoxine (vitamin $B_6$) |
| (5) Any other changes in usual patterns, such as drowsiness, dizziness, decreased urine output, skin rash, or fever | These may indicate adverse reactions to drugs that must be evaluated by the physician because they may be caused by other conditions as well. |

## Nursing Actions

## Rationale/Explanation

**b.** If taking PAS, discard any tablets that turn brownish or purplish.

PAS deteriorates rapidly in contact with water, heat, and sunlight. Deterioration is manifested by discoloration of the tablets.

**c.** If taking rifampin, urine, tears, saliva, and other body secretions become red. Discoloration of secretions is harmless, except that contact lenses may be permanently stained.

## Review and Application Exercises

1. How do tuberculosis infections differ from most other bacterial infections?
2. Why are AIDS patients at high risk of developing tuberculosis?
3. What are the main risk factors for developing drug-resistant tuberculosis?
4. Who should receive INH to prevent tuberculosis? Who should not be given INH? Why?
5. When INH is given alone for prophylaxis, how long should it be taken?
6. If you worked in a health department with clients on INH prophylaxis, what are some interventions to promote client adherence to the drug regimen?
7. Why is active, symptomatic tuberculosis always treated with multiple drugs?
8. In a client with tuberculosis newly started on drug therapy, how could you explain the emergence of drug-resistant organisms and the importance of preventing this problem?
9. What are advantages and disadvantages of short-course (6–9 months) treatment programs?
10. For which clients would intermittent, direct administration of antitubercular drugs be preferred?
11. What are adverse effects associated with INH, rifampin, pyrazinamide, and ethambutol, and how may they be prevented or minimized?
12. In a client with multidrug-resistant tuberculosis, what are nursing implications?

## Selected References

Abrutyn, E. (1992). Multidrug-resistant nosocomial TB: Newest facet of the HIV epidemic. *Hospital Practice, 11,* 15–17.

Alford, R. H. (1990). Antimycobacterial agents. In G. L. Mandell, R. D. Douglas Jr., & J. E. Bennett (Eds.), *Principles and practice of infectious diseases* (3rd ed.) (pp. 350–360). New York: Churchill Livingstone.

Boutotte, J. (1993). TB. The second time around . . . and how you can help control it. *Nursing 93, 23,* 42–49.

Centers for Disease Control and Prevention (1993). Initial therapy for tuberculosis in the era of multidrug resistance. Recommendations of the Advisory Council for the Elimination of Tuberculosis. *Morbidity and Mortality Weekly Report, 42*(No. RR-7), 1–7.

DeBarge, J. E. (1992). Nursing management of adults with disorders of the lung and pleurae. In L. O. Burrell, (Ed.), *Adult nursing in hospital and community settings* (pp. 762–802). Norwalk, CT: Appleton & Lange.

Ellner, J. J., & Toosi, Z. (1992). Tuberculosis. In W. N. Kelley (Ed.), *Textbook of internal medicine* (2nd ed.) (pp. 1426–1434). Philadelphia: J.B. Lippincott.

Porth, C. M. (1990). *Pathophysiology: Concepts of altered health states* (3rd ed.) (pp. 439–441). Philadelphia: J.B. Lippincott.

Van Scoy, R. E., & Wilkowski, C. J. (1992). Antituberculous agents. *Mayo Clinic Proceedings, 67,* 179–187.

Ward, E. S. (1992). Tuberculosis. In M. A. Koda-Kimble & L. Y. Young (Eds.), *Applied therapeutics: The clinical use of drugs* (5th ed.) (pp. 39-1–39-15). Vancouver, WA: Applied Therapeutics.

# CHAPTER 42

# Antiviral Drugs

## General characteristics of viruses and viral infections

Viruses produce many diseases, including hepatitis, encephalitis, pneumonia, rhinitis, skin and mucous membrane diseases, and other disorders that affect almost every body system. Many potentially pathogenic viral strains exist. For example, more than 150 distinct viruses infect the human respiratory tract, including about 100 types of rhinovirus that cause the common cold. Viruses are spread by secretions from infected people, ingestion of contaminated food or water, breaks in skin or mucous membrane, blood transfusions, sexual contact, pregnancy, breast-feeding, and organ transplantation. Viral infections vary from mild, localized disease with few symptoms to severe systemic illness and death. Severe infections are more common when host defense mechanisms are impaired by disease or drugs. Additional characteristics of viruses and viral infections include the following:

1. Viruses are intracellular parasites that can live and reproduce only while inside other living cells. They gain entry to human host cells by binding to specific receptors on cell membranes. The locations and numbers of the receptors determine which host cells can be infected by a particular virus. For example, the mucous membranes lining the tracheobronchial tree have receptors for the influenza A virus.
2. Once inside host cells, viruses use cellular metabolic activities for their own survival and replication. Viral replication involves dissolution of the protein coating and subsequent exposure of the genetic material (de-oxyribonucleic acid [DNA] or ribonucleic acid [RNA]). Next, viral DNA enters the host cell's nucleus, where it becomes incorporated into the host cells' chromosomal DNA. Then, host cell genes are coded to produce new viruses. The new viruses accumulate and eventually cause lysis of the cell. When the cell is destroyed, the viruses are released into the blood and surrounding tissues, from which they can transmit the viral infection to other host cells. In addition, the viral DNA incorporated with host DNA is transmitted to the host's daughter cells during host cell mitosis and becomes part of the inherited genetic information of the host cell and its progeny.
3. Viruses induce antibodies and immunity. Antibodies are proteins that defend against microbial or viral invasion. They are very specific; that is, an antibody will protect only against a specific virus or other antigen. For instance, a person who has had measles develops antibody protection (immunity) against future infection by the measles virus but does not develop immunity against other viral infections, such as chickenpox or hepatitis.

   The protein coat of the virus allows the immune system of the host to recognize the virus as a "foreign invader" and to produce antibodies against it. This system works efficiently for most viruses but does not work for the influenza A virus. Apparently, the influenza A virus can alter its protein covering so much and so often that the immune system does not recognize it as foreign to the body. Thus, last year's antibody cannot recognize and neutralize this year's virus.

   Antibodies against infecting viruses can function to prevent their reaching the bloodstream, or if they have reached the bloodstream, prevent their invasion

Anne Collins Abrams: CLINICAL DRUG THERAPY, Fourth Edition.
© 1995 J.B. Lippincott Company.

of host cells. Once the virus has penetrated the cell, it is protected from antibody action, and the host depends on cell-mediated immunity (lymphocytes and macrophages) to eradicate the virus along with the cell harboring it.

4. Viral infection may occur without signs and symptoms of illness. If illness does occur, the clinical course is usually short and self-limited. Recovery occurs as the virus is eliminated from the body. Some viruses, however, can survive in host cells for a long time and can cause chronic infection. Also, autoimmune diseases may be caused by viral alteration of host cells so that lymphocytes are fooled into thinking the host's own tissues are foreign.

5. Symptoms usually associated with acute viral infections include fever, headache, cough, malaise, muscle pain, nausea and vomiting, diarrhea, insomnia, and photophobia. White blood cell count is usually normal. Other signs and symptoms vary with the type of virus and the body organs involved.

# Antiviral drugs

Drug therapy for viral infections is limited and primarily geared toward relieving symptoms or slowing progress of the disease. Development of effective antiviral drugs is extremely difficult owing to the relationship between viruses and their host cells. Viruses depend on the enzymatic, genetic, and nutritional systems of the host cells for all their own vital functions. Consequently, few drugs suppress multiplication or transmission of viruses without being excessively toxic to host tissues. The drugs inhibit viral reproduction (i.e., are virustatic) but do not kill or eliminate viruses. Available antiviral drugs are expensive, relatively toxic, and effective in a limited number of specific infections. They are of potential use in treating an established infection if given promptly and in chemoprophylaxis if given before, or as soon as possible after, exposure. Protection conferred by chemoprophylaxis is immediate but lasts only while the drug is being taken.

## MECHANISMS OF ACTION

Amantadine interferes with viral penetration of host cells; other antiviral drugs inhibit viral protein synthesis and replication. More specifically, acyclovir and ganciclovir are activated by a viral enzyme found in virus-infected cells, after which they inhibit viral DNA reproduction. Zidovudine, didanosine, and dideoxycytidine inhibit reverse transcriptase, an enzyme required by retroviruses to convert RNA to DNA and allow replication.

# Individual antiviral drugs

Clinically useful antiviral drugs are described below and summarized in Table 42-1.

**Acyclovir** (Zovirax) is a synthetic agent used in the treatment of mucosal and cutaneous infections caused by herpes simplex virus. The major use is for genital herpes, in which acyclovir decreases viral shedding and the duration of skin lesions and pain. The drug does not eliminate inactive virus in the body and thus does not prevent transmission or recurrence of the disease unless oral drug therapy is continued. Acyclovir is also indicated for treatment of herpes labialis ("cold sores" or "fever blisters") or other herpes simplex infections in immunocompromised clients. Prolonged or repeated courses of acyclovir therapy may result in the emergence of acyclovir-resistant viral strains. This is most likely to occur in immunocompromised clients.

Acyclovir can be given orally, intravenously, or applied topically to lesions. Intravenous use is recommended only for severe genital herpes in nonimmunocompromised clients and any herpes infections in immunocompromised clients. The drug is excreted through the kidneys, and dosage must be reduced in the presence of renal failure. Safety and effectiveness of acyclovir during pregnancy and lactation have not been established.

**Amantadine** (Symmetrel) is a synthetic agent that prevents viral penetration into human host cells. It is most effective in preventing infections caused by the influenza A virus. It may be given to clients having contact with active influenza cases. In confirmed epidemics of influenza A infections, amantadine is recommended for clients at high risk who have not been vaccinated. The high-risk population includes older adults, those who have chronic lung disease, and those who have immunodeficiency disorders. Amantadine may be given daily throughout the epidemic (5–6 weeks) or, if the client is vaccinated at the beginning of amantadine therapy, for 10 to 14 days. The drug also may be useful in the treatment of influenza A infections if started as early as possible after onset and continued for 5 to 7 days.

Amantadine is excreted in the urine unchanged; it accumulates in the body when renal function is impaired. Dosage should be reduced with renal impairment. The drug is contraindicated during pregnancy and must be used cautiously in clients with cerebral atherosclerosis, psychiatric disorders, or a history of epilepsy.

**Ganciclovir** (Cytovene) and **foscarnet** (Foscavir) are approved only for treatment of cytomegalovirus (CMV) retinitis in immunocompromised clients, including those with acquired immunodeficiency syndrome (AIDS). CMV retinitis is characterized by a progressive loss of vision. Ganciclovir may improve, but does not cure, the disease. Long-term maintenance therapy may be useful if granulocytopenia and thrombocytopenia do not require that the drug be stopped or interrupted until

**TABLE 42-1.   ANTIVIRAL DRUGS**

| Generic/Trade Name | Indications for Use | Routes and Dosage Ranges | |
|---|---|---|---|
| | | **Adults** | **Children** |
| **Acyclovir** (Zovirax) | Oral mucocutaneous lesions (*e.g.*, cold sores, fever blisters) Genital herpes Herpes simplex encephalitis Varicella (chickenpox) in immunocompromised hosts Herpes zoster (shingles) in normal and immunocompromised hosts | Genital herpes, PO 200 mg q4h, five times daily for 10 d for initial infection; 400 mg two times daily to prevent recurrence of chronic infection; 200 mg q4h five times daily for 5 d to treat recurrence Herpes zoster, PO 800 mg q4h five times daily for 7–10 d Chickenpox PO 20 mg/kg (maximum dose 800 mg) four times daily for 5 d Mucosal and cutaneous herpes simplex virus (HSV) infections in immunocompromised hosts (ICH), IV 5 mg/kg infused at constant rate over 1 h, q8h for 7 d Varicella-zoster infections in ICH IV 10 mg/kg, infused as above, q8h for 7 d HSV encephalitis IV 10 mg/kg infused as above, q8h for 10 d Topically to lesions q3h, six times daily for 7 d | Children under 12 years: IV 250 mg/m$^2$ q8h for 7 d |
| **Amantadine** (Symmetrel) | Prophylaxis of influenza A for contacts of infected people and for high-risk people during outbreaks of influenza A Treatment of influenza A infection | PO 200 mg/d in one or two doses | PO 200 mg/d in one or two doses for children over 9 y; 4.4–8.8 mg/kg per day for children 1–9 y (maximum dose, 150 mg/d) |
| **Didanosine (ddI)** (Videx) | Advanced human immunodeficiency virus (HIV) infection in people who cannot tolerate zidovudine or whose condition worsens while receiving zidovudine | 35–49 kg: PO 125 mg q12h 50–74 kg: PO 200 mg q12h 75 kg or more: PO 300 mg q12h | <0.4 m$^2$ body surface area (BSA): PO 25 mg q12h 0.5–0.7 m$^2$ BSA: 50 mg q12h 0.8–1 m$^2$ BSA: 75 mg q12h 1.1–1.4 m$^2$ BSA: PO 100 mg q12h |
| **Dideoxycytidine (ddC)** (Zalcitabine) | Advanced HIV infection in people whose condition worsens while receiving zidovudine. Given concurrently with zidovudine | PO 0.75 mg q8h (2.25 mg/d) with zidovudine 200 mg q8h (600 mg/d) | Children weighing 30 kg or more: PO same as adults Children weighing <30 kg: PO reduce doses proportionately |
| **Foscarnet** (Foscavir) | Cytomegalovirus (CMV) retinitis in people with acquired immunodeficiency syndrome (AIDS) | Normal renal function: Induction, IV infusion 60 mg/kg, through infusion pump over 1 h, q8h for 14–21 d, depending on clinical response Maintenance, IV infusion 90–120 mg/kg per day, using infusion pump over 2 h | |
| **Ganciclovir** (Cytovene) | CMV retinitis in people with AIDS or other conditions of immunosuppression | Induction, IV infusion 5 mg/kg q12h for 14–21 d Maintenance, IV infusion 5 mg/kg each day, or 6 mg/kg per day for 5 d of each week | |
| **Idoxuridine** (Herplex) | Keratoconjunctivitis caused by herpes viruses | Topically to eye, 0.1% solution, 1 drop q1h daytime and q2h during the night until improvement, then 1 drop q2h daytime and q4h during the night; 0.5% ointment, apply q4h during the day and at bedtime. Continue for 5 d after healing is complete. | |
| **Ribavirin** (Virazole) | Pneumonia caused by respiratory syncytial virus (RSV) | | Inhalation, diluted to a concentration of 20 mg/ml for 12 to 18 h/d for 3–7 d |
| **Trifluridine** (Viroptic) | Keratoconjunctivitis caused by herpes viruses | Topically to eye, 1% ophthalmic solution, 1 drop q2h while awake (maximum 9 drops/d) until re-epithelialization of corneal ulcer occurs; then 1 drop q4h (maximum 5 drops/d) for 7 d | |
| **Vidarabine** (Vira-A) | Keratoconjunctivitis caused by herpes viruses | IV 15 mg/kg per day, dissolved in 2500 ml of fluid and given over 12–24 h daily for 10 d Topically to eye, 3% ophthalmic ointment, applied q3h until re-epithelialization, then twice daily for 7 d | |
| **Zidovudine** (Retrovir) | HIV infection (AIDS and AIDS-related complex) | PO 200 mg q4h around the clock IV 1–2 mg/kg q4h around the clock | Children 3 mo to 12 y: 180 mg/m$^2$ q6h (not to exceed 200 mg q6h) |

bone marrow recovery occurs. Foscarnet causes renal impairment in most recipients; thus, renal function must be assessed periodically during treatment. Dosage of both drugs must be reduced with renal impairment (see manufacturers' literature for specific instructions).

**Idoxuridine** (Herplex), **trifluridine** (Viroptic), and **vidarabine** (Vira-A) are applied topically to treat infections of the eye, such as keratoconjunctivitis and corneal ulcers caused by the herpes simplex virus (herpetic keratitis). Trifluridine may promote more rapid healing of corneal ulcers than other drugs but should not be used longer than 21 days because of possible ocular toxicity. Vidarabine is as effective as idoxuridine for keratoconjunctivitis and causes less tissue irritation. Vidarabine also is given intravenously to treat herpes zoster infections in clients whose immune systems are impaired and encephalitis caused by herpes simplex viruses. Intravenous dosage must be reduced with impaired renal function.

**Ribavirin** (Virazole) is used for the treatment of respiratory tract infections caused by the respiratory syncytial virus. It has been used mainly in infants and children. It is given only by inhalation with the Viratek Small Particle Aerosol Generator. The drug is not recommended for clients on ventilators because it precipitates and blocks tubes, including endotracheal tubes. Deterioration of pulmonary function is a common adverse effect.

**Zidovudine** (Retrovir), **didanosine** or ddI (Videx), and **dideoxycytidine** or ddC (Zalcitabine) are used for the treatment of symptomatic human immunodeficiency virus (HIV) infection (AIDS) and advanced AIDS-related complex (ARC). Zidovudine is the first drug of choice. The drug slows progression but does not cure the disease. In addition, it does not prevent transmission of the virus through sexual contact or blood contamination. Granulocytopenia and anemia are common adverse effects. If severe, drug therapy should be interrupted until bone marrow recovery occurs.

Didanosine is considered a second-line drug. It is approved for treatment of adults and children older than 6 months who have advanced HIV infection and either cannot tolerate zidovudine or whose condition continues to deteriorate while receiving zidovudine. The drug causes a high incidence of adverse effects, including peripheral neuropathy and pancreatitis.

Dideoxycytidine is approved for combination therapy with zidovudine in advanced HIV infection in adults whose condition continues to deteriorate while receiving zidovudine.

## Nursing Process

### Assessment

- Assess for AIDS, ARC, influenza or other viral infections of the respiratory tract, genital herpes, viral infections of the eye, and other viral disorders for which antiviral drugs are indicated.
- Assess renal function and adequacy of fluid intake.

### Nursing diagnoses

- Self-Care Deficit related to systemic infection
- Anxiety related to a medical diagnosis of AIDS or genital herpes
- Altered Sexuality Patterns related to sexually transmitted viral infections (AIDS, genital herpes)
- Body Image Disturbance related to sexually transmitted infection
- Social Isolation related to a medical diagnosis of AIDS or genital herpes
- Knowledge Deficit: Disease process and methods of spread
- High Risk for Injury: Recurrent infection
- High Risk for Injury: Adverse drug effects
- High Risk for Injury: Infections and other problems associated with compromised immune systems in AIDS

### Planning/Goals

*The client will:*

- Receive or take antiviral drugs as prescribed
- Be safeguarded against new or recurrent infection
- Act to prevent spread of viral infection to others and recurence in self
- Avoid preventable adverse drug effects
- Receive emotional support and counseling to assist in coping with AIDS or genital herpes

### Interventions

- Follow recommended policies and procedures for preventing spread of viral infections.
- For clients receiving systemic antiviral drugs, monitor serum creatinine and other tests of renal function, complete blood count, and fluid balance.
- Spend time with the client when indicated to reduce anxiety and support usual coping mechanisms.

*Teach clients:*

- Ways to control spread and recurrence of viral infection
- To maintain immunizations against viral infections as indicated
- That drug therapy for genital herpes and AIDS does not prevent the causative virus from being transmitted to other people
- That zidovudine for AIDS does not prevent opportunistic infections or other disorders associated with the disease

### Evaluation

- Observe for improvement in signs and symptoms of the viral infection for which a drug is given.
- Interview outpatients regarding their compliance with instructions for taking antiviral drugs.
- Interview and observe for use of infection-control measures.
- Interview and observe for adverse drug effects.
- Observe mood and psychological status in clients with AIDS or genital herpes.

# Principles of therapy

1. Drug therapy has a limited place in treating viral infections. Management mainly involves preventive measures, such as vaccination, handwashing, teaching infected clients to cover their mouth and nose when coughing or sneezing, treatment of symptoms, and recognition and treatment of complications.
2. Viral vaccines are used for active immunization of clients before exposure or to control epidemics of viral disease in a community. Vaccines for prevention of poliomyelitis, measles, rubella, mumps, smallpox, and yellow fever and for protection against influenza and rabies are available (see Chap. 46).
3. Live attenuated viral vaccines are generally quite safe and nontoxic. However, they probably should not be used in clients who are pregnant, immunodeficient, or receiving corticosteroids, antineoplastic or immunosuppressive drugs, or irradiation.
4. Influenza vaccines prevent infection in most clients. If infection does occur, less virus is shed in respiratory secretions. Thus, vaccination reduces transmission of influenza by decreasing the number of susceptible people and by decreasing transmission by immunized people who still become infected.
5. The multiplicity of rhinoviruses (common cold), enteroviruses, and respiratory viruses precludes imminent development of practical vaccines for these common diseases.
6. Antiviral drugs are available to prevent or treat a few specific viral infections. They should not be used unless the etiologic diagnosis is certain.
7. Antibacterial drugs should not be used in viral infections in the hope of preventing complications. They do have a role, however, in treating bacterial complications of viral infections.

## USE IN CHILDREN

Most systemic antiviral drugs have not been established as safe and effective for use in children. Amantadine is given to prevent or treat influenza A in children 1 year old or older. Safety and effectiveness have not been established for use in children under 1 year old. Zidovudine is approved for treatment of HIV infection in children.

## USE IN OLDER ADULTS

Most of the systemic antiviral drugs are excreted by the kidneys. Because renal impairment is common in older adults, there probably are greater risks of toxicity. These risks may be minimized by close monitoring of renal function and maintaining adequate fluid intake. When amantadine is given to prevent or treat influenza A, dosage should be reduced with renal impairment, and older adults must be monitored closely for central nervous system effects (*e.g.*, hallucinations, depression, confusion) and cardiovascular effects (*e.g.*, congestive heart failure, orthostatic hypotension).

# NURSING ACTIONS: ANTIVIRAL DRUGS

| *Nursing Actions* | *Rationale/Explanation* |
|---|---|
| **1. Administer accurately** | |
| **a.** With intravenous acyclovir, dissolve contents in 10 ml of sterile water for injection, add to 50 to 100 ml of an appropriate intravenous solution, and infuse over at least 1 hour. | A concentration of 7 mg/ml or lower is recommended, and infusion over at least 1 hour helps prevent precipitation of drug in the renal tubules and the possible renal damage that may occur with a bolus or rapid administration. Renal damage also is less likely to occur if the client is well hydrated. |
| **b.** With topical acyclovir, wear a glove to apply. | To prevent spread of infection, because lesions contain herpesvirus |
| **c.** Give amantadine in two divided doses. | To reduce adverse reactions, which are more likely if the full daily dose is given at one time |
| **d.** Give the second daily dose of amantadine at least 6 hours before bedtime. | To decrease the insomnia that may occur during amantadine therapy |
| **e.** With ribavarin, follow the manufacturer's instructions for dilution and administration. | Specific techniques are required for accurate usage. |
| **f.** With zidovudine, give q4h around the clock. | To maintain therapeutic blood levels |

## Nursing Actions

## Rationale/Explanation

**2. Observe for therapeutic effects**

**a.** With acyclovir, observe for healing of lesions and decreased pain and itching.

**b.** When amantadine is given for influenza A prophylaxis, absence of symptoms indicates therapeutic benefit.

**c.** When amantadine is given in active influenza A infection, observe for decreased fever, cough, muscle aches, and malaise.

**d.** With idoxuridine and ophthalmic vidarabine, observe for decreased signs of eye infection.

**e.** With parenteral vidarabine, observe for decreased fever and headache and increased mental alertness.

Vidarabine is not effective in clients with herpes simplex encephalitis who are comatose when drug therapy is initiated.

**3. Observe for adverse effects**

**a.** With acyclovir, observe for nausea, vomiting, diarrhea, headache, dizziness, skin rash, itching and burning, and increased serum creatinine. Rare but potentially serious encephalopathy may be manifested by lethargy, confusion, tremors, seizures, or coma.

Adverse effects are usually infrequent and mild. Gastrointestinal effects and headache are most common; central nervous system (CNS) effects are most likely to occur with intravenous administration.

**b.** With amantadine, observe for CNS effects—insomnia, hyperexcitability, ataxia, dizziness, slurred speech, mental confusion.

Symptoms may be similar to those caused by atropine and amphetamines. Adverse reactions are more likely to occur in older adults and those with renal impairment.

**c.** With ganciclovir and zidovudine, observe for anemia, neutropenia, thrombocytopenia, nausea, vomiting, diarrhea, headache, skin rash, and CNS effects (confusion, dizziness).

Severe hematologic effects may require that drug therapy be stopped, at least until the white blood count recovers. Transfusions may be needed for anemia.

**d.** With ribavarin, observe for increased respiratory distress.

Pulmonary function may deteriorate.

**e.** With ophthalmic antiviral preparations, observe for pain, itching, edema, or inflammation of eyelids.

These symptoms are more likely to occur with idoxuridine than vidarabine. They result from tissue irritation or hypersensitivity reactions.

**4. Observe for drug interactions**

**a.** With acyclovir, probenecid *increases* effects.

Prolongs half-life and slows renal excretion of acyclovir

**b.** Drugs that *alter* effects of amantadine:

(1) Anticholinergics (*e.g.*, atropine)

Increased anticholinergic effects, such as blurred vision, mouth dryness, urine retention, constipation

(2) CNS stimulants and psychotropic drugs

Amantadine has CNS and psychic effects ranging from stimulation (insomnia, nervousness, hyperexcitability) to depression (decreased ability to concentrate, confusion, mental depression). Therefore, other drugs with these effects potentiate amantadine.

**c.** Drugs that *alter* effects of idoxuridine:

(1) Boric acid

Boric acid and idoxuridine ophthalmic solutions should not be administered at the same time or close together because the combination may irritate tissues.

*(continued)*

| *Nursing Actions* | *Rationale/Explanation* |
|---|---|
| (2) Corticosteroids | These drugs may accelerate the spread of a viral infection, such as herpes simplex keratitis. Therefore, they should not be used with idoxuridine unless necessary. |
| (3) Other medications | To ensure stability, do not mix idoxuridine ophthalmic solution with other ophthalmic drugs. |
| **d.** Drugs that *increase* effects of zidovudine: | |
| (1) Acetaminophen, aspirin, indomethacin | These drugs inhibit glucuronidation, the chemical reaction by which zidovudine is metabolized in the liver, and may increase adverse effects. |
| (2) Doxorubicin, vincristine, vinblastine | Increased bone marrow depression, including neutropenia |
| (3) Amphotericin B, flucytosine | Increased nephrotoxicity |
| (4) Ganciclovir | Increased neutropenia |
| (5) Pentamidine | Increased neutropenia |
| **5. Teach clients**<br>**a.** With acyclovir:<br><br>(1) Avoid sexual intercourse when visible lesions are present.<br><br>(2) Always wash hands after touching any lesion.<br><br>(3) Start oral acyclovir for recurrent genital herpes as soon as signs and symptoms begin.<br><br>(4) Use gloves to apply ointment to lesions. | |
| **b.** With amantadine, do not operate machinery of any kind if feeling dizzy or drowsy. | Amantadine causes CNS changes that may impair physical and mental responses, and thus safety may be impaired. |
| **c.** Report insomnia, ataxia, and other adverse effects with amantadine. | |
| **d.** With zidovudine, take q4h around the clock, including during the night. | For therapeutic effects |
| **e.** Correct administration of eye medications (*e.g.*, wash hands before and after instilling eye drops or ointments; do not touch the tip of the medication container to the eye or any other surface) | To avoid spreading infection and contaminating medications |

## Review and Application Exercises

1. Are antiviral drugs virucidal or virustatic?
2. What are the clinical indications for use of acyclovir, amantadine, ganciclovir and foscarnet, and zidovudine?
3. How do zidovudine, didanoside, and dideoxycytidine act against HIV?
4. What are the major adverse effects associated with zidovudine, didanoside, and dideoxycytidine? How would you assess for each of the adverse effects?

5. What nursing interventions may help prevent or minimize adverse effects of anti-AIDS drugs?
6. Why is it important to monitor renal function in any client receiving a systemic antiviral drug?

## Selected References

Bullock, B. L. (1992). Infectious agents. In B. L. Bullock & P. P. Rosendahl, (Eds.), *Pathophysiology: Adaptations and alterations in function* (3rd ed.) (pp. 264–280). Philadelphia: J.B. Lippincott.
(1993). *Drug facts and comparisons*. St. Louis: Facts and Comparisons.

Hayden, F. G., & Douglas, R. G. Jr. (1990). Antiviral agents. In G. L. Mandell, R. G. Douglas Jr., & J. E. Bennett (Eds.), *Principles and practice of infectious diseases* (3rd ed.) (pp. 370–393). New York: Churchill Livingstone.

Jordan, M. C. (1992). Cytomegalovirus. In W. N. Kelley (Ed.), *Textbook of internal medicine* (2nd ed.) (pp. (1497–1499). Philadelphia: J.B. Lippincott.

Kapusnik-Uner, J. E. (1992). Acquired immunodeficiency syndrome. In M. A. Koda-Kimble & L. Y. Young (Eds.), *Applied therapeutics: The clinical use of drugs* (5th ed.) (pp. 47-1–47-29). Vancouver, WA: Applied Therapeutics.

Keating, M. R. (1992). Antiviral agents. *Mayo Clinic Proceedings, 67,* 160–178.

Kohl, S., & Bonik, B. (1992). Herpes simplex virus infections. In W. N. Kelley (Ed.), *Textbook of internal medicine* (2nd ed.) (pp. 1491–1496). Philadelphia: J.B. Lippincott.

Nahata, M. C. (1992). Viral infections. In M. A. Koda-Kimble & L. Y. Young (Eds.), *Applied therapeutics: The clinical use of drugs* (5th ed.) (pp. 48-1–48-11). Vancouver, WA: Applied Therapeutics.

Pomerantz, R. J., & Hirsch, M. S. (1992). Infections caused by retroviruses. In W. N. Kelley (Ed.), *Textbook of internal medicine* (2nd ed.) (pp. 1514–1517). Philadelphia: J.B. Lippincott.

### CHAPTER 43

# Antifungal Drugs

## Fungi and fungal infections

Fungi are plant-like, parasitic microorganisms that are widely dispersed in the environment. Humans are often unavoidably exposed to fungi; conditions in which exposure is followed by infection are not fully known. Mechanisms of infection include inhalation of airborne spores, oral ingestion, and implantation of the fungus under the skin as a result of injury. Fungal infections (mycoses) range from mild, superficial infections to life-threatening systemic infections. Serious systemic fungal infections have become more common, largely because of acquired immunodeficiency syndrome (AIDS), the use of immunosuppressant drugs to treat cancer and organ transplant recipients, the use of indwelling intravenous catheters for prolonged drug therapy or parenteral nutrition, more frequent implantation of prosthetic devices, and widespread use of broad-spectrum antibacterial drugs. Additional characteristics of fungi and fungal infections include the following:

1. Fungi that cause superficial infections of the skin, hair, and nails are called *dermatophytes*. These fungi are often present on the body without causing infection. They obtain nourishment from keratin, a protein in skin, hair, and nails. Dermatophytic infections include tinea pedis (athlete's foot) and tinea capitis (ringworm of the scalp) (see Chap. 69).
2. *Candida albicans* is usually part of the indigenous microbial flora of the skin, mouth, intestine, and vagina. It causes infection in certain circumstances. Vaginal candidiasis is common in women who are pregnant, have diabetes mellitus, or take oral contraceptives. Oral candidiasis (thrush) is common in newborns. Oral, intestinal, vaginal, and systemic candidiasis can occur with antibiotic, antineoplastic, corticosteroid, and immunosuppressant drug therapy. Systemic candidiasis also occurs in clients receiving parenteral nutrition and in those with burn wounds, organ transplants, and immune disorders, such as AIDS. *Candida* may cause endocarditis after insertion of a prosthetic heart valve.
3. Fungi that cause other serious infections are not part of the indigenous microbial flora. These fungi grow independently in soil and decaying organic matter. Fungal infections, such as histoplasmosis, coccidioidomycosis, and blastomycosis, usually occur as pulmonary disease but may be systemic. Severity of disease increases with intensity of exposure.
   a. Histoplasmosis is endemic in many parts of the world. Most infections are asymptomatic or produce minimal symptoms for which treatment is not sought. Clinically evident symptoms are usually those of an acute, influenza-like respiratory infection. The disease occasionally occurs as a rapidly fatal infection involving the liver, spleen, and other organs. Healed lung lesions may calcify and be confused with the lesions of tuberculosis. The fungus causing histoplasmosis is found in soil and organic debris, especially around chicken houses, bird roosts, and caves inhabited by bats.
   b. Coccidioidomycosis usually occurs as an acute, self-limiting respiratory infection but may occur as a chronic, diffuse disease involving almost any body part.
   c. Blastomycosis most often causes respiratory infection that resembles pneumonia or tuberculosis. Other organs may be involved, however, espe-

Anne Collins Abrams: CLINICAL DRUG THERAPY, Fourth Edition.
© 1995 J.B. Lippincott Company.

cially the skin. Skin pustules, ulcerations, and abscesses may occur.

# Antifungal drugs

Drugs for superficial fungal infections of skin and mucous membranes are usually applied topically. Numerous preparations are available, many without a prescription. Drugs for systemic infections are most often given intravenously, and only a few relatively toxic agents are available.

## MECHANISM OF ACTION

Most antifungal drugs bind with essential components in fungal cell membranes. This binding increases permeability of the cell membrane and allows intracellular contents to leak out.

# Individual antifungal drugs

See Table 43-1.

## *Nursing Process*

### Assessment

Assess for fungal infections. Specific signs and symptoms vary with location and type of infection.
* Superficial lesions of skin, hair, and nails are usually characterized by pain, burning, and itching. Some lesions are moist; others are dry and scaling. They also may appear inflamed or discolored.
* Candidiasis occurs in warm, moist areas of the body. Skin lesions are likely to occur in perineal and intertriginous areas. They are usually moist, inflamed, pruritic areas with vesicles and pustules. Oral lesions are white patches that adhere to the buccal mucosa. Vaginal infection causes a cheesy vaginal discharge, burning, and itching. Intestinal infection causes diarrhea.
* Histoplasmosis, coccidioidomycosis, and blastomycosis often simulate influenza, pneumonia, or tuberculosis, with cough, fever, malaise, and other manifestations.
* Systemic mycoses are confirmed by recovery of organisms from specimens of body tissues or fluids.

### Nursing diagnoses
* Self-Care Deficit related to systemic infection
* Knowledge Deficit: Prevention and treatment of fungal infection
* Knowledge Deficit: Accurate drug usage

* High Risk for Noncompliance related to the need for long-term therapy
* High Risk for Injury: Adverse drug effects with systemic antifungal drugs

### Planning/Goals
*The client will:*
* Receive systemic antifungal drugs as prescribed
* Apply topical drugs accurately
* Act to prevent recurrence of fungal infection
* Avoid preventable adverse effects from systemic drugs

### Interventions

Use measures to prevent spread of fungal infections. Superficial infections (*e.g.*, ringworm or tinea) are highly contagious and can be spread by sharing towels and hairbrushes. Systemic mycoses are not contagious.

With neutropenic and other immunocompromised clients, try to decrease exposure to environmental fungi. For example, do not allow soil-containing plants and request regular cleaning and inspection of air conditioning systems. Aspergillosis has occurred following inhalation of airborne spores from air conditioning units.

*Teach clients:*
* With skin lesions, wash hands often; do not share towels, hairbrushes, or other personal items.
* With histoplasmosis and other potentially serious fungal infections, avoid or minimize future exposure to chicken, pigeon, and bat excreta.

### Evaluation
* Observe for relief of symptoms for which an antifungal drug was prescribed.
* Interview outpatients regarding their compliance with instructions for using antifungal drugs.
* Interview and observe for adverse drug effects with systemic antifungal agents.

# Principles of therapy

## DIAGNOSTIC AND THERAPEUTIC FACTORS

1. An etiologic diagnosis should be made before an antifungal drug is used. Local infections can be caused by bacteria, fungi, or both. Most antifungal drugs are ineffective in bacterial infections. Antifungal drugs effective in candidiasis are not usually effective in dermatophytic infections and vice versa.
2. Candidal infections of blood or urine often respond to the removal of predisposing factors, such as antibiotics, corticosteroids or other immunosuppressive drugs, and indwelling intravenous or bladder catheters. Candidal endocarditis, which may occur after prosthetic heart valve replacement, is best treated by surgical removal of the infected prosthesis and administration of amphotericin B.

**TABLE 43-1.  SELECTED ANTIFUNGAL DRUGS**

| Generic/ Trade Name | Clinical Indications | Routes and Dosage Ranges | |
| --- | --- | --- | --- |
| | | **Adults** | **Children** |
| **Amphotericin B** (Fungizone) | Systemic mycoses (*e.g.*, candidiasis, histoplasmosis, blastomycosis, others) Cutaneous candidiasis | Intravenous individualized according to disease severity and client tolerance. Average dose, 0.25–0.5 mg/kg per day Topically to skin lesions, two to four times daily for 1–4 wk | Same as for adults |
| **Butoconazole** (Femstat) | Vaginal candidiasis | Intravaginally, once daily for 3 d | |
| **Ciclopirox** (Loprox) | Tinea infections, cutaneous candidiasis | Topically to skin lesions, twice daily for 2–4 wk | |
| **Clotrimazole** (Lotrimin, Mycelex, Gyne-Lotrimin) | Cutaneous dermatophytosis; oral, cutaneous, and vaginal candidiasis | Orally 1 troche dissolved in mouth five times daily Topically to skin twice daily Intravaginally once daily | Same as for adults  Dosage not established |
| **Econazole** (Spectazole) | Tinea infections, cutaneous candidiasis | Topically to skin lesions once or twice daily for 2–4 wk | |
| **Fluconazole** (Diflucan) | Oropharyngeal, esophageal, and systemic candidiasis; cryptococcal meningitis | Oral or esophageal infection, PO, IV 200 mg on first day, then 100 mg daily for 2–3 wk Systemic infection, PO, IV 400 mg on first day, then 200 mg daily for at least 4 wk and 2 wk after symptoms subside Cryptococcal meningitis, PO, IV 400 mg on first day, then 200 mg daily for 10–12 wk after cultures of cerebrospinal fluid become negative | |
| **Flucytosine** (Ancobon) | Systemic mycoses due to *Candida* species or *Cryptococcus neoformans* | PO 50–150 mg/kg per day in divided doses q6h. Dosage must be decreased with impaired liver function | Same as for adults |
| **Griseofulvin** (Fulvicin) | Dermatophytosis (skin, hair, nails) | Microsize, PO 500 mg–1 g daily in divided doses q6h Ultramicrosize, PO 250–500 mg daily | Microsize, PO 10 mg/kg in divided doses q6h Ultramicrosize, PO 5–7 mg/kg per day |
| **Haloprogin** (Halotex) | Dermatophytosis, mainly tinea pedis (athlete's foot), cutaneous candidiasis | Topically to skin, 1% cream or solution twice daily for 2–4 wk | Dosage not established |
| **Itraconazole** (Sporanox) | Systemic fungal infections, including aspergillosis, in neutropenic and immunocompromised hosts | PO 200 mg once or twice daily | |
| **Ketoconazole** (Nizoral) | Candidiasis, histoplasmosis, coccidioidomycosis, paracoccidioidomycosis | PO 200 mg once daily, increased to 400 mg once daily if necessary in severe infections | Weight above 40 kg: PO 200 mg once daily Weight 20–40 kg: PO 100 mg (1/2 tablet) once daily Weight under 20 kg: PO 50 mg (1/4 tablet) once daily |
| **Miconazole** (Monistat) | Systemic mycoses Dermatophytosis, cutaneous and vulvovaginal candidiasis | IV 600 mg–1 g q8h Topically to skin, once or twice daily for 4 wk Intravaginally once daily for 1–2 wk | IV 20–40 mg/kg per day in divided infusions |
| **Naftifine** (Naftin) | Tinea infections (athlete's foot, jock itch, ringworm) | Topically to skin, once daily (cream) or twice daily (gel) | Safety and efficacy not established |
| **Natamycin** (Natacyn) | Fungal infections of the eye | Topically to eye, 1 drop q1–2h for 3–4 d, then 1 drop six to eight times daily for 14–24 d | |
| **Nystatin** (Mycostatin) | Candidiasis of skin, mucous membrane, and intestinal tract | Oral or intestinal infection, PO 400,000–600,000 U four times daily Topically to skin lesions, two or three times daily, continued for 1 wk after cure Intravaginally, 1 vaginal tablet once daily for 14 d | Oral infection, PO 100,000 U three or four times daily |
| **Oxiconazole** (Oxistat) | Tinea infections | Topically to skin lesions, once daily in evening, for 2–4 wk | |
| **Sulconazole** (Exelderm) | Tinea infections | Topically to skin lesions once or twice daily for 3 to 4 wk | Safety and efficacy not established |
| **Terconazole** (Terazol) | Vaginal candidiasis | Intravaginally, 1 applicator once daily at bedtime for 7 doses | |
| **Tioconazole** (Vagistat) | Vaginal candidiasis | Intravaginally, 1 applicator at bedtime | |
| **Tolnaftate** (Tinactin) | Cutaneous mycoses (dermatophytosis) | Topically to skin lesions, twice daily for 2–6 wk | Same as for adults |
| **Triacetin** (Fungoid) | Dermatophytosis (*e.g.*, athlete's foot), cutaneous candidiasis | Topically to skin lesions, twice daily until 1 wk after symptoms are relieved | Same as for adults |
| **Zinc undecylenate** (Desenex) | Dermatophytosis | Topically to skin twice daily for 2–4 wk | Same as for adults |

3. Most antifungal drug therapy is long term (several weeks to months).

## USE IN CHILDREN

Antifungal drugs are used in children for the same indications as for adults. With oral and parenteral drugs, few studies have been done in children. Dosages are often listed for children older than 1 or 2 years.

No pediatric guidelines have been established for intravenous amphotericin B (Fungizone), a highly toxic drug often used for serious systemic infections. As with adults, children receiving this drug must be monitored closely to reduce the incidence and severity of nephrotoxicity, hypokalemia, and other adverse effects.

Guidelines for topical agents are the same as those for adults.

## USE IN OLDER ADULTS

No geriatric guidelines have been established for antifungal drugs. The main concern is with oral or parenteral drugs, because topical agents produce few adverse effects.

Virtually all adults receiving intravenous amphotericin B experience kidney damage and other adverse effects. With the impaired renal and cardiovascular functions that usually accompany aging, older adults are especially vulnerable to serious adverse effects. They must be monitored closely to reduce the incidence and severity of nephrotoxicity, hypokalemia, and other adverse drug reactions.

## NURSING ACTIONS: ANTIFUNGAL DRUGS

| Nursing Actions | Rationale/Explanation |
|---|---|
| 1. Administer accurately | |
| a. Check the package insert for complete instructions before giving intravenous amphotericin B. Some major points of administration include the following: | |
| (1) Use sterile water without a bacteriostatic agent for initial dissolution of the powdered drug; use 5% dextrose in water for further dilution to a 0.1 to 0.2 mg/ml concentration. | Use of any other solution causes precipitation of amphotericin B. |
| (2) Use a large vein and a scalp vein needle to administer. | To decrease phlebitis and pain at the venipuncture site. In addition, heparin and hydrocortisone may be added to the infusion solution to prevent local reactions. |
| (3) Administer each day's dose over a 6-hour period. | To decrease adverse reactions |
| b. For intravenous miconazole, dilute in at least 200 ml of 0.9% saline or 5% dextrose and infuse over 60 minutes or longer. | To prevent cardiorespiratory toxicity during infusion |
| c. For ketoconazole, do not give antacids, anticholinergics, or cimetidine within 2 hours of administration of ketoconazole. For clients with achlorhydria, dissolve ketoconazole tablets in 4 ml aqueous solution of 0.2 N hydrochloric acid, and have them drink the mixture through a straw and then drink 8 oz of tap water. | The drug is dissolved and absorbed only in an acid environment. |
| d. For nystatin, the suspension should be swished in the mouth for a few minutes before swallowing. | To increase contact with oral lesions |
| 2. Observe for therapeutic effects | |
| a. Decreased fever and malaise with systemic mycoses | |
| b. Healing of lesions on skin and mucous membranes | |
| c. Diminished diarrhea with intestinal candidiasis | |
| d. Decreased vaginal discharge and discomfort with vaginal candidiasis | |

(continued)

| *Nursing Actions* | *Rationale/Explanation* |
|---|---|
| **3. Observe for adverse effects** | |
| **a.** With amphotericin B, observe for fever, chills, anorexia, nausea, vomiting, renal damage (elevated blood urea nitrogen and serum creatinine), hypokalemia, hypomagnesemia, headache, stupor, coma, convulsions, anemia from bone marrow depression, phlebitis at venipuncture sites, anaphylaxis. | Amphotericin B is a highly toxic drug, and most recipients develop some adverse reactions, including some degree of renal damage. Antipyretic and antiemetic drugs may be given to help minimize adverse reactions and promote patient comfort. Adequate hydration may decrease renal damage. |
| **b.** With flucytosine, observe for nausea, vomiting, and diarrhea. | These are common effects. Hepatic, renal, and hematologic functions also may be affected. Drug resistance often develops when flucytosine is used alone. |
| **c.** With intravenous miconazole, observe for nausea, phlebitis, anemia, thrombocytopenia, and pruritus. | |
| **d.** With ketoconazole, observe for nausea, vomiting, pruritus, and abdominal pain. | Adverse effects are mild and transient. |
| **e.** With griseofulvin, observe for gastrointestinal symptoms, hypersensitivity (urticaria, photosensitivity, skin rashes, angioedema), headache, mental confusion, fatigue, dizziness, peripheral neuritis, and blood dyscrasias (leukopenia, neutropenia, granulocytopenia). | Incidence of serious reactions is very low. |
| **f.** With topical drugs, observe for skin rash and irritation. | Adverse reactions are usually minimal with topical drugs, although hypersensitivity may occur. |
| **4. Observe for drug interactions** | |
| **a.** Drugs that alter effects of amphotericin B: | |
| (1) Antibiotics, especially nephrotoxic ones, such as aminoglycosides | Additive nephrotoxicity because each drug alone is nephrotoxic |
| (2) Antineoplastic drugs | Increased bone marrow depression and blood dyscrasias. However, clients receiving antineoplastic drugs are highly susceptible to systemic fungal infections, and amphotericin B may be required concomitantly. The combination is indicated only if the illness is more life-threatening than the drug toxicity. |
| (3) Corticosteroids | Systemic mycoses sometimes develop in clients receiving corticosteroids because corticosteroids depress the immune system. They should not be given with amphotericin B unless absolutely necessary to control reactions to the drug or to treat the underlying disease. |
| (4) Potassium-losing diuretics, corticosteroids | Additive hypokalemia |
| (5) Minocycline, rifampin, flucytosine | Potentiate antifungal activity of amphotericin B |
| **b.** Drugs that alter effects of griseofulvin: Barbiturates and other drugs that induce liver enzymes | Enzyme inducers inhibit effects of griseofulvin by increasing its rate of metabolism. |
| **c.** Drugs that alter effects of ketoconazole: Antacids, anticholinergics, and cimetidine | These drugs decrease dissolution and absorption of ketoconazole by decreasing gastric acidity. |
| **5. Teach clients** | |
| **a.** Take drugs as prescribed. | To avoid recurrence of the infection. Drugs often must be taken several weeks after symptoms subside. |
| **b.** Report severe adverse effects. | Drug administration may need to be altered or discontinued. |

## Review and Application Exercises

1. What environmental factors predispose clients to develop fungal infections?
2. What signs and symptoms occur with candidiasis, and how would you assess for these?
3. What are the clinical indications for use of intravenous amphotericin B?
4. What are nursing interventions to decrease adverse effects of intravenous amphotericin B?
5. What are the clinical indications for use of oral antifungal drugs?

## Selected References

Armstrong, D. (1993). Treatment of opportunistic fungal infections. *Clinical Infectious Diseases, 16,* 1–9.

Bennett, J. E. (1990). Antifungal agents. In G. L. Mandell, R. G. Douglas Jr., & J. E. Bennett (Eds.), *Principles and practice of infectious diseases* (3rd ed.) (pp. 361–370). New York: Churchill Livingstone.

Clark, A. M. (1992). The need for new antifungal drugs. In P. B. Fernardes (Ed.), *New approaches for antifungal drugs* (pp. 1–19). Boston: Birkhauser.

(1993). *Drug facts and comparisons.* St. Louis: Facts and Comparisons.

Edwards, J. E. Jr. (1992). Opportunistic fungal infections. In W. N. Kelley (Ed.), *Textbook of internal medicine* (2nd ed.) (pp. 1458–1462). Philadelphia: J.B. Lippincott.

Mandler, H. D., & Dudley, M. N. (1992). Immunocompromised host infections. In M. A. Koda-Kimble & L. Y. Young (Eds.), *Applied therapeutics: The clinical use of drugs* (5th ed.) (pp. 46-1–46-23). Vancouver, WA: Applied Therapeutics.

# CHAPTER 44

# Antiparasitics

A parasite is a living organism that survives at the expense of another organism, called the host. Parasitic infestations are common human ailments worldwide. The effects of parasitic diseases on human hosts vary from minor and annoying to major and life-threatening. Parasitic diseases in this chapter are those caused by protozoa, helminths (worms), the itch mite, and pediculi (lice). Protozoa and helminths can infect the digestive tract and other body tissues; the itch mite and pediculi affect the skin.

## Protozoal infections

### AMEBIASIS

Amebiasis is a common disease in Africa, Asia, and Latin America, but it can occur in any geographic region. In the United States it is most likely to occur in residents of institutions for the mentally retarded, homosexual and bisexual men, and residents or travelers in countries with poor sanitation.

Amebiasis is caused by the pathogenic protozoan *Entamoeba histolytica*, which exists in two forms. The cystic form is inactive and resistant to drugs, heat, cold, and drying and can live outside the body for long periods. Amebiasis is transmitted by the fecal–oral route, such as ingesting food or water contaminated with human feces containing amebic cysts. Once ingested, some cysts break open in the ileum to release amebae, which produce trophozoites. Other cysts remain intact to be expelled in feces and continue the chain of infection. Trophozoites are active amebae that feed, multiply, move

about, and produce clinical manifestations of amebiasis. Trophozoites produce an enzyme that allows them to invade body tissues. They may form erosions and ulcerations in the intestinal wall and cause diarrhea (this form of the disease is called *intestinal amebiasis* or *amebic dysentery*), or they may penetrate blood vessels and be carried to other organs, where they form abscesses. These abscesses are usually found in the liver (hepatic amebiasis), but they also may occur in the lungs or brain.

Drugs used to treat amebiasis (amebicides) are classified according to their site of action. Some drugs (*e.g.*, iodoquinol, paromomycin) are called *intestinal amebicides* because they act within the lumen of the bowel. Other drugs (*e.g.*, chloroquine, emetine) are called *tissue* or *extraintestinal amebicides* because they act in the bowel wall, liver, and other tissues. Metronidazole (Flagyl) is effective in intestinal and extraintestinal amebiasis. No available amebicides are recommended for prophylaxis of amebiasis.

### MALARIA

Malaria is a common cause of morbidity and mortality in many parts of the world, especially in tropical regions. In the United States, malaria is rare and affects travelers or immigrants from malarious areas.

Malaria is caused by four species of protozoa of the genus *Plasmodium*. The human being is the only natural reservoir of these parasites. All types of malaria are transmitted only by *Anopheles* mosquitoes. *Plasmodium vivax*, *Plasmodium malariae*, and *Plasmodium ovale* cause recurrent malaria by forming reservoirs in the human host. In these types of malaria, signs and symptoms may occur months or years after the initial attack. *Plasmodium falciparum* causes the most life-threatening type of malaria but does not form a reservoir. This type of malaria may be cured and prevented from recurring.

Plasmodia have a life cycle in which one stage of development occurs within the human body. When a mosquito bites a person with malaria, it ingests blood that contains gametocytes (male and female forms of the protozoan parasite). From these forms, sporozoites are produced and transported to the mosquito's salivary glands. When the mosquito bites the next person, the sporozoites are injected into that person's bloodstream. From the bloodstream, the organisms lodge in the liver and other tissues, where they reproduce asexually and form merozoites. The liver cells containing the parasite eventually rupture and release the merozoites into the bloodstream, where they invade red blood cells. After a period of growth and asexual reproduction, merozoites rupture red blood cells, invade other erythrocytes, form gametocytes, and continue the cycle. After several cycles, clinical manifestations of malaria occur because of the large numbers of parasites. The characteristic cycles of chills and fever correspond to the release of merozoites from erythrocytes.

Antimalarial drugs act at different stages in the life cycle of plasmodial parasites. Some drugs (*e.g.*, chloroquine) are effective against erythrocytic forms and are therefore useful in preventing or treating acute attacks of malaria. These drugs do not prevent infection with the parasite, but they do prevent clinical manifestations. Other drugs (*e.g.*, primaquine) act against exoerythrocytic or tissue forms of the parasite to prevent initial infection and recurrent attacks or to cure some types of malaria. Combination drug therapy, administered concomitantly or consecutively, is common with antimalarial drugs.

### TRICHOMONIASIS

The most common form of trichomoniasis is a vaginal infection caused by the protozoan *Trichomonas vaginalis*. The disease is usually spread by sexual intercourse. Antitrichomonal drugs may be administered systemically (*i.e.*, metronidazole) or applied locally as douche solutions or vaginal creams.

### MISCELLANEOUS PROTOZOAL INFECTIONS

*Giardiasis* is a protozoal infection caused by *Giardia lamblia*. This disease is similar to amebiasis in that it is spread by food or water contaminated with human feces containing encysted forms of the organism. This disease may occur in people who camp or hike in wilderness areas or who drink untreated well water in areas where sanitation is poor.

*Pneumocystis carinii pneumonia* (PCP) is an acute, life-threatening respiratory infection. It rarely occurs in the general population but is not uncommon in people whose immune systems are impaired. Groups at risk include those with acquired immunodeficiency syndrome (AIDS) and those receiving corticosteroids, antineoplastics, and other immunosuppressive drugs. It is often the cause of death in people with AIDS.

## Helminthiasis

Helminthiasis, an infestation with parasitic worms, is a major disease in many parts of the world. Helminths are most often found in the gastrointestinal tract. However, several types of parasitic worms penetrate body tissues or produce larvae, which migrate to the blood, lymph channels, lungs, liver, and other body tissues. Specific types of helminthiasis include the following:

1. *Hookworm infections* are caused by *Necator americanus*, a species found in the United States, and *Ancylostoma duodenale*, a species found in Europe, the Middle East, and North Africa. Hookworm is spread by ova-containing feces from infected people. Ova develop into larvae when deposited on the soil. Larvae burrow through the skin (*e.g.*, if the person walks on the soil with bare feet), enter blood vessels, and migrate through the lungs to the pharynx, where they are swallowed. Larvae develop into adult hookworms in the small intestine and attach themselves to the intestinal mucosa.

2. *Pinworm infections* (enterobiasis), caused by *Enterobius vermicularis*, are the most common parasitic worm infections in the United States. Pinworm infections are highly communicable; they often involve school children and household contacts. Infection occurs from contact with ova in food or water or on bed linens. The female pinworm migrates from the bowel to the perianal area to deposit eggs, especially at night. Touching or scratching the perianal area deposits ova on hands and any objects touched by the contaminated hands.

3. *Roundworm infections* (ascariasis), caused by *Ascaris lumbricoides*, are the most common parasitic worm infections in the world. They occur most often in tropical regions but may occur wherever sanitation is poor. The infection is transmitted by ingesting food or water contaminated with feces from infected people. Ova are swallowed and hatch into larvae in the intestine. Like the hookworm larvae, roundworm larvae penetrate blood vessels and migrate through the lungs before returning to the intestines, where they develop into adult worms.

4. *Tapeworms* attach themselves to the intestinal wall and may grow as long as several yards. Segments called proglottids, which contain tapeworm eggs, are

expelled in feces. Tapeworms are transmitted by ingestion of contaminated, raw, or improperly cooked beef, pork, or fish. Beef and fish tapeworm infections are not usually considered serious illnesses. Pork tapeworm, which is uncommon in the United States, is more serious because it produces larvae that enter the bloodstream and migrate to other body tissues (*i.e.*, muscles, liver, lungs, and brain).

5. *Threadworm infections* (strongyloidiasis), caused by *Strongyloides stercoralis*, are potentially serious infections. This parasitic worm burrows into the mucosa of the small intestine, where the female lays eggs. The eggs hatch into larvae that can penetrate all body tissues.

6. *Trichinosis*, a parasitic worm infection caused by *Trichinella spiralis*, occurs worldwide. It is caused by inadequately cooked meat, especially pork. Encysted larvae are ingested in infected pork. In the intestine, the larvae excyst, mature, and produce eggs that hatch into new larvae. The larvae enter blood and lymphatic vessels and are transported throughout the body. They penetrate various body tissues (*e.g.*, muscles and brain) and evoke inflammatory reactions. Eventually, the larvae are re-encysted or walled off in the tissues and may remain for 10 years or longer.

7. *Whipworm infections* (trichuriasis) are caused by *Trichuris trichiura*. Whipworms attach themselves to the wall of the colon.

Drugs used for treatment of helminthiasis are called *anthelmintics*. Most anthelmintics act locally to kill or cause expulsion of parasitic worms from the intestines; some anthelmintics act systemically against parasites that have penetrated various body tissues. The goal of anthelmintic therapy may be to eradicate the parasite completely or to decrease the magnitude of infestation ("worm burden").

## Scabies and pediculosis

Scabies and pediculosis are parasitic infestations of the skin. Scabies is caused by the itch mite (*Sarcoptes scabiei*), which burrows into the skin and lays eggs that hatch in 4 to 8 days. The burrows may produce visible skin lesions, most often between the fingers and on the wrists, but other parts of the body may be affected as well.

Pediculosis is caused by three types of lice, which are blood-sucking insects. Pediculosis capitis (head lice) is the most common type of pediculosis in the United States. It is diagnosed by finding louse eggs (nits) attached to hair shafts close to the scalp. Pediculosis corporis (body lice) is diagnosed by finding lice in clothing, especially in seams. Body lice can transmit typhus and other diseases. Pediculosis pubis (pubic or crab lice) is

diagnosed by finding lice in the pubic and genital areas. Occasionally, these lice infest the axillae, mustache, or eyelashes.

Although scabies and pediculosis are caused by different parasites, the conditions have several characteristics in common:

1. Scabies and pediculosis are more likely to occur in areas of poverty, overcrowding, and poor sanitation. However, they may occur in any geographic area and socioeconomic group.

2. Scabies and pediculosis are highly communicable. The diseases are transmitted by direct contact with an infected person or the person's personal effects (*e.g.*, clothing, combs and hairbrushes, bed linens).

3. Pruritus is usually the major symptom of scabies and pediculosis. It results from an allergic reaction to parasite secretions and excrement. In addition to the intense discomfort associated with pruritus, scratching is likely to cause skin excoriation with secondary bacterial infection and formation of vesicles, pustules, and crusts.

4. Some of the same medications, applied topically, are used in both scabies and pediculosis.

## Individual antiparasitic drugs

### AMEBICIDES

**Chloroquine** (Aralen) is a drug used primarily for its antimalarial effects. When used as an amebicide, the drug is effective in extraintestinal amebiasis (*i.e.*, hepatic amebiasis) but generally ineffective in intestinal amebiasis. The phosphate salt is given orally. When the oral route is contraindicated, severe nausea and vomiting occur, or the infection is severe, the hydrochloride salt can be given intramuscularly. Treatment is usually combined with an intestinal amebicide.

Chloroquine phosphate

#### *Route and dosage ranges*

*Adults:* PO 1 g/d for 2 d, then 500 mg/d for 2–3 wk
*Children:* PO 20 mg/kg per day, in two divided doses, for 2 d, then 10 mg/kg per day for 2–3 wk

Chloroquine hydrochloride

#### *Route and dosage ranges*

*Adults:* IM 200–250 mg/d for 10–12 d
*Children:* IM 15 mg/kg per day for 2 days, then 7.5 mg/kg per day for 2–3 wk

**Emetine hydrochloride** is an effective but highly toxic tissue amebicide. It acts against amebae in the intestinal wall and extraintestinal sites, such as the liver and lungs. It is more effective against active amebae (trophozoites) than against the cystic form. Emetine is used with other drugs for treatment of severe amebic dysentery and amebic hepatitis. Adverse effects occur in about 50% to 75% of emetine recipients. During emetine therapy, clients are hospitalized and maintained on bed rest. Emetine accumulates in the body, and the risk of serious adverse reactions increases with repeated courses of therapy. Therefore, a course of therapy should be followed by an interval of at least 6 weeks before starting a second course. Emetine is generally contraindicated in pregnant, elderly, or debilitated clients and in those with cardiac or renal disease.

### Routes and dosage ranges

*Adults:* IM, SC 1 mg/kg per day for up to 5 d (10 d in hepatitis); maximum dose, 60 mg/d

*Children:* IM, SC 1 mg/kg per day for up to 5 d; maximum dose, 10 mg/d for children under 8 years and 20 mg/d for children over 8 years

**Iodoquinol** or diiodohydroxyquin (Yodoxin) is an iodine compound that acts against active amebae (trophozoites) in the intestinal lumen. Iodoquinol may be used alone in asymptomatic intestinal amebiasis to decrease the number of amebic cysts passed in the feces. When given for symptomatic intestinal amebiasis (*e.g.,* amebic dysentery), iodoquinol is usually given with other amebicides in concurrent or alternating courses. Iodoquinol is ineffective in amebic hepatitis and abscess formation. Its use is contraindicated with iodine allergy and liver disease. A related drug, clioquinol or iodochlorhydroxyquin (Vioform), is also an effective amebicide, but clioquinol tablets for oral administration are not marketed in the United States. Iodoquinol and clioquinol are ingredients in various dermatologic and vaginal preparations for topical application.

### Route and dosage ranges

*Adults:* Asymptomatic carriers, PO 650 mg/d

Symptomatic intestinal amebiasis, PO 650 mg three times per day after meals for 20 d. If necessary, the 20-d course of therapy may be repeated after a drug-free interval of 2–3 wk.

*Children:* PO 30–40 mg/kg per day in two or three divided doses for 20 d (maximum dose, 2 g/d); repeat after 2–3 wk if necessary

**Metronidazole** (Flagyl) is effective against protozoa that cause amebiasis, giardiasis, and trichomoniasis and against anaerobic bacilli, such as *Bacteroides* and *Clostridia* (see Chap. 39). In amebiasis, metronidazole is amebicidal at intestinal and extraintestinal sites of infection. It is probably the drug of choice for all forms of amebiasis except asymptomatic intestinal amebiasis (in which

amebic cysts are expelled in the feces). In trichomoniasis, metronidazole is the only systemic trichomonacide available, and it is more effective than any locally active agent.

Because trichomoniasis is transmitted by sexual intercourse, some authorities recommend simultaneous treatment of both partners to prevent reinfection. Metronidazole is given orally for protozoal infections and intravenously for anaerobic bacterial infections. It is generally contraindicated during the first trimester of pregnancy and must be used with caution in clients with central nervous system or blood disorders. Because the drug is carcinogenic in rodents and mutagenic in bacteria, it should be used only when necessary.

### Route and dosage ranges

*Adults:* Amebiasis, PO 500–750 mg three times per day for 5–10 d

Trichomoniasis, PO 250 mg three times per day for 7 d, 1 g twice daily for 1 d, or 2 g in a single dose. If necessary, the course of treatment may be repeated after 4–6 wk.

*Gardnerella vaginalis* vaginitis, PO 500 mg twice daily for 7 d

*Children:* Amebiasis, PO 35–50 mg/kg per day in three divided doses, for 10 d

**Tetracycline** (Achromycin) and **oxytetracycline** (Terramycin) are broad-spectrum antibiotics (see Chap. 37) that act against amebae in the intestinal lumen. These drugs are not directly amebicidal; instead, they exert their effects by altering the bacterial flora required for amebic viability. One of these drugs may be used with other amebicides in the treatment of all forms of amebiasis except asymptomatic intestinal amebiasis.

### Route and dosage ranges

*Adults:* PO 250–500 mg q6h, up to 14 d

*Children:* PO 25–50 mg/kg per day in four divided doses for 7–10 d

## ANTIMALARIAL AGENTS

**Chloroquine** (Aralen) is one of the most widely used antimalarial agents. Chloroquine acts against erythrocytic forms of plasmodial parasites to prevent or treat malarial attacks. When used for prophylaxis, chloroquine is given before, during, and after travel or residence in endemic areas. When used for treatment of malaria caused by *P. vivax, P. malariae,* or *P. ovale,* chloroquine relieves symptoms of the acute attack. However, chloroquine does not prevent recurrence of malarial attacks because the drug does not act against the tissue (exoerythrocytic) forms of the parasite. When used for treatment of malaria caused by *P. falciparum,* chloroquine relieves symptoms of the acute attack and because *P. falciparum* does not have tissue reservoirs, eliminates the parasite from the body. However, chloroquine-resistant strains of *P. falciparum* have developed in some geographic areas.

Chloroquine also is used in protozoal infections other than malaria, including extraintestinal amebiasis and giardiasis. Chloroquine should be used with caution in clients with hepatic disease or severe neurologic, gastrointestinal, or blood disorders.

**Hydroxychloroquine sulfate** (Plaquenil) is a derivative of chloroquine with essentially the same actions, uses, and adverse effects as chloroquine. It is also used to treat rheumatoid arthritis and lupus erythematosus.

### Chloroquine phosphate

#### Route and dosage ranges

***Adults:*** Prophylaxis of malaria, PO 5 mg/kg (base) weekly (maximum of 300 mg of chloroquine base weekly), starting 2 wk before entering a malarious area and continuing for 8 wk after return
Treatment of an acute attack of malaria, PO 1 g (600 mg of base) initially, then 500 mg (300 mg of base) after 6–8 h, then 500 mg daily for 2 d (total of 2.5 g in four doses)

***Children:*** Treatment of an acute attack of malaria, PO 10 mg/kg of chloroquine base initially, then 5 mg/kg after 6 h, then 5 mg/kg per day for 2 d (total of four doses)

### Chloroquine hydrochloride

#### Route and dosage ranges

***Adults:*** Treatment of malarial attacks, IM 250 mg (equivalent to 200 mg of chloroquine base) initially, repeated q6h if necessary, to a maximal dose of 800 mg of chloroquine base in 24 h

***Children:*** Treatment of malarial attacks, IM 5 mg/kg chloroquine base initially, repeated after 6 h if necessary; maximal dose, 10 mg/kg/24 h

### Hydroxychloroquine sulfate

#### Route and dosage ranges

***Adults:*** Prophylaxis, PO 5 mg/kg, not to exceed 310 mg (of hydroxychloroquine base), once weekly for 2 wk before entry to and 8 wk after return from malarious areas
Treatment of acute malarial attacks, PO 620 mg initially, then 310 mg 6 h later, and 310 mg/d for 2 d (total of four doses)

***Children:*** Prophylaxis, PO 5 mg/kg (of hydroxychloroquine base) once weekly for 2 wk before entry to and 8 wk after return from malarious areas
Treatment of acute malarial attacks, PO 10 mg/kg

initially, then 5 mg/kg 6 h later, and 5 mg/kg per day for two doses (total of four doses)

**Chloroquine phosphate** (Aralen) with **primaquine phosphate** is a mixture available in tablets containing chloroquine phosphate 500 mg (equivalent to 300 mg of chloroquine base) and primaquine phosphate 79 mg (equivalent to 45 mg of primaquine base). This combination is effective for prophylaxis of malaria and may be more acceptable to clients. It also may be more convenient for use in children, because no pediatric formulation of primaquine is available.

#### Route and dosage ranges

***Adults:*** Prophylaxis of malaria, PO 1 tablet weekly on the same day each week for 2 wk before entering and 8 wk after leaving malarious areas

***Children:*** PO same as adults for children weighing over 45 kg; one-half tablet for children weighing 25–45 kg. For younger children, a suspension is prepared, using the tablets and chocolate syrup or fruit juice. The usual concentration is 40 mg of chloroquine base and 6 mg of primaquine base in 5 ml of suspension. Dosages are then 2.5 ml for children weighing 5–7 kg, 5 ml for 8–11 kg, 7.5 ml for 12–15 kg, 10 ml for 16–20 kg, and 12.5 ml for 21–24 kg. These dosages are administered weekly, on the same day of the week, for 2 wk before entering and 8 wk after leaving malarious areas.

**Halofantrine** (Halfan) is a newer drug indicated for treatment of malaria caused by *P. falciparum* or *P. vivax*, including chloroquine-resistant strains.

#### Route and dosage ranges

***Adults:*** PO 500 mg q6h for three doses, repeat in 1 wk for clients without previous exposure to malaria (*e.g.*, travelers)

***Children less than 40 kg:*** PO 8 mg/kg according to the schedule for adults

**Mefloquine** (Lariam) is used to prevent *P. falciparum* malaria, including chloroquine-resistant strains, and to treat acute malaria caused by *P. falciparum* or *P. vivax*.

#### Route and dosage ranges

***Adults:*** Prophylaxis, PO 250 mg 1 wk before travel, then 250 mg weekly during travel and for 4 wk after leaving a malarious area
Treatment, 1250 mg (5 tablets) as a single dose

***Children:*** Prophylaxis, PO 1/4 tablet for 15–19 kg weight; 1/2 tablet for 20–30 kg; 3/4 tablet for 31–45 kg; and 1 tablet for more than 45 kg, according to the schedule for adults

**Primaquine phosphate** is an antimalarial agent used to prevent the initial occurrence of malaria; to prevent recurrent attacks of malaria caused by *P. vivax*, *P. malariae*, and *P. ovale*; and to achieve "radical cure" of these three types of malaria. (Radical cure involves eradicating the exoerythrocytic forms of the plasmodium and preventing the survival of the blood forms.) The clinical usefulness of primaquine stems primarily from its ability to destroy tissue (exoerythrocytic) forms of the malarial parasite. Primaquine is especially effective in vivax malaria. Thus far, plasmodial strains causing the three relapsing types of malaria have not developed resistance to primaquine. When used to prevent initial occurrence of malaria (causal prophylaxis), primaquine is given concurrently with a suppressive agent (*e.g.*, chloroquine or hydroxychloroquine) after the client has returned from a malarious area. Primaquine is not effective for treatment of acute attacks of malaria.

### Route and dosage ranges

*Adults:* Prophylaxis, PO 26.3 mg (equivalent to 15 mg of primaquine base) daily for 14 d, beginning immediately after leaving a malarious area, or 79 mg (45 mg of base) once a week for 8 wk. To prevent relapse (*i.e.*, acute malarial attacks), the same dose is given with chloroquine or a related drug daily for 14 d.

*Children:* Prophylaxis of the disease and relapse, PO 0.3 mg of base/kg per day for 14 d, according to the schedule outlined above, or 0.9 mg of base/kg per week for 8 wk

**Pyrimethamine** (Daraprim) is a folic acid antagonist used to prevent malaria caused by susceptible strains of plasmodial parasites. Pyrimethamine is sometimes used with a sulfonamide and quinine to treat chloroquine-resistant strains of *P. falciparum*. Folic acid antagonists and sulfonamides act synergistically against plasmodial parasites because they block different steps in the synthesis of folic acid, a nutrient required by the parasites.

### Route and dosage ranges

*Adults:* Prophylaxis, PO 25 mg once weekly, starting 2 wk before entering and continuing for 8 wk after returning from malarious areas

*Children:* Prophylaxis, PO 25 mg once weekly, as above, for children over 10 years; 6.25–12.5 mg once weekly for children under 10 years

**Quinine sulfate** (Quinamm) is a naturally occurring alkaloid derived from the bark of the cinchona tree. Quinine was the primary antimalarial drug for many years but has been largely replaced by synthetic agents that cause fewer adverse reactions. However, it may still be used in the treatment of chloroquine-resistant falciparum malaria, usually in conjunction with pyrimethamine and a sulfonamide. Quinine also relaxes skeletal

muscles and is used for prevention and treatment of nocturnal leg cramps.

### Route and dosage ranges

*Adults:* Treatment of malaria, PO 650 mg q8h for 10–14 d

Leg cramps, PO 260–300 mg at bedtime

*Children:* Treatment of malaria, PO 25 mg/kg per day in divided doses q8h for 10–14 d

## ANTITRICHOMONAL AGENTS

For information about **Metronidazole** (Flagyl), see amebicides above.

**Povidone-iodine** (Betadine) is an antiseptic (see Chap. 69) available in a douche solution for treatment of vaginal infections in general, possibly including trichomoniasis.

### Route and dosage range

*Adults:* Topically to vagina, as a vaginal douche each morning for 10–15 d. Treatment should be continued through menstruation if it occurs.

## ANTI–*PNEUMOCYSTIS CARINII* AGENTS

**Atovaquone** (Mepron) is a newer drug used for treatment of PCP. Adverse effects include nausea, vomiting, diarrhea, fever, insomnia, and elevated hepatic enzymes.

### Routes and dosage ranges

*Adults:* PO 750 mg three times daily with food

**Pentamidine isethionate** (Pentam 300, NebuPent) is an antiprotozoal agent used to prevent or treat PCP. Pentamidine interferes with production of ribonucleic acid and deoxyribonucleic acid by the protozoa. The drug is given parenterally for treatment of PCP and by inhalation for prophylaxis. It is excreted by the kidneys and accumulates in the presence of renal failure, so dosage should be reduced with renal failure.

### Routes and dosage ranges

*Adults:* IM, IV 4 mg/kg once daily for 14 d

Inhalation, 300 mg every 4 wk (see manufacturer's instructions)

*Children:* IM, IV same as adults

Inhalation, dosage not established

## ANTHELMINTICS

**Mebendazole** (Vermox) is a broad-spectrum anthelmintic drug that is effective in the treatment of parasitic infections by hookworms, pinworms, roundworms, and whipworms. It is also useful but somewhat less effective in tapeworm infection. Mebendazole kills helminths by preventing uptake of the glucose necessary for parasitic metabolism. The helminths become immobilized and die slowly, so they may be expelled from the gastrointestinal tract up to 3 days after drug therapy is completed. Mebendazole acts locally within the gastrointestinal tract, and less than 10% of the drug is absorbed systemically.

Mebendazole is usually the drug of choice for single or mixed infections caused by the above parasitic worms. The drug is contraindicated during pregnancy because of teratogenic effects in rats; it is relatively contraindicated in children under 2 years of age because it has not been extensively investigated for use in this age group.

### Route and dosage range

*Adults and children:* Most infections, PO 100 mg morning and evening for 3 consecutive days. For pinworms, a single 100-mg dose may be sufficient. A second course of therapy may be administered in 3 wk, if necessary.

**Niclosamide** (Niclocide) is an anthelmintic effective against beef, fish, and dwarf tapeworm infestations of the intestine. Clients are not considered cured until the stool has been negative for at least 3 months.

### Route and dosage ranges

*Adults:* Beef and fish tapeworm, PO 2 g (4 tablets) as a single dose
  Dwarf tapeworm, PO 2 g as a single daily dose for 7 d
*Children over 34 kg (75 lb):* Beef and fish tapeworm, PO 1.5 g as a single dose
  Dwarf tapeworm, PO 1.5 g the first day, then 1 g daily for 6 d
*Children 11–34 kg (25–75 lb):* Beef and fish tapeworm, PO 1 g as a single dose
  Dwarf tapeworm, PO 1 g the first day, then 0.5 g daily for 6 d

**Piperazine citrate** (Antepar) is an anthelmintic agent that is highly effective against roundworm and pinworm infestations. The drug is not parasiticidal; it causes expulsion of the parasitic worms. Roundworms are alive but paralyzed when expelled by peristalsis. Pinworms are alive and active and may cause reinfection if not disposed of properly. Good personal and environmental hygienic practices are necessary to prevent reinfection.

Piperazine citrate forms piperazine hexahydrate in solution, and the hexahydrate salt exerts anthelmintic action. The drug is well absorbed after oral administration; a portion is metabolized in the liver, and the remainder is excreted in the urine. Piperazine is contraindicated in people with liver, kidney, or convulsive disorders.

### Route and dosage ranges

*Adults:* Roundworms, PO 3.5 g/d for 2 d
  Pinworms, PO 65 mg/kg per day for 7 d (maximum dose, 2.5 g/d of hexahydrate equivalent). In severe roundworm or pinworm infestations, the course of therapy may be repeated after 1 wk.
*Children:* Roundworms, PO 75 mg/kg per day for 2 d (maximum dose, 3.5 g/d of hexahydrate equivalent)
  Pinworms, same as adults

**Pyrantel pamoate** (Antiminth) is effective in parasitic infestation of roundworms, pinworms, and hookworms. The drug acts locally to paralyze worms in the intestinal tract. Pyrantel is poorly absorbed from the gastrointestinal tract, and most of an administered dose may be recovered in feces. Pyrantel is contraindicated in pregnancy and is not recommended for children under 1 year of age.

### Route and dosage range

*Adults and children:* Roundworms and pinworms, PO 11 mg/kg (maximal dose, 1 g) as a single dose; for hookworms, the same dose is given daily for 3 consecutive days. The course of therapy may be repeated in 1 mo, if necessary.

**Pyrvinium pamoate** (Povan) is a type of dye that is effective for treatment of pinworm infestations. The drug kills the worms by preventing absorption of the glucose required for metabolism. Pyrvinium acts locally within the intestinal tract; little drug is absorbed systemically. Because the drug is a dye, it colors vomitus, feces, or clothing a bright red. The tablets should be swallowed immediately, without chewing, to avoid staining of teeth.

### Route and dosage range

*Adults and children:* Pinworms, PO 5 mg/kg in a single dose (maximal dose, 350 mg of pyrvinium base), repeated after 2–3 wk to eliminate worms that have developed after the first dose

**Thiabendazole** (Mintezol) is an anthelmintic agent that is most effective against threadworms and pinworms. It is useful but less effective against hookworms, roundworms, and whipworms. Because of the broad spectrum of anthelmintic activity, thiabendazole may be especially useful in mixed parasitic infestations. In trichinosis, thiabendazole decreases symptoms and eosinophilia but apparently does not eliminate larvae from muscle tissues. The mechanism of anthelmintic action is uncertain but probably involves interference with parasitic metabolism. The drug is relatively toxic compared to other anthelmintic agents.

Thiabendazole is a first drug of choice for threadworm infestations. For other types of helminthiasis, it is usually considered an alternative drug. Thiabendazole is rapidly absorbed after oral administration. Most of the drug is excreted in urine within 24 hours. Thiabendazole should be used with caution in clients with liver or kidney disease.

### Route and dosage range

*Adults and children:* PO 22 mg/kg (maximal single dose, 3 g) twice daily after meals; 1 d for pinworms, repeated after 1–2 wk; 2 d for other infections, except trichinosis, which requires about 5 d

## SCABICIDES AND PEDICULICIDES

**Lindane** or **gamma benzene hexachloride** (Kwell, Gamene) is a frequently prescribed drug for scabies and pediculosis. It is applied topically, and substantial amounts are absorbed through intact skin. Central nervous system toxicity has been reported with excessive use, especially in infants and children. The drug is available in a 1% concentration in a cream, lotion, and shampoo. A single application is usually sufficient to kill parasites and ova.

### Route and dosage range

*Adults and children:* Scabies, apply topically to entire skin except the face, neck, and scalp, leave in place for 24 h, then remove by shower
Pediculosis, use the cream or lotion (rub into the affected area, leave in place for 12 h, then wash thoroughly) or shampoo (rub into the affected area for 4 min and rinse thoroughly)

**Malathion** (Ovide) is a pediculicide used in the treatment of head lice. It is sprinkled on the hair and rubbed in until the hair is thoroughly moistened. Allow the hair to dry naturally; keep uncovered and do not apply heat or a hair dryer. After 8 to 12 hours, the hair should be shampooed, rinsed, and combed with a fine-toothed comb to remove dead lice and eggs. If necessary, treatment can be repeated in 7 to 9 days.

**Crotamiton** (Eurax) is used as a 10% cream or lotion for scabies. **Pyrethrin** preparations (*e.g.*, A-200-Pyrinate, Barc) are available as gels, shampoos, and liquid suspensions for treatment of pediculosis. These topical agents are applied in the same manner as lindane.

## Nursing Process

### Assessment

Assess for conditions in which antiparasitic drugs are used.
- Assess for exposure to parasites. Although exposure is influenced by many variables (*e.g.*, geographic location, personal hygiene, environmental sanitation), some useful questions may include the following:
  - Does the person live in an institution, an area of poor sanitation, an underdeveloped country, a tropical region, or an area of overcrowded housing? All these conditions predispose to parasitic infestations with lice, the itch mite, protozoa, and worms.
- Are parasitic diseases present in the person's environment? For example, head lice, scabies, and pinworm infestations often affect school children and their families.
- Has the person recently traveled (within the previous 1–3 weeks) in malarious regions? If so, were prophylactic measures used appropriately?
- With vaginal trichomoniasis, assess in relation to sexual activity. The disease is spread by sexual intercourse, and men may need treatment to prevent reinfection of women.
- With pubic (crab) lice, assess sexual activity. Lice may be transmitted by sexual and other close contact and by contact with infested bed linens.
- Assess for signs and symptoms. These vary greatly, depending on the extent of parasitic infestation.
  - *Amebiasis.* The person may be asymptomatic, have nausea, vomiting, diarrhea, abdominal cramping, and weakness or experience symptoms from ulcerations of the colon or abscesses of the liver (amebic hepatitis) if the disease is severe, prolonged, and untreated. Amebiasis is diagnosed by identifying cysts or trophozoites of *E. histolytica* in stool specimens.
  - *Malaria.* Initial symptoms may resemble those produced by influenza (*e.g.*, headache, myalgia). Characteristic paroxysms of chills, fever, and copious perspiration may not be present in early malaria. During acute malarial attacks, the cycles occur every 36 to 72 hours. Additional symptoms include nausea and vomiting, splenomegaly, hepatomegaly, anemia, leukopenia, thrombocytopenia, and hyperbilirubinemia. Malaria is diagnosed by identifying the plasmodial parasite in peripheral blood smears (by microscopic examination).
  - *Trichomoniasis.* Females usually have vaginal burning, itching, and yellowish discharge; males are usually asymptomatic. The condition is diagnosed by finding *T. vaginalis* organisms in a wet smear of vaginal exudate, semen, prostatic fluid, or urinary sediment (by microscopic examination). Cultures may be necessary.
  - *Helminthiasis.* Light infestations may be asymptomatic. Heavy infestations produce symptoms according to the particular parasitic worm. Hookworm, roundworm, and threadworm larvae migrate through the lungs and may cause symptoms of pulmonary congestion. The hookworm may cause anemia by sucking blood from the intestinal mucosa; the fish tapeworm may cause megaloblastic or pernicious anemia by absorbing folic acid and vitamin $B_{12}$. Large masses of roundworms or tapeworms have caused intestinal obstruction. The major symptom usually associated with pinworms is intense itching in the perianal area (pruritus ani). Helminthiasis is diagnosed by microscopic identification of parasites or ova in stool specimens. Pinworm infestation is diagnosed by identifying ova on anal swabs, obtained by touching the sticky side of cellophane tape to the anal area. (Early morning swabs are best because the female pinworm deposits eggs during sleeping hours.)
  - *Scabies and pediculosis.* Pruritus is usually the primary symptom. Secondary symptoms result from scratching and often include skin excoriation and infection (*i.e.*, vesi-

cles, pustules, and crusts). Pediculosis is diagnosed by visual identification of lice or ova (nits) on the client's body or clothing.

### Nursing diagnoses

- Knowledge Deficit: Management of disease process and prevention of recurrence
- Knowledge Deficit: Accurate drug administration
- High Risk for Altered Nutrition: Less than Body Requirements related to parasitic disease or drug therapy
- High Risk for Self-Esteem Disturbance related to a medical diagnosis of parasitic infestation
- High Risk for Noncompliance related to need for hygienic and other measures to prevent and treat parasitic infestations

### Planning/Goals

*The client will:*
- Experience relief of symptoms for which therapeutic antiparasitic drugs were taken
- Self-administer drugs accurately
- Avoid preventable adverse effects
- Act to prevent recurrent infestation
- Keep appointments for follow-up care

### Interventions

Use measures to avoid exposure to or prevent transmission of parasitic diseases.
- Environmental health measures often attempt to interrupt the life cycle of parasites. Specific measures include the following:
  - Sanitary sewers to prevent deposition of feces on surface soil and the resultant exposure to helminths
  - Monitoring of community water supplies, food handling establishments, and food handling personnel
  - Follow-up examination and possibly treatment of household and other close contacts of people with helminthiasis, amebiasis, trichomoniasis, scabies, and pediculosis
  - Mosquito control in malarious areas and prophylactic drug therapy for travelers to malarious areas
- Personal and other health measures include the following:
  - Maintain personal hygiene (*i.e.*, regular bathing and shampooing, handwashing before eating or handling food and after defecation or urination).
  - Avoid raw fish and undercooked pork products. Smoking, pickling, or other processing of pork does not prevent trichinosis.
  - Avoid contaminating streams or other water sources with feces.

- Control flies and avoid foods exposed to flies.
- With scabies and pediculosis infestations, drug therapy must be accompanied by adjunctive measures to avoid reinfection or transmission to others. For example, clothes, bed linens, and towels should be washed and dried on hot cycles. Clothes that cannot be washed should be dry cleaned. With head lice, combs and brushes should be cleaned and disinfected; carpets and upholstered furniture should be vacuumed.
- With pinworms, clothing, bed linens, and towels should be washed daily on hot cycles. Toilet seats should be disinfected daily.
- Ensure follow-up measures, such as stool specimens, vaginal examinations, anal swabs, smears, and cultures.
- With vaginal infections, avoid sexual intercourse, or have the male partner use a condom.

### Evaluation

- Interview and observe for relief of symptoms.
- Interview outpatients regarding compliance with instructions for taking antiparasitic drugs and measures to prevent recurrence of infestation.
- Interview and observe for adverse drug effects.
- Interview and observe regarding food intake or changes in weight.

## Principles of therapy

1. Many of the drugs described in this chapter are quite toxic; they should be used only when clearly indicated (*i.e.*, laboratory documentation of parasitic infestation or infection).
2. Atavaquone and pentamidine are usually considered second-line drugs, after trimethoprim-sulfamethoxazole (Bactrim, Septra), for treatment of PCP because of severe adverse effects. However, one of these drugs may be preferred in clients with AIDS, in whom the adverse effects of trimethoprim-sulfamethoxazole may be especially severe. When pentamidine is used, especially parenterally, appropriate tests should be performed before, during, and after treatment (*e.g.*, complete blood count, platelet count, serum creatinine, blood urea nitrogen, blood glucose, serum calcium, and electrocardiogram).

# NURSING ACTIONS: ANTIPARASITICS

| *Nursing Actions* | *Rationale/Explanation* |
|---|---|

**1. Administer accurately**

**a.** Give chloroquine and related drugs, iodoquinol, and oral metronidazole with or after meals.

To decrease gastrointestinal irritation

**b.** Check manufacturer's instructions before giving IV metronidazole.

The drug requires specific techniques for preparation and administration.

**c.** With pentamidine:

(1) For IM administration, dissolve the drug in 3 ml of sterile water for injection and inject deeply in a large muscle mass.

IM administration is painful and may cause sterile abscesses.

(2) For IV administration, dissolve the calculated dose in 3 to 5 ml of sterile water or 5% dextrose in water. Dilute further with 50 to 250 ml of 5% dextrose solution and infuse over 60 minutes.

**d.** Give anthelmintics without regard to mealtimes or food ingestion. Mebendazole tablets may be chewed, swallowed, or crushed and mixed with food. Niclosamide tablets should be chewed or crushed.

Food in the gastrointestinal tract does not decrease effectiveness of most anthelmintics.

**e.** For scabicides, use the following sequence:

(1) Have the client bathe.

(2) Wearing gown and gloves, apply scabicide thinly to all skin surfaces except the face, neck, and scalp.

Because scabies is highly infectious, most of these procedures are aimed toward preventing reinfection of the client (*i.e.*, wearing clean clothes, laundering soiled clothing) or infection of the nurse (*i.e.*, wearing gloves with direct contact). Isolation is unnecessary. Gloves are unnecessary after 24 hours.

(3) Have the client don clean clothing; remove soiled clothing for laundering.

(4) Leave the medication in place for 12 to 24 hours; have the client bathe and again don clean clothing.

(5) Wear gloves if direct contact is required while the medication is in place.

**f.** For pediculicides, rub cream or lotion into the affected area, leave in place for 12 hours, then wash thoroughly; rub shampoo into the scalp for 4 minutes, then rinse thoroughly.

These methods of administration are used for treatment of head and pubic lice. Skin treatment is not necessary with body lice because the parasites live in the clothing, especially in undergarments and seams.

**2. Observe for therapeutic effects**

**a.** With chloroquine for acute malaria, observe for relief of symptoms and negative blood smears.

Fever and chills usually subside within 24 to 48 hours, and blood smears are negative for plasmodia within 48 to 72 hours.

**b.** With amebicides, observe for relief of symptoms and negative stool examinations.

Relief of symptoms does not indicate cure of amebiasis; laboratory evidence is required. Stool specimens should be examined for amebic cysts and trophozoites periodically for about 6 months.

**c.** With anthelmintics, observe for relief of symptoms, absence of the parasite in blood or stool for three consecutive examinations, or a reduction in the number of parasitic ova in the feces.

The goal of anthelmintic drug therapy may be complete eradication of the parasite or reduction of the "worm burden."

*(continued)*

| Nursing Actions | Rationale/Explanation |
|---|---|
| **d.** With pediculicides, inspect affected areas daily for lice or nits for 1 to 2 weeks. | For most clients, one treatment is effective. For others, a second treatment may be necessary about 1 week after the first (to eliminate newly hatched lice). |
| **3. Observe for adverse effects** | |
| **a.** With amebicides, observe for anorexia, nausea, vomiting, epigastric burning, diarrhea. | Gastrointestinal effects may occur with all amebicides. |
| (1) With iodoquinol, observe for agitation, amnesia, peripheral neuropathy, and optic neuropathy. | These effects are most likely to occur with large doses or long-term drug administration. |
| (2) With emetine, observe for cardiovascular effects (*e.g.*, hypotension, chest pain, dyspnea, tachycardia, electrocardiogram abnormalities) and local tissue reactions at injection sites (*e.g.*, pain, tenderness, weakness). | Emetine is a highly toxic drug. Adverse effects may be minimized by close observation during emetine therapy. The client is hospitalized and maintained on bed rest. |
| **b.** With antimalarial agents, observe for nausea, vomiting, diarrhea, pruritus, skin rash, headache, central nervous system (CNS) stimulation. | These effects may occur with most antimalarial agents. However, adverse effects are usually mild because small doses are used for prophylaxis, and the larger doses required for treatment of acute malarial attacks are given only for short periods. When chloroquine and related drugs are used for long-term treatment of rheumatoid arthritis or lupus erythematosus, adverse effects increase (*e.g.*, blood dyscrasias, retinal damage). |
| (1) With pyrimethamine, observe for anemia, thrombocytopenia, and leukopenia. | This drug interferes with folic acid metabolism. |
| (2) With quinine, observe for signs of cinchonism (headache, tinnitus, decreased auditory acuity, blurred vision). | These effects occur with usual therapeutic doses of quinine. They do not usually necessitate discontinuance of quinine therapy. |
| **c.** With metronidazole, observe for convulsions, peripheral paresthesias, nausea, diarrhea, unpleasant taste, vertigo, headache, and vaginal and urethral burning sensation. | CNS effects are most serious; gastrointestinal effects are most common. |
| **d.** With parenteral pentamidine, observe for leukopenia, thrombocytopenia, hypoglycemia, hypocalcemia, hypotension, acute renal failure, ventricular tachycardia, and Stevens-Johnson syndrome. | Severe hypotension may occur after a single parenteral dose. Deaths from hypotension, hypoglycemia, and cardiac arrhythmias have been reported. |
| **e.** With aerosol pentamidine, observe for fatigue, shortness of breath, bronchospasm, cough, dizziness, rash, anorexia, nausea, vomiting, chest pain. | These are the most common adverse effects. |
| **f.** With topical antitrichomonal agents, observe for hypersensitivity reactions (*e.g.*, rash, inflammation), burning, and pruritus | Hypersensitivity reactions are the major adverse effects. Other effects are minor and rarely require that drug therapy be discontinued. |
| **g.** With scabicides and pediculicides, observe for irritation and allergic reactions (*e.g.*, rash, inflammation). In addition, gamma benzene hexachloride may cause CNS stimulation (nervousness, tremors, insomnia, convulsions). | Hypersensitivity reactions necessitate discontinuation of the drug. Inflammation should be allowed to subside before other topical scabicides and pediculicides are applied. CNS stimulation may occur with gamma benzene hexachloride because the drug is absorbed systemically through intact skin. Adverse effects are uncommon if the drug is used correctly. They are more likely to occur with excessive application (*i.e.*, increased amounts, leaving in place longer than prescribed, or applying more frequently than prescribed). |

| *Nursing Actions* | *Rationale/Explanation* |
|---|---|
| **4. Observe for drug interactions** | Few clinically significant drug interactions occur because many antiparasitic agents are administered for local effects in the gastrointestinal tract or on the skin. The drugs also are given for short periods. |
| **a.** Drugs that alter effects of chloroquine: | |
| (1) Acidifying agents (*e.g.*, ascorbic acid) | Inhibit chloroquine by increasing the rate of urinary excretion |
| (2) Alkalinizing agents (*e.g.*, sodium bicarbonate) | Potentiate chloroquine by decreasing the rate of urinary excretion |
| (3) MAO inhibitors | Increase risk of toxicity and retinal damage by inhibiting hepatic enzymes |
| **b.** Drugs that alter effects of metronidazole: | |
| (1) Phenobarbital, phenytoin | These drugs induce hepatic enzymes and decrease effects of metronidazole by accelerating its rate of hepatic metabolism |
| (2) Cimetidine | May increase effects by inhibiting hepatic metabolism of metronidazole |
| **5. Teach clients** <br> **a.** Use antiparasitic drugs as prescribed | To achieve therapeutic effects without adverse effects |
| **b.** Measures to prevent parasitic infection or reinfection | |

## Review and Application Exercises

1. What groups are at risk of developing parasitic infections (*e.g., amebiasis, malaria, pediculosis, helminthiasis)?*
2. What interventions are needed to prevent parasitic infections?
3. How would you assess for a parasitic infection in a client who has been in an environment associated with a particular infestation?
4. How can you assess a client's personal hygiene practices and environmental sanitation facilities?
5. How would you instruct a mother about treatment and prevention of reinfection with head lice or pinworms?
6. What are adverse effects of commonly used antiparasitic drugs, and how may they be prevented or minimized?

## Selected References

Anandan, J. V. (1992). Parasitic infections. In M. A. Koda-Kimble & L. Y. Young (Eds.), *Applied therapeutics: The clinical use of drugs* (5th ed.) (pp. 49-1–49-15). Vancouver, WA: Applied Therapeutics.

(1993). *Drug facts and comparisons.* St. Louis: Facts and Comparisons.

Krogstad, D. J. (1992). Malaria. In W. N. Kelley (Ed.), *Textbook of internal medicine* (2nd ed.) (pp. 1521–1524). Philadelphia: J.B. Lippincott.

Navin, T. R. (1992). Intestinal protozoa. In W. N. Kelley (Ed.), *Textbook of internal medicine* (2nd ed.) (pp. 1517–1521). Philadelphia: J.B. Lippincott.

Rosenblatt, J. E. (1992). Antiparasitic agents. *Mayo Clinic Proceedings, 67,* 276–287.

# Drugs Affecting the Immune System

# CHAPTER 45

# Physiology of the Immune System

## Overview of body defense mechanisms

The immune system is one of several mechanisms that protect the body from potentially harmful substances, including pathogenic microorganisms. The body's primary external defense mechanism is intact skin, which prevents entry of foreign substances and produces secretions that inhibit microbial growth. The mucous membranes lining the gastrointestinal and respiratory tracts are internal defense mechanisms that act as physical barriers and produce mucus that traps foreign substances so that they may be expelled from the body. Mucous membranes also produce other secretions (*e.g.*, gastric acid) that kill ingested microorganisms. Additional internal mechanisms include the normal microbial population, which is usually nonpathogenic and controls potential pathogens, and secretions (*e.g.*, perspiration, tears, and saliva) that contain lysozyme, an enzyme that destroys the cell walls of gram-positive bacteria.

If a foreign substance gets through the above defenses and penetrates body tissues, an inflammatory response begins immediately. Inflammation is a generalized reaction to cellular injury from any cause. It involves phagocytic leukocytes and chemical substances that destroy the foreign invader.

The final defense mechanism is the immune response, a specific reaction that stimulates production of antibodies and activated lymphocytes, which then destroy foreign invaders. Immune responses occur more slowly than inflammatory responses. Inflammatory and immune re-

sponses interact in complex ways and share a number of processes, including phagocytosis. As a result, understanding inflammation promotes understanding of immunity and vice versa. Cellular physiology and inflammation as a response to cellular injury are discussed in Chapter 1.

## Immunity

Immunity indicates protection from a disease, and the major function of the immune system is to detect and eliminate foreign substances that may cause tissue injury or disease. To perform this function, the immune system must be able to differentiate body tissues (self) from foreign substances (nonself). Self tissues are recognized by distinctive protein molecules on the surface membranes of essentially all body cells. These molecules or markers (sometimes called self antigens or autoantigens) are encoded by a group of genes called the major histocompatibility complex (MHC). MHC markers are essential to immune system function because they regulate the antigens to which a person responds and allow immune cells (*e.g.*, lymphocytes and macrophages) to recognize and communicate with each other. Nonself or foreign substances are also recognized by distinctive molecules, called epitopes, on their surfaces. Epitopes vary widely in type, number, and ability to elicit an immune response.

A normally functioning immune system does not attack body tissues labeled as self but attacks nonself sub-

Anne Collins Abrams: CLINICAL DRUG THERAPY, Fourth Edition.
© 1995 J.B. Lippincott Company.

stances. In most instances, a normally functioning immune system is highly desirable. With organ or tissue transplants, however, the system responds appropriately but undesirably when it attacks the nonself grafts. An abnormally functioning immune system causes numerous diseases. When the system is hypoactive, immunodeficiency disorders develop in which the person is highly susceptible to infectious and neoplastic diseases. When the system is hyperactive, it perceives ordinarily harmless environmental substances (*e.g.*, foods, plant pollens) as harmful and induces allergic reactions. When the system is inappropriately activated (it loses its ability to distinguish between self and nonself, so an immune response is aroused against the host's own body tissues), the result is autoimmune disorders, such as systemic lupus erythematosus and rheumatoid arthritis. Many other disorders, including diabetes mellitus and myasthenia gravis, are thought to involve autoimmune mechanisms. To aid understanding of the immune response and drugs used to alter immune response, more specific characteristics, processes, and functions of the immune system are described.

## TYPES OF IMMUNITY

**Innate immunity**, which includes the general protective mechanisms described above, is not produced by the immune system. It is often described as species dependent. Thus, humans have an inborn resistance to many infectious diseases that affect other species because human tissues do not provide a suitable environment for growth of the causative microorganisms.

**Acquired immunity** develops during gestation or after birth and may be active or passive. *Active immunity* is produced by the person's own immune system in response to a disease caused by a specific antigen or administration of an antigen (*e.g.*, a vaccine) from a source outside the body, usually by injection. The immune response stimulated by the antigen produces activated lymphocytes and antibodies against the antigen. When an antigen is present for the first time, production of antibodies requires several days. As a result, the serum concentration of antibodies does not reach protective levels for about 7 to 10 days, and the host develops the disease. When the antigen is eliminated, the antibody concentration gradually decreases over several weeks.

The duration of active immunity may be relatively brief (*e.g.*, to influenza viruses), or it may last for years or a lifetime. Long-term active immunity has a unique characteristic called *memory*. When the host is re-exposed to the antigen, lymphocytes are activated and antibodies are produced rapidly, and the host does not develop the disease. This characteristic allows "booster" doses of antigen to increase antibody levels and maintain active immunity against some diseases.

*Passive immunity* occurs when antibodies are formed by the immune system of another person or animal and transferred to the host. For example, an infant is normally protected for several months by maternal antibodies received through the placenta during gestation. Also, antibodies previously formed by a donor can be transferred to the host by an injection of immune serum. These antibodies act against antigens immediately. Passive immunity is short term, lasting only a few weeks or months.

Types of acquired immunity have traditionally been separated into cellular immunity (mainly involving activated T lymphocytes in body tissues) and humoral immunity (mainly involving B lymphocytes and antibodies in the blood). However, it is now known that the two types are closely connected, that virtually all antigens elicit cellular and humoral responses, and that most humoral (B cell) responses require cellular (T cell) stimulation.

Although most humoral immune responses occur when antibodies or B cells encounter antigens in blood, some occur when antibodies or B cells encounter antigens in other body fluids (*e.g.*, tears, sweat, saliva, mucus, and breast milk). The antibodies in body fluids other than blood are produced by a part of humoral immunity sometimes called the secretory or mucosal immune system. The B cells of the mucosal system migrate through lymphoid tissues of tear ducts, salivary glands, breasts, bronchi, intestines, and genitourinary structures. The antibodies (mostly immunoglobulin A [IgA], some IgM and IgG) secreted at these sites act locally rather than systemically. This local protection combats foreign substances, especially pathogenic microorganisms, that are inhaled, swallowed, or otherwise come in contact with external body surfaces. When the foreign substances bind to local antibodies, they are unable to attach to and invade mucosal tissue.

## ANTIGENS

Antigens are the foreign (nonself) substances, usually microorganisms, other proteins, or polysaccharides, that initiate immune responses. Antigens have specific sites that interact with immune cells to induce the immune response. The number of antigenic sites on a molecule depends largely on its molecular weight. Large protein and polysaccharide molecules are complete antigens because of their complex chemical structures and multiple antigenic sites. Smaller molecules (*e.g.*, animal danders, plant pollens, and most drugs) are incomplete antigens (called haptens) and cannot act as antigens by themselves. However, they have antigenic sites and can combine with carrier substances to become antigenic. Antigens also may be called immunogens, which is a more accurate term because an antigen may be too weak to arouse an immune response. In discussions of allergic conditions, antigens are often called allergens.

## Immune responses to antigens

The immune response involves antigens that induce the formation of antibodies or sensitized T lymphocytes. The initial response occurs when an antigen is first introduced into the body. B lymphocytes recognize the antigen as foreign and develop antibodies against it. Antibodies are proteins called immunoglobulins that interact with specific antigens. Antigen–antibody interactions may result in formation of antigen–antibody complexes, agglutination or clumping of cells, neutralization of bacterial toxins, destruction of pathogens or cells, attachment of antigen to immune cells, activation of complement (a group of plasma proteins essential to normal inflammatory and immunologic responses), and coating of the antigen so that it is more readily phagocytized (opsonization). With a later exposure to the antigen, antibody is rapidly produced.

The exact number of exposures required to produce enough antibodies to bind a significant amount of antigen is unknown. Thus, an allergic reaction may occur with the second exposure or after several exposures, when sufficient antibodies have been produced. Antigen–T lymphocyte interactions stimulate production and function of other T lymphocytes and help to regulate immunoglobulin production by B lymphocytes. T cells are involved in delayed hypersensitivity reactions, rejection of tissue or organ transplants, and response to neoplasms and some infections.

## Immune cells

Immune cells (Fig. 45-1) are white blood cells (WBCs) found throughout the body in lymphoid tissues (bone

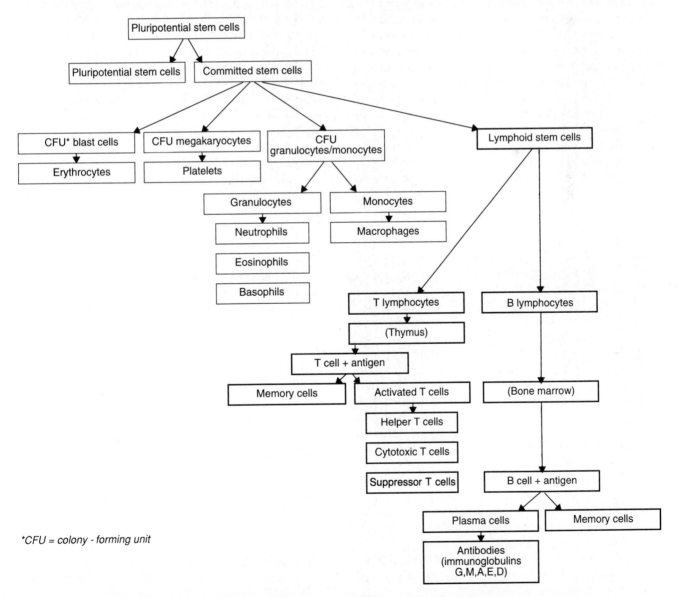

*CFU = colony - forming unit

**FIGURE 45-1.** Hematopoiesis and formation of immune cells.

marrow, spleen, thymus, tonsils and adenoids, Peyer's patches in the small intestine, lymph nodes, and blood and lymphatic vessels that transport the cells). When exposure to an antigen occurs and an immune response is aroused, WBCs are attracted to the antigen in a process called chemotaxis. Once WBCs reach the area, they phagocytize the antigen. Specific WBCs are granulocytes (neutrophils, eosinophils, basophils), monocytes, and lymphocytes. Although all WBCs play a role, neutrophils, monocytes, and lymphocytes are especially important in phagocytic and immune processes.

*Neutrophils* arrive first and start phagocytosis; *monocytes* arrive several hours later. In comparison to neutrophils, monocytes are larger, can ingest larger amounts of antigen, and have a much longer life span. In addition to their activity in the bloodstream, monocytes can enter tissue spaces (then called tissue macrophages). Tissue macrophages are widely distributed throughout the body and form the mononuclear phagocyte system (formerly called the reticuloendothelial system). Both mobile monocytes and fixed monocyte–macrophages can initiate the immune response by activating lymphocytes. They perform this function as part of phagocytosis in which they engulf a circulating antigen, break it into fragments, and return antigenic fragments to the cell surface. The antigenic fragments are recognized as foreign material by circulating T and B lymphocytes, and an immune response is initiated. Because the monocytes prepare the antigen to interact with T and B lymphocytes, they are called antigen-processing and antigen-presenting cells.

*Lymphocytes* are the main immunocytes, and those in tissues are in dynamic equilibrium with those in circulating blood. These cells continuously travel through blood and lymph vessels from one lymphoid organ to another. The three types of lymphocytes are natural killer cells, T cells, and B cells.

Natural killer cells, so called because they do not need to interact with a specific antigen to become activated, destroy infectious microorganisms and malignant cells by releasing powerful chemicals. T lymphocytes are especially able to combat intracellular infections (*e.g.*, virally infected cells), whereas B lymphocytes secrete antibodies that can neutralize pathogens prior to their entry into host cells. Both T and B cells must be activated by antigens before they can fulfill their immune functions, and both have proteins on their cell membrane surfaces that act as receptors for antigens.

Each T or B lymphocyte reacts only with a specific type of antigen and is capable of forming only one type of antibody or one type of T cell. When a specific antigen attaches to the cell membrane receptors to form an antigen–antibody complex, the complex activates the lymphocyte to form tremendous numbers of duplicate lymphocytes (clones) that are exactly like the parent cell. Clones of a B lymphocyte eventually secrete antibodies that circulate throughout the body. Clones of a T lymphocyte are sensitized T cells that are released into lymphatic ducts, carried to the blood, circulated through all tissue fluids, then returned to lymphatic ducts and recirculated. Additional participants in the activation process are phagocytic macrophages and helper T cells, which secrete substances called cytokines that regulate the growth, reproduction, and function of lymphocytes.

## T LYMPHOCYTES

T lymphocytes are the primary regulators of immune responses because they direct the activities of B cells and macrophages. They originate in pluripotential stem cells in the bone marrow and differentiate into immune cells in the thymus gland. The thymus produces a substance called thymosin, which is necessary for T cell maturation. When T cells bind with an antigen, specific genes are activated to produce substances that direct T cell proliferation and differentiation. One such substance is interleukin-2 (IL-2), which stimulates T cell deoxyribonucleic acid replication and mitosis. Cell division is necessary for production of large numbers of antigen-reactive cells and for cellular changes associated with the different subgroups of T cells. Specific types and functions of T cells include the following:

- *Helper T cells* (also called T4 or CD4 cells), the largest subgroup, regulate virtually all immune functions by producing protein substances called lymphokines (cytokines produced by lymphocytes). Lymphokines generally stimulate the growth of bone marrow and other cells of the immune system (*e.g.*, cytotoxic and suppressor T cells and B cells). They also activate macrophages and facilitate phagocytosis. Important lymphokines include IL-2, -3, -4, -5, and -6 and granulocyte-macrophage colony-stimulating factor (CSF) and interferon-gamma. The devastating effects of acquired immunodeficiency syndrome (AIDS) result primarily from the ability of the human immunodeficiency virus to destroy helper T cells.
- *Cytotoxic T cells* (also called killer T cells) are recruited and activated by helper T cells. More specifically, helper T cells secrete IL-2, which is necessary for activation and proliferation (clonal expansion) of cytotoxic T cells. Once activated by antigen and IL-2, cytotoxic T cells bind to antigens on surfaces of target cells and release substances that form large holes in the target cell membrane. The damaged cell membrane allows water, electrolytes, and other molecules to enter the cell, resulting in cellular edema and death. Once these cytotoxic cells have damaged the target cells, they can detach themselves and attack other target cells.

Cytotoxic T cells are especially lethal to virally infected tissue cells because virus particles become entrapped in the membranes of the cells and act as strong antigens that attract the T cells. These cells persist in tissues for months, even after destruction of all the invaders that elicited the original cytotoxic activity. Thus, T cells are especially important in killing body cells that have been invaded by foreign microorganisms or cells that have become malignant. Cytotoxic T cells also play a role in the destruction of transplanted organs and delayed hypersensitivity reactions.

- *Suppressor T cells* (also called T8 or CD8 cells) stop the immune response when an antigen has been destroyed by decreasing the activities of B cells and other T cells. This function is important in preventing further tissue damage. In autoimmune disorders, suppressor T cell function is impaired, and extensive tissue damage may result.

## B LYMPHOCYTES

B lymphocytes originate in stem cells in the bone marrow, differentiate into cells capable of forming antibodies (also in the bone marrow), and migrate to the spleen, lymph nodes, or other lymphoid tissue. In lymphoid tissue, the cells may be dormant until exposed to an antigen. In response to an antigen and IL-2 from helper T cells, B cells multiply rapidly, enlarge, and differentiate into plasma cells, which then produce antibodies (immunoglobulins) to oppose the antigen. Immunoglobulins are secreted into lymph and transported to the bloodstream for circulation throughout the body. There are five main classes of immunoglobulins:

- *IgG* is the most abundant immunoglobulin, constituting about 80% of the antibodies in human serum. Molecules of IgG combine with molecules of antigen, and the antigen–antibody complex activates complement. Activated complement causes an inflammatory reaction, promotes phagocytosis, and inactivates or destroys the antigen. IgG also crosses the placenta to provide maternally acquired antibodies (passive immunity) to the infant.
- *IgA* is located primarily in secretions of the respiratory and gastrointestinal tracts, where it acts against antigens entering those areas.
- *IgM* constitutes about 10% of serum antibodies and reacts with antigens in the bloodstream because its large molecular size prevents transport through capillary walls. It activates complement to destroy microorganisms.
- *IgE* is located mainly in tissues and is thought to be responsible for allergic reactions, including anaphylaxis. IgE sensitizes mast cells, which then release histamine and other chemical mediators that cause bronchoconstriction, edema, urticaria, and other manifestations of allergic reactions. IgE does not activate complement. The production of IgE is stimulated by T lymphocytes and lymphokines (mainly IL-4, -5, and -6) and inhibited by the interferons. Small amounts of IgE are present in the serum of nonallergic people; larger amounts are produced by people with allergies.
- *IgD* is present in serum in trace amounts and probably functions in recognition of antigens.

## CYTOKINES

Cytokines are protein growth factors secreted by WBCs that act on the secreting cells or other leukocytes to stimulate leukocyte replication and function. Generally, cytokines act as messengers between cells through receptors on cell surfaces and interact synergistically with other growth factors. More specifically, cytokines regulate tissue inflammation and repair and immune responses.

In the immune system, they regulate growth, mobility and differentiation of leukocytes. Although the process is not completely clear, it appears that cytokines formed by activated macrophages enter the bone marrow where they induce the synthesis and release of other cytokines that activate resting stem cells to produce more granulocytes and monocyte–macrophages. Newly formed granulocytes and monocytes leave the bone marrow and enter the circulating blood in about 3 days. Cytokines produced by lymphocytes are called lymphokines, and those produced by monocyte–macrophages are called monokines.

Lymphokines enhance macrophage activity by two main mechanisms. First, they cause macrophages to accumulate in damaged tissues by delaying or stopping macrophage migration from the area. Second, they increase the capacity and effectiveness of phagocytosis. Some lymphokines, especially IL-2, directly stimulate helper T cells and enhance their antiantigenic activity. They also enhance the antiantigenic activity of the entire immune system. Several types of cytokines have been identified, including CSFs, interferons, interleukins, and tumor necrosis factor. Cytokines are described further below and in Table 45-1.

### Colony-stimulating factors

**Colony-stimulating factors** stimulate the growth and function of hematopoietic cells. All blood cells originate in bone marrow in stem cells that are capable of becoming different types of blood cells. As these pluripotential stem cells reproduce during the life of the host, some

**TABLE 45-1.  CYTOKINES**

| Type | Name | Main Source | Main Functions |
|------|------|-------------|----------------|
| Colony-stimulating factors (CSF) | G-CSF | Leukocytes | Stimulates growth of bone marrow<br>Generates neutrophils |
| | M-CSF | | Generates macrophages<br>Stimulates growth of macrophages |
| | GM-CSF | | Stimulates growth of monocyte–macrophages |
| Interferons (IFN) | IFN-alpha | Leukocytes | Antiviral, antiproliferative, and immunomodulating effects<br>Stimulates macrophages and natural killer (NK) cells |
| | IFN-beta | Fibroblasts | Antiviral and immunoregulatory effects |
| | IFN-gamma | Circulating T cells and NK cells | Induces cell membrane antigens (*e.g.*, major histocompatibility complex)<br>Influences functions of basophils and mast cells by increasing their ability to release histamine and decreasing their capacity for growth |
| Interleukins (IL) | IL-1 | Monocytes | Interacts with tumor necrosis factor to induce other growth factors<br>Stimulates growth of blood cells, especially B and T lymphocytes<br>Enhances interactions between monocytes and lymphocytes<br>Causes inflammation<br>Causes fever |
| | IL-2 | T lymphocytes | Promotes growth of T cells<br>Activates T and B cells and NK cells<br>Augments production of other lymphokines, such as interferon-gamma<br>Influences the expression of histocompatibility antigens<br>May inhibit granulocyte–macrophage colony-formation and erythropoiesis. |
| | IL-3 (Multi-CSF) | T lymphocytes | Stimulates bone marrow; growth factor for all blood cells<br>Stimulates growth of macrophages, eosinophils, and mast cells |
| | IL-4 | Helper T cells | Stimulates growth of T and B cells and mast cells<br>Promotes immunoglobulin synthesis and reactions<br>Interacts with other cytokines to stimulate granulocytes, macrophages, mast cells, and other cells |
| | IL-5 | Helper T cells | Stimulates B cell growth, differentiation, and antibody secretion<br>Stimulates eosinophils; promote eosinophilia<br>Stimulates T cell replacement |
| | IL-6 | Fibroblasts and others | Interacts with other growth factors to stimulate growth and differentiation of B and T cells and production of antibodies<br>Augments inflammatory and immune responses<br>Augments colony-formation induced by other growth factors<br>Stimulates granulocyte–macrophage and megakaryocyte colony formation |
| | IL-7 (lymphopoietin-1) | Stromal cells | Generates pre–B and pre–T cells<br>Stimulates lymphocyte growth<br>Activates B and T cells |
| | IL-8 | Macrophages and others | Regulates growth and movement of neutrophils and lymphocytes<br>Induces immediate inflammatory responses |
| | IL-9 | | Stimulates production of red blood cells and platelets |
| | IL-10 | | ? |
| | IL-11 | | Stimulates growth of megakaryocytes, B cells and blast cells |
| Tumor necrosis factor (TNF) | TNF-alpha | Monocytes | Inflammatory, immunoenhancing, and tumoricidal<br>Causes vascular thromboses and tumor necrosis |
| | TNF-beta (lymphotoxin) | T lymphocytes | ? |
| T lymphocyte growth factor (TGF) | TGF-beta | Platelets, bone, other tissue | Fibroplasia and immunosuppression<br>Wound healing and bone remodeling |

reproduced cells are exactly like the original multicapacity cells and are retained in bone marrow to maintain a continuing supply. However, most reproduced stem cells differentiate to form other types of cells. The early offspring are committed to become a particular type of cell, and a committed stem cell that will produce a cell type is called a colony-forming unit (CFU), such as CFU-erythrocyte or CFU-granulocyte. CSFs control the growth, differentiation and reproduction of the CFUs.

Four major CSFs have been identified. One (multiCSF or IL-3) promotes the growth of virtually all types of stem cells; the other three induce the growth of specific types of committed stem cells, such as granulocytes and macrophages. Although most cytokines were initially defined by their action on one lineage, they actually act on different lineages. For example, G-CSF was initially labeled as a granulocyte-colony stimulator, but it also affects erythrocyte, megakaryocyte (platelet precursors), macrophage, and pre–B cell lineages. These growth factors also may stimulate cell division in neoplastic counterparts of their target cells, including the cancerous cells of acute myelocytic leukemia, lymphomas, and multiple myeloma.

## Interferons

**Interferons** "interfere" with the ability of viruses in infected cells to replicate and spread to uninfected cells. They also inhibit reproduction and growth of other cells, including tumor cells, and activate natural killer cells. These antiproliferative and immunomodulatory activities play important roles in normal host defense mechanisms.

## Interleukins

**Interleukins** stimulate growth and differentiation of early lymphoid and multilineage stem cells into lymphocytes, for the most part. IL-3, also known as multiCSF, stimulates pluripotential stem cells to produce all types of blood cells. Most interleukins stimulate B lymphocyte activity, but IL-4, -5, and -6 are especially important in B cell activities.

## Tumor necrosis factor

**Tumor necrosis factor** is produced by activated macrophages and other cells and acts on many immune and nonimmune target cells. It participates in the inflammatory response and causes hemorrhagic necrosis in several types of tumor cells. It is structurally the same as cachectin, a substance associated with debilitation and weight loss in patients with cancer.

# Patient-related factors that influence immune function

## AGE

### Immune function during fetal and neonatal periods

During the first few months of gestation, the fetal immune system is deficient in antibody production and phagocytic activity. During the last trimester, the fetal immune system may be able to respond to infectious antigens, such as cytomegalovirus, rubella virus, and toxoplasmosis. However, most fetal protection against infectious microorganisms is by maternal antibodies that reach the fetal circulation through the placenta. In the placenta, maternal blood and fetal blood are separated only by a layer of specialized cells called trophoblasts. Because antibodies are too large to diffuse across the trophoblastic layer, they are actively transported from the maternal to the fetal circulation by the trophoblastic cells.

At birth, the neonatal immune system is still immature, but IgG levels (from maternal blood) are near adult levels in umbilical cord blood. However, the source of maternal antibodies is severed at birth. Antibody titers in infants decrease over approximately 6 months as maternal antibodies are catabolized. Although the infant does start producing IgG, the rate of production is lower than the rate of breakdown of maternal antibodies. Cellmediated immunity is probably completely functional at birth.

### Immune function in older adults

Both humoral and cell-mediated immune functions decline with aging, and this decline is probably a major factor in the older adult's increased susceptibility to infections and tumors. The regulation of immunologic functions also declines with age, which may account for the greater frequency of autoimmune diseases in this age group. Lymphocytes are less able to proliferate in response to antigenic stimulation and a relative state of immunodeficiency prevails. With T lymphocytes, function is impaired, and the numbers are possibly decreased in peripheral blood. The functional impairment includes decreased activity of helper T cells and increased activity of suppressor T cells. With B lymphocytes, the numbers probably do not decrease, but the cells are less able to form antibodies in response to antigens. Abnormal antibody production results from impaired function of B cells and helper T cells. In addition, older adults have increased blood levels of antibodies against their own tissues (autoantibodies).

Impaired immune mechanisms have several implications for clinicians who care for elderly patients, including the following:

- Older adults are more susceptible to develop infections and less able to recover from them. Therefore, older adults need protective measures, such as rigorous personal hygiene; good nutrition; adequate exercise, rest, and sleep; minimal exposure to potential pathogens, when possible; and appropriate immunizations (e.g., influenza, pneumonia, tetanus). When older adults develop an infection, signs and symptoms (e.g., fever and drainage) may be absent or less pronounced than in younger adults.
- Older adults have impaired immune responses to antigens. Thus, higher doses of immunizing antigens may be needed in older adults to achieve protective antibody titers than in younger adults.
- Older adults often exhibit a less intense positive reaction in skin tests for tuberculosis (indicating a decreased delayed hypersensitivity response).

## NUTRITIONAL STATUS

Nutritional status can have profound effects on immune function. Adequate nutrient intake contributes to immunocompetence (ability of the immune system to function effectively). Malnutrition contributes to immunodeficiency. A severe lack of calories or protein decreases numbers and functions of T cells, complement activity, neutrophil chemotaxis, and phagocytosis. An inadequate zinc intake can depress the functions of T and B cells. Zinc is a cofactor for many enzymes, some of which are found in lymphocytes and are required for lymphocyte function. Zinc deficiency also may result from inadequate absorption in the gastrointestinal tract or excessive losses in urine, feces, or through the skin with such disorders as chronic renal disease, chronic diarrhea, burns, or severe psoriasis. Vitamin deficiencies may also depress T and B cell function because several (e.g., A, E, folic acid, pantothenic acid, and pyridoxine) also are enzyme cofactors in lymphocytes.

## STRESS

There is evidence that stress depresses immune function and therefore increases risks of developing infection and cancer. The connection between the stress response and the immune response is thought to involve neuroendocrine mechanisms. The stress response is characterized by increased activity of catecholamine neurotransmitters in the central and autonomic nervous systems (e.g., norepinephrine, epinephrine) and increased secretion of cortisol from the adrenal cortex. Cortisol and other corticosteroids are well known to suppress immune function

and are used therapeutically for that purpose. The immune response is affected by these neuroendocrine influences on lymphoid organs and lymphocyte functions because lymphocytes have receptors for many neurotransmitters and hormones.

## Immune disorders

Dysfunction of the immune system is related to many different disease processes, including allergic, autoimmune, immunodeficiency, and neoplastic disorders. Each of these is described below to promote an understanding of the use of exogenous naturally occurring substances or drug formulations to alter immune functions:

- In *allergic disorders*, the body erroneously perceives normally harmless substances (e.g., foods, pollens) as antigens and mounts an immune response. More specifically, IgE binds to antigen on the surface of mast cells and causes the release of chemical mediators (e.g., histamine) that produce the allergic manifestations. This reaction may cause tissue damage ranging from mild skin rashes to life-threatening anaphylaxis.
- In *autoimmune disorders*, the body erroneously perceives the person's own body tissues as antigens and elicits an immune response, often inflammatory in nature. Rheumatoid arthritis and systemic lupus erythematosus have long been considered autoimmune disorders. More recently, insulin-dependent diabetes mellitus, myasthenia gravis, and several other disorders have been added to the list. Autoimmune processes may damage virtually every body tissue.
- In *immunodeficiency disorders*, the body is especially susceptible to infections and neoplastic disease. Primary deficiency states are serious but uncommon. The best known disorder is AIDS, which is caused by a virus. AIDS decreases the numbers and almost all functions of T lymphocytes and several functions of B lymphocytes and monocytes. Secondary immunodeficiency also is induced by severe malnutrition, cancer, and immunosuppressant drugs.
- In *neoplastic disease*, immune cells apparently lose their ability to destroy mutant cells (which, left alone, may become malignant) or early malignant cells. This effect could logically result either from immunodeficiency states or from cancer cells that are overwhelming in number or highly malignant. Mutant cells constantly occur during cell division, but few survive or lead to cancer. Most mutant cells simply die; some survive but retain the normal controls that prevent excessive growth; and some

are destroyed by immune processes activated by abnormal proteins found in most mutant cells.

## Immunotherapy

Immunotherapy involves alteration of the immune response for therapeutic purposes. Immunotherapy is mainly used to prevent or treat rejection of transplanted tissues or organs and to treat immunodeficiency disorders and some cancers. Methods include administering exogenous antigens (*e.g.*, immunizations and desensitization procedures), strengthening antigens (*e.g.*, an antigen that is too weak to elicit an immune response), or suppressing the normal response to an antigen. In desensitization procedures, weak extracts of antigenic substances (*e.g.*, foods, plant pollens, penicillin) are prepared as drugs and administered in small, increasing amounts so that the patient develops a tolerance for the substances and avoids serious allergic reactions.

Drugs can be given to stimulate immune responses (immunizing agents [see Chap. 46] and other immunostimulants [see Chap. 47]) or to suppress the normal response (immunosuppressants [see Chap. 48]).

## Review and Application Exercises

1. What is the difference between innate and acquired immunity?
2. What are methods of producing active acquired immunity?
3. Which WBCs are phagocytes?
4. Describe phagocytosis.
5. Where are T lymphocytes formed, and what are their functions?
6. Where are B lymphocytes formed, and what are their functions?
7. What are antigens, and how do they elicit an immune response?
8. What are cytokines, and how do they function in the immune response?
9. What is complement, and how does it function in the immune response?

## Selected References

Ashman, R. F. (1992). B-lymphocytes and immunoglobulins. In W. N. Kelley (Ed.), *Textbook of internal medicine* (2nd ed.) (pp. 885–891). Philadelphia: J.B. Lippincott.

Boon, T. (1993). Teaching the immune system to fight cancer. *Scientific American, 266*(3) 82–89.

DiPiro, J. T., & Stafford, C. T. (1992). Allergic and pseudoallergic drug reactions. In J. T. DiPiro, R. L. Talbert, P. E. Hayes, G. C. Yee, G. R. Matzke, & L. M. Posey (Eds.), *Pharmacotherapy: A pathophysiologic approach* (2nd ed.) (pp. 1279–1291). New York: Elsevier.

Flannery, J. C. (1992). Immunologic disorders. In L. O. Burrell (Ed.), *Adult nursing in hospital and community settings* (pp. 141–175). Norwalk, CT: Appleton & Lange.

Guyton, A. C. (1991). *Textbook of medical physiology* (8th ed.). Philadelphia: W.B. Saunders.

Kamani, N. R., & Douglas, S. D. (1991). Structure and development of the immune system. In D. P. Stites & A. I. Terr (Eds.), *Basic and clinical immunology* (7th ed.) (pp. 9–33). Norwalk, CT: Appleton & Lange.

O'Hanley, P. D., Tam, J. Y., Holodniy, M. (1992). Infectious disorders. In K. L. Melmon, H. F. Morrelli, B. B. Hoffman & D. W. Nierenberg (Eds.), *Clinical pharmacology: Basic principles in therapeutics* (3rd ed.) (pp. 642–720). New York: McGraw-Hill.

Oppenheim, J. J., Ruscetti, F. W., & Faltynek, C. (1991). Cytokines. In D. P. Stites & A. I. Terr (Eds.), *Basic and clinical immunology* (7th ed.) (pp. 78–100). Norwalk, CT: Appleton & Lange.

Porth, C. M. (1990). *Pathophysiology: Concepts of altered health states* (3rd ed.). Philadelphia: J.B. Lippincott.

Quesenberry, P. J. (1992). Normal hematopoiesis. In W. N. Kelley (Ed.), *Textbook of internal medicine* (2nd ed.) (pp. 1052–1058). Philadelphia: J.B. Lippincott.

Rote, N. S. (1990). Immunity. In K. L. McCance & S. E. Huether (Eds.), *Pathophysiology: The biologic basis for disease in adults and children* (pp. 192–216). St. Louis: C.V. Mosby.

Sahai, J., & Louie, S. G. (1993). Overview of the immune and hematopoietic systems. *American Journal of Hospital Pharmacy, 50*(Suppl. 3), S4–9.

Smith, K. A. (1992). T-Lymphocytes. In W. N. Kelley (Ed.), *Textbook of internal medicine* (2nd ed.) (pp. 880–885). Philadelphia: J.B. Lippincott.

Tami, J. A., & DiPiro, J. T. (1992). Function and evaluation of the immune system. In J. T. DiPiro, R. L. Talbert, P. E. Hayes, G. C. Yee, G. R. Matzke, & L. M. Posey (Eds.), *Pharmacotherapy: A pathophysiologic approach* (2nd ed.) (pp. 1251–1262). New York: Elsevier.

# CHAPTER 46

# Immunizing Agents

Immune responses and types of immunity are described in Chapter 45. Many antigens that activate the immune response are microorganisms that cause infectious diseases. Early scientists observed that people who developed certain diseases were thereafter protected despite repeated exposure to the disease. As knowledge evolved, it was discovered that protection stemmed from body substances called antibodies and that antibodies could also be induced by deliberate, controlled exposure to the antigen. Subsequently, immunization techniques were developed.

## Immunization

Immunization or vaccination involves administration of an antigen to induce antibody formation (for active immunity) or serum from immune people or animals (for passive immunity). Preparations used for immunization are biologic products prepared by pharmaceutical companies and regulated by the Food and Drug Administration.

## Agents for active immunity

The biologic products used for active immunity are vaccines and toxoids. *Vaccines* are suspensions of microorganisms that have been killed or attenuated (weakened or reduced in virulence) so that they can induce antibody formation while preventing or causing very mild forms of the disease. *Toxoids* are bacterial toxins that have been modified to destroy toxicity while retaining antigenic properties (*i.e.*, ability to induce antibody formation). For maximum effectiveness, vaccines and toxoids must be given before exposure to the pathogenic microorganism.

## INDICATIONS FOR USE

Clinical indications for use of vaccines and toxoids include the following:

1. Routine immunization of all children against diphtheria, tetanus, pertussis (whooping cough), rubeola ("red" measles), rubella (German measles), mumps, and poliomyelitis
2. Immunization of adults against tetanus
3. Immunization of prepubertal girls or women of childbearing age against rubella. Rubella during the first trimester of pregnancy is associated with a high incidence of birth defects in the newborn.
4. Immunization of people at high risk of serious morbidity or mortality from a particular disease. For example, hepatitis B, influenza, and pneumococcal vaccines are recommended for selected groups of people (Table 46-1).
5. Immunization of adults and children at high risk of exposure to a particular disease. For example, several diseases (*e.g.*, yellow fever, cholera) rarely occur in most parts of the world. Thus, immunization is recommended only for people who live in or travel to geographic areas where the disease can be contracted.

(*Text continues on p. 478*)

472

## TABLE 46-1. VACCINES AND TOXOIDS FOR ACTIVE IMMUNITY

| Generic/Trade Name | Characteristics | Clinical Indications | Routes and Dosage Ranges | |
|---|---|---|---|---|
| | | | *Adults* | *Children* |
| **Cholera vaccine** | Sterile suspension of killed cholera organisms<br>Protects about 50% of recipients for 3–6 mo. Does not prevent transmission of cholera.<br>Protection begins about 1 wk after the initial dose. | Travel to endemic areas (Asia, Africa, Middle East)<br>Living in endemic areas | IM, SC 0.5 ml initially, 0.5 ml 4 wk later, then 0.5 ml every 6 mo if indicated | Over age 10 y, same as adults<br>Age 5–10 y, IM, SC 0.3 ml initially, 0.3 ml 4 wk later, then 0.3 ml every 6 mo if indicated<br>Age 6 mo–4 y, IM, SC 0.2 ml initially, 0.2 ml 4 wk later, then 0.2 ml every 6 mo if indicated |
| **Haemophilus b conjugate vaccine**<br>(HibTITER<br>Pedvax HIB<br>ProHibit) | Formed by conjugating a derivative of the organism with a protein | To prevent infection with Hib, a common cause of serious bacterial infections, including meningitis, in children under 5 years of age | | HibTITER age 2–6 mo, IM 0.5 ml q2 mo for 3 doses; age 15 mo, 0.5 ml as a single booster dose<br>Age 7–11 mo, IM 0.5 ml q2 mo for 2 doses; age 15 mo, 0.5 ml as a single booster dose<br>Age 12–14 mo, IM 0.5 ml as single dose; age 15 mo, 0.5 ml as a single booster dose, at least 2 mo after the first dose<br>Age 15–59 mo, IM 0.5 ml as a single dose (no additional booster dose)<br>Pedvax HIB age 2–6 mo, IM 0.5 ml q2 mo for 2 doses; age 12 mo, 0.5 ml as a booster dose<br>Age 7–11 mo, IM 0.5 ml q2 mo for 2 doses; age 15 mo, 0.5 ml as booster dose<br>Age 12–14 mo, IM 0.5 ml as single dose; age 15 mo, 0.5 ml as a single booster dose, at least 2 mo after the first dose<br>Age 15–59 mo, IM 0.5 ml as a single dose (no additional booster dose)<br>ProHIBit Age 15–59 mo, IM 0.5 ml as a single dose (no additional booster dose) |
| **Hepatitis B vaccine (recombinant)**<br>(Recombivax HB<br>Engerix B) | Prepared by recombinant DNA techniques of inserting the gene coding for production of hepatitis B surface antigen (HBsAG) into yeast cells<br>Contains no blood or blood products<br>About 96% effective in children and young adults; about 88% effective in adults >40 years | Pre-exposure immunization of high-risk groups, such as health-care providers (nurses, physicians, dentists, laboratory workers); clients with cancer, organ transplants, hemodialysis, immunosuppressant drug therapy, or multiple infusions of blood or blood products; male homosexuals; intra- | Engerix, IM 20 μg (1 ml) × three doses, initially and at 1 mo and 6 mo after the first dose.<br>Booster, IM 20 μg × 1 dose<br>Dialysis patients, IM 40 μg (2 ml) × 4 doses, initially and at 1, 2, and 6 mo after the first dose<br>Recombivax, IM 10 μg (1 ml) × 3 doses, ini- | Engerix, neonates to 10 y, IM 10 μg (0.5 ml) × 3 doses, initially and at 1 mo and 6 mo after first dose<br>Booster, IM 10 μg × 1 dose<br>Children >10 years, IM 20 μg (1 ml) × 3 doses, same schedule as above<br>Booster, IM 20 μg × 1 dose<br>Recombivax, birth to 10 |

(continued)

**TABLE 46-1.   VACCINES AND TOXOIDS FOR ACTIVE IMMUNITY** *(Continued)*

| Generic/Trade Name | Characteristics | Clinical Indications | Routes and Dosage Ranges | |
|---|---|---|---|---|
| | | | *Adults* | *Children* |
| | Duration of protection unknown; can measure serum antibody levels periodically (protective levels about 10 million U/ml) | venous drug abusers; residents and staff of institutions for mentally handicapped people | tially and at 1 mo and 6 mo after the first dose<br>Booster 10 μg × 1 dose<br>Dialysis formulation, IM 40 μg (1 ml) × three doses, initially and at 1 mo and 6 mo after the first dose<br>Booster 40 μg × 1 dose if antibody level <10 million U/ml 1–2 mo after third dose of above schedule | years, IM 2.5 μg (0.25 ml) × 3 doses, initially and at 1 mo and 6 mo after the first dose<br>11–19 y, IM 5 μg (0.5 ml) × 3 doses, same schedule as above |
| **Influenza vaccine** (Fluogen) | Inactivated strains of A and B influenza viruses, reformulated annually to include current strains<br>Protects 60%–75% of recipients for a few months. Maximal antibody production occurs the second week after vaccination; the titer remains constant about 1 mo, then gradually declines.<br>Grown in chick embryos; therefore, contraindicated in clients who are highly allergic to eggs | Recommended annually for health-care providers; older adults; and people chronically ill with pulmonary, cardiovascular, or renal disorders, diabetes mellitus, or adrenocortical insufficiency | IM 0.5 ml as single dose | <3 years, IM 0.25 ml as single dose<br>>3 years, IM 0.5 ml as single dose<br>Note: Children <9 years not previously immunized need 2 doses, at least 1 mo apart |
| **Measles vaccine** (Attenuvax) | Sterile preparation of live, attenuated measles (rubeola) virus<br>Protects approximately 95% of recipients for several years or lifetime<br>Usually given with mumps and rubella vaccines. A combination product containing all three antigens is available and preferred.<br>Measles vaccine should not be given for 3 mo after administration of immune serum globulin, plasma, or whole blood | Routine immunization of children 1 y of age or older<br>Immunization of adults not previously immunized | SC 0.5 ml in a single dose | SC, same as adults |
| **Measles and rubella vaccine** (M-R-Vax II) | A mixture of live attenuated rubeola virus (Attenuvax) and rubella (German measles) virus | Immunization of 15-mo-old children against rubeola and rubella | | SC, total volume of reconstituted vial |
| **Measles, mumps, and rubella vaccine** (M-M-R II) | A mixture of three vaccines (rubeola, rubella, mumps)<br>Usually preferred over single immunizing agents | Immunization from age 15 mo to puberty | | SC, total volume of reconstituted vial |
| **Meningitis vaccine** (Menomune A/C Menomune A/C/Y/W-135) | A suspension prepared from groups A and C or A, C, Y, and W-135 of *Neisseria meningitidis* | Immunization of people at risk in epidemic or endemic areas<br>Type A only should be given to infants and | SC, 0.5 ml | |

*(continued)*

**TABLE 46-1.  VACCINES AND TOXOIDS FOR ACTIVE IMMUNITY**  *(Continued)*

| Generic/Trade Name | Characteristics | Clinical Indications | Routes and Dosage Ranges | |
| --- | --- | --- | --- | --- |
| | | | *Adults* | *Children* |
| **Mumps vaccine** (Mumpsvax) | Sterile suspension of live, attenuated mumps virus Provides active immunity in about 97% of children and 93% of adults for at least 10 y Most often given in combination with measles and rubella vaccines | children under 2 y of age. Routine immunization of children (1 y and older) and adults | SC, 0.5 ml in a single dose of reconstituted vaccine. (Reconstituted vaccine retains potency for 8 h if refrigerated. Discard if not used within 8 h.) | Over 1 y, same as adults (vaccination not indicated in children under 1 y) |
| **Plague vaccine** | A sterile suspension of killed plague bacilli | Immunization of high-risk people (*e.g.*, laboratory workers, people in disaster areas) | IM 1.0 ml initially, then 0.2 ml after 1–3 mo and 3–6 mo (total of 3 doses) Booster doses of 0.1–0.2 ml every 6 mo during active exposure | Age 5–10 y, 3/5 adult dose Age 1–4 y, 2/5 adult dose Age under 1 y, 1/5 adult dose |
| **Pneumococcal vaccine, polyvalent** (Pneumovax 23 Pnu-Imune 23) | Consists of 23 strains of pneumococci, which cause approximately 85%–90% of the serious pneumococcal infections in the United States Protection begins about the third week after vaccination and lasts years. Not recommended for children under 2 y old because they may be unable to produce adequate antibody levels | Adults with chronic cardiovascular or pulmonary diseases Adults with chronic disease associated with increased risk of pneumococcal infection (*e.g.*, splenic dysfunction, Hodgkin's disease, multiple myeloma, cirrhosis, alcohol dependence, renal failure, immunosuppression) Adults 65 y or older who are otherwise healthy Children 2 y or older with chronic disease associated with increased risk of pneumococcal infection (*e.g.*, asplenia, nephrotic syndrome, immunosuppression) | SC, IM 0.5 ml as a single dose | Same as adults |
| **Poliomyelitis vaccine, inactivated** (IPOL) | A suspension of inactivated poliovirus types I, II, and III | Children not previously immunized Adults not previously immunized and at high risk of exposure (*e.g.*, health-care or laboratory workers) | SC, 0.5 ml × 3 doses initially, second dose 1–2 mo after first, third dose 6–12 mo after second dose | SC, 0.5 ml × 3 doses with first at 2 mo of age, second at 4 mo, third at 10–16 mos (6–12 mo after second dose) Booster 0.5 ml × 1 dose at 4–6 y of age |
| **Poliovirus vaccine, trivalent, oral (Sabin)** (Orimune) | A suspension of live, attenuated poliovirus types I, II, and III Effective in >90% of recipients | Routine immunization of all infants and children Immunization of high-risk adults (*e.g.*, health-care workers, people who live in or travel to epidemic or endemic areas) | Same as children and adolescents | Infants, PO 0.5 ml at 2, 4, and 6 mo, followed by a fourth dose at approximately 15–18 mo Children and adolescents, PO 0.5 ml for 2 doses, 6–8 wk apart, followed by a third dose of 0.5 ml 8–12 mo after the second dose. All children who have received the series should be given a single booster dose at 4–6 y of age. |

*(continued)*

**TABLE 46-1. VACCINES AND TOXOIDS FOR ACTIVE IMMUNITY** *(Continued)*

| Generic/Trade Name | Characteristics | Clinical Indications | Routes and Dosage Ranges | |
|---|---|---|---|---|
| | | | *Adults* | *Children* |
| **Rabies vaccine (human diploid cell rabies vaccine [HDCV])** (Imovax) | An inactivated virus vaccine<br>Immunity develops in 7–10 d and lasts 1 year or longer | Pre-exposure immunization in people at high risk of exposure (veterinarians, animal handlers, laboratory personnel who work with rabies virus)<br>Postexposure prophylaxis in people who have been bitten by potentially rabid animals or who have skin scratches or abrasions exposed to animal saliva (*e.g.*, animal licking of wound), urine, or blood | Pre-exposure prophylaxis, IM 1.0 ml for 3 doses. The second dose is given 1 wk after the first; the third dose is given 4 wk after the first. Thereafter, booster doses (1 ml) are given every 2 y in high-risk people.<br>Postexposure, IM 1 ml for 5 doses. After the initial dose, remaining doses are given 3, 7, 14, and 28 d later. Rabies immunoglobulin is administered at the same time as the initial dose of HDVC vaccine | |
| **Rubella vaccine** (Meruvax II) | Sterile suspension of live, attenuated rubella virus<br>Protects about 95% of recipients at least 15 y, probably for lifetime<br>Should not be given for 3 mo after receiving immune serum globulin, plasma, or whole blood<br>Usually given with measles and mumps vaccines. A combination product containing all three antigens is available and preferred. | Routine immunization of children 1 y of age or older<br>Initial or repeat immunization of adolescent girls or women of child-bearing age *if* serum antibody levels are low | SC, 0.5 ml in a single dose | SC, same as adults |
| **Rubella and mumps vaccine** (Biavax-II) | A mixture of mumps and rubella virus strains<br>Less frequently used than measles, mumps, and rubella vaccine | Immunization of children | | Age 1 y and older, SC, total volume of reconstituted vial |
| **Smallpox vaccine** | Preparation of live (cowpox) virus<br>Protection lasts 3–10 y, beginning 8 d after vaccination<br>Not recommended for routine immunization in United States<br>Available from Centers for Disease Control and Prevention | Foreign travel to Africa, Asia, Central America, and South America | Intradermal, by multiple puncture technique, of one capillary tube | |
| **Tuberculosis vaccine (Bacillus Calmette-Guérin)** (TICEBCG) | Suspension of attenuated tubercle bacillus<br>Converts negative tuberculin reactors to positive reactors. Therefore, precludes use of the tuberculin skin test for screening or early diagnosis of tuberculosis.<br>Contraindicated in clients who have not had a (negative) tuberculin | People at high risk for exposure, including newborns of women with tuberculosis | Percutaneous, by multiple puncture disk, 0.2–0.3 ml | Newborns, percutaneous, by multiple puncture disk, 0.1 ml<br>Children >1 mo of age, same as adults |

*(continued)*

## TABLE 46-1. VACCINES AND TOXOIDS FOR ACTIVE IMMUNITY (Continued)

| Generic/Trade Name | Characteristics | Clinical Indications | Routes and Dosage Ranges | |
|---|---|---|---|---|
| | | | **Adults** | **Children** |
| | skin test within the preceding 2 wk; who are actually ill or suspected of having respiratory tract, skin, or other infection; who have dysgammaglobulinemia; and who have a positive tuberculin skin test | | | |
| **Typhoid vaccine** (Vivotif Berna) | Sterile suspension of attenuated or killed typhoid bacilli Protects >70% of recipients | High-risk people (household contacts of typhoid carriers or people whose occupation or travel predisposes to exposure) | SC 0.5 ml for 2 doses at least 4 wk apart, then a booster dose of 0.5 ml (or 0.1 ml intradermal) at least every 3 y for repeated or continued exposure PO 1 capsule every other day × 4 doses; repeat every 4 y as a booster dose with repeated or continued exposure | Age over 10 y, SC 0.5 ml for 2 doses at least 4 wk apart, then a booster dose of 0.5 ml at least every 3 y for repeated or continued exposure Age 6 mo–10 y, SC 0.25 ml for 2 doses, at least 4 wk apart, then a booster dose of 0.25 ml (or 0.1 ml intradermal) every 3 y if indicated Children >6 y of age, same as adults |
| **Yellow fever vaccine** (YF-Vax) | Suspension of live, attenuated yellow fever virus Protects approximately 95% of recipients for 10 y or longer | Laboratory personnel at risk of exposure Travel to endemic areas (Africa, South America) | SC 0.5 ml; booster dose of 0.5 ml every 10 y if in endemic areas | Age over 6 mo, SC same as adults |
| **Diphtheria and tetanus toxoids and whole-cell pertussis vaccine (DTwP)** (Tri-Immunol) | Diphtheria component is a preparation of detoxified growth products of *Corynebacterium diphtheriae* Pertussis component is killed, whole bacterial cells | Routine immunization of infants and children 6 y of age or younger | | IM 0.5 ml for 3 doses at 4- to 6-wk intervals, beginning at 2 mo of age, followed by a reinforcing dose 7–12 mo later and a booster dose when the child is 5–6 y of age |
| **Diphtheria and tetanus toxoids and acellular pertussis vaccine (DTaP)** (Acel-Imune, Tripedia) | Differs from Tri-Immunol in that the pertussis component is acellular bacterial particles, formulated to decrease serious adverse reactions associated with the whole-cell vaccine | As fourth or fifth dose, after initial immunization with whole cell vaccine, in children at least 15 mo of age | | IM 0.5 ml at approximately 18 mo of age; repeat at 4–6 y of age |
| **Diphtheria and tetanus toxoids and whole-cell pertussis and *Haemophilus influenzae* type B conjugate vaccines (DTwP-HibTITER)** (Tetramune) | A mixture of DTwP (Tri-Immunol) and Hib vaccine (HibTITER) | Immunization of children 2 mo to 5 y of age when indications for diphtheria, tetanus, pertussis (DTP) and *Haemophilus* b conjugate vaccine coincide (usually at 2, 4, 6, and 15 mo of age) | | IM 0.5 ml at age 2, 4, 6, and 15 mo (total of 4 doses) |
| **Diphtheria and tetanus toxoids adsorbed (pediatric type)** | Also called DT Contains a larger amount of diphtheria antigen than tetanus and diphtheria toxoids, adult type (Td) | Routine immunization of infants and children up to 6 y of age in whom pertussis vaccine is contraindicated (*i.e.*, those who have adverse reactions to initial doses of DTP) | | Infants and children up to 6 y of age, IM 0.5 ml for 2 doses at least 4 wk apart, followed by a reinforcing dose 1 y later and at the time the child starts school |
| **Tetanus toxoid, adsorbed** | Preparation of detoxified growth products of *Clostridium tetani* | Routine immunization of infants and young children | Primary immunization in adults not previously immunized, IM 0.5 ml | Primary immunization and prophylaxis, same as adults |

(continued)

**TABLE 46-1.   VACCINES AND TOXOIDS FOR ACTIVE IMMUNITY   (Continued)**

| Generic/Trade Name | Characteristics | Clinical Indications | Routes and Dosage Ranges | |
| --- | --- | --- | --- | --- |
| | | | Adults | Children |
| | Protects approximately 100% of recipients for 10 y or more Usually given in combination with DTP or diphtheria toxoid (DT) for primary immunization of infants and children up to 6 y of age Usually given alone or combined with diphtheria toxoid (Td, adult type) for primary immunization of adults | Primary immunization of adults Prevention of tetanus in previously immunized people who sustain a potentially contaminated wound | initially, followed by 0.5 ml in 4–8 wk, followed by 0.5 ml 6–12 mo later (total of 3 doses). Then, 0.5 ml booster dose every 10 y. Prophylaxis, IM, 0.5 ml if wound severely contaminated and no booster dose received for 5 y; 0.5 ml if wound clean and no booster dose received for 10 y | |
| **Tetanus and diphtheria toxoids, adsorbed (adult type)** | Also called Td Contains a smaller amount of diphtheria antigen than diphtheria and tetanus toxoids, pediatric type | Primary immunization or booster doses in adults and children over 6 y of age | IM 0.5 ml for 2 doses, at least 4 wk apart, followed by a reinforcing dose 6–12 mo later and every 10 y thereafter | Age above 6 y, same as adults |

## CONTRAINDICATIONS FOR USE

Vaccines and toxoids are generally contraindicated during febrile illnesses; immunosuppressive drug therapy (see Chap. 48); immunodeficiency states; leukemia, lymphoma, or generalized malignancy; and pregnancy.

## Agents for passive immunity

The biologic products used for passive immunity are immune serums and antitoxins. These substances may be obtained from human or animal sources, and they may consist of whole serum or the immunoglobulin portion of serum in which the specific antibodies are concentrated. When possible, human serum is preferred to animal serum because risks of severe allergic reactions are reduced. Also, immunoglobulin fractions are preferred over whole serum because they are more likely to be effective. Human immunoglobulins are available for measles, hepatitis, rabies, rubella, tetanus, and varicella-zoster infections.

To obtain antitoxins or animal immune serums, an animal such as a horse is injected with a purified toxin or toxoid. After antibodies have had time to develop, blood is withdrawn from the animal and prepared for clinical use. Antitoxins are available for rabies, botulism, diphtheria, gas gangrene, and tetanus. A major disadvantage of antitoxins is that a relatively high number of people are allergic to horse serum.

Immune serums and antitoxins are used to provide temporary immunity in people exposed to or experiencing a particular disease. The goal of therapy is to prevent or modify the disease process (i.e., decrease incidence and severity of symptoms). Antitoxins are contraindicated in clients allergic to horse serum.

## Individual immunizing agents

Vaccines and toxoids are listed in Table 46-1; immune serums and antitoxins are listed in Table 46-2.

## Nursing Process

### Assessment

Assess the client's immunization status by obtaining the following information:
- Determine the client's previous history of diseases for which immunizing agents are available (e.g., measles, influenza).
- Ask if the client has had previous immunizations.
  - For which diseases were immunizations received?
  - Which immunizing agent was received?
  - Were any adverse effects experienced? If so, what symptoms occurred, and how long did they last?
  - Was tetanus toxoid given for any cuts or wounds?
  - Did any foreign travel require immunizations?
- Determine whether the client has any conditions that contraindicate administration of immunizing agents (e.g., malignancy, pregnancy, immunosuppressive drug therapy).
- For pregnant women not known to be immunized against rubella, serum antibody titer should be measured to determine resistance or susceptibility to the disease.

**TABLE 46-2. IMMUNE SERUMS AND ANTITOXINS FOR PASSIVE IMMUNITY**

| Generic/Trade Name | Characteristics | Clinical Indications | Routes and Dosage Ranges |
|---|---|---|---|
| *Immune Serums* | | | |
| **Cytomegalovirus immune globulin, IV, human (CMV-IGIV)** (CytoGam) | Contains antibodies against CMV | Treat CMV infection in renal transplant patients | IV infusion, 150 mg/kg within 72 h of transplant; 100 mg/kg 2–8 wks after transplant; 50 mg/kg 12–16 weeks after transplant |
| **Hepatitis B immune globulin, human** (H-BIG, Hyper-Hep, Hep-B-Gammagee) | A solution of immunoglobulins that contains antibodies to hepatitis B surface antigen | To prevent hepatitis after exposure | Adults and children: IM 0.06 ml/kg as soon as possible after exposure. Repeat dose in 1 mo. |
| **Immune serum globulin (human) (ISG)** (Gammar) | Commonly called gamma globulin Obtained from pooled plasma of normal donors Consists primarily of immunoglobulin G (IgG), which contains concentrated antibodies Produces adequate serum levels of IgG in 2–5 d | To decrease the severity of hepatitis A, measles, and varicella after exposure To treat immunoglobulin deficiency Adjunct to antibiotics in severe bacterial infections and burns To lessen possibility of fetal damage in pregnant women exposed to rubella virus (however, routine use in early pregnancy is not recommended) | Adults and children: Exposure to hepatitis A, IM 0.02–0.04 ml/kg Exposure to measles, IM 0.25 ml/kg given within 6 d of exposure Exposure to varicella, IM 0.6–1.2 ml/kg Exposure to rubella (pregnant women only), IM 0.55 ml/kg Immunoglobulin deficiency, IM 1.3 ml/kg initially, then 0.6 ml/kg every 3–4 wk Bacterial infections, IM 0.5–3.5 ml/kg |
| **Immune serum globulin IV (IGIV)** (Gamimune, Sandoglobulin) | Given IV only Provides immediate antibodies Half-life about 3 wk Mechanism of action in idiopathic thrombocytopenic purpura (ITP) unknown | Immunodeficiency syndrome ITP | Gamimune: IV infusion 100–200 mg/kg once a month. May be given more often or increased to 400 mg/kg if clinical response or serum level of IgG is insufficient. ITP, IV infusion, 400 mg/kg daily for 5 consecutive days Sandoglobulin: IV infusion, 200 mg/kg once a month. May be given more often or increased to 300 mg/kg if clinical response or level of IgG is inadequate. ITP, IV infusion, 400 mg/kg daily for 5 consecutive days |
| **Rabies immune globulin (human)** (Hyperab, Imogam) | Gamma globulin obtained from plasma of people hyperimmunized with rabies vaccine Not useful in treatment of clinical rabies infection | Postexposure prevention of rabies, in conjunction with rabies vaccine | Adults and children: IM 20 U/kg (half the dose may be infiltrated around the wound) as soon as possible after possible exposure (*e.g.*, animal bite) |
| **Rh₀(D) immune globulin (human)** (Gamulin Rh, HypRho-D, RhoGAM) | Prepared from fractionated human plasma A sterile concentrated solution of specific immunoglobulin (IgG) containing anti-Rh₀(D) For IM use only | To prevent sensitization in a subsequent pregnancy to the Rh₀(D) factor in an Rh-negative mother who has given birth to an Rh-positive infant by an Rh-positive father To prevent Rh₀(D) sensitization in Rh-negative clients accidently transfused with Rh-positive blood Also available in microdose form (MICRhoGAM) for the prevention of maternal Rh immunization following abortion or miscarriage up to 12 weeks' gestation | Obstetric use: inject contents of 1 vial IM for every 15 ml fetal packed red cell volume within 72 h following delivery, miscarriage, or abortion. Transfusion accidents: inject contents of 1 vial IM for every 15 ml of Rh-positive packed red cell volume Consult package instructions for blood typing and drug administration procedures. |
| **Tetanus immune globulin (human)** (Hyper-Tet) | Solution of globulins from plasma of people hyperimmunized with tetanus toxoid Tetanus toxoid should be given at the same time (in a different syringe and injection site) to initiate active immunization. | To prevent tetanus in clients with wounds possibly contaminated with *Clostridium tetani* and whose immunization history is uncertain or included less than 2 immunizing doses of tetanus toxoid Treatment of tetanus | Adults and children: Prophylaxis, IM 250 units as a single dose Treatment of clinical disease, IM 3000–6000 U |

*(continued)*

**TABLE 46-2. IMMUNE SERUMS AND ANTITOXINS FOR PASSIVE IMMUNITY** (*Continued*)

| Generic/Trade Name | Characteristics | Clinical Indications | Routes and Dosage Ranges |
|---|---|---|---|
| **Varicella-zoster immune globulin (human) (VZIG)** (Varicella-zoster immune globulin) | The globulin fraction of human plasma<br>Antibodies last 1 mo or longer. | To prevent or decrease severity of varicella infections (chicken-pox, shingles) in children under 15 y of age who are immuno-deficient because of illness (*e.g.*, leukemia, lymphoma) or drug therapy (*e.g.*, corticoste-roids, antineoplastics) and who have had significant exposure to chickenpox or herpes zoster (*i.e.*, playmate, household or hospital contact)<br>May be used in other children under 15 and adults on an individualized basis | IM 125 U/10 kg up to a maxi-mum of 625 U as soon as pos-sible after exposure, up to 96 h after exposure. Minimal dose, 125 U |
| *Animal Serums (Antitoxins)* | | | |
| **Antirabies serum, equine** | A hyperimmune horse serum used only if human rabies im-mune globulin is not available | To prevent rabies after severe ex-posure (*e.g.*, multiple, deep ani-mal bites, especially around the head). Used in conjunction with rabies vaccine. | Adults and children: IM 55 U/kg (half the dose may be infiltrated around the wound) as soon as possible. A test for hypersen-sitivity to horse serum should precede administration. |
| **Botulism antitoxin** | 1. Obtained from blood of horses immunized against toxins of *Clostridium botulinum*<br>2. The only specific agent avail-able for treatment of botulism. Prompt use markedly de-creases mortality<br>3. May be obtained from the Centers for Disease Control and Prevention | For treatment of suspected botu-lism (a severe form of food poi-soning that develops from raw or improperly preserved foods such as home-canned vegeta-bles). Botulism has a 20% to 35% mortality. | Adults and children: Consult the manufacturer's instructions re-garding dosages and routes of administration. Testing for hyper-sensitivity to horse serum should precede administration of the antitoxin. |
| **Diphtheria antitoxin** | 1. Obtained from blood of horses hyperimmunized against diph-theria toxin<br>2. Used in conjunction with anti-biotics (*e.g.*, penicillin, tetra-cycline, erythromycin), which eliminate bacteria but do not eliminate bacterial toxins | 1. To prevent diphtheria in ex-posed, nonimmunized clients<br>2. For treatment of diphtheria in-fection (based on clinical diag-nosis, without waiting for bacteriologic confirmation of *Corynebacterium diphtheriae*) | Adults and children: Prophylaxis, IM 10,000 U<br>Treatment, IV 20,000–120,000 U |

- For clients with wounds, assess the type of wound and determine how, when, and where it was sustained. Such information may reveal whether tetanus immunization is needed.
- For clients exposed to infectious diseases, try to determine the extent of exposure (*e.g.*, household or brief, casual contact) and when it occurred.

**Nursing diagnoses**

- Knowledge Deficit: Importance of maintaining immuniza-tions for both children and adults
- Knowledge Deficit: Risk of disease development versus risk of immunization
- High Risk for Fluid Volume Deficit related to inadequate intake and febrile reactions to immunizing agent
- High Risk for Noncompliance in obtaining recommended immunizations related to fear of adverse effects
- High Risk for Injury related to disease development
- High Risk for Injury related to hypersensitivity, fever, and other adverse drug effects

**Planning/Goals**

*The client will:*

- Avoid diseases for which immunizations are given
- Obtain recommended immunizations for children and self
- Keep appointments for immunizations

**Interventions**

Use measures to prevent infectious diseases, and provide information about the availability of immunizing agents. Gen-eral measures include those to promote health and resistance to disease (*e.g.*, nutrition, rest, and exercise). Additional mea-sures include the following:

- Education of the public, especially parents of young children, regarding the importance of immunizations to personal and public health. Include information about the diseases that can be prevented and where immunizations can be obtained.
- Prevention of disease transmission. The following are help-ful measures:
  - Handwashing (probably the most effective method)

- Avoiding contact with people who have known or suspected infectious diseases, when possible
- Using isolation techniques when appropriate
- Using medical and surgical aseptic techniques
- For someone exposed to rubeola, administration of measles vaccine within 48 hours to prevent the disease
- For someone with a puncture wound or a dirty wound, administration of tetanus immune globulin to prevent tetanus, a life-threatening disease
- For someone with an animal bite, washing the wound immediately with large amounts of soap and water. Health care should then be sought. Administration of rabies vaccine may be needed to prevent rabies, a life-threatening disease.
- Explaining to the client that contracting rubella or undergoing rubella immunization during pregnancy, especially during the first trimester, may cause severe birth defects in the infant. The goal of immunization is to prevent congenital rubella syndrome. Current recommendations are to immunize children against rubella at 12 to 15 months of age.

It is recommended that previously unimmunized girls ages 11 to 13 years be immunized. Further, nonpregnant women of childbearing age should have rubella antibody tests. If antibody concentrations are low, the women should be immunized. Pregnancy should be avoided for 3 months after immunization.

*Teach clients:*

- To maintain immunization records for themselves and their children. This is important because immunizations are often obtained at different places and over a period of years. Written, accurate, up-to-date records help to prevent diseases and unnecessary immunizations.
- That if a physician recommends immunization and it is uncertain whether the client has had a particular immunization or disease, it is probably safer to take the immunization than to risk having the disease. Immunization after a client has been previously immunized or has had the disease is generally not harmful.
- That to avoid rubella-induced abnormalities in fetal development, women of childbearing age who receive a rubella immunization must avoid becoming pregnant (*i.e.*, must use effective contraceptive methods) for 3 months

#### Evaluation

- Interview and observe for symptoms.
- Interview and observe for adverse drug effects.
- Check immunization records when indicated.

## Principles of therapy

### SOURCES OF INFORMATION

Recommendations regarding immunizations change periodically as additional information and new immunizing agents become available. Consequently, health-care personnel should update their knowledge at least annually. The best sources of information regarding current recommendations are the local health department and the Centers for Disease Control and Prevention, U.S. Public Health Service, Department of Health and Human Services, Atlanta, Georgia. Local health departments can be consulted on routine immunizations and those required for foreign travel.

### SELECTION OF PREPARATION

For routine immunizations, combined antigen preparations are preferred (*e.g.*, diphtheria, tetanus, and pertussis [DTP] and measles, mumps, and rubella [MMR]). Single antigens are recommended only when other components are contraindicated.

### STORAGE OF VACCINES

To maintain effectiveness of vaccines and other biologic preparations, the products must be stored properly. Most products require refrigeration at 2°C to 8°C (35.6°F–46.4°F); some (*e.g.*, MMR) require protection from light. Follow the manufacturer's instructions for storage.

### USE IN CHILDREN

Routine immunization of children has greatly reduced the prevalence of many common childhood diseases. However, many children are not being immunized appropriately, and diseases for which vaccines are available still occur. Standards of practice, aimed toward increasing immunizations, have been established and are supported by most pediatric provider groups (Box 46-1).

Guidelines for children whose immunizations begin in early infancy are listed below. Different schedules are recommended for children ages 1 to 5 years and for those over 6 years of age who are being immunized for the first time.

1. DTP and trivalent oral poliovirus vaccine (TOPV) at ages 2 months, 4 months, 6 months, 18 months, and 4 to 6 years
2. MMR at 12 to 15 months of age, usually as a combined vaccine. These vaccines are given later than DTP and TOPV because sufficient antibodies may not be produced until passive immunity acquired from the mother dissipates (at 12–15 months of age).
3. Tetanus-diphtheria (adult type) at 14 to 16 years of age and every 10 years thereafter
4. For children with acquired immunodeficiency syndrome (AIDS), live viral and bacterial vaccines (MMR, OPV, Bacillus Calmette-Guérin) are contraindicated because they may cause the disease rather than prevent it. However, immunizations with DTP, inactivated polio vaccine, and *Haemophilus influenzae* type b are recommended even though they may be less effective than in children with competent immune systems. Also recommended are annual administra-

# BOX 46-1. STANDARDS FOR PEDIATRIC IMMUNIZATION PRACTICES

The following standards are recommended for use by all health professionals in the public and private sector who administer vaccines to or manage immunization services for infants and children.

Standard 1. . . . Immunization services are *readily* available.

Standard 2. . . . There are no barriers or unnecessary prerequisites to the receipt of vaccines.

Standard 3. . . . Immunization services are available free or for a minimal fee.

Standard 4. . . . Providers use all clinical encounters to screen and, when indicated, immunize children.

Standard 5. . . . Providers educate parents and guardians about pediatric immunizations in general terms.

Standard 6. . . . Providers question parents or guardians about contraindications and, before immunizing a child, inform them in specific terms about the risks and benefits of the immunizations their child is to receive.

Standard 7. . . . Providers follow only true contraindications.

Standard 8. . . . Providers administer simultaneously all vaccine doses for which a child is eligible at the time of each visit.

Standard 9. . . . Providers use accurate and complete recording procedures.

Standard 10. . . . Providers coschedule immunization appointments in conjunction with appointments for other child health services.

Standard 11. . . . Providers report adverse events following immunization promptly, accurately, and completely.

Standard 12. . . . Providers operate a tracking system.

Standard 13. . . . Providers adhere to appropriate procedures for vaccine management.

Standard 14. . . . Providers conduct semiannual audits to assess immunization coverage levels and to review immunization records in the patient population they serve.

Standard 15. . . . Providers maintain up-to-date, easily retrievable medical protocols at all locations where vaccines are administered.

Standard 16. . . . Providers operate with patient-oriented and community-based approaches.

Standard 17. . . . Vaccines are administered by properly trained individuals.

Standard 18. . . . Providers receive ongoing education and training on current immunization recommendations.

---

tion of inactivated influenza vaccine for children over 6 months old and one-time administration of pneumococcal vaccine for children over 2 years of age.

## USE IN HEALTHY YOUNG AND MIDDLE-AGED ADULTS

Healthy adults should maintain immunizations against tetanus. For most other diseases (hepatitis, poliomyelitis, rabies, influenza), immunization is recommended primarily for people at high risk of exposure, such as health-care providers and laboratory workers.

## USE IN OLDER ADULTS

Annual influenza vaccine and one-time administration of pneumococcal vaccine are recommended for healthy older adults and those with chronic respiratory, cardiovascular, and other diseases. As with younger adults, immunization for most other diseases is recommended for older adults at high risk of exposure.

## USE IN IMMUNOSUPPRESSION

Live, attenuated viral vaccines (MMR, oral polio) should not be given to people with AIDS, other immune diseases, or impaired immune systems due to leukemia, lymphoma, corticosteroid or anticancer drugs, or radiation therapy. The virus may be able to reproduce and cause infection in these individuals. If exposed to measles or varicella, immune globulin or varicella-zoster immune globulin may be given for passive immunization.

# NURSING ACTIONS: IMMUNIZING AGENTS

| *Nursing Actions* | *Rationale/Explanation* |
|---|---|

**1. Administer accurately**

**a.** Read the package insert, and check the expiration date on all biologic products (*e.g.*, vaccines, toxoids, human immune serums, and antitoxins).

Concentration, dosage, and administration of biologic products often vary with the products. Fresh products are preferred; avoid administration of expired products. Also, use reconstituted products within designated time limits because they are usually stable for only a few hours.

**b.** Give trivalent oral poliovirus vaccine into the side of an infant's mouth with a dropper, by placing on a child's tongue or a sugar cube or by mixing with milk, distilled water, or chlorine-free water.

Several methods of administration are effective and can be varied to meet the needs of individual infants or children. Avoid administering TOPV to a crying child because the dose may be lost or aspirated into the lungs.

**c.** Check the child's temperature before giving diphtheria, tetanus, pertussis (DTP) vaccine.

If the temperature is elevated, do not give the vaccine.

**d.** Give DTP in the lateral thigh muscle of the infant.

The vastus lateralis is the largest skeletal muscle mass in the infant and the preferred site for all IM injections.

**e.** With measles, mumps, rubella (MMR) vaccine, use only the diluent provided by the manufacturer, and administer the vaccine SC, within 8 hours after reconstitution.

The reconstituted preparation is stable for approximately 8 hours. If not used within 8 hours, discard the solution.

**f.** Give hepatitis B vaccine IM in the anterolateral thigh of infants and young children and in the deltoid of older children and adults. Although the IM route is preferred, the drug can be given SC in people at high risk of bleeding from IM injections (*e.g.*, hemophiliacs).

Higher blood levels of protective antibodies are produced when the vaccine is given in the thigh or deltoid than when it is given in the buttocks, probably because of injection into fatty tissue rather than gluteal muscles.

**g.** Give IM human immune serum globulin with an 18- to 20-gauge needle, preferably in gluteal muscles. If the dose is 5 ml or more, divide it and inject it into two or more IM sites. Follow manufacturer's instruction for preparation and administration of IV formulations.

To promote absorption and minimize tissue irritation and other adverse reactions

**h.** Test for sensitivity to horse serum before administering any antitoxin (*e.g.*, botulism, diphtheria). This test is preferably performed by the physician. If done by the nurse, a physician should be in close proximity. Also, a syringe with 1 ml of epinephrine 1:1000 should be prepared *before* testing.

Anaphylactic shock may occur. Epinephrine aqueous solution 1:1000 is used for emergency treatment of anaphylaxis. Epinephrine is injected subcutaneously in a dose of 0.5 ml for adults and 0.01 ml/kg for children.

    If sensitivity tests are positive and antitoxins are deemed necessary, special desensitization procedures may be performed. Follow the manufacturer's recommendations for desensitization.

    **(1)** For the intradermal test, inject 0.1 to 0.2 ml of a 1:1000 dilution of horse serum into the forearm. The test is positive (*i.e.*, indicates allergy to horse serum) if a wheal appears at the injection site within 30 minutes.

    **(2)** For the conjunctival test, 1 drop of a 1:10 dilution of horse serum in isotonic saline solution is instilled in one eye. The test is positive if lacrimation and conjunctivitis appear within 30 minutes.

**i.** Aspirate carefully before IM or SC injection of any immunizing agent.

To avoid inadvertent IV administration and greatly increased risks of severe adverse effects

**j.** Have aqueous epinephrine 1:1000 readily available before administering any vaccine.

For immediate treatment of allergic reactions

*(continued)*

| *Nursing Actions* | *Rationale/Explanation* |
|---|---|
| **k.** After administration of an immunizing agent in a clinic or office setting, have the client stay in the area for at least 30 minutes. | To be observed for allergic reactions, which usually occur within 30 minutes |
| **2. Observe for therapeutic effects**<br>**a.** Absence of diseases for which immunized<br><br>**b.** Decreased incidence and severity of symptoms when given to modify disease processes | |
| **3. Observe for adverse effects** | Immunizing agents may cause adverse, life-threatening reactions. The risk of serious adverse effects from immunization is usually much smaller than the risk of the disease immunized against. Adverse effects may be caused by the immunizing agent or by foreign protein incorporated with the immunizing agent (*e.g.*, egg protein in viral vaccines grown in chick embryos). |
| **a.** Pain, tenderness, redness at injection sites | Local tissue irritation may occur with an injected immunizing agent. It is especially likely to occur with adsorbed DTP or tetanus toxoid. With DTP, a nodule or lump may persist for months but eventually resolves. |
| **b.** Fever, malaise, myalgia | These adverse effects are relatively common with vaccines and toxoids. They rarely occur with human immune serums given for passive immunity. |
| **c.** Severe fever, shock, somnolence, convulsions, encephalopathy | These are rare adverse reactions to DTP. If they occur, they are thought to be caused by the pertussis antigen, and further administration of pertussis vaccine or DTP is contraindicated. |
| **d.** Paralysis (Guillain-Barré syndrome) | This is a rare reaction to oral poliovirus vaccine. |
| **e.** Anaphylaxis (cardiovascular collapse, shock, laryngeal edema, urticaria, angioneurotic edema, severe respiratory distress) | Anaphylaxis is most likely to occur with injections of antitoxins (horse serum) but may occasionally occur with other immunizing agents. Anaphylaxis is a medical emergency that requires immediate treatment with SC epinephrine (0.5 ml for adults; 0.01 ml/kg for children). Anaphylaxis is most likely to occur within 30 minutes after immunizing agents are injected. |
| **f.** Serum sickness (urticaria, fever, arthralgia, enlarged lymph nodes) | Serum sickness is a delayed hypersensitivity reaction that occurs several days or weeks after an injection of serum. It is most likely to occur with antitoxins (horse serum). Treatment is symptomatic. Symptoms are usually relieved by aspirin, antihistamines, and corticosteroids. |
| **4. Observe for drug interactions**<br>Drugs that alter effects of vaccines: Immunosuppressant agents (*e.g.*, corticosteroids, antineoplastic drugs, phenytoin [Dilantin]) | Vaccines may be contraindicated in clients receiving immunosuppressive drugs. These clients cannot produce sufficient amounts of antibodies for immunity and may develop the illness produced by the particular organism contained in the vaccine. The disease is most likely to occur with the live virus vaccines (measles, mumps, rubella). Similar effects occur when the client is receiving irradiation and phenytoin, an anticonvulsant drug that suppresses both cellular and humoral immune responses. |

## Nursing Actions

## Rationale/Explanation

**5. Teach clients**

**a.** Give acetaminophen (Tylenol) every 4 to 6 hours to children who develop fever 24 to 48 hours after DTP injection.

For symptomatic relief and comfort

**b.** Report adverse reactions other than discomfort at the injection site, minor fever, malaise, and muscle aches.

This is especially important when vaccines are given in serial doses or booster doses. Subsequent doses may need to be reduced.

## Review and Application Exercises

1. What is the difference between active immunity and passive immunity?
2. How do vaccines act to produce active immunity?
3. What are the sources and functions of immune serums?
4. List common childhood diseases for which immunizing agents are available.
5. Which immunizations are recommended for adults?
6. What are advantages of administering a combination of immunizing agents rather than single agents?
7. What are common adverse reactions to immunizing agents, and how may they be prevented or minimized?
8. Why should live vaccines not be given to people whose immune systems are suppressed by drugs or diseases?

## Selected References

Ad hoc working group for the development of standards for pediatric immunization practices (1993). Standards for pediatric immunization practices. *Journal of the American Medical Association, 269,* 1817–1822.

Bertino, J. S. (1992). Vaccines, toxoids, and other immunobiologics. In J. T. DiPiro, R. L. Talbert, P. E. Hayes, G. C. Yee, G. R. Matzke, & L. M. Posey (Eds.), *Pharmacotherapy: A pathophysiologic approach* (2nd ed.) (pp. 1817–1836). New York: Elsevier.

Bolinger, A. M., Murphy, V. A., & Bubica, G. (1992). General pediatric therapy. In M. A. Koda-Kimble & L. Y. Young (Eds.), *Applied therapeutics: The clinical use of drugs* (5th ed.) (pp. 77-1–77-24). Vancouver, WA: Applied Therapeutics.

(1994). *Drug facts and comparisons.* St. Louis: Facts and Comparisons.

Eickhoff, T. C. (1992). Immunizations. In W. N. Kelley (Ed.), *Textbook of internal medicine* (2nd ed.) (pp. 1653–1656). Philadelphia: J.B. Lippincott.

Hinman, A. R., Orenstein, W. A., Bart, K. J., & Preblud, S. R. (1990). Immunization. In G. L. Mandell, R. D. Douglas Jr., & J. E. Bennett (Eds.), *Principles and practice of infectious diseases* (3rd ed.) (pp. 2320–2334). New York: Churchill Livingstone.

(1993). *Physicians' Desk Reference.* Montvale, NJ: Medical Economics Company.

Porth, C. M. (1990). *Pathophysiology: Concepts of altered health states* (3rd ed.). Philadelphia: J.B. Lippincott

Streit, L. A. (1992). Nursing management of adults with infections. In L. O. Burrell (Ed.), *Adult nursing in hospital and community settings* (pp. 79–99). Norwalk, CT: Appleton & Lange.

### CHAPTER 47

# Immunostimulants

## Description

Activating or enhancing a person's own immune system to fight infection and cancer is a recently developed and still evolving concept. Immunostimulant drug therapy is a type of immunotherapy in which the goal is to restore normal function or increase the ability of the immune system to eliminate potentially harmful invaders. Most immunostimulant drugs are facsimiles of natural endogenous protein substances (see Chap. 45). Techniques of molecular biology are used to delineate the type and sequence of amino acids and to identify the genes responsible for producing the substances. These genes are then inserted into bacteria (usually *Escherichia coli*) or yeasts capable of producing the substances exogenously (called recombinant deoxyribonucleic acid [DNA] biotechnology, genetic engineering, or gene splicing). Laboratory production greatly increased the available amounts of these substances and therefore facilitated their development as drugs for prevention and treatment of disease.

Immunostimulants currently available as pharmaceutical agents include colony-stimulating factors (CSFs), interferons, and an interleukin. These drugs are the primary focus of this chapter. Bacillus Calmette-Guérin (BCG) vaccine, used in the treatment of bladder cancer, is also discussed. Other drugs with immunostimulant properties are discussed in other chapters. These include traditional immunizing agents (see Chap. 46); levamisole (Ergamisol), which restores functions of macrophages and T cells and is used with fluorouracil in the treatment of intestinal cancer (see Chap. 67); lithium, a mood-stabilizing agent used in the treatment of bipolar affective disorder (see Chap. 10), which mobilizes neutro-

phils and other granulocytes from bone marrow and is sometimes given to patients with neutropenia induced by cancer chemotherapy; and antiviral drugs used in the treatment of acquired immunodeficiency syndrome (AIDS) (see Chap. 42). Levamisole and antiviral drugs are more accurately called immunorestoratives because they help a compromised immune system regain normal function rather than stimulating "supranormal" function. In AIDS, the human immunodeficiency virus causes immune system malfunction, so the antiviral drugs indirectly improve immunologic function.

### COLONY-STIMULATING FACTORS

*Epoetin alfa* (Epogen, Procrit) is a recombinant DNA version of erythropoietin, a hormone that stimulates bone marrow production of red blood cells. This drug, classified as a blood modifier rather than an immunostimulant, was the first CSF used clinically. It is used to treat anemia caused by chronic renal failure, by the anti-AIDS drug zidovudine, or by cancer chemotherapy. *Filgrastim* and *sargramostim* are the only other Food and Drug Administration (FDA)-approved CSFs currently available. These drugs stimulate bone marrow production of white blood cells (WBCs). Although they have similar effects and are considered relatively safe and effective for short-term treatment of patients with bone marrow deficiency associated with cancer chemotherapy or bone marrow transplantation, they are FDA-approved for different uses.

Filgrastim stimulates granulocyte (*e.g.*, neutrophil) production and is used in patients with cancer to prevent infection. These patients are often at risk for infection

Anne Collins Abrams: CLINICAL DRUG THERAPY, Fourth Edition.
© 1995 J.B. Lippincott Company.

because of the debilitating disease process and antineoplastic drugs that depress the immune system, including bone marrow production of WBCs. In an immunocompromised patient, infections often result from the normal microbial flora of the patient's body or environmental microorganisms, and they may involve bacteria, fungi, and viruses. The client is most vulnerable to infection when the neutrophil count falls below 500/mm$^3$.

Treatment of infections in neutropenic patients consists primarily of antimicrobial therapy, with drugs chosen according to probable organisms, likely effectiveness, the patient's signs and symptoms, and other factors. Antimicrobial drugs are usually given intravenously and may cause adverse effects, including the emergence of drug resistant microorganisms. Obviously, it is desirable to prevent infections in neutropenic patients rather than treat them. Filgrastim helps to prevent infection by reducing the incidence, severity, and duration of neutropenia associated with several chemotherapy regimens. Most patients taking filgrastim have fewer days of fever, infection, and antimicrobial drug therapy. In addition, by promoting bone marrow recovery after a course of cytotoxic antineoplastic drugs, filgrastim also may allow higher doses or more timely administration of subsequent antitumor drugs.

Sargramostim stimulates production of granulocytes and macrophages and is used in patients undergoing bone marrow transplant. Before receiving a bone marrow transplant, the patient's immune system is suppressed by chemotherapeutic drugs or irradiation. After the transplant, it takes 2 to 4 weeks for the engrafted bone marrow cells to mature and begin producing blood cells. During this time, the patient has virtually no functioning granulocytes and is at high risk for infection. Sargramostim promotes engraftment and function of the transplanted bone marrow, thereby decreasing risks of infection. If the graft is successful, the granulocyte count starts to rise in about 2 weeks. Sargramostim also is used to treat graft failure.

## INTERFERONS

Interferons are drugs with antiviral, antiproliferative, and immunoregulatory activities. They are designated as alfa, beta, or gamma according to specific characteristics. Interferon-alfa is the most studied and most clinically useful thus far. Interferon-alfa-2a and interferon-alfa-2b, structurally the same except for one amino acid, are both FDA approved to treat hairy cell leukemia and Kaposi's sarcoma associated with AIDS. Interferon-alfa-2b is also approved for the treatment of viral infections, such as chronic hepatitis and condylomata acuminata (genital warts associated with infection by human papillomavirus). Interferon-alfa-n3 is manufactured from pooled human leukocytes and approved only for the treatment of refractory or recurring condylomata.

Interferon-gamma is approved for the treatment of chronic granulomatous disease; interferon-beta is approved for the treatment of multiple sclerosis.

Interferons are being investigated for additional uses, especially in cancer and viral infections, including AIDS. In cancer, for example, interferon-alfa has demonstrated antitumor effects in non-Hodgkin's lymphoma, chronic myelogenous leukemia, multiple myeloma, malignant melanoma, and renal cell carcinoma. Common solid tumors of the breast, lung, and colon are unresponsive. In chronic hepatitis C, interferon improves liver function in about 50% of patients, but relapse often occurs when drug therapy is stopped. In condylomata, interferons are injected directly into the lesions for several weeks, and a majority of the lesions disappear completely.

Interferons are given only by injection because they are proteins and would be destroyed by digestive enzymes if given orally. Systemic interferons are generally well absorbed, widely distributed, and eliminated primarily by the kidneys.

## INTERLEUKIN

Although numerous interleukins have been identified (see Chap. 45), only interleukin-2 (IL-2, aldesleukin) is available for clinical use. Human recombinant aldesleukin is somewhat different from native IL-2, but it has the same biologic activity. Pharmacologic effects include activation of cellular immunity (e.g., produces leukocytosis); production of cytokines, such as tumor-necrosis factor, IL-1, and interferon-gamma; and inhibition of tumor growth. Aldesleukin is approved for treatment of metastatic renal cell carcinoma, and approximately 15% to 25% of patients experience objective therapeutic responses. The best responses occur in patients with prior nephrectomy and low tumor burden. The drug is being investigated for use in malignant melanoma, alone and combined with other antineoplastic drugs known to have antimelanoma activity. When used alone, about 18% of patients show objective responses; when combined with other drugs, somewhat higher response rates occur.

Various approaches are being researched to elucidate additional clinical uses of aldesleukin. In cancer, for example, cancer-fighting T cells are found within tumors. These T cells, called tumor-infiltrating lymphocytes (TIL), can be removed from the tumors, incubated in vitro with aldesleukin, and reinjected into the patient. These reinjected TIL cells return to the tumor and are more active in killing malignant cells than untreated T cells.

Aldesleukin is a protein that is not absorbed after oral administration. It is given by intravenous infusion, after which it is rapidly distributed to extravascular, extracellular spaces and eliminated by metabolism in the kidneys.

## BACILLUS CALMETTE-GUÉRIN

BCG vaccine is a suspension of attenuated *Mycobacterium bovis*, long used as an immunizing agent against tuberculosis (see Chap. 46). The drug's immunostimulant properties stem from its ability to stimulate cell-mediated immunity. It is used as a topical agent to treat superficial cancers of the urinary bladder, in which approximately 80% of patients achieve a therapeutic response.

## MECHANISMS OF ACTION

Exogenous immunostimulant drugs have the same mechanisms of action as the endogenous products described in Chapter 45. Thus, CSFs bind to receptors on the cell surfaces of immature WBCs in the bone marrow and thereby increase the number, maturity, and functional ability of the cells. Interferons also bind to specific cell surface receptors. In viral infections, interferons induce enzymes that inhibit protein synthesis and degrade viral RNA. As a result, viruses are less able to enter uninfected cells, reproduce, and release new viruses.

In cancer, immunostimulant effects enhance activities of immune cells (*i.e.*, natural killer cells, T cells, B cells, and macrophages), induce tumor cell antigens (which make tumor cells more easily recognized by immune cells), or alter the expression of oncogenes (genes that can cause a normal cell to change to a cancer cell). Interleukins increase the response of lymphocytes and other WBCs to antigens and other foreign substances. In cancer, interleukins stimulate cytotoxic cells, including lymphokine-activated killer cells, natural killer cells, and TIL. The exact mechanisms by which interferons and interleukins exert antineoplastic effects are unknown. BCG vaccine is thought to act against cancer of the urinary bladder by stimulating the immune system and eliciting a local inflammatory response, but its exact mechanism of action is unknown.

## INDICATIONS FOR USE

Immunostimulants are used primarily to prevent or treat infection, neutropenia, and some types of cancer (Table 47-1). In cancer, a major reason for using CSFs is to stimulate the bone marrow to regenerate normal numbers of WBCs. An increased WBC increases the ability of patients with cancer to fight infection and to tolerate higher doses or more frequent administration of antineoplastic drugs that depress bone marrow function.

The drugs also are used to treat patients who undergo bone marrow transplant for Hodgkin's disease, non-Hodgkin's lymphoma, or acute lymphoblastic leukemia.

In these patients, CSFs promote engraftment and function of the transplanted bone marrow. They are also effective in treating graft failure. Interferons are used primarily to treat viral infections and some specific cancers. Aldesleukin is used in the treatment of metastatic renal cell carcinoma. These drugs and similar ones are undergoing intensive investigation for use in other conditions. Thus, the number of immunostimulant drugs and their indications for use are expected to expand during the next few years.

## CONTRAINDICATIONS FOR USE

All of the drugs are contraindicated for use in clients who have previously experienced hypersensitivity reactions to any component of the pharmaceutical preparations. In addition, aldesleukin should not be given initially to patients who have had an organ transplant or those with serious cardiovascular disease (*e.g.*, an abnormal thallium stress test, which reflects coronary artery disease) or serious pulmonary disease (*e.g.*, abnormal pulmonary function tests). Also, with aldesleukin, repeated courses of therapy are contraindicated in patients who developed serious toxicity during earlier courses, including the following:

- Cardiac—arrhythmias unresponsive to treatment or ventricular tachycardia lasting for five beats or more, recurrent episodes of chest pain with electrocardiographic evidence of angina or myocardial infarction, pericardial tamponade
- Renal—impairment requiring dialysis for longer than 72 hours
- Gastrointestinal—bleeding requiring surgery, bowel ischemia or perforation
- Respiratory—intubation required longer than 72 hours
- Central nervous system—coma or toxic psychosis lasting longer than 72 hours, repetitive or hard to control seizures

BCG is contraindicated in immunosuppressed patients, because the live tubercular organism may cause tuberculosis in this high-risk population.

## Individual immunostimulants

See Table 47-1 for names, uses, and dosages.

## *Nursing Process*

### Assessment

- Assess the client's status in relation to infection or cancer.
- Assess nutritional status, including appetite and weight.

## TABLE 47-1. IMMUNOSTIMULANTS

| Generic/Trade Name | Indications for Use | Routes and Dosage Ranges | Comments |
|---|---|---|---|
| **Aldesleukin (interleukin-2)** (Proleukin) | Metastatic renal cell carcinoma in adults* | IV infusion over 15 min 600,000 IU or 0.037 mg/kg q8h for 14 doses; after 9 d, repeat q8h for 14 doses | Adverse reactions are common and may be serious or fatal. Drug administration must be interrupted or stopped for serious toxicity. |
| **Bacillus Calmette-Guérin** (TICE BCG, TheraCys) | Bladder cancer | Intravesical instillation by urinary catheter, three vials, reconstituted according to manufacturer's instructions, then diluted further in 50 ml of sterile, preservative-free saline solution (total volume per dose, 53 ml). Repeat once weekly for 6 wk, then give 1 dose monthly for 6–12 mo (TICE BCG) or 1 dose at 3, 6, 12, 18, and 24 mo (TheraCys). | Start 7–14 d after bladder biopsy or transurethral resection |
| **Filgrastim (G-CSF)** (Neupogen) | Reduce infection in neutropenic patients | SC, IV 5 μg/kg per day as a single injection, up to 2 wk. Increase by 5 μg/kg each course of chemotherapy if necessary to raise white blood cells enough. | Do not give 24 h before or after a dose of cytotoxic chemotherapy |
| **Interferon-alfa-2a** (Roferon-A) | Hairy cell leukemia in adults* AIDS-related Kaposi's sarcoma in adults* | Hairy cell leukemia SC, IM Induction, 3 million IU daily for 16–24 wk Maintenance, 3 million IU three times weekly Kaposi's sarcoma SC, IM Induction, 36 million IU daily for 10–12 wk Maintenance, 36 million IU three times weekly | SC recommended for patients with platelet counts <50,000/mm³ or who are at risk for bleeding Omit single doses or reduce dosage by 50% if severe adverse reactions occur. |
| **Interferon-alfa 2b** (Intron-A) | Hairy cell leukemia in adults AIDS-related Kaposi's sarcoma in adults Condylomata (genital warts) Chronic hepatitis (B and non-A, non-B/C) | Hairy cell leukemia SC, IM Induction and maintenance, 2 million IU/m² three times weekly Kaposi's sarcoma SC, IM Induction and maintenance, 30 million IU/m² three times weekly Chronic hepatitis C SC, IM 3 million IU three times weekly Chronic hepatitis B SC, IM 5 million IU daily or 10 million IU three times weekly (total of 30–35 million IU per wk) for 16 wk Condylomata intralesionally 1 million IU/lesion (maximum of five lesions) three times weekly for 3 wk | Omit single doses, or reduce dosage by 50% if severe adverse reactions occur. |
| **Interferon-alfa-n3** (Alferon N) | Condylomata | Intralesionally 250,000 IU/wart, two times weekly up to 8 wk | |
| **Interferon-gamma-1b** (Actimmune) | Chronic granulomatous disease | SC 50 μg/m² if body surface area (BSA) is >0.5 m²; 1.5 μg/kg if BSA <0.5 m² three times weekly (e.g., Mon., Wed., Fri.) | |
| **Sargramostim (GM-CSF)** (Leukine, Prokine) | After bone marrow transplantation to promote bone marrow function or to treat graft failure or delayed function | Bone marrow reconstitution, IV infusion over 2 h, 250 μg/m² per day, starting 2–4 h after bone marrow infusion, and continuing for 21 d Graft failure or delay, IV infusion over 2 h, 250 μg/m² per day, for 14 d. Course of treatment may be repeated after 7 d off therapy if engraftment has not occurred. | |

* = 18 years and older

- Assess functional abilities in relation to activities of daily living (ADL).
- Assess adequacy of support systems for outpatients (e.g., transportation for clinic visits).
- Assess ability and attitude toward planned drug therapy and associated monitoring and follow-up.
- Assess coping mechanisms of client and significant others in stressful situations.
- Assess client (e.g., skin integrity, invasive devices, cigarette smoking) for factors predisposing to infection.
- Assess environment for factors predisposing to infection (e.g., family or health care providers with infections).
- Assess baseline values of laboratory and other diagnostic test reports to aid monitoring of responses to immunostimulant drug therapy.

**Nursing diagnoses**

- High Risk for Injury: Infection related to drug-induced neutropenia, immunosuppression, malnutrition, chronic disease
- High Risk for Injury: Adverse drug effects
- Altered Nutrition: Less than Body Requirements related to disease process or drug therapy
- Activity Intolerance related to weakness, fatigue from debilitating disease, or drug therapy

- Anxiety related to the diagnosis of cancer or AIDS, disease progression, and treatment
- Self-Care Deficit related to debilitation from disease process or drug therapy
- Self-Esteem Disturbance related to illness, inability to perform usual ADLs
- Knowledge Deficit: Disease process
- Knowledge Deficit: Immunotherapy
- Ineffective Individual Coping related to a medical diagnosis of life-threatening illness
- Ineffective Family Coping related to illness and treatment of a family member

### Planning/Goals

*The client will:*
- Participate in interventions to prevent or decrease infection
- Remain afebrile during immunostimulant therapy
- Experience increased immunocompetence as indicated by increased WBCs (if initially leukopenic) or tumor regression
- Avoid preventable infections
- Experience relief or reduction of disease symptoms
- Maintain independence in ADLs when able; be assisted appropriately when unable
- Maintain adequate levels of nutrition and fluids, rest and sleep, and exercise
- Maintain or increase appetite and weight if initially anorectic and underweight
- Be assisted to cope with stresses of the disease process and drug therapy
- Learn to self-administer medications accurately when indicated

### Interventions

- Practice and promote good handwashing techniques by patients and all others in contact with the patient.
- Use sterile technique for all injections, intravenous site care, wound dressing changes, and any other invasive diagnostic or therapeutic measures.
- Allow patients to perform hygienic care when able, or provide assistance when unable.
- Screen staff and visitors for signs and symptoms of infection; if infection is noted, do not allow contact with the patient.
- Allow patients to participate in self-care and decision-making when possible and appropriate.
- Use isolation procedures when indicated, usually when the neutrophil count is below 500/mm$^3$.
- Promote adequate nutrition, with nutritious fluids, supplements, and snacks when indicated.
- Promote adequate rest, sleep, and exercise (*e.g.*, schedule frequent rest periods, avoid interrupting sleep when possible, individualize exercise or activity according to the patient's condition).
- Inform patients about diagnostic test results, planned changes in therapeutic regimens, and evidence of progress.
- Allow family members or significant others to visit patients when feasible.
- Monitor complete blood count (CBC) and other diagnostic test reports for normal or abnormal values.
- Schedule and coordinate drug administration, diagnostic tests, and other elements of care to conserve clients' energy and decrease stress.

- Consult other health-care providers (*e.g.*, physician, dietitian, social worker) on the client's behalf when indicated.

*Teach clients:*
- Ways to prevent or reduce the incidence of infections (*e.g.*, meticulous personal hygiene, avoiding contact with infected people)
- To enhance immune mechanisms and other body defenses by healthy life-style habits, such as a nutritious diet, adequate rest and sleep, and avoidance of tobacco and alcohol
- Ways to maintain or improve intake of food and fluids
- Stress management techniques
- The importance of taking the drugs as prescribed
- The importance of keeping appointments for monitoring response to drug therapy and follow-up care
- To inform any other physician, dentist, or health-care provider of the disease process and therapeutic plan
- Techniques of preparation, self-administration, and disposal of medications

### Evaluation

- Determine the number and type of infections that have occurred in neutropenic patients.
- Compare current CBC reports with baseline values for changes toward normal levels (*e.g.*, WBCs 5000–10,000/mm$^3$).
- Compare weight and nutritional status to baseline values for maintenance or improvement.
- Observe and interview for decreased numbers or severity of disease symptoms.
- Observe for increased energy and ability to participate in ADLs.
- Observe and interview outpatients regarding compliance with follow-up care.
- Observe and interview regarding the mental and emotional status of the client and family members.

# Principles of therapy

## INPATIENT VERSUS OUTPATIENT SETTINGS FOR DRUG ADMINISTRATION

Choosing inpatient or outpatient immunostimulant therapy depends on many factors, including the condition of the client, route of drug administration, expected duration of therapy, and potential severity of adverse drug reactions. Most of the immunostimulants are proteins, and anaphylactic or other allergic reactions may occur, especially with parenteral administration. Thus, initial doses should be given where appropriate supplies and personnel are available to treat allergic reactions. Because severe, life-threatening adverse effects may occur with high-dose aldesleukin, this drug should be given only in a hospital with intensive care facilities, under the supervision of health-care providers experienced in critical care.

## DOSAGE

Because drug therapy with interferon and aldesleukin continues to be evaluated, optimally effective and maximally safe dosages have not been established. For patients who experience severe adverse reactions with interferon-alfa, dosage should be reduced by 50% or administration stopped until the reaction abates. For patients who experience severe reactions to aldesleukin, dosage reduction is not recommended. Instead, one or more doses should be withheld, or the drug should be discontinued. Withhold the dose for cardiac arrhythmias, hypotension, chest pain, agitation or confusion, sepsis, renal impairment (oliguria, increased serum creatinine), hepatic impairment (encephalopathy, increasing ascites), positive stool guaiac test, or severe dermatitis until the condition is resolved. The drug should be discontinued for the occurrence of any of the conditions listed as contraindications (see the section Contraindications for Use, above) for repeat courses of aldesleukin therapy (e.g., sustained ventricular tachycardia, angina, myocardial infarction, pulmonary intubation, renal dialysis, coma, and gastrointestinal bleeding).

## LABORATORY MONITORING

CBC with WBC differential and platelet count should be done before initiating immunostimulant drug therapy and regularly during therapy to monitor response to drug therapy and prevent avoidable adverse drug reactions. With CSFs, CBC, WBC differential, and platelet count are recommended twice weekly during drug administration. With aldesleukin, the above tests plus electrolytes and renal and liver function tests are recommended daily during drug administration.

## USES IN PATIENTS WITH CANCER

### Colony-stimulating factors

When filgrastim is given to prevent infection in neutropenic cancer patients, the drug should be started at least 24 hours after the last dose of the antineoplastic agent. It should then be continued during the period of maximum bone marrow depression and the lowest neutrophil count (nadir) and during bone marrow recovery, until the neutrophil count exceeds 10,000/mm³. CBC and platelet counts should be performed twice weekly during therapy. When the neutrophil count rises, continued CBCs are needed to avoid excessive leukocytosis (above 20,000/mm³). When sargramostim is given to cancer patients who have had bone marrow transplantation, the drug should be started 2 to 4 hours after the bone marrow infusion and at least 24 hours after the last dose of antineoplastic chemotherapy or 12 hours after the last radiotherapy treatment. Administration should

be continued until the neutrophil count reaches approximately 20,000/mm³.

### Interferons

In hairy cell leukemia, interferons normalize WBC counts in 70% to 90% of patients, with or without prior splenectomy. Drug therapy must be continued indefinitely to avoid relapse, which usually develops rapidly after the drug is discontinued. In AIDS-related Kaposi's sarcoma, larger doses are required than in other clinical uses, with resultant increases in toxicity. Interferon-alfa is recommended for patients with CD4 cell counts higher than 200/ml (CD4 cells are the helper T cells especially attacked by the AIDS virus), who have no systemic symptoms, and who have had no opportunistic infections. About 40% of these patients achieve a therapeutic response that lasts an average of 1 to 2 years. In addition to antineoplastic effects, data indicate that viral replication is suppressed in responding patients. Research studies suggest a combination of interferon-alfa and zidovudine, an antiviral drug used in the treatment of AIDS, may have synergistic antineoplastic and antiviral effects. Lower doses of interferon must be used when the drug is combined with zidovudine to minimize neutropenia.

### Interleukins

Aldesleukin is a highly toxic drug and contraindicated in patients with preexisting, serious cardiovascular or pulmonary impairment. Therefore, patients must be carefully selected, evaluated, and monitored. One way to decrease toxicity is to give the drug by continuous infusion rather than bolus injection. Another method is to combine aldesleukin with cytotoxic tumor infiltrating lymphocytes harvested from the patient's tumor, which allows lower and therefore less toxic doses of aldesleukin. Although corticosteroids can decrease toxicity, they are not recommended for use because they also decrease the antineoplastic effects of aldesleukin.

In addition, aldesleukin may impair neutrophil function and increase the risk of infections, including septicemia and bacterial endocarditis. Therefore, any preexisting infection should be treated and resolved prior to initiating aldesleukin therapy. Patients with indwelling central intravenous devices should be given prophylactic antibacterials that are effective against Staphylococcus aureus (e.g., nafcillin [Unipen], vancomycin [Vancocin]).

### Bacillus Calmette-Guérin

BCG, when instilled into the urinary bladder of patients with superficial bladder cancer, causes remission in up to 82% of patients for an average of 4 years. Early and successful treatment of carcinoma-in-situ also prevents development of invasive bladder cancer. A specific protocol has been developed for administration of BCG solution, and it should be followed accurately.

## USE IN CHILDREN

There has been limited experience with immunostimulants in children (younger than 18 years), and the drugs' safety and effectiveness have not been established. The CSFs (filgrastim, sargramostim) have been used in children with therapeutic and adverse effects similar to those seen in adults. In clinical trials, filgrastim produced a greater incidence of subclinical spleen enlargement in children than in adults, but whether this affects growth and development or has other long-term consequences is unknown. Little information is available about the use of interferons in children. Aldesleukin has been used but has not yet demonstrated effectiveness. Adverse effects were similar to those seen in adults.

## USE IN OLDER ADULTS

Generally, immunostimulants have the same uses and responses in older adults as in younger adults. As with many other drugs, older adults may be at greater risk of adverse effects, especially if large doses are used.

## NURSING ACTIONS: IMMUNOSTIMULANTS

| *Nursing Actions* | *Rationale/Explanation* |
|---|---|
| **1. Administer accurately** | For hospitalized clients, the drugs may be prepared for administration in a pharmacy. When nurses prepare the drugs, they should consult the manufacturer's instructions.<br><br>    Outpatients may be taught self-administration techniques. |
| **a.** Give filgrastim SC or IV as a single daily injection. Do not add diluent or shake the vial, and do not save unused portions for later use. | These are the manufacturer's recommendations. The drug has not been tested for compatibility with IV solutions or other diluents. |
| **b.** Give sargramostim by IV infusion over 2 hours, after reconstitution with 1 ml sterile water for injection and addition to 0.9% sodium chloride. | |
| **c.** Inject interferon for condylomata intralesionally into the base of each wart with a small-gauge needle. For large warts, inject at several points. | Manufacturer's recommendation |
| **d.** With intravesical *Bacillus Calmette-Guérin (BCG)*, | |
| (1) Reconstitute solution (see Table 47-1). | Reconstituted solution should be used immediately or refrigerated. Discard if not used within two hours. |
| (2) Wear gown and gloves. | |
| (3) Insert a sterile urethral catheter and drain bladder. | |
| (4) Instill medication slowly by gravity. | |
| (5) Remove catheter. | |
| (6) Have the patient lie on abdomen, back, and alternate sides for 15 minutes in each position. Then, allow to ambulate but ask to retain solution for a total of 2 hours before urinating, if able. | |
| (7) Dispose of all equipment in contact with BCG solution appropriately. | BCG contains live mycobacterial organisms and is therefore infectious material. |
| (8) Do not give if catheterization causes trauma (*e.g.*, bleeding), and wait 1 week before a repeat attempt. | |

## Nursing Actions

## Rationale/Explanation

**2. Observe for therapeutic effects**

    **a.** With aldesleukin, observe for tumor regression (improvement in signs and symptoms).

Tumor regression may occur as early as 4 weeks after the first course of therapy and may continue up to 12 months.

    **b.** With parenteral interferons, observe for improvement in signs and symptoms.

With hairy cell leukemia, hematologic tests may improve within 2 months, but optimal effects may require 6 months of drug therapy. With acquired immunodeficiency syndrome (AIDS)-related Kaposi's sarcoma, skin lesions may resolve or stabilize over several weeks. With chronic hepatitis, liver function tests may improve within a few weeks.

    **c.** With intralesional interferons, observe for disappearance of genital warts.

Lesions usually disappear after several weeks of treatment.

**3. Observe for adverse effects**

Colony-stimulating factors (CSFs) are well tolerated overall. Adverse effects occur more often with sargramostim than filgrastim.

    **a.** With filgrastim, observe for bone pain, erythema at SC injection sites, and increased serum lactate dehydrogenase (LDH), alkaline phosphatase, and uric acid levels.

Bone pain reportedly occurs in 20% to 25% of patients and can be treated with acetaminophen or a nonsteroidal anti-inflammatory drug (NSAID).

    **b.** With sargramostim, observe for bone pain, fever, headache, myalgias, generalized maculopapular skin rash, and fluid retention (peripheral edema, pleural effusion, pericardial effusion).

Pleural and pericardial effusions are more likely at doses greater than 20 μg/kg per day.

    **c.** With interferons, observe for acute flu-like symptoms (*e.g.*, fever, chills, fatigue, muscle aches, headache), chronic fatigue, depression, leukopenia, and increased liver enzymes.

Acute effects occur in most patients, increasing with higher doses and decreasing with continued drug administration. Symptoms can be relieved by acetaminophen. Fatigue and depression occur with long-term administration and are dose-limiting effects.

    **d.** With aldesleukin, observe for capillary leak syndrome (hypotension, shock, angina, myocardial infarction, arrhythmias, edema, respiratory distress, gastrointestinal bleeding, renal insufficiency, mental status changes). Other effects may involve most body systems, such as chills and fever, blood (anemia, thrombocytopenia, eosinophilia), and central nervous system (CNS) (seizures, psychiatric symptoms), skin (erythema, burning, pruritus), hepatic (cholestasis), endocrine (hypothyroidism), and bacterial infections. In addition, drug-induced tumor breakdown may cause hypocalcemia, hyperkalemia, hyperphosphatemia, hyperuricemia, renal failure, and electrocardiogram changes.

Adverse effects are frequent, often serious and sometimes fatal. Most subside within 2 to 3 days after stopping the drug. Capillary leak syndrome, which may begin soon after treatment starts, is characterized by a loss of plasma proteins and fluids into extravascular space. Signs and symptoms result from decreased organ perfusion, and most patients can be treated with vasopressor drugs, cautious fluid replacement, diuretics, and supplemental oxygen.

    **e.** With intravesical BCG, assess for symptoms of bladder irritation (*e.g.*, frequency, urgency, dysuria, hematuria) and systemic symptoms of fever, chills, and malaise.

These effects occur in more than 50% of patients, usually starting a few hours after administration and lasting 2 to 3 days. They can be decreased by phenazopyridine (Pyridium), an analgesic; propantheline (Pro-Banthine) or oxybutynin (Ditropan), antispasmodics; and acetaminophen (Tylenol) or ibuprofen (Motrin), analgesics and antipyretics.

**4. Observe for drug interactions**

    **a.** Drugs that *increase* effects of sargramostim

        Corticosteroids, lithium

These drugs have myeloproliferative (bone marrow stimulating) effects of their own, which may add to those of sargramostim.

(*continued*)

| *Nursing Actions* | *Rationale/Explanation* |
|---|---|
| **b.** Drugs that *alter* effects of interferons | |
| Other antineoplastic agents | Additive therapeutic and myelosuppressive effects. |
| **c.** Drugs that *increase* effects of aldesleukin | All of the listed drug groups may potentiate adverse effects of aldesleukin. |
| (1) Aminoglycoside antibiotics (*e.g.,* gentamicin, others | Increased nephrotoxicity |
| (2) Antihypertensives | Increased hypotension |
| (3) Antineoplastics (*e.g.,* asparaginase, doxorubicin, methotrexate) | Increased toxic effects on bone marrow, heart, and liver. Aldesleukin is usually given as a single antineoplastic agent; its use in combination with other antineoplastic drugs is being evaluated. |
| (4) Narcotic analgesics | Increased CNS adverse effects |
| (5) NSAIDs (*e.g.,* ibuprofen) | Increased nephrotoxicity |
| (6) Sedative-hypnotics | Increased CNS adverse effects |
| **d.** Drugs that *decrease* effects of aldesleukin | |
| Corticosteroids | These drugs should not be given concurrently with aldesleukin. Although they decrease some adverse effects, such as fever, renal impairment, confusion, and others, they also decrease the drug's therapeutic antineoplastic effects. |
| **5. Teach clients** | |
| **a.** Report signs of infection, bleeding, weight loss, severe fatigue, and so forth. | These are potential problems that can be managed more effectively if recognized early. |
| **b.** Maintain a fluid intake of 2 to 3 quarts daily. | This is adequate for normal metabolic needs; more may be needed with fever or tumor lysis to excrete products of cellular metabolism and maintain kidney function. |
| **c.** Drug preparation, administration, and disposal | These drugs are often taken on an outpatient basis, and a client or family member must be taught accurate administration, including injection techniques. |

## Review and application exercises

1. What are cytokines, and how do they function in normal immunity?
2. What are the clinical uses of interferons and aldesleukin?
3. What are the adverse effects of interferons and aldesleukin, and how can they be prevented or minimized?
4. Describe the origin, functions, and clinical uses of CSFs.
5. What are adverse effects of CSFs, and how may they be prevented or minimized?

## Selected References

Balmer, C., & Valley, A. W. (1992). Basic principles of cancer treatment and cancer chemotherapy. In J. T. DiPiro, R. L. Talbert, P. E. Hayes, G. C. Yee, G. R. Matzke, & L. M. Posey (Eds.), *Pharmacotherapy: A pathophysiologic approach* (2nd ed.) (pp. 1879–1929). New York: Elsevier.

(1994). *Drug facts and comparisons*. St. Louis: Facts and Comparisons.

Feldmann, M., June, C. H., & McMichael, D. E. (1992). T-cell-targeted immunotherapy. *Immunology Today, 13*(3), 84–85.

Finley, R. S., & La Civita, C. L.(1992). Neoplastic diseases. In M. A. Koda-Kimble & L. Y. Young (Eds.), *Applied therapeutics: The clinical use of drugs* (5th ed.) (pp. 52-1–52-48). Vancouver, WA: Applied Therapeutics.

Hadden, J. W., & Smith, D. L. (1992). Immunopharmacology: Immunomodulation and immunotherapy. *Journal of the American Medical Association, 268,* 2964–2969.

Krown, S. E., & Paredes, J. (1992). Approach to the management of Kaposi's sarcoma. In W. N. Kelley (Ed.), *Textbook of internal medicine* (2nd ed.) (pp. 1157–1159). Philadelphia: J.B. Lippincott.

Lara, A. E. (1993). Biologic response modifiers. In J. L. Kee & E. R. Hayes (Eds.), *Pharmacology: A nursing process approach* (pp. 337–348). Philadelphia: W.B. Saunders.

Longo, D. L., & Urba, W. J. (1992). Principles of cancer treatment. In W. N. Kelley (Ed.), *Textbook of internal medicine* (2nd ed.) (pp. 1113–1126). Philadelphia: J.B. Lippincott.

Louie, S. G., & Jung, B. (1993). Clinical effects of biologic response modifiers. *American Journal of Hospital Pharmacy, 50*(Suppl. 3), S10–S18.

Mandler, H. D., & Dudley, M. N. (1992). Immunocompromised host infections. In M. A. Koda-Kimble & L. Y. Young (Eds.), *Applied therapeutics: The clinical use of drugs* (5th ed.) (pp. 46-1–46-25). Vancouver, WA: Applied Therapeutics.

Michaeli, J. (1992). Approach to the management of plasma cell disorders. In W. N. Kelley (Ed.), *Textbook of internal medicine* (2nd ed.) (pp. 1200–1205). Philadelphia: J.B. Lippincott.

Nemunaitis, J. (1993). Colony-stimulating factors: A new step in clinical practice. Part II. *Annals of Medicine, 25,* 25–29.

Perillo, R. P., & Regenstein, F. G. (1992). Viral and immune hepatitis. In W. N. Kelley (Ed.), *Textbook of internal medicine* (2nd ed.) (pp. 550–560). Philadelphia: J.B. Lippincott.

Seaman, W. (1991). Approaches to immune response modulation. In D. P. Stites & A. I. Terr (Eds.), *Basic and clinical immunology* (7th ed.) (pp. 717–722). Norwalk, CT: Appleton & Lange.

Steward, W. P. (1993). Granulocyte and granulocyte-macrophage colony stimulating factors. *The Lancet, 342,* 153–157.

Wiernik, P. H., & Canellos, G. P. (1992). Approach to the management of leukemia. In W. N. Kelley (Ed.), *Textbook of internal medicine* (2nd ed.) (pp. 1177–1185). Philadelphia: J.B. Lippincott.

## CHAPTER 48

# Immunosuppressants

## Description

Immunosuppressant drugs interfere with the production or function of immune cells. The drugs are used therapeutically to decrease an inappropriate or undesirable immune response. The immune response is normally a protective mechanism that helps the body defend itself against potentially harmful external (*e.g.*, microorganisms) and internal agents (*e.g.*, cancer cells). However, numerous disease processes are thought to be caused or aggravated when the immune system perceives one's own body tissues as harmful invaders and tries to eliminate them. This inappropriate activation of the immune response is a major factor in a growing list of serious diseases believed to involve autoimmune processes, including rheumatoid arthritis, systemic lupus erythematosus, membranous glomerulonephritis, chronic active hepatitis, inflammatory bowel disease, multiple sclerosis, myasthenia gravis, and others.

An appropriate but undesirable immune response is elicited when foreign tissue is transplanted into the body. If the immune response is not sufficiently suppressed, the body reacts as with other antigens and attempts to destroy (reject) the foreign organ or tissue. Although numerous advances have been made in transplant technology, the immune response remains a major factor in determining the success or failure of a tissue or organ transplant.

A major goal of research is to develop pharmacologic agents that suppress the immune response to specific antigens. However, available drugs provide nonspecific inhibition of the immune response. Drugs used therapeutically as immunosuppressants comprise a diverse group, several of which also are used for other purposes.

These include corticosteroids (see Chap. 24) and certain cytotoxic antineoplastic drugs (see Chap. 67). These drugs are discussed here primarily in relation to their effects on the immune response. Four drugs, azathioprine, cyclosporine, antithymocyte globulin, and muromonab-CD3, used mainly to prevent or treat transplant rejection reactions (solid organ and bone marrow transplants), are the main focus of this chapter. These drugs are described below and listed in Table 48-1. To aid understanding of immunosuppressive drug therapy, autoimmune disorders, tissue and organ transplants, and rejection reactions are briefly discussed.

## Autoimmune disorders

Autoimmune disorders occur when a person's immune system loses its tolerance to its own body tissues (self antigens), perceives body tissues as "nonself" antigens, initiates an immune reponse, and destroys host tissues. Although much remains to be learned about autoimmunity, disease processes involving virtually every body cell or tissue are associated with autoimmune reactions. The major mechanism of tissue inflammation and destruction is thought to be a cell-mediated immune response in which T lymphocytes either destroy tissue directly or produce substances that recruit and activate phagocytes, especially macrophages, which then destroy antigen-containing cells.

In most instances, the perceived antigen is thought to be a protein. Thus, in rheumatoid arthritis, the antigen is a protein found in joint tissue; in autoimmune thyroiditis, the antigen is a protein found on thyroid cells;

Anne Collins Abrams: CLINICAL DRUG THERAPY, Fourth Edition.

**TABLE 48-1. IMMUNOSUPPRESSANTS**

| Generic/Trade Name | Indications for Use | Contraindications | Routes and Dosage Ranges |
|---|---|---|---|
| **Azathioprine** (Imuran) | Prevent renal transplant rejection Severe rheumatoid arthritis unresponsive to other treatment | Pregnancy Allergy to azathioprine | Renal transplant: PO, IV 3–5 mg/kg per day initially, decreased (1–3 mg/kg per day) for maintenance and in presence of renal impairment Rheumatoid arthritis: PO 1 mg/kg per day (50–100 mg), increased by 0.5 mg/kg per day after 8 wks, then every 5 wk to a maximum dose of 2.5 mg/kg per day. Decrease dosage for maintenance. |
| **Cyclosporine** (Sandimmune) | Prevent rejection of solid organ (*e.g.*, heart, kidney, liver) transplant Prevent and treat graft-versus-host disease (GVHD) in bone marrow transplant | Allergy to cyclosporine or polyoxyethylated castor oil (in IV preparation only) Cautious use during pregnancy or lactation | PO 15 mg/kg 4–12 h before transplant surgery, then 15 mg/kg once daily for 1–2 wk, then decrease by 5% per week to a maintenance dose of 5–10 mg/kg per day IV 5–6 mg/kg infused over 2–6 h |
| **Lymphocyte immune globulin, antithymocyte globulin (Equine)** (Atgam) | Prevent or treat renal rejection Treat aplastic anemia | Allergy to horse serum or prior allergic reaction to ATG | IV 15 mg/kg per day for 14 d, then every other day for 14 d (21 doses) |
| **Methotrexate (MTX)** (Rheumatrex) | Severe rheumatoid arthritis unresponsive to other therapy | Allergy to MTX Pregnancy, lactation, liver disease Blood dyscrasias | PO 7.5 mg/wk as single dose, or 2.5 mg q12h for 3 doses once weekly |
| **Muromonab-CD3** (Orthoclone OKT3) | Treatment of renal transplant rejection | Allergy to muromonab-CD3 Signs of fluid overload (*e.g.*, heart failure, weight gain during week before starting drug therapy) Cautious use during pregnancy | IV 5 mg bolus injection once daily for 10–14 d |

and in insulin-dependent diabetes mellitus, only recently thought to have an autoimmune component in its etiology, the antigen is a protein on the pancreatic beta cells that normally produce insulin. Systemic lupus erythematosus, a chronic inflammatory disease involving connective tissue of the skin, kidneys, joints, and nervous sytem, is considered the classic autoimmune disease.

## Tissue and organ transplants

Tissue and organ transplantation involves replacing diseased host tissue with healthy donor tissue. The goal of such treatment is to save or enhance the quality of the host's life. Skin and renal grafts are commonly and sucessfully performed; heart, liver, lung, pancreas, and bone marrow transplants are increasing. Although numerous factors affect graft survival, including the degree of matching between donor tissues and recipient tissues, drug-induced immunosuppression is a major part of transplant technology. The goal is to provide adequate, but not excessive, immunosuppression. If immunosuppression is inadequate, graft rejection reactions occur

with solid organ transplants, and graft-versus-host disease (GVHD) occurs with bone marrow transplants. If immunosuppression is excessive, the client is likely to develop serious, perhaps fatal, infections.

## REJECTION REACTIONS WITH SOLID ORGAN TRANSPLANTS

A rejection reaction occurs when the host's immune system is stimulated to destroy the transplanted organ. In a few specific instances (*e.g.*, transfer of skin from one site to another on the same host or when the donor and the recipient are identical twins), an immune response does not occur. In most instances, however, the immune cells (primarily T lymphocytes) of the recipient react against the antigens of the donor organ. This reaction usually destroys the solid organ graft within 2 weeks unless the recipient's immune system is adequately suppressed by immunosuppressant drugs.

Rejection reactions are designated as hyperacute, acute, or chronic, depending on the time lapse between transplantation and rejection. Hyperacute reactions occur as soon as blood from the recipient perfuses the grafted organ. This type of reaction is rare and usually occurs in recipients who have previously formed anti-bodies against antigens in the graft. The antibodies bind to the graft and induce inflammation.

Acute reactions occur about 2 weeks following trans-plantation. These reactions involve an immune response that may be delayed or less intense in clients receiving immunosuppressant drugs.

Chronic reactions may occur after months or years of normal function. They are characterized by slow, progressive organ failure.

Rejection reactions produce general manifestations of inflammation and specific manifestations depending on the organ involved. With renal transplants, for example, acute rejection reactions produce fever, flank tenderness over the graft organ site, and symptoms of renal failure (*e.g.*, increased serum creatinine, decreased urine out-put, edema and weight gain, hypertension).

## Bone marrow transplants and graft-versus-host disease

With bone marrow transplants, the donor bone marrow mounts an immune response (mainly by stimulating T lymphocytes) against antigens on the host's tissues, pro-ducing GVHD. Acute GVHD occurs in 30% to 50% of patients (about 70% in adults over 40 years and 10% in children under 10 years of age), usually within 6 weeks. Signs and symptoms include delayed recovery of bone marrow production of blood cells, skin rash, liver dys-function (indicated by increased alkaline phosphatase, transaminase, and bilirubin), and diarrhea. Chronic GVHD occurs more than 100 days after bone marrow transplant.

## Corticosteroids

Corticosteroids have long been used to suppress inflam-mation and immune reactions. In many disorders, they relieve signs and symptoms by decreasing the accumula-tion of lymphocytes and macrophages and the produc-tion of cell-damaging chemicals at sites of inflammatory reactions. Because inflammation is a common response to chemical mediators or antigens that cause tissue in-jury, the anti-inflammatory and immunosuppressive actions of corticosteroids often overlap and are indis-tinguishable. Despite this somewhat arbitrary separa-tion, corticosteroid effects on the immune response are emphasized here. Generally, the drugs suppress growth of all lymphoid tissue and therefore decrease formation

and function of antibodies and T cells. Specific effects include the following:

- Increased numbers of circulating neutrophils (more are released from bone marrow and fewer leave the circulation to enter inflammatory exu-dates). In terms of neutrophil functions, corticoste-roids increase chemotaxis and release of lysosomal enzymes but decrease the release of non-lysosomal proteolytic enzymes, such as collagenase and plas-minogen activator.
- Decreased numbers of circulating basophils, eosin-ophils, and monocytes. The reduced availability of monocytes is thought to be a major factor in the anti-inflammatory activity of corticosteroids. Func-tions of monocyte–macrophages are also impaired. Corticosteroids suppress phagocytosis and initial antigen processing (necessary to initiate an im-mune response), impair migration to areas of tissue injury, and block the differentiation of monocytes to macrophages.
- Decreased numbers of circulating lymphocytes (immune cells), resulting from impaired produc-tion (*i.e.*, inhibition of deoxyribonucleic acid [DNA], ribonucleic acid [RNA], and protein synthesis), se-questration in lymphoid tissues, or lysis of the cells. T cells are markedly reduced, with the CD4 subset (helper T cells) reduced more than the CD8 (sup-pressor T cells). B cells are moderately reduced.
- Impaired function of cellular (mainly T cells) and humoral (B cells) immunity. Corticosteroids in-hibit the production of immunostimulant cyto-kines (*e.g.*, interleukins 1 and 2) required for acti-vation and clonal expansion of lymphocytes and cytotoxic cytokines, such as tumor necrosis factor, lymphotoxin, and interferons. When administered for 2 to 3 weeks, the drugs also inhibit immune reactions to antigenic skin tests and reduce serum concentrations of some antibodies (immunoglobu-lins G and A but not IgM).

## Cytotoxic agents

Cytotoxic drugs damage or kill cells that are able to reproduce, such as immunologically competent lym-phocytes. These drugs are used primarily in cancer che-motherapy. However, in small doses, some also exhibit immunosuppressive activities and are used to treat auto-immune disorders (*e.g.*, methotrexate) and to prevent rejection reactions in organ transplants (azathioprine). These drugs cause generalized suppression of the im-mune system and can kill lymphocytes and nonlymphoid proliferating cells (*e.g.*, bone marrow blood cells, gastrointestinal mucosal cells, and germ cells in gonads).

*Azathioprine* is a cytotoxic antimetabolite that interferes with production of DNA and RNA and thus blocks cellular reproduction, growth, and development. Once ingested into the body, azathioprine is metabolized by the liver to 6-mercaptopurine, a purine analog, and incorporated into the DNA of proliferating cells in place of the natural purine bases to produce abnormal DNA. Rapidly proliferating cells are most affected, including lymphocytes, which normally reproduce rapidly in response to stimulation by an antigen. The drug acts especially on T cells to block cell division, clonal proliferation, and differentiation. Azathioprine is well absorbed following oral administration, with peak serum concentrations occurring in 1 to 2 hours and a half-life of less than 5 hours. The mercaptopurine resulting from initial biotransformation is inactivated mainly by the enzyme xanthine oxidase. Although the drug is not thought to be excreted by the kidneys, doses are usually reduced in patients with renal impairment. It is used mainly to prevent organ graft rejection and has little effect on established rejection reactions. It is also used to treat severe rheumatoid arthritis not responsive to conventional treatment.

*Methotrexate* is a cytotoxic folate antagonist. It inhibits dihydrofolate reductase, the enzyme that converts dihydrofolate to the tetrahydrofolate required for biosynthesis of DNA and cell reproduction. The resultant DNA impairment inhibits production and function of immune cells, especially T cells. Methotrexate has long been used in the treatment of cancer. Other uses have evolved from its immunosuppressive effects, including treatment of autoimmune or inflammatory disorders, such as severe arthritis and psoriasis, that do not respond to other treatment measures. It is also used (with cyclosporine) to prevent GVHD associated with bone marrow transplantation, but it is not FDA-approved for this purpose. Much lower doses are given for these conditions than for cancers. Thus, adverse drug effects are minimal.

## CYCLOSPORINE

Cyclosporine is a powerful drug used only as an immunosuppressant, primarily in organ transplants. The drug inhibits cellular and humoral immunity but affects T lymphocytes more than B lymphocytes. With T cells, cyclosporine reduces proliferation of helper and cytotoxic T cells and synthesis of several lymphokines (*e.g.*, interleukin-2, interferons). Suppressor T cells seem to be less affected by cyclosporine. With B cells, cyclosporine reduces production and function to some extent, but considerable activity is retained.

Cyclosporine is used to prevent rejection reactions

(destruction of the transplanted tissues by the body's immune system) following solid organ transplants (*e.g.*, kidney, liver, heart) or to treat chronic rejection in patients previously treated with other immunosuppressive agents. Transplant rejection reactions mainly involve cellular immunity or T cells. With cyclosporine-induced deprivation of interleukin-2, T cells stimulated by the graft antigen do not undergo clonal expansion and differentiation, and graft destruction is inhibited. In addition to its use in solid organ transplants, cyclosporine is used to prevent and treat GVHD, a potential complication of bone marrow transplant. In GVHD, T lymphocytes from the transplanted marrow of the donor arouse an immune response against the tissues of the recipient.

Absorption of cyclosporine is slow and incomplete with oral administration. The drug is highly bound to plasma proteins (90%), and about 50% is distributed in erythrocytes, so drug levels in whole blood are significantly higher than those in plasma. Peak plasma levels occur 4 to 5 hours after a dose, and the elimination half-life is about 10 to 27 hours. Cyclosporine is metabolized in the liver and excreted in bile; less than 10% is excreted unchanged in urine. Because the drug is insoluble in water, other solvents are used in commercial formulations. Thus, it is prepared in alcohol and olive oil for oral administration and in alcohol and polyoxyethylated castor oil for intravenous administration. Anaphylactic reactions, attributed to the polyoxyethylated castor oil, have occurred with the intravenous formulation.

## ANTILYMPHOCYTE ANTIBODY PREPARATIONS

Antilymphocyte antibody preparations are derived from animals injected with human lymphoid tissue to stimulate an immune response. The antibodies may be nonspecific polyclonal or specific monoclonal. Polyclonal preparations are a mixture of antibodies (*e.g.*, IgA, IgD, IgE, IgG, or IgM) produced by several clones of B lymphocytes. Each clone produces a structurally and functionally different antibody, even though the humoral immune response was induced by a single antigen. Monoclonal antibodies are produced by DNA recombinant techniques that combine B lymphocytes from animals (usually mice) that have been injected with a specific antigen and B lymphocytes (plasma cells) from malignant myelomas (plasma cell tumors). The resulting "hybridoma" is a clone of B lymphocytes that produces antibody against a specific antigen and proliferates indefinitely. Hybridomas are capable of producing relatively large amounts of monoclonal antibodies.

*Lymphocyte immune globulin, antithymocyte globulin* (ATG) is a nonspecific polyclonal antibody with activity against all blood cells, although it acts mainly against T lymphocytes. ATG is obtained from the serum of horses immunized with human thymus tissue or T lymphocytes. It contains antibodies that destroy lymphoid tissues and decrease the number of circulating T cells, thereby suppressing cellular and humoral immune responses. In addition to its high concentration of antibodies against T lymphocytes, the preparation contains low concentrations of antibodies against other blood cells. A skin test is recommended prior to administration to determine whether the patient is allergic to horse serum. Because there is a high risk of anaphylactic reactions in recipients previously sensitized to horse serum, patients with positive skin tests should be desensitized before drug therapy is begun. ATG is usually given for a few weeks to treat rejection reactions following solid organ transplants, and it may be used to treat aplastic anemia.

*Muromonab-CD3* (OKT3) is a monoclonal antibody that acts specifically against an antigenic receptor called cell differentiation cluster 3 (CD3) found on the surface membrane of most T cells in blood and body tissues. The CD3 molecule is associated with the antigen recognition structure of T cells and is essential for T-cell activation. Muromonab-CD3 binds with its antigen (CD3) and therefore blocks all known functions of T cells containing the CD3 molecule. Because rejection reactions are mainly T-cell mediated immune responses against antigenic (nonself) tissues, the drug's ability to suppress such reactions accounts for its therapeutic effects in treating renal transplant rejection. It is usually given for 10 to 14 days. After treatment, CD3-positive T cells reappear rapidly and reach pretreatment levels within 1 week. The drug's name is derived from its source (murine or mouse cells) and its action (monoclonal antibody against the CD3 antigen). Because the drug is a protein and induces antibodies in most patients, decreased effectiveness and serious allergic reactions may occur if it is readministered later. Second courses of treatment must be undertaken cautiously.

## Nursing Process

### Assessment

- Assess clients receiving or anticipating immunosuppressant drug therapy for signs and symptoms of current infection.
- Assess clients receiving or anticipating immunosuppressant drug therapy for factors predisposing them to potential infection (*e.g.*, skin integrity, invasive devices, cigarette smoking).
- Assess environment for factors predisposing to infection (*e.g.*, family or health-care providers with infections, contact with young children, and potential exposure to childhood infectious diseases).
- Assess nutritional status, including appetite and weight.
- Assess response to planned drug therapy and associated monitoring and follow-up.

- Assess coping mechanisms of client and significant others in stressful situations.
- Assess baseline values of laboratory and other diagnostic test reports to aid monitoring of responses to immunosuppressant drug therapy. With pretransplant patients, this includes assessing for impaired function of the diseased organ and for abnormalities that need treatment prior to surgery.
- Assess adequacy of support systems for transplant recipients.
- Assess post-transplant patients for surgical wound healing and manifestations of organ rejection.

### Nursing diagnoses

- High Risk for Injury: Infection related to immunosuppression and increased susceptibility
- High Risk for Injury: Cancer related to immunosuppression and increased susceptibility
- High Risk for Injury: Adverse drug effects
- Knowledge Deficit: Disease process or planned treatment
- Knowledge Deficit: Immunosuppressant therapy
- Anxiety related to the diagnosis of serious disease or need for organ transplant
- Body Image Disturbance: Cushingoid changes with long-term corticosteroid therapy; alopecia with azathioprine
- Ineffective Individual Coping related to chronic illness and long-term treatment
- Ineffective Family Coping related to illness and treatment of a family member
- Fear related to potential transplant complications, disease progression, or death
- Social Isolation related to activities to reduce exposure to infection

### Planning/Goals

*The client will:*

- Participate in decision making about the treatment plan
- Receive or take immunosuppressant drugs correctly
- Verbalize or demonstrate essential drug information
- Participate in interventions to prevent infection (*e.g.*, avoid known sources of infection) while immunosuppressed
- Experience relief or reduction of disease symptoms
- Maintain adequate levels of nutrition and fluids, rest and sleep, and exercise
- Be assisted to cope with anxiety and fear related to the disease process and drug therapy
- Keep appointments for follow-up care
- Have adverse drug effects prevented or recognized and treated as soon as possible
- Maintain diagnostic test values within acceptable limits
- Maintain family and other emotional or social support systems
- Receive optimal instructions and information about the treatment plan, self-care in activities of daily living, reporting adverse drug effects, and other concerns
- Before and after tissue or organ transplant, receive appropriate care, including prevention or early recognition and treatment of rejection reactions

## Interventions

- Practice and emphasize good personal hygiene and hand-washing techniques by patients and all others in contact with the patient.
- Use sterile technique for all injections, intravenous site care, wound dressing changes, and any other invasive diagnostic or therapeutic measures.
- Screen staff and visitors for signs and symptoms of infection; if infection is noted, do not allow contact with the patient.
- Report fever and other manifestations of infection *immediately*.
- Allow patients to participate in decision making when possible and appropriate.
- Use isolation techniques according to institutional policies, usually after transplants or when the neutrophil count is below 500/mm³.
- Assist clients to maintain adequate nutrition, rest and sleep, and exercise.
- Inform patients about diagnostic test results, planned changes in therapeutic regimens, and evidence of progress.
- Allow family members or significant others to visit patients when feasible.
- Monitor complete blood count (CBC) and other diagnostic test reports related to blood, liver, and kidney function throughout drug therapy. Specific tests vary with the client's health or illness status and the immunosuppressant drug(s) being taken.
- Schedule and coordinate drug administration to maximize therapeutic effects and minimize adverse effects.
- Consult other health-care providers (*e.g.*, physician, dietitian, social worker) on the client's behalf when indicated. Multidisciplinary consultation is essential for transplant patients.

*Teach clients on long-term*
*immunosuppressant drug therapy:*

- Ways to prevent or reduce the incidence of infections (*e.g.*, meticulous personal hygiene, avoiding contact with infected people)
- To report any signs or symptoms of infection to a health-care provider immediately
- To enhance immune mechanisms and other body defenses by maintaining healthy life-style habits, such as a nutritious diet, adequate rest and sleep, and avoiding tobacco and alcohol
- Stress management techniques
- The importance of taking the drugs as prescribed
- The importance of keeping appointments for monitoring response to drug therapy and other follow-up care
- To carry identification that states the drug(s) being taken; the dosage; the physician's name, address, and telephone number; and instructions for emergency treatment. This information is needed if an accident or emergency situation occurs.
- To inform all health-care providers that immunosuppressant drug therapy is being taken and must be considered in any treatment plan
- To maintain regular medical supervision. This is extremely important so that the physician can detect adverse reactions, evaluate disease status, and evaluate drug response and indications for dosage change, as well as other responsibilities that can be carried out only with personal contact between the physician and the client. Periodic blood tests and other diagnostic or monitoring studies are needed.
- To take no other drugs, prescription or nonprescription, without notifying the physician who is managing immunosuppressant therapy. Immunosuppressant drugs may influence reactions to other drugs, and other drugs may influence reactions to the immunosuppressants. Thus, taking other drugs may decrease therapeutic effects or increase adverse effects.
- To practice effective contraceptive techniques during immunosuppressive drug therapy if sexually active

## Evaluation

- Interview and observe for accurate drug administration.
- Interview and observe for personal hygiene practices and infection-avoiding maneuvers.
- Interview and observe for adverse drug effects with each patient contact.
- Interview regarding knowledge and attitude toward the drug therapy regimen, including follow-up care and symptoms to report to health-care providers.
- Determine the number and type of infections that have occurred in the neutropenic patient.
- Compare current CBC and other reports with baseline values for acceptable levels, according to the client's condition.
- Observe and interview outpatients regarding compliance with follow-up care.
- Observe and interview regarding the mental and emotional status of clients and family members or significant others.
- Interview and observe for organ function and absence of rejection reactions in post-transplant patients.

# Principles of therapy

The use of immunosuppressant drugs in autoimmune disorders and tissue and organ transplantation is relatively recent and still evolving in drug selection, dosages, routes of administration, scheduling, and protocols for particular purposes. These drugs are often used in highly technical, complex circumstances to manage life-threatening illness. Consequently, except for corticosteroids, the drugs should be used only by specialist physicians who are adept in their management. In addition, all health-care providers need to review research studies and other current literature regularly for ways to maximize safety and effectiveness and minimize adverse effects of immunosuppression.

## RISK—BENEFIT FACTORS

Immunosuppression is a serious, life-threatening condition that may result from disease processes or drug therapy. At the same time, most immunosuppressant drugs are used to treat life-threatening illnesses, and their use may therefore be justified. Rational use of immunosuppressant drugs requires thorough assessment of a client's health or illness status, clear cut indications for use, a lack of more effective and safer alternative treatments, analysis of potential risks versus potential benefits, cautious administration, and vigilant monitoring of the patient's response. If a decision is then made that immunosuppressant drug therapy is indicated and benefits outweigh risks, the therapeutic plan must be discussed with the client (*i.e.*, reasons, expected benefits, consequences for the client's health, behavior, and life-style).

In addition to the specific risks or adverse effects of individual immunosuppressant drugs, general risks of immunosuppression include infection and cancer. Infection is a major cause of morbidity and mortality, especially in patients who are neutropenic (neutrophil count less than 1000/mm$^3$) from cytotoxic immunosuppressant drugs or who have had bone marrow or solid organ transplant. For the latter group who must continue lifelong immunosuppression to avoid graft rejection, serious infection is a constant hazard. Extensive efforts are made to prevent infections; if these efforts are unsuccessful and infections occur, they may be fatal unless recognized promptly and treated vigorously. Common infections include bacterial (gram-positive, such as *Staphylococcus aureus* or *epidermidis*, and gram-negative, such as *Escherichia coli*, *Klebsiella*, and *Pseudomonas* species), fungal (candiasis, aspergillosis), viral (cytomegalovirus, herpes simplex or zoster), and protozoal (*Pneumocystis carinii*).

Cancer, most commonly lymphoma or skin cancer, may result from immunosuppression. The normal immune system is thought to recognize and destroy malignant cells as they develop, as long as they can be differentiated from normal cells. With immunosuppression, the malignant cells are no longer destroyed and thus are allowed to proliferate.

## DRUG CHOICES AND COMBINATIONS

Choice of an immunosuppressant drug is limited, and available drugs are relatively toxic. Thus, when feasible, less toxic drugs and nondrug treatment measures should be used to avoid or delay immunosuppressant drug therapy. In many instances, though, there are no acceptable alternatives, and such therapy is required. Moreover, combinations of drugs are often used. For example, most organ transplant centers use a combination regimen for prevention and treatment of rejection reactions. Generally, once the transplanted tissue is functioning and rejection has been successfully prevented or treated, it is often possible to maintain the graft with fewer drugs or lower drug dosages. Some recommendations to increase safety or effectiveness of drug combinations include the following:

- *Antithymocyte globulin* is usually given concomitantly with azathioprine and a corticosteroid.
- *Azathioprine* may be given alone to treat rheumatoid arthritis but is often combined with other drugs to treat organ transplant rejection reactions. For example, azathioprine, cyclosporine, and prednisone are coadministered for treatment of liver or pancreatic graft rejection.
- *Corticosteroids* may be given alone or included in multidrug regimens with cyclosporine and muromonab-CD3. A corticosteroid should always accompany cyclosporine administration to enhance immunosuppression. In prophylaxis of organ transplant rejection, the combination seems more effective than azathioprine alone or azathioprine and a corticosteroid.
- *Cyclosporine* should be used cautiously with immunosuppressants other than corticosteroids to decrease risks of excessive immunosuppression and its complications.
- *Methotrexate* may be used alone for rheumatoid arthritis and alone or with cyclosporine for prophylaxis of GVHD following bone marrow transplantation.
- *Muromonab-CD3* may be given cautiously with reduced numbers or dosages of other immunosuppressants. When coadministered with prednisone and azathioprine, the maximum daily dose of prednisone is 0.5 mg/kg, and the maximum for azathioprine is 25 mg. When muromonab-CD3 is coadministered with cyclosporine, cyclosporine dosage should be reduced or temporarily discontinued. Cyclosporine is then restarted 3 days before completing the course of muromonab-CD3 therapy to resume a maintenance level of immunosuppression.

## DOSAGE FACTORS

Currently available immunosuppressant drugs are relatively toxic, and adverse effects occur more often and are likely to be more severe with higher doses. Thus, the general principle of using the smallest effective dose for the shortest period of time is especially important with immunosuppressant drug therapy. Generally, dosage must be individualized according to the patient's clinical response (*i.e.*, improvement in signs and symptoms or occurrence of adverse effects). Specifically, some factors to be considered in drug dosage decisions include the following:

- *Azathioprine* dosage should be reduced or the drug discontinued if severe bone marrow depression occurs (*e.g.*, reduced erythrocytes, leukocytes, and platelets on CBC). If necessary to stop the drug, administration usually may be resumed at a smaller dosage once the bone marrow has recovered. With renal transplant recipients, the dosage required to prevent rejection and minimize toxicity varies. When given long-term for maintenance of immunosuppression, the lowest effective dose is recommended. If given concomitantly with muromonab-CD3, reduce dosage to 25 mg daily.

- *Corticosteroid* dosages vary widely, depending on the disease process and the goal of treatment. For long-term treatment of chronic diseases, such as many immunologic disorders, the smallest dose that will partially relieve symptoms is indicated. For short-term use and rapid symptom control in such serious disorders as autoimmune hemolytic anemia, idiopathic thrombocytopenic purpura, or immune-induced glomerulonephritis, larger doses are required. For short-term, rapid treatment of life-threatening illness or organ graft rejection reactions, very large doses are given intravenously. When given in combination with other immunosuppressant drugs, corticosteroid dosage may be reduced. In addition, the doses used concomitantly with cyclosporine are often less than those given with azathioprine.

- *Cyclosporine* dosage should be individualized according to blood levels of drug and serum creatinine. When a patient receiving cyclosporine is given muromonab-CD3, cyclosporine is stopped temporarily. If continued, cyclosporine dosage should be reduced. Dosage of cyclosporine also is reduced for long-term maintenance of immunosuppression following solid organ transplant.

- *Methotrexate* dosages, both initial and maintenance, are much lower for autoimmune disorders than for antineoplastic indications. When given for severe, disabling rheumatoid arthritis, small doses are usually given weekly.

- *Muromonab-CD3* dosage should follow established amounts and protocols.

## DRUG ADMINISTRATION SCHEDULES

The effectiveness of immunosuppressant drug therapy may be enhanced by appropriate timing of drug administration. For example, corticosteroids are most effective when given just before exposure to the antigen, while the cytotoxic agents (*e.g.*, azathioprine, methotrexate) are most effective when given soon after exposure (*i.e.*, during the interval between exposure to the antigen and the production of sensitized T cells or antibodies).

## LABORATORY MONITORING

With *azathioprine*, bone marrow depression (*e.g.*, severe leukopenia or thrombocytopenia) may occur. To monitor bone marrow function, CBC and platelet counts should be checked weekly during the first month, every 2 weeks during the second and third months, then monthly. If dosage is changed or a client's health status worsens at any time during therapy, more frequent blood tests are needed.

With oral *cyclosporine*, monitor blood levels of the drug periodically for low or high values. Low or subtherapeutic levels may occur because the drug is poorly absorbed (about 30%) and may lead to organ transplant rejection, especially with liver transplants. High levels increase adverse effects. The blood levels can be used to regulate dosage. Drug levels are higher in whole blood than in plasma, so the laboratory technique must be known to interpret reported values accurately. In addition, renal (serum creatinine, blood urea nitrogen) and liver (bilirubin, enzymes) function tests should be performed regularly to monitor for nephrotoxicity and hepatotoxicity.

With *methotrexate*, CBC and platelet counts should be checked periodically to monitor for bone marrow depression.

With *muromonab-CD3*, WBC and differential counts should be performed periodically.

## USE IN CHILDREN

Corticosteroids and cytotoxic immunosuppressant drugs have long been used in children, generally for the same disorders as in adults. Cyclosporine has been safely and effectively given to children as young as 6 months old, but extensive studies have not been performed. Muromonab-CD3 has been sucessfully in children as young as 2 years old; however, safety and efficacy for use in children have not been established. Adverse effects of immunosuppressants are similar in children to those in adults, except that corticosteroids may impair growth in children.

## USE IN OLDER ADULTS

Immunosuppressants are generally used for the same purposes and produce similar therapeutic and adverse effects in older adults as in younger adults. Because older adults often have multiple disorders and organ impairments, it is especially important that drug choices, dosages, and monitoring tests are individualized.

# NURSING ACTIONS: IMMUNOSUPPRESSANTS

| *Nursing Actions* | *Rationale/Explanation* |
|---|---|
| **1. Administer accurately**<br>**a.** Give oral azathioprine in divided doses, after meals; give IV drug by infusion, usually over 30 to 60 minutes. | To decrease nausea and vomiting with oral drug |
| **b.** Measure oral cyclosporine solution with the pipette supplied by the manufacturer, and mix in a glass container with 4 to 8 oz of water, milk, or juice. Administer immediately. Rinse the glass, and have the patient drink the rinse solution. Dilute IV cyclosporine in 20 to 100 ml of 0.9% sodium chloride or 5% dextrose and infuse over 2 to 6 hours | The amount of fluid should be large enough to increase palatability, especially for children, but small enough to be consumed quickly. Rinsing ensures that the entire dose is taken.<br>Oral administration is preferred. If necessary to give IV temporarily, resume oral use when able. Oral cyclosporine may be given to clients who have had anaphylactic reactions to the IV preparation, because the reaction is attributed to the oil diluent rather than the drug. |
| **c.** Give muromonab-CD3 in an IV bolus injection once daily. Do not give by IV infusion or mix with other drug solutions. | Manufacturer's recommendations |
| **d.** Dilute lymphocyte immune globulin, antithymocyte globulin in 0.9% sodium chloride or 5% dextrose and sodium chloride (0.225% or 0.45%) to a concentration of 1 mg/ml. Using an in-line filter, infuse IV into a large or central vein over at least 4 hours. Once diluted, use within 24 hours. | Manufacturer's recommendations. Using a high-flow vein decreases phlebitis and thrombosis at the IV site. The filter is used to remove any insoluble particles. |
| **2. Observe for therapeutic effects**<br>**a.** When a drug is given to suppress the immune response to organ transplants, therapeutic effect is the absence of signs and symptoms indicating rejection of the transplanted tissue. | |
| **b.** When azathioprine or methotrexate is given for rheumatoid arthritis, observe for decreased pain. | With azathioprine, therapeutic effects usually occur after 6 to 8 weeks. If no response occurs within 12 weeks, other treatment measures are indicated. With methotrexate, therapeutic effects usually occur within 3 to 6 weeks. |
| **3. Observe for adverse effects**<br>**a.** Observe for infection (fever, sore throat, wound drainage, productive cough, dysuria, and so forth). | Frequency and severity increase with higher drug dosages. Risks are high in immunosuppressed patients. Infections may be caused by almost any microorganism and may affect any part of the body, although respiratory and urinary tract infections may occur more often. |
| **b.** With azathioprine, observe for | The incidence of adverse effects is high in renal transplant recipients. |
| (1) Bone marrow depression (anemia, leukopenia, thrombocytopenia, abnormal bleeding). | |
| (2) Nausea and vomiting | Can be reduced by dividing the daily dosage and giving after meals |
| **c.** With cyclosporine, observe for | |
| (1) Nephrotoxicity (increased serum creatinine and blood urea nitrogen [BUN], decreased urine output, edema, hyperkalemia) | This is a major adverse effect, and it may produce signs and symptoms that are difficult to distinguish from those caused by renal graft rejection. Rejection usually occurs within the first month after surgery. If it occurs, dosage must be reduced and the patient observed for improved renal function. |

## Nursing Actions

## Rationale/Explanation

Also, note that graft rejection and drug-induced nephrotoxicity may be present simultaneously. The latter may be decreased by reducing dosage. The reported incidence of nephrotoxicity is 25% in clients with kidney transplants, 38% in those with heart transplants, and 37% in those with liver transplants. It often occurs 2 to 3 months after transplantation and results in a stable but decreased level of renal function (BUN of 35–45 mg/dl and serum creatinine of 2.0–2.5 mg/dl).

(2) Hepatotoxicity (increased serum enzymes and bilirubin)

The reported incidence is less than 8% after kidney, heart, or liver transplantation. It usually occurs during the first month, when high doses are used, and decreases with dosage reduction.

(3) Hypertension

This is especially likely to occur in patients with heart transplant and may require antihypertensive drug therapy. Do not give a potassium-sparing diuretic as part of the antihypertensive regimen because of increased risk of hyperkalemia.

(4) Anaphylaxis (with IV cyclosporine) (urticaria, hypotension or shock, respiratory distress)

This is rare but may occur. The allergen is thought to be the polyoxyethylated castor oil because people who had allergic reactions with the IV drug have later taken oral doses without allergic reactions. During IV administration, observe the patient continuously for the first 30 minutes and often thereafter. Stop the infusion if a reaction occurs, and give emergency care (e.g., epinephrine 1:1000).

(5) Central nervous system toxicity (confusion, depression, hallucinations, seizures, tremor)

These effects are relatively uncommon and may be caused by factors other than cyclosporine (e.g., nephrotoxicity).

(6) Other (gingival hyperplasia, hirsutism)

Gingival hyperplasia can be minimized by thorough oral hygiene.

d. With muromonab-CD3, observe for

(1) Acute (first dose) reactions—fever, chills, dyspnea, pulmonary edema

These reactions are most likely to occur during the first 6 hours, especially chills and fever. Pulmonary edema has occurred only in patients who were already overloaded with fluid. The first two to three doses should be given only in an inpatient setting with resuscitation supplies readily available and when fluid overload has been ruled out (by chest x-ray, assessing weight, fluid intake, and urine output). These effects may be prevented or minimized by premedicating with acetaminophen, an antihistamine, and a corticosteroid (e.g., hydrocortisone or methylprednisolone).

(2) Nausea, vomiting, diarrhea

e. With lymphocyte immune globulin, antithymocyte globulin, observe for

(1) Anaphylaxis (chest pain, respiratory distress, hypotension or shock)

An uncommon but serious allergic reaction to the animal protein in the drug that may occur anytime during therapy. If it occurs, stop the drug infusion, inject 0.3 ml epinephrine 1:1000, and provide other supportive emergency care as indicated.

(2) Chills and fever

Fever occurs in about 50% of patients; it may be decreased by premedicating with acetaminophen, an antihistamine, or a corticosteroid.

(continued)

| *Nursing Actions* | *Rationale/Explanation* |
|---|---|
| **4. Observe for drug interactions**<br>**a.** Drugs that *increase* effects of azathioprine<br><br>(1) Allopurinol | Inhibits hepatic metabolism, thereby increasing pharmacologic effects. If the two drugs are given concomitantly, the dose of azathioprine should be reduced drastically to 25% to 35% of the usual dose. |
| (2) Corticosteroids | Increased immunosuppression and risk of infection |
| **b.** Drugs that *increase* effects of cyclosporine<br><br>(1) Aminoglycoside antibiotics (*e.g.*, gentamicin), antifungals (amphotericin B, ketoconazole) | Increased risk of nephrotoxicity. Avoid other nephrotoxic drugs when possible. |
| (2) Antifungals (fluconazole, itraconazole), calcium channel-blockers (diltiazem, nicardipine, verapamil), cimetidine | Decreased hepatic metabolism, increased serum drug levels, and increased risk of toxicity |
| (3) Erythromycin, metoclopramide | Increased gastrointestinal absorption of cyclosporine |
| **c.** Drugs that *decrease* effects of cyclosporine<br><br>Enzyme inducers, including anticonvulsants (carbamazepine, phenobarbital, phenytoin), rifampin, sulfamethoxazole-trimethoprim | Enzyme-inducing drugs stimulate hepatic metabolism of cyclosporine, thereby reducing blood levels. If concurrent administration is necessary, monitor cyclosporine blood levels to avoid subtherapeutic levels and decreased effectiveness. |
| **5. Teach clients on long-term immunosuppressant drug therapy:**<br>**a.** Take drugs as directed. | This is extremely important with these drugs. Missing doses, stopping the drug, changing the amount or time of administration, or taking extra drug or any other alterations may result in the occurrence of the condition the drugs are given to prevent (*e.g.*, rejection of a transplanted organ) or adverse effects of the drugs. |
| **b.** Report to the prescribing physician if unable to take a dose orally because of vomiting or some other illness or problem. | |
| **c.** Avoid exposure to infection when possible (*e.g.*, avoid crowds and people with infections). Also, wash hands frequently and thoroughly. | These drugs increase the likelihood of infection, so preventive measures are needed. |
| **d.** Wear protective clothing, and use sunscreens to decrease exposure of skin to sunlight. | To decrease risks of skin cancers (squamous cell carcinoma, malignant melanoma). In addition, methotrexate may cause photosensitivity reactions. |
| **e.** Obtain regular physical examinations and screening tests for cancers of the breast, cervix, colon, and lung. | For early recognition and treatment, especially important in patients who have had solid organ transplants. |
| **f.** Report to a health-care provider:<br><br>(1) Sore throat, fever, or other signs of infection<br><br>(2) Decreased urine output (with cyclosporine)<br><br>(3) Easy bruising or bleeding (with azathioprine and methotrexate) | These are symptoms of adverse reactions. If they occur, they need to be assessed by a health-care provider who can determine whether changes in immunosuppressant therapy are indicated. |
| **g.** Use the manufacturer's pipette to measure oral cyclosporine solution. | For accurate dosage |
| **h.** Take immunosuppressants about the same time each day. | For more consistent blood levels, possibly improving therapeutic effects and decreasing adverse effects |

## Review and Application Exercises

1. List clinical indications for use of immunosuppressant drug therapy.
2. How do corticosteroids, antineoplastic drugs, azathioprine, cyclosporine, and muromonab-CD3 exert their immunosuppressant effects?
3. What are major adverse effects of immunosuppressant drugs?
4. When assessing a client receiving one or more immunosuppressant drugs, what specific signs and symptoms indicate adverse drug effects?
5. What are the similarities and differences between solid organ and bone marrow transplants?
6. For a client taking one or more immunosuppressant drugs, prepare a teaching plan related to safe and effective drug therapy.

## Selected references

(1994). *Drug facts and comparisons*. St. Louis: Facts and Comparisons.

Flannery, J. C. (1992). Nursing management of adults with immunologic disorders. In L. O. Burrell (Ed.), *Adult nursing in hospital and community settings* (pp. 141–175). Norwalk, CT: Appleton & Lange.

Guyton, A. C. (1991). *Textbook of medical physiology* (8th ed.). Philadelphia: W.B. Saunders.

Handschumacher, R. E. (1990). Immunosuppressive agents. In A. G. Gilman, T. W. Rall, A. S. Nies, & P. Taylor (Eds.), *The pharmacological basis of therapeutics* (8th ed.) (pp. 1264–1276). New York: Pergamon Press.

Marsh, J. W., Vehe, K. L., & White, H. M. (1992). Immunosuppressants. *Gastroenterology Clinics of North America, 21* (3), 679–693.

(1993). *Physicians' Desk Reference*. Montvale, NJ: Medical Economics.

Pinals, R.S. (1992). Management of chronic inflammatory and degenerative joint diseases. In W. N. Kelley (Ed.), *Textbook of internal medicine* (2nd ed.) (pp. 1020–1028). Philadelphia: J.B. Lippincott.

Rote, N. S. (1990). Alterations in immunity and inflammation. In K. L. McCance & S. E. Huether (Eds.), *Pathophysiology: The biologic basis for disease in adults and children*. St. Louis: C.V. Mosby.

Shaefer, M. S. (1992). Solid organ transplantation. In M. A. Koda-Kimble & L. Y. Young (Eds.), *Applied therapeutics: The clinical use of drugs* (5th ed.) (pp. 24-1–24-24). Vancouver, WA: Applied Therapeutics.

Turka, L. A. (1992). Transplantation immunology. In W. N. Kelley (Ed.), *Textbook of internal medicine* (2nd ed.) (pp. 698–702). Philadelphia: J.B. Lippincott.

Vanoli, M. (1992). Drug-induced immunodeficiencies. *Pharmacological Research, 26*(Suppl. 2), 88–93.

Winkelstein, A. (1991). Immunosuppressive therapy. In D. P. Stites & A. I. Terr (Eds.), *Basic and clinical immunology* (7th ed.) (pp. 766–775). Norwalk, CT: Appleton & Lange.

# Drugs Affecting the Respiratory System

### CHAPTER 49

# Physiology of the Respiratory System

## The respiratory system

The respiratory system helps meet the basic human need for oxygen ($O_2$). Oxygen is necessary for the oxidation of foodstuffs, by which energy for cellular metabolism is produced. When the oxygen supply is inadequate, cell function is impaired; when oxygen is absent, cells die. Permanent brain damage occurs within 4 to 6 minutes of anoxia. In addition to providing oxygen to all body cells, the respiratory system also removes carbon dioxide ($CO_2$), a major waste product of cell metabolism. Excessive accumulation of $CO_2$ damages or kills body cells.

The efficiency of the respiratory system depends on the quality and quantity of air inhaled, the patency of air passageways, the ability of the lungs to expand and contract, and the ability of $O_2$ and $CO_2$ to cross the alveolar–capillary membrane. In addition to the respiratory system itself, the circulatory, nervous, and musculoskeletal systems have important functions in respiration.

Some characteristics of the respiratory system and the process of respiration include the following:

1. *Respiration* is the process of gas exchange by which $O_2$ is obtained and $CO_2$ eliminated. This gas exchange occurs between the lung and the blood across the alveolar–capillary membrane and between the blood and body cells. The first phase of respiration depends on the adequacy of air flow to and from alveoli in the lungs (ventilation). The second phase depends on the adequacy of the circulatory system.
2. The respiratory tract is a series of branching tubes with progressively smaller diameters. These tubes (nose, pharynx, larynx, trachea, bronchi, and bronchioles) function as air passageways and air "conditioners" that filter, warm, and humidify incoming air. Most of the conditioning is done by the ciliated mucous membrane that lines the entire respiratory tract except the pharynx and alveoli. *Cilia* are tiny, hairlike projections that sweep mucus toward the pharynx to be expectorated or swallowed. The mucous membrane secretes mucus, which forms a protective blanket and traps foreign particles, such as bacteria or dust.
   a. When air is inhaled through the nose, it is conditioned by the nasal mucosa. When the nasal passages are blocked, the mouth serves as an alternate airway. The oral mucosa may warm and humidify air but cannot filter it.
   b. Air passes from the nasal cavities to the *pharynx* (throat). Its walls are composed of skeletal muscle, and its lining is composed of mucous membrane. The pharynx contains the palatine tonsils, which are large masses of lymphatic tissue. The pharynx is a passageway for food, fluids, and air. Food and fluids go from the pharynx to the esophagus, and air passes from the pharynx into the trachea.
   c. The *larynx* is composed of nine cartilages joined by ligaments and controlled by skeletal muscles. It contains the vocal cords and forms the upper end of the trachea. It closes on swallowing to prevent aspiration of food and fluids into the lungs.

Anne Collins Abrams: CLINICAL DRUG THERAPY, Fourth Edition.
© 1995 J.B. Lippincott Company.

d. The *trachea* is the passageway between the upper respiratory tract and the lungs. It divides into right and left primary or mainstem *bronchi*, which branch into secondary and smaller bronchi, then into bronchioles. *Bronchioles* are about the size of broom straws. The walls of the bronchioles contain smooth muscle, which is controlled by the autonomic nervous system. Parasympathetic nerves cause constriction; sympathetic nerves cause relaxation or dilation. The bronchioles give rise to the *alveoli*, which are grape-like clusters of air sacs surrounded by capillaries.

e. Gas exchange occurs across the alveolar–capillary membrane by passive diffusion. $O_2$ enters the bloodstream to be transported to body cells; $CO_2$ enters the alveoli to be exhaled from the lungs.

3. Beginning with the bronchi, the respiratory structures are contained in the *lungs*.

a. Each lung is divided into lobes. The right lung has three lobes, the left has two. Each lobe is supplied by a secondary bronchus. The lobes are further subdivided into bronchopulmonary segments, supplied by smaller bronchi. The bronchopulmonary segments contain lobules, which are the functional units of the lung (the site where gas exchange takes place). Each lobule is supplied by a bronchiole and by an arteriole, a venule, and a lymphatic vessel.

b. The lungs are encased in a membrane called the *pleura*, which is composed of two layers. The inner layer, which adheres to the surface of the lung, is called the *visceral pleura*. The outer layer, which lines the thoracic cavity, is called the *parietal pleura*. The potential space between the layers is called the pleural cavity. It contains fluid that allows the layers to glide over each other and minimizes friction.

c. The lungs expand and relax in response to changes in pressure relationships (intrapulmonic and intrapleural pressures). Elastic tissue in the bronchioles and alveoli allows the lungs to stretch or expand to accommodate incoming air. This ability is called *compliance*. The lungs also recoil (like a stretched rubber band) to expel air. Some air remains in the lungs after expiration, which allows gas exchange to continue between respirations.

4. The nervous system regulates the rate and depth of respiration by the respiratory center in the medulla oblongata, the pneumotaxic center in the pons, and the apneustic center in the reticular formation. The respiratory center is stimulated primarily by increased $CO_2$ in the fluids of the center. (However, excessive $CO_2$ will depress the respiratory center.) When the center is stimulated, the rate and depth of breathing are increased, and excessive $CO_2$ is exhaled. A lesser stimulus to the respiratory center is decreased oxygen in arterial blood.

The nervous system also operates several reflexes important to respiration. The cough reflex is especially important because it helps protect the lungs from foreign particles, air pollutants, bacteria, and other potentially harmful substances. A cough occurs when nerve endings in the respiratory tract mucosa are stimulated by dryness, pressure, cold, irritant fumes, and excessive secretions.

5. The circulatory system transports $O_2$ and $CO_2$. After oxygen enters the bloodstream across the alveolar–capillary membrane, it combines with hemoglobin in red blood cells for transport to body cells, where it is released. $CO_2$ combines with hemoglobin in the cells for return to the lungs and elimination from the body.

6. The musculoskeletal system participates in chest expansion and contraction. Normally, the diaphragm and external intercostal muscles expand the chest cavity and are called muscles of inspiration. The abdominal and internal intercostal muscles are the muscles of expiration.

7. Normal respiration requires:

a. Atmospheric air containing at least 21% $O_2$

b. Adequate ventilation. Ventilation, in turn, requires patent airways, expansion and contraction of the chest, expansion and contraction of the lungs, and maintenance of a normal range of intrapulmonic and intrapleural pressures.

c. Adequate diffusion of $O_2$ and $CO_2$ through the alveolar–capillary membrane. Factors influencing diffusion include the thickness and surface area of the membrane and pressure differences between gases on each side of the membrane.

d. Adequate perfusion or circulation of blood and sufficient hemoglobin to carry needed $O_2$

8. Normal breathing occurs 16 to 20 times per minute and is quiet, rhythmic, and effortless. About 500 ml of air is inspired and expired with a normal breath (tidal volume); deep breaths or "sighs" occur six to 10 times per hour to ventilate more alveoli. Fever, exercise, pain, and emotions such as anger tend to increase respirations. Sleep or rest and various medications, such as tranquilizers, sedatives, and narcotic analgesics, tend to slow respiration.

## Disorders of the respiratory system

The respiratory system is subject to many disorders that interfere with respiration. Common disorders include respiratory tract infections, allergic disorders, inflammatory disorders, and conditions that obstruct air flow (*e.g.*, excessive respiratory tract secretions, emphysema, and other chronic obstructive pulmonary diseases). Common signs and symptoms of respiratory disorders include cough, increased secretions, mucosal congestion, and bronchospasm.

## Drug therapy

As a general rule, drug therapy is more effective in relieving symptoms than in curing the underlying disorders that cause the symptoms. Major drug groups used to treat respiratory symptoms are bronchodilating and antiasthmatic agents (see Chap. 50), antihistamines (see Chap. 51), and nasal decongestants, antitussives, and cold remedies (see Chap. 52).

## Review and Application Exercises

1. What is the main function of the respiratory system?

2. Where does the exchange of oxygen and carbon dioxide occur?
3. List factors that stimulate rate and depth of respiration.
4. List factors that depress rate and depth of respiration.
5. What are common signs and symptoms of respiratory disorders for which drug therapy is often used?

## Selected References

Burrell, L. O. (1992). Overview of anatomy, physiology, and pathophysiology of the respiratory system. In L. O. Burrell (Ed.), *Adult nursing in hospital and community settings* (pp. 622–635). Norwalk, CT: Appleton & Lange.

Guyton, A. C. (1991). *Textbook of medical physiology* (8th ed.). Philadelphia: W.B. Saunders.

Renfroe, D. H. (1992). Normal respiratory function. In B. L. Bullock & P. P. Rosendahl (Eds.), *Pathophysiology: Adaptations and alterations in function* (3rd ed.) (pp. 554–578). Philadelphia: J.B. Lippincott.

# CHAPTER 50

# Bronchodilating and Antiasthmatic Drugs

## Respiratory disorders

Bronchodilating and antiasthmatic agents are used in the treatment of respiratory disorders characterized by bronchoconstriction or bronchospasm, inflammation, mucosal edema, and excessive mucus production (asthma, bronchitis, and emphysema). Bronchoconstriction involves narrowing of the airways, which is aggravated by the inflammation, mucosal edema, and excessive mucus. Resultant symptoms include dyspnea, wheezing, coughing, and other signs of respiratory distress.

Bronchoconstriction may be precipitated by respiratory infections, odors, smoke, chemical fumes or other air pollutants, cold air, exercise, emotional upsets, tartrazine (a yellow dye found in many foods and drugs), and some drugs (*e.g.*, beta-adrenergic blocking agents, aspirin, and nonsteroidal anti-inflammatory agents). When lung tissues are exposed to these stimuli, mast cells release histamine and other substances that cause bronchoconstriction and inflammation. Mast cells are found throughout the body in connective tissues and are abundant in tissues surrounding capillaries in the lungs.

Bronchoconstrictive substances include acetylcholine, cyclic guanosine monophosphate (GMP), histamine, leukotrienes, prostaglandins, serotonin, and others. These substances are antagonized by adenosine 3′ : 5′-cyclic monophosphate (cyclic AMP). Cyclic AMP is an intracellular substance that initiates various intracellular activities, depending on the type of cell. In lung cells, cyclic AMP inhibits release of bronchoconstrictive substances and promotes bronchodilation.

### ASTHMA

The two major characteristics of *asthma* are inflammation and bronchoconstriction. Bronchoconstriction is attributed to hyperactive responses of smooth muscle in the trachea and bronchi to certain stimuli. Bronchoconstriction is usually reversible, either spontaneously or with drug therapy, and clients may be symptom free between periodic attacks. Asthma may occur at any age but is especially common in childhood and early adulthood.

### CHRONIC BRONCHITIS AND EMPHYSEMA

In *chronic bronchitis* and *emphysema*, commonly called chronic obstructive pulmonary disease (COPD), bronchoconstriction is more constant and less reversible than with asthma. Anatomic and physiologic changes occur over several years and lead to increasing dyspnea and activity intolerance. These conditions usually affect middle-aged or older adults.

## Drug therapy

Drug therapy of these disorders involves dilating the airways, reducing inflammation, and stabilizing mast cells. Several types of drugs are used, including bronchodilators, corticosteroids, and others.

## MECHANISMS OF ACTION

### Bronchodilators

*Adrenergics* (see Chap. 18) stimulate beta$_2$-adrenergic receptors in bronchial smooth muscle. The receptors, in turn, stimulate the enzyme adenylate cyclase to increase production of cyclic AMP. The increased cyclic AMP produces bronchodilation. Some beta-adrenergic drugs (*e.g.*, epinephrine) also stimulate beta$_1$-receptors in the heart to increase the rate and force of contraction. Cardiac stimulation is an adverse effect when the drugs are given for bronchodilation. Newer beta-adrenergic bronchodilators (*e.g.*, albuterol, metaproterenol, pirbuterol, terbutaline) act more selectively on beta$_2$-receptors and cause fewer cardiac effects.

*Xanthines* were formerly thought to increase cyclic AMP by inhibiting the enzyme phosphodiesterase, which metabolizes cyclic AMP. However, several other mechanisms (*e.g.*, increasing endogenous catecholamines, inhibiting calcium ion movement into smooth muscle, inhibiting prostaglandin synthesis and release, or inhibiting the release of bronchoconstrictive substances from mast cells and leukocytes) have been proposed. In addition to their bronchodilating effects, xanthines also increase cardiac output, cause peripheral vasodilation, exert a mild diuretic effect, and stimulate the central nervous system (CNS). The cardiovascular and CNS effects are considered adverse effects.

*Anticholinergics* (see Chap. 21) block the action of acetylcholine in bronchial smooth muscle when given by inhalation. This action reduces intracellular GMP, a bronchoconstrictive substance.

### Corticosteroids

In bronchoconstrictive disorders, corticosteroids have two major actions. First, the drugs have potent anti-inflammatory effects, which reduce inflammation and mucus secretion. Second, they increase the number and sensitivity of beta-adrenergic receptors, which restores or increases the effectiveness of adrenergic bronchodilators. Because systemic corticosteroids may cause severe adverse effects, especially with high dosage or prolonged use, several drugs (beclomethasone, flunisolide, triamcinolone) have been developed for topical administration by oral inhalation.

### Mast cell stabilizers

Cromolyn and nedocromil stabilize mast cells and prevent the release of bronchoconstrictive and inflammatory substances when mast cells are confronted with allergens and other stimuli.

## INDICATIONS FOR USE

The drugs are used to prevent and treat bronchoconstriction associated with asthma, acute and chronic bronchitis, and emphysema. Adrenergic bronchodilators, usually given by inhalation, are used in acute and chronic bronchoconstrictive disorders. Intravenous aminophylline is used for acute bronchoconstriction; oral theophylline preparations are used for long-term treatment of chronic disorders. Inhaled anticholinergic bronchodilators are used primarily for chronic disorders.

Corticosteroids are useful in the treatment of acute and chronic disorders. Cromolyn and nedocromil are indicated only for prophylaxis of asthma attacks.

## CONTRAINDICATIONS FOR USE

*Adrenergics* are contraindicated in clients with cardiac tachyarrhythmias and severe coronary artery disease; they should be used cautiously in clients with hypertension, hyperthyroidism, diabetes mellitus, and seizure disorders. *Xanthines* are contraindicated in clients with acute gastritis and peptic ulcer disease; they should be used cautiously in those with cardiovascular disorders that could be aggravated by drug-induced cardiac stimulation. Inhaled *anticholinergics* should be used with caution in clients with narrow-angle glaucoma and prostatic hypertrophy. *Corticosteroids* should be used with caution in clients with peptic ulcer disease, inflammatory bowel disease, hypertension, congestive heart failure, and thromboembolic disorders. *Mast cell stabilizers* are contraindicated in clients who are hypersensitive to the drugs. They should be used with caution in clients with impaired renal or hepatic function. Also, the propellants in the aerosol may aggravate coronary artery disease or arrhythmias.

## Individual bronchodilating and antiasthmatic drugs

### ADRENERGIC BRONCHODILATORS

**Epinephrine** (Adrenalin, Bronkaid) is administered subcutaneously in an acute attack of bronchoconstriction. Therapeutic effects may occur within 5 minutes and last for 4 hours. Epinephrine is available in a pressurized aerosol form without a physician's prescription (*e.g.*, Primatene). When given by inhalation, epinephrine rapidly relieves bronchoconstriction associated with asthma, bronchitis, or emphysema. Almost all over-the-counter aerosol products promoted for use in asthma contain epinephrine. These products are often abused and may delay the client from seeking medical attention.

Clients should be cautioned that excessive use may produce tolerance and hazardous adverse effects.

### Routes and dosage ranges

*Adults:* Aqueous solution (epinephrine 1 : 1000), SC 0.2–0.5 ml; dose may be repeated after 20 minutes if necessary

> Aqueous suspension (Sus-Phrine 1 : 200), SC 0.1–0.3 ml; dose may be repeated after 4 h if necessary

> Inhalation by inhaler, 1 or 2 inhalations four to six times per day

> Inhalation by nebulizer, 0.25–0.5 ml of 2.25% racemic epinephrine in 2.5 ml normal saline

*Children:* Aqueous solution (epinephrine 1 : 1000), SC 0.01 ml/kg q4h as needed. A single dose should not exceed 0.5 ml.

> Aqueous suspension (Sus-Phrine 1 : 200), SC 0.005 ml/kg q8–12h if necessary

> Inhalation, same as adults for both inhaler and nebulizer

**Albuterol** (Proventil), **bitolterol** (Tornalate), and **pirbuterol** (Maxair) are relatively selective beta$_2$-adrenergic agents used for prevention and treatment of bronchoconstriction. Although they have less effect on the cardiovascular system than epinephrine or isoproterenol, they should be used with caution in clients with cardiac disorders.

Albuterol

### Routes and dosage ranges

*Adults:* PO 2–4 mg three or four times per day
> Inhalation, 1 or 2 inhalations (90 µg/puff) q4–6h
*Children:* Safety and effectiveness in children younger than 12 years have not been established.

Bitolterol

### Route and dosage ranges

*Adults and children over 12 years:* Treatment, 2 inhalations (0.37 mg/puff) at least 1–3 min apart, followed by a third if necessary
> Prophylaxis, 2 inhalations q8h; maximum recommended dose, 3 inhalations q6h or 2 inhalations q4h

Pirbuterol

### Route and dosage range

*Adults:* Inhalation, 2 puffs (0.4 mg/dose), four to six times per day; maximum dose, 12 inhalations/d
*Children over 12 years:* Inhalation, same as adults; not recommended for use in children younger than 12 years

**Ephedrine** is an adrenergic drug occasionally used in the treatment of asthma. It has a long duration of action and is effective with oral administration. Ephedrine stimulates alpha and beta receptors (causing cardiac stimulation and increased blood pressure) and the CNS (causing insomnia and nervousness). Because of these adverse effects and the availability of selective beta$_2$-adrenergic agonists, the use of ephedrine has declined.

### Route and dosage ranges

*Adults:* PO 25–50 mg q3–4h
> Sustained-release preparations, 30–60 mg q8–12h
*Children:* PO 3 mg/kg per day in four to six divided doses

**Isoetharine** (Bronkosol, Bronkometer) is used to treat acute attacks of asthma. Although the drug acts more selectively on beta$_2$-adrenergic receptors than on beta$_1$-receptors, cardiac and CNS stimulation may occur with high doses. Isoetharine is relatively short acting (duration of 1–3 hours). It is available as a solution for nebulization or in a pressurized container for inhalation.

### Route and dosage ranges

*Adults and children:* Inhalation by nebulizer, 0.25–0.5 ml of 1% isoetharine in 2.5 ml of normal saline
> Inhalation by inhaler, 1 or 2 inhalations (0.34 mg/dose) four times per day

**Isoproterenol** (Isuprel) is a potent bronchodilator and cardiac stimulant. When used for treatment of bronchospasm, isoproterenol is given by inhalation, alone or in combination with other agents. Isoproterenol is a short-acting agent (approximate duration of 1–3 hours).

### Route and dosage ranges

*Adults and children:* Inhalation by nebulizer, 0.25–0.5 ml of 1 : 200 Isuprel solution in 2.5 ml saline
> Inhalation by inhaler, 1 or 2 inhalations (0.075–0.125 mg/puff) four times per day; maximum dose, 3 inhalations per attack of bronchospasm

**Metaproterenol** (Alupent) is a relatively selective, intermediate-acting beta$_2$-adrenergic agonist that may be given orally or by metered-dose inhaler. Metaproterenol is used to treat acute bronchospasm and to prevent exercise-induced asthma. In high doses, metaproterenol loses some of its selectivity and may cause cardiac and CNS stimulation.

### Routes and dosage ranges

*Adults:* Inhalation, 1–3 puffs (0.65 mg/dose), four times per day; maximum dose, 12 inhalations/d
> PO 10–20 mg q6–8h
*Children:* Inhalation, not recommended for use in children younger than 12 years

Under 9 years or weight under 27 kg, PO 10 mg q6–8h

Over 9 years or weight over 27 kg, PO 20 mg q6–8h

**Terbutaline** (Brethine, Bricanyl) is a relatively selective beta$_2$-adrenergic agonist that is a long-acting bronchodilator. When given subcutaneously, terbutaline loses its selectivity and has little advantage over epinephrine. Muscle tremor is the most frequent side effect with this agent.

### Routes and dosage ranges

*Adults:* PO 2.5–5 mg q6–8h; maximum dose, 15 mg/d
SC 0.25 mg, repeated in 15–30 min if necessary, q4–6h
Inhalation, 2 inhalations (400 μg/dose) q4–6h
*Children:* PO 2.5 mg three times per day for children 12 years and older; maximum dose, 7.5 mg/d
SC dosage not established
Inhalation, same as adults for children 12 years and older

## ANTICHOLINERGIC BRONCHODILATORS

**Atropine** (Dey-Dose Atropine Sulfate) is the prototype anticholinergic drug with multiple indications for use. It is given by inhalation for prevention and treatment of bronchospasm associated with asthma, bronchitis, and emphysema. Systemic absorption is variable and more likely to occur with higher doses.

### Route and dosage ranges

*Adults:* Inhalation, 0.025 mg/kg diluted with 3 to 5 ml of saline and given by nebulizer three or four times per day; maximum dose, 2.5 mg/d
*Children:* Inhalation, 0.05 mg/kg diluted in saline and given by nebulizer three or four times per day

**Ipratropium bromide** (Atrovent) is similar to atropine in its actions, uses, and effects. It is ineffective in acute bronchospasm when a rapid response is required. It is used in maintenance therapy of bronchoconstriction associated with chronic bronchitis and emphysema. Improved pulmonary function usually occurs within 15 minutes, peaks in 1 to 2 hours, and lasts about 4 hours. The most common adverse effects are cough, nervousness, nausea, gastrointestinal upset, headache, and dizziness. Ipratropium acts synergistically with adrenergic bronchodilators and may be used concomitantly.

### Route and dosage range

*Adults:* 2 inhalations (36 μg) from the metered-dose inhaler four times per day
*Children:* Dosage not established

## XANTHINE BRONCHODILATORS

**Theophylline** is widely used in the prevention and treatment of bronchoconstriction associated with asthma, bronchitis, and emphysema. Numerous dosage forms are availabile, including tablets, capsules, long-acting or sustained-release tablets and capsules, elixirs, suspensions, enemas, and rectal suppositories. Most formulations contain anhydrous theophylline (100% theophylline) as the active ingredient; some contain theophylline salts. For example, theophylline ethylenediamine (aminophylline) is frequently used and contains approximately 85% theophylline; it is the only theophylline preparation that can be given intravenously. In addition to the single-drug formulations, many combination products are available. These products contain other active ingredients, such as an adrenergic drug (*e.g.,* ephedrine), an expectorant (*e.g.,* guaifenesin), or a sedative (*e.g.,* phenobarbital, hydroxyzine). Selected theophylline preparations are listed in Table 50-1.

## CORTICOSTEROIDS

**Beclomethasone** (Beclovent, Vanceril), **flunisolide** (Aerobid), and **triamcinolone** (Azmacort) are topical corticosteroids for inhalation. Topical administration minimizes systemic absorption and adverse effects. These preparations may substitute for or allow reduced dosage of systemic corticosteroids.

In asthmatics taking an oral corticosteroid, the oral dosage is reduced slowly (over weeks to months) when an inhaled corticosteroid is added. The goal is to give the lowest oral dose necessary to control symptoms. Beclomethasone and flunisolide also are available in nasal solutions for treatment of allergic rhinitis that does not respond to other treatment.

Beclomethasone

### Routes and dosage ranges

*Adults:* Oral inhalation, 2 inhalations (0.84 mg/dose) three or four times daily; maximum dose, 20 inhalations/24 h
Nasal inhalation (Vanceril nasal inhaler), 1 inhalation (0.42 mg) in each nostril two to four times per day
*Children 6–12 years:* Oral inhalation, 1 or 2 inhalations three or four times per day; maximum dose, 10 inhalations/24 h
*Children over 12 years:* Nasal inhalation, same as adults

Flunisolide

### Routes and dosage ranges

*Adults:* Oral inhalation, 2 inhalations (0.50 mg/dose) twice daily, morning and evening; maximum dose, 4 inhalations twice daily (2 mg)

**TABLE 50-1.  THEOPHYLLINE PREPARATIONS**

| Generic/Trade Name | Routes and Dosage Ranges | |
| --- | --- | --- |
| | *Adults* | *Children* |
| *Short-Acting Preparations* | | |
| **Theophylline anhydrous (100% theophylline)** (Elixophyllin, Theolair, others) | PO 100–250 mg q6h | PO 50–100 mg q6h |
| **Theophylline ethylenediamine (85% theophylline) (aminophylline)** (Aminophylline, others) | PO 500 mg initially, then 200–300 mg q6–8h Acute bronchospasm, IV 6 mg/kg over 20–30 min, followed by a maintenance infusion of 0.1–1.2 mg/kg per hour. Dilute the dose in 5% dextrose injection or 0.9% sodium chloride injection to a concentration of 2 mg of aminophylline/ml of IV solution. | PO 7.5 mg/kg initially, then 5–6 mg/kg q6–8h Acute bronchospasm, IV 6 mg/kg over 30 min as a loading dose, followed by a maintenance infusion of 0.6–0.9 mg/kg per hour |
| **Theophylline monothanolamine (75% theophylline)** (Fleet Theophylline) | Rectally, as a retention enema, 250–500 mg twice daily | Not recommended |
| **Oxtriphylline (64% theophylline)** (Choledyl) | PO 200 mg four times daily | PO 15 mg/kg daily, in four divided doses |
| *Long-Acting Preparations* | | |
| **Theophylline anhydrous (100% theophylline)** (Theo-Dur, Theobid, Theoclear LA, Theolair-SR) | PO 150–300 mg q8–12h; maximal dose, 13 mg/kg or 900 mg daily, whichever is less | PO 100–200 mg q8–12h; maximal dose, 24 mg/kg per day |
| *Theophylline Mixtures* | | |
| **Theophylline 130 mg, ephedrine sulfate 25 mg, hydroxyzine hydrochloride 10 mg** (Marax) | PO 1 tablet two to four times daily | Age over 5 years, PO ½ tablet two to four times daily |
| **Theophylline 150 mg, guaifenesin 90 mg** (Quibron) | Tablets, PO 1–2 capsules q6–8h Elixir, PO 15–30 ml q6–8h | PO 4–6 mg/kg q6–8h |
| **Theophylline 18 mg, ephedrine hydrochloride 24 mg, phenobarbital 8 mg** (Tedral) | PO 1–2 tablets q4h | Weight over 60 lb, PO ½–1 tablet q4h |

Nasal inhalation (Nasalide), 2 sprays in each nostril twice daily; maximum dose, 8 sprays in each nostril per day

*Children 6–15 years:* Oral inhalation, 2 inhalations twice daily

Nasal inhalation, 1 spray in each nostril three times per day, or 2 sprays twice daily; maximum dose, 4 sprays in each nostril per day

Triamcinolone

### Route and dosage ranges

*Adults:* Oral inhalation, 2 inhalations three or four times per day; maximum dose, 16 inhalations/24 h

*Children 6–12 years:* 1 or 2 inhalations three or four times per day; maximum dose, 12 inhalations/24 h

**Hydrocortisone**, **prednisone**, and **methylprednisolone** (Solu-Medrol) are systemic corticosteroids given to clients who do not respond adequately to bronchodilator therapy. Corticosteroids are given intravenously in acute, severe attacks of asthma or bronchospasm; they are given orally or topically in chronic asthma or bronchospasm.

Hydrocortisone sodium phosphate and sodium succinate

### Route and dosage ranges

*Adults:* IV 100–200 mg q4–6h initially, then decreased or switched to an oral dosage form

*Children:* IV 1–5 mg/kg q4–6h

Methylprednisolone sodium succinate

### Route and dosage ranges

*Adults:* IV 2–60 mg q4–6h
*Children:* IV 1–4 mg/kg q4–6h

Prednisone

### Route and dosage ranges

*Adults:* PO 20–60 mg/d
*Children:* PO 2 mg/kg per day initially

## MAST CELL STABILIZERS

**Cromolyn** (Intal) and **nedocromil** (Tilade) are used to prevent acute asthma attacks in clients with chronic asthma, including allergic and exercise-induced asthmas. Use of one of these drugs may allow reduced dosage of bronchodilators and corticosteroids. The drugs are used only for prophylaxis; they are not effective in acute bronchospasm or status asthmaticus and should not be used in these conditions.

Cromolyn is available in a capsule and a solution for inhalation. The capsule is placed in a turboinhaler (Spinhaler) that punctures the capsule. When the client places the turboinhaler in the mouth and inhales, the capsule spins and vibrates, causing the micronized powder to be inhaled. The solution is for use with a power-operated nebulizer; hand-operated nebulizers are unsuitable.

Occasionally, the client may experience cough or bronchospasm following cromolyn inhalation. If a significant amount of bronchospasm occurs, the drug should be discontinued. Also, the drug should be discontinued if a therapeutic response is not obtained within 4 weeks of therapy.

A nasal solution (Nasalcrom) is available for prevention and treatment of allergic rhinitis; an ophthalmic solution (Opticrom) is available for prevention and treatment of allergic conjunctivitis and keratitis.

Intal

### Route and dosage range

*Adults:* 20 mg (capsule or solution) inhaled four times per day
*Children 5 years and older for capsules, 2 years and older for nebulizer solution:* Same as adults

Nasalcrom

### Route and dosage range

*Adults and children 6 years and older:* 1 spray in each nostril three to six times per day at regular intervals

Opticrom

### Route and dosage range

*Adults and children:* 1 or 2 drops (cromolyn 1.6 mg/drop) in each eye four to six times per day at regular intervals

Nedocromil

### Route and dosage range

*Adults and children over 12 years:* Inhalation, 4 mg q6–12h

## *Nursing Process*

### Assessment

Assess the client's pulmonary function:

- General assessment factors include rate and character of respiration, skin color, arterial blood gas analysis, and pulmonary function tests. Abnormal breathing patterns (*e.g.,* rate below 12 or above 24 per minute, dyspnea, cough, orthopnea, wheezing, "noisy" respirations) may indicate respiratory distress. Severe respiratory distress is characterized by tachypnea, dyspnea, use of accessory muscles of respiration, and hypoxia. Early signs of hypoxia include mental confusion, restlessness, anxiety, and increased blood pressure and pulse rate. Late signs include cyanosis and decreased blood pressure and pulse. Hypoxemia is confirmed if arterial blood gas analysis shows decreased partial pressure of oxygen ($PO_2$).
- In acute bronchospasm, a medical emergency, the client is in obvious and severe respiratory distress. A characteristic feature of bronchospasm is forceful expiration or wheezing.
- If the client has chronic asthma, try to determine the frequency and severity of acute attacks, factors that precipitate or relieve acute attacks, antiasthmatic medications taken occasionally or regularly, allergies, and condition between acute attacks, such as restrictions in activities of daily living due to asthma.
- If the client has chronic bronchitis or emphysema, assess for signs of respiratory distress, hypoxia, cough, amount and character of sputum, exercise tolerance (*e.g.,* dyspnea on exertion, dyspnea at rest), medications, and nondrug treatment measures (*e.g.,* breathing exercises, chest physiotherapy).

### Nursing diagnoses

- Impaired Gas Exchange related to bronchoconstriction and excessive mucus production
- Ineffective Breathing Pattern related to bronchoconstriction
- Activity Intolerance related to fatigue
- Self-Care Deficit related to impaired gas exchange
- High Risk for Altered Nutrition: Less than Body Requirements related to fatigue
- High Risk for Injury: Respiratory infection
- Anxiety related to chronic illness
- High Risk for Altered Tissue Perfusion related to bronchodilator-induced cardiac stimulation and arrhythmias

- High Risk for Noncompliance: Overuse of adrenergic bronchodilators
- Sleep Pattern Disturbance: Insomnia with adrenergic and xanthine bronchodilators
- Altered Thought Processes: Confusion and nervousness related to CNS stimulation with adrenergic and xanthine bronchodilators
- Knowledge Deficit: Factors precipitating bronchoconstriction
- Knowledge Deficit: Measures to avoid precipitating factors and respiratory infection
- Knowledge Deficit: Accurate self-administration of drugs, including use of inhalers

## Planning/Goals

*The client will:*
- Self-administer bronchodilating and other drugs accurately
- Experience relief of symptoms
- Avoid preventable adverse drug effects
- Avoid overusing bronchodilating drugs
- Avoid exposure to stimuli that cause bronchospasm when possible
- Avoid respiratory infections when possible

## Interventions

Use measures to prevent, relieve, or decrease bronchoconstriction when possible. General measures include those to prevent respiratory disease or promote an adequate airway. Some specific measures include the following:
- Use mechanical measures for removing respiratory tract secretions and preventing their retention. Effective measures include coughing, deep breathing, percussion, and postural drainage.
- Help the client identify and avoid exposure to conditions that precipitate bronchoconstriction. For example, allergens may be removed from the home, school, or work environment. When bronchospasm is precipitated by exercise, prophylaxis by prior inhalation of bronchodilating agents is better than avoiding exercise, especially in children.
- Try to prevent or reduce anxiety, which may cause or aggravate bronchospasm. Stay with the client during an acute asthma attack if feasible. Clients experiencing severe and prolonged bronchospasm (status asthmaticus) should be admitted or transferred to a hospital intensive care unit.

*Teach clients:*
- To drink 2000 to 3000 ml of fluids daily to help thin respiratory tract secretions and make them easier to remove.
- To stop smoking and avoid other bronchial irritants (*e.g.,* aerosol hair spray, antiperspirants, and cleaning products) when possible.
- To avoid excessive intake of coffee, tea, and cola drinks. These caffeine-containing beverages may increase bronchodilation but also may increase nervousness and insomnia with bronchodilating drugs.
- To take influenza vaccine annually and pneumococcal vaccine once if they have chronic lung disease.

## Evaluation

- Observe for relief of symptoms and improved arterial blood gas values.

- Interview and observe for correct drug administration, including use of inhalers.
- Interview and observe for tachyarrhythmias, nervousness, insomnia, and other adverse drug effects.
- Interview about and observe behaviors to avoid stimuli that cause bronchoconstriction and respiratory infections.

# Principles of therapy

## DRUG SELECTION AND ADMINISTRATION

Choice of drug and route of administration are determined largely by the severity of the disease process and the client's response to therapy. Some guidelines include the following:

1. An inhaled beta$_2$-agonist or subcutaneous epinephrine is the initial drug of choice for an acute attack of bronchospasm.
2. Because aerosol products act directly on the lungs, drugs given by inhalation can usually be given in smaller doses and produce fewer adverse effects than oral drugs.
3. The more selective beta$_2$-agonists (*e.g.,* albuterol, metaproterenol) are preferred when adrenergic bronchodilators are prescribed for clients who are elderly or who have heart disease or a history of cardiac arrhythmias.
4. Theophylline preparations are most often given orally. Aminophylline may be given intravenously for rapid drug action.
5. Anticholinergic bronchodilators are ineffective in relieving acute bronchospasm. They are most useful in the long-term management of COPD.
6. Cromolyn and nedocromil are used prophylactically; they are ineffective in acute bronchospasm.
7. Because inflammation has been established as a major component of asthma and other bronchoconstrictive respiratory disorders, corticosteroids are being used earlier in the disease process, along with bronchodilators or mast cell stabilizers. In acute bronchoconstriction, a corticosteroid is often given for approximately 1 week. A continuous intravenous infusion may be used initially; oral therapy is substituted when feasible. In chronic bronchoconstriction, inhaled corticosteroids are preferred. These drugs may be effective when used alone or with relatively small doses of an oral corticosteroid.
8. Using several drugs concurrently may be more effective than using a single agent. One advantage of a multiple drug regimen is that smaller doses of each agent usually can be given. This may decrease adverse effects and allow dosages to be increased when exacerbation of symptoms occurs.

## DOSAGE FACTORS

Dosage of bronchodilators, corticosteroids, and mast cell stabilizers must be individualized so that the smallest effective amounts are given. With theophylline preparations, guidelines include the following:

1. Dosage should be individualized to maintain serum drug concentrations of 10 to 20 μg/ml. Serum levels should be monitored because of individual differences in hepatic metabolism. Serum levels above 20 μg/ml are associated with a high incidence of toxicity. Blood for serum levels should be drawn 1 to 2 hours after immediate-release dosage forms and 4 hours after sustained-release forms.
2. Children and cigarette smokers usually need higher doses to maintain therapeutic blood levels because they metabolize theophylline rapidly.
3. Clients who have liver disease, congestive heart failure, chronic pulmonary disease, or acute viral infections usually need smaller doses because these conditions impair theophylline metabolism.
4. For obese clients, the theophylline dosage should be calculated on the basis of lean or ideal body weight, because theophylline is not highly distributed in fatty tissue.
5. Other factors, such as absorption and bioavailability of particular dosage forms, also affect serum drug levels and therefore affect drug toxicity.
6. A rational way to optimize dosage is to start with a low dose and gradually increase the amount according to symptom relief and serum theophylline levels.

## USE IN CHILDREN

Bronchodilators are used in children for the same indications as for adults. Adrenergic bronchodilators are discussed in Chapter 18; pediatric use of xanthines is discussed below.

Theophylline use in children should be closely monitored because dosage needs and rates of metabolism vary widely. In children younger than 6 months, especially premature infants and neonates, drug elimination may be prolonged due to immature liver function. Except for preterm infants with apnea, theophylline preparations are not recommended for use in this age group.

Children aged 6 months to 16 years, approximately, metabolize theophylline more rapidly than younger or older clients. Thus, they may need higher doses than adults in proportion to size and weight. If the child is obese, the dosage should be calculated on the basis of lean or ideal body weight because the drug is not highly distributed in fatty tissue.

Children are generally more sensitive to the CNS-stimulating effects of theophylline than adults. When the drug is given to asthmatic children, they may become hyperactive and disruptive. Tolerance to these effects usually develops with continued use of the drug.

Long-acting dosage forms are not recommended for children younger than 6 years.

## USE IN OLDER ADULTS

Adrenergic bronchodilators are discussed in Chapter 18; xanthines are discussed below.

Theophylline use in older adults must be carefully monitored because drug effects are somewhat unpredictable with a given dose. On one hand, cigarette smoking and drugs that stimulate drug-metabolizing enzymes in the liver (*e.g.*, phenobarbital, phenytoin) increase the rate of metabolism and therefore dosage requirements. On the other hand, impaired liver function, decreased blood flow to the liver, and some drugs (*e.g.*, cimetidine, erythromycin) impair metabolism and therefore decrease dosage requirements.

Adverse effects include cardiac and CNS stimulation. Safety can be increased by taking periodic measurements of serum drug levels and adjusting dosage to maintain therapeutic levels of 10 to 20 μg/ml. If the client is obese, the dosage should be based on lean or ideal body weight because theophylline is not highly distributed in fatty tissue.

## NURSING ACTIONS: BRONCHODILATING AND ANTIASTHMATIC DRUGS

*Nursing Actions*

*Rationale/Explanation*

1. **Administer accurately**

   **a.** Give oral theophylline preparations at regular intervals around the clock.

   To maintain therapeutic serum drug levels

   **b.** Give oral theophylline preparations before meals and with a full glass of water. If gastrointestinal (GI) upset occurs, give with food.

   To promote dissolution and absorption. Taking with food may help to decrease nausea and vomiting. However, these symptoms are primarily due to stimulation of the vomiting center in the brain rather than to local irritation of the GI tract.

   **c.** For a continuous IV infusion of aminophylline, dilute the drug in 5% dextrose in water or 0.9% sodium chloride injection to a concentration of 1 or 2 mg/ml (*e.g.*, 500 mg of aminophylline in 500 ml of IV fluid). Infuse a loading dose (about 6 mg/kg) over 20 to 30 minutes; infuse a maintenance dose of 0.5 to 0.9 mg/kg per hour.

   Dosage for maintenance therapy is based on serum drug concentrations and appearance of adverse effects (*e.g.*, tachycardia, premature ventricular contractions, nausea, vomiting, seizures).

2. **Observe for therapeutic effects**

   **a.** Decreased dyspnea and wheezing

   Relief of bronchospasm and wheezing should be evident within a few minutes after giving SC epinephrine, IV aminophylline, or aerosolized adrenergic bronchodilators.

   **b.** Reduced rate and improved quality of respirations

   **c.** Reduced anxiety and restlessness

   **d.** Therapeutic serum levels of theophylline (10–20 $\mu$g/ml)

   **e.** Improved arterial blood gas levels (normal values: $PO_2$, 80 to 100 mm Hg; $PCO_2$, 35 to 45 mm Hg; pH, 7.35 to 7.45)

   **f.** Improved exercise tolerance

   **g.** Decreased incidence and severity of acute attacks of bronchospasm with chronic administration of drugs

3. **Observe for adverse effects**

   **a.** With adrenergic bronchodilators, observe for tachycardia, arrhythmias, palpitations, restlessness, agitation, insomnia.

   These signs and symptoms result from cardiac and central nervous system (CNS) stimulation.

   **b.** With anticholinergic bronchodilators, observe for dry mouth, blurred vision, headache, nervousness, nausea. Ipratropium also may cause cough or exacerbation of symptoms.

   When atropine is given by inhalation, a variable amount of systemic absorption occurs. Adverse effects are increased with greater systemic absorption. Ipratropium is not absorbed systemically.

   **c.** With xanthine bronchodilators, observe for tachycardia, arrhythmias, palpitations, restlessness, agitation, insomnia, nausea, vomiting, convulsions.

   Theophylline causes cardiac and CNS stimulation. Convulsions occur at toxic serum concentrations (above 20 $\mu$g/ml). They may occur without preceding symptoms of toxicity and may result in death. IV diazepam (Valium) may be used to control seizures. Theophylline also stimulates the chemoreceptor trigger zone in the medulla oblongata to cause nausea and vomiting.

   **d.** With inhaled corticosteroids, observe for hoarseness, cough, throat irritation, and fungal infection of mouth and throat.

   Inhaled corticosteroids are unlikely to produce the serious adverse effects of long-term systemic therapy (see Chap. 24).

## Nursing Actions

## Rationale/Explanation

**e.** With cromolyn, observe for arrhythmias, hypotension, chest pain, restlessness, dizziness, convulsions, CNS depression, anorexia, nausea and vomiting. Sedation and coma may occur with overdosage.

Some of the cardiovascular effects are thought to be caused by the propellants used in the aerosol preparation.

**4. Observe for drug interactions**

**a.** Drugs that *increase* effects of bronchodilators:

    (1) MAO inhibitors

These drugs inhibit the metabolism of catecholamines. The subsequent administration of bronchodilators may increase blood pressure. Severe hypertensive reactions have been reported with ephedrine.

    (2) Erythromycin, clindamycin, cimetidine

These drugs may decrease theophylline clearance and thereby increase plasma levels.

**b.** Drugs that *decrease* effects of bronchodilators:

    (1) Lithium

Lithium may increase excretion of theophylline and therefore decrease therapeutic effectiveness.

    (2) Phenobarbital

This drug may increase the metabolism of theophylline by way of enzyme induction.

    (3) Propranolol, other nonselective beta-blockers

These drugs may cause bronchoconstriction and oppose effects of bronchodilators.

**5. Teach clients**

**a.** Take the drugs only as prescribed. If desired effects are not achieved or if symptoms worsen, inform the physician. Do not increase dosage or frequency of taking medication.

Tolerance may develop to bronchodilators after repeated use or abuse. It is most commonly seen with the inhalers. Continued use in this manner may lead to serious cardiac side effects.

**b.** Use inhalers correctly:

    (1) Shake well immediately before each use.

To disperse medication evenly

    (2) Remove the cap from the mouthpiece.

    (3) Exhale fully, expelling as much air from the lungs as possible.

To increase drug effectiveness.

    (4) With the inhaler in the upright position, place the mouthpiece just inside the mouth, and use the lips to form a tight seal.

    (5) While inhaling deeply, fully depress the top of the inhaler with the index finger.

    (6) Hold the breath as long as possible. Before exhaling, remove the mouthpiece from the mouth and the finger from the canister.

    (7) Wait 3 to 5 minutes before taking a second inhalation of the drug.

    (8) Rinse the mouthpiece and store the inhaler away from heat.

Inhaler contents are pressurized and may explode if heated.

**c.** If a bronchodilator and a corticosteroid are prescribed for inhalation, use the bronchodilator first.

To increase penetration of the corticosteroid

## Review and Application Exercises

1. What are some causes of bronchoconstriction, and how can they be prevented or minimized?
2. How do beta-adrenergic agonists and theophylline act as bronchodilators?
3. Which beta-adrenergic agonists act more selectively on beta$_2$-adrenergic receptors than on beta$_1$-receptors?
4. What adverse effects are associated with bronchodilators, and how can they be prevented or minimized?
5. What is an adverse effect associated with theophylline toxicity?
6. What is the therapeutic range of serum theophylline levels?
7. How do cromolyn and nedocromil act to prevent acute asthma attacks?
8. For what effects are corticosteroids used in the treatment of bronchoconstrictive respiratory disorders?

## Selected References

Barnes, P. J. (1992). Pulmonary disorders. In K. L. Melmon, H. F. Morrelli, B. B. Hoffman, & D. W. Nierenberg (Eds.), *Clinical pharmacology: Basic principles in therapeutics* (3rd ed.) (pp. 186–218). New York: McGraw-Hill.

(1993). *Drug facts and comparisons*. St. Louis: Facts and Comparisons.

Gotz, V. P. (1992). Chronic obstructive airways disease. In M. A. Koda-Kimble & L. Y. Young (Eds.), *Applied therapeutics: The clinical use of drugs* (5th ed.) (pp. 16-1–16-17). Vancouver, WA: Applied Therapeutics.

Guyton, A. C. (1991). *Textbook of medical physiology* (8th ed.). Philadelphia: W.B. Saunders.

Kelly, H. W. (1992). Asthma. In M. A. Koda-Kimble & L. Y. Young (Eds.), *Applied theratpeutics: The clinical use of drugs* (5th ed.) (pp. 15-1–15-24). Vancouver, WA: Applied Therapeutics.

Lidell, K. O., & Mazzocco, M. C. (1990). Breaking bronchospasm's grip with MDIs. *American Journal of Nursing, 90*, 34–39.

Porth, C. M. (1990). *Pathophysiology: Concepts of altered health states* (3rd ed.). Philadelphia: J.B. Lippincott.

CHAPTER **51**

# Antihistamines

## Antihistamines

Antihistamines are drugs that antagonize the action of histamine, an important chemical mediator stored in almost every body tissue, especially connective tissue (mast cells) and blood (basophils). To understand the use of antihistamines, it is necessary to understand the action of histamine in the body. Histamine is derived from histidine, an amino acid, and discharged from mast cells into the vascular system in response to certain stimuli (*e.g.*, antigen–antibody reactions, tissue injury, extreme cold, and specific drugs). Once released, histamine exerts various effects on body tissues, as listed below:

1. It contracts smooth muscles, such as those of the bronchi, gastrointestinal tract, and uterus. Histamine-induced bronchoconstriction may play a role in the cause of bronchial asthma.
2. It acts on capillaries to cause vasodilation and subsequent hypotension. In addition, the skin on the face and upper parts of the body may become flushed.
3. It increases capillary permeability to fluid, resulting in outflow of fluid into subcutaneous tissues and edema formation. Local edema in nasal mucosa produces the nasal congestion characteristic of allergic reactions and the common cold.
4. It dilates cerebral blood vessels, which may cause severe headache.
5. It stimulates secretion of gastric juice in large amounts and with high acidity. It also increases bronchial, intestinal, and salivary secretions.
6. It stimulates sensory nerve endings to cause pain and itching.

Many antihistamines are available for clinical use. These agents are similar in effectiveness as histamine antagonists but differ in potency, dosage, incidence of adverse effects, and dosage forms available. Antihistamines can be divided into the following groups:

1. *Alkylamines* are effective in relatively low dosage and are the most suitable agents for daytime use. The members of this group are among the most commonly used antihistamines. Individual responses to these drugs vary, and central nervous system (CNS) depression or stimulation may occur. Prototype: chlorpheniramine (Chlor-Trimeton).
2. *Ethanolamines* are strong CNS depressants and cause a high incidence of drowsiness. Incidence of gastrointestinal distress is low. Prototype: diphenhydramine (Benadryl).
3. *Ethylenediamines* have weak CNS depressant effects and therefore cause less drowsiness than most other antihistamines, but they often cause gastrointestinal distress. Prototype: pyrilamine.
4. *Phenothiazines* are used mainly for CNS depressant and antiemetic effects. They are related to the phenothiazine antipsychotic drugs discussed in Chapter 9. Prototype: promethazine (Phenergan).
5. *Piperazines* have prolonged antihistaminic activity with a relatively low incidence of drowsiness. However, mental alertness is decreased, and operation of machinery may be hazardous.
6. *Nonsedating* agents include astemizole (Hismanal), loratadine (Claritin), and terfenadine (Seldane). These drugs were developed specifically to produce less sedation.
7. A *miscellaneous* agent is hydroxyzine (Vistaril), which

Anne Collins Abrams: CLINICAL DRUG THERAPY, Fourth Edition.
© 1995 J.B. Lippincott Company.

is often used as an antiemetic and a preoperative sedative.

Antihistamines are well absorbed following oral and parenteral administration. They are primarily metabolized by the liver and excreted within 24 hours by the kidneys. When given orally, effects occur within 15 to 60 minutes and last about 4 to 6 hours. Enteric-coated or sustained-release preparations last 8 to 12 hours. Long-acting dosage forms may be less effective owing to inadequate dissolution and absorption. When given parenterally, antihistaminic effects occur more rapidly.

## MECHANISM OF ACTION

Antihistamines prevent histamine from acting on target tissues. Because antihistamines are structurally related to histamine, the drugs occupy the same receptor sites as histamine and competitively antagonize its actions. They do not prevent histamine release or reduce the amount released. The two types of histamine receptors are $H_1$ and $H_2$. Conventional antihistamines act on $H_1$ receptors and may be called $H_1$ blockers. These are the antihistamines discussed in this chapter. Cimetidine (Tagamet), ranitidine (Zantac), famotidine (Pepcid), and nizatidine (Axid) are $H_2$ blocking agents used to prevent or treat peptic ulcer disease. These are discussed in Chapter 63.

Antihistamines are effective in inhibiting vascular permeability, edema formation, bronchoconstriction, and pruritus associated with histamine release. Except for the nonsedating drugs, most antihistamines cause sedation and anticholinergic effects. Terfenadine and similar drugs do not produce sedation and anticholinergic effects because they bind more specifically with $H_1$ receptors in peripheral tissues than with $H_1$ receptors in the brain. In a few people, particularly children, antihistamines may produce paradoxical restlessness and hyperactivity.

## INDICATIONS FOR USE

Clinical indications for the use of antihistamines include:

1. **Allergic rhinitis and other hypersensitivity reactions**. Of people with hay fever (seasonal allergic rhinitis), 75% to 95% experience some relief of sneezing, rhinorrhea, nasal airway obstruction, and conjunctivitis with the use of antihistamines. People with perennial allergic rhinitis (nonseasonal) usually experience decreased nasal congestion and drying of nasal mucosa. With anaphylaxis and other serious allergic reactions, antihistamines are helpful in treating urticaria and pruritus but are less effective in treating bronchoconstriction and hypotension. Epinephrine, rather than an antihistamine, is the drug of choice for treating anaphylaxis and other serious allergic reactions. With pruritus, trimeprazine (Temaril) and cyproheptadine (Periactin) are especially effective. In addition to *treatment* of allergic disorders, antihistamines may be given to *prevent* allergic reactions to blood transfusions and contrast media (*e.g.*, iodine preparations) used for various diagnostic tests.

2. **Dermatologic conditions**. Antihistamines are the drugs of choice for treatment of acute urticaria but are less effective in chronic urticaria. Other indications for use include contact dermatitis, atopic dermatitis, drug-induced allergic skin reactions, pruritus ani, and pruritus vulvae. However, topical preparations containing antihistamines are not recommended because they may induce dermatologic allergic reactions (*e.g.*, skin rashes).

3. **Vascular disorders**. Antihistamines may be useful in treating angioedema, but they are second-choice drugs, after epinephrine.

4. **Miscellaneous**. Some antihistamines are commonly used for nonallergic disorders, such as motion sickness (*e.g.*, dimenhydrinate, meclizine), nausea and vomiting (*e.g.*, promethazine, hydroxyzine), and sleep (the active ingredient in over-the-counter products, such as Compoz and Sominex, is a sedating antihistamine). Antihistamines are also common ingredients in over-the-counter cold remedies (see Chap. 52). However, such usage should be discouraged because there is no evidence of efficacy in treatment of this viral infection.

## CONTRAINDICATIONS FOR USE

Antihistamines are contraindicated or must be used with caution in clients with hypersensitivity to the drugs, narrow-angle glaucoma, prostatic hypertrophy, stenosing peptic ulcer, and bladder neck obstruction and during pregnancy. The nonsedating antihistamines (astemizole, loratadine, terfenadine) are generally contraindicated in clients who are receiving macrolide antibiotics (*e.g.*, erythromycin, azithromycin, clarithromycin) or members of the imidazole group of antifungal agents (*e.g.*, itraconazole, ketoconazole). Ventricular fibrillation, ventricular tachycardia, and torsades de pointes have been reported with concurrent use of astemizole or terfenadine and erythromycin or ketoconazole. Apparently, the interacting drugs interfere with metabolism and increase blood concentrations of the antihistamines to toxic levels. Although life-threatening arrhythmias have not been reported thus far with loratadine or the newer macrolides, the drugs are similar to the interacting drugs.

## Individual antihistamines

For individual antihistamines, see Table 51-1.

## TABLE 51-1. COMMONLY USED ANTIHISTAMINES

| Generic/Trade Name | Routes and Dosage Ranges | | Comments |
|---|---|---|---|
| | **Adults** | **Children** | |
| **Alkylamines** | | | |
| **Chlorpheniramine maleate** (Chlor-Trimeton) | PO 2–4 mg t.i.d.–q.i.d. Sustained-release preparation, PO 8–12 mg q.d.–t.i.d. IM, IV, SC 5–40 mg | Age 6–12 years, PO, SC 0.35 mg/kg per day in four divided doses Age 7 years and over, sustained-release preparation, PO 8 mg q12h Not recommended for children under 6 years of age | Overall, low incidence of adverse effects; drowsiness is the most common. Given parenterally for amelioration of allergic reactions to blood or plasma and in anaphylaxis. Only preparations without preservatives may be given IV, and the drug should be injected over 1 minute. A common ingredient in over-the-counter products for cold and allergy symptoms. |
| **Brompheniramine maleate** (Dimetane) | PO 4–8 mg t.i.d.–q.i.d. Sustained-release preparation, PO 8–12 mg b.i.d. IM, IV, SC 10 mg q6–12h; maximal daily dose, 40 mg | Infant to 6 years, PO 0.5 mg/kg per day or 15 mg/m² per day in divided doses Age over 6 years, PO, half of adult dose Age under 12, IM, IV, SC 0.5 mg/kg per day or 15 mg/m² per day in divided doses | Mild drowsiness is the most common reaction. Do not use solution containing preservatives for IV injection. |
| **Dexchlorpheniramine maleate** (Polaramine) | PO 2 mg t.i.d. or q.i.d. Sustained-release preparation, PO 4–6 mg b.i.d. | Infants, PO, one fourth of adult dose or 0.15 mg/kg per day in four divided doses. Under 12 years, PO, half of adult dose Do not use sustained-release preparation. | Incidence of adverse effects is low. Most common reaction is mild drowsiness. |
| **Triprolidine hydro-chloride** (Actidil) | PO 2.5 mg t.i.d.–q.i.d. | Age over 6 years, PO 1.25 mg t.i.d.–q.i.d. Age 4–6 years, PO 0.9 mg t.i.d.–q.i.d. Age 2–4 years, 0.6 mg t.i.d.–q.i.d. Age 4 months–2 years, 0.3 mg t.i.d.–q.i.d. In children up to 6 years, use syrup only. | Rapid onset with low incidence of adverse effects; drowsiness is the most common. Others include dizziness, GI distress, paradoxical excitation, hyper-irritability. |
| **Ethanolamines** | | | |
| **Carbinoxamine maleate** (Clistin) | PO 12–32 mg daily in divided doses Long-acting preparation, PO 8–12 mg q6–12h | PO 0.2 mg/kg in three or four divided doses or 2–4 mg t.i.d.–q.i.d. | Lowest incidence of drowsiness of the ethanolamines. Anti-cholinergic effect very weak. Causes some drowsiness, dizziness, dryness of mouth, and GI distress. |
| **Clemastine fumarate** (Tavist) | PO 2.68 mg one to three times daily, not to exceed 8.04 mg/d Long-acting preparation, initially, PO 1.34 mg b.i.d., not to exceed 8.04 mg/d | Safety and efficacy in children under 12 years of age have not been established. | Drowsiness is the most frequent side effect, but central sedative effects are generally low in occurrence. Anticholinergic effect very weak. |
| **Dimenhydrinate** (Dramamine) | PO 50–100 mg q4h Rectal 100 mg q.d.–b.i.d. IM, IV 50 mg | Age 8–12 years, 25–50 mg t.i.d. | Often used to prevent motion sickness. May cause drowsiness. May mask ototoxicity caused by aminoglycoside antibiotics. |
| **Diphenhydramine hydro-chloride** (Benadryl) | PO 25–50 mg t.i.d.–q.i.d. IM, IV 10–50 mg to a maximal single dose of 100 mg; maximal daily dose, 400 mg | PO 12.5–25 mg t.i.d. or 5 mg/kg per day IM, IV 5 mg/kg or 150 mg/m² per day in four divided doses during a 24-h period, to a maximum of 300 mg/d | Topical preparation also available. May affect blood pressure when given parenterally. Also used in motion sickness and for emotionally disturbed children. Drowsiness decreases with continued usage. Protect from light. |
| **Ethylenediamines** | | | |
| **Pyrilamine maleate** | PO 75–200 mg daily in three or four divided doses | Age 6–12 years, PO 12.5–25 mg q.i.d. | Low incidence of drowsiness |

*(continued)*

**TABLE 51-1.   COMMONLY USED ANTIHISTAMINES   (Continued)**

| Generic/Trade Name | Routes and Dosage Ranges | | Comments |
| --- | --- | --- | --- |
| | **Adults** | **Children** | |
| **Tripelennamine hydro-chloride** (PBZ) | PO tablets and elixir 25–50 mg q4–6h; maximal daily dose, 600 mg<br>PO sustained-release tablets, 100 mg q12h | PO tablets and elixir 5 mg/kg per 24 h in four to six divided doses or 150 mg/m² per day in four to six divided doses<br>Do not use sustained-release tablets in children. | Elixir contains 37.5 mg of tripe-lennamine citrate (equivalent to 25 mg hydrochloride) per 5 ml. |
| *Phenothiazines* | | | |
| **Methdilazine, meth-dilazine hydrochloride** (Tacaryl, Tacaryl hydro-chloride) | PO 8 mg b.i.d.–q.i.d. | Infants, PO 2 mg b.i.d.<br>Age over 3 years, PO 4 mg b.i.d.–q.i.d. | Used as an antipruritic in allergic and nonallergic pruritus. Drowsi-ness less prominent than with other phenothiazines used as antihistamines. Most serious ad-verse reactions seen with anti-psychotic phenothiazines have not been reported with this agent. Chewable tablet must be chewed and swallowed promptly. |
| **Promethazine hydro-chloride** (Phenergan) | PO 25 mg at bedtime or 12.5 mg q.d.–b.i.d.<br>Rectal 25 mg, may be repeated in 4–6 h<br>IM, IV 12.5–25 mg, may be re-peated in 2 h | PO 0.13 mg/kg in AM and, when necessary, 0.5 mg/kg at bed-time; or 25 mg at bedtime and 6.25–12.5 mg t.i.d.<br>IM no more than half of adult dose | Very potent antihistamine with pronounced sedative effects that limit its use in ambulatory clients. Also used as sedative and in motion sickness. Photo-sensitization is a contraindication to further use. All precautions applicable to phenothiazines should be observed (see Chap. 9). |
| **Trimeprazine tartrate** (Temaril) | PO 2.5 mg q.i.d.<br>Sustained-release preparation, PO 5 mg q12h | Age under 3 years, PO 1.25 mg t.i.d.; maximal daily dose, 5 mg<br>Age 3–12 years, PO 2.5 mg q.i.d.; maximal daily dose, 10 mg | Used for symptomatic relief of acute and chronic pruritus. Drowsiness is the most com-mon reaction. Dizziness and dry mouth may occur (see also phe-nothiazines in Chap. 9). |
| *Piperazines* | | | |
| **Meclizine hydrochloride** (Antivert) | Motion sickness, PO 25–50 mg q.d. 1 h before traveling<br>Vertigo, 25–100 mg daily in divided doses | | Used mostly in motion sickness. May cause drowsiness, dry mouth, blurred vision. |
| **Cyclizine hydrochloride** (Marezine hydrochloride) | PO 50 mg ½ h before travel; repeat q4–6h; maximal daily dose, 300 mg<br>IM 50 mg t.i.d.–q.i.d. or as required | Age 6–10 years, PO, half of adult dose, IM 1 mg/kg t.i.d. | Widely used as an antiemetic. Contraindicated in pregnancy. May cause drowsiness, dizzi-ness, irritability. |
| *Nonsedating Antihistamines* | | | |
| **Astemizole** (Hismanal) | PO 10 mg/d | Age above 12 years, PO 10 mg/d<br>Age below 12 years, safety and efficacy not established | This group is chemically different from other antihistamines. High doses of astemizole and ter-fenadine have been associated with serious cardiac arrhythmias |
| **Loratadine** (Claritin)<br>**Terfenadine** (Seldane) | PO 10 mg/d<br>PO 60 mg q12h | Dosage not established<br>Age above 12 years, PO 60 mg twice daily<br>Age 6–12 years, PO 30–60 mg twice daily<br>Age 3–5 years, PO 15 mg twice daily | |

*(continued)*

**TABLE 51-1. COMMONLY USED ANTIHISTAMINES** (*Continued*)

| Generic/Trade Name | Routes and Dosage Ranges | | Comments |
|---|---|---|---|
| | *Adults* | *Children* | |
| *Miscellaneous Antihistamines* | | | |
| **Azatadine maleate** (Optimine) | PO 1–2 mg b.i.d. Use lower dosage in older adults. | Dosage not established | Chemically similar to cyproheptadine. Has prolonged action. Used in allergic rhinitis and chronic urticaria. Drowsiness is the most common side effect. Should not be used in clients with asthma, in children under 12 years of age, or during pregnancy or lactation. |
| **Cyproheptadine** (Periactin) | PO 4 mg t.i.d., not to exceed 0.5 mg/kg per day | Age 2–6 years, PO 2 mg b.i.d.–t.i.d., not to exceed 12 mg daily<br>Age 6–14 years, 4 mg t.i.d., not to exceed 16 mg daily | Particularly used in treatment of pruritic dermatoses, angioedema, and migraine. Weight gain has been reported. Sometimes used therapeutically as an appetite stimulant in children. May cause drowsiness and dry mouth. Contraindicated in glaucoma, urinary retention, and premature and full-term infants. |
| **Hydroxyzine hydrochloride, hydroxyzine pamoate** (Atarax, Vistaril) | PO 75–100 mg daily in three or four divided doses<br>Preoperative and postoperative sedation, prepartum and postpartum sedation, IM 25–100 mg as a single dose<br>Serious psychiatric conditions, IM 50–100 mg q4–6h PRN | PO 2 mg/kg per day in four divided doses<br>Preoperative and postoperative sedation, IM 0.6 mg/kg in a single dose | Has antihistaminic, antiemetic, antianxiety, and sedative effects and is used for all these actions. Low incidence of adverse effects; drowsiness is usually transient. |

## Nursing Process

### Assessment

Assess the client's condition in relation to disorders in which antihistamines are used. For the client with known allergies, try to determine the factors that precipitate or relieve allergic reactions and specific signs and symptoms experienced during a reaction.

### Nursing diagnoses

- Ineffective Airway Clearance related to thick respiratory secretions
- High Risk for Injury related to drowsiness and dizziness
- Knowledge Deficit: Safe and accurate drug use
- Knowledge Deficit: Ways of preventing conditions for which antihistamines are used

### Planning/Goals

*The client will:*
- Experience relief of symptoms
- Take antihistamines accurately
- Avoid hazardous activities if sedated from antihistamines
- Avoid preventable adverse drug effects
- Avoid taking sedative-type antihistamines with alcohol or other sedative drugs

### Interventions

- Monitor the client closely for excessive drowsiness during the first few days of therapy with antihistamines known to cause sedation.

- Encourage a fluid intake of 2000 to 3000 ml daily, if not contraindicated.

*Teach clients:*
- With astemizole, terfenadine, and probably loratadine, do not take more than the prescribed dose, and avoid taking erythromycin (an antibacterial drug), itraconazole, or ketoconazole (antifungal drugs) concurrently. Serious cardiac arrhythmias may result.
- Antihistamines are most effective before exposure to the stimulus that causes histamine release.
- Antihistamines may thicken respiratory tract secretions and make them more difficult to remove.
- Avoid using sedating antihistamines with other sedative-type drugs.

### Evaluation

- Observe for relief of symptoms.
- Interview and observe for correct drug usage.
- Interview and observe for excessive drowsiness.

## Principles of therapy

1. When specific allergens or precipitating factors are identified, allergic reactions may be prevented by avoiding exposure to them.

2. Antihistamines are more effective when given before exposure to allergens because the drugs can then occupy receptor sites before histamine is released.
3. Choice of antihistamine is based on the desired effect, duration of action, and adverse effects.
   a. *For treatment of acute allergic reactions*, a rapid-acting agent of short duration is preferred.
   b. *For chronic allergic symptoms* (*e.g.*, allergic rhinitis), long-acting preparations provide more consistent relief.
   c. *For clients who are sensitive to the sedative effects* of antihistamines or who must stay alert, a non-sedating antihistamine may be indicated.
   d. Some clients respond better to certain antihistamines than to others. Consequently, if one antihistamine does not relieve symptoms or produces excessive sedation, another may be effective.
   e. An antihistamine is often included in prescription and over-the-counter combination products for the common cold. Several studies have demonstrated that antihistamines do not relieve cold symptoms any better than a placebo. Therefore, their usage exposes the client to adverse effects without expected benefit and is considered irrational.

## USE IN CHILDREN

Conventional antihistamines (histamine$_1$-receptor antagonists), such as diphenhydramine, may cause drowsiness and decreased mental alertness in children as in adults. Young children may experience paradoxical excitement. These reactions may occur with therapeutic dosages. In overdosage, hallucinations, convulsions, and death may occur. Close supervision and appropriate dosages are required for safe drug usage in children.

Three newer antihistamines do not cause drowsiness in recommended dosages. With terfenadine, dosages are recommended for children as young as 3 years. Safety and efficacy of astemizole and loratadine have not been established, and dosages are not listed for children under 12 years old.

## USE IN OLDER ADULTS

Histamine$_1$-receptor antagonists, such as diphenhydramine may cause dizziness, sedation, syncope, confusion, paradoxical CNS stimulation, and hypotension in older adults. Older men with prostatic hypertrophy may have difficulty voiding while taking these drugs. Despite the increased risk of adverse effects, however, diphenhydramine is sometimes prescribed as a sleep aid and may be safer than other hypnotics in older adults.

# NURSING ACTIONS: ANTIHISTAMINES

| *Nursing Actions* | *Rationale/Explanation* |
|---|---|
| **1. Administer accurately** | |
| **a.** Give most oral antihistamines with meals; give astemizole 2 hours before a meal and instruct to avoid eating for 1 hour after taking the medication. | To decrease gastrointestinal (GI) effects of the drugs. Absorption of astemizole is reduced by 60% when taken with meals. |
| **b.** Give IM antihistamines deeply into a large muscle mass. | To decrease tissue irritation |
| **c.** Inject IV antihistamines slowly, over a few minutes. | Severe hypotension may result from rapid IV injection. |
| **d.** When a drug is used to prevent motion sickness, give it 30 to 60 minutes before travel. | |
| **2. Observe for therapeutic effects** | Therapeutic effects depend on the reason for use. |
| **a.** A verbal statement of therapeutic effect (relief of symptoms) | |
| **b.** Decreased nausea and vomiting when given for antiemetic effects | |
| **c.** Decreased dizziness and nausea when taken for motion sickness | |
| **d.** Drowsiness or sleep when given for sedation | |

| *Nursing Actions* | *Rationale/Explanation* |
|---|---|
| **3. Observe for adverse effects**<br>**a.** Sedation—ranging from mild drowsiness to deep sleep | Due to central nervous system (CNS) depression, which occurs with most antihistamines. Sedation is the most common adverse effect. |
| **b.** Paradoxical excitation—restlessness, insomnia, tremors, nervousness, palpitations | This reaction is more likely to occur in children. It may result from the anticholinergic effects of antihistamines. |
| **c.** Convulsive seizures | Antihistamines, particularly the phenothiazines, may lower the seizure threshold. |
| **d.** Dryness of mouth, nose, and throat, blurred vision, urinary retention, constipation | Due to antihistamines' anticholinergic effects |
| **e.** GI distress—anorexia, nausea, vomiting | These symptoms are especially likely to occur with the ethylenediamine group of antihistamines. |
| **f.** Allergic reactions—skin rashes, photosensitivity | These are more likely to occur with topical antihistamine preparations. |
| **g.** Teratogenicity | Piperazine antihistamines are teratogenic. |
| **h.** Cardiac arrhythmias | Serious ventricular arrhythmias (fibrillation, tachycardia, torsades de pointes) have been reported with higher than recommended doses of astemizole and terfenadine or concurrent administration with erythromycin, itraconazole, or ketoconazole. |
| **4. Observe for drug interactions**<br>Drugs that *increase* effects of antihistamines: | |
| (1) Ethyl alcohol, CNS depressants (*e.g.*, antianxiety and antipsychotic agents, narcotic analgesics, sedative-hypnotics) | Additive CNS depression. Concomitant use may lead to drowsiness, lethargy, stupor, respiratory depression, coma, and death. |
| (2) MAO inhibitors | Inhibit metabolism of antihistamines, leading to an increased duration of action; increased incidence and severity of anticholinergic adverse effects |
| (3) Tricyclic antidepressants | Additive anticholinergic side effects |
| (4) Erythromycin, itraconazole, and ketoconazole | These antimicrobials increase the risks of serious cardiac arrhythmias with astemizole and terfenadine, probably by interfering with their metabolism and thereby increasing their blood levels. |
| **5. Teach clients**<br>**a.** Take antihistamines only as prescribed or as instructed on packages of over-the-counter preparations. | To maximize therapeutic benefit and minimize adverse effects |
| **b.** Do not drink alcohol or take other drugs without the physician's knowledge and consent. | To avoid adverse effects and dangerous drug interactions. Alcohol and other drugs with CNS-depressant effects may cause excessive sedation, respiratory depression, and death. |
| **c.** Do not smoke, drive a car, or operate machinery until drowsiness has worn off. | To avoid injury. Drowsiness usually decreases after a few days of continuous drug administration. |
| **d.** Report adverse effects, such as excessive drowsiness. | The physician may be able to change drugs or dosages to decrease adverse effects. |
| **e.** Store antihistamines out of reach of children. | To avoid accidental ingestion |
| **f.** Do not exceed prescribed dosage of astemizole or terfenadine. | To avoid potentially serious irregularities of the heart beat |
| **g.** Inform any health-care provider if taking astemizole or terfenadine. | To increase safety by avoiding possible adverse drug interactions |

## Review and Application Exercises

1. Describe several factors that cause histamine release from cells.
2. What signs and symptoms are produced by the release of histamine?
3. How do antihistamines act to block the effects of histamine?
4. Differentiate between histamine$_1$- and histamine$_2$-receptor antagonists in terms of pharmacologic effects and clinical indications for use.
5. In general, when should an antihistamine be taken to prevent or treat allergic disorders?
6. Describe advantages and disadvantages of the newer, nonsedating antihistamines in comparison with the older antihistamines.
7. In a client taking terfenadine or astemizole, what would you teach about safe usage?

## Selected References

(1993). *Drug facts and comparisons*. St. Louis: Facts and Comparisons.

Hendeles, L. (1993). Efficacy and safety of antihistamines and expectorants in nonprescription cough and cold preparations. *Pharmacotherapy, 13*(2), 154–158.

Porth, C. M. (1990). *Pathophysiology: Concepts of altered health states* (3rd ed.). Philadelphia: J.B. Lippincott.

Reese, G. L., & Kelly, H. W. (1992). Pediatric respiratory diseases: Cystic fibrosis, bronchopulmonary dysplasia, chronic rhinitis, and common cold. In M. A. Koda-Kimble & L. Y. Young (Eds.), *Applied therapeutics: The clinical use of drugs* (5th ed.) (pp. 17-1–17-20). Vancouver, WA: Applied Therapeutics.

(1993). Reports of dangerous cardiac arrhythmias prompt new contraindications for the drug Hismanal. *FDA Medical Bulletin, 23*(1), 2.

### CHAPTER 52

# Nasal Decongestants, Antitussives, Mucolytics, and Cold Remedies

## Description

Common signs and symptoms of respiratory disorders are nasal congestion, cough, and increased secretions. Characteristics of these signs and symptoms include the following:

1. *Nasal congestion* is manifested by obstructed nasal passages ("stuffy nose") and nasal drainage ("runny nose"). It is a prominent symptom of the common cold and allergic rhinitis. Nasal congestion results from dilation of the blood vessels in the nasal mucosa and engorgement of the mucous membranes with blood. At the same time, nasal membranes are stimulated to increase mucus secretion. Related symptomatic terms are *rhinorrhea* (the discharge of mucus from the nose), *rhinitis* (inflammation of the mucous membrane of the nose), and *coryza* (profuse discharge from the mucous membrane of the nose).
2. *Cough* is a forceful expulsion of air from the lungs. It is normally a protective reflex for removing foreign bodies, environmental irritants, or accumulated secretions from the respiratory tract. The cough reflex involves central and peripheral mechanisms. Centrally, the cough center in the medulla oblongata receives stimuli and initiates the reflex response (deep inspiration, closed glottis, buildup of pressure within the lungs, and forceful exhalation). Periph-

erally, "cough receptors" in the pharynx, larynx, trachea, or lungs may be stimulated by air, dryness of mucous membranes, or excessive secretions. A cough is described as "productive" when secretions are expectorated; it is "nonproductive" when it is dry, and no sputum is expectorated.

Cough is a prominent symptom of respiratory tract infections (*e.g.*, influenza, bronchitis, pharyngitis) and chronic obstructive pulmonary diseases (*e.g.*, emphysema, chronic bronchitis).
3. *Increased secretions* may result from excessive production or decreased ability to cough or otherwise remove secretions from the respiratory tract. Secretions may seriously impair respiration by obstructing airways and preventing air flow to and from alveoli, where gas exchange occurs. Secretions also may cause atelectasis and cause or aggravate infections by supporting bacterial growth.

Respiratory disorders characterized by retention of secretions include influenza, pneumonia, upper respiratory infections, acute and chronic bronchitis, emphysema, and acute attacks of bronchial asthma. Nonrespiratory conditions that predispose to secretion retention include immobility, debilitation, cigarette smoking, and postoperative status. Surgical procedures involving the chest or abdomen are most likely to be associated with retention of secretions because pain may decrease the client's ability to cough, breathe deeply, and ambulate.

Numerous drugs are available and widely used to treat these symptoms. Many are nonprescription drugs and can be obtained alone or in combination products. Available products include nasal decongestants, antitussives, and expectorants.

## NASAL DECONGESTANTS

Nasal decongestants are used to relieve nasal obstruction and discharge. Adrenergic (sympathomimetic) drugs are most often used for this purpose (see Chap. 18). These agents relieve nasal congestion by constricting arterioles and reducing blood flow to nasal mucosa. Some nasal decongestants are applied topically to the nasal mucosa as nasal sprays or solutions. Some (*e.g.*, ephedrine, phenylephrine) may be used orally or topically; phenylpropanolamine is prepared only for oral use. Nasal decongestants are most often used to relieve rhinitis associated with respiratory infections or allergies. They also may be used to reduce local blood flow before nasal surgery and to aid visualization of the nasal mucosa during diagnostic examinations.

Nasal decongestants are contraindicated in clients with severe hypertension or coronary artery disease because of their cardiac stimulating and vasoconstricting effects. They also are contraindicated for clients with narrow-angle glaucoma and those taking tricyclic antidepressants or monoamine oxidase inhibitors. They must be used with caution in the presence of cardiac arrhythmias, hyperthyroidism, diabetes mellitus, glaucoma, and prostatic hypertrophy.

## ANTITUSSIVES

Antitussive agents suppress cough by depressing the cough center in the medulla oblongata or the cough receptors in the throat, trachea, or lungs. Centrally acting antitussives include narcotics (codeine, hydrocodone, hydromorphone, and morphine) and non-narcotics (benzonatate, dextromethorphan). Peripherally acting agents (*e.g.*, glycerin, ammonium chloride) usually contain demulcents or local anesthetics to decrease irritation of pharyngeal mucosa. These agents are used as gargles, lozenges, and syrups. Flavored syrups are often used as vehicles for other drugs. Lozenges and hard candy increase the flow of saliva, which also soothes pharyngeal mucosa and may suppress cough.

The major clinical indication for use of antitussives is a dry, hacking, nonproductive cough that interferes with rest and sleep. It is usually not desirable to suppress a productive cough.

## EXPECTORANTS

Expectorants are agents given orally to liquefy respiratory secretions and allow for their easier removal. Guai-

fenesin is an ingredient in many combination cough and cold remedies.

## MUCOLYTICS

Mucolytics are administered by inhalation to liquefy mucus in the respiratory tract. Solutions of mucolytic drugs may be nebulized into a face mask or mouthpiece or instilled directly into the respiratory tract through a tracheostomy. Sodium chloride solution and acetylcysteine (Mucomyst) are the only agents currently recommended for use as mucolytics. Acetylcysteine is effective within 1 minute after inhalation, and maximal effects occur within 5 to 10 minutes. It is effective immediately after direct instillation. Oral acetylcysteine is widely used in the treatment of acetaminophen overdosage (see Chap. 6).

## COLD REMEDIES

Many combination products are available for treating symptoms of the common cold. Most of the products contain an antihistamine, a nasal decongestant, and an analgesic. Some contain antitussives, expectorants, and other agents as well. Although some cold remedies require a physician's prescription, many are proprietary over-the-counter (OTC) formulations. Commonly used ingredients include chlorpheniramine (antihistamine), phenylephrine or phenylpropanolamine (adrenergic nasal decongestants), acetaminophen (analgesic), codeine or dextromethorphan (antitussives), and guaifenesin (expectorant). Specific ingredients and amounts of each vary; several proprietary products come in several formulations; for example, see Novahistine, Phenergan, and Robitussin in Table 52-2.

# Individual drugs

Individual decongestants, antitussives, expectorants, and mucolytics are listed in Table 52-1; combination cold, cough, and allergy remedies are listed in Table 52-2.

## *Nursing Process*

### Assessment

Assess the client's condition in relation to disorders for which the drugs are used.
- With nasal congestion, observe for decreased ability to breathe through the nose. If nasal discharge is present, note the amount, color, and thickness. Question the client about the duration and extent of nasal congestion and factors that precipitate or relieve the symptom.

**TABLE 52-1.   NASAL DECONGESTANTS, ANTITUSSIVES, AND EXPECTORANTS**

| Generic/Trade Name | Routes and Dosage Ranges | |
| --- | --- | --- |
| | *Adults* | *Children* |
| ***Nasal Decongestants*** | | |
| **Ephedrine sulfate** | PO 25–50 mg q3–4h<br>Topically, 1–2 drops of 1%–3% solution as needed | |
| **Naphazoline hydro-chloride** (Privine hydro-chloride) | Topically, 1–2 drops or 2 spray inhalations no more often than q4–6h | Age over 6 years, topically, same as adults<br>Age under 6 years, not recommended |
| **Oxymetazoline hydro-chloride** (Afrin) | Topically, 2–4 drops or 2–3 spray inhalations in each nostril, morning and bedtime | Age over 6 years, topically, same as adults<br>Age under 6 years, 2–3 drops of 0.025% solution twice daily |
| **Phenylephrine hydro-chloride** (Neo-Synephrine) | PO 10 mg three times daily<br>Topically, 2–3 drops of 0.25%–1% solution in each nostril as needed | Age over 6 years, PO 5 mg three times daily; topically, same as adults<br>Infants, topically, 1–2 drops of 0.125% solution as needed |
| **Phenylpropanolamine hydrochloride** (Propagest) | PO 25 mg q3–4h or 50 mg q6–8h | Age 8–12 years, PO 20–25 mg three times daily |
| **Propylhexedrine** (Benzedrex) | Topically, 2 inhalations (0.6–0.8 mg) in each nostril as needed | |
| **Pseudoephedrine hydro-chloride** (Sudafed) | PO 60 mg three or four times daily<br>Sustained-release preparations, PO 120 mg twice daily | Age over 6 years, PO 60 mg three or four times daily<br>Age 4 months–6 years, PO 30 mg three or four times daily |
| **Tetrahydrozoline hydro-chloride** (Tyzine) | Topically, 2–3 drops or 1–2 sprays of 0.1% solution instilled in each nostril, no more often than q3h | Age 6 years and over, topically, 1–3 drops of 0.05% solution in each nostril q4–6h<br>Age under 6 years, not recommended |
| **Xylometazoline hydro-chloride** (Otrivin hydro-chloride) | Topically, 2–4 drops or inhalations of 0.1% solution in each nostril two or three times daily | Age 6 months–12 years, topically, 2–3 drops of 0.05% solution in each nostril two or three times daily<br>Age under 6 months, topically, 1 drop of 0.05% solution in each nostril two to three times daily |
| ***Narcotic Antitussives*** | | |
| **Codeine phosphate or sulfate** | PO 15 mg q4h as needed; maximal dose, 120 mg/24 h | PO 1–1.5 mg/kg per day in six divided doses as necessary |
| **Hydrocodone bitartrate** | PO 5–10 mg three or four times daily | PO 0.6 mg/kg per day in three or four divided doses |
| **Hydromorphone hydro-chloride** (Dilaudid) | PO 1 mg q3–4h | |
| **Morphine sulfate** | PO 2–4 mg three or four times daily | Age over 1 year, PO 0.06 mg/kg three or four times daily |
| ***Nonnarcotic Antitussives*** | | |
| **Benzonatate** (Tessalon) | PO 100 mg three times daily; maximal dose, 600 mg/d | Age over 10 years, PO same as adults<br>Age under 10 years, PO 8 mg/kg per day in 3–6 divided doses |
| **Dextromethorphan** (Benylin DM, others) | PO 10–30 mg three or four times daily. Maximum dose 120 mg/24 h | Age 2–6 years, PO 2.5–7.5 mg q4–8h. Maximum dose, 30 mg/24 h<br>Age 6–12 years, PO 5–10 mg q4h or 15 mg q6–8h. Maximum dose 60 mg/24 h |
| ***Expectorant*** | | |
| **Guaifenesin (glyceryl guaiacolate)** (Robitussin) | PO 200 mg (2 tsp) q4h | Age 12 years or over, PO 200 mg (2 tsp) q4h<br>Age 6–12 years, PO 100 mg (1 tsp) q4h<br>Age 2–6 years, PO 50 mg (1/2 tsp) q4h |
| ***Mucolytic*** | | |
| **Acetylcysteine** (Mucomyst) | Nebulization, 1–10 ml of a 20% solution or 2–20 ml of a 10% solution three or four times daily<br>Instillation, 1–2 ml of a 10% or 20% solution q1–4h<br>Acetaminophen overdosage, PO 140 mg/kg initially, then 70 mg/kg q4h for 17 doses; dilute a 10% or 20% solution to a 5% solution with cola, fruit juice, or water | |

**TABLE 52-2.  REPRESENTATIVE COMBINATION COLD, COUGH, AND ALLERGY REMEDIES***

| Trade Name | Ingredients | | | | | | Comments |
|---|---|---|---|---|---|---|---|
| | Antihistamine | Nasal Decongestant | Analgesic | Antitussive | Expectorant | Other | |
| Actifed | Triprolidine HCl 2.5 mg/tab or cap; 1.25 mg/5 ml of syrup | Pseudoephedrine HCl 60 mg/tab or cap; 30 mg/5 ml of syrup | | | | | OTC |
| Actifed with codeine cough syrup | Triprolidine HCl 1.25 mg/5 ml | Pseudoephedrine HCl 30 mg/5 ml | | Codeine 10 mg/5 ml | | Alcohol 4.3% | ℞ |
| Allerest | Chlorpheniramine maleate 2 mg/tab | Phenylpropanolamine HCl 18.7 mg/tab | | | | | OTC |
| Allerest (children's preparation) | Chlorpheniramine maleate 1 mg/tab | Phenylpropanolamine HCl 9.4 mg/tab | | | | | OTC |
| Cheracol Syrup | | | | Codeine 10 mg/5 ml | Guaifenesin 100 mg/5 ml | Alcohol 4.75% | |
| Cheracol D Cough Liquid | | | | Dextromethorphan 10 mg/5 ml | Guaifenesin 100 mg/5 ml | Alcohol 4.75% | OTC |
| Comtrex | Chlorpheniramine maleate 2 mg/tab or cap | Phenylpropanolamine HCl 12.5 mg/tab or cap | Acetaminophen 325 mg/tab or cap | Dextromethorphan 10 mg/tab or cap | | | OTC |
| Contac | Chlorpheniramine maleate 8 mg/cap | Phenylpropanolamine HCl 75 mg/cap | | | | | OTC, long-acting (timed-release capsule) |
| Coricidin | Chlorpheniramine maleate 2 mg/tab | | Acetaminophen 325 mg/tab | | | | OTC |
| Coricidin D | Chlorpheniramine maleate 2 mg/tab | Phenylpropanolamine 12.5 mg/tab | Acetaminophen 325 mg/tab | | | | OTC |
| CoTylenol cold formula | Chlorpheniramine maleate 2 mg/tab or cap | Pseudoephedrine HCl 30 mg/tab or cap | Acetaminophen 325 mg/tab or cap | Dextromethorphan 15 mg/tab or cap | | | OTC |
| CoTylenol liquid (children's preparation) | Chlorpheniramine maleate 1 mg/5 ml | Phenylpropanolamine HCl 6.25 mg/5 ml | Acetaminophen 160 mg/5 ml | | | Alcohol 8.5% | OTC |
| Dimetapp Elixir | Brompheniramine maleate 2 mg/5 ml | Phenylpropanolamine HCl 12.5 mg/5 ml | | | | Alcohol 2.3% | |
| Dimetapp Tablets | Brompheniramine maleate 4 mg/tab | Phenylpropanolamine HCl 25 mg/tab | | | | | OTC |
| Dimetapp Extentabs | Brompheniramine maleate 12 mg/tab | Phenylpropanolamine HCl 75 mg/tab | | | | | OTC, frequently prescribed, long-acting (10–12 h) preparation |
| Dristan | Chlorpheniramine maleate 2 mg/cap or tab | Phenylephrine HCl 5 mg/cap or tab | Acetaminophen 325 mg/cap or tab | | | | OTC |

(continued)

## TABLE 52-2. REPRESENTATIVE COMBINATION COLD, COUGH, AND ALLERGY REMEDIES* (Continued)

| Trade Name | Ingredients | | | | | | Comments |
|---|---|---|---|---|---|---|---|
| | Antihistamine | Nasal Decongestant | Analgesic | Antitussive | Expectorant | Other | |
| Drixoral | Dexbrompheniramine maleate 6 mg/tab | Pseudoephedrine sulfate 120 mg/tab | | | | | OTC, timed-release tablets, long-acting |
| Novahistine Elixir | Chlorpheniramine maleate 2 mg/5 ml | Phenylephrine HCl 5 mg/5 ml | | | | Alcohol 5% | OTC |
| Novahistine DH | Chlorpheniramine maleate 2 mg/5 ml | Pseudoephedrine HCl 30 mg/5 ml | | Codeine 10 mg/5 ml | | Alcohol 5% | ℞ |
| Novahistine DMX | | Pseudoephedrine HCl 30 mg/5 ml | | Dextromethorphan 10 mg/5 ml | Guaifenesin 100 mg/5 ml | Alcohol 10% | OTC |
| Novahistine Expectorant | | Pseudoephedrine HCl 30 mg/5 ml | | Codeine 10 mg/5 ml | Guaifenesin 100 mg/5 ml | Alcohol 7.5% | ℞ |
| Phenergan VC | Promethazine HCl 6.25 mg/5 ml | Phenylephrine HCl 5 mg/5 ml | | | | Alcohol 7% | ℞ |
| Phenergan VC with codeine | Promethazine HCl 6.25 mg/5 ml | Phenylephrine HCl 5 mg/5 ml | | Codeine 10 mg/5 mL | | Alcohol 7% | ℞ |
| Robitussin A-C | | | | Codeine 10 mg/5 ml | Guaifenesin 100 mg/5 ml | Alcohol 3.5% | ℞ |
| Robitussin-CF | | Phenylpropanolamine HCl 12.5 mg/5 ml | | Dextromethorphan 10 mg/5 ml | Same as Robitussin A-C | Alcohol 4.75% | OTC |
| Robitussin-DAC | | Pseudoephedrine HCl 30 mg/5 ml | | Codeine 10 mg/5 ml | Same as Robitussin A-C | Alcohol 1.4% | ℞ |
| Robitussin-DM | | | | Dextromethorphan 15 mg/5 ml | Same as Robitussin A-C | Alcohol 1.4% | OTC |
| Robitussin-PE | | Pseudoephedrine HCl 30 mg/5 ml | | | Same as Robitussin A-C | Alcohol 1.4% | OTC |
| Sine-Off | Chlorpheniramine maleate 2 mg/tab | Phenylpropanolamine HCl 12.5 mg/tab | Aspirin 325 mg/tab | | | | OTC |
| Sinutab | Chlorpheniramine maleate 2 mg/tab | Pseudoephedrine HCl 30 mg/tab | Acetaminophen 325 mg/tab | | | | OTC |
| Sinutab II | | Pseudoephedrine HCl 30 mg/tab or cap | Acetaminophen 500 mg/tab or cap | | | | OTC |

* OTC indicates nonprescription products.

- With coughing, a major assessment factor is whether the cough is productive of sputum or dry and hacking. If the cough is productive, note the color, odor, viscosity, and amount of sputum. In addition, assess factors that stimulate or relieve cough and the client's ability and willingness to cough effectively.

### Nursing diagnoses

- High Risk for Injury related to cardiac arrhythmias, hypertension, and other adverse effects of nasal decongestants
- High Risk for Noncompliance: Overuse of nasal decongestant and antitussive drugs

- Ineffective Airway Clearance related to suppression of a productive cough
- Constipation with narcotic antitussives
- Knowledge Deficit: Appropriate use of single- and combination-drug formulations

### Planning/Goals

*The client will:*
- Experience relief of symptoms
- Take drugs accurately and safely
- Avoid overuse of nasal decongestants and narcotic antitussives
- Avoid preventable adverse drug effects
- Act to avoid recurrence of symptoms

### Interventions

Encourage clients to use measures to prevent or minimize the incidence and severity of symptoms:
- With allergic disorders, avoid exposure to allergens when possible. Common allergens include plant pollens, dust, animal dander, and medications.
- Avoid smoking cigarettes. Cigarette smoke irritates respiratory tract mucosa, and this irritation causes cough, increased secretions, and decreased effectiveness of cilia in cleaning the respiratory tract.
- Avoid exposure to crowds, especially during winter when the incidence of influenza is high.
- Avoid contact with people who have colds or other respiratory infections. This is especially important for clients with chronic lung disease, because upper respiratory infections may precipitate acute attacks of asthma or bronchitis.
- Maintain a fluid intake of 2000 to 3000 ml daily unless contraindicated by cardiovascular or renal disease.
- Maintain nutrition, rest, activity, and other general health measures.
- Practice good handwashing techniques.
- Annual vaccination for influenza is recommended for clients who are elderly or have chronic respiratory, cardiovascular, or renal disorders.

*Teach clients:*
- That drugs may relieve symptoms but do not cure the disorder causing the symptoms
- That an adequate fluid intake, humidification of the environment, and sucking on hard candy or throat lozenges can help to relieve mouth dryness and cough
- To avoid using OTC cold remedies longer than 1 week
- Not to increase drug dosage if symptoms are not relieved by recommended amounts
- To see a health-care provider if symptoms persist longer than 1 week
- To read the labels of OTC allergy and cold remedies for information about indications for use, contraindications, and adverse effects

### Evaluation

- Interview and observe for relief of symptoms.
- Interview and observe for tachycardia, hypertension, drowsiness, and other adverse drug effects.
- Interview and observe for compliance with instructions about drug usage.

# Principles of therapy

## DRUG SELECTION AND ADMINISTRATION

Choice of drugs and routes of administration are influenced by several client- and drug-related variables. Some guidelines include the following:

1. Single-drug formulations are usually preferred over combination products because they allow flexibility and individualization of dosage. Combination products may contain unneeded or ineffective components and less-than-optimum dosages of individual ingredients.
2. With nasal decongestants, topical preparations (*i.e.,* nasal solutions or sprays) are often preferred for short-term use. They are rapidly effective because they come into direct contact with nasal mucosa. If used longer than 7 days or in excessive amounts, these products may produce rebound nasal congestion. Oral drugs are preferred for long-term use (more than 7 days). Phenylephrine (Neo-Synephrine), phenylpropanolamine, and pseudoephedrine (Sudafed) are commonly used nasal decongestants in prescription and OTC products. For clients with cardiovascular disease, topical nasal decongestants are preferred. Oral agents are generally contraindicated because of cardiovascular effects (*e.g.,* increased force of myocardial contraction, increased heart rate, increased blood pressure).
3. Most antitussives are given orally as tablets or cough syrups. Syrups serve as vehicles for antitussive drugs and may exert antitussive effects of their own by soothing irritated pharyngeal mucosa. Narcotic antitussives are controlled substances. Strong narcotic agents (*e.g.,* morphine, hydromorphone) should be used as antitussives only in severe, painful cough that cannot be controlled by milder narcotics (*e.g.,* codeine, hydrocodone) or non-narcotic antitussives.

   Dextromethorphan is probably the antitussive drug of choice in most circumstances. Compared with codeine, dextromethorphan is similarly effective without the disadvantages of a narcotic preparation. Dextromethorphan has no analgesic effect, does not produce tolerance or dependence, and does not depress respiration. Further, dextromethorphan is the only non-narcotic antitussive for which efficacy has been demonstrated by extensive research studies. A dose of 15 to 30 mg reportedly equals 8 to 15 mg of codeine in antitussive effectiveness.
4. For treatment of excessive respiratory tract secretions, mechanical measures (*e.g.,* coughing, deep breathing, ambulation, chest physiotherapy, forcing fluids) are more likely to be effective than expectorant drug therapy.

## USE IN CHILDREN

Upper respiratory infections with nasal congestion, cough, and increased secretions are common in children. The drugs described in this chapter are often used, and general principles apply.

Nasal congestion may interfere with an infant's ability to nurse. Phenylephrine nasal solution, applied just before feeding time, is usually effective.

Excessive amounts or too frequent administration of topical agents may result in rebound nasal congestion and systemic effects of cardiac and central nervous system stimulation. Despite these potential difficulties, topical drugs are less likely to cause systemic effects than oral agents.

## USE IN OLDER ADULTS

Older adults are at high risk of adverse effects (*e.g.*, hypertension, arrhythmias, nervousness, insomnia) from oral nasal decongestants. Adverse effects from topical agents are less likely, but rebound nasal congestion and systemic effects may occur with overuse. Older adults with significant cardiovascular disease should generally avoid the drugs.

With codeine and other narcotic antitussives, older adults may experience drowsiness or paradoxical excitement. Serious adverse effects are uncommon with the small doses used to relieve cough but may occur with excessive amounts.

# NURSING ACTIONS: NASAL DECONGESTANTS, ANTITUSSIVES, AND COLD REMEDIES

| *Nursing Actions* | *Rationale/Explanation* |
|---|---|
| **1. Administer accurately** <br> **a.** With topical nasal decongestants: | |
| (1) Use only preparations labeled for intranasal use. | Intranasal preparations are usually dilute, aqueous solutions prepared specifically for intranasal use. Some agents (*e.g.*, phenylephrine) are available in ophthalmic solutions as well. The two types of solutions *cannot* be used interchangeably. |
| (2) Use the drug concentration ordered. | Some drug preparations are available in several concentrations. For example, phenylephrine preparations may contain 0.125%, 0.25%, 0.5%, or 1% of drug. |
| (3) For instillation of nose drops, have the client lie down or sit with the neck hyperextended. Instill medication without touching the dropper to the nares. Rinse the medication dropper after each use. | To avoid contamination of the dropper and medication |
| (4) For nasal sprays, have the client sit, squeeze the container once to instill medication, avoid touching the spray tip to the nares, and rinse the spray tip after each use. | Most nasal sprays are designed to deliver one dose when used correctly. If necessary, secretions may be cleared and a second spray used. Correct usage and cleansing prevents contamination and infection. |
| (5) Give nasal decongestants to infants 20 to 30 minutes before feeding. | Nasal congestion interferes with an infant's ability to suck. |
| **b.** Administer cough syrups undiluted, and instruct the client to avoid eating and drinking for about 30 minutes. | Part of the therapeutic benefit of cough syrups stems from soothing effects on pharyngeal mucosa. Food or fluid removes the medication from the pharynx. |
| **c.** Instruct clients to swallow benzonatate perles without chewing. | If perles are chewed, local anesthetic effects numb oral mucosa. |
| **2. Observe for therapeutic effects** | Therapeutic effects depend on the reason for use. |
| **a.** When nasal decongestants are given, observe for decreased nasal obstruction and drainage. | |

(*continued*)

| *Nursing Actions* | *Rationale/Explanation* |
|---|---|
| **b.** With antitussives, observe for decreased coughing. | The goal of antitussive therapy is to suppress nonpurposeful coughing, not productive coughing. |
| **c.** With cold and allergy remedies, observe for decreased nasal congestion, rhinitis, muscle aches, and other symptoms. | |

**3. Observe for adverse effects**

**a.** With nasal decongestants, observe for:

| | |
|---|---|
| (1) Tachycardia, cardiac arrhythmias, hypertension | These effects may occur with any of the adrenergic drugs (see Chap. 18). When adrenergic drugs are used as nasal decongestants, cardiovascular effects are more likely to occur with oral agents. However, topically applied drugs also may be systemically absorbed through the nasal mucosa or by being swallowed and absorbed through the gastrointestinal tract. |
| (2) Rebound nasal congestion, chronic rhinitis, and possible ulceration of nasal mucosa | Adverse effects on nasal mucosa are more likely to occur with excessive or long-term (more than 10 days) use. |

**b.** With antitussives, observe for:

| | |
|---|---|
| (1) Excessive suppression of the cough reflex (inability to cough effectively when secretions are present) | This is a potentially serious adverse effect because retained secretions may lead to atelectasis, pneumonia, hypoxia, hypercarbia, and respiratory failure. |
| (2) Nausea, vomiting, constipation, dizziness, drowsiness, pruritus, and drug dependence | These are adverse effects associated with narcotic agents (see Chap. 5). When narcotics are given for antitussive effects, however, they are given in relatively small doses and are unlikely to cause adverse reactions. |
| (3) Nausea, drowsiness, and dizziness with non-narcotic antitussives | Adverse effects are infrequent and mild with these agents. |

| | |
|---|---|
| **c.** With combination products (*e.g.,* cold remedies), observe for adverse effects of individual ingredients (*i.e.,* antihistamines, adrenergics, analgesics, and others) | Adverse effects are rarely significant when the products are used as prescribed. There may be subtherapeutic doses of one or more component drugs, especially in over-the-counter formulations. Also, the drowsiness associated with antihistamines may be offset by stimulating effects of adrenergics. Ephedrine, for example, has central nervous system (CNS)-stimulating effects. |

**4. Observe for drug interactions**

| | |
|---|---|
| **a.** Drugs that *increase* effects of nasal decongestants: | These interactions are more likely to occur with oral decongestants than topically applied drugs. |
| (1) Cocaine, digitalis, general anesthetics, MAO inhibitors, other adrenergic drugs, thyroid preparations, and xanthines | Increased risks of cardiac arrhythmias |
| (2) Antihistamines, epinephrine, ergot alkaloids, MAO inhibitors, methylphenidate | Increased risks of hypertension due to vasoconstriction |
| **b.** Drugs that *increase* antitussive effects of codeine: | |
| CNS depressants (alcohol, antianxiety agents, barbiturates, and other sedative-hypnotics) | Additive CNS depression. Codeine is given in small doses for antitussive effects, and risks of significant interactions are minimal. |
| **c.** Drugs that alter effects of dextromethorphan: | |
| MAO inhibitors | This combination is contraindicated. Apnea, muscular rigidity, hyperpyrexia, laryngospasm, and death may occur. |

## Nursing Actions

## Rationale/Explanation

**d.** Drugs that may alter effects of combination products for coughs, colds, and allergies:

(1) Adrenergic (sympathomimetic) agents (see Chap. 18)

(2) Antihistamines (see Chap. 51)

(3) CNS depressants (see Chaps. 5, 7, 8, and 13)

(4) CNS stimulants (see Chap. 16)

Interactions depend on the individual drug components of each formulation. Risks of clinically significant drug interactions are increased with use of combination products.

**5. Teach clients**

**a.** Do not use nose drops more often than recommended or for longer than 7 consecutive days.

Excessive or prolonged use may damage nasal mucosa and produce chronic nasal congestion.

**b.** Blow the nose gently before instilling nasal solutions or sprays.

To clear nasal passages and increase effectiveness of medications

**c.** Do not touch the dropper tip to the nostrils when instilling nasal solutions.

To prevent contamination of the solution

**d.** Rinse the dropper or spray tip after each use.

To prevent bacterial contamination of the medication

**e.** Report palpitations, dizziness, drowsiness, rapid pulse.

These effects may occur with nasal decongestants and cold remedies and may indicate excessive dosage.

## Review and Application Exercises

1. How do adrenergic drugs relieve nasal congestion?
2. Who should generally avoid OTC nasal decongestants and cold remedies?
3. What are advantages and disadvantages of multi-ingredient cold remedies?
4. What is usually the antitussive of choice?
5. When is an antitussive generally contraindicated or undesirable?
6. Given a client with a productive cough, what are nondrug interventions to promote removal of secretions?

## Selected References

Barnes, P. J. (1992). Pulmonary disorders. In K. L. Melmon, H. F. Morrelli, B. B. Hoffman, & D. E. Nierenberg (Eds.), *Clinical pharmacology: Basic principles in therapeutics* (3rd ed.) (pp. 186–218). New York: McGraw-Hill.

(1993). *Drug facts and comparisons*. St. Louis: Facts and Comparisons.

Guyton, A. C. (1991). Textbook of medical physiology (8th ed.). Philadelphia: W.B. Saunders.

Hendeles, L. (1993). Efficacy and safety of antihistamines and expectorants in nonprescription cough and cold preparations. *Pharmacotherapy, 13*(2), 154–158.

Porth, C. M. (1990). *Pathophysiology: Concepts of altered health states* (3rd ed.). Philadelphia: J.B. Lippincott.

Reese, G. L., & Kelly, H. W. (1992). Pediatric respiratory diseases: Cystic fibrosis, bronchopulmonary dysplasia, chronic rhinitis, and common cold. In M. A. Koda-Kimble & L. Y. Young (Eds.), *Applied therapeutics: The clinical use of drugs* (5th ed.) (pp. 17-1–17-20). Vancouver, WA: Applied Therapeutics.

(1993). Reports of dangerous cardiac arrhythmias prompt new contraindications for the drug Hismanal. *FDA Medical Bulletin, 23*(1), 2.

# Drugs Affecting the Cardiovascular System

# CHAPTER 53

# Physiology of the Cardiovascular System

The cardiovascular or circulatory system is composed of the heart, blood vessels, and blood. The general functions of the system are to carry oxygen, nutrients, hormones, antibodies, and other substances to all body cells and to remove waste products of cell metabolism ($CO_2$ and others). The efficiency of the system depends on the heart's ability to pump blood, the patency of blood vessels, and the quality and quantity of blood.

## Heart

The heart is a hollow, muscular organ that functions as a double pump to circulate 5 to 6 liters of blood through the body every minute.

1. The heart has four chambers: two atria and two ventricles. The *atria* are receiving chambers. The right atrium receives deoxygenated blood from the upper part of the body by way of the superior vena cava, from the lower part of the body by way of the inferior vena cava, and from veins and sinuses within the heart itself. The left atrium receives oxygenated blood from the lungs through the pulmonary veins. The *ventricles* are distributing chambers. The right ventricle sends deoxygenated blood through the pulmonary circulation. It is small and thin-walled because it contracts against minimal pressure. The left ventricle pumps oxygenated blood through the systemic circuit. It is much more muscular and thick-walled be-

cause it contracts against relatively high pressure. The right atrium and right ventricle form one pump, and the left atrium and left ventricle form another. The right and left sides of the heart are separated by a strip of muscle called the *septum*.

2. The layers of the heart are the endocardium, myocardium, and epicardium. The *endocardium* is the membrane lining the heart chambers. It is continuous with the lining of blood vessels entering and leaving the heart and covers the heart valves. The *myocardium* is the strong muscular layer of the heart that provides the pumping power of the circulation. The *epicardium* is the outer, serous layer of the heart. The heart is enclosed in a fibroserous sac called the *pericardium*.

3. Heart valves function to guide the one-way flow of blood and prevent backflow. The *mitral* valve separates the left atrium and left ventricle. The *tricuspid* valve separates the right atrium and right ventricle. The *pulmonic* valve separates the right ventricle and pulmonary artery. The *aortic* valve separates the left ventricle and aorta.

4. The heart contains special cells that can carry electrical impulses much more rapidly than ordinary muscle fibers. This special conduction system consists of the sinoatrial (SA) node, the atrioventricular node, bundle of His, right and left bundle branches, and Purkinje fibers. The SA node, the normal pacemaker of the heart, can be compared to a battery. It originates a burst of electrical energy about 70 to 80 times each minute under normal circumstances. The electrical current flows over the heart in an orderly way to produce contraction of both atria, then both ventricles.

Anne Collins Abrams: CLINICAL DRUG THERAPY, Fourth Edition.
© 1995 J.B. Lippincott Company.

A unique characteristic of the heart is that each part can generate its own electrical impulse to contract. For example, the ventricles can beat independently but at a rate of only 30 to 40 beats per minute. In addition, the heart does not require nervous stimulation to contract. However, the autonomic nervous system does influence heart rate. Sympathetic nerves increase heart rate; parasympathetic nerves (by way of the vagus nerve) decrease heart rate.

5. The heart receives its blood supply from the coronary arteries. Coronary arteries branch off the aorta and fill during *diastole*, the resting or filling phase of the cardiac cycle. Coronary arteries branch into "end arteries," which supply certain parts of the myocardium without an overlapping supply from other branches. However, there are many artery-to-artery anastomoses between adjacent vessels. The anastomotic arteries do not supply sufficient blood to the heart if a major artery is suddenly occluded, but they may dilate into arteries of considerable size when disease (usually coronary atherosclerosis) develops slowly. The resultant *collateral circulation* may provide sufficient blood for myocardial function, at least during rest.

## Blood vessels

The three types of blood vessels are arteries, veins, and capillaries. Arteries and veins are similar in that they have three layers. The *intima* is the smooth inner lining of endothelium. The *media* is the middle layer of muscle and elastic tissue. The *adventitia* is the outer layer of connective tissue.

1. *Arteries* and *arterioles* have a thick media and control peripheral vascular resistance. They are sometimes called "resistance" vessels. Their efficiency depends on patency and ability to constrict or dilate in response to various stimuli. The degree of constriction or dilation (vasomotor tone) determines peripheral vascular resistance, which is a major determinant of blood pressure.
2. *Veins* have a thin media and valves that assist blood flow against gravity. They are sometimes called "capacitance" vessels, because blood may accumulate in various parts of the venous system. Their efficiency depends on patency, competency of valves, and the pumping action of muscles around veins.
3. *Capillaries* are very thin-walled vessels. Exchange of gases, nutrients, and waste products occurs across capillary walls.
4. *Lymphatic vessels* parallel the veins and drain tissue fluids. They carry lymphocytes and large molecules of protein and fat. They empty into the venous system.

## Blood

Blood generally functions to nourish and oxygenate all body cells, protect the body from invading microorganisms, and initiate hemostasis when a blood vessel is injured. Specific functions and components include the following:

1. Functions
   a. Transports oxygen to cells and carbon dioxide from cells to lungs for removal from the body
   b. Carries absorbed food products from the gastrointestinal tract to tissues; at the same time, it carries metabolic wastes from tissues to the kidneys, skin, and lungs for excretion
   c. Carries hormones from endocrine glands to other parts of the body
   d. Carries leukocytes and antibodies to sites of injury, infection, and inflammation
   e. Helps regulate body temperature by transferring heat produced by cell metabolism to the skin, where it can be released
   f. Carries platelets to injured areas for hemostasis
2. Components
   a. Plasma comprises about 55% of the total blood volume, and it is more than 90% water. Other ingredients are:
      (1) Serum albumin, which helps maintain blood volume by exerting colloid osmotic pressure
      (2) Fibrinogen, which is necessary for hemostasis
      (3) Gamma globulin, which is necessary for defense against microorganisms
      (4) Less than 1% antibodies, nutrients, metabolic wastes, respiratory gases, enzymes, and inorganic salts
   b. Solid particles comprise about 45% of total blood volume. Solid particles are erythrocytes, also called red blood cells (RBCs); leukocytes, also called white blood cells (WBCs); and thrombocytes, also called platelets. The bone marrow produces all RBCs, 60% to 70% of WBCs, and all platelets. Lymphatic tissues (spleen and lymph nodes) produce 20% to 30% of the WBCs, and reticuloendothelial tissues (spleen, liver, lymph nodes) produce 4% to 8% of WBCs. Characteristics of solid particles include the following:
      (1) Erythrocytes function mainly to transport oxygen. Almost all oxygen (95%–97%) is transported in combination with hemoglobin; very little is dissolved in blood. The life span of a normal RBC is about 120 days.
      (2) Leukocytes function mainly as a defense mechanism against microorganisms. They leave the bloodstream to enter injured tissues and phagocytize the injurious agent. They

also produce antibodies. The life span of a normal WBC is a few hours.

(3) Platelets are fragments of large cells, called megakaryocytes, found in the red bone marrow. Platelets are essential to blood coagulation.

# Drug therapy in cardiovascular disorders

Cardiovascular disorders are leading causes of morbidity and mortality. They may involve any structure or function of the cardiovascular system. Generally, a disorder in one part of the system eventually disturbs the function of all other parts. Cardiovascular disorders that are usually responsive to drug therapy include congestive heart failure, cardiac arrhythmias, angina pectoris, hypertension, hypotension, and shock. Disorders that are relatively unresponsive to drug therapy include atherosclerosis, peripheral vascular disease, and valvular disease. Blood disorders that respond to drug therapy include certain types of anemia and coagulation disorders.

Cardiovascular drugs may be given to increase or decrease cardiac output, blood pressure, and heart rate; to alter heart rhythm; increase or decrease blood clotting; alter the quality of blood; and decrease chest pain of cardiac origin. Cardiovascular drugs are often given for palliation of symptoms. For example, in disorders caused or aggravated by atherosclerosis (*e.g.*, angina pectoris, hypertension, congestive heart failure), the drugs relieve symptoms but do not alter the underlying disease process.

## Review and Application Exercises

1. How does the heart muscle differ from skeletal muscle?
2. What is the normal pacemaker of the heart?
3. In what circumstances do other parts of the heart take over as pacemaker?
4. What is the effect of parasympathetic (vagal) stimulation on the heart?
5. What is the effect of sympathetic stimulation on the heart and blood vessels?
6. How does low or high blood volume influence blood pressure?

## Selected References

Burrell, L. O. (1992). Overview of anatomy, physiology, and pathophysiology of the heart. In L. O. Burrelll (Ed.), *Adult nursing in hospital and community settings* (pp. 341–350). Norwalk, CT: Appleton & Lange.

Guyton, A. C. (1991). *Textbook of medical physiology* (8th ed.). Philadelphia: W.B. Saunders.

Pless, B. S. (1992). Overview of anatomy, physiology, and pathophysiology of the vascular system. In L. O. Burrell (Ed.), *Adult nursing in hospital and community settings* (pp. 464–471). Norwalk, CT: Appleton & Lange.

Porth, C. M. (1990). *Pathophysiology: Concepts of altered health states* (3rd ed.). Philadelphia: J.B. Lippincott.

### CHAPTER 54

# Cardiotonic-Inotropic Agents Used in Congestive Heart Failure

Cardiotonic-inotropic agents increase the force of myocardial contraction and thereby improve the heart's pumping ability. Drugs with cardiotonic-inotropic effects include adrenergics, digitalis glycosides, amrinone, and milrinone. Adrenergics (*e.g.,* epinephrine) also increase cardiac workload and oxygen consumption (see Chap. 18). Digitalis glycosides, amrinone, and milrinone are the focus of this chapter. A major clinical use of these agents is the treatment of congestive heart failure (CHF); digitalis glycosides also are used to treat atrial tachyarrhythmias.

## Congestive heart failure

CHF is a common condition that occurs when the heart cannot pump enough blood to meet tissue needs for oxygen and nutrients. Most CHF is caused by hypertension, coronary artery disease, or valvular disorders. Other causative factors include hyperthyroidism, excessive intravenous fluids or blood transfusions, and drugs that decrease the force of myocardial contraction (*e.g.,* beta-adrenergic blocking agents) or cause retention of sodium and water (*e.g.,* corticosteroids, estrogens, nonsteroidal anti-inflammatory agents). These factors impair the pumping ability or increase the workload of the heart so that an adequate cardiac output cannot be maintained.

When cardiac output falls, compensatory mechanisms help the body maintain blood flow to tissues. One mechanism is increased sympathetic activity, which increases the force of myocardial contraction, increases heart rate, and causes vasoconstriction. Another mechanism involves increased volume of blood and increased pressure within the heart chambers, which stretches muscle fibers and results in ventricular hypertrophy. A third mechanism is activation of the renin-angiotensin-aldosterone system. Renin is an enzyme produced in the kidney in response to impaired blood flow and tissue perfusion. When released into the bloodstream, it stimulates the production of angiotensin II, a powerful vasoconstrictor. The adrenal cortex is also stimulated to increase production of aldosterone, and aldosterone increases reabsorption of sodium and water in renal tubules.

As a result of these compensatory mechanisms, preload (amount of venous blood returning to the heart), workload of the heart, and afterload (amount of resistance in the aorta and peripheral blood vessels that the heart must overcome to pump effectively) are increased. All these mechanisms act to increase blood pressure. Although initially effective, the compensatory mechanisms themselves increase the workload of the heart, and they are limited in extent and duration of action. Eventually, signs and symptoms of CHF occur when, despite these compensatory mechanisms, an adequate

Anne Collins Abrams: CLINICAL DRUG THERAPY, Fourth Edition.
© 1995 J.B. Lippincott Company.

cardiac output can no longer be maintained, and failure or decompensation occurs.

## DRUG THERAPY

Drug therapy for CHF is aimed toward improving circulation and altering the compensatory mechanisms. In addition to cardiotonic-inotropic agents, diuretics, vasodilators, and angiotensin-converting enzyme (ACE) inhibitors are used.

1. **Diuretics** are often used in the treatment of CHF. They act to decrease plasma volume (extracellular fluid volume) and increase excretion of sodium and water, thereby decreasing preload. Intravenous furosemide (Lasix) also has a vasodilatory effect that helps to relieve vasoconstriction (afterload) in acute CHF (pulmonary edema). Diuretics are discussed in greater detail in Chapter 59.
2. **Vasodilators** also are frequently used, often with diuretics and digitalis glycosides. Venous dilators (*e.g.*, nitroglycerin and other nitrates) decrease preload; arterial dilators (*e.g.*, hydralazine [Apresoline]) decrease afterload; and prazosin (Minipress) dilates veins and arteries to decrease preload and afterload. Nitrates are discussed in Chapter 56; other vasodilators are discussed primarily in Chapter 58.
3. **ACE inhibitors**, such as captopril (Capoten) and others prevent the pharmacologically inactive angiotensin I from being converted to the powerful vasoconstrictor, angiotensin II. Although the mechanism of action differs, the overall effect of these agents is that of vasodilation.

## Digitalis glycosides

Digitalis glycosides are frequently prescribed drugs. In CHF, the drugs exert a cardiotonic or positive inotropic effect. Increased myocardial contractility allows the ventricles to empty more completely with each heart beat. With improved cardiac output, heart size, heart rate, end-systolic and end-diastolic pressures, vasoconstriction, sympathetic nerve stimulation, and venous congestion decrease.

Digitalis glycosides are distributed to most body tissues, including red blood cells, skeletal muscle, and the heart. To achieve therapeutic effects, cardiac tissue must maintain an adequate concentration of digitalis. Maximum drug effect is exerted when a steady-state tissue concentration has been achieved. This occurs in about five drug half-lives when loading doses are not given (approximately 1 week for digoxin and 1 month for digitoxin); if more rapid drug effects are required, a loading dose may be given.

Traditionally, a loading dose is called a digitalizing dose. Digitalization (administration of an amount sufficient to produce therapeutic effects) may be accomplished rapidly by giving about 0.75 to 1 mg of digoxin in divided doses 6 to 8 hours apart over a 24-hour period. Because rapid digitalization engenders higher risks of toxicity, it is usually done for atrial tachyarrhythmias rather than for CHF. Slow digitalization may be accomplished by initiating digitalis therapy with a maintenance dose.

Digitalis has a low therapeutic index; that is, a dose adequate for therapeutic effect may be accompanied by signs of toxicity. Digitalis toxicity may result from many contributing factors:

1. Accumulation of larger than necessary maintenance doses
2. Rapid loading or digitalization, whether by one or more large doses or frequent administration of small doses
3. Impaired renal function, which delays excretion of digoxin
4. Impaired liver function, which delays metabolism and excretion of digitoxin
5. Age extremes (young or old)
6. Electrolyte imbalance (*e.g.*, hypokalemia, hypomagnesemia, hypercalcemia)
7. Hypoxia, whether resulting from heart or lung disease, which increases myocardial sensitivity to digitalis
8. Hypothyroidism, which slows metabolism and causes drug accumulation
9. Concurrent treatment with other drugs affecting the heart, such as quinidine, verapamil, or nifedipine

All digitalis glycosides have the same pharmacologic actions (*i.e.*, therapeutic and adverse effects). However, digitalis preparations used clinically vary in potency, rate of absorption, onset of action, and rate of elimination.

## MECHANISMS OF ACTION

The mechanism by which digitalis increases the force of myocardial contraction is thought to be inhibition of Na,K-ATPase, an enzyme in cardiac cell membranes that decreases the movement of sodium out of myocardial cells after contraction. As a result, calcium enters the cell in exchange for sodium and causes additional calcium to be released from intracellular binding sites. With the increased intracellular concentration of free calcium ions, more calcium is available to activate the contractile proteins, actin and myosin, and increase myocardial contractility.

In atrial arrhythmias, digitalis slows the rate of ventricular contraction (negative chronotropic effect). Negative chronotropic effects are probably caused by several factors. First, digitalis has a direct depressant effect on cardiac conduction tissues, especially the atrioventricular node. This action decreases the number of electrical impulses allowed to reach the ventricles from supraventricular sources. Second, digitalis indirectly stimulates the vagus nerve. Third, increased efficiency of myocardial contraction and vagal stimulation decrease compensatory tachycardia resulting from the sympathetic nervous system response to inadequate circulation.

## Indications for use

The clinical uses of digitalis are treatment of CHF and atrial tachyarrhythmias (atrial fibrillation, atrial flutter, paroxysmal atrial tachycardia).

## Contraindications for use

Digitalis glycosides are contraindicated in severe myocarditis, ventricular tachycardia, or ventricular fibrillation and must be used cautiously in clients with acute myocardial infarction, heart block, Adams-Stokes syndrome, Wolff-Parkinson-White syndrome (risk of fatal arrhythmias), electrolyte imbalances (hypokalemia, hypomagnesemia, hypercalcemia), and renal impairment.

## Individual cardiotonic-inotropic agents

### DIGITALIS PREPARATIONS

**Digoxin** (Lanoxin) is by far the most prescribed digitalis preparation. A versatile drug, digoxin may be used in acute or chronic conditions, for digitalization, or for maintenance therapy. It is only 20% to 30% protein bound and can be given by oral or parenteral routes. Additional characteristics of digoxin include the following:

1. Digoxin has a *rapid onset of action*. When given intravenously, onset of action occurs within 10 to 30 minutes, and maximal effects occur in 1 to 5 hours. This rapid onset of action allows digoxin to be used in emergency situations when rapid digitalization is desired. When given orally, onset of action occurs in 30 minutes to 2 hours, and maximal effects occur in about 6 hours.
2. Digoxin has a *serum half-life of 1 to 2 days*. When

digoxin therapy is initiated with maintenance doses, therapeutic serum levels and maximal drug benefit are achieved in about 1 week. When digoxin is discontinued, the drug is eliminated from the body in about 1 week. This characteristic is advantageous in titrating dosage to achieve optimal therapeutic effects without toxicity. In addition, if toxicity does occur, toxic effects are not prolonged.

3. The *absorption of oral preparations* is influenced by several factors:
   a. The most efficiently absorbed oral digoxin preparations are the liquid-filled capsules (Lanoxicaps) and the elixir used for children. Lanoxicaps are reportedly close to intravenous digoxin in bioavailability. Capsules containing 0.1 mg are equivalent to 0.125-mg tablets, and 0.2-mg capsules are equivalent to 0.25-mg tablets. The elixir dosage form is approximately 90% absorbed.
   b. Digoxin tablets vary in rate of absorption from 40% to 75%. Differences in bioavailability may be a significant clinical problem, because a person may be stabilized on a particular brand of digoxin but underdosed or overdosed if another brand is taken. Differences are attributed to rate and extent of tablet dissolution rather than amounts of digoxin.
   c. Digoxin absorption is delayed or decreased by the presence of food in the gastrointestinal tract, delayed gastric emptying, malabsorption syndromes, and concurrent administration of some drugs (*e.g.*, antacids, cholestyramine, colestipol).
4. Most (60%–70%) of digoxin is *excreted unchanged by the kidneys*. Dosage must be reduced in the presence of renal failure to prevent drug accumulation and toxicity. The remainder is metabolized or excreted by nonrenal routes.
5. *Serum levels*. Therapeutic serum levels of digoxin are 0.5 to 2 ng/ml; toxic serum levels are above 2 ng/ml. However, toxicity may occur at virtually any serum level.
6. *Routes*. The preferred routes of administration for digoxin are oral and intravenous. Although the parenteral solution can be given intramuscularly, this route may cause severe pain and muscle necrosis at the site of injection.
7. *Available preparations* include *tablets* containing 0.125 mg, 0.25 mg, or 0.5 mg; *capsules* (Lanoxicaps) containing 0.05 mg, 0.1 mg, or 0.2 mg; *solutions for injection* containing 0.1 mg/ml in a 1-ml ampule or 0.25 mg/ml in a 2-ml ampule; and a *pediatric elixir* containing 0.05 mg/ml.

### Routes and dosage ranges

*Adults and children over 10 years:* Digitalizing dose, PO 0.75–1 mg in three or four divided doses over 24 h; IV 0.5–0.75 mg in divided doses over 24 h Maintenance dose, PO, IV 0.125–0.5 mg/d (average, 0.25)

*Children 2–10 years:* Digitalizing dose, PO 0.02–0.04 mg/kg in four divided doses q6h; IV 0.015–0.035 mg/kg in four divided doses q6h

Maintenance dose, PO, IV about 20%–35% of the digitalizing dose

*Children 1 month–2 years:* Digitalizing dose, PO 0.035–0.06 mg/kg in four divided doses q6h; IV 0.035–0.05 mg/kg in four divided doses q6h

Maintenance dose, PO, IV about 20%–35% of the digitalizing dose

*Newborns:* Digitalizing dose, PO 0.025–0.035 mg/kg in four divided doses q6h; IV 0.02–0.03 mg/kg in four divided doses q6h

Maintenance dose, PO, IV about 20%–35% of the digitalizing dose

**Digitoxin** (Crystodigin) has a slow onset of action, a long interval to peak action time, a long half-life, and is 90% to 95% protein bound. It is used for maintenance therapy rather than rapid digitalization. Compared to digoxin, digitoxin has the following characteristics:

1. *Slower onset of action.* When given intravenously, onset of action occurs in 30 to 120 minutes with maximal effects in 4 to 8 hours. When given orally, onset of action occurs in 3 to 6 hours with maximal effects in 8 to 12 hours.
2. *Half-life of 7 days.* If digitoxin therapy is initiated with maintenance doses, therapeutic serum levels and maximal effects do not occur for about 1 month. This delay may be somewhat minimized by initiating therapy with loading doses. When digitoxin is discontinued, about 1 month is required for elimination of the drug from the body. The longer duration of action may be an advantage for clients who are unable or unwilling to take digitoxin daily, because therapeutic effects persist for several days after a dose. However, if toxicity occurs, the delay in drug elimination prolongs toxic effects.
3. *Absorption.* Digitoxin tablets are well absorbed from the intestinal tract (90%–100%). However, absorption is delayed or decreased by the presence of food in the gastrointestinal tract, delayed gastric emptying, and malabsorption syndromes.
4. *Metabolism.* Digitoxin is metabolized in the liver, excreted in bile, reabsorbed from the gastrointestinal tract, and eventually excreted in the urine as inactive metabolites. For this reason, digitoxin may be the digitalis preparation of choice in clients with renal failure.
5. *Serum levels.* Therapeutic serum levels of digitoxin are 10–35 ng/ml. Toxic serum levels are above 35 ng/ml.

### Route and dosage range

*Adults and children over 12 years:* PO 0.1–0.2 mg daily

**Deslanoside** (Cedilanid-D) is occasionally used for rapid digitalization (onset of action, 10–30 minutes; maximal effects, 2–3 hours). If used, another digitalis glycoside must be given for maintenance therapy because no oral dosage form is available.

### Routes and dosage range

*Adults:* Digitalizing dose IM, IV 0.8–1.6 mg in divided doses over 24 h

## AMRINONE AND MILRINONE

**Amrinone** (Inocor) and **milrinone IV** (Primacor) are cardiotonic-inotropic agents used in short-term management of severe CHF that is not controlled by digitalis, diuretics, and vasodilators. The drugs increase levels of cyclic adenosine monophosphate (cAMP) in myocardial cells by inhibiting phosphodiesterase, the enzyme that normally metabolizes cAMP. They also relax vascular smooth muscle to produce vasodilation and decrease preload and afterload. In CHF, inotropic and vasodilator effects increase cardiac output. Compared to amrinone, milrinone is reportedly more potent as an inotropic agent and causes fewer adverse effects. A high incidence of serious adverse effects was observed with oral preparations of both drugs. Consequently, both drugs are given only by intravenous infusions.

Amrinone

### Route and dosage ranges

*Adults:* IV injection (loading dose), 0.75 mg/kg slowly, over 2–3 min

IV infusion (maintenance dose), 5–10 μg/kg per minute, diluted in 0.9% or 0.45% NaCl solution to a concentration of 1–3 mg/ml; maximum dosage, 10 mg/kg per day

Milrinone

### Route and dosage ranges

*Adults:* IV bolus infusion (loading dose), 50 μg/kg over 10 min

IV continuous infusion (maintenance dose), 0.375–0.75 μg/kg per minute, diluted in 0.9% or 0.45% NaCl solution or 5% dextrose injection

## Nursing Process

### Assessment

Assess clients for current or potential CHF:
• Identify risk factors for CHF:
  • *Cardiovascular disorders*: atherosclerosis, hypertension, coronary artery disease, myocardial infarction, cardiac arrhythmias, cardiac valvular disease. Hypertension is one of the most frequent causes of CHF, especially if it is longstanding and inadequately treated.

- *Noncardiovascular disorders*: severe infections, hyperthyroidism, pulmonary disease (*e.g.*, cor pulmonale—right-sided heart failure resulting from lung disease)
- *Other factors*: excessive amounts of intravenous fluids, rapid infusion of intravenous fluids or blood transfusions, advanced age
- A *combination* of any of the above factors
- Interview and observe for signs and symptoms of chronic CHF. Within the clinical syndrome of CHF, clinical manifestations vary from few and mild to many and severe, depending on the heart's pumping ability. Specific signs and symptoms include the following:
  - *Mild CHF.* Common signs and symptoms of mild CHF are ankle edema, dyspnea on exertion, and easy fatigue with exercise. Edema results from increased venous pressure, which allows fluids to leak into tissues; dyspnea and fatigue result from tissue hypoxia.
  - *Moderate or severe CHF.* More extensive edema, dyspnea, and fatigue at rest are likely to occur. Additional signs and symptoms include orthopnea, postnocturnal dyspnea, and cough (from congestion of the respiratory tract with venous blood); mental confusion (from cerebral hypoxia); oliguria and decreased renal function (from decreased blood flow to the kidneys); and anxiety.
- Observe for signs and symptoms of acute heart failure. Acute pulmonary edema indicates acute heart failure and is a medical emergency. Causes include acute myocardial infarction, cardiac arrhythmias, severe hypertension, acute fluid or salt overload, and certain drugs (*e.g.*, quinidine and other cardiac depressants, propranolol and other antiadrenergics, and phenylephrine, norepinephrine, and other alpha-adrenergic stimulants). Pulmonary edema occurs when left ventricular failure causes blood to accumulate in pulmonary veins and tissues. As a result, the person experiences severe dyspnea, hypoxia, hypertension, tachycardia, hemoptysis, frothy respiratory tract secretions, and anxiety.

Assess clients for signs and symptoms of atrial tachyarrhythmias:

- Record the rate and rhythm of apical and radial pulses. Atrial fibrillation, the most common atrial arrhythmia, is characterized by tachycardia, pulse deficit (faster apical rate than radial rate), and a very irregular rhythm. Fatigue, dizziness, and fainting may occur.
- Check the electrocardiogram (ECG) for abnormal P waves, rapid rate of ventricular contraction, and QRS complexes of normal configuration but irregular intervals.

Assess baseline vital signs; weight; edema; laboratory reports of potassium, magnesium, and calcium levels; and other tests of cardiovascular function when available.

Assess a baseline ECG before digitalis therapy when possible. If a client is in normal sinus rhythm, later ECGs may aid recognition of digitalis toxicity (*i.e.*, drug-induced arrhythmias). If a client has an atrial tachyarrhythmia and is receiving digitalis to slow the ventricular rate, later ECGs may aid recognition of therapeutic and adverse effects. For clients who are already receiving digitalis at the initial contact, a baseline ECG can still be valuable because changes in later ECGs may promote earlier recognition and treatment of drug-induced arrhythmias.

## Nursing diagnoses

- Altered Tissue Perfusion related to decreased cardiac output
- Activity Intolerance related to decreased cardiac output
- Self-Care Deficit related to dyspnea and fatigue
- Anxiety related to chronic illness and life-style changes
- Impaired Gas Exchange related to venous congestion and fluid accumulation in lungs
- High Risk for Decreased Cardiac Output related to drug-induced arrhythmias
- Sensory-Perceptual Alterations related to drug-induced changes in vision
- High Risk for Altered Nutrition: Less than Body Requirements related to digoxin-induced anorexia, nausea, and vomiting
- High Risk for Noncompliance related to the need for long-term drug therapy and regular medical supervision
- Knowledge Deficit: Managing drug therapy regimen safely and effectively

## Planning/Goals

*The client will:*
- Take drugs safely and accurately
- Experience improved breathing and less fatigue and edema
- Maintain serum digoxin levels within therapeutic ranges
- Be closely monitored for therapeutic and adverse effects, especially during digitalization, when dosage is being changed, and when other drugs are added to or removed from the treatment regimen
- Keep appointments for follow-up monitoring of vital signs, serum potassium levels, serum digoxin level, and renal function

## Interventions

Use measures to prevent or minimize CHF and atrial arrhythmias. In the broadest sense, preventive measures include sensible eating habits (a balanced diet, avoiding excess saturated fat and salt, weight control), avoiding cigarette smoking, and regular exercise. In the client at risk for developing CHF and arrhythmias, preventive measures include the following:

- Treatment of hypertension
- Avoidance of hypoxia
- Weight control
- Avoidance of excess sodium in the diet
- Avoidance of fluid overload, especially in elderly clients
- Maintenance of treatment programs for CHF, atrial arrhythmias, and other cardiovascular or noncardiovascular disorders

Monitor vital signs, weight, urine output, and serum potassium regularly, and compare with baseline values.

Monitor ECGs when available, and compare with baseline or previous tracings.

## Teach clients:

- The importance of taking digitalis preparations as prescribed. *Do not* miss a dose. *Do not* take an extra dose. *Do not* take other prescription or nonprescription drugs without consulting the physician who prescribed digoxin. All these precautions are necessary to increase the drug's safety and effectiveness. The drug must be taken regularly to maintain therapeutic blood levels, but overuse may cause serious adverse effects. Also, several drugs interact with digoxin to increase or decrease its effects.

- That when taking a diuretic and a potassium supplement with a digitalis preparation, the drugs should not be altered in dosage or frequency of administration or discontinued without consulting the physician. The balance among these drugs must be maintained for safety. If the diuretic is continued and the potassium stopped, hypokalemia may occur and precipitate cardiac arrhythmias. If the diuretic is stopped, edema is likely to recur or worsen. If the diuretic is stopped but the potassium is continued, hyperkalemia may occur.
- That important adverse drug effects should be reported to the physician or nurse, such as undesirable changes in heart rate or rhythm, gastrointestinal upset, or visual problems.
- *Not* to use salt substitutes without consulting a health-care provider. Salt substitutes contain potassium, which may be contraindicated, especially if a potassium supplement is being taken. Excessive potassium is cardiotoxic.

### Evaluation

- Interview and observe for relief of symptoms (weight loss, increased urine output, less extremity edema, easier breathing, improved activity tolerance and self-care ability, slower heart rate).
- Observe serum drug levels for normal or abnormal values, when available.
- Interview regarding compliance with instructions for taking the drug.
- Interview and observe for adverse drug effects, especially cardiac arrhythmias.

# Principles of therapy

## TREATMENT OF CONGESTIVE HEART FAILURE

The main treatment measures for CHF consist of drug therapy and diet therapy.

1. *Drug therapy* for CHF has become controversial in relation to choice of drug and duration of administration. Until recent years, a digitalis preparation and a diuretic were considered the best treatment. Now, however, many previous assumptions and practices are being challenged, and opinions differ about the role of digitalis and other drugs. Factors influencing the viewpoints include the high incidence of adverse drug effects, greater understanding of the basic pathophysiology of CHF, and the development of new drugs or new uses for older drugs. More specifically:

   a. Some authorities recommend monotherapy with either digitalis or a diuretic, or a combination of the two, for initial treatment. Other drugs are added only if signs and symptoms persist or recur despite treatment.

   b. Some authorities suggest that digitalis is indicated when CHF is accompanied by atrial tachyarrhythmias (to slow ventricular response and decrease the workload of the heart), but it may not be needed with normal sinus rhythm. These physicians may use a diuretic as the initial drug of choice, with digitalis as a second choice if needed or even as a third-choice drug after a vasodilator.

   c. For both groups, vasodilators have assumed greater importance. Even with these, however, some cardiologists recommend vasodilator therapy early in the course of the disease, while others recommend it only for severe CHF that is not controlled by other drugs.

   d. ACE inhibitors are being increasingly used as monotherapy or as part of a multidrug regimen with digitalis, a diuretic, or both. All three types of drugs may be indicated for severe CHF. ACE inhibitors prevent formation of angiotensin II, a strong vasoconstrictor and stimulator of aldosterone release. Beneficial effects of ACE inhibitors stem mainly from the vasodilation and decreased retention of sodium and water that result from decreased formation of angiotensin II. In addition, studies indicate improved survival rates and relief of symptoms in clients with CHF.

   e. Another challenge to traditional therapy is whether digitalis should be continued throughout the client's life or whether it can be safely stopped. Some studies indicate that digitalis can be discontinued in some clients without recurrence of heart failure, but no clear-cut criteria exist for selecting these clients.

   f. At present, amrinone and milrinone are indicated only for short-term treatment of CHF that does not respond to other measures.

2. *Diet therapy.* Dietary sodium restriction may reduce edema and allow a decrease in dosage of diuretics. For most clients, sodium restriction need not be severe. A common order, "no added salt," may be accomplished by avoiding obviously salty food (*e.g.*, ham, potato chips, snack foods) and by not adding salt during cooking or eating. A major source of sodium intake is table salt: A level teaspoonful contains 2300 mg of sodium.

## GUIDELINES FOR DIGITALIS THERAPY

1. **Choice of digitalis preparation** and route of administration depend primarily on the client's condition and the rapidity with which therapeutic effects are desired.

   a. Digoxin is the drug of choice in most situations because it can be used for rapid or slow digitalization, and if toxicity occurs, the drug leaves the body within a few days. It is the most commonly used digitalis preparation for adults and children.

b. Digitoxin may be the drug of choice in clients with renal disease, because it is excreted primarily by the liver rather than by the kidneys.

c. Deslanoside may be given parenterally for rapid digitalization, but it offers no significant advantage over digoxin.

d. Preferred routes of digitalis administration are oral and intravenous. The intramuscular route is not recommended because pain and muscle necrosis may occur at intramuscular injection sites.

2. **Dosage of digitalis preparations** must be individualized.

a. Digitalis dosages are usually stated as the average amounts needed for digitalization and maintenance therapy. These dosages must be interpreted with consideration of specific client characteristics. Digitalizing or loading doses are safe *only* for a short period, usually 24 hours. In addition, loading doses should be used cautiously in clients who have taken digitalis preparations within the previous 2 or 3 weeks. Maintenance doses, which are much smaller than digitalizing doses, may be safely used to initiate digitalis therapy and are always used for long-term digitalis therapy.

b. Generally, larger doses are needed to slow the heart rate in atrial arrhythmias than to increase myocardial contractility in CHF.

c. Smaller doses (loading and maintenance) should be given to clients who are elderly or who have hypothyroidism. Because metabolism and excretion of digitalis preparations are delayed in such people, the drugs may accumulate and cause toxicity if dosage is not reduced. Dosage also should be reduced in clients with hypokalemia, extensive myocardial damage, or cardiac conduction disorders. These conditions increase risks of digitalis-induced arrhythmias.

d. Dosage can be titrated according to client response. In CHF, severity of symptoms, ECGs, and serum drug concentrations are useful. In atrial fibrillation, dosage can be altered to produce the desired decrease in the ventricular rate of contraction. Optimal dosage is the lowest amount that relieves signs and symptoms of heart failure or alters heart rate and rhythm toward normal without producing toxicity.

e. Intravenous dosage of digoxin should be 20% to 30% less than oral dosage.

f. Dosage of digoxin must be reduced by about half in the presence of renal failure or when certain drugs are given concurrently.

(1) With renal failure, digoxin dosage should be based on signs and symptoms of toxicity, creatinine clearance, and serum drug levels. Because most digoxin is excreted renally, failure to reduce dosage in clients with renal failure leads to drug accumulation in the body, with resultant toxicity.

(2) When given concurrently with digoxin, quinidine, nifedipine (Procardia), and verapamil (Calan) slow digoxin excretion and increase serum digoxin levels. As a result, digoxin may accumulate and cause toxicity.

3. **Maintenance therapy in the hospitalized client** must be individualized. Hospitalized clients may be unable to take a daily maintenance dose of digitalis at the scheduled time owing to diagnostic tests, treatment measures, or other reasons. As a general rule, the dose should be given later rather than omitted. If the client is having surgery, the nurse often must ask the physician whether the drug should be given on the day of surgery (*i.e.*, orally with a small amount of water or parenterally) and whether the drug should be reordered postoperatively. Many clients require continued digitalis therapy. However, if a dose is missed, probably no ill effects will occur, because the pharmacologic actions of both digoxin and digitoxin persist longer than 24 hours.

4. **Electrolyte balance** must be monitored and maintained during digitalis therapy, particularly normal serum levels of potassium (3.5–5 mEq/L), magnesium (1.5–2.5 mg/100 ml), and calcium (8.5–10 mg/100 ml). Hypokalemia and hypomagnesemia increase cardiac excitability and ectopic pacemaker activity, leading to arrhythmias; hypercalcemia enhances digitalis effects. These electrolyte abnormalities increase the risk of digitalis toxicity. Hypocalcemia increases excitability of nerve and muscle cell membranes and causes myocardial contraction to be weak (leading to a decrease in digitalis effect).

The most common electrolyte abnormality is hypokalemia because potassium-losing diuretics are often given concurrently with digitalis preparations in the treatment of CHF. Supplemental potassium may be given to maintain normal serum levels.

5. **Identification and treatment of digitalis toxicity** require attention to several factors.

a. *Identification.* A persistent difficulty in digitalis therapy is the similarity between the signs and symptoms of heart disease for which digitalis is given and the signs and symptoms of digitalis intoxication. Continued atrial fibrillation with a rapid ventricular response may indicate inadequate dosage. However, other arrhythmias may indicate toxicity. Premature ventricular contractions commonly occur. Serum drug levels and ECGs may be helpful in verifying suspected toxicity. Serum digoxin levels should be drawn just before a dose. Drug distribution to tissues requires about 6 hours after a dose is given; if the blood is drawn before 6 hours, the level may be high.

b. *Discontinued dose.* When signs and symptoms of digitalis toxicity occur, digitalis should be discontinued, not just reduced in dosage. Most clients with mild or early toxicity recover completely within a few days after the drug is discontinued. If serious cardiac arrhythmias are present, more aggressive treatment measures may be indicated.

c. *Drug therapy.* Drugs used to treat cardiac arrhythmias resulting from digitalis intoxication include:

(1) *Potassium chloride*, a myocardial depressant that acts to decrease myocardial excitability. The dose depends on the severity of toxicity, serum potassium level, and client response. Potassium is contraindicated in renal failure and should be used with caution in the presence of cardiac conduction defects.

(2) *Lidocaine*, an antiarrhythmic local anesthetic agent commonly used in the treatment of digitalis-induced arrhythmias. It acts to decrease myocardial irritability.

(3) *Atropine* or *isoproterenol*, used in the treatment of bradycardia or conduction defects

(4) *Other antiarrhythmic drugs.* These may be used but are generally less effective in digitalis-induced arrhythmias than in arrhythmias due to other causes.

(5) *Digoxin immune fab* (Digibind, Digidote) is a digitalis-binding antidote derived from specific antidigoxin antibodies produced in sheep. It is recommended only for life-threatening toxicity. See manufacturers' instructions for dosage calculation and administration.

## USE IN CHILDREN

Digoxin is commonly used in children for the same indications as for adults. The response to a given dose varies with age, size, and renal and hepatic function. There may be little difference between a therapeutic dose and a toxic dose. Very small amounts are often given to children. These factors increase the risks of dosage errors in children, and each dose should be verified with an-other nurse before it is administered. ECG monitoring is desirable when digoxin therapy is started.

As in adults, dosage of digoxin should be individualized and carefully titrated. Digoxin is primarily excreted by the kidneys, and dosage must be reduced with impaired renal function. Divided daily doses should be given to infants and children under 10 years, and adult dosages adjusted to their weight should be given to children older than 10. Larger doses are usually needed to slow a too-rapid ventricular rate in children with atrial fibrillation or flutter. Differences in bioavailability of different preparations (parenterals, capsules, elixirs, and tablets) must be considered when switching from one preparation to another.

Neonates vary in tolerance of digoxin, depending on their degree of maturity. Premature and immature infants are especially sensitive to drug effects. Dosage must be reduced and digitalization should be even more individualized and cautiously approached than in more mature infants and children. Early signs of toxicity in newborns are undue slowing of sinus rate, sinoatrial arrest, and prolongation of the PR interval.

## USE IN OLDER ADULTS

Digoxin is widely used and a frequent cause of adverse effects in older adults. The usual recommended dose is 0.125 to 0.25 mg daily. Reduced dosages are usually required because of decreased liver or kidney function, decreased lean body weight, and advanced cardiac disease. All of these characteristics are common in older adults. Impaired renal function leads to slower drug excretion and increased risk of accumulation, so smaller doses are needed. Dosage must be reduced by about 50% with renal failure or concurrent administration of quinidine, nifedipine, or verapamil. These drugs increase serum digoxin levels and increase risks of toxicity if dosage is not reduced. Antacids decrease absorption of oral digoxin and should not be given at the same time.

A client's need for digoxin should be reevaluated periodically. Dosage needs may change, or the drug may no longer be needed.

Digitoxin, which is excreted by the liver, is rarely used but may be preferred if renal function is impaired.

## NURSING ACTIONS: CARDIOTONIC-INOTROPIC DRUGS

**Nursing Actions**

**Rationale/Explanation**

1. **Administer accurately**
   **a.** With digitalis preparations:

   (1) Read the drug label and the physician's order carefully when preparing a dose of any digitalis preparation.

   Owing to name similarity, especially digoxin and digitoxin, special care must be taken to avoid giving one for the other, because dose and potency differ.

   (2) Check the apical pulse before each dose. If the rate is below 60 in adults or 100 in children, omit the dose, and notify the physician.

   Bradycardia is an adverse effect.

   (3) Have the same nurse give digitalis to the same clients when possible because it is important to detect *changes* in rate and rhythm (see *Observe for therapeutic effects* and *Observe for adverse effects*, below).

   (4) Give oral digitalis preparations with food or after meals.

   This may minimize gastric irritation and symptoms of anorexia, nausea, and vomiting. However, these symptoms probably arise from drug stimulation of chemoreceptors in the medulla rather than a direct irritant effect of the drug on the gastrointestinal (GI) tract.

   (5) Inject IV digitalis preparations slowly (over at least 5 minutes).

   Digoxin should be given slowly because the diluent, propylene glycol, has toxic effects on the cardiac conduction system if given too rapidly. Digoxin may be given undiluted or diluted with a fourfold or greater volume of sterile water for injection, 0.9% sodium chloride injection, or 5% dextrose injection. If diluted, use the solution immediately.

   **b.** With amrinone:

   (1) Give undiluted or diluted to a concentration of 1 mg/ml to 3 mg/ml.

   (2) Dilute with 0.9% or 0.45% sodium chloride solution, and use the diluted solution within 24 hours. Do not dilute with solutions containing dextrose.

   Amrinone may be injected into IV tubing containing a dextrose solution because contact is brief. However, a chemical interaction occurs with prolonged contact.

   (3) Give bolus injections into the tubing of an IV infusion, over 2 to 3 minutes.

   (4) Administer maintenance infusions at a rate of 5 to 10 µg/kg per minute.

   **c.** With milrinone, consult manufacturer's instructions.

2. **Observe for therapeutic effects**
   **a.** When the drugs are given in congestive heart failure (CHF), observe for:

   (1) Fewer signs and symptoms of pulmonary congestion (dyspnea, orthopnea, cyanosis, cough, hemoptysis, rales, anxiety, restlessness)

   The pulmonary symptoms that develop with CHF are a direct result of events initiated by inadequate cardiac output. The left side of the heart is unable to accommodate incoming blood flow from the lungs. The resulting back pressure in pulmonary veins and capillaries causes leakage of fluid from blood vessels into tissue spaces and alveoli. Fluid accumulation may result in severe respiratory difficulty and pulmonary edema, a life-threatening development. The improved strength of myocardial contraction resulting from cardiotonic-inotropic drugs reverses this potentially fatal chain of events.

## Nursing Actions

## Rationale/Explanation

(2) Decreased edema—absence of pitting, decreased size of ankles or abdominal girth, decreased weight

Diuresis and decreased edema result from improved circulation and increased renal blood flow.

(3) Increased tolerance of activity

Indicates a more adequate supply of blood to tissues

**b.** When digitalis is given in atrial arrhythmias, observe for:

(1) Gradual slowing of the heart rate to 70 to 80 beats per minute

(2) Elimination of the pulse deficit

In clients with atrial fibrillation, slowing of the pulse rate and elimination of the pulse deficit are rough guides that digitalization has been achieved.

(3) Change in rhythm from irregular to regular

**3. Observe for adverse effects**
  **a.** With digitalis, observe for:

There is a high incidence of adverse effects with digitalis therapy. Therefore, every client receiving a digitalis preparation requires close observation. Severity of adverse effects can be minimized with early detection and treatment.

(1) Cardiac arrhythmias:

Digitalis toxicity may cause any type of cardiac arrhythmia. These are the most serious adverse effects associated with digitalis therapy. They are detected as abnormalities in ECGs and in pulse rate or rhythm.

(a) Premature ventricular contractions (PVCs)

PVCs are among the most common digitalis-induced arrhythmias. They are not specific for digitalis toxicity because there are many possible causes. They are usually perceived as "skipped" heartbeats.

(b) Bradycardia

Excessive slowing of the pulse rate is an extension of the drug's therapeutic action of slowing conduction through the AV node and probably depressing the SA node as well.

(c) Paroxysmal atrial tachycardia with heart block

(d) AV nodal tachycardia

(e) AV block (second- or third-degree heart block)

(2) Anorexia, nausea, vomiting

These GI effects commonly occur with digitalis therapy. Because they are caused, at least in part, by stimulation of the vomiting center in the brain, they occur with parenteral and oral administration. The presence of these symptoms raises suspicion of digitalis toxicity, but they are not specific because many other conditions may cause anorexia, nausea, and vomiting. Also, clients receiving digitalis are often taking other medications that cause these side effects, such as diuretics and potassium supplements.

(3) Headache, drowsiness, confusion

These CNS effects are most common in older adults.

(4) Visual disturbances (*e.g.*, blurred vision, photophobia, altered perception of colors, flickering dots)

These are due mainly to drug effects on the retina and may indicate acute toxicity.

**b.** With amrinone, observe for:

(1) Thrombocytopenia

Thrombocytopenia is more likely to occur with prolonged therapy and is usually reversible if dosage is reduced or the drug is discontinued.

(2) Anorexia, nausea, vomiting, abdominal pain

GI symptoms can be decreased by reducing drug dosage

*(continued)*

| Nursing Actions | Rationale/Explanation |
|---|---|
| (3) Hypotension | Hypotension probably results from vasodilatory effects of amrinone |
| (4) Hepatotoxicity | If marked changes in liver enzymes occur in conjunction with clinical symptoms, the drug should be discontinued |
| **c.** With milrinone, observe for ventricular arrhythmias, hypotension, and headache | Ventricular arrhythmias reportedly occur in 12% of clients, hypotension and headache in about 3% of clients. |
| **4. Observe for drug interactions** | Most significant drug interactions increase risks of toxicity. Some alter absorption or metabolism to produce under-digitalization and decreased therapeutic effect. |
| **a.** Drugs that *increase* effects of digitalis glycosides | |
| (1) Adrenergic drugs (*e.g.*, ephedrine, epinephrine, isoproterenol), succinylcholine | Increase risks of cardiac arrhythmias |
| (2) Antiarrhythmics (*e.g.*, amiodarone, propafenone, quinidine) | Decrease clearance of digoxin, thereby increasing serum digoxin levels and risks of toxicity. Dosage of digoxin should be reduced if one of these drugs is given concurrently (about 25% with propafenone and about 50% with amiodarone and quinidine). |
| (3) Anticholinergics | Increase absorption of oral digitalis preparations by slowing transit time through the GI tract |
| (4) Calcium preparations | Increase risks of cardiac arrhythmias. IV calcium salts are contraindicated in digitalized clients. |
| (5) Calcium channel blockers (*e.g.*, diltiazem, felodipine, nifedipine, verapamil) | Decrease clearance of digoxin, thereby increasing serum digoxin levels and risks of toxicity. Dosage of digoxin should be reduced about 25% if verapamil is given concurrently. |
| **b.** Drugs that *decrease* effects of digitalis glycosides | |
| (1) Antacids, cholestyramine, colestipol, laxatives, oral aminoglycosides (*e.g.*, neomycin) | Decrease absorption of oral digitalis preparations |
| (2) Barbiturates, phenytoin, rifampin | Activate liver enzymes and accelerate metabolism of digitoxin |
| **5. Teach clients about digitalis**<br>**a.** Name of drug, dose, reason receiving | |
| **b.** Teach the client or a family member to check the radial pulse at least once daily. Omit digitalis and report to the physician if the pulse is below 60 or unusually irregular in adults or under approximately 100 in children. | Changes in the pulse may indicate adverse drug effects and a need to discontinue the drug. |
| **c.** Take the drug about the same time each day. | To maintain more even blood levels and to assist in remembering to take the drug |

## Review and Application Exercises

1. What signs and symptoms usually occur with CHF? How would you assess for these?
2. What are the physiologic effects of digitalis on the heart?
3. What is digoxin's mechanism of action?
4. How does digoxin produce diuresis?
5. What is digitalization?
6. Differentiate between a digitalizing dose of digoxin and a daily maintenance dose.
7. Why do nurses need to check heart rate and rhythm before giving digoxin?
8. When is it appropriate to withhold a dose of digoxin?
9. What are adverse effects associated with digoxin, and how may they be prevented or minimized?

10. For clients with renal failure who need digitalis, what are the options for safe, effective therapy?
11. Why is it important to maintain a therapeutic serum potassium level during digitalis therapy?
12. Which commonly used cardiovascular drugs increase blood levels of digoxin and risks of toxicity?
13. What is the antidote for severe digitalis toxicity?

## Selected References

Beare, P. G., & Myers, J. L. (Eds.) (1990). *Principles and practice of adult health nursing*. St. Louis: C.V. Mosby.

Brater, D. C. (1992). Clinical pharmacology of cardiovascular drugs. In W. N. Kelley (Ed.), *Textbook of internal medicine* (2nd ed.) (pp. 315–335). Philadelphia: J.B. Lippincott.

Brown, B. M. (1992). Nursing management of adults with heart failure. In L. O. Bullock (Ed.), *Adult nursing in hospital and community settings* (pp. 407–418). Norwalk, CT: Appleton & Lange.

Brown, K. K. (1993). Boosting the failing heart with inotropic drugs. *Nursing 93, 23*, 34–44.

Bullock, B. L. (1992). Compromised pumping ability of the heart. In B. L. Bullock & P. P. Rosendahl (Eds.), *Pathophysiology: Adaptations and alterations in function* (3rd ed.) (pp. 479–495). Philadelphia: J.B. Lippincott.

Cohn, J. N. (1992). Approach to the patient with heart failure. In W. N. Kelley (Ed.), *Textbook of internal medicine* (2nd ed.) (pp. 340–347). Philadelphia: J.B. Lippincott.

(1993). *Drug facts and comparisons*. St. Louis: Facts and Comparisons.

Francis, G. S., & Alpert, J. S. (Eds.) (1990). *Modern coronary care*. Boston: Little, Brown.

Guyton, A. C. (1991). *Textbook of medical physiology* (8th ed.). Philadelphia: W.B. Saunders.

Kradjan, W. A. (1992). Congestive heart failure. In M. A. Koda-Kimble & L. Y. Young (Eds.), *Applied therapeutics: The clinical use of drugs* (5th ed.) (pp. 9-1–9-37). Vancouver, WA: Applied Therapeutics.

# CHAPTER 55

# Antiarrhythmic Drugs

## Description

Antiarrhythmic agents are diverse drugs used for prevention and treatment of cardiac arrhythmias. Arrhythmias, also called dysrhythmias, are irregularities in heart rate or rhythm. They become significant when they interfere with cardiac function. To aid in understanding of arrhythmias and antiarrhythmic drug therapy, the physiology of cardiac conduction and contractility is reviewed.

## Cardiac electrophysiology

The heart is an electrical pump. The "electrical" activity resides primarily in the specialized tissues that can generate and conduct an electrical impulse. Although impulses are conducted through muscle cells, the rate is much slower. The mechanical or "pump" activity resides in contractile tissue. Normally, these activities result in effective cardiac contraction and distribution of blood throughout the body. Each heart beat or cardiac cycle occurs at regular intervals and consists of four events. These are *stimulation* from an electrical impulse, *transmission* of the electrical impulse to adjacent conductive or contractile tissue, *contraction* of atria and ventricles, and *relaxation* of atria and ventricles, during which they refill with blood in preparation for the next contraction.

### AUTOMATICITY

Automaticity is the heart's ability to generate an electrical impulse. Any part of the conduction system can spontaneously start an impulse, but the sinoatrial (SA)

node normally has the highest degree of automaticity and therefore the highest rate of spontaneous impulse formation. With its faster rate of electrical discharge or depolarization, the SA node serves as pacemaker and controls heart rate and rhythm.

Initiation of an electrical impulse depends on the movement of sodium and calcium ions into a myocardial cell and the movement of potassium ions out of the cell. Normally, the cell membrane becomes more permeable to sodium and opens pores or channels to allow its rapid movement into the cell. Calcium ions follow sodium ions into the cell at a slower rate. As sodium and calcium ions move into cells, potassium moves out of cells. The movement of the ions changes the membrane from its resting state of electrical neutrality to an activated state of electrical energy buildup. When the electrical energy is discharged (depolarization), muscle contraction occurs.

The ability of a cardiac muscle cell to respond to an electrical stimulus is called *excitability* or *irritability*. The stimulus must reach a certain intensity or threshold to cause contraction. Following contraction, there is a period of decreased excitability (called the *refractory period*) during which the cell cannot respond to a new stimulus. During the refractory period, sodium and calcium ions return to the extracellular space, potassium ions return to the intracellular space, muscle relaxation occurs, and the cell prepares for the next electrical stimulus and contraction.

### CONDUCTIVITY

Conductivity is the ability of cardiac tissue to transmit electrical impulses. Although the electrophysiology of a single myocardial cell can assist understanding of the

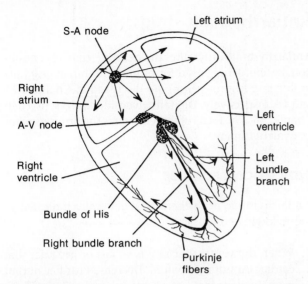

**FIGURE 55-1.** The conducting system of the heart. Impulses originating in the SA node are transmitted through the atria, into the AV node to the bundle of His, and by way of Purkinje fibers through the ventricles.

process, the orderly, rhythmic transmission of impulses to all cells results in effective myocardial contraction.

Normally, electrical impulses originate in the SA node and are transmitted to atrial muscle, where they cause atrial contraction, and then to the atrioventricular (AV) node, bundle of His, bundle branches, Purkinje fibers, and ventricular muscle, where they cause ventricular contraction. The cardiac conduction system is shown in Figure 55-1.

# Cardiac arrhythmias

Cardiac arrhythmias result from disturbances in electrical impulse formation (automaticity), conduction (conductivity), or both. The characteristic of automaticity allows myocardial cells other than the SA node to depolarize and initiate the electrical impulse that culminates in atrial and ventricular contraction. This may occur when the SA node fails to initiate an impulse or does so too slowly. When the electrical impulse arises anywhere other than the SA node, it is an abnormal or ectopic focus. If the ectopic focus depolarizes at a rate faster than the SA node, the ectopic focus becomes the dominant pacemaker. Ectopic pacemakers may arise in the atria, AV node, Purkinje fibers, or ventricular muscle. They may be activated by hypoxia, ischemia, or hypokalemia. Ectopic foci indicate myocardial irritability (increased responsiveness to stimuli) and potentially serious impairment of cardiac function.

A common mechanism by which abnormal conduction causes arrhythmias is called *re-entry excitation*. With

normal conduction, the electrical impulse moves freely down the conduction system until it reaches recently excited tissue that is refractory to stimulation. This causes the impulse to be extinguished. The SA node then recovers, fires spontaneously, and the conduction process starts over again.

Re-entry excitation means that an impulse continues to re-enter an area of the heart rather than becoming extinguished. For this to occur, the impulse must encounter an obstacle in the normal conducting pathway. The obstacle is usually an area of damage, such as myocardial infarction. The damaged area allows conduction in only one direction and causes a circular movement of the impulse.

## TYPES OF ARRHYTHMIAS

Arrhythmias may be mild or severe, acute or chronic, episodic or relatively continuous. They are clinically significant if they interfere with cardiac function (*i.e.*, the heart's ability to pump sufficient blood to all body tissues). The normal heart can maintain an adequate cardiac output with ventricular rates ranging from 40 to 180 beats per minute. The diseased heart, however, may not be able to maintain an adequate cardiac output with heart rates below 60 or above 120.

Arrhythmias are usually categorized by rate, location, or patterns of conduction. They may originate in the SA node (sinus arrhythmias), atria, AV node (nodal arrhythmias), bundle branches, or ventricles. Commonly occurring arrhythmias include sinus tachycardia, sinus bradycardia, premature atrial contractions (PACs), paroxysmal atrial tachycardia (PAT), atrial fibrillation, atrial flutter, AV nodal rhythm, paroxysmal nodal tachycardia, heart block, premature ventricular contractions (PVCs), ventricular fibrillation, and bundle branch blocks.

1. *Sinus arrhythmias* are usually significant only if they are severe or prolonged. Tachycardia increases the workload of the heart and may lead to congestive heart failure or angina pectoris. Sinus tachycardia may cause anginal pain (myocardial ischemia) by two related mechanisms. One mechanism involves increased myocardial oxygen consumption. The other mechanism involves a shortened diastole so that coronary arteries may not have adequate filling time between heart beats. Thus, additional blood flow to the myocardium is required at the same time that a decreased blood supply is delivered.

2. *Atrial arrhythmias* are usually significant only in the presence of underlying heart disease. In coronary artery disease, atrial tachycardia increases myocardial oxygen consumption and shortens diastole. As a result, anginal pain may occur. In aortic valvular disease or hypertrophic myopathies, atrial fibrillation

or flutter may decrease ventricular filling by as much as 30%, so that cardiac output may be severely impaired. Atrial fibrillation and flutter also may lead to the formation of thrombi in the atria.

3. *Nodal arrhythmias* may involve tachycardia and increased workload of the heart or bradycardia from heart block. Either tachycardia or bradycardia may decrease cardiac output. Heart block involves impaired conduction of the electrical impulse through the AV node. With first-degree heart block, conduction is slowed but not significantly. With second-degree heart block, every second, third, or fourth atrial impulse is blocked and does not reach the ventricles (2:1, 3:1, or 4:1 block). Thus, atrial and ventricular rates differ. Second-degree heart block may interfere with cardiac output or progress to third-degree block. Third-degree is the most serious type of heart block because no impulses reach the ventricles. As a result, ventricles beat independently at a rate of 30 to 40 per minute. This slow ventricular rate severely reduces cardiac output.

4. *Ventricular arrhythmias*, the most serious, include PVCs, ventricular tachycardia, and ventricular fibrillation. PVCs occasionally may occur in anyone and are rarely significant. However, PVCs often occur after acute myocardial infarction and with ischemic heart disease. These may be life-threatening or may lead to ventricular tachycardia, ventricular fibrillation, or asystole. PVCs are considered serious if they occur more than five times per minute, are coupled or grouped, are multifocal, or occur during the resting phase of the cardiac cycle.

Ventricular tachycardia increases myocardial oxygen consumption and shortens diastole. Ventricular fibrillation produces ineffective myocardial contraction so that there is no cardiac output. Death results unless effective cardiopulmonary resuscitation (CPR) or defibrillation is instituted within about 4 to 6 minutes.

## NONPHARMACOLOGIC TREATMENT OF ARRHYTHMIAS

Nonpharmacologic treatment is preferred, at least initially, for several arrhythmias. For example, sinus tachycardia usually results from such disorders as infection, dehydration, or hypotension, and treatment should be aimed toward relieving the underlying cause. For paroxysmal supraventricular tachycardia (PSVT) with mild or moderate symptoms, the Valsalva's maneuver, carotid sinus massage, or other measures to increase vagal tone are preferred. For ventricular fibrillation, immediate defibrillation by electrical countershock is the initial treatment of choice.

# Antiarrhythmic drugs

Antiarrhythmic drugs alter the heart's electrical conduction system. Drugs used for bradyarrhythmias (*e.g.*, atropine and isoproterenol) are discussed in Chapters 21 and 18, respectively. Digitalis glycosides are discussed in Chapter 54. The focus of this chapter is the drugs used for tachyarrhythmias.

## INDICATIONS FOR USE

Antiarrhythmic drug therapy is generally indicated in the following conditions:

1. When the ventricular rate is so fast or irregular that cardiac output is impaired. Decreased cardiac output leads to symptoms of decreased systemic, cerebral, and coronary circulation.
2. When PVCs may develop into serious episodes of ventricular tachycardia
3. When dangerous arrhythmias have already developed and may be fatal if not quickly terminated. For example, ventricular tachycardia may cause cardiac arrest.

## MECHANISMS OF ACTION

Drugs used for rapid arrhythmias mainly *reduce automaticity* (spontaneous depolarization of myocardial cells, including ectopic pacemakers), *slow conduction* of electrical impulses through the heart, and *prolong the refractory period* of myocardial cells (so they are less likely to be prematurely activated by adjacent cells). Several different groups of drugs perform one or more of these actions. They are classified according to their mechanisms of action and effects on the conduction system, even though they differ in other respects.

# Classifications and individual drugs

## CLASS I

Class I drugs block the movement of sodium into cells of the cardiac conducting system. This results in a membrane-stabilizing effect and decreased formation and conduction of electrical impulses. These drugs are sometimes called sodium channel-blockers or local anesthetics.

## Class IA

**Quinidine**, the prototype of class IA, exerts antiarrhythmic effects by reducing automaticity, slowing conduction, and prolonging the refractory period. It is used for chronic therapy of supraventricular and ventricular tachyarrhythmias. For clients with atrial fibrillation or flutter who have converted to normal sinus rhythm with digitalis glycosides or electrical cardioversion, quinidine may be used to maintain normal sinus rhythm. It is also used to prevent frequent PVCs, paroxysmal tachycardia, and postcountershock arrhythmias.

Quinidine is well absorbed after oral administration. Therapeutic serum levels (2–6 µg/ml) are attained within 1 hour and persist for 6 to 8 hours. Quinidine is highly bound to serum albumin, which probably accounts for its relatively long duration of action and its half-life of about 6 hours. Quinidine is metabolized by the liver (about 80%) and excreted in the urine (about 20%). In alkaline urine (*i.e.*, pH above 7), renal excretion of quinidine decreases, and serum levels may rise. Serum levels greater than 8 µg/ml are toxic.

Quinidine's low therapeutic ratio and high incidence of adverse effects limit its clinical usefulness. The drug is usually contraindicated in clients with severe, uncompensated congestive heart failure or with heart block because it depresses myocardial contractility and conduction through the AV node.

**Quinidine salts** used clinically include quinidine gluconate (Quinaglute), quinidine sulfate (Quinora), and quinidine polygalacturonate (Cardioquin). These salts differ in the amount of active drug (quinidine base) they contain and the rate of absorption with oral administration. The sulfate salt contains 83% quinidine base, and peak effects occur in 0.5 to 1.5 hours (4 hours for sustained-release forms). The gluconate salt contains 62% active drug, and peak effects occur in 3 to 4 hours. The polygalacturonate salt contains 60% active drug, and peak effects occur in about 6 hours. Quinidine preparations are usually given orally. The gluconate and polygalacturonate salts reportedly cause less gastrointestinal irritation than quinidine sulfate; this is probably related to their lower quinidine content. Oral extended-action preparations of quinidine (Quinidex Extentabs, Quinaglute Dura-Tabs) also are available.

### Routes and dosage ranges

*Adults:* PO 200–600 mg q6h; maximum dose, 3–4 g/d
 Maintenance dose, PO 200–600 mg q6h, or 1 or 2 extended-action tablets, two or three times per day
 IM (quinidine gluconate) 600 mg initially, then 400 mg q4–6h
 IV (quinidine gluconate) 200 mg in 100 ml of solution, given over 20–30 min with continuous electrocardiogram (ECG) and blood pressure monitoring
*Children:* PO 6 mg/kg q4–6h

**Disopyramide** (Norpace), which is similar to quinidine in pharmacologic actions, is given orally to adults with ventricular tachyarrhythmias. It is well absorbed after oral administration and reaches peak serum levels (2–8 µg/ml) within 30 to 60 minutes. Drug half-life is 5 to 8 hours. Disopyramide is excreted by the kidneys and the liver in almost equal proportions. Dosage must be reduced in renal insufficiency.

### Route and dosage range

*Adults:* PO 300 mg loading dose, followed by 150 mg q6h; usual dose, PO 400–800 mg/d in four divided doses

**Procainamide** (Pronestyl, Procan) is related to the local anesthetic procaine and is similar to quinidine in actions and uses. Quinidine may be preferred for long-term use because procainamide produces a high incidence of adverse effects, including a syndrome resembling lupus erythematosus. Procainamide has a short duration of action (3–4 hours); sustained-release tablets (Procan SR) prolong action to about 6 hours. Therapeutic serum levels are 4 to 8 µg/ml.

### Routes and dosage ranges

*Adults:* PO 1 g loading dose initially, then 250–500 mg q3–4h (q6h for sustained-release tablets)
 IM 500–1000 mg as a single loading dose for rapid drug action, followed by oral maintenance doses
 IV 25–50 mg/min; maximum dose, 1000 mg
*Children:* PO 50 mg/kg per day in four to six divided doses

## Class IB

**Lidocaine** (Xylocaine), a local anesthetic (see Chap. 14), is the prototype of class IB. It is the drug of choice for treating serious ventricular arrhythmias associated with acute myocardial infarction, cardiac surgery, cardiac catheterization, and electrical cardioversion. Lidocaine decreases myocardial irritability (automaticity) in the ventricles. It has little effect on atrial tissue and is not useful in treating atrial arrhythmias. It differs from quinidine in that:

1. It must be given by injection.
2. It does not decrease AV conduction or myocardial contractility with usual therapeutic doses.
3. It has a rapid onset and short duration of action. After intravenous administration of a bolus dose, therapeutic effects occur within 1 to 2 minutes and last about 20 minutes. This characteristic is advantageous in emergency treatment but limits lidocaine usage to intensive care settings.
4. It is metabolized in the liver. Dosage must be reduced in clients with hepatic insufficiency or congestive heart failure to avoid drug accumulation and toxicity.

5. It is less likely to cause heart block, cardiac asystole, ventricular arrhythmias, and congestive heart failure.

Therapeutic serum levels of lidocaine are 2 to 5 μg/ml. Lidocaine may be given intramuscularly in emergencies when intravenous administration is impossible. When given intramuscularly, therapeutic effects occur in about 15 minutes and last about 90 minutes. Lidocaine is contraindicated in clients allergic to related local anesthetics (*e.g.*, procaine). Anaphylactic reactions may occur in sensitized people.

### Routes and dosage ranges

*Adults:* IV 1–2 mg/kg, usually not to exceed 50–100 mg, as a single bolus injection over 2 min, followed by a continuous infusion (1 g of lidocaine in 500 ml of 5% dextrose in water) at a rate to deliver 1–4 mg/min; maximum dose, 300 mg/h.
  IM 4–5 mg/kg as a single dose; may repeat in 60–90 min
*Children:* IV injection 1 mg/kg, followed by IV infusion of 20–50 μg/kg per minute

**Mexiletine** (Mexitil) and **tocainide** (Tonocard) are oral analogs of lidocaine with similar pharmacologic actions. They are used to suppress ventricular arrhythmias, including frequent PVCs and ventricular tachycardia. They are well absorbed from the gastrointestinal tract, and peak serum levels are obtained within 3 hours. Taking the drug with food delays but does not decrease absorption.

Mexiletine

### Route and dosage range

*Adults:* PO 200 mg q8h initially, increased by 50–100 mg every 2 or 3 days if necessary to a maximum of 1200 mg/d

Tocainide

### Route and dosage range

*Adults:* PO 400 mg q8h initially, increased up to 1800 mg/d in three divided doses if necessary

**Phenytoin** (Dilantin), an anticonvulsant (see Chap. 11), may be used to treat arrhythmias produced by digitalis intoxication. Phenytoin decreases automaticity and improves conduction through the AV node. Decreased automaticity helps control arrhythmias, while enhanced conduction may improve cardiac function. Further, because heart block may result from digitalis, quinidine, or procainamide, phenytoin may relieve arrhythmias without intensifying heart block. Phenytoin is not a cardiac depressant. Its only quinidine-like action is to suppress automaticity; otherwise, it counteracts the effects of quinidine and procainamide largely by increasing the rate of conduction. Phenytoin also has a longer half-life (22–36 hours) than other antiarrhythmic drugs. Given intravenously, a therapeutic plasma level (10–20 μg/ml) can be obtained rapidly. Given orally, however, the drug may not reach a steady-state concentration for about 1 week unless loading doses are given initially.

### Routes and dosage ranges

*Adults:* PO, loading dose 13 mg/kg (about 1000 mg) first day, 7.5 mg/kg second and third days; maintenance dose, 4–6 mg/kg per day (average 400 mg) in one or two doses starting on the fourth day of phenytoin therapy
  IV 100 mg every 5 min until the arrhythmia is reversed or toxic effects occur; maximum dose, 1 g/24 h
  IM not recommended for treatment of serious arrhythmias because absorption is delayed

## Class IC

**Flecainide** (Tambocor), and **propafenone** (Rythmol) are oral agents that greatly decrease conduction in the ventricles. They may initiate new arrhythmias or aggravate preexisting arrhythmias, sometimes causing sustained ventricular tachycardia or ventricular fibrillation. These effects are more likely to occur with high doses and rapid dose increases. The drugs are recommended for use only in life-threatening ventricular arrhythmias.

Flecainide

### Route and dosage range

*Adults:* PO 100 mg q12h initially, increased by 50 mg q12h every 4 days until effective; maximum dose, 400 mg/d

Propafenone

### Route and dosage range

*Adults:* PO 150 mg q8h initially, increased to a maximum dose of 1200 mg/d if necessary; usual maintenance dose 150–300 mg q8h

**Moricizine** (Ethmozine) is a newer class I agent with properties of all three subclasses (*i.e.*, IA, IB, and IC), but it is most similar to the class IC agents. It is indicated for treatment of life-threatening ventricular arrhythmias, such as sustained ventricular tachycardia, and contraindicated in clients with heart block, cardiogenic shock, and hypersensitivity reactions to the drug. Following oral administration, onset of action occurs within 2 hours, and duration of action is 10 to 24 hours. The drug is 95% protein bound, extensively metabolized in the liver, and excreted in the urine. Because moricizine may cause new arrhythmias or aggravate preexisting arrhythmias, therapy should be initiated in hospitalized clients with continuous electrocardiographic monitoring.

### Route and dosage range

*Adults:* PO 200–300 mg q8h

## CLASS II

These are the beta-adrenergic blocking agents (see Chap. 19), which exert antiarrhythmic effects by blocking sympathetic nervous system stimulation of beta receptors in the heart. Blockage of receptors in the SA node and ectopic pacemakers decreases automaticity, and blockage of receptors in the AV node increases the refractory period. Beta-blocking agents are most often used to slow the ventricular rate of contraction in supraventricular tachyarrhythmias (*e.g.*, atrial fibrillation, atrial flutter, paroxysmal supraventricular tachycardia). Only four of the beta-blockers marketed in the United States are Food and Drug Administration-approved for treatment of arrhythmias. Acebutolol and propranolol may be used for chronic therapy to prevent ventricular arrhythmias, especially those precipitated by exercise. Beta-blockers are contraindicated in the presence of congestive heart failure unless the arrhythmia being treated is the cause of the heart failure.

**Acebutolol** (Sectral) may be given orally for ventricular arrhythmias. **Esmolol** (Brevibloc) has a rapid onset and short duration of action. It is given intravenously for supraventricular tachyarrhythmias, especially during anesthesia, surgery, or other emergency situation when the ventricular rate must be reduced rapidly. It is not used for chronic therapy. **Propranolol** (Inderal) may be given intravenously for life-threatening arrhythmias or those occurring during anesthesia or orally for chronic therapy. **Sotalol** (Betapace) is a noncardioselective beta-blocker (class II) that also has properties of class III antiarrhythmic drugs. Because its Class III characteristics are considered more important in its antiarrhythmic effects, it is a class III drug (see below).

Acebutolol

### Route and dosage range

*Adults:* PO 200 mg twice daily, increased gradually until optimal response is obtained (usually 600–1200 mg/d)

Esmolol

### Route and dosage range

*Adults:* IV infusion 500 μg/kg per minute initially as a loading dose, followed by a maintenance dose of 50 μg/kg per minute over 4 min. Repeat the same loading dose, and increase maintenance doses in 50-μg/kg increments every 5–10 min until therapeutic effects are obtained. Average maintenance dose, 100 μg/kg per minute.

Propranolol

### Routes and dosage ranges

*Adults:* IV injection 1–3 mg at a rate of 1 mg/min
PO 10–20 mg three or four times per day

## CLASS III

These drugs act to slow repolarization and prolong the refractory period. Because of their adverse effects, they are considered second- or third-line agents and recommended for use only when other drugs are ineffective.

**Amiodarone** (Cordarone) may be effective in supraventricular tachycardia, atrial fibrillation and flutter, and ventricular tachycardia. The drug has a long serum half-life, and therapeutic effects may be delayed 5 to 30 days unless loading doses are given. Effects may persist for several weeks after the drug is discontinued.

Adverse effects include hypothyroidism, hyperthyroidism, pulmonary fibrosis, myocardial depression, hypotension, bradycardia, hepatic dysfunction, central nervous system (CNS) disturbances (depression, insomnia, nightmares, hallucinations), peripheral neuropathy and muscle weakness, bluish discoloration of skin and corneal deposits that may cause photosensitivity, appearance of colored halos around lights, and reduced visual acuity. Most adverse effects are considered dose dependent and reversible.

### Route and dosage ranges

*Adults:* Loading dose, PO 800–1600 mg/d for 1–3 wk, with a gradual decrease to 600–800 mg/d for 1 mo
Maintenance dose, PO 400 mg/d

**Bretylium** (Bretylol) is given parenterally, and its use should be limited to ventricular arrhythmias in the intensive care setting. Because it is excreted almost entirely by the kidney, drug half-life is prolonged with renal insufficiency, and dosage must be reduced. Adverse effects include hypotension and arrhythmias.

### Routes and dosage ranges

*Adults:* IM 5 mg/kg, repeated in 1–2 h then q6–8h
IV 5–10 mg/kg, diluted (10-ml ampule of drug solution in at least 50 ml of IV fluid) and infused over 10–20 min
During CPR, IV 5 mg/kg given by direct injection (undiluted); may be repeated q15–30 min to a maximum total dose of 30 mg/kg

**Sotalol** is well absorbed after oral administration, and peak serum level is reached in 2 to 4 hours. It has an elimination half-life of about 12 hours, and 80% to 90% is excreted unchanged by the kidneys. Sotalol is approved for treatment of life-threatening ventricular arrhythmias refractory to other antiarrhythmic drugs. It is contraindicated in clients with asthma, sinus bradycardia, heart block, cardiogenic shock, heart failure, and previous hypersensitivity to sotalol. Dosage should be individualized, reduced with renal impairment, and increased slowly (*e.g.,* every 2–3 days with normal renal function, at longer intervals with impaired renal function). Arrhythmogenic effects are most likely to occur when therapy is started or when dosage is increased. Most adverse effects are attributed to beta-blocking activity.

### Route and dosage range

*Adults:* PO 80 mg q12h initially, titrated to response; average dose, 160 to 320 mg daily. See manufacturer's recommendations for dosing in renal failure.

## CLASS IV

Class IV drugs are the calcium channel-blockers, which block the movement of calcium into conductile and contractile myocardial cells. As a result, they reduce automaticity of the SA node and ectopic pacemakers, slow conduction through the AV node, and prolong the refractory period in the AV node.

**Diltiazem** (Cardizem) and **verapamil** (Calan, Isoptin) are the only calcium channel-blockers approved for treatment of arrhythmias. Both drugs may be given intravenously to slow the rate of ventricular response and improve cardiovascular function in acute paroxysmal supraventricular tachycardia and in atrial fibrillation and flutter. When given intravenously, the drugs act within 15 minutes and last up to 6 hours. Oral verapamil may be used in the chronic treatment of the above arrhythmias. Diltiazem and verapamil are metabolized by the liver, and metabolites are primarily excreted by the kidneys. The drugs are contraindicated in digitalis toxicity because they may worsen heart block. If used with propranolol or digitalis, caution must be exercised to avoid further impairment of myocardial contractility. *Do not* use intravenous verapamil with intravenous propranolol; potentially fatal bradycardia and hypotension may occur.

Diltiazem

### Route and dosage range

*Adults:* IV injection 0.25 mg/kg (average dose 20 mg) over 2 min. A second dose of 0.35 mg/kg (average, 25 mg) may be given in 15 min, and an IV infusion of 5–15 mg/h may be given up to 24 h, if necessary.

Verapamil

### Routes and dosage ranges

*Adults:* PO 40–120 mg q6–8h
IV 5–10 mg initially, then 10 mg 30 min later if necessary
*Children up to 1 year:* IV injection 0.1–0.2 mg/kg (usual range, 0.75–2.0 mg for a single dose) over 2 min with continuous ECG monitoring
*Children 1–15 years:* IV injection 0.1–0.3 mg/kg (usual range 2–5 mg for a single dose) over 2 min with continuous ECG monitoring; repeat in 30 min if necessary

## UNCLASSIFIED

**Adenosine**, a naturally occurring component of all body cells, is an antiarrhythmic drug (Adenocard) that differs chemically from other agents. Adenosine is used only for treatment of paroxysmal supraventricular tachycardia; it is ineffective in other arrhythmias. It is thought to act by decreasing calcium movement into cells or increasing vagal tone. The drug has a very short duration of action (serum half-life is less than 10 seconds) and a high degree of effectiveness.

### Route and dosage range

*Adults:* IV 6 mg given rapidly over 1–2 sec. If first dose does not slow the supraventricular tachycardia within 1–2 min, give 12 mg rapidly, and repeat one time if necessary.

## *Nursing Process*

### Assessment

Assess the client's condition in relation to cardiac arrhythmias:
- Identify conditions or risk factors that may precipitate arrhythmias. These include the following:
  - Hypoxia
  - Electrolyte imbalances
  - Acid-base imbalances
  - Myocardial infarction, coronary artery disease
  - Cardiac valvular disease
  - Febrile illness
  - Respiratory disorders (*e.g.,* chronic lung disease)
  - Exercise
  - Emotional upset
  - Excessive ingestion of caffeine-containing beverages (*e.g.,* coffee, tea, colas)
  - Cigarette smoking
  - Drug therapy with digitalis glycosides, antiarrhythmic drugs, CNS stimulants, anorexiants, and tricyclic antidepressants
  - Hyperthyroidism
- Observe for clinical signs and symptoms of arrhythmias. Mild or infrequent arrhythmias may be perceived by the

client as palpitations or skipped heart beats. More severe arrhythmias may produce manifestations that reflect decreased cardiac output and other hemodynamic changes, as follows:

- Hypotension, bradycardia or tachycardia, and irregular pulse
- Shortness of breath, dyspnea, and cough from impaired respiration
- Syncope or mental confusion from reduced cerebral blood flow
- Chest pain from decreased coronary artery blood flow. Angina pectoris or myocardial infarction may occur.
- Oliguria from decreased renal blood flow
- When ECGs are available (e.g., 12-lead ECG or continuous ECG monitoring), assess for indications of arrhythmias.

### Nursing diagnoses

- Decreased Cardiac Output related to ineffective pumping action of the heart
- Altered Tissue Perfusion related to decreased cardiac output
- Altered Tissue Perfusion related to drug-induced hypotension
- Activity Intolerance related to weakness and fatigue
- Self-Care Deficit related to decreased tissue perfusion and fatigue
- Impaired Gas Exchange related to decreased tissue perfusion
- Anxiety related to potentially serious illness
- Knowledge Deficit: Pharmacologic and nonpharmacologic management of arrhythmias
- High Risk for Fluid Volume Excess: Peripheral edema and pulmonary congestion related to decreased cardiac output
- High Risk for Noncompliance: Underuse of drugs related to adverse drug effects

### Planning/Goals

*The client will:*
- Receive or take antiarrhythmic drugs accurately
- Avoid conditions that precipitate arrhythmias, when feasible
- Experience improved heart rate, circulation, and activity tolerance
- Be closely monitored for therapeutic and adverse drug effects
- Avoid preventable adverse drug effects
- Have adverse drug effects promptly recognized and treated if they occur
- Keep follow-up appointments for monitoring responses to treatment measures

### Interventions

Use measures to prevent or minimize arrhythmias:
- Treat underlying disease processes that contribute to arrhythmia development. These include cardiovascular (e.g., acute myocardial infarction) and noncardiovascular (e.g., chronic lung disease) disorders.
- Prevent or treat other conditions that predispose to arrhythmias (e.g., hypoxia, electrolyte imbalance).
- Help the client avoid cigarette smoking, overeating, excessive coffee drinking, and other habits that may cause or aggravate arrhythmias. Long-term supervision and counseling may be needed.
- For the client receiving antiarrhythmic drugs, implement the above measures to minimize the incidence and severity

of acute arrhythmias, and help the client comply with drug therapy.

Monitor heart rate and rhythm and blood pressure every 4 to 6 hours.

Check laboratory reports of serum electrolytes and serum drug levels when available. Report abnormal values.

*Teach clients:*
- Ways to prevent or decrease the incidence and severity of fast arrhythmias
- The importance of periodic blood tests, ECGs, and medical supervision
- To avoid over-the-counter cold and asthma remedies, appetite suppressants, and antisleep preparations. These drugs are stimulants that can cause or aggravate irregular heart beats.

### Evaluation

- Check vital signs for improved heart rate and rhythm.
- Interview and observe for relief of symptoms and improved functioning in activities of daily living.
- Interview and observe for hypotension and other adverse drug effects.
- Interview and observe for compliance with instructions for taking antiarrhythmic drugs and other aspects of care.

# Principles of therapy

## REQUIREMENTS FOR DRUG THERAPY

Rational drug therapy for cardiac arrhythmias requires accurate identification of the arrhythmia, understanding of the basic mechanisms causing the arrhythmia, observation of the hemodynamic and ECG effects of the arrhythmia, and knowledge of the pharmacologic actions of specific antiarrhythmic drugs.

## GOALS OF THERAPY

The goals of antiarrhythmic drug therapy are to abolish the abnormal rhythm, restore normal sinus rhythm, and prevent recurrence of the arrhythmia.

## CHOICE OF DRUG

In symptomatic arrhythmias that require drug therapy, choice of antiarrhythmic drug is largely empirical. Although some arrhythmias usually respond to particular drugs, different drugs or combinations of drugs are often required.

1. Atropine and isoproterenol (Isuprel) are drugs of choice for sinus bradycardia or heart block.
2. A digitalis glycoside is the initial drug of choice in atrial fibrillation and atrial flutter.

3. Quinidine, procainamide, and disopyramide are useful in long-term prevention or acute treatment of atrial and ventricular arrhythmias (*e.g.*, PACs, PAT, atrial fibrillation, atrial flutter, AV nodal premature contractions, AV nodal tachycardia, PVCs, ventricular tachycardia).

4. Lidocaine is the drug of choice for treating digitalis-induced arrhythmias; phenytoin is a second-line agent for this purpose.

5. Lidocaine is the drug of choice for treating PVCs and ventricular tachycardia. Mexiletine and tocainide may be useful because they can be given orally.

6. Propranolol and other beta-blockers are not drugs of choice for initial treatment of most arrhythmias but may be useful in treating a variety of arrhythmias, often in combination with other antiarrhythmic drugs.

7. Amiodarone, bretylium, flecainide, propafenone, and sotalol are approved for use only in refractory life-threatening ventricular arrhythmias, such as sustained ventricular tachycardia.

8. Verapamil is effective only in atrial arrhythmias.

## TREATMENT OF ATRIAL FIBRILLATION OR FLUTTER

Quinidine and procainamide have a vagal blocking action on the AV node and should *not* be used to treat atrial fibrillation unless digitalis has been given. Without the digitalis action of blocking AV conduction, these drugs may allow a 1:1 ventricular response at a dangerously rapid rate.

## USE IN CHILDREN

Antiarrhythmic drugs are less often needed in children than in adults. Supraventricular tachycardias are the most common arrhythmias in children, and propranolol, quinidine, or verapamil may be used to prevent or treat them. Lidocaine may be used to treat ventricular arrhythmias precipitated by cardiac surgery or digitalis toxicity. As with adults, the drugs should be used only when clearly indicated, and children should be monitored closely because all of the drugs can cause adverse effects, including hypotension and arrhythmias.

## USE IN OLDER ADULTS

Cardiac arrhythmias are common in older adults, but generally only those causing symptoms of circulatory impairment should be treated with antiarrhythmic drugs. Compared with younger adults, older adults are more likely to experience serious adverse drug effects, including aggravation of existing arrhythmias, production of new arrhythmias, hypotension, and congestive heart failure. Cautious use is required, and dosage generally needs to be reduced to compensate for heart disease or impaired drug elimination processes.

# NURSING ACTIONS: ANTIARRHYTHMIC DRUGS

| Nursing Actions | Rationale/Explanation |
| --- | --- |
| **1. Administer accurately** | |
| **a.** Check apical and radial pulses before each dose. Withhold the dose and report to the physician if marked changes are noted in rate, rhythm, or quality of pulses. | Bradycardia may indicate impending heart block or cardiovascular collapse. |
| **b.** Check blood pressure at least once daily in hospitalized clients. | To detect hypotension. Hypotension is most likely to occur when antiarrhythmic drug therapy is being initiated or altered. |
| **c.** During IV administration of antiarrhythmic drugs, maintain continuous cardiac monitoring and check blood pressure about every 5 minutes. | For early detection of hypotension and impending cardiac collapse. These drug side effects are more likely to occur with IV use. |
| **d.** Give oral drugs at evenly spaced time intervals. | To maintain adequate blood levels |
| **e.** Give mexiletine, quinidine, and tocainide with food. | To decrease gastrointestinal (GI) symptoms |
| **f.** Follow undiluted IV phenytoin with an injection of sterile saline through the same needle or catheter. *Do not* mix parenteral phenytoin with any other drug, and *do not* add to IV solutions other than normal saline (0.9% NaCl) for intermittent IV infusion. | Phenytoin is strongly alkaline, with a pH of 11 to 12. Saline is used to flush the vein and avoid local venous irritation. Solubility of the drug is pH dependent, and mixing with other drugs or solutions other than normal saline causes a white precipitate. IM injection is not recommended owing to pain and delayed absorption. |

## Nursing Actions

## Rationale/Explanation

**g.** Give lidocaine parenterally only, as a bolus injection or a continuous drip. Use only solutions labeled "For cardiac arrhythmias," and *do not* use solutions containing epinephrine. Give an IV bolus over 2 minutes.

Lidocaine solutions that contain epinephrine are used for local anesthesia only. They should *never* be given intravenously in cardiac arrhythmias because the epinephrine can cause or aggravate arrhythmias. Rapid injection (within about 30 seconds) produces transient blood levels several times greater than therapeutic range limits. Therefore, there is increased risk of toxicity without a concomitant increase in therapeutic effectiveness.

**h.** Give in a peripheral vein

To allow mixing with blood. Injection into the central circulation (through a central venous pressure line, for example) is hazardous because a high drug concentration develops locally within the heart.

**i.** *Do not* add to a blood transfusion assembly.

**2. Observe for therapeutic effects**
   **a.** Conversion to normal sinus rhythm

   **b.** Improvement in rate, rhythm, and quality of apical and radial pulses and the ECG

   **c.** Signs of increased cardiac output—blood pressure near normal range, urine output more adequate, no complaints of dizziness

After a single oral dose, peak plasma levels are reached in about 1 to 4 hours with quinidine, procainamide, and propranolol and in 6 to 12 hours with phenytoin. A state of equilibrium between plasma and tissue levels is reached in 1 or 2 days with quinidine, procainamide, and propranolol; in about 1 week with phenytoin; in several weeks with amiodarone (unless loading doses are given); and in just a few minutes with IV lidocaine. Although this information may be helpful in determining when therapeutic effects are most likely to appear, remember that many other factors influence therapeutic effects, such as dose, frequency of administration, presence of conditions that alter drug metabolism, arterial blood gases, serum electrolyte levels, and myocardial status.

   **d.** Serum drug levels within therapeutic ranges:

Serum drug levels must be interpreted in light of the client's clinical status.

| | | |
|---|---|---|
| Class IA | | |
| Quinidine | 2–6 | μg/ml |
| Disopyramide | 2–8 | μg/ml |
| Procainamide | 4–8 | μg/ml |
| Class IB | | |
| Lidocaine | 1.5–6 | μg/ml |
| Mexiletine | 0.5–2 | μg/ml |
| Phenytoin | 10–20 | μg/ml |
| Tocainide | 4–10 | μg/ml |
| Class IC | | |
| Flecainide | 0.2–1 | μg/ml |
| Propafenone | 0.06–1 | μg/ml |
| Class II | | |
| Propranolol | 0.05–0.1 | μg/ml |
| Class III | | |
| Amiodarone | 0.5–2.5 | μg/ml |
| Bretylium | 0.5–1.5 | μg/ml |
| Class IV | | |
| Verapamil | 0.08–0.3 | μg/ml |

**3. Observe for adverse effects**
   **a.** Heart block—may be indicated on the ECG by a prolonged P-R interval, prolonged QRS complex, or absence of P waves

Owing to depressant effects on the cardiac conduction system

*(continued)*

| *Nursing Actions* | *Rationale/Explanation* |
|---|---|
| **b.** Arrhythmias—aggravation of existing arrhythmia, tachycardia, bradycardia, PVCs, ventricular tachycardia or fibrillation | Tachycardia is probably caused by the anticholinergic effect of the drugs plus the response of the sympathetic nervous system to the mild hypotension induced by the drug. Bradycardia may occur with propranolol. |
| **c.** Hypotension | Owing to decreased cardiac output |
| **d.** Additional adverse effects with specific drugs: | |
| (1) Disopyramide—mouth dryness, blurred vision, urinary retention, other anticholinergic effects | These effects commonly occur. |
| (2) Lidocaine—drowsiness, paresthesias, muscle twitching, convulsions, changes in mental status (*e.g.*, confusion), hypersensitivity reactions (*e.g.*, urticaria, edema, anaphylaxis) | Most adverse reactions result from drug effects on the central nervous system (CNS). Convulsions are most likely to occur with high doses. Hypersensitivity reactions may occur in people who are allergic to related local anesthetic agents. |
| (3) Phenytoin—nystagmus, ataxia, slurring of speech, tremors, drowsiness, confusion, gingival hyperplasia | CNS changes are caused by depressant effects. |
| (4) Propranolol—weakness or dizziness, especially with activity or exercise | The beta-adrenergic blocking action of propranolol blocks the normal sympathetic nervous system response to activity and exercise. Clients may have symptoms caused by deficient blood supply to body tissues. |
| (5) Quinidine—hypersensitivity and cinchonism (tinnitus, vomiting, severe diarrhea, vertigo, headache) | |
| (6) Tocainide—lightheadedness, dizziness, nausea, paresthesia, tremor | These are the most frequent adverse effects. They may be reversed by decreasing dosage, administering with food, or discontinuing the drug. |
| **4. Observe for drug interactions** | |
| **a.** Drugs that *increase* effects of antiarrhythmics: | These drugs may potentiate therapeutic effects or increase risk of toxicity. |
| (1) Antiarrhythmic agents | When antiarrhythmic drugs are combined, there are additive cardiac depressant effects. |
| (2) Anticholinergics | Additive anticholinergic effects |
| (3) Antihypertensives, diuretics, phenothiazine antipsychotic agents | Additive hypotension |
| (4) Digitalis preparations | Additive bradycardia with propranolol |
| (5) Chloramphenicol (Chloromycetin), isoniazid (INH) | These drugs inhibit metabolism of phenytoin and may produce phenytoin toxicity. |
| **b.** Drugs that *decrease* effects of antiarrhythmic agents: | |
| Atropine sulfate | Atropine is used to reverse propranolol-induced bradycardia. |
| **5. Teach clients** | |
| **a.** Name, dose, and reason for receiving drug | |
| **b.** Report ankle edema, fatigue, dyspnea, weight gain. | These symptoms may indicate drug-induced congestive heart failure because these cardiac depressant drugs decrease myocardial contractility. |
| **c.** Space activities and rest at intervals. | With these drugs, there is decreased tolerance of activity and exercise. |
| **d.** Check pulse at least once daily for irregularity or excessive slowness. | Antiarrhythmic drugs may cause arrhythmias. Bradycardia is a side effect of propranolol. |
| **e.** Maintain regular time intervals in taking medication. | To maintain therapeutic blood levels |
| **f.** Phenytoin may color urine pink to reddish brown. | This color change is harmless. |

## Review and Application Exercises

1. Which tissues in the heart are able to generate an electrical impulse and therefore serve as a pacemaker?
2. What are risk factors that predispose a client to developing arrhythmias?
3. Name interventions that clients or health-care providers can perform to decrease risks of arrhythmias.
4. Differentiate the hemodynamic effects of common arrhythmias.
5. What are the classes of antiarrhythmic drugs?
6. Explain why antiarrhythmic drugs can be called "cardiac depressants."
7. How do quinidine and related drugs and beta-adrenergic blocking agents act on the conduction system to slow heart rate?
8. When is intravenous lidocaine the drug of choice?
9. What is the main difference between lidocaine and tocainide in treatment of arrhythmias?
10. Why is flecainide reserved for serious ventricular arrhythmias?
11. What are common and potentially serious adverse effects associated with antiarrhythmic drugs?

## Selected References

Auricchio, R. J. (1992). Cardiac arrhythmias. In M. A. Koda-Kimble & L. Y. Young (Eds.), *Applied therapeutics: The clinical use of drugs* (5th ed.) (pp. 10-1–10-40). Vancouver, WA: Applied Therapeutics.

Burke, L. J. (1990). Alterations in cardiac function. In C. M. Porth (Ed.), *Pathophysiology: Concepts of altered health states* (3rd ed.) (pp. 331–376). Philadelphia: J.B. Lippincott.

Burrell, L. O., & Streit, L. A. (1992). Nursing management of adults with cardiac dysrhythmias. In L. O. Burrell (Ed.), *Adult nursing in hospital and community settings* (pp. 367–406). Norwalk, CT: Appleton & Lange.

Clark, J. B., Queener, S. F., & Karb, V. B. (1993). *Pharmacologic basis of nursing practice* (4th ed.) (pp. 296–315). St. Louis: C.V. Mosby.

(1993). *Drug facts and comparisons*. St. Louis: Facts and Comparisons.

Fenster, P. E., & Nolan, P. E., Jr. (1993). Antiarrhythmic drugs. In R. Bressler & M. D. Katz (Eds.), *Geriatric pharmacology* (pp. 105–149). New York: McGraw-Hill.

Francis, G. S., & Alpert, J. S. (Eds.) (1990). *Modern coronary care*. Boston: Little, Brown.

Funck-Brentano, C., Kroemer, H. K., Lee, J. T., & Roden, D. M. (1990). Propafenone. *New England Journal of Medicine, 322,* 518–525.

Nappi, J. M., & McCollam, P. L. (1993). Sotalol: A breakthrough antiarrhythmic? *The Annals of Pharmacotherapy, 27,* 1359–1368.

(1993). New drug approved for life-threatening arrhythmias. *FDA Medical Bulletin, 23*(1), 5.

Roden, D. M. (1992). Treatment of cardiovascular disorders: Arrhythmias. In K. L. Melmon, H. G. Morrelli, B. B. Hoffman, & D. W. Nierenberg (Eds.), *Clinical pharmacology: Basic principles in therapeutics* (3rd ed.) (pp. 151–185). New York: McGraw-Hill.

Zipes, D. P. (1992). Cardiac arrhythmias. In W. N. Kelley (Ed.), *Textbook of internal medicine* (2nd ed.) (pp. 157–182). Philadelphia: J.B. Lippincott.

### CHAPTER 56

# Antianginal Drugs

## Angina pectoris

*Angina pectoris* is a clinical syndrome characterized mainly by chest pain or pressure. It occurs when there is a deficit in myocardial oxygen supply (myocardial ischemia) in relation to myocardial oxygen demand. It is most often caused by atherosclerotic plaque formation in the coronary arteries. Atherosclerotic plaque narrows the lumen, decreases elasticity, and impairs dilation of coronary arteries. The result is impaired blood flow to the myocardium, especially with exercise or other factors that increase the cardiac workload and need for oxygen.

### TYPES OF ANGINA

Angina pectoris is generally described as a dull, heavy substernal pain that radiates into the left shoulder and down the left arm. The pain also may radiate to the back, neck, or lower jaw. There are several types of angina pectoris. *Stable angina* is the typical chest pain that is usually precipitated by exercise and relieved by rest or nitroglycerin. It also may be precipitated by stress, anxiety, cigarette smoking, or cold weather. Recurrent episodes of stable angina usually have the same pattern of onset, duration, and intensity of symptoms. *Unstable angina* results from progressive atherosclerosis and produces increased frequency, intensity, and duration of symptoms. Unstable angina is less responsive to rest, nitroglycerin, and other medical therapy. In *vasospastic angina* (also called Prinzmetal's or variant angina), chest pain occurs at rest. It is attributed to spasm in a coronary artery.

## NONPHARMACOLOGIC TREATMENT OF ANGINA

Nonpharmacologic measures for prevention and treatment of angina include rest, cessation of smoking, weight control, relaxation or stress-management techniques, and avoidance of circumstances known to precipitate acute attacks.

## Antianginal drugs

Drugs used in angina pectoris are the organic nitrates, the beta-adrenergic blocking agents, and the calcium channel-blocking agents. Generally, these drugs relieve anginal pain by decreasing myocardial demand for oxygen or increasing blood supply to the myocardium.

### ORGANIC NITRATES

Organic nitrates relax smooth muscle in blood vessel walls. This action produces vasodilation, which relieves anginal pain by several mechanisms. First, dilation of veins reduces venous pressure and venous return to the heart. This decreases blood volume and pressure within the heart (preload), which in turn decreases cardiac workload and oxygen demand. Second, nitrates dilate coronary arteries and can increase blood flow to ischemic areas of the myocardium. Third, nitrates dilate arterioles, which lowers peripheral vascular resistance (afterload). This results in lower systolic blood pressure

Anne Collins Abrams: CLINICAL DRUG THERAPY, Fourth Edition.
© 1995 J.B. Lippincott Company.

and, consequently, reduced cardiac workload. The prototype and most widely used nitrate is nitroglycerin.

Clinical indications for nitroglycerin and other nitrates are treatment and prevention of acute chest pain caused by myocardial ischemia. For acute angina and prophylaxis before a situation deemed likely to precipitate acute angina, fast-acting preparations (sublingual or chewable tablets, transmucosal spray or tablet) are used. For management of recurrent angina, long-acting preparations (oral and sustained-release tablets or transdermal ointment and discs) are used. Intravenous nitroglycerin is used to treat angina that is unresponsive to organic nitrates or beta-adrenergic blocking agents. It also may be used to control blood pressure in perioperative or emergency situations and to reduce preload and afterload in severe congestive heart failure.

Contraindications include hypersensitivity reactions, severe anemia, hypotension, and hypovolemia. The drugs should be used cautiously in the presence of head injury or cerebral hemorrhage because they may increase intracranial pressure.

## BETA-ADRENERGIC BLOCKING AGENTS

Beta-adrenergic blocking agents, of which propranolol is the prototype, are often prescribed in a variety of clinical conditions. Their actions, uses, and adverse effects are discussed in Chapter 19. In this chapter, the drugs are discussed only in relation to their use in angina pectoris.

Sympathetic stimulation of beta receptors in the heart increases heart rate and force of myocardial contraction, both of which increase myocardial oxygen demand and may precipitate acute anginal attacks. Beta-blocking drugs prevent or inhibit sympathetic stimulation. Thus, the drugs reduce heart rate and myocardial contractility, particularly when sympathetic output is increased during exercise. Beta-blockers also reduce blood pressure, which in turn decreases myocardial workload and oxygen demand. In angina pectoris, beta-adrenergic blocking agents are used in long-term management to decrease the frequency and severity of anginal attacks, decrease the need for sublingual nitroglycerin, and increase exercise tolerance.

## CALCIUM CHANNEL-BLOCKING AGENTS

Calcium channel-blockers act on contractile and conductive tissues of the heart and on vascular smooth muscle. For these cells to function normally, the concentration of intracellular calcium must be increased. This is usually accomplished by movement of extracellular calcium ions into the cell (through calcium channels or pores in the cell membrane) and release of bound calcium from the sarcoplasmic reticulum in the cell. Thus, calcium plays an important role in maintaining vasomotor tone, myocardial contractility, and conduction. Calcium channel-blocking agents prevent the movement of extracellular calcium into the cell. As a result, coronary and peripheral arteries are dilated, myocardial contractility is decreased, and the conduction system is depressed in relation to impulse formation (automaticity) and conduction velocity.

In angina pectoris, the drugs improve the blood supply to the myocardium by dilating coronary arteries and decrease the workload of the heart by dilating peripheral arteries. In atrial fibrillation or flutter and other supraventricular tachyarrhythmias, diltiazem and verapamil slow the rate of ventricular response. In hypertension, the drugs lower blood pressure primarily by dilating peripheral arteries.

Calcium channel-blockers are well absorbed after oral administration but undergo extensive first-pass metabolism in the liver. Most of the drugs are more than 90% protein bound and reach peak plasma levels within 1 to 2 hours (6 hours or longer for sustained-release forms). Most also have short elimination half-lives (less than 5 hours), so doses must be given three or four times daily unless sustained-release formulations are used. Amlodipine (30–50 hours), bepridil (24 hours), and felodipine (11–16 hours) have long elimination half-lives and therefore can be given once daily. The drugs are metabolized in the liver, and dosage should be reduced in clients with severe liver disease. Dosage reductions are not required with renal disease.

The calcium channel-blockers approved for use in the United States vary in their chemical structures and effects on body tissues. Six of these are chemically dihydropyridines, of which nifedipine is the prototype. Bepridil, diltiazem, and verapamil differ chemically from the dihydropyridines and each other. Generally, nifedipine and related drugs have greater vasodilating effects, while verapamil and diltiazem have greater effects on the cardiac conduction system.

The drugs also vary in clinical indications for use; most are used for angina or hypertension, and only diltiazem and verapamil are used to treat supraventricular tachyarrhythmias (Table 56-1). In addition, nimodipine is approved for use only in subarachnoid hemorrhage to decrease spasm in cerebral blood vessels and thereby limit the extent of brain damage. In animal studies, nimodipine exerted greater effects on cerebral arteries than on other arteries, probably because it is highly lipid soluble and penetrates the blood-brain barrier.

Contraindications include second- or third-degree heart block, cardiogenic shock, and severe bradycardia, congestive heart failure, or hypotension. The drugs should be used cautiously with milder bradycardia, congestive heart failure, or hypotension and with renal or hepatic impairment.

## TABLE 56-1.   CALCIUM CHANNEL-BLOCKERS

| Generic/Trade Name | Indications | Routes and Dosage Ranges |
|---|---|---|
| **Amlodipine** (Norvasc) | Angina<br>Hypertension | PO 5–10 mg once daily |
| **Bepridil** (Vascor) | Angina | PO 200 mg/d initially, increased to 300 mg daily after 10 d if necessary; maximum dose, 400 mg daily |
| **Diltiazem** (Cardizem) | Angina<br>Hypertension<br>Atrial fibrillation and flutter<br>PSVT* | Angina or hypertension, immediate release, PO 60–90 mg four times daily before meals and at bedtime<br>Hypertension, sustained-release only, PO 120–180 mg twice daily<br>Arrhythmias (Cardizem IV only) IV injection 0.25 mg/kg (average dose 20 mg) over 2 min with a second dose of 0.35 mg/kg (average dose 25 mg) in 15 min if necessary, followed by IV infusion of 5–15 mg/h up to 24 h |
| **Felodipine** (Plendil) | Hypertension | PO 5–10 mg once daily |
| **Isradipine** (DynaCirc) | Hypertension | PO 2.5–5 mg twice daily |
| **Nicardipine** (Cardene) | Angina<br>Hypertension | Angina, immediate-release only, PO 20–40 mg three times daily<br>Hypertension, immediate release, same as for angina, above; sustained-release, PO 30–60 mg twice daily |
| **Nifedipine** (Adalat, Procardia) | Angina<br>Hypertension | Angina, immediate release, PO 10–30 mg three times daily; sustained release, PO 30–60 mg once daily<br>Hypertension, sustained release only, 30–60 mg once daily |
| **Nimodipine** (Nimotop) | Subarachnoid hemorrhage | PO 60 mg q4h for 21 consecutive days. If patient unable to swallow, aspirate contents of capsule into a syringe with an 18-gauge needle, administer by nasogastric tube, and follow with 30 ml normal saline. |
| **Verapamil** (Calan, Isoptin) | Angina<br>Atrial fibrillation or flutter, PSVT*<br>Hypertension | Angina, PO 80–120 mg three times daily<br>Arrhythmias, PO 80–120 mg three to four times daily; IV injection, 5–10 mg over 2 min or longer, with continuous monitoring of ECG and blood pressure<br>Hypertension, PO 80 mg three times daily or 240 mg (sustained release) once daily |

* PSVT = paroxysmal supraventricular tachycardia.

# Individual antianginal drugs

Specific nitrates and beta-blockers used for angina are described below; calcium channel-blockers are listed in Table 56-1.

## ORGANIC NITRATES

**Nitroglycerin** (Nitro-Bid, others), the prototype drug, is used to relieve acute angina pectoris, prevent exercise-induced angina, and decrease the frequency and severity of acute anginal episodes. Oral dosage forms are rapidly metabolized in the liver, and relatively small proportions of doses reach the systemic circulation. In addition, oral doses act slowly and do not help relieve acute chest pain.

For these reasons, several alternative dosage forms have been developed, including transmucosal tablets and sprays administered sublingually or buccally, transdermal ointments and adhesive discs applied to the skin, and an intravenous preparation. When given sublingually, nitroglycerin is absorbed directly into the systemic circulation. It acts within 1 to 3 minutes and lasts about 30 to 60 minutes. When applied topically to the skin, nitroglycerin is also absorbed directly into the systemic circulation. However, absorption occurs at a slower rate, and topical nitroglycerin has a longer duration of action than other forms. It is available in an ointment, which is effective for 4 to 8 hours, and a transdermal disc, which is effective for about 18 to 24 hours. An intravenous form of nitroglycerin is used to relieve acute anginal pain that does not respond to other agents.

### Routes and dosage ranges

*Adults:* PO 2.5–9 mg two or three times per day; sustained-release tablets or capsules, 2.5 mg three or four times per day

SL 0.15–0.6 mg PRN for chest pain

Translingual spray, one or two metered doses (0.4 mg/dose) sprayed onto oral mucosa at onset of anginal pain, to a maximum of three doses in 15 min

Transmucosal tablet, 1 mg q3–5h while awake, placed between lip and gum or cheek and gum

Topical ointment, 1/2–2 inches q4–8h; do not rub in

Topical transdermal disc, applied once daily

IV 5–10 µg/min initially, increased in 10- to 20-µg/min increments up to 100 µg/min or more if necessary to relieve pain

**Amyl nitrite** (Vaporole) is dispensed in a container that is crushed to release vapors; the vapors are inhaled. Onset of action and pain relief are rapid, but amyl nitrite is more likely to cause headache and hypotension than other nitrates used in angina pectoris.

### Route and dosage range

*Adults:* Inhalation, 0.18–0.3 ml (one container)

**Erythrityl tetranitrate** (Cardilate) is used for the long-term management or prophylaxis of angina pectoris. The drug is unsuitable for acute episodes of anginal pain, because onset of action occurs after 5 to 10 minutes. Beneficial effects last 3 to 4 hours.

### Routes and dosage ranges

*Adults:* SL 10 mg three times per day or before stress
PO 5–15 mg three times per day

**Isosorbide dinitrate** (Isordil, Sorbitrate) is used to reduce the frequency and severity of acute anginal episodes. When given sublingually, isosorbide dinitrate acts in about 2 minutes, and its effects last about 1 to 2 hours. When higher doses are given orally, more drug escapes metabolism in the liver and produces systemic effects in about 30 minutes. Lower doses may be relatively ineffective. Therapeutic effects last about 4 hours after oral administration. The effective oral dose is usually determined by increasing the dose until headache occurs, indicating the maximum tolerable dose. Sustained-release capsules also are available.

### Routes and dosage ranges

*Adults:* SL 2.5–10 mg PRN or q2–4h
PO 10–60 mg q4–6h
Sustained-release capsules, PO 40 mg q6–12h

**Isosorbide mononitrate** (Ismo) is the metabolite and active component of isosorbide dinitrate. It is well absorbed after oral administration and about 100% bioavailable. Unlike other oral nitrates, this drug is not subject to first-pass hepatic metabolism. Onset of action occurs within 1 hour, peak effects occur between 1 and 4 hours, and the elimination half-life is about 5 hours. It is used only for prophylaxis of angina; it does not act rapidly enough to relieve acute attacks.

### Route and dosage range

*Adults:* PO 20 mg twice daily, with first dose on arising and the second dose 7 h later

**Pentaerythritol tetranitrate** (Peritrate) is similar to erythrityl tetranitrate in actions and uses. It is used prophylactically in the long-term management of angina pectoris. It is available in short-acting and sustained-release dosage forms.

### Route and dosage range

*Adults:* PO 10–40 mg four times daily

Sustained-release PO 30–80 mg q12h

## BETA-ADRENERGIC BLOCKING AGENTS

**Propranolol** (Inderal), the prototype beta-blocker, is used in the treatment of angina pectoris to reduce the frequency and severity of acute attacks. Propranolol is usually added to the antianginal drug regimen when nitrates do not prevent anginal episodes. Propranolol is especially useful in preventing exercise-induced tachycardia, which can precipitate anginal attacks.

Propranolol is well absorbed following oral administration. It is then metabolized extensively in the liver; a relatively small proportion of an oral dose (about 30%) reaches the systemic circulation. For this reason, oral doses of propranolol are much higher than intravenous doses. Onset of action is 30 minutes after oral administration and 1 to 2 minutes after intravenous injection. Because of variations in the degree of hepatic metabolism, clients vary widely in the dosages required to maintain a therapeutic response.

### Routes and dosage ranges

*Adults:* PO 10–80 mg two to four times per day
IV 0.5–3 mg q4h until desired response is obtained

**Atenolol** (Tenormin) and **nadolol** (Corgard) have the same actions, uses, and adverse effects as propranolol, but they have long half-lives and can be given once daily. They are excreted by the kidneys, and dosage must be reduced in clients with renal impairment.

Atenolol

### Route and dosage range

*Adults:* PO 50 mg once daily, initially, increased to 100 mg/d after 1 week if necessary

Nadolol

### Route and dosage range

*Adults:* PO 40–240 mg/d in a single dose

## Nursing Process

### Assessment

Assess the client's condition in relation to angina pectoris. Specific assessment data vary with each client but usually should include the following:
- During the initial nursing history interview, try to answer the following questions:
  - How long has the client been taking antianginal drugs? For what purpose are they being taken (prophylaxis, treatment of acute attacks, or both)?

- What is the frequency and duration of acute anginal attacks?
- Do symptoms other than chest pain occur during acute attacks (*e.g.*, sweating, nausea)?
- Are there particular activities or circumstances that provoke acute attacks? Do attacks ever occur when the client is at rest?
- What relieves symptoms of acute angina?
- If the client takes nitroglycerin, ask how often it is required, how many tablets are needed for relief of pain, how often the supply is replaced, and where the client stores or carries the drug.
- Assess blood pressure and pulse, electrocardiogram reports, presence of symptoms other than chest pain, posture, and facial expression for baseline values.
- During an acute attack, assess the following:
  - Location and quality of the pain. Chest pain is nonspecific. It may be a symptom of numerous disorders, such as pulmonary embolism, esophageal spasm or inflammation (heartburn), costochondritis, or anxiety. Chest pain of cardiac origin is caused by myocardial ischemia and may indicate angina pectoris or myocardial infarction.
  - Precipitating factors. For example, what was the client doing, thinking, or feeling just before the onset of chest pain?

### Nursing diagnoses

- Decreased Cardiac Output related to disease process or drug therapy
- Altered Tissue Perfusion: Cerebral and peripheral, related to drug-induced hypotension
- Pain in chest related to inadequate perfusion of the myocardium
- Pain (headache) related to vasodilating effects of nitrate antianginal drugs
- Activity Intolerance related to chest pain
- High Risk for Injury related to hypotension and syncope from antianginal drugs
- High Risk for Noncompliance related to drug therapy and life-style changes
- Impaired Tissue Integrity related to skin irritation from topical nitroglycerin preparations
- Constipation related to drug therapy with calcium channel-blockers
- Knowledge Deficit related to management of disease process and drug therapy
- High Risk for Ineffective Individual Coping related to chronic disease process
- Social Isolation related to activity intolerance
- Body Image Disturbance related to inability to perform usual activities of daily living
- Sexual Dysfunction related to fear of precipitating chest pain

### Planning/Goals

*The client will:*

- Receive or take antianginal drugs accurately
- Experience relief of acute chest pain
- Have fewer episodes of acute chest pain
- Have increased activity tolerance

- Identify and avoid or learn to manage situations that precipitate anginal attacks
- Be closely monitored for therapeutic and adverse effects, especially when drug therapy is started
- Avoid preventable adverse effects
- Verbalize essential information about the disease process, needed dietary and life-style changes to improve health status, and drug therapy
- Keep appointments for follow-up care and monitoring

### Interventions

Use the following measures to prevent acute anginal attacks:
- Assist in preventing, recognizing, and treating contributory disorders, such as atherosclerosis, hypertension, hyperthyroidism, hypoxia, and anemia.
- Help the client recognize and avoid precipitating factors (*e.g.*, heavy meals, cigarette smoking, strenuous exercise) when possible. If anxiety is a factor, relaxation techniques or psychological counseling may be helpful.
- Help the client to develop a more healthful life-style in terms of diet, adequate rest and sleep, and regular exercise. A supervised exercise program helps to develop collateral circulation.

During an acute anginal attack in a client known to have angina or coronary artery disease:
- Assume that any chest pain may be of cardiac origin.
- Have the client lie down or sit down to reduce cardiac workload and provide rest.
- Check vital signs and compare them with baseline values.
- Record characteristics of chest pain and the presence of other signs and symptoms.
- Have the client take a fast-acting nitroglycerin preparation (previously prescribed), up to three sublingual tablets or three oral sprays within 15 minutes, if necessary.
- If chest pain is not relieved with rest and nitroglycerin, assume that a myocardial infarction has occurred until proven otherwise. Keep the client at rest and notify the physician immediately.

Leave sublingual nitroglycerin at the bedside of hospitalized clients. The tablets or spray should be within reach so they can be used immediately. Record the number of tablets used daily, and be sure an adequate supply is available.

*Teach clients:*
- To seek medical attention immediately if acute chest pain is not relieved by rest and three sublingual tablets or oral sprays 5 minutes apart
- To keep family members or support people informed about the location and use of antianginal medications in case help is needed
- That long-acting forms of nitrates and beta-blocking agents should be tapered and discontinued gradually to avoid rebound angina
- To avoid over-the-counter decongestants, cold remedies, and diet pills, which stimulate the heart and constrict blood vessels and thus may cause angina
- That various dosage forms of nitroglycerin were developed for specific routes of administration and are not interchangeable. Also, that transdermal discs vary in the amount of drug released in a particular time interval.

### Evaluation

- Observe and interview for relief of acute chest pain.
- Observe and interview regarding the number of episodes of acute chest pain.
- Interview regarding diet and life-style factors that relate to angina.
- Interview regarding compliance with drug therapy.

## Principles of therapy

### GOALS OF THERAPY

The goals of drug therapy are to relieve acute anginal pain, reduce the number and severity of acute anginal attacks, and improve exercise tolerance and quality of life.

### CHOICE OF DRUG AND DOSAGE FORM

For relief of acute angina and prophylaxis before events that cause acute angina, nitroglycerin (sublingual tablets or translingual spray) is usually the first drug of choice. Sublingual or chewable tablets of isosorbide dinitrate or amyl nitrite also may be used. For long-term prevention or management of recurrent angina, oral or topical nitrates, beta-adrenergic blocking agents, or calcium channel-blocking agents are used. Combination drug therapy with a nitrate and one of the other drugs is common. Clients taking one or more long-acting antianginal drugs usually carry a short-acting drug as well to be used for acute attacks.

### TITRATION OF DOSAGE

Dosage of all antianginal drugs should be individualized to achieve optimal benefit and minimal adverse effects. This is usually accomplished by starting with relatively small doses and increasing them at appropriate intervals if necessary. Generally, doses may vary widely among individuals.

### TOLERANCE TO LONG-ACTING NITRATES

Clients who take long-acting dosage forms of nitrates on a regular schedule develop tolerance to the vasodilating (antianginal) effects of the drug. While this decreases the adverse effects of hypotension, dizziness, and headache, therapeutic effects also may be decreased. As a result, episodes of chest pain may occur more often or be more severe than expected. In addition, short-acting nitrates may be less effective in relieving acute pain.

Opinions seem divided about the best way to prevent or manage nitrate tolerance. Some authorities recommend using short-acting nitrates when needed and avoiding the long-acting forms. Others recommend using the long-acting forms for 16 to 18 hours daily during active periods and omitting them during inactive periods or sleep. Thus, a dose of an oral nitrate or topical ointment would be given every 6 hours for three doses daily, allowing a rest period of 6 hours without a dose. Transdermal discs should be removed at bedtime.

### USE IN CHILDREN

The safety and effectiveness of antianginal drugs have not been established for children. Nitroglycerin has been given intravenously for congestive heart failure and intraoperative control of blood pressure, with the initial dose adjusted for weight and later doses titrated to response. Verapamil (Calan, Isoptin) has been used to treat supraventricular tachycardias in children (see Chap. 55).

### USE IN OLDER ADULTS

Antianginal drugs are often used because cardiovascular disease and myocardial ischemia are common problems in older adults. Adverse drug effects, such as hypotension and syncope, are likely to occur, and they may be more severe than in younger adults. Blood pressure and ability to ambulate safely should be closely monitored, especially when drug therapy is started. Ambulatory clients also should be monitored for their ability to take the drugs correctly.

## NURSING ACTIONS: ANTIANGINAL DRUGS

| *Nursing Actions* | *Rationale/Explanation* |
|---|---|

**1. Administer accurately**

**a.** Check blood pressure and heart rate before each dose of an antianginal drug. Withhold the drug if systolic blood pressure is below 90 mm Hg. If the dose is omitted, record and report to the physician.

Hypotension is an adverse effect of antianginal drugs. Bradycardia is an adverse effect of propranolol and nadolol. Dosage adjustments may be necessary if these effects occur.

**b.** Give antianginal drugs on a regular schedule, at evenly spaced intervals.

To increase effectiveness in preventing acute attacks of angina

**c.** If oral nitrates and topical nitroglycerin are being used concurrently, stagger times of administration.

To minimize risks of additive hypotension and headache

**d.** For sublingual nitroglycerin and isosorbide dinitrate, instruct the client to place the tablets under the tongue until they dissolve.

**e.** For oral isosorbide dinitrate, regular and chewable tablets are available. Be sure each type of tablet is taken appropriately.

**f.** For sublingual nitroglycerin, check the expiration date on the container.

Sublingual tablets of nitroglycerin are volatile. Once the bottle has been opened, they become ineffective after about 6 months and should be replaced.

**g.** To apply nitroglycerin ointment, use the special paper to measure the dose. Place the ointment on a nonhairy part of the body, and apply with the applicator paper. Cover the area with plastic wrap or tape. Rotate application sites.

The measured paper must be used for accurate dosage. The paper is used to apply the ointment because the drug is readily absorbed through the skin. Skin contact should be avoided except on the designated area of the body. Plastic wrap or tape aids absorption and prevents removal of the drug. It also prevents soiling of clothes and linens. Application sites should be rotated because the ointment can irritate the skin.

**h.** For nitroglycerin patches, apply at the same time each day to clean, dry, hairless areas on the upper body or arms. Rotate sites. Avoid applying below the knee or elbow or in areas of skin irritation or scar tissue.

To promote effective and consistent drug absorption. The drug is not as well absorbed from distal portions of the extremities because of decreased blood flow. Rotation of sites decreases skin irritation.

**i.** For IV nitroglycerin, dilute the drug and give by continuous infusion, with frequent monitoring of blood pressure and heart rate. Use only with the special administration set supplied by the manufacturer to avoid drug adsorption onto tubing.

The drug should not be given by direct IV injection. The drug is potent and may cause hypotension. Dosage (flow rate) is adjusted according to response (pain relief or drop in systolic blood pressure of 20 mm Hg).

**j.** With IV verapamil, inject slowly, over 2 to 3 minutes.

To decrease hypotension and other adverse effects

**2. Observe for therapeutic effects**

**a.** Relief of chest pain with acute attacks

Sublingual nitroglycerin usually relieves pain within 5 minutes. If pain is not relieved, two additional tablets may be given, 5 minutes apart. If pain is not relieved after 3 tablets, report to the physician.

**b.** Reduced incidence and severity of acute attacks with prophylactic antianginal drugs

**c.** Increased exercise tolerance

## Nursing Actions

## Rationale/Explanation

**3. Observe for adverse effects**

**a.** With nitrates, observe for hypotension, dizziness, lightheadedness, tachycardia, palpitations, and headache.

Adverse effects are extensions of pharmacologic action. Vasodilation causes hypotension, which in turn causes dizziness from cerebral hypoxia and tachycardia from compensatory sympathetic nervous system stimulation. Hypotension can decrease blood flow to coronary arteries and precipitate angina pectoris or myocardial infarction. Hypotension is most likely to occur within an hour after drug administration. Vasodilation also causes headache, the most common adverse effect of nitrates.

**b.** With beta-adrenergic blocking agents, observe for hypotension, bradycardia, bronchospasm, and congestive heart failure.

Beta-blockers lower blood pressure by decreasing myocardial contractility and cardiac output. Excessive bradycardia may contribute to hypotension and cardiac dysrhythmias. Bronchospasm is more likely to occur in clients with asthma or other chronic respiratory problems.

**c.** With calcium channel-blockers, observe for hypotension, dizziness, lightheadedness, weakness, peripheral edema, headache, congestive heart failure, pulmonary edema, nausea, and constipation. Bradycardia may occur with verapamil and diltiazem; tachycardia may occur with nifedipine and nicardipine.

Adverse effects result primarily from reduced smooth muscle contractility. These effects, except constipation, are much more likely to occur with nifedipine and other dihydropyridines. Nifedipine may cause profound hypotension, which activates the compensatory mechanisms of the sympathetic nervous system and the renin-angiotensin-aldosterone system. Peripheral edema may require the administration of a diuretic. Constipation is more likely to occur with verapamil. Diltiazem reportedly causes few adverse effects.

**4. Observe for drug interactions**

**a.** Drugs that *increase* effects of antianginal drugs:

(1) Antiarrhythmics, antihypertensive drugs, diuretics, phenothiazine antipsychotic agents

Additive hypotension

(2) Cimetidine

May increase beta-blocking effects of propranolol by slowing its hepatic clearance and elimination. Increases effects of all calcium channel-blockers by inhibiting hepatic metabolism and increasing serum drug levels.

(3) Digitalis glycosides

Additive bradycardia when given with beta-blocking agents

**b.** Drugs that *decrease* effects of antianginal drugs:

(1) Adrenergic drugs (*e.g.*, epinephrine, isoproterenol)

Adrenergic drugs, which stimulate beta receptors, can reverse bradycardia induced by beta-blockers.

(2) Anticholinergic drugs

Drugs with anticholinergic effects can increase heart rate, offsetting slower heart rates produced by beta-blockers.

(3) Calcium salts

May decrease therapeutic effectiveness of calcium channel-blockers

(4) Carbamazepine, phenobarbital, phenytoin, rifampin

May decrease effects of calcium channel-blockers by inducing hepatic enzymes and thereby increasing their rate of metabolism

**5. Teach clients**

**a.** Take the drugs only as prescribed. Do not increase dosage or discontinue the drugs without specific instructions from the physician.

Dosage of antianginal drugs must be individualized to maximize therapeutic effects and minimize adverse effects. Discontinuing antianginal drugs abruptly has been associated with increased anginal episodes and possibly myocardial infarctions.

*(continued)*

## Nursing Actions

## Rationale/Explanation

**b.** With sublingual nitroglycerin, keep tablets in the original container, carry them so that they are always within reach but not where they are exposed to body heat, and replace them about every 6 months.

The tablets lose their potency after about 6 months, or more rapidly if exposed to light and heat. Tablets should be readily accessible if chest pain occurs.

**c.** With sublingual or buccal tablets, hold under the tongue or between the cheek and gum until they dissolve. Do not chew the tablets.

Chewing the tablets increases risks of hypotension and headache.

**d.** Correct application of topical or transdermal preparations (see 1g and 1h). Areas may be shaved.

**e.** Record the number and severity of anginal episodes daily, along with the number of nitroglycerin tablets required to relieve the attack and the total number of tablets taken daily.

Antianginal drugs are most often given on an outpatient basis. Information from the client is necessary to monitor therapeutic and adverse effects of drug therapy.

**f.** Headaches and dizziness may occur when antianginal drugs are started. These effects are usually transient and dissipate with continued therapy. If they persist or prevent normal activities of daily living, report to the physician.

Dosage may need to be reduced.

**g.** If dizziness occurs, avoid strenuous activity, and assume an upright position slowly for about 1 hour after taking the drugs.

Dizziness is caused by a temporary decrease in blood pressure. It is most likely to occur when changing position from lying or sitting to standing and during the first hour after drug administration.

## Review and Application Exercises

1. What is angina pectoris, and what is its cause?
2. How do nitrates relieve angina?
3. Develop a teaching plan for a client who is beginning nitrate therapy.
4. How do beta-blockers relieve angina?
5. Why should beta-blockers be tapered and discontinued slowly in clients with angina?
6. How do calcium channel-blockers relieve angina?
7. Develop a teaching plan for a client taking a calcium channel-blocker.

## Selected References

Beare, P. G., & Myers, J. L. (Eds) (1990). *Principles and practice of adult health nursing.* St Louis: C.V. Mosby.

Brater, D. C. (1992). Clinical pharmacology of cardiovascular drugs. In W. N. Kelley (Ed.), *Textbook of internal medicine* (2nd ed.) (pp. 315–335). Philadelphia: J.B. Lippincott.

Burke, L. J. (1990). Alterations in cardiac function. In C. M. Porth (Ed.), *Pathophysiology: Concepts of altered health states* (3rd ed.) (pp. 331–376). Philadelphia: J.B. Lippincott.

Debusk, R. F. (1992). Treatment of cardiovascular disorders: Ischemic heart disease. In K. L. Melmon, H. F. Morrelli, B. B. Hoffman, & D. W. Nierenberg (Eds.), *Clinical pharmacology: Basic principles in therapeutics* (3rd ed.) (pp. 132–150). New York: McGraw-Hill.

(1994). *Drug facts and comparisons.* St. Louis: Facts and Comparisons.

Francis, G. S., & Alpert, J. S. (Eds) (1990). *Modern coronary care.* Boston: Little, Brown.

Glasser, S. P., & Arnett, D. K. (1990). Update on nitrate therapy: Reexamination of tolerance issues and efficacy endpoints of long-acting products. *Hospital Formulary, 25,* 42–49.

Gollub, S. B. (1993). Combination medical therapy in the treatment of angina pectoris. *Hospital Formulary, 28,* 34–44.

Raehl, C. L., & Nolan, P. E., Jr. (1992). Angina pectoris. In M. A. Koda-Kimble & L. Y. Young (Eds.), *Applied therapeutics: The clinical use of drugs* (5th ed.) (pp. 11-1–11-24). Vancouver, WA: Applied Therapeutics.

### CHAPTER 57

# Drugs Used in Hypotension and Shock

## Hypotension and shock

*Shock* is a clinical syndrome characterized by decreased blood supply to tissues. Clinical symptoms depend on the degree of impaired perfusion of vital organs (*e.g.*, brain, heart, and kidneys). Common signs and symptoms include oliguria, heart failure, disorientation, clouded sensorium, mental confusion, seizures, cool extremities, and coma. Most, but not all, people in shock are hypotensive. In a previously hypertensive person, shock may be present if a drop in blood pressure of greater than 50 mm Hg has occurred, even if current blood pressure readings are "normal."

### TYPES OF SHOCK

*Hypovolemic shock* is characterized by a decreased circulating blood volume and may occur with acute blood loss, severe burns, or dehydration.

*Cardiogenic shock* is characterized by decreased cardiac output and may result from myocardial infarction, arrhythmias, or valvular disease.

*Septic shock* is characterized by decreased peripheral vascular resistance. It most often results from gram-negative bacterial infections but may occur with gram-positive infections as well.

*Anaphylactic shock* is characterized by decreased peripheral vascular resistance. It may result from a hyper-sensitivity (allergic) reaction to drugs or other substances (see Chap. 18).

## Antishock drugs

Drugs used in the treatment of shock are primarily the adrenergic drugs, which are discussed more extensively in Chapter 18. In this chapter, the drugs are discussed only in relation to their usage in hypotension and shock. In hypotension and shock, drugs with alpha-adrenergic activity (*e.g.*, norepinephrine, phenylephrine, methoxamine) are used to increase peripheral vascular resistance and raise blood pressure. Drugs with beta-adrenergic activity (*e.g.*, dobutamine, isoproterenol) are used to increase myocardial contractility and heart rate, which in turn raises blood pressure. Several drugs have both alpha- and beta-adrenergic activity (*e.g.*, dopamine, epinephrine, metaraminol). In many cases, a combination of drugs is used, depending on the type of shock and the client's response to treatment.

Adrenergic drugs with beta activity may be relatively contraindicated in shock states precipitated or complicated by cardiac arrhythmias. Beta-stimulating drugs also should be used cautiously in cardiogenic shock following myocardial infarction, because increased contractility and heart rate can increase myocardial oxygen consumption and extend the area of infarction.

# Individual drugs used in hypotension and shock

**Dopamine** (Intropin) is a naturally occurring catecholamine that functions as a neurotransmitter. Dopamine exerts its actions by stimulating alpha, beta, or dopaminergic receptors, depending on the dose being used. In addition, dopamine acts indirectly by releasing norepinephrine from sympathetic nerve endings and the adrenal glands. Peripheral dopamine receptors are located in splanchnic and renal vascular beds. Stimulation of dopamine receptors produces vasodilation in the renal circulation and increases urine output. At low doses (2–5 μg/kg per minute), dopamine stimulates dopaminergic receptors. At moderate doses (5–10 μg/kg per minute), dopamine also stimulates beta receptors and increases heart rate, myocardial contractility, and blood pressure. At rates higher than 10 μg/kg per minute, beta activity remains, but increasing alpha stimulation (vasoconstriction) may overcome the dopaminergic actions.

Dopamine is useful in hypovolemic and cardiogenic shock. Adequate fluid therapy is necessary for the maximal pressor effect of dopamine. Acidosis decreases the effectiveness of dopamine.

### Route and dosage range

*Adults and children:* IV 2–5 μg/kg per minute initially, gradually increasing to 10–15 μg/kg per minute if necessary. Prepare by adding 200 mg of dopamine to 250 ml of IV fluid for a final concentration of 800 μg/ml or to 500 ml IV fluid for a final concentration of 400 μg/ml.

**Dobutamine** (Dobutrex) is a synthetic catecholamine developed to provide an agent with little vascular activity. Dobutamine acts mainly on beta$_1$ receptors in the heart to increase the force of myocardial contraction with minimal increase in heart rate. Dobutamine also may increase blood pressure with large doses. Dobutamine is less likely to induce tachycardia and arrhythmias than dopamine and isoproterenol. It is most useful in cases of shock that require increases in cardiac output without the need for blood pressure support. Dobutamine has a short plasma half-life and therefore must be administered by continuous intravenous (IV) infusion. It is rapidly metabolized to inactive metabolites. It is recommended for short-term use only.

### Route and dosage range

*Adults:* IV 2.5–10 μg/kg per minute, increased to 40 μg/kg per minute if necessary. Reconstitute the 250-mg vial with 10 ml of sterile water or 5% dextrose injection. The resulting solution should be diluted to at least 50 ml with IV solution before administering (5000 μg/ml). Add 250 mg of drug to 500 ml of diluent for a concentration of 500 μg/ml.

**Epinephrine** (Adrenalin) is a naturally occurring catecholamine produced by the adrenal glands. At low doses, epinephrine stimulates beta receptors, which results in increased cardiac output and bronchodilation. Larger doses act on alpha receptors to increase blood pressure. Epinephrine is the drug of choice for treatment of anaphylactic shock because of its rapid onset of action and its antiallergic effects (it prevents the release of histamine and other mediators that cause symptoms of anaphylaxis). Its use in other types of shock is limited because it may produce excessive cardiac stimulation, ventricular arrhythmias, and reduced renal blood flow. In addition, more potent vasoconstrictors are available (*e.g.*, norepinephrine). Epinephrine is rapidly inactivated to metabolites, which are excreted by the kidneys. It is usually given by continuous IV infusion to treat shock. A single IV dose may be given in emergencies, such as cardiac arrest.

### Routes and dosage ranges

*Adults:* IV 1–4 μg/min. Prepare the solution by adding 2 mg (2 ml) of epinephrine injection 1 : 1000 to 250 or 500 ml of IV fluid. The final concentration is 8 or 4 μg/ml, respectively.
  IV direct injection, 100–1000 μg of 1 : 10,000 injection, q5–15 min, injected slowly. Prepare the solution by adding 1 ml epinephrine 1 : 1000 to 9 ml sodium chloride injection. The final concentration is 100 μg/ml.

*Children:* IV infusion, 0.025–0.3 μg/kg per minute
  IV direct injection, 5–10 μg/kg, slowly

**Isoproterenol** (Isuprel) is a synthetic catecholamine that acts exclusively on beta receptors to increase heart rate, myocardial contractility, and systolic blood pressure. However, it also stimulates vascular beta$_2$ receptors, which causes vasodilation and may decrease diastolic blood pressure. For this reason, isoproterenol has limited usefulness as a pressor agent. It also may increase myocardial oxygen consumption and decrease coronary artery blood flow, which in turn causes myocardial ischemia. Cardiac arrhythmias may result from excessive beta stimulation. Because of these limitations, use of isoproterenol is limited to shock associated with slow heart rates and myocardial depression.

### Route and dosage ranges

*Adults:* IV infusion, 0.5–10 μg/min. Prepare solution by adding 2 mg to 250 ml of IV fluid. Final concentration is 8 μg/ml.
*Children:* IV infusion, 0.05–0.3 μg/kg per minute

**Metaraminol** (Aramine), occasionally used in hypotensive states, acts indirectly by releasing norepinephrine from sympathetic nerve endings. Its actions are similar to those of norepinephrine, except that metaraminol is less potent and has a longer duration of action.

## Routes and dosage ranges

*Adults:* IM 2–10 mg
    IV injection, 2–5 mg
    IV infusion, add 100–500 mg of metaraminol to 500 ml of IV fluid. Adjust flow rate (dosage) to maintain the desired blood pressure.
*Children:* IM 0.1 mg/kg
    IV injection, 0.01 mg/kg
    IV infusion, 1 mg/25 ml of diluent. Adjust flow rate to maintain the desired blood pressure.

**Methoxamine** (Vasoxyl) acts on alpha-adrenergic receptors to cause vasoconstriction, increase peripheral vascular resistance, and raise blood pressure. The drug acts similarly to phenylephrine and is used occasionally in hypotension.

## Routes and dosage ranges

*Adults:* IM 10–20 mg
    IV 3–5 mg, slowly
*Children:* IM 0.25 mg/kg
    IV 0.08 mg/kg, slowly

**Norepinephrine**, also called **levarterenol** (Levophed) is a pharmaceutical preparation of the naturally occurring catecholamine norepinephrine. Norepinephrine increases blood pressure primarily by vasoconstriction. It also increases heart rate and force of myocardial contraction. It is useful in cardiogenic and septic shock, but reduced renal blood flow limits its prolonged use. Norepinephrine is used mainly with clients who are unresponsive to dopamine or dobutamine.

## Route and dosage ranges

*Adults:* IV infusion, 2–4 μg/min, to a maximum of 20 μg/min. Prepare solution by adding 2 mg to 500 ml of IV fluid. Final concentration is 4 μg/ml.
*Children:* IV infusion, 0.03–0.1 μg/kg/min

**Phenylephrine** (Neo-Synephrine) is an adrenergic drug that stimulates alpha-adrenergic receptors. As a result, phenylephrine constricts arterioles and raises systolic and diastolic blood pressures. Phenylephrine resembles epinephrine but has fewer cardiac effects and a longer duration of action. Reduction of renal and mesenteric blood flow limits prolonged usage.

## Routes and dosage ranges

*Adults:* IV infusion, 100–180 μg/min initially, then 40–60 μg/min. Prepare solution by adding 10 or 20 mg of phenylephrine to 500 ml of IV fluid. Final concentration is 20 or 40 μg/ml, respectively.
    IV injection, 100–500 μg
*Children:* SC, IM 0.1 mg/kg

# Nursing Process

## Assessment

Assess the client's condition in relation to hypotension and shock.
- Check blood pressure; heart rate; urine output; skin temperature of extremities; level of consciousness; orientation to person, place, and time; and adequacy of respiration. Abnormal values are not specific indicators of hypotension and shock, but they may indicate a need for further evaluation. Generally, report blood pressure below 90/60, heart rate above 100, and urine output below 50 ml/h.
- Check electrocardiogram and other assessment data if available.

## Nursing diagnoses

- Decreased Cardiac Output related to hypotension and vasoconstriction
- Altered Tissue Perfusion: Decreased related to decreased cardiac output
- Fluid Volume Deficit related to fluid loss or vasodilation
- Anxiety related to potentially life-threatening illness
- High Risk for Injury: Myocardial infarction, stroke, or renal damage related to decreased blood flow to vital organs

## Planning/Goals

*The client will:*
- Have improved tissue perfusion and relief of symptoms
- Have improved vital signs
- Be guarded against recurrence of hypotension and shock if possible
- Be monitored for therapeutic and adverse effects of adrenergic drugs
- Avoid preventable adverse effects of adrenergic drugs

## Interventions

Use measures to prevent or minimize hypotension and shock.
- General measures include those to maintain fluid balance, control hemorrhage, treat infections, prevent hypoxia, and control other causative factors.
- Learn to recognize *impending* shock so that treatment can be initiated early. *Do not wait* until symptoms are severe.

Monitor clients during shock and vasopressor drug therapy.
- Titrate adrenergic drug infusion to maintain blood pressure and tissue perfusion without causing hypertension.
- Check blood pressure and pulse constantly or at least every 5 to 15 minutes during acute shock and vasopressor drug therapy.
- Monitor distal pulses, urine output, and skin temperature closely to assess tissue perfusion.
- Check venipuncture site frequently for infiltration or extravasation.

*Teach clients and family:*
- Descriptions and purposes of drug therapy and monitoring equipment
- The need for close observation of vital signs, IV infusion site, urine output, and so forth

## Evaluation

Observe for improved vital signs, color and temperature of skin, and urine output.

# Principles of therapy

## GOAL OF THERAPY

The goal of adrenergic drug therapy in hypotension and shock is to restore and maintain adequate tissue perfusion.

## CHOICE OF DRUG

The choice of drug depends primarily on the pathophysiology involved. For cardiogenic shock and decreased cardiac output, dopamine or dobutamine is given. With severe congestive heart failure characterized by decreased cardiac output and high peripheral vascular resistance, vasodilator drugs (*e.g.*, nitroprusside, nitroglycerin) may be given along with the cardiotonic drug. The combination increases cardiac output and decreases the heart's workload by decreasing preload and afterload. However, vasodilators should not be used alone because of the risk of severe hypotension and further compromising tissue perfusion.

For anaphylactic or neurogenic shock characterized by severe vasodilation and decreased peripheral vascular resistance, a vasoconstrictor or vasopressor drug, such as norepinephrine, is the first drug of choice. Drug dosage must be carefully titrated to avoid excessive vasoconstriction and hypertension, which causes impairment rather than improvement in tissue perfusion.

## GUIDELINES FOR TREATMENT OF HYPOTENSION AND SHOCK

1. Vasopressor drugs are less effective in the presence of inadequate blood volume, electrolyte abnormalities, and acidosis. These conditions also must be treated if present. Dopamine, dobutamine, or norepinephrine IV infusions may be titrated to maintain a low normal blood pressure.
2. Septic shock requires appropriate antibiotic therapy in addition to other treatment measures. If an abscess is the source of infection, it must be surgically drained.
3. Hypovolemic shock is most effectively treated by IV fluids that replace the type of fluid lost; that is, blood loss should be replaced with whole blood, and gastrointestinal losses should be replaced with solutions containing electrolytes (*e.g.*, Ringer's lactate or sodium chloride solutions with added potassium chloride).
4. Cardiogenic shock may be complicated by pulmonary congestion, for which diuretic drugs are indicated.
5. Anaphylactic shock is often treated by nonadrenergic drugs as well as epinephrine. For example, the histamine-induced cardiovascular symptoms (*e.g.*, vasodilation and increased capillary permeability) are thought to be mediated through both types of histamine receptors. Consequently, treatment may include a histamine$_1$ receptor blocker (*e.g.*, diphenhydramine 1 mg/kg IV) and histamine$_2$ receptor blocker (*e.g.*, cimetidine 4 mg/kg IV), given over at least 5 minutes. In addition, IV corticosteroids are frequently given, such as methylprednisolone (20–100 mg) or hydrocortisone (100–500 mg). Doses may need to be repeated every 2 to 4 hours. Corticosteroids increase tissue responsiveness to adrenergic drugs in about 2 hours but do not produce anti-inflammatory effects for several hours.

## USE IN CHILDREN

Little information is available about adrenergic drugs for the treatment of hypotension and shock in children. Generally, treatment is the same as for adults, with drug dosages adjusted for weight.

## USE IN OLDER ADULTS

The use of adrenergic drugs to manage hypotension and shock in the older adult is essentially the same as for younger adults. Older adults often have disorders such as atherosclerosis, peripheral vascular disease, and diabetes mellitus. When adrenergic drugs are given, their vasoconstricting effects may decrease blood flow and increase risks of tissue ischemia and thrombosis. Careful monitoring of pulses and skin color and temperature, especially in the extremities, is required.

# NURSING ACTIONS: DRUGS USED IN HYPOTENSION AND SHOCK

| *Nursing Actions* | *Rationale/Explanation* |
|---|---|
| **1. Administer accurately** | |
| **a.** Use a large vein for the venipuncture site (*e.g.*, the antecubital vein). Tape the needle or catheter securely. Use arm boards and other devices to restrict movement if necessary. | To decrease risks of extravasation |
| **b.** Dilute drugs for continuous infusion in 250 or 500 ml of IV fluid. A 5% dextrose injection is compatible with all of the drugs and is most often used. For use of other IV fluids, consult drug manufacturers' literature. Dilute drugs for bolus injections to at least 10 ml with sodium chloride or water for injection. | To avoid adverse effects, which are more likely to occur with concentrated drug solutions |
| **c.** Use a separate IV line or a "piggyback" IV setup. | This allows the adrenergic drug solution to be regulated or discontinued without disruption of other IV lines. |
| **d.** Use an infusion pump. | To administer the drug at a consistent rate. This helps to prevent wide fluctuations in blood pressure and other cardiovascular functions. |
| **e.** Discard any solution with a brownish color or precipitate. | Most of the solutions are stable for 24 to 48 hours. Epinephrine and isoproterenol decompose on exposure to light, producing a brownish discoloration. |
| **f.** Start the adrenergic drug slowly, and increase as necessary to obtain desired responses in blood pressure and other parameters of cardiovascular function. | Flow rate (dosage) is titrated according to client response. |
| **g.** Stop the drug gradually. | Abrupt discontinuance of pressor drugs may cause rebound hypotension. |
| **2. Observe for therapeutic effects** | |
| **a.** Systolic blood pressure of 80 to 100 mm Hg | These levels are adequate for tissue perfusion. Higher levels may increase cardiac workload, resulting in reflex bradycardia and decreased cardiac output. However, higher levels may be necessary to maintain cerebral blood flow in older adults. |
| **b.** Heart rate of 60 to 100; improved quality of peripheral pulses | These indicate improved tissue perfusion and cardiovascular function. |
| **c.** Improved urine output | Increased urine output indicates improved blood flow to the kidneys. |
| **d.** Improved skin color and temperature | |
| **e.** Pulmonary-capillary wedge pressure between 15 and 20 mm Hg in cardiogenic shock | Normal pulmonary-capillary wedge pressure is 6 to 12 mm Hg. Higher levels are required to maintain cardiac output in cardiogenic shock. |
| **3. Observe for adverse effects** | |
| **a.** Bradycardia | Reflex bradycardia may occur with levarterenol, metaraminol, methoxamine, and phenylephrine. |
| **b.** Tachycardia | This is most likely to occur with isoproterenol but may occur with dopamine and epinephrine. |

*(continued)*

## *Nursing Actions*

## *Rationale/Explanation*

**c.** Arrhythmias

Fatal arrhythmias due to excessive adrenergic stimulation of the heart may occur with any of the agents used in hypotension and shock.

**d.** Hypertension

This is most likely to occur with high doses of levarterenol, metaraminol, methoxamine, and phenylephrine.

**e.** Hypotension

This is most likely to occur with low doses of dopamine and isoproterenol, owing to vasodilation.

**f.** Angina pectoris—chest pain, dyspnea, palpitations

All pressor agents may increase myocardial oxygen consumption and induce myocardial ischemia.

**g.** Tissue necrosis if extravasation occurs

This may occur with extravasation of solutions containing dopamine, levarterenol, metaraminol, and phenylephrine, owing to local vasoconstriction and impaired blood supply. Tissue necrosis may be prevented by injecting 5 to 10 mg of phentolamine (Regitine), subcutaneously, around the area of extravasation. Regitine is most effective if injected within 12 hours after extravasation.

**4. Observe for drug interactions**
  **a.** Drugs that *increase* effects of pressor agents:

    (1) General anesthetics (*e.g.,* halothane)

Halothane and other halogenated anesthetics increase cardiac sensitivity to sympathomimetic drugs and increase the risks of cardiac arrhythmias.

    (2) Anticholinergic drugs (*e.g.,* atropine)

Atropine and other drugs with anticholinergic activity may potentiate the tachycardia that often occurs with pressor agents, especially isoproterenol.

    (3) MAO inhibitors (*e.g.,* tranylcypromine)

All effects of exogenously administered adrenergic drugs are magnified in clients taking MAO inhibitors because MAO is the circulating enzyme responsible for metabolism of adrenergic agents.

    (4) Oxytocics (*e.g.,* oxytocin)

The risk of severe hypertension is increased.

  **b.** Drugs that *decrease* effects of pressor agents:

    Beta-blocking agents (*e.g.,* propranolol)

Beta-blocking agents antagonize the cardiac stimulation produced by some pressor agents (*e.g.,* dobutamine, isoproterenol). Decreased heart rate, myocardial contractility, and blood pressure may result.

**5. Teach clients**
  **a.** Report pain, edema, or cool skin around the venipuncture site

These symptoms may indicate leakage of the drug solution into surrounding tissues. If extravasation occurs, prompt treatment may prevent severe tissue damage.

  **b.** That frequent measurements of blood pressure and pulse and other observations are necessary

Knowing what to expect will decrease the client's anxiety.

## Review and Application Exercises

1. How do adrenergic drugs improve circulation in hypotension and shock?
2. Which adrenergic drug improves renal blood flow?
3. Which adrenergic drug should be readily available for treatment of anaphylactic shock?
4. What are adverse effects of adrenergic drugs?
5. How would you assess the client for therapeutic or adverse effects of an adrenergic drug being given by continuous IV infusion?
6. Why is it important to prevent extravasation of adrenergic drug infusions into tissues surrounding the vein?
7. In hypovolemic shock, should fluid volume be replaced before or after an adrenergic drug is given?

## Selected References

Arrigoni, L. W., & Depew, C. C. (1992). Intensive care therapeutics. In M. A. Koda-Kimble & L. Y. Young (Eds.), *Applied therapeutics: The clinical use of drugs* (5th ed.) (pp. 12-1–12-33). Vancouver, WA: Applied Therapeutics.

Cohn, J. N. (1990). Pharmacologic support of the failing circulation in acute myocardial infarction. In G. S. Francis & J. S. Alpert (Eds.), *Modern coronary care* (pp. 255–265). Boston: Little, Brown.

Dolan, J. T. (1991). *Critical care nursing: Clinical management through the nursing process.* Philadelphia: F.A. Davis.

Leier, C. V. (1992). Approach to the patient with hypotension and shock. In W. N. Kelley (Ed.), *Textbook of internal medicine* (2nd ed.) (pp. 353–361). Philadelphia: J.B. Lippincott.

McLean, J. A. (1992). Treatment of anaphylaxis. In W. N. Kelley (Ed.), *Textbook of internal medicine* (2nd ed.) (pp. 75–77). Philadelphia: J.B. Lippincott.

Tatro, E. H., & Burrell, L. O. (1992). Major principles of shock and related nursing management. In L. O. Burrell (Ed.), *Adult nursing in hospital and community settings* (pp. 208–222). Norwalk, CT: Appleton & Lange.

Urban, N. (1990). Circulatory shock. In Porth, C. M. (Ed.), *Pathophysiology: Concepts of altered health states* (3rd ed.) (pp. 389–402). Philadelphia: J.B. Lippincott.

### CHAPTER 58

# Antihypertensive Drugs

Antihypertensive drugs are used to treat hypertension, a common, chronic disorder affecting an estimated 60 million people in the United States. Hypertension increases risks of myocardial infarction, congestive heart failure, cerebral infarction and hemorrhage, and renal disease. To understand hypertension and antihypertensive drug therapy, one must first understand the physiologic mechanisms that normally control blood pressure, characteristics of hypertension, and characteristics of antihypertensive drugs.

## Regulation of arterial blood pressure

Arterial blood pressure reflects the force exerted on arterial walls by blood flow. Blood pressure normally stays relatively constant because of homeostatic mechanisms that adjust blood flow. The two major determinants of arterial blood pressure are cardiac output (systolic pressure) and peripheral vascular resistance (diastolic pressure). Cardiac output equals the product of the heart rate and stroke volume ($CO = HR \times SV$). Stroke volume is the amount of blood ejected with each heart beat (about 60–90 ml). Thus, cardiac output depends on the force of myocardial contraction, blood volume, and other factors. Peripheral vascular resistance is determined by the degree of constriction or dilation in arterioles (vascular tone). Any condition that affects heart rate, stroke volume, or peripheral resistance affects arterial blood pressure.

Regulation of blood pressure involves a complex network of nervous, hormonal, and renal mechanisms. The nervous and hormonal mechanisms act rapidly; renal mechanisms act more slowly. When hypotension occurs, the sympathetic nervous system (SNS) is stimulated, the hormones epinephrine and norepinephrine are secreted by the adrenal medulla, angiotensin II and aldosterone are formed, and the kidneys retain fluid. These compensatory mechanisms raise the blood pressure. Specific effects include the following:

1. Constriction of arterioles, which increases peripheral vascular resistance
2. Constriction of veins and increased venous tone
3. Stimulation of cardiac beta-adrenergic receptors, which increases heart rate and force of myocardial contraction
4. Secretion of renin by the kidneys. In the bloodstream, renin acts on a plasma protein to produce angiotensin I, which is converted to angiotensin II by the enzyme peptidyl dipeptidase. Angiotensin II is a potent vasoconstrictor that constricts arterioles and increases peripheral resistance. It also stimulates secretion of aldosterone by the adrenal cortex. Aldosterone causes the kidneys to retain sodium and water.
5. Retention of fluid by the kidneys, which increases blood volume and cardiac output

When arterial blood pressure is elevated, the following sequence of events occurs:

1. Kidneys excrete more fluid (increase urine output).
2. Fluid loss reduces both extracellular fluid volume and blood volume.
3. Decreased blood volume reduces venous blood flow to the heart and therefore decreases cardiac output.

Anne Collins Abrams: CLINICAL DRUG THERAPY, Fourth Edition.
© 1995 J.B. Lippincott Company.

4. Decreased cardiac output reduces arterial blood pressure.

# Hypertension

Hypertension is persistently high blood pressure that results from abnormalities in the regulatory mechanisms described above. It is usually defined as a systolic pressure above 140 mm Hg or a diastolic pressure above 90 mm Hg on multiple blood pressure measurements.

Primary or essential hypertension (that for which no cause can be found) makes up about 90% of known cases. Secondary hypertension may result from renal, endocrine, or central nervous system disorders and from drugs that stimulate the SNS or cause retention of sodium and water. Primary hypertension can be controlled with appropriate therapy; secondary hypertension can sometimes be cured by surgical therapy.

The Fifth Report of the Joint National Committee on Detection, Evaluation, and Treatment of High Blood Pressure, published in 1993, describes a new classification of blood pressures in adults (in mm of Hg), as follows:

- Normal = systolic 130 or below; diastolic 85 or below
- High normal = systolic 130 to 139; diastolic 85 to 89
- Stage 1 hypertension (mild) = systolic 140 to 159; diastolic 90 to 99
- Stage 2 hypertension (moderate) = systolic 160 to 179; diastolic 100 to 109
- Stage 3 hypertension (severe) = systolic 180 to 209; diastolic 110 to 119
- Stage 4 hypertension (very severe) = systolic 210 or above; diastolic 120 or above

A systolic pressure of 140 or above with a diastolic pressure below 90 is usually called isolated systolic hypertension.

Hypertension profoundly alters cardiovascular function by increasing the workload of the heart and causing thickening and sclerosis of arterial walls. As a result of increased cardiac workload, the myocardium hypertrophies as a compensatory mechanism. However, heart failure eventually occurs. As a result of arterial changes, the lumen is narrowed, blood supply to tissues is decreased, and risks of thrombosis are increased. In addition, necrotic areas may develop in arteries, and these may rupture with sustained high blood pressure. The areas of most serious damage are the heart, brain, kidneys, and eyes. These are often called "target organs."

Initially and perhaps for years, primary hypertension may produce no symptoms. If symptoms occur, they are usually vague and nonspecific. Hypertension may go undetected, or it may be incidentally discovered when blood pressure measurements are taken as part of a routine physical examination, screening test, or assessment of other disorders. Eventually, symptoms reflect target organ damage. Not infrequently, hypertension is discovered after a person experiences angina pectoris, myocardial infarction, congestive heart failure, stroke, or renal disease.

Hypertensive emergencies are episodes of severely elevated blood pressure that may be an extension of malignant hypertension or caused by cerebral hemorrhage, dissecting aortic aneurysm, renal disease, pheochromocytoma, or eclampsia. These require immediate treatment, usually intravenous antihypertensive drugs, to lower blood pressure. Symptoms include severe headache, nausea, vomiting, visual disturbances, neurologic disturbances, disorientation, and decreased level of consciousness (drowsiness, stupor, coma). Hypertensive urgencies are episodes of less severe hypertension that often may be managed with oral drugs. The goal of treatment is to lower blood pressure within 24 hours. In most instances, it is better to lower blood pressure gradually (rather than precipitously) and to avoid wide fluctuations in blood pressure.

# Antihypertensive drugs

Drugs used in the treatment of primary hypertension belong to several different groups, including angiotensin-converting enzyme (ACE) inhibitors, antiadrenergics (alpha receptor blocking agents, beta receptor blocking agents, centrally acting agents), calcium channel-blockers, diuretics, and direct vasodilators. These drugs generally act to decrease blood pressure by decreasing cardiac output or peripheral vascular resistance.

## ANGIOTENSIN-CONVERTING ENZYME INHIBITORS

Captopril (Capoten) and other ACE inhibitors interfere with the renin-angiotensin-aldosterone system of blood pressure control. More specifically, they block the enzyme that normally converts the physiologically inactive angiotensin I to the potent vasoconstrictor angiotensin II. This action also results in decreased aldosterone production.

In clients with normal renal function, ACE inhibitors may be used alone or in combination with other antihypertensive agents, such as thiazide diuretics. In clients with impaired renal function, the drugs are recommended for those who fail to respond or who experience intolerable adverse effects with other antihypertensive agents.

Captopril and enalapril also are used in the treatment of congestive heart failure; they decrease vasoconstriction and peripheral vascular resistance, thereby reducing cardiac workload.

## ANTIADRENERGICS

Antiadrenergic (sympatholytic) drugs inhibit activity of the SNS. When the SNS is stimulated (see Chap. 17), the nerve impulse travels from the brain and spinal cord to the ganglia. From the ganglia, the impulse travels along postganglionic fibers to effector organs (*e.g.*, heart, blood vessels). Although SNS stimulation produces widespread effects in the body, the effects relevant to this discussion are the increases in heart rate, force of myocardial contraction, cardiac output, and blood pressure that occur. When the nerve impulse is inhibited or blocked at any location along its pathway, the result is decreased blood pressure.

Alpha$_1$ receptor blocking agents (*e.g.*, prazosin) dilate blood vessels and decrease peripheral vascular resistance. Alpha$_2$-blocking agents (*e.g.*, clonidine) block SNS impulses in the brain. Beta-adrenergic blocking agents (*e.g.*, propranolol) decrease heart rate, force of myocardial contraction, cardiac output, and renin release from the kidneys. Other antiadrenergic drugs include trimethaphan, which acts at ganglionic sites; guanethidine and related drugs, which act at postganglionic nerve endings; and two other alpha-blockers (phentolamine and phenoxybenzamine), which occasionally are used in hypertension resulting from catecholamine excess. The latter two drugs are discussed in Chapter 19.

## CALCIUM CHANNEL-BLOCKING AGENTS

Calcium channel-blockers (*e.g.*, verapamil) are used for several cardiovascular disorders. Their mechanism of action and use in the treatment of tachyarrhythmias and angina pectoris are discussed in Chapters 55 and 56, respectively. In hypertension, they mainly decrease peripheral vascular resistance. The decrease in peripheral vascular resistance stems largely from their ability to dilate peripheral arteries.

Most of the available drugs are approved for use in hypertension. Nifedipine is often used to treat hypertensive emergencies or urgencies. Because it is available only in a capsule, various methods have been used to obtain rapid drug action; these methods include puncturing the capsule and squeezing the contents under the tongue. Studies indicate that the drug is not absorbed through oral mucosa and that its effects result from the swallowed drug. Thus, clients should bite and swallow the capsule when rapid lowering of blood pressure is the desired effect. Do *not* give a long-acting form of nifedipine by this method; toxicity may result.

## DIURETICS

Antihypertensive effects of diuretics are usually attributed to sodium and water depletion. In fact, diuretics generally produce the same effects as severe dietary sodium restriction. In many cases of hypertension, diuretic therapy alone may lower blood pressure. When diuretic therapy is begun, blood volume and cardiac output decrease. With long-term administration of a diuretic, cardiac output returns to normal, but there is a persistent decrease in peripheral vascular resistance. This has been attributed to a persistent small reduction in extracellular water and plasma volume, decreased receptor sensitivity to vasopressor substances such as angiotensin, direct arteriolar vasodilation, and arteriolar vasodilation secondary to electrolyte depletion in the vessel wall.

In moderate or severe hypertension that does not respond to a diuretic alone, the diuretic may be continued and another antihypertensive drug added, or monotherapy with a different type of antihypertensive drug may be tried.

The most commonly used diuretics are the thiazides (*e.g.*, hydrochlorothiazide [HydroDiuril]). Others are useful in particular circumstances; see Chapter 59 for more information regarding diuretic drugs.

## VASODILATORS (DIRECT ACTING)

Vasodilator antihypertensive drugs act directly on blood vessels to cause dilation and decreased peripheral vascular resistance. Hydralazine, diazoxide, and minoxidil act mainly on arterioles; nitroprusside acts on arterioles and venules. These drugs have a limited effect on hypertension when used alone because the vasodilating action that lowers blood pressure also stimulates the SNS and arouses reflexive compensatory mechanisms (vasoconstriction, tachycardia, and increased cardiac output), which raise blood pressure. This effect can be prevented during long-term therapy by also giving a drug that prevents excessive sympathetic stimulation (*e.g.*, propranolol). These drugs also cause sodium and water retention, which may be minimized by giving a diuretic concomitantly.

# Individual drugs

Diuretics are discussed in Chapter 59 and listed in Table 59-1. Antihypertensive agents are shown in Table 58-1; antihypertensive–diuretic combination products are listed in Table 58-2.

## TABLE 58-1. ANTIHYPERTENSIVE DRUGS

| Generic/Trade Name | Routes and Dosage Ranges | |
| --- | --- | --- |
| | **Adults** | **Children** |
| ***Angiotensin-Converting Enzyme Inhibitors*** | | |
| **Benazepril** (Lotensin) | PO 10 mg once daily initially, increased to 40 mg daily if necessary, in one or two doses | |
| **Captopril** (Capoten) | PO 25 mg two to three times daily initially, increased after 1–2 wk if necessary to 50 mg two to three times daily, then to 100 mg two to three times daily, then to 150 mg two to three times daily. Maximal dose, 450 mg/d. | |
| **Enalapril** (Vasotec) | PO 5 mg once daily, increased to 10–40 mg daily, in one or two doses, if necessary | |
| **Fosinopril** (Monopril) | Same as benazepril, above | |
| **Lisinopril** (Prinivil, Zestril) | PO 10 mg once daily, increased to 40 mg if necessary | |
| **Quinapril** (Accupril) | PO 10 mg once daily initially, increased to 20, 40, or 80 mg daily if necessary, in one or two doses. Wait at least 2 wk between dose increments. | |
| **Ramipril** (Altace) | PO 2.5 mg once daily, increased to 20 mg daily if necessary, in one or two doses | |
| ***Antiadrenergic Agents*** | | |
| ***Alpha₁-Blocking Agents*** | | |
| **Doxazosin** (Cardura) | PO 1 mg once daily initially, increased to 2 mg, then to 4, 8, and 16 mg if necessary | |
| **Prazosin** (Minipress) | PO 1 mg two to three times daily initially, increased if necessary to a total daily dose of 20 mg in divided doses. Average maintenance dose, 6–15 mg/d. | |
| **Terazosin** (Hytrin) | PO 1 mg at bedtime initially, increased gradually to maintenance dose, usually 1–5 mg once daily | |
| ***Alpha₂-Blocking Agents*** | | |
| **Clonidine** (Catapres) | PO 0.1 mg two times daily initially, gradually increased if necessary up to 2.4 mg/d. Average maintenance dose, 0.2–0.8 mg/d. | |
| **Guanabenz** (Wytensin) | PO 4 mg twice daily, increased by 4–8 mg daily every 1–2 wk if necessary to a maximal dose of 32 mg twice daily | |
| **Guanfacine** (Tenex) | PO 1 mg daily at bedtime, increased to 2 mg after 3–4 wk, then to 3 mg if necessary | |
| **Methyldopa** (Aldomet) | PO 250 mg two or three times daily initially, increased gradually at intervals of not less than 2 d until blood pressure is controlled or a daily dose of 3 g is reached | PO 10 mg/kg per day in two to four divided doses initially, increased or decreased according to response. Maximal dose, 65 mg/kg per day or 3 g daily, whichever is less. |
| ***Ganglionic-Blocking Agent*** | | |
| **Trimethaphan camsylate** (Arfonad) | Hypertensive crisis, IV diluted in 5% dextrose injection to a concentration of 1 mg/ml and given as a continuous infusion at an initial flow rate of 3–4 mg/min, then individualize rate depending on blood pressure. Rates vary from 0.3–6 mg/min. | |
| ***Postganglionic-Active Drugs*** | | |
| **Guanadrel** (Hylorel) | PO 10 mg daily initially. Usual dosage range, 20–75 mg daily in divided doses. | |
| **Guanethidine sulfate** (Ismelin) | PO 10 mg daily initially, increased every 5–7 d to a maximal daily dose of 300 mg if necessary. Usual daily dose, 25–50 mg. For hospitalized clients, therapy may be initiated with 25–50 mg daily and increased every 1–2 d. | PO 0.2 mg/kg per day initially, increased by the same amount every 7–10 d if necessary to a maximum dose of 3 mg/kg per day Safety has not been established for use in children. |
| **Reserpine** (Serpasil) | PO 0.25–0.5 mg daily initially for 1–2 wk, reduced slowly to 0.1–0.25 mg daily for maintenance | |
| ***Beta-Adrenergic Blocking Agents*** | | |
| **Acebutolol** (Sectral) | PO 400 mg once daily initially, increased to 800 mg daily if necessary | |
| **Atenolol** (Tenormin) | PO 50 mg once daily initially, increased in 1–2 wk to 100 mg once daily, if necessary | |

*(continued)*

**TABLE 58-1. ANTIHYPERTENSIVE DRUGS** *(Continued)*

| | Routes and Dosage Ranges | |
| Generic/Trade Name | *Adults* | *Children* |
| --- | --- | --- |
| **Betaxolol** (Kerlone) | PO 10–20 mg daily | |
| **Carteolol** (Cartrol) | PO 2.5 mg once daily initially, gradually increased to a maximum daily dose of 10 mg if necessary. Usual maintenance dose, 2.5–5 mg once daily. Extend dosage interval to 48 h for a creatinine clearance of 20–60 ml/min and to 72 h for a creatinine clearance below 20 ml/min. | |
| **Metoprolol** (Lopressor) | PO 50 mg twice daily, gradually increased in weekly or longer intervals if necessary, to a maximal daily dose of 450 mg | |
| **Nadolol** (Corgard) | PO 40 mg daily initially, gradually increased if necessary, by 40–80 mg daily. Average daily dose, 80–320 mg. | |
| **Penbutolol** (Levatol) | PO 20 mg once daily | |
| **Pindolol** (Visken) | PO 5 mg two or three times daily initially, increased by 10 mg/d at 3- to 4-wk intervals to a maximal daily dose of 60 mg | |
| **Propranolol** (Inderal) | PO 40 mg twice daily initially, gradually increased to 160–640 mg daily | PO 1 mg/kg per day initially, gradually increased to a maximum dose of 10 mg/kg per day |
| **Timolol** (Blocadren) | PO 10 mg twice daily initially, increased gradually if necessary. Average daily dose, 20–40 mg; maximal daily dose, 60 mg. | |

### *Alpha–Beta-Adrenergic Blocking Agent*

| | | |
| --- | --- | --- |
| **Labetalol** (Trandate, Normodyne) | PO 100 mg twice daily, increased by 100 mg twice daily every 2–3 d if necessary. Usual maintenance dose, 200–400 mg twice daily. Severe hypertension may require 1200–2400 mg daily. IV injection, 20 mg slowly over 2 minutes, followed by 40–80 mg every 10 minutes until the desired blood pressure is achieved or 300 mg has been given. IV infusion, add 200 mg to 250 ml of 5% dextrose or 0.9% sodium chloride solution (concentration 2 mg/3 ml) and infuse at a rate of 3 ml/min. Adjust flow rate according to blood pressure, and substitute oral labetalol when blood pressure is controlled. | |

### *Calcium Channel-Blocking Agents*

| | | |
| --- | --- | --- |
| **Amlodipine** (Norvasc) | PO 5–10 mg once daily | |
| **Diltiazem (sustained-release)** (Cardizem SR) | PO 60–120 mg twice daily | |
| **Felodipine** (Plendil) | PO 5–10 mg once daily. Extended-release tablets; swallow whole, do not crush or chew. | |
| **Isradipine** (DynaCirc) | PO 2.5–5 mg twice daily | |
| **Nicardipine** (Cardene, Cardene SR) | PO 20–40 mg three times daily; Sustained-release, PO 30–60 mg twice daily | |
| **Nifedipine** (Adalat, Procardia) | PO 10 mg for hypertensive crisis (Have client bite and swallow capsule.) | |
| **Nifedipine (sustained-release)** (Procardia XL) | PO 30–60 mg once daily, increased over 1–2 wk if necessary | |
| **Verapamil** (Calan, Isoptin) | PO 80 mg three times daily | |
| **Verapamil (sustained-release)** (Calan SR, Isoptin SR) | PO 240 mg once daily | |

### *Vasodilators, Direct Acting*

| | | |
| --- | --- | --- |
| **Diazoxide** (Hyperstat) | Hypertensive crisis, IV 1–3 mg/kg (up to 150 mg) by rapid injection (within 30 seconds), repeated as necessary at 5- to 15-min intervals | Hypertensive crisis, same as for adults |
| **Hydralazine** (Apresoline) | Chronic hypertension, PO 10 mg four times daily for 2–4 d, increased to 25 mg four times daily for 2–4 d if necessary, then increased to 50 mg four times daily if necessary, to a maximal dose of 300 mg/d. Hypertensive crisis, IM, IV 10–20 mg, increased to 40 mg if necessary. Repeat dose as needed. | Chronic hypertension, 0.75 mg/kg per day initially in four divided doses. Gradually increased over 3–4 wk to a maximal dose of 7.5 mg/kg per day if necessary |

**TABLE 58-1. ANTIHYPERTENSIVE DRUGS** *(Continued)*

| Generic/Trade Name | Routes and Dosage Ranges | |
|---|---|---|
| | **Adults** | **Children** |
| **Minoxidil** (Loniten) | PO 5 mg once daily initially, increased gradually until blood pressure is controlled. Average daily dose, 10–40 mg; maximal daily dose, 100 mg in single or divided doses | Hypertensive crisis, IM, IV 0.1–0.2 mg/kg per dose every 4–6 h as needed Age under 12 years, PO 0.2 mg/kg per day initially as a single dose, increased gradually until blood pressure is controlled. Average daily dose, 0.25–1.0 mg/kg; maximal dose, 50 mg/d. |
| **Sodium nitroprusside** (Nipride) | IV infusion at a flow rate to deliver 0.5–10 μg/kg per minute. Average dose is 3 μg/kg per minute. Prepare solution by adding 50 mg of sodium nitroprusside to 250–1000 ml of 5% dextrose in water, and wrap promptly in aluminum foil to protect from light. | Same as for adults. |

## Nursing Process

### Assessment

Assess the client's condition in relation to hypertension.
- Identify conditions and risk factors that may lead to hypertension. These include:
  - Obesity
  - Elevated serum cholesterol and triglycerides
  - Cigarette smoking
  - Sedentary life-style
  - Family history of hypertension or other cardiovascular disease
  - African-American race
  - Renal disease (*e.g.*, renal artery stenosis)
  - Adrenal disease (*e.g.*, hypersecretion of aldosterone, pheochromocytoma)
  - Other cardiovascular disorders (*e.g.*, atherosclerosis, left ventricular hypertrophy)
  - Diabetes mellitus

**TABLE 58-2. REPRESENTATIVE ANTIHYPERTENSIVE-DIURETIC COMBINATION PRODUCTS**

| Trade Name | Antihypertensive Component | Diuretic Component | Route and Dosage Range |
|---|---|---|---|
| Aldoril-15 | Methyldopa 250 mg | Hydrochlorothiazide 15 mg | PO 1 tablet two or three times daily for 48 h, then increased or decreased according to response |
| Aldoril-25 | Methyldopa 250 mg | Hydrochlorothiazide 25 mg | Same as Aldoril-15 |
| Aldoril D30 | Methyldopa 500 mg | Hydrochlorothiazide 30 mg | Same as Aldoril-15 |
| Aldoril D50 | Methyldopa 500 mg | Hydrochlorothiazide 50 mg | Same as Aldoril-15 |
| Capozide | Captopril 25 mg | Hydrochlorothiazide 15 mg | PO 1 tablet two or three times daily |
| | Captopril 25 mg | Hydrochlorothiazide 25 mg | PO 1 tablet two or three times daily |
| | Captopril 50 mg | Hydrochlorothiazide 15 mg | PO 1 tablet two or three times daily |
| | Captopril 50 mg | Hydrochlorothiazide 25 mg | PO 1 tablet two or three times daily |
| Combipres 0.1 mg | Clonidine 0.1 mg | Chlorthalidone 15 mg | PO 1 tablet twice daily |
| Combipres 0.2 mg | Clonidine 0.2 mg | Chlorthalidone 15 mg | PO 1 tablet twice daily |
| Combipres 0.3 mg | Clonidine 0.3 mg | Chlorthalidone 15 mg | PO 1 tablet twice daily |
| Corzide 40/5 | Nadolol 40 mg | Bendroflumethiazide 5 mg | PO 1 tablet daily |
| Corzide 80/5 | Nadolol 80 mg | Bendroflumethiazide 5 mg | PO 1 tablet daily |
| Inderide 40/25 | Propranolol 40 mg | Hydrochlorothiazide 25 mg | PO 1–2 tablets twice daily |
| Inderide 80/25 | Propranolol 80 mg | Hydrochlorothiazide 25 mg | PO 1–2 tablets twice daily |
| Lopressor HCT 100/50 | Metoprolol 100 mg | Hydrochlorothiazide 50 mg | PO 1 tablet daily |
| Lopressor HCT 100/25 | Metoprolol 100 mg | Hydrochlorothiazide 25 mg | PO 1–2 tablets daily |
| Lopressor HCT 50/25 | Metoprolol 50 mg | Hydrochlorothiazide 25 mg | PO 1–2 tablets daily |
| Minizide 1 | Prazosin 1 mg | Polythiazide 0.5 mg | PO 1 capsule two or three times daily |
| Minizide 2 | Prazosin 2 mg | Polythiazide 0.5 mg | PO 1 capsule two or three times daily |
| Minizide 5 | Prazosin 5 mg | Polythiazide 0.5 mg | PO 1 capsule two or three times daily |
| Tenoretic 50 | Atenolol 50 mg | Chlorthalidone 25 mg | PO 1 tablet daily |
| Tenoretic 100 | Atenolol 100 mg | Chlorthalidone 25 mg | PO 1 tablet daily |
| Timolide | Timolol 10 mg | Hydrochlorothiazide 25 mg | PO 1–2 tablets one or two times daily |
| Vaseretic | Enalapril 10 mg | Hydrochlorothiazide 25 mg | PO 1–2 tablets daily |

- Oral contraceptives, corticosteroids, appetite suppressants, decongestants, nonsteroidal anti-inflammatory agents
- Neurologic disorders (*e.g.*, brain damage)
- Observe for signs and symptoms of hypertension.
  - Check blood pressure accurately and repeatedly. As a rule, multiple measurements in which systolic pressure is above 140 mm Hg, diastolic pressure is above 90 mm Hg, or both are necessary to establish a diagnosis of hypertension. Single measurements provide little useful information.

    The importance of accurate blood pressure measurements cannot be overemphasized because there are many possibilities for errors. Some ways to improve accuracy and validity include using correct equipment (*e.g.*, proper cuff size), having the client in the same position each time blood pressure is measured (*e.g.*, sitting or supine with arm at heart level), using the same arm for repeated measurements, and having the same person do successive recordings on a particular client.
  - In most cases of early hypertension, elevated blood pressure is the only clinical manifestation. If symptoms do occur, they are usually nonspecific (*e.g.*, headache, weakness, fatigue, tachycardia, dizziness, palpitations, epistaxis).
  - Eventually, signs and symptoms occur as target organs are damaged. Heart damage is often reflected as angina pectoris, myocardial infarction, or congestive heart failure. Chest pain, tachycardia, dyspnea, fatigue, and edema may occur. Brain damage may be indicated by transient ischemic attacks or strokes of varying severity with symptoms ranging from syncope to hemiparesis. Renal damage may be reflected by proteinuria, increased blood urea nitrogen, and increased serum creatinine. Ophthalmoscopic examination may reveal hemorrhages, sclerosis of arterioles, and inflammation of the optic nerve (papilledema). Because arterioles can be visualized in the retina of the eye, damage to retinal vessels may indicate damage to arterioles in the heart, brain, and kidneys.

### Nursing diagnoses

- Decreased Cardiac Output related to disease process or drug therapy
- Anxiety related to fear of myocardial infarction or stroke
- Ineffective Individual Coping related to long-term life-style changes and drug therapy
- Noncompliance related to lack of knowledge about hypertension and its management, costs and adverse effects of drug therapy, and psychosocial factors
- Body Image Disturbance related to the need for long-term treatment and medical supervision
- Fatigue related to antihypertensive drug therapy
- Knowledge Deficit related to hypertension, antihypertensive drug therapy, and nondrug life-style changes
- Sexual Dysfunction related to adverse drug effects
- High Risk for Injury related to drug-induced hypotension and dizziness

### Planning/Goals

*The client will:*

- Receive or take antihypertensive drugs correctly

- Be monitored closely for therapeutic and adverse drug effects, especially when drug therapy is started and when changes are made in drugs or dosages
- Use nondrug measures to assist in blood pressure control
- Avoid, manage, or report adverse drug reactions
- Verbalize or demonstrate knowledge of prescribed drugs and recommended life-style changes
- Keep follow-up appointments

### Interventions

Implement measures to prevent or minimize hypertension. Preventive measures are mainly life-style changes to reduce risk factors. These measures should be started in childhood and continued throughout life. Once hypertension is diagnosed, lifetime adherence to a therapeutic regimen may be necessary to control the disease and prevent complications. The nurse's role is important in the prevention, early detection, and treatment of hypertension. Some guidelines for intervention at community, family, and personal levels include the following:

- Participate in programs to promote healthful life-styles (*e.g.*, improving eating habits, increasing exercise, managing stress more effectively, and decreasing cigarette smoking).
- Participate in community screening programs, and make appropriate referrals when abnormal blood pressures are detected. If hypertension develops in women taking oral contraceptives, the drug is usually discontinued for 3 to 6 months to see whether blood pressure decreases without antihypertensive drugs.
- Help the hypertensive client comply with prescribed therapy. Noncompliance is high among clients with hypertension. Reasons often given for noncompliance include lack of symptoms, lack of motivation and self-discipline to make needed life-style changes (*e.g.*, lose weight, stop smoking, restrict salt intake), perhaps experiencing more symptoms from medications than from hypertension, the cost of therapy, and the client's failure to realize the importance of treatment, especially as related to prevention of major cardiovascular diseases (myocardial infarction, stroke, and death). In addition, several studies have shown that compliance decreases as the number of drugs and number of doses increase.

    The nurse can help increase compliance by teaching the client about hypertension, helping the client make necessary life-style changes, and maintaining supportive interpersonal relationships. Losing weight, stopping smoking, and other changes are most likely to be effective if attempted one at a time.

*Teach clients:*

- About the disease process of hypertension, including factors thought to cause or aggravate it
- That hypertension can be controlled by appropriate treatment
- That hypertension rarely causes symptoms unless complications occur
- That uncontrolled hypertension may lead to stroke, myocardial infarction, and kidney failure
- That antihypertensive drug therapy is usually long term, may require more than one drug, and produces side effects. Inform the client that he or she may not feel well when a medication is started or when dosage is increased, that drugs must be taken as prescribed for optimal benefits, and

that changes in drugs or dosages may be needed to increase effectiveness or decrease side effects.

### Evaluation

- Observe for blood pressure measurements within goal or more nearly normal ranges.
- Observe and interview regarding compliance with instructions about drug therapy and life-style changes.
- Observe and interview regarding adverse drug effects.

## Principles of therapy

### THERAPEUTIC REGIMENS

Once the diagnosis of hypertension is established, a therapeutic regimen must be designed and implemented.

The goal of treatment for most clients is to achieve and maintain normal blood pressure range (below 140/90). If this goal cannot be achieved, lowering blood pressure to any extent is still considered beneficial in decreasing the incidence of coronary artery disease and stroke.

The Joint National Committee on Detection, Evaluation, and Treatment of High Blood Pressure recommends a treatment algorithm in which initial interventions are life-style modifications (i.e., reduction of weight and sodium intake, regular physical activity, moderate alcohol intake, and no smoking). If these modifications do not produce goal blood pressure or substantial progress toward goal blood pressure within 3 to 6 months, they should be continued along with an antihypertensive drug. Although the Committee recommends monotherapy (use of one antihypertensive drug) with a diuretic or a beta-blocker because research studies demonstrate reduced morbidity and mortality with these agents, a drug from another classification (e.g., ACE inhibitors, calcium channel-blockers, alpha₁-adrenergic blockers) may also be used effectively.

If the initial drug (and dose) does not produce the desired blood pressure, options for further treatment include increasing the drug dose, substituting another drug, or adding a second drug from a different group. If the response is still inadequate, a second or third drug may be added, including a diuretic if not previously prescribed. When current treatment is ineffective, reassess the client's compliance with life-style modifications or drug therapy. In addition, review other factors that may be sabotaging the therapeutic regimen, such as over-the-counter appetite suppressants or nasal decongestants, which raise blood pressure.

### DRUG SELECTION

Because many effective antihypertensive drugs are available, choices depend primarily on client character-

istics and responses. Some general guidelines include the following:

1. **ACE inhibitors** may be effective alone in white hypertensive clients or in combination with a diuretic in African-American hypertensive clients.
2. **Antiadrenergics** may be effective in any hypertensive population. **Alpha-blockers** are most often used in multidrug regimens for stages 2, 3, or 4, because they may cause postural hypotension and syncope. **Beta-blockers** may be the drugs of first choice for clients under 50 years old with high renin hypertension, tachycardia, angina pectoris, or left ventricular hypertrophy. Most beta-blockers are approved for use in hypertension and are probably equally effective. However, the cardioselective drugs (see Chap. 19) are preferred for hypertensive clients who also have asthma, peripheral vascular disease, or insulin-dependent diabetes mellitus.

   **Other antiadrenergic drugs** are usually added in stages 3 or 4 because of drowsiness, postural hypotension, and other adverse effects. Clonidine also may cause severe hypertension if discontinued abruptly. Clonidine is available in a skin patch that is applied once a week and reportedly reduces adverse effects.
3. **Calcium channel-blockers** may be used for monotherapy or in combination with other drugs. They may be especially useful for hypertensive clients who also have angina pectoris or other cardiovascular disorders.
4. **Diuretics** are usually preferred for initial therapy in older clients and African-American hypertensive clients. They are usually included in any multidrug regimen for other populations. Thiazide and related diuretics are equally effective. Hydrochlorothiazide is commonly used.
5. **Vasodilators** are usually used in combination with a beta-blocker and a diuretic to prevent hypotension-induced compensatory mechanisms (stimulation of the SNS and fluid retention) that raise blood pressure.
6. **Combination products** usually contain an antiadrenergic drug (*e.g.*, alpha-blocker, beta-blocker, clonidine, or methyldopa) as the antihypertensive component and a thiazide or related diuretic as the diuretic component. Most are available in various formulations (see Table 58-2). Combination products may allow smaller doses of individual components and therefore cause fewer adverse effects.

   Combination products are not recommended for initial treatment of hypertension because the dosage of each ingredient should be individualized. However, if individualized dosages of ingredients are comparable to a combination product, the combination product may be used for long-term maintenance therapy. A combination product may aid compliance by reducing the number of doses taken daily.

## DOSAGE FACTORS

1. Dosage of antihypertensive drugs must be titrated according to individual response. Generally, dosage is started at minimal levels and increased if necessary. Several drugs, including thiazide diuretics, are effective at lower doses than formerly used. Lower doses decrease the incidence and severity of adverse effects.
2. For many clients, it may be more beneficial to add another drug rather than increase dosage. Two or three drugs in small doses may be effective and cause fewer adverse effects than a single drug in large doses. When two or more drugs are given, the dose of each drug may need to be reduced.

## DURATION OF THERAPY

Clients who maintain control of their blood pressure for 1 year or so may be candidates for reduced dosages or reduced numbers of drugs. Any such adjustments must be gradual and carefully supervised by a health-care provider. Expected benefits include fewer adverse effects and greater compliance.

## SODIUM RESTRICTION

Any therapeutic regimen for hypertension includes sodium restriction. Severe restrictions are not generally acceptable to clients; however, moderate restrictions (avoiding heavily salted foods, such as cured meats, sandwich meats, pretzels, and potato chips, and not adding salt to food at the table) are beneficial and more easily implemented. These statements are based on research studies that indicate the following:

1. Sodium restriction alone reduces blood pressure.
2. Sodium restriction potentiates the antihypertensive actions of diuretics and other antihypertensive drugs. Conversely, excessive sodium intake decreases the antihypertensive actions of all antihypertensive drugs. Patients with unrestricted salt intake who are taking thiazides may lose excessive potassium and become hypokalemic.
3. Sodium restriction may decrease dosage requirements of antihypertensive drugs, thereby decreasing the incidence and severity of adverse effects.

## GENETIC/ETHNIC CONSIDERATIONS

For most antihypertensive drugs, there have been few reasearch studies comparing their effects in different genetic or ethnic groups. However, several studies indicate that beta-blockers have greater effects in people of Asian heritage, compared with their effects in white people. For hypertension, Asians generally need much smaller doses because they metabolize and excrete beta-blockers slowly. In African-Americans, diuretics are effective and recommended as initial drug therapy; calcium channel-blockers, alpha$_1$ receptor blockers, and the alpha–beta-blocker labetalol are reportedly equally effective in African-American and white people. ACE inhibitors and beta-blockers are less effective as monotherapy in African-Americans. When beta-blockers are used, they are usually one component of a multidrug regimen, and higher doses may be required. Overall, African-Americans are more likely to have severe hypertension and require multiple drugs.

## USE IN SURGICAL CLIENTS

The Joint National Committee on Detection, Evaluation, and Treatment of High Blood Pressure recommends that drug therapy be continued until surgery and restarted as soon as possible after surgery. If clients cannot take drugs orally, parenteral diuretics, antiadrenergic agents, ACE inhibitors, calcium blockers, or vasodilators may be given to avoid the rebound hypertension associated with abrupt discontinuance of some antiadrenergic antihypertensive agents. Transdermal clonidine also may be used. The anesthesiologist and surgeon must be informed about the client's medication status.

## USE IN RENAL IMPAIRMENT

In hypertensive clients with primary renal disease or diabetic nephropathy, drug therapy may slow progression of renal impairment. Sodium retention may be a causative factor, so diuretics are important in treatment. Thiazides should be used cautiously if at all; metolazone (Zaroxolyn) is the only thiazide or related drug with significant diuretic activity if serum creatinine is above 2 mg/dl, and relatively large doses may be required. Loop diuretics, such as furosemide (Lasix) or bumetanide (Bumex), are more often used, and relatively large doses may be required. Antiadrenergics, vasodilators, and ACE inhibitors are usually effective in renal disease. Dosage of ACE inhibitors should be reduced in clients with renal impairment.

## USE IN CHILDREN

Most principles of managing adult hypertension apply to managing childhood and adolescent hypertension; some additional elements that should be considered include the following:

1. Children may have primary or secondary hypertension, but the incidence is unknown, and treatment is not well defined. The Joint National Committee on Detection, Evaluation, and Treatment of High Blood

Pressure recommends annual blood pressure measurement in well children, from 3 years of age through adolescence. This is especially important for children who have a hypertensive parent.

2. Blood pressure is probably more labile in children and adolescents. Therefore, multiple accurate measurements are especially important in diagnosing hypertension.

3. Children have a greater incidence of secondary hypertension than adults. Generally, the higher the blood pressure and the younger the child, the greater the likelihood of secondary hypertension. Diagnostic tests may be needed to rule out renovascular disease or coarctation of the aorta in those under 18 years of age with blood pressure above 140/90 and young children with blood pressures above the 95th percentile for their age group. Oral contraceptives may cause secondary hypertension in adolescents.

4. For most antihypertensive drugs, safety and effectiveness in children under 12 years old are not established, and long-term effects on growth and development are unknown. Therefore, sodium restriction and weight reduction, if needed, may be preferred initially. If this approach is unsuccessful, diuretics, antiadrenergics, and vasodilators are indicated, especially for those with significantly elevated blood pressures or target organ involvement. The fewest drugs and the lowest doses should be used. Thus, if an initial drug is ineffective, it may be better to give a different single drug than to add a second drug to the regimen.

5. Some guidelines for choosing drugs are as follows:
   a. Thiazide diuretics do not commonly produce hyperglycemia, hyperuricemia, or hypercalcemia in children as they do in adults.
   b. Beta-blocking drugs should probably not be given to children with resting pulse rates under 60.
   c. Captopril (Capoten) has been used to treat neonatal hypertension and children aged 2 months to 15 years with secondary hypertension and renal insufficiency. It is recommended for use only when other measures for controlling blood pressure have been ineffective.
   d. Verapamil (Calan, Isoptin) has been given for tachyarrhythmias in infants and children, but no controlled studies have been done regarding the use of calcium channel-blockers for hypertension in children.
   e. Hydralazine (Apresoline) seems to be less effective in childhood and adolescent hypertension than in adult disease.

6. Although all clients with primary hypertension need regular supervision and assessment of blood pressure, this is especially important with young children and adolescents because of growth and developmental changes.

## USE IN OLDER ADULTS

Management of hypertension in adults over 65 years requires consideration of the following factors:

1. There are basically two types of hypertension in older adults. One is systolic hypertension, in which systolic blood pressure is above 160 mm Hg, but diastolic pressure is below 95 mm Hg or normal. The other type, systolic-diastolic hypertension, involves elevations of both systolic and diastolic pressures.

   Until recently, systolic hypertension was considered a normal aspect of aging that did not require treatment. However, ample evidence indicates that both types of hypertension increase cardiovascular morbidity and mortality, especially congestive heart failure and stroke, and should be treated.

2. If the hypertensive geriatric client is obese and hypertension is not severe, weight reduction and moderate sodium restriction may be the initial treatment of choice.

3. If antihypertensive drug therapy is required, drugs used for younger adults may be used alone or in combination. ACE inhibitors, calcium channel-blocking agents, and diuretics may be effective as a single drug (monotherapy); beta-adrenergic blocking agents are usually less effective as monotherapy. Additional guidelines for antihypertensive drug therapy include the following:
   a. The goal of drug therapy may be partial reduction of blood pressure rather than achievement of normal levels.
   b. Older adults may be especially susceptible to the adverse effects of antihypertensive drugs; one reason is that their homeostatic mechanisms are less efficient. For example, if hypotension occurs, the mechanisms that raise blood pressure are less efficient. Therefore, syncope may occur. In addition, renal and liver function may be reduced, making accumulation of drugs more likely. Also, an older adult already prone to mental depression could be more sensitive to this adverse effect of antihypertensive drugs.
   c. Lower drug doses are often effective in older adults. For example, the recommended dose for hydrochlorothiazide is 12.5 to 25 mg daily or equivalent doses of other thiazides and related drugs. Doses above 25 mg daily are usually no more effective and increase risks of adverse effects. Generally, treatment should be started with smaller doses, and increases should be smaller and spaced at longer intervals.
   d. Blood pressure should be reduced *slowly* to facilitate adequate blood flow through arteriosclerotic vessels. Rapid lowering of blood pressure may produce cerebral insufficiency (syncope, transient ischemic attacks, stroke).

# NURSING ACTIONS: ANTIHYPERTENSIVE DRUGS

| *Nursing Actions* | *Rationale/Explanation* |
|---|---|
| **1. Administer accurately** | |
| **a.** Check blood pressure before each dose, preferably with the client in supine and standing positions. | To monitor therapeutic and adverse responses to drug therapy. This is especially important when initiating drug therapy, changing medications, or changing dosages. |
| **b.** Give oral captopril on an empty stomach. | Food decreases drug absorption. |
| **c.** Give other oral antihypertensive agents with or after food intake. | To decrease gastric irritation |
| **d.** For IV injection of propranolol or labetalol, the client should be attached to a cardiac monitor. In addition, parenteral atropine and isoproterenol (Isuprel) must be readily available. | For early detection and treatment of excessive myocardial depression and arrhythmias. Atropine may be used to treat excessive bradycardia. Isoproterenol may be used to stimulate myocardial contractility and increase cardiac output. |
| **e.** Inject diazoxide into an established peripheral IV line. Monitor the client closely for 15 minutes after the injection; observe for excessive hypotension, cerebral ischemia, or myocardial ischemia.<br><br>   Discontinue the drug immediately if extravasation occurs. | Diazoxide is a potent drug, and constant supervision is required initially to detect adverse reactions. After about 15 minutes, blood pressure gradually increases to the original level.<br>The solution is very alkaline and irritating to tissues. |
| **f.** For nitroprusside administration, consult the manufacturer's instructions. | Nitroprusside is unstable in solution. It requires special mixing procedures and additional dilution in IV fluids. |
| **2. Observe for therapeutic effects**<br>   Decreased blood pressure. The usual goal is a normal blood pressure (that is, below 140/90). | The choice of drugs and drug dosages often requires adjustment to maximize beneficial effects and minimize adverse effects. Thus, optimal therapeutic effects may not occur immediately after drug therapy is begun. |
| **3. Observe for adverse effects** | Adverse effects are most likely to occur in clients who are elderly, have impaired renal function, and are receiving multiple antihypertensive drugs or large doses of antihypertensive drugs. |
| **a.** Postural hypotension, dizziness, weakness | This is an extension of the expected pharmacologic action. Postural hypotension results from drug blockage of compensatory reflexes (vasoconstriction, decreased venous pooling in extremities, and increased venous return to the heart) that normally maintain blood pressure in the upright position. This adverse reaction may be aggravated by other conditions that cause vasodilation (*e.g.*, exercise, heat or hot weather, and alcohol consumption). Postural hypotension is more likely to occur with guanethidine, methyldopa, and reserpine. |
| **b.** Sodium and water retention, increased plasma volume, perhaps edema and weight gain | These effects result from decreased renal perfusion. This reaction can be prevented or minimized by concurrent administration of a diuretic. |
| **c.** Prolonged atrioventricular conduction, bradycardia | Owing to increased vagal tone and stimulation |
| **d.** Gastrointestinal disturbances, including nausea, vomiting, and diarrhea | These effects are more likely to occur with hydralazine, methyldopa, propranolol, and captopril. |
| **e.** Mental depression (with reserpine) | Apparently caused by decreased levels of catecholamines and serotonin in the brain |

## *Nursing Actions*

## *Rationale/Explanation*

**f.** Bronchospasm or cardiac failure (with propranolol and other beta-adrenergic blocking agents)

Caused by bronchoconstriction and depression of myocardial contractility. These drugs are contraindicated in asthma, other bronchoconstrictive lung diseases, and congestive heart failure.

**g.** Hypertensive crisis (with abrupt withdrawal of clonidine or guanabenz)

This may be prevented by tapering the prescribed dosage over a period of at least 2 to 4 days before discontinuing the drug.

**4. Observe for drug interactions**
   **a.** Drugs that *increase* effects of antihypertensives:

   (1) Alcohol, phenothiazine antipsychotic agents, peripheral vasodilators

Because these drugs have hypotensive effects when used alone, additive hypotension occurs when they are combined with antihypertensive agents.

   (2) Digitalis glycosides

Additive bradycardia with propranolol

   **b.** Drugs that *decrease* effects of antihypertensives:

   (1) Adrenergics

These drugs stimulate the sympathetic nervous system and raise blood pressure. They include over-the-counter nasal decongestants, cold remedies, bronchodilators, and appetite suppressants.

   (2) Amphetamines

When given with guanethidine, amphetamines displace guanethidine from its site of action. When given with methyldopa, amphetamines decrease antihypertensive effects by increasing sympathetic activity.

   (3) Tricyclic antidepressants

These drugs inhibit the action of clonidine and guanethidine.

   (4) MAO inhibitors

Caused by antagonistic effects, which are apparently most significant with guanethidine

   (5) Oral contraceptives

Oral contraceptives tend to increase blood pressure, probably by causing retention of sodium and water. When they are given concurrently with antihypertensive agents, dosage of antihypertensives may need to be increased.

   (6) Nonsteroidal anti-inflammatory drugs

Aspirin, ibuprofen, and related drugs may cause retention of sodium and water.

**5. Teach clients**

In few other conditions is client education as important as with hypertension. Every effort must be made to aid understanding and compliance with the treatment regimen.

   **a.** Name and purpose of each drug

   **b.** Adverse effects to be reported

Adverse effects can sometimes be prevented or minimized by nondrug measures, by changing drugs, or by reducing drug dosage.

   **c.** Measures to control orthostatic hypotension and dizziness. These include the following: move from supine or sitting positions to a standing position slowly; sleep with the head of the bed elevated; wear elastic stockings; exercise legs; avoid prolonged standing; avoid hot baths.

These measures allow adaptation of normal homeostatic mechanisms, avoid vasodilation, and avoid pooling of blood in the extremities. If symptoms still occur, the person should sit or lie down immediately to avoid a fall and possible injury.

   **d.** Do not stop any antihypertensive drug abruptly or without discussion with the prescribing physician.

Several of the drugs may cause rebound hypertension that may be as severe or worse than the original levels. To avoid this phenomenon, antihypertensive drugs should be tapered in dosage and discontinued gradually.

## Review and Application Exercises

1. Describe the physiologic mechanisms that control blood pressure.
2. What are common factors that raise blood pressure?
3. What signs and symptoms occur with hypertension, and how would you assess for them?
4. Why is it important to measure blood pressure accurately and repeatedly?
5. Does all hypertension require nonpharmacologic or pharmacologic treatment? Justify your answer.
6. What are the potential consequences of untreated or inadequately treated hypertension?
7. How do ACE inhibitors, alpha- and beta-adrenergic blockers, calcium channel-blockers, and direct vasodilators lower blood pressure?
8. What are adverse effects of each group of antihypertensive drugs, and how may they be prevented or minimized?
9. For a client newly diagnosed with hypertension, outline a teaching plan for life-style and pharmacologic interventions.
10. List interventions by health-care providers that may help hypertensive clients adhere to their treatment regimens and maintain "quality of life."
11. In a client being treated for hypertension, how would you assess for compliance with the prescribed life-style and drug therapy regimen?

## Selected References

Applegate, W. B. (1992). Hypertension in the elderly. In W. N. Kelley (Ed.), *Textbook of internal medicine* (2nd ed.) (pp. 2359–2362). Philadelphia: J.B. Lippincott.

Brater, D. C. (1992). Clinical pharmacology of cardiovascular drugs. In W. N. Kelley (Ed.), *Textbook of internal medicine* (2nd ed.) (pp. 315–335). Philadelphia: J.B. Lippincott.

Burke, L. J. (1990). Alterations in cardiac function. In C. M. Porth (Ed.), *Pathophysiology: Concepts of altered health states* (3rd ed.) (pp. 331–376). Philadelphia: J.B. Lippincott.

Clark, J. B., Queener, S. F., & Karb, V. B. (1993). *Pharmacologic basis of nursing practice* (4th ed.). St. Louis: C.V. Mosby.

(1993). *Drug facts and comparisons*. St. Louis: Facts and Comparisons.

Francis, G. S., & Alpert, J. S. (Eds.) (1990). *Modern coronary care*. Boston: Little, Brown.

Guyton, A. C. (1991). *Textbook of medical physiology* (8th ed.) Philadelphia: W.B. Saunders.

Joint National Committee on Detection, Evaluation, and Treatment of High Blood Pressure (1993). *The Fifth Report: NIH Publication No. 93-1088*. Bethesda, MD: National Institutes of Health.

Jones, W. N., & Fagan, T. C. (1993). Hypertension. In R. Bressler & M. D. Katz (Eds.), *Geriatric pharmacology* (pp. 79–103). New York: McGraw-Hill.

May, D. B., Young, L. Y., & Wiser, T. H. (1992). Essential hypertension. In M. A. Koda-Kimble & L. Y. Young (Eds.), *Applied therapeutics: The clinical use of drugs* (5th ed.) (pp. 7-1–7-32). Vancouver, WA: Applied Therapeutics.

Onrot, J., & Rangno, R. E. (1992). Treatment of cardiovascular disorders: Hypertension. In K. L. Melmon, H. F. Morrelli, B. B. Hoffman, & D. W. Nierenberg (Eds.), *Clinical pharmacology: Basic principles in therapeutics* (3rd ed.) (pp. 52–83). New York: McGraw-Hill.

Pfeffer, M. A. (1990). Angiotensin-converting enzyme inhibition. In E. J. Topol (Ed.), *Textbook of interventional cardiology* (pp. 66–75). Philadelphia: W.B. Saunders.

Pless, B. S. (1992). Overview of the anatomy, physiology, and pathophysiology of the vascular system. In L. O. Burrell (Ed.), *Adult nursing in hospital and community settings* (pp. 464–471). Norwalk, CT: Appleton & Lange.

Sharp, D. S., & Benowitz, N. L. (1990). Pharmacoepidemiology of the effect of caffeine on blood pressure. *Clinical Pharmacology and Therapeutics, 47*, 57–60.

Shlafer, M. (1993). *The nurse, pharmacology, and drug therapy* (2nd ed.). Redwood City, CA: Addison-Wesley.

### CHAPTER 59

# Diuretics

## Description

Diuretics are drugs that increase renal excretion of water, sodium, and other electrolytes, thereby increasing urine formation and output. Diuretics are important therapeutic agents widely used in the treatment of edematous (*e.g.*, congestive heart failure, renal and hepatic disease) and nonedematous (*e.g.*, hypertension, ophthalmic surgery) conditions. To aid understanding of diuretic drug therapy, renal physiology related to drug action and characteristics of edema are reviewed before further discussion of the drugs. Individual diuretics are listed in Table 59-1.

## Renal physiology

The primary function of the kidneys is to regulate the volume, composition, and pH of body fluids. The kidneys receive about 25% of the cardiac output. From this large amount of blood flowing through it, the normally functioning kidney is efficient in retaining substances needed by the body and eliminating those not needed.

### THE NEPHRON

The nephron is the functional unit of the kidney; each kidney contains about 1 million nephrons. Each nephron is composed of a glomerulus and a tubule (Fig. 59-1). The glomerulus is a network of capillaries that receives blood from the renal artery. Bowman's capsule is a thin-walled structure that surrounds the glomerulus,

then narrows and continues as the tubule. The tubule is a thin-walled structure of epithelial cells surrounded by peritubular capillaries. The tubule is divided into three segments (the proximal tubule, loop of Henle, and distal tubule), which differ in structure and function. The tubules are often called "convoluted" tubules because of their many twists and turns. The convolutions provide a large surface area of close proximity between the blood flowing through the peritubular capillaries and the glomerular filtrate flowing through the tubular lumen. Consequently, substances can be readily exchanged through the walls of the tubules.

The nephron functions by three processes: glomerular filtration, tubular reabsorption, and tubular secretion. These processes normally maintain the fluid volume, electrolyte concentration, and pH of body fluids within a relatively narrow range. They also remove waste products of cellular metabolism. A minimum daily urine output of about 400 ml is required to remove normal amounts of metabolic end-products.

### GLOMERULAR FILTRATION

Arterial blood enters the glomerulus by the afferent arteriole at the relatively high pressure of about 70 mm Hg. This pressure "pushes" water, electrolytes, and other solutes out of the capillaries into Bowman's capsule and then to the proximal tubule. This fluid, called *glomerular filtrate*, contains the same components as blood except for blood cells, fats, and proteins.

The glomerular filtration rate is about 180 L/d, or 125 ml/min. Most of this fluid is reabsorbed as the glomerular filtrate travels through the tubules. The end-product is about 2 L of urine daily. Urine flows into collecting

Anne Collins Abrams: CLINICAL DRUG THERAPY, Fourth Edition.
© 1995 J.B. Lippincott Company.

## TABLE 59-1.  DIURETIC AGENTS

| Generic/Trade Name | Routes and Dosage Ranges | |
| --- | --- | --- |
| | **Adults** | **Children** |

*Thiazide and Related Diuretics*

| | | |
| --- | --- | --- |
| **Bendroflumethiazide** (Naturetin) | PO 5 mg daily initially. For maintenance, 2.5–20 mg daily or intermittently | PO up to 0.4 mg/kg per day initially, in two divided doses. For maintenance, 0.05–0.1 mg/kg per day in a single dose. |
| **Benzthiazide** (Exna) | PO 50–200 mg daily for several days initially, depending on response. For maintenance, dosage is gradually reduced to the minimal effective amount. | PO 1–4 mg/kg per day initially, in three divided doses. For maintenance, dosage is reduced to the minimal effective amount. |
| **Chlorothiazide** (Diuril) | PO 500–1000 mg one or two times daily<br>IV 500 mg twice daily | PO 22 mg/kg per day in two divided doses<br>Infants under age 6 months, up to 33 mg/kg per day in two divided doses<br>IV not recommended |
| **Chlorthalidone** (Hygroton) | PO 25–100 mg daily | PO 3 mg/kg three times weekly, adjusted according to response |
| **Hydrochlorothiazide** (HydroDiuril, Esidrix, Oretic) | PO 25–100 mg one or two times daily<br>Elderly adults, 12.5–25 mg daily | PO 2 mg/kg per day in two divided doses<br>Infants under age 6 months, up to 3.3 mg/kg per day in two divided doses |
| **Hydroflumethiazide** (Saluron) | PO 25–200 mg daily | PO 1 mg/kg per day |
| **Indapamide** (Lozol) | PO 2.5–5 mg daily | Dosage not established |
| **Methyclothiazide** (Enduron) | PO 2.5–10 mg daily | PO 0.05–0.2 mg/kg per day |
| **Metolazone** (Zaroxolyn, Mykrox) | PO 5–20 mg daily, depending on severity of condition and response | |
| **Polythiazide** (Renese) | PO 1–4 mg daily, depending on severity of condition and response | PO 0.02–0.08 mg/kg per day |
| **Quinethazone** (Hydromox) | PO 50–200 mg daily | Dosage not established |
| **Trichlormethiazide** (Metahydrin, Naqua) | PO 2–4 mg one or two times daily initially. For maintenance, 1–4 mg once daily | PO 0.07 mg/kg per day in single or divided doses |

*Loop Diuretics*

| | | |
| --- | --- | --- |
| **Bumetanide** (Bumex) | PO 0.5–2 mg daily as a single dose. May be repeated q4–6h to a maximal dose of 10 mg, if necessary. Giving on alternate days or for 3–4 d with rest periods of 1–2 d is recommended for long-term control of edema.<br>IV, IM 0.5–1 mg, repeated in 2–3 h if necessary, to a maximal daily dose of 10 mg. Give IV injections over 1–2 min. | Not recommended for children under age 18 years |
| **Ethacrynic acid** (Edecrin) | Edema, PO 50–100 mg daily, increased or decreased according to severity of condition and response; maximal daily dose, 400 mg<br>Rapid mobilization of edema, IV 50 mg or 0.5–1 mg/kg injected slowly to a maximum of 100 mg/dose | PO 25 mg daily<br><br><br>No recommended parenteral dose in children |
| **Furosemide** (Lasix) | Edema, PO 20–80 mg as a single dose initially. If an adequate diuretic response is not obtained, dosage may be gradually increased by 20- to 40-mg increments at intervals of 6–8 h. For maintenance, dosage range and frequency of administration vary widely and must be individualized. Maximal daily dose, 600 mg.<br>Hypertension, PO 40 mg twice daily, gradually increased if necessary<br>Rapid mobilization of edema, IV 20–40 mg initially, injected slowly. This dose may be repeated in 2 h. With acute pulmonary edema, initial dose is usually 40 mg, which may be repeated in 60–90 min.<br>Acute renal failure, IV 40 mg initially, increased if necessary. Maximum dose, 1–2 g/24 h<br>Hypertensive crisis, IV 40–80 mg injected over 1–2 min. With renal failure, much larger doses may be needed. | PO 2 mg/kg one or two times daily initially, gradually increased by increments of 1–2 mg/kg per dose if necessary at intervals of 6–8 h. Maximal daily dose, 6 mg/kg<br>IV 1 mg/kg initially. If diuretic response is not adequate, increase dosage by 1 mg/kg no sooner than 2 h after previous dose. Maximal dose, 6 mg/kg |

*Potassium-Sparing Diuretics*

| | | |
| --- | --- | --- |
| **Amiloride** (Midamor) | PO 5–20 mg daily | Dosage not established |
| **Spironolactone** (Aldactone) | PO 25–200 mg daily | PO 3.3 mg/kg per day in divided doses |

*(continued)*

**TABLE 59-1.   DIURETIC AGENTS** *(Continued)*

| Generic/Trade Name | Routes and Dosage Ranges | |
| --- | --- | --- |
| | **Adults** | **Children** |
| **Triamterene** (Dyrenium) | PO 100–300 mg daily in divided doses | PO 2–4 mg/kg per day in divided doses |
| *Osmotic Agents* | | |
| **Glycerin** (Osmoglyn) | PO 1–1.5 g/kg of body weight, usually given as a 50% or 75% solution, 1–2 h before ocular surgery | Same as adults |
| **Isosorbide** (Ismotic) | PO 1.5–3 g/kg, up to four times daily if necessary for glaucoma or ocular surgery | |
| **Mannitol** (Osmitrol) | Diuresis, IV infusion 50–200 g over 24 h, flow rate adjusted to maintain a urine output of 30–50 ml/h<br>Oliguria and prevention of renal failure, IV 50–100 g<br>Reduction of intracranial or intraocular pressure,<br>  IV 1.5–2 g/kg, given as a 20% solution, over 30–60 min | Same as adults |
| *Combination Diuretic Products* | | |
| **Hydrochlorothiazide** 50 mg and **amiloride** 5 mg (Moduretic) | PO 1–2 tablets daily | |
| **Hydrochlorothiazide** 25 mg and **spironolactone** 25 mg (Aldactazide 25/25) | PO 1–8 tablets daily | |
| **Hydrochlorothiazide** 50 mg and **spironolactone** 50 mg (Aldactazide 50/50) | PO 1–4 tablets daily | |
| **Hydrochlorothiazide** 25 mg and **triamterene** 50 mg (Dyazide) | Hypertension, PO 1 capsule twice daily initially, then adjusted according to response<br>Edema, 1–2 capsules twice daily | |
| **Hydrochlorothiazide** 50 mg and **triamterene** 75 mg (Maxzide) | PO 1 tablet daily | |

tubules, which carry it to the renal pelvis. From the renal pelvis, urine flows through the ureters, bladder, and urethra for elimination from the body.

Blood that does not become part of the glomerular filtrate travels out of the glomerulus through the efferent arteriole. The efferent arteriole branches into the peritubular capillaries, which eventually empty into veins and return the blood to the systemic circulation.

## TUBULAR REABSORPTION

The term *reabsorption*, in relation to renal function, indicates movement of substances from the tubule (glomerular filtrate) to the blood in the peritubular capillaries. Most reabsorption occurs in the proximal tubule. Almost all glucose and amino acids are reabsorbed; about 80% of water, sodium, potassium, chloride, and most other substances is reabsorbed. As a result, only some of the glomerular filtrate (about 20%) enters the loop of Henle. In the descending limb of the loop of Henle, water is reabsorbed; in the ascending limb, sodium is reabsorbed. A large fraction of the total amount of sodium (up to 30%) filtered by the glomeruli is reabsorbed in the loop of Henle. Additional sodium is reabsorbed in the

distal tubule, primarily by the exchange of sodium ions for potassium ions secreted by epithelial cells of tubular walls. Final reabsorption of water occurs in the distal tubule and small collecting tubules. The remaining water and solutes are now correctly called urine.

Antidiuretic hormone from the posterior pituitary gland promotes reabsorption of water from the distal tubules and the collecting ducts of the kidneys. This conserves water needed by the body and produces a more concentrated urine. Aldosterone, a hormone from the adrenal cortex, promotes sodium–potassium exchange mainly in the distal tubule and collecting ducts. Thus, aldosterone promotes sodium reabsorption and potassium loss.

## TUBULAR SECRETION

The term *secretion*, in relation to renal function, indicates movement of substances from blood in the peritubular capillaries to glomerular filtrate flowing through the renal tubules. Secretion occurs in the proximal and distal tubules, across the epithelial cells that line the tubules. In the proximal tubule, uric acid, creatinine, hydrogen ions, and ammonia are secreted; in the distal tubule,

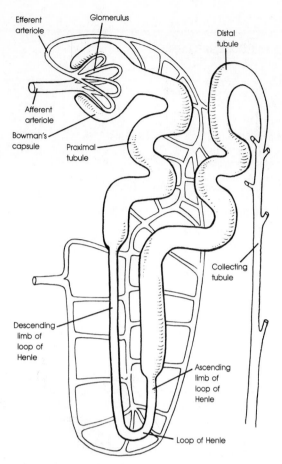

*FIGURE 59-1.* The nephron is the functional unit of the kidney.

potassium ions, hydrogen ions, and ammonia are se-creted. Secretion of hydrogen ions is important in main-taining acid-base balance in body fluids.

## Alterations in renal function

Many clinical conditions alter renal function. In some conditions, excessive amounts of substances (*e.g.*, so-dium and water) are retained; in others, needed sub-stances (*e.g.*, potassium, proteins) are eliminated. These conditions include cardiovascular, renal, hepatic, and other disorders that may be treated with diuretic drugs.

### EDEMA

*Edema* is the excessive accumulation of fluid in body tissues. It is a symptom of many disease processes and may occur in any part of the body. Additional character-istics include the following:

1. Edema formation results from one or more of the following mechanisms that allow fluid to leave the bloodstream (intravascular compartment) and enter interstitial spaces.
   a. *Increased capillary permeability* occurs as part of the response to tissue injury. Thus, edema may occur with burns and trauma or allergic and inflamma-tory reactions.
   b. *Increased capillary hydrostatic pressure* results from a sequence of events in which increased blood vol-ume (from fluid overload or sodium and water retention) or obstruction of venous blood flow causes a high venous pressure and a high capillary pressure. This is the primary mechanism for edema formation in congestive heart failure, pulmonary edema, and renal failure.
   c. *Decreased plasma oncotic pressure* may occur with decreased synthesis of plasma proteins (caused by liver disease or malnutrition) or increased loss of plasma proteins (caused by burn injuries or the nephrotic syndrome). Plasma proteins are impor-tant in keeping fluids within the bloodstream. When plasma proteins are lacking, fluid leaves the capillaries and accumulates in tissues.
2. Edema interferes with blood flow to tissues. Thus, it interferes with delivery of oxygen and nutrients and removal of metabolic waste products. If severe, edema may distort body features, impair movement, and interfere with activities of daily living.
3. Specific manifestations of edema are determined by its location and extent. A common type of localized edema occurs in the feet and ankles (dependent edema), especially with prolonged sitting or stand-ing. A less common but more severe type of localized edema is pulmonary edema, a life-threatening condi-tion that occurs with circulatory overload (of intra-venous fluids or blood transfusions, for example) or acute heart failure. Generalized massive edema (an-asarca) interferes with the functions of many body organs and tissues.

## Diuretic drugs

Diuretic drugs act on the kidneys to decrease reabsorp-tion of sodium, chloride, water, and other substances. Major subclasses are the thiazides and related diuretics, loop diuretics, and potassium-sparing diuretics. These groups differ from each other primarily because they act at different sites in the nephron.

Major clinical indications for diuretics are edema and hypertension. In edematous states, diuretics mobilize tissue fluids by decreasing plasma volume. In hyperten-sion, the exact mechanism by which diuretics lower blood pressure is unknown, but antihypertensive action is usually attributed to sodium depletion. Initially, diuretics decrease blood volume and cardiac output. With chronic use, cardiac output returns to normal, but there is a persistent decrease in plasma volume and peripheral vascular resistance. Sodium depletion may have a vasodilating effect on arterioles.

Use of diuretic agents in the treatment of congestive heart failure and hypertension is discussed further in Chapters 54 and 58, respectively.

## THIAZIDE AND RELATED DIURETICS

Thiazide diuretics are synthetic drugs that are chemically related to the sulfonamides. Chlorothiazide (Diuril) is the prototype of thiazide diuretics, but hydrochlorothiazide (HydroDiuril), a more potent derivative, is more commonly used. Related diuretics are nonthiazides whose pharmacologic actions are essentially the same as those of the thiazides; they include chlorthalidone (Hygroton), metolazone (Zaroxolyn), and quinethazone (Hydromox).

Thiazides and related drugs are the most frequently prescribed diuretic agents. They decrease reabsorption of sodium and water in the ascending limb of the loop of Henle and in the distal tubule. They also decrease reabsorption of chloride and bicarbonate.

Thiazides and related drugs are well absorbed from the gastrointestinal tract following oral administration. They are widely distributed in body fluids but accumulate only in the kidneys. With most of the drugs, diuretic effects occur within 2 hours, peak at 4 to 6 hours, and last 6 to 24 hours. Most of the drugs are excreted unchanged by the kidneys within 3 to 6 hours. Some of the newer drugs (e.g., polythiazide [Renese] and chlorthalidone) have longer durations of action (about 48–72 hours), attributed to slower excretion.

These drugs are especially useful in long-term treatment of congestive heart failure and hypertension. They are ineffective when immediate diuresis is required and are relatively ineffective with decreased renal function. Because they cross the placenta and may have adverse effects on the fetus, usage during pregnancy must be based on careful consideration of potential benefits versus potential harm. Thiazides and related drugs are contraindicated in clients allergic to sulfonamide drugs.

## LOOP DIURETICS

Loop diuretics exert their primary pharmacologic actions in the ascending limb of the loop of Henle. They also are called high-ceiling diuretics because their dosage can be increased to produce greater diuretic effects (in contrast to the thiazides; increasing the dosage of these beyond a certain point does not increase diuretic effects). Loop diuretics are the most effective and versatile diuretics available for clinical use.

Loop diuretics inhibit sodium and chloride reabsorption primarily in the loop of Henle. Their saluretic (sodium-losing) effect is up to 10 times greater than that of thiazide diuretics. These drugs may be given orally or intravenously. After oral administration, diuretic effects occur within 30 to 60 minutes, peak in 1 to 2 hours, and last 6 to 8 hours. After intravenous administration, diuretic effects occur within 5 minutes, peak within 30 minutes, and last about 2 hours. Thus, the drugs produce extensive diuresis for short periods of time, after which the kidney tubules regain their ability to reabsorb sodium. Actually, the kidneys reabsorb more sodium than usual during this postdiuretic phase, so a high dietary intake of sodium can cause sodium retention and reduce or cancel the diuretic-induced sodium loss. Thus, dietary sodium restriction is required to achieve optimum therapeutic benefits. The drugs are rapidly excreted by the kidneys, and drug accumulation does not occur even with repeated doses.

The loop diuretics are the diuretics of choice when rapid effects are required (e.g., in pulmonary edema) and when renal function is impaired (creatinine clearance less than 30 ml/min). The drugs are contraindicated during pregnancy unless necessary.

Furosemide is the most commonly used loop diuretic. Bumetanide may be used to produce diuresis in some clients who are allergic to or no longer respond to furosemide. It is more potent than furosemide on a weight basis, and large doses can be given in small volumes. Ethacrynic acid is uncommonly used because it produces more ototoxicity and gastrointestinal symptoms than the other drugs. These drugs differ mainly in potency and produce similar effects at equivalent doses (furosemide 40 mg = bumetanide 1 mg = ethacrynic acid 50 mg).

## POTASSIUM-SPARING DIURETICS

Potassium-sparing diuretics include three drugs. One is spironolactone (Aldactone), an aldosterone antagonist. Aldosterone is a hormone secreted by the adrenal cortex. It promotes retention of sodium and water and excretion of potassium by stimulating the sodium–potassium exchange mechanism in the distal tubule and collecting ducts. The other two drugs, amiloride and triamterene, are chemically unrelated to spironolactone but are similar to each other in diuretic activity.

Potassium-sparing diuretics are usually given in combination with potassium-losing diuretics to increase diuretic activity and decrease potassium loss. Amiloride and triamterene act directly on the distal renal tubule to decrease the exchange of sodium for potassium. Spironolactone blocks the sodium-retaining effects of aldosterone, and aldosterone must be present for spirono-lactone to be effective.

Potassium-sparing diuretics are contraindicated in the presence of renal insufficiency because their use may cause hyperkalemia. Hyperkalemia is the major adverse effect of these drugs; clients receiving potassium-sparing diuretics should *not* be given potassium supplements, encouraged to eat foods high in potassium, or allowed to use salt substitutes. Salt substitutes contain potassium chloride rather than sodium chloride.

## OSMOTIC DIURETICS

Osmotic agents produce rapid diuresis by increasing the solute load (osmotic pressure) of the glomerular filtrate. The increased osmotic pressure causes water to be pulled from extravascular sites into the bloodstream, thereby increasing blood volume and decreasing reabsorption of water and electrolytes in the renal tubules. Mannitol (Osmitrol) is useful in treating oliguria or anuria, and it may prevent acute renal failure during prolonged surgery, trauma, or infusion of cisplatin, an antineoplastic agent. Mannitol is effective even when renal circulation and glomerular filtration rate are reduced (*e.g.*, in hypovolemic shock, trauma, or dehydration). Other important clinical uses of hyperosmolar agents include reduction of intracranial pressure before or after neurosurgery, reduction of intraocular pressure before certain types of ophthalmic surgery, and urinary excretion of toxic substances. Other osmotic agents are listed in Table 59-1.

## *Nursing Process*

### Assessment

Assess the client's status in relation to baseline data and conditions in which diuretic drugs are used.
- Useful baseline data include serum electrolytes, uric acid, blood glucose, creatinine, and urea nitrogen, because diuretics may alter these values. Other data are blood pressure readings, weight, amount and appearance of urine output, and measurement of edematous areas, such as ankles or abdomen.
- Observe for edema. Visible edema often occurs in the feet and legs of ambulatory clients. Rapid weight gain may indicate fluid retention.
  - With congestive heart failure, numerous signs and symptoms result from edema of various organs and tissues. For example, congestion in the gastrointestinal tract may cause nausea and vomiting, liver congestion may cause abdominal pain and tenderness, and congestion in the lungs (pulmonary edema) causes rapid, labored breathing, hypoxemia, frothy sputum, and other manifestations of severe respiratory distress.
  - Cerebral edema may be manifested by confusion, headache, dizziness, convulsions, unconsciousness, bradycardia, or failure of the pupils to react to light.

- Ascites, which occurs with hepatic cirrhosis, is an accumulation of fluid in the abdominal cavity. The abdomen appears much enlarged.
- With congestive heart failure, fatigue and dyspnea, in addition to edema, are common symptoms.
- Hypertension (blood pressure above 140/90 mm Hg on several measurements) may be the only clinical manifestation present.

### Nursing diagnoses
- Fluid Volume Excess in edematous clients related to retention of sodium and water
- Fluid Volume Deficit related to increased urine output after a diuretic drug is begun
- Altered Urinary Elimination: Increased frequency
- High Risk for Altered Nutrition: Less than Body Requirements related to excessive loss of potassium
- High Risk for Injury: Hypotension and dizziness as adverse drug effects
- Knowledge Deficit related to the need for and correct usage of diuretics
- Sexual Dysfunction related to adverse drug effects

### Planning/Goals

*The client will:*
- Take or receive diuretic drugs as prescribed
- Experience reduced edema and improved control of blood pressure
- Reduce dietary intake of sodium and increase dietary intake of potassium
- Avoid preventable adverse drug effects
- Keep appointments for follow-up monitoring of blood pressure, edema, and serum electrolytes

### Interventions

Promote measures to prevent or minimize conditions for which diuretic drugs are used.
- With edema, helpful measures include the following:
  - Decreasing dietary sodium intake
  - Losing weight, if obese
  - Elevating legs when sitting
  - Avoiding prolonged standing or sitting
  - Wearing support hose or elastic stockings
  - Treating the condition causing edema
- With congestive heart failure and in older adults, administer intravenous fluids or blood transfusions carefully to avoid fluid overload and pulmonary edema. Fluid overload may occur with rapid administration or excessive amounts of intravenous fluids.
- With hypertension, helpful measures include decreasing dietary sodium intake and losing weight, if obese.

*Teach clients:*
- That reducing dietary sodium intake will help diuretic drugs be more effective and allow smaller doses to be given. Smaller doses are less likely to cause adverse effects.
- To avoid excessive table salt and obviously salty foods (*e.g.*, ham, packaged sandwich meats, potato chips, dill pickles, most canned soups). These foods may aggravate edema or hypertension by causing sodium and water retention.

- Not to use salt substitutes unless recommended by a health-care provider. These preparations contain potassium instead of sodium, and excessive potassium in the blood may have serious adverse effects on the heart.
- To maintain regular medical supervision so that drug effects can be monitored and dosages adjusted when indicated

### Evaluation

- Observe for reduced edema and body weight.
- Observe for reduced blood pressure.
- Observe for increased urine output.
- Monitor serum electrolytes for normal values.
- Interview regarding compliance with instructions for diet and drug therapy.
- Monitor compliance with follow-up appointments in outpatients.

## Principles of therapy

### DRUG SELECTION

The choice of diuretic drug depends primarily on the client's condition.

1. *Thiazides and related diuretics* are the drugs of choice for most clients who require diuretic therapy. They are especially useful in conditions that require long-term use of diuretics (*e.g.*, congestive heart failure and hypertension). All the drugs in this group have similar effects and differ mainly in duration of action. For most clients, short-acting (*e.g.*, bendroflumethiazide, trichlormethiazide) or intermediate-acting (*e.g.*, hydrochlorothiazide, hydroflumethiazide, indapamide) agents are preferred. Although long-acting drugs (*e.g.*, remaining thiazides and metolazone) may increase client compliance by requiring less frequent administration, they also may cause more hypokalemia. Some of the drugs are also more expensive than others.
2. *Furosemide* is the drug of choice when rapid diuretic effects are required or when renal insufficiency is present.
3. A *potassium-sparing diuretic* may be given concurrently with a potassium-losing diuretic to prevent or treat hypokalemia and to augment the diuretic effect.
4. *Combination products* (see Table 59-1) containing a potassium-losing and a potassium-sparing diuretic are often prescribed because of client convenience and compliance. However, for initial therapy, it is better to titrate the dosage of each drug separately. If titrated doses are similar to the amounts in the combination products, the combination products may then be used.

### DOSAGE FACTORS

Dosage of diuretics depends largely on the client's condition and response and should always be individualized to administer the minimal effective amount. With hydrochlorothiazide, for example, research studies indicate that smaller doses (*e.g.*, 25 mg daily) are usually as effective as the larger doses formerly used and are less likely to cause hypokalemia and other adverse effects.

In liver disease, electrolyte imbalances produced by diuretics may precipitate or aggravate hepatic coma. For renal disease, furosemide is often given in large doses to achieve a diuretic response. Bumetanide may be a useful alternative, because it can be given in smaller doses.

### USE IN EDEMA

When diuretics are used to treat patients with edema, the underlying cause of the edema should be addressed, not just the edema itself. When treating such patients, it is preferable to aim for a weight loss of about 2 lb (about 1 kg) per day. Rapid and excessive diuresis may cause dehydration and decreased blood volume with circulatory collapse.

### USE WITH DIGITALIS

When digitalis preparations and diuretics are given concomitantly, as is common when treating patients with congestive heart failure, the risk of digitalis toxicity is increased. Digitalis toxicity is related to diuretic-induced hypokalemia. Potassium is a myocardial depressant and antiarrhythmic; it has essentially opposite cardiac effects to those of digitalis. In other words, extracellular potassium decreases the excitability of myocardial tissue, but digitalis increases excitability. The higher the serum potassium, the less effective a given dose of digitalis will be. Conversely, decreased serum potassium increases the likelihood of digitalis-induced cardiac arrhythmias, even with "small" doses and therapeutic serum levels of digitalis.

Supplemental potassium chloride, a potassium-sparing diuretic, and other measures to prevent hypokalemia are often used to maintain normal serum potassium levels (3.5–5.0 mEq/L).

### PREVENTION AND TREATMENT OF POTASSIUM IMBALANCES

Potassium imbalances (see Chap. 32) may occur with diuretic therapy. Hypokalemia and hyperkalemia are cardiotoxic and should be prevented when possible.

1. *Hypokalemia* (serum potassium level under 3.5 mEq/L) may occur with potassium-losing diuretics (*e.g.,* hydrochlorothiazide, furosemide). Measures to prevent or treat hypokalemia include the following:
   a. Giving supplemental potassium, usually potassium chloride, in an average dosage range of 20 to 60 mEq daily
   b. Giving a potassium-sparing diuretic along with the potassium-losing drug
   c. Increasing food intake of potassium. Many texts advocate this approach as preferable to supplemental potassium or combination diuretic therapy, but the effectiveness of this approach is not clearly established. Although the minimal daily requirement of potassium is unknown, usual recommendations are 40 to 50 mEq daily for the healthy adult. Potassium loss with diuretics may be several times this amount.

      Some foods (*e.g.,* bananas) have undeserved reputations for having high potassium content; actually, large amounts must be ingested. To provide 50 mEq of potassium daily, estimated amounts of certain foods include 1000 ml of orange juice, 1600 ml of apple or grape juice, 1200 ml of pineapple juice, four to six bananas, or 30 to 40 prunes. Some of these foods are high in calories and may be contraindicated, at least in large amounts, for obese clients.
   d. Using salt substitutes. One teaspoonful of salt substitute contains about 60 to 70 mEq of potassium chloride.
   e. Restricting dietary sodium intake. This reduces potassium loss by decreasing the amount of sodium available for exchange with potassium in renal tubules.
2. *Hyperkalemia* (serum potassium level above 5 mEq/L) may occur with potassium-sparing diuretics (spironolactone, triamterene, amiloride). The following measures prevent hyperkalemia:
   a. Avoiding use of potassium-sparing diuretics and potassium supplements in clients with renal insufficiency
   b. Avoiding excessive amounts of potassium chloride supplements and salt substitutes

   c. Maintaining urine output, the major route for eliminating potassium from the body

## USE IN CHILDREN

Thiazides are used for treatment of edema in children, and they do not commonly cause hyperglycemia, hyperuricemia, or hypercalcemia in children as they do in adults. Pediatric doses of hydrochlorothiazide are about 1 mg/lb per day (2.2 mg/kg per day).

Furosemide (Lasix) is the loop diuretic that has been used most extensively in children. Oral therapy is preferred when feasible, and doses above 6 mg/kg per day are not recommended. Furosemide stimulates production of prostaglandin $E_2$ in the kidneys and may therefore increase the incidence of patent ductus arteriosus and neonatal respiratory distress syndrome if given to premature infants. Potassium-sparing diuretics are not usually indicated for use in children.

## USE IN OLDER ADULTS

Thiazide diuretics are often prescribed for the treatment of hypertension and congestive heart failure, which are common in older adults. Older adults are especially sensitive to adverse drug effects, such as hypotension and electrolyte imbalance. Thiazides may aggravate renal or hepatic insufficiency. With rapid or excessive diuresis, myocardial infarction, renal impairment, or cerebral thrombosis may occur from fluid volume depletion and hypotension. The smallest effective dose is recommended, usually a daily dose of 12.5 to 25 mg of hydrochlorothiazide or equivalent doses of other thiazides and related drugs. Risks of adverse effects may exceed benefits at doses greater than 25 mg.

With loop diuretics, older adults are at greater risk of excessive diuresis, hypotension, fluid volume deficit, and possibly thrombosis or embolism. Rapid diuresis may cause urinary incontinence. With potassium-sparing diuretics, hyperkalemia is more likely to occur in older adults because of the renal impairment that occurs with aging.

## NURSING ACTIONS: DIURETICS

| *Nursing Actions* | *Rationale/Explanation* |
|---|---|

**1. Administer accurately**

**a.** Give in the early morning if ordered daily.

So that peak action will occur during waking hours and not interfere with sleep

**b.** Take safety precautions. Keep a bedpan or urinal within reach. Keep the call light within reach, and be sure the client knows how to use it. Assist to the bathroom anyone who is elderly, weak, dizzy, or unsteady in walking.

Mainly to avoid falls

**2. Observe for therapeutic effects**

Decrease or absence of edema, increased urine output, decreased blood pressure

Most oral diuretics start their action within about 2 hours; IV diuretics act within minutes. Antihypertensive effects may not be evident for several days.

(1) Weigh the client daily while edema is present and two or three times weekly thereafter. Weigh under standard conditions: early morning before eating or drinking, after urination, with the same amount of clothing, and using the same scales.

Body weight is a very good indicator of fluid gain or loss. A weight change of 2.2 lb (1 kg) may indicate a gain or loss of 1000 ml of fluid. Also, weighing assists in dosage regulation to maintain therapeutic benefit without excessive or too rapid fluid loss.

(2) Record fluid intake and output every shift.

Normally, oral fluid intake approximates urinary output (1500 ml/24 h). With diuretic therapy, urinary output may exceed intake, depending on the amount of edema or fluid retention, renal function, and diuretic dosage. All sources of fluid gain, including IV fluids, must be included; all sources of fluid loss (perspiration, fever, wound drainage, gastrointestinal [GI] tract drainage) are important. Clients with abnormal fluid losses have less urine output with diuretic therapy. Oliguria (decreased excretion of urine) may require stopping the drug. Output greater than 100 ml/h may indicate that side effects are more likely to occur.

(3) Observe and record characteristics of urine.

Excessively dilute urine may indicate excessive fluid intake or greater likelihood of fluid and electrolyte imbalance due to rapid diuresis. Concentrated urine may mean oliguria or decreased fluid intake.

(4) Check daily for edema: ankles for the ambulatory client, sacral area and posterior thighs for clients at bed rest. Also, it is often helpful to measure abdominal girth, ankles, and calves to monitor gain or loss of fluid.

Expect a decrease in visible edema and size of measured areas. If edema reappears or worsens, a thorough reassessment of the client is in order. Questions to be answered include the following:
(1) Is the prescribed diuretic being taken correctly?
(2) What type of diuretic and what dosage is ordered?
(3) Is there worsening of the underlying condition(s) that contributed to edema formation in the first place?
(4) Has other disease developed?

(5) In clients with congestive heart failure or acute pulmonary edema, observe for decreased dyspnea, rales, cyanosis, and cough.

Decreased fluid in the lungs leads to dramatic improvement in respirations as more carbon dioxide and oxygen gas exchange takes place and greater tissue oxygenation occurs.

(6) Record blood pressure two to four times daily when diuretic therapy is initiated.

Although thiazide diuretics apparently do not lower normal blood pressure, other diuretics may, especially with excessive or rapid diuresis.

*(continued)*

*Nursing Actions*                                                  *Rationale/Explanation*

**3. Observe for adverse effects**                              Major adverse effects are fluid and electrolyte imbalances.

**a.** With potassium-losing diuretics (thiazides, bumetanide, furosemide, ethacrynic acid), observe for:

    (1) Hypokalemia                            Potassium is required for normal muscle function. Thus, potassium depletion causes weakness of cardiovascular, respiratory, digestive, and skeletal muscles. Clients most likely to develop hypokalemia are those who are taking large doses of diuretics, potent diuretics (*e.g.,* furosemide), or adrenal corticosteroids; those who have decreased food and fluid intake; or those who have increased potassium losses through vomiting, diarrhea, chronic laxative or enema use, or GI suction. Clinically significant symptoms are most likely to occur with a serum potassium level below 3 mEq/L.

        (a) Serum potassium levels below 3.5 mEq/L

        (b) ECG changes (*e.g.,* low voltage, flattened T wave, depressed ST segment)

        (c) Cardiac arrhythmias; weak, irregular pulse

        (d) Hypotension

        (e) Weak, shallow respirations

        (f) Anorexia, nausea, vomiting

        (g) Decreased peristalsis or paralytic ileus

        (h) Skeletal muscle weakness

        (i) Confusion, disorientation

    (2) Hyponatremia, hypomagnesemia, hypochloremic alkalosis, changes in serum and urinary calcium levels        In addition to potassium, sodium, chloride, magnesium, and bicarbonate also are lost with diuresis. Thiazides and related diuretics cause hypercalcemia and hypocalciuria. They have been used to prevent calcium nephrolithiasis (kidney stones). Furosemide and other loop diuretics tend to cause hypocalcemia and hypercalciuria.

    (3) Dehydration                            Fluid volume depletion occurs with excessive or rapid diuresis. If it is prolonged or severe, hypovolemic shock may occur.

        (a) Poor skin turgor, dry mucous membranes

        (b) Oliguria; urine of high specific gravity

        (c) Thirst

        (d) Tachycardia; hypotension

        (e) Decreased level of consciousness

        (f) Elevated hematocrit (above 45%)

    (4) Hyperglycemia—blood glucose above 120 mg/100 ml, polyuria, polydipsia, polyphagia, glycosuria        Hyperglycemia is more likely to occur in clients with known or latent diabetes mellitus. Larger doses of hypoglycemic agents may be required. The hyperglycemic effect may be reversible when diuretic therapy is discontinued.

    (5) Hyperuricemia—serum uric acid above 7.0 mg/100 ml        Hyperuricemia is usually asymptomatic except for clients with gout, a predisposition toward gout, or chronic renal failure. Apparently, decreased renal excretion of uric acid allows its accumulation in the blood.

    (6) Pulmonary edema (with osmotic diuretics)        Pulmonary edema is most likely to occur in clients with congestive heart failure who cannot tolerate the increased blood volume produced by the drugs.

    (7) Ototoxicity (with furosemide and ethacrynic acid)        Reversible or transient hearing impairment, tinnitus, and dizziness are more common, although irreversible deafness may occur. Ototoxicity is more likely to occur when the drugs are injected rapidly in clients with severe renal impairment, or when other ototoxic drugs (*e.g.,* aminoglycoside antibiotics) are being taken concurrently.

## Nursing Actions                                    Rationale/Explanation

(8) Hypersensitivity reactions (skin rash, dermatitis) and hematologic reactions (leukopenia, thrombocytopenia)

These effects rarely occur.

**b.** With potassium-sparing diuretics (spironolactone, triamterene, amiloride), observe for:

Hyperkalemia

(a) Serum potassium levels above 5 mEq/L

(b) ECG changes (*i.e.*, prolonged P-R interval; wide QRS complex; tall, peaked T wave; depressed ST segment)

Hyperkalemia is most likely to occur in clients with impaired renal function or those who are ingesting additional potassium (*e.g.*, salt substitutes)

(c) Cardiac arrhythmias, which may progress to ventricular fibrillation and asystole

**4. Observe for drug interactions**
 **a.** Drugs that *increase* effects of diuretics:

(1) Aminoglycoside antibiotics

Additive ototoxicity with ethacrynic acid

(2) Antihypertensive agents

Additive hypotensive effects

(3) Corticosteroids

Additive hypokalemia

**b.** Drugs that *decrease* effects of diuretics:

(1) Nonsteroidal anti-inflammatory drugs (*e.g.*, aspirin, ibuprofen, others)

These drugs cause retention of sodium and water.

(2) Oral contraceptives

Retention of sodium and water

(3) Vasopressors (*e.g.*, epinephrine, norepinephrine)

These drugs may antagonize hypotensive effects of diuretics by decreasing responsiveness of arterioles.

**5. Teach clients**
 **a.** Take diuretics in the early morning.

To avoid nocturia

**b.** Expect increased frequency of urination, decreased edema, and weight loss.

Polyuria lasts only a few days or weeks in nonedematous clients.

**c.** Weigh periodically, under standardized conditions.

Weighing is most helpful in edematous conditions.

**d.** If the client is taking digitalis, a potassium-losing diuretic, and a potassium supplement, emphasize that these drugs must be taken as prescribed.

This is a frequently ordered combination of drugs for clients with congestive heart failure. To increase therapeutic effectiveness and avoid hypokalemia and digitalis toxicity, the balance among these drugs must be maintained.

**e.** Report adverse effects.

So that the treatment regimen can be altered, if indicated.

## Review and Application Exercises

1. What are clinical indications for the use of diuretics?
2. What is the general mechanism by which all diuretics act?
3. How can you assess a client for therapeutic effects of a diuretic?
4. Compare and contrast the main groups of diuretics in terms of adverse effects.
5. Why should serum potassium levels be monitored regularly during diuretic therapy?
6. Which prescription and over-the-counter drugs may decrease the effects of a diuretic?
7. For a client who is starting diuretic therapy, what are important points to teach the client about safe and effective drug usage?

**8.** For a client who is taking a potassium-losing diuretic and a potassium chloride supplement, explain the possible consequences of discontinuing one drug while continuing the other.

## Selected References

Applegate, W. B. (1992). Hypertension in the elderly. In W. N. Kelley (Ed.), *Textbook of internal medicine* (2nd ed.) (pp. 2359–2362). Philadelphia: J.B. Lippincott.

Brater, D. C. (1992). Clinical pharmacology of cardiovascular drugs. In W. N. Kelley (Ed.), *Textbook of internal medicine* (2nd ed.) (pp. 315–335). Philadelphia: J.B. Lippincott.

Clark, J. B., Queener, S. F., & Karb, V. B. (1993). *Pharmacologic basis of nursing practice* (4th ed.). St. Louis: C.V. Mosby.

(1993). *Drug facts and comparisons*. St. Louis: Facts and Comparisons.

Francis, G. S., & Alpert, J. S. (Eds.) (1990). *Modern coronary care*. Boston: Little, Brown.

Guyton, A. C. (1991). *Textbook of medical physiology* (8th ed.). Philadelphia: W.B. Saunders.

Joint National Committee on Detection, Evaluation, and Treatment of High Blood Pressure (1993). *The Fifth Report*: NIH Publication No. 93-1088. Bethesda, MD: National Institutes of Health.

May, D. B., Young, L. Y., & Wiser, T. H. (1992). Essential hypertension. In M. A. Koda-Kimble & L. Y. Young (Eds.), *Applied therapeutics: The clinical use of drugs* (5th ed.) (pp. 7-1–7-32). Vancouver, WA: Applied Therapeutics.

Porth, C. M. (1990). *Pathophysiology: Concepts of altered health states* (3rd ed.). Philadelphia: J.B. Lippincott.

# CHAPTER 60

# Anticoagulant, Antiplatelet, and Thrombolytic Agents

## Description

Anticoagulant, antiplatelet, and thrombolytic drugs are used in the prevention and treatment of thrombotic and thromboembolic disorders. Thrombosis involves the formation (thrombogenesis) or presence of a blood clot (thrombus) within the vascular system. Blood coagulation is a normal body defense mechanism to prevent blood loss. Thus, thrombogenesis may be life saving when it occurs as a response to hemorrhage; however, it may be life threatening when it occurs at other times, because the thrombus can obstruct a blood vessel and impair the blood supply of tissues beyond the clot. When part of a thrombus breaks off and travels to another part of the body, it is called an *embolus*. Ultimate consequences of thrombi and emboli depend primarily on location and size. Thrombi and emboli that lodge in vital organs are major causes of morbidity and mortality from such disorders as myocardial infarction, stroke, and pulmonary embolism.

Under normal circumstances, thrombi are constantly being formed and dissolved (thrombolysis), but the blood stays fluid, and blood flow is not significantly obstructed. If the balance between thrombogenesis and thrombolysis is upset, thrombotic or bleeding disorders result. Thrombotic disorders occur much more often than bleeding disorders. To aid understanding of drug therapy for thrombotic disorders, normal blood coagula-

tion and characteristics of arterial and venous thrombosis are discussed.

## Blood coagulation

Normal blood coagulation is a complex process involving numerous interacting elements. It is initiated by injury to a blood vessel and followed by two successive phases or series of events that result in clot formation.

### PLATELET OR VASCULAR PHASE

*Platelets*, also called thrombocytes, are produced in the bone marrow and released into the bloodstream, where they circulate for about 7 to 10 days before they are removed by the spleen. Platelets are fragments of large cells called *megakaryocytes;* they contain no nuclei and therefore cannot repair or replicate themselves. Their only known function in the body is related to hemostasis (the control of bleeding by blood coagulation).

When injury occurs to a blood vessel wall, platelets elongate and become "sticky" so that they adhere to the vessel wall and to other platelets (platelet aggregation). At the same time, the fragile cell membrane disintegrates and allows leakage of platelet contents (*e.g.*, thromboplastin and other clotting factors, calcium, serotonin, epinephrine, adenosine diphosphate, and thromboxane $A_2$), which serve various functions to stop bleeding. Thromboplastin activates prothrombin. Serotonin and epinephrine cause vasoconstriction. Thromboxane $A_2$ (a prostaglandin synthesized by platelets) is a potent stimulus of vasoconstriction and platelet aggregation.

Platelets act within seconds to form a platelet plug and stop bleeding. Platelets usually disappear from a blood clot within 24 hours and are replaced by fibrin.

### BLOOD COAGULATION PHASE

Blood coagulation acts more slowly (within 1–2 minutes) to cause hemostasis. It involves sequential activation of clotting factors that are normally present in blood and tissues as inactive precursors. Characteristics and functions of coagulation factors are listed in Table 60-1. Major steps in the coagulation process are the following:

1. Release of thromboplastin by disintegrating platelets and damaged tissue
2. Conversion of prothrombin to thrombin, which requires thromboplastin and calcium ions
3. Conversion of fibrinogen to fibrin by thrombin

## Thrombotic and thromboembolic disorders

Thrombosis may occur in both arteries and veins. Arterial thrombosis is usually associated with atherosclerotic plaque, hypertension, and turbulent blood flow. These conditions damage the inner lining of the artery so that platelets adhere, aggregate, and release thromboplastin to initiate the coagulation process. Arterial thrombi cause disease by obstructing blood flow. If the obstruction is incomplete or temporary, local tissue ischemia (deficient blood supply) occurs. If the obstruction is complete or prolonged, local tissue death or infarction occurs.

Venous thrombosis is usually associated with venous stasis. When blood flows very slowly, thrombin and other coagulant substances present in the blood become sufficiently concentrated in local areas to initiate the clotting process. With a normal rate of blood flow, these substances are rapidly removed from the blood, primarily by Kupffer's cells in the liver. A venous thrombus is less cohesive than an arterial thrombus. Consequently, an embolus can easily become detached and travel to other parts of the body.

Venous thrombi cause disease by two mechanisms. First, thrombosis causes local congestion, edema, and perhaps inflammation by impairing normal outflow of venous blood (*e.g.*, thrombophlebitis, deep vein thrombosis [DVT]). Second, embolization causes obstruction of blood supply when the embolus becomes lodged. The pulmonary arteries are common sites of embolization.

## Drugs used in thrombotic and thromboembolic disorders

Drugs given to prevent or treat thrombosis alter some aspect of the blood coagulation process. Anticoagulants are widely used in thrombotic disorders. They are more effective in preventing venous thrombosis than arterial thrombosis. Antiplatelet drugs are used to prevent arterial thrombosis. Thrombolytic agents are used to dissolve thrombi and limit tissue damage in selected thromboembolic disorders.

### ANTICOAGULANTS

Anticoagulant drugs are given to prevent formation of new clots and extension of clots already present. They do not dissolve formed clots, improve blood flow in tissues

---

**TABLE 60-1.  BLOOD COAGULATION FACTORS**

| Number | Name | Functions |
|---|---|---|
| I | Fibrinogen | Forms fibrin, the insoluble protein strands that compose the supporting framework of a blood clot. Thrombin and calcium are required for the conversion. |
| II | Prothrombin | Forms thrombin, which catalyzes the conversion of fibrinogen to fibrin |
| III | Thromboplastin | Converts prothrombin to thrombin |
| IV | Calcium | Catalyzes the conversion of prothrombin to thrombin |
| V | Labile factor | Required for formation of active thromboplastin |
| VII | Proconvertin or stable factor | Accelerates action of tissue thromboplastin |
| VIII | Antihemophilic factor | Promotes breakdown of platelets and formation of active platelet thromboplastin |
| IX | Christmas factor | Similar to factor VIII |
| X | Stuart factor | Promotes action of thromboplastin |
| XI | Plasma thromboplastin antecedent | Promotes platelet aggregation and breakdown, with subsequent release of platelet thromboplastin |
| XII | Hageman factor | Similar to factor XI |
| XIII | Fibrin-stabilizing factor | Converts fibrin meshwork to the dense, tight mass of the completely formed clot |

around the clot, or prevent ischemic damage to tissues beyond the clot. The two most commonly used anticoagulants are heparin and warfarin sodium (Coumadin). These drugs act by different mechanisms to interfere with certain coagulation factors and prevent thrombus formation (see discussions of the individual drugs).

Clinical indications for anticoagulants include prevention or treatment of thromboembolic disorders, such as thrombophlebitis, DVT, and pulmonary embolism. Heparin is also used for other purposes.

## ANTIPLATELET DRUGS

Antiplatelet drugs prevent platelet aggregation and thereby interfere with the initial phase of blood coagulation. Increased platelet aggregation is associated with atherosclerosis and thromboembolic disorders. For example, arterial thrombi, which are composed primarily of platelets, may embolize from abnormal heart valves, mural thrombi, or atherosclerotic plaque.

Drugs used clinically for antiplatelet effects are aspirin, dipyridamole (Persantine), and ticlopidine (Ticlid). They are used to prevent myocardial infarction, stroke in clients with transient ischemic attacks (TIAs), and thromboembolism in clients with prosthetic heart valves.

## THROMBOLYTIC AGENTS

Thrombolytic agents are given to dissolve thrombi. They stimulate conversion of plasminogen to plasmin (also called fibrinolysin). Plasmin is a proteolytic enzyme that breaks down fibrin, the framework of a thrombus. The main use of thrombolytic agents is for treatment of acute, severe thromboembolic disease, such as myocardial infarction, pulmonary embolism, and iliofemoral thrombosis. The goal of thrombolytic therapy is to reestablish blood flow and prevent or limit tissue damage. The drugs also are used to dissolve clots in intravascular catheters. Currently approved thrombolytics are alteplase (Activase), anistreplase (Eminase), streptokinase (Streptase), and urokinase (Abbokinase).

## Individual drugs

### ANTICOAGULANTS AND THEIR ANTIDOTES

**Heparin sodium** (Lipo-Hepin, Liquaemin) is a pharmaceutical preparation of the natural anticoagulant produced primarily by mast cells in pericapillary connective tissue. Endogenous heparin is found in various body tissues, most abundantly in the liver and lungs. Exogenous heparin is obtained from bovine lung or porcine intestinal mucosa and standardized in units of biologic activity.

Heparin combines with antithrombin III to inactivate several clotting factors (IX, X, XI, XII) and thrombin so that thrombus formation is prevented. Antithrombin III is an alpha globulin normally present in the blood as a natural anticoagulant substance. Antithrombin III must be present for heparin action.

Heparin acts immediately after intravenous administration and within 20 to 30 minutes after subcutaneous injection. It is metabolized in the liver and excreted in the urine, primarily as inactive metabolites. Heparin does not cross the placental barrier and is not secreted in breast milk. Disadvantages of heparin are its short duration of action and the subsequent need for frequent administration, the necessity for parenteral injection (because it is not absorbed from the gastrointestinal tract), its relatively high cost, and local tissue reactions at injection sites.

Prophylactically, low doses of heparin are given to prevent DVT and pulmonary embolism in clients at risk of developing these disorders, such as the following:

1. Those having abdominal or thoracic surgery who are over age 40 or have additional risk factors for DVT (*e.g.*, obesity, varicose veins)
2. Those with a history of thrombophlebitis or pulmonary embolism
3. Those having gynecologic surgery, especially if they have been taking estrogens or oral contraceptives or have other risk factors for DVT
4. Those expected to be on bed rest or to have limited activity for longer than 5 days, especially if debilitating conditions are also present (*e.g.*, severe congestive heart failure, stroke, malignant disease)

Low-dose heparin prophylaxis is either ineffective or contraindicated in major orthopedic surgery, abdominal prostatectomy, and brain surgery.

Therapeutically, heparin is used for treatment of acute thromboembolic disorders (*e.g.*, DVT, thrombophlebitis, pulmonary embolism). In these conditions, the aim of therapy is to prevent further thrombus formation and embolization. Heparin is also used in disseminated intravascular coagulation (DIC), a life-threatening condition characterized by widespread clotting, which depletes the blood of coagulation factors. The depletion of coagulation factors then produces widespread bleeding. The goal of heparin therapy in DIC is to prevent blood coagulation long enough for clotting factors to be replenished and thus be able to control hemorrhage.

Although sometimes used in arterial occlusive disease, myocardial infarction, and stroke, heparin therapy has not been proven effective in preventing further thromboembolic problems. However, heparin may be effective in preventing embolization from prosthetic heart valves.

Heparin is also used to prevent clotting during cardiac and vascular surgery, extracorporeal circulation, hemodialysis, and blood transfusions and in blood samples to be used in laboratory tests. It has been used to maintain patency of intermittent intravenous infusion devices (*e.g.*, catheters and heparin locks). With heparin locks, several studies have indicated that normal saline flushes are effective, and use of heparin for this purpose has declined.

**Enoxaparin** (Lovenox) is a low molecular weight formulation of heparin. Other heparin preparations are a mixture of high and low molecular weights. Most anticoagulant activity is attributed to the low molecular weight heparin. Some studies indicate that subcutaneous enoxaparin may be as effective as intravenous heparin in treating thrombotic disorders. In addition, enoxaparin does not require close monitoring of blood coagulation tests. These characteristics may allow outpatient treatment for disorders that have required hospitalization.

Contraindications to heparin therapy include gastrointestinal ulcerations (*e.g.*, peptic ulcer disease, ulcerative colitis), blood dyscrasias, severe kidney or liver disease, severe hypertension, polycythemia vera, and recent surgery of the eye, spinal cord, or brain. It should be used with caution in clients with mild hypertension, renal or hepatic disease, alcoholism, history of gastrointestinal ulcerations, drainage tubes (*e.g.*, nasogastric tubes, indwelling urinary catheters), and any occupation with high risks of traumatic injury.

Heparin sodium

### Routes and dosage ranges

*Adults:* IV injection, 5000 units initially, followed by 5000–10,000 units q4–6h, to a maximum dose of 25,000 units/d

DIC, IV injection, 50–100 units/kg q4h

IV infusion, 20,000–40,000 units/d at initial rate of 0.25 units/kg per minute, then adjusted according to blood clotting tests (activated partial thromboplastin time [APTT])

SC 10,000–12,000 units q8h, or 14,000–20,000 units q12h

Low-dose prophylaxis, SC 5000 units 2 h before surgery, then q12h until discharged from hospital or fully ambulatory

*Children:* DIC, IV injection, 25–50 units/kg q4h

IV infusion, 50 units/kg initially, followed by 100 units/kg q4h or 20,000 units/m$^2$ over 24 h

Enoxaparin

### Route and dosage range

*Adults:* SC 30 mg twice daily, with first dose soon after surgery but not more than 24 hours postoperatively. Usual duration, 7–10 d

**Protamine sulfate** is an antidote or antagonist for heparin. Heparin is an acid; protamine sulfate is a base. Thus, protamine neutralizes heparin activity. Protamine dosage depends on the amount of heparin administered during the previous 3 or 4 hours. Each milligram of protamine neutralizes 80 to 100 units of heparin. A single dose should not exceed 50 mg. The drug is injected intravenously over 1 to 3 minutes. Protamine effects occur immediately and last for about 2 hours. A second dose may be required, because heparin activity lasts about 4 hours.

**Warfarin** (Panwarfin) is the prototype and most commonly used coumarin anticoagulant. Warfarin acts in the liver to prevent synthesis of vitamin K-dependent clotting factors (*i.e.*, factors II, VII, IX, and X). Warfarin is similar to vitamin K in structure and therefore acts as a competitive antagonist to hepatic use of vitamin K. Anticoagulant effects do not occur for about 3 to 5 days after warfarin is started because clotting factors already in the blood follow their normal pathway of elimination. Warfarin has no effect on circulating clotting factors or on platelet function.

Warfarin is well absorbed after oral administration. Although it can be given parenterally, there is no advantage in therapeutic effect. Warfarin is highly bound to plasma proteins (about 98%), mainly albumin. It is metabolized in the liver and primarily excreted as inactive metabolites by the kidneys.

Warfarin is most useful in long-term prevention or treatment of venous thromboembolic disorders. It is also used to prevent embolization from prosthetic heart valves. Warfarin has sometimes been advocated for use after myocardial infarction (to prevent reinfarction) and in strokes caused by cerebral thrombosis. However, the usefulness of anticoagulant therapy in these conditions is not clearly established. As a general rule, warfarin is not indicated in arterial thrombosis because arterial thrombi are composed primarily of platelets, and warfarin has no effect on platelet functions.

Contraindications to warfarin therapy include gastrointestinal ulcerations (*e.g.*, peptic ulcer disease, ulcerative colitis), blood dyscrasias (*e.g.*, hemophilia, thrombocytopenia), severe kidney or liver disease, severe hypertension, and recent surgery of the eye, spinal cord, or brain. Warfarin crosses the placenta and is contraindicated during pregnancy. Warfarin should be used cautiously with hypertension, renal or hepatic disease, alcoholism, history of gastrointestinal ulcerations, drainage tubes (*e.g.*, nasogastric tubes, indwelling urinary catheters), and occupations with high risks of traumatic injury.

### Route and dosage range

*Adults:* PO 10 mg/day for 2–3 d, then adjusted according to prothrombin time (PT); average maintenance dose, 2–10 mg/d

**Phytonadione** (vitamin K, Mephyton) is the antidote for warfarin overdosage. An oral dose of 10 to 20 mg will usually stop minor bleeding and return the prothrombin time to a normal range within 24 hours.

## ANTIPLATELET AGENTS

**Aspirin** is a commonly used analgesic–antipyretic–anti-inflammatory drug (see Chap. 6) with potent antiplatelet effects. Aspirin exerts pharmacologic actions by inhibiting synthesis of prostaglandins. In this instance, aspirin acetylates the enzyme in platelets that normally synthesizes thromboxane $A_2$, a prostaglandin that causes platelet aggregation. Thus, aspirin prevents formation of thromboxane $A_2$, thereby preventing platelet aggregation and thrombus formation. Antithrombotic effects persist for the life of the platelet (about 10 days). Aspirin may be used as an antiplatelet agent for prevention of myocardial infarction and in clients with prosthetic heart valves or TIAs. Adverse effects are uncommon with the small doses used for antiplatelet effects. However, there is an increased risk of bleeding.

### Route and dosage range

*Adults:* PO 80–325 mg/d

**Dipyridamole** is an antiplatelet drug used for prevention of thromboembolism after cardiac valve replacement, usually with warfarin, and for prevention of myocardial reinfarction, usually with aspirin.

### Route and dosage range

*Adults:* PO 25–75 mg three times per day, 1 h before meals

**Ticlopidine** inhibits platelet aggregation irreversibly and effects persist for the life span of the platelet. The drug is indicated for prevention of thrombotic stroke in people with premonitory symptoms, such as TIAs or previous thrombotic strokes. Because ticlopidine may cause neutropenia or agranulocytosis, it is considered a second-line drug for use in clients who cannot take aspirin. Contraindications include active bleeding disorders (*e.g.,* gastrointestinal bleeding from peptic ulcer or intracranial bleeding), neutropenia, thrombocytopenia, severe liver disease, and hypersensitivity to the drug.

Ticlopidine is rapidly absorbed after oral administration and reaches peak plasma levels about 2 hours after a dose. It is highly protein bound (98%), extensively metabolized in the liver, and excreted in urine and feces. As with other antiplatelet drugs, there is increased risk of bleeding with ticlopidine.

### Route and dosage range

*Adults:* PO 250 mg twice daily with food

## THROMBOLYTIC AGENTS AND THEIR ANTIDOTES

**Alteplase** is a thrombolytic agent produced by recombinant DNA. It is a tissue plasminogen activator and is often called tPA. It is used in acute myocardial infarction to dissolve clots obstructing coronary arteries and reestablish perfusion of tissues beyond the thrombotic area. The drug binds to fibrin in a clot and acts locally to dissolve the clot with less systemic effect than streptokinase.

The most common adverse effect is bleeding, which may be internal (intracranial, from gastrointestinal or genitourinary sites) or external (from venous or arterial puncture sites or surgical incisions). The drug is contraindicated in the presence of bleeding, a history of cerebrovascular accident, central nervous system surgery or trauma within the previous 2 months, and severe hypertension.

### Route and dosage range

*Adults:* IV infusion, 100 mg over 3 h (first hour, 60 mg with a bolus of 6–10 mg over 1–2 min initially; second hour, 20 mg; third hour 20 mg)

**Anistreplase** is a combination of human plasminogen and streptokinase. Like alteplase, it breaks down fibrin and is used to lyse coronary artery clots in acute myocardial infarction. Adverse effects and contraindications are the same as for other thrombolytic agents. An advantage is that anistreplase can be given in a single intravenous injection.

### Route and dosage range

IV injection, 30 units over 2–5 min

**Streptokinase**, a protein derived from streptococci, promotes dissolution of blood clots by interacting with a plasminogen proactivator. The resulting substance catalyzes the conversion of plasminogen to plasmin. Plasmin (fibrinolysin) breaks down fibrin. Streptokinase may be used for treatment of acute pulmonary emboli or iliofemoral thrombophlebitis when these conditions are severe and life threatening. Bleeding, fever, and allergic reactions may occur. Heparin and warfarin are given after streptokinase therapy is finished.

Streptokinase also may be injected directly into a coronary artery to dissolve a thrombus if done within 6 hours of onset of symptoms. An additional use is to dissolve clots in arterial or venous lines.

### Route and dosage range

*Adults:* IV 250,000 units over 30 min, then 100,000 units/h for 24–72 h

**Urokinase** is a proteolytic enzyme that catalyzes the conversion of plasminogen to plasmin. Plasmin breaks down fibrin and thereby promotes dissolution of blood clots. Urokinase is recommended for use in clients allergic to streptokinase. Urokinase is contraindicated in children, pregnant women, and clients with wounds, malignancies, and recent strokes. In addition, all other contraindications to heparin and warfarin therapy apply to urokinase. Incidence of bleeding is high with urokinase. Heparin and warfarin are started after urokinase therapy is completed.

### Route and dosage range

*Adults:* IV 4400 units/kg over 10 min, followed by continuous infusion of 4400 units/kg per hour for 12 h

**Aminocaproic acid** (Amicar) and **tranexamic acid** (Cyklokapron) are antidotes for overdoses of thrombolytic agents that inhibit fibrinolysis (clot dissolution). The drugs are used to control bleeding induced by thrombolytic agents. Aminocaproic acid also may be used in other bleeding disorders caused by hyperfibrinolysis (*e.g.*, cardiac surgery, blood disorders, hepatic cirrhosis, prostatectomy, neoplastic disorders). Tranexamic acid also is used for short periods (2–8 days) in hemophiliacs to prevent or decrease bleeding from tooth extraction. Dosage of tranexamic acid should be reduced in the presence of moderate or severe renal impairment.

Aminocaproic acid

### Route and dosage range

*Adults:* PO, IV infusion, 5 g initially, followed by 1.0 to 1.25 g/h for 8 h or until bleeding is controlled; maximum dose, 30 g/24 h

Tranexamic acid

### Route and dosage range

*Adults:* Hemophiliacs having dental extraction, PO 25 mg/kg three to four times daily, starting 1 d prior to surgery or IV 10 mg/kg immediately before surgery, followed by 25 mg/kg PO three to four times daily for 2 to 8 d

## Nursing Process

### Assessment

Assess the client's status in relation to thrombotic and thromboembolic disorders.
- Risk factors for thromboembolism include:
  - Immobility (*e.g.*, limited activity or bed rest for more than 5 days)
  - Obesity
  - Cigarette smoking

- History of varicose veins, thrombophlebitis, or pulmonary emboli
- Congestive heart failure
- Pedal edema
- Lower limb trauma
- Myocardial infarction
- Atrial fibrillation
- Mitral or aortic stenosis
- Prosthetic heart valves
- Abdominal, thoracic, pelvic, or major orthopedic surgery
- Atherosclerotic heart disease or peripheral vascular disease
- Use of oral contraceptives
- Signs and symptoms of thrombotic and thromboembolic disorders depend on the location and size of the thrombus.
  - DVT and thrombophlebitis usually occur in the legs. The conditions may be manifested by edema (the affected leg is often measurably larger than the other) and pain, especially in the calf when the foot is dorsiflexed (positive Homan's sign). If thrombophlebitis is superficial, it may be visible as a red, warm, tender area following the path of a vein.
  - Pulmonary embolism, if severe enough to produce symptoms, is manifested by chest pain, cough, hemoptysis, tachypnea, and tachycardia. Massive emboli cause hypotension, shock, cyanosis, and death.
  - DIC is usually manifested by bleeding, which may range from petechiae or oozing from a venipuncture site to massive internal bleeding or bleeding from all body orifices.

### Nursing diagnoses

- Altered Tissue Perfusion related to thrombus or embolus
- Pain related to tissue ischemia
- Impaired Physical Mobility related to bed rest and pain
- Altered Tissue Perfusion related to drug-induced bleeding
- Decreased Cardiac Output related to hemorrhage and volume depletion
- Anxiety related to fear of myocardial infarction or stroke
- Ineffective Individual Coping related to the need for long-term prophylaxis of thromboembolic disorders or fear of excessive bleeding
- Noncompliance related to anxiety, the need for periodic blood tests, and lack of knowledge about anticoagulant therapy
- Knowledge Deficit related to anticoagulant or antiplatelet drug therapy
- High Risk for Injury related to drug-induced impairment of blood coagulation

### Planning/Goals

*The client will:*
- Receive or take anticoagulant and antiplatelet drugs correctly
- Be monitored closely for therapeutic and adverse drug effects, especially when drug therapy is started and when changes are made in drugs or dosages
- Use nondrug measures to decrease venous stasis and prevent thromboembolic disorders
- Act to prevent trauma from falls and other injuries
- Inform any health-care provider when taking an anticoagulant

- Avoid or report adverse drug reactions
- Verbalize or demonstrate knowledge of safe management of anticoagulant drug therapy
- Keep follow-up appointments for tests of blood coagulation and drug dosage regulation

### Interventions

Use measures to prevent thrombotic and thromboembolic disorders.
- Have the client ambulate and exercise legs regularly, especially postoperatively.
- For clients who cannot ambulate or do leg exercises, do passive range-of-motion and other leg exercises several times daily when changing the client's position or performing other care.
- Have the client wear elastic stockings. Elastic stockings should be removed every 8 hours and replaced after inspecting the skin. Improperly applied elastic stockings can impair circulation rather than aid it.
- Avoid trauma to lower extremities.
- Maintain adequate fluid intake (1500–3000 ml/day) to avoid dehydration and hemoconcentration.

For the client receiving anticoagulant therapy, implement safety measures to prevent trauma and bleeding.
- For clients who cannot ambulate safely due to weakness, sedation, or other conditions, keep the call light within reach, keep bedrails elevated, and assist in ambulation.
- Provide an electric razor for shaving.
- Avoid intramuscular injections, venipunctures, and arterial punctures when possible.
- Avoid intubations when possible (*e.g.*, nasogastric tubes, indwelling urinary catheters).

*Teach clients:*
- To exercise legs periodically, especially if walking and other activities are limited
- To avoid situations that impair blood circulation, such as wearing tight clothing; crossing the legs at the knees; prolonged sitting, standing, and bed rest; and placing pillows under the knees when in bed
- Risks of thromboembolic disorders
- The importance of continued supervision and monitoring by a health-care provider

### Evaluation

- Observe for signs and symptoms of thromboembolic disorders or bleeding.
- Check blood coagulation tests for therapeutic ranges.
- Observe and interview regarding compliance with instructions about drug therapy.
- Observe and interview regarding adverse drug effects.

# Principles of therapy

## DRUG SELECTION

The choice of anticoagulant or antiplatelet drug depends mainly on the reason for use.

1. Heparin is the drug of choice in acute thromboembolic disorders because the anticoagulant effect begins immediately with intravenous administration.
2. Warfarin is the drug of choice for long-term maintenance therapy (*i.e.*, several weeks or months), since it can be given orally.
3. Aspirin is the most widely used antiplatelet drug for prevention of myocardial reinfarction and arterial thrombosis in clients with TIAs and prosthetic heart valves.
4. When anticoagulation is required during pregnancy, heparin is used because it does not cross the placenta. Warfarin is contraindicated during pregnancy.

## DOSAGE FACTORS

Dosage of anticoagulant drugs must be individualized, primarily according to blood coagulation tests, client characteristics, and concomitant drug therapy.

### Heparin

Dosage is regulated by the activated partial thromboplastin time (APTT), a modification of the PTT test that is reportedly more sensitive and requires less time to perform. The APTT is sensitive to changes in blood clotting factors, except factor VII. Thus, normal or control values indicate normal blood coagulation; therapeutic values indicate low levels of clotting factors and delayed blood coagulation. During heparin therapy, the APTT should be maintained at about 1.5 to 2.5 times the control or baseline value. The normal control value is 25 to 35 seconds; therefore, therapeutic values are 35 to 85 seconds, approximately. With continuous IV infusion, blood for the APTT may be drawn anytime; with intermittent administration, blood for the APTT should be drawn about 1 hour before a dose of heparin is scheduled. APTT is not necessary with low-dose heparin given subcutaneously for prophylaxis of thromboembolism.

### Warfarin

Dosage is regulated according to the prothrombin time (PT) or the international normalized ratio (INR) system. PT is sensitive to changes in three of the four vitamin K–dependent coagulation factors (*i.e.*, II, VII, IX, and X). Thus, normal or control values indicate normal levels of these blood coagulation factors; therapeutic values indicate low levels of the factors and delayed blood coagulation. A normal baseline or control PT is about 12 seconds; a therapeutic value is about 1.5 times the control, or 18 seconds.

When warfarin is started, PT should be measured daily until a stable daily dose is reached (the dose that maintains PT within therapeutic values and does not cause bleeding). Often, the daily dose is ordered after the physician obtains the PT report. This process may require 1 to 2 weeks. Thereafter, PT is measured every 2 to 4 weeks for the duration of oral anticoagulant drug therapy.

The PT test is performed by adding a mixture of thromboplastin and calcium to citrated plasma and measuring the time (in seconds) it takes for the blood to clot. A major problem in using the PT to monitor warfarin therapy is that values vary among laboratories according to the type of thromboplastin (*e.g.*, rabbit or human) and the instrument used to measure PT. The INR system standardizes the PT by comparing a particular thromboplastin with a standard thromboplastin designated by the World Health Organization (WHO). When laboratories report the INR (therapeutic values are 2.0–3.0 in most conditions requiring warfarin therapy), advantages include consistent values among laboratories, more consistent warfarin dosage with less risk of bleeding or thrombosis, and more consistent reports of clinical trials and other research studies.

For laboratories that still report PT rather than INR, the nurse must know the values used by a particular laboratory to interpret PT test results accurately. Also, the nurse must instruct the client receiving long-term therapy to use the same laboratory for PT tests or to notify the physician when this is impossible.

Warfarin dosage may need to be reduced in clients with biliary tract disorders (*e.g.*, obstructive jaundice), liver disease (*e.g.*, hepatitis, cirrhosis), malabsorption syndromes (*e.g.*, steatorrhea), and hyperthyroidism or fever. These conditions increase anticoagulant drug effects by reducing absorption of vitamin K, decreasing hepatic synthesis of blood-clotting factors, or increasing the rate of degradation of clotting factors. Despite these influencing factors, however, the primary determinant of dosage is the PT.

Warfarin and other coumarin anticoagulants interact with many other drugs to cause increased, decreased, or unpredictable anticoagulant effects. Thus, warfarin dosage may need to be increased or decreased when other drugs are given concomitantly. Most drugs can be given if warfarin dosage is carefully titrated according to the PT or INR and altered appropriately when an interacting drug is added or stopped. INR or PT measurements and vigilant observation are needed whenever a drug is added to or removed from a drug therapy regimen containing warfarin.

## THROMBOLYTIC THERAPY

1. Thrombolytic therapy should be performed only by experienced personnel in an intensive care setting with cardiac and other monitoring devices in place.
2. All of the available agents are effective with recommended uses. Thus, the choice of a thrombolytic agent depends mainly on risks of adverse effects and costs. All of the drugs may cause bleeding. The two newer agents, alteplase and anistreplase, reportedly act more specifically on the fibrin in a clot and cause less systemic depletion of fibrinogen, but these agents are very expensive. Streptokinase, the least expensive agent, may cause allergic reactions since it is a foreign protein. Combination therapy (*e.g.*, with alteplase and streptokinase) is being investigated for safety, efficacy, and cost.
3. Before a thrombolytic agent is begun, PT (or INR), PTT, platelet count, and fibrinogen should be checked to establish baseline values and to determine if a blood coagulation disorder is present. Two or three hours after thrombolytic therapy is started, the fibrinogen level can be measured to determine that fibrinolysis is occurring. Alternatively, PT and/or PTT can be checked for increased values since the breakdown products of fibrin exert anticoagulant effects.
4. Major factors in decreasing risks of bleeding are selecting recipients carefully, avoiding invasive procedures when possible, and omitting anticoagulant or antiplatelet drugs while thrombolytics are being given. If bleeding does occur, it is most likely from a venipuncture or invasive procedure site, and local pressure may control it. If bleeding cannot be controlled or involves a vital organ, the thrombolytic drug should be stopped and fibrinogen replaced with whole blood plasma or cryoprecipitate. Aminocaproic acid or tranexamic acid may also be given.
5. When the drugs are used in acute myocardial infarction, cardiac arrhythmias may occur when blood flow is reestablished. Therefore, antiarrhythmic drugs should be readily available.

## USE IN CHILDREN

Little information is available about the use of anticoagulants in children. Heparin solutions containing benzyl alcohol as a preservative should not be given to premature infants because fatal reactions have been reported. When given for systemic anticoagulation, heparin dosage should be based on the child's weight (about 50 units/kg).

Warfarin is given to children after cardiac surgery to prevent thromboembolism, but doses and guidelines for safe, effective usage have not been developed. Accurate drug administration, close monitoring of blood coagulation tests, safety measures to prevent trauma and bleeding, avoiding interacting drugs, and informing others in the child's environment (*e.g.*, teachers, babysitters, health-care providers) are necessary.

Antiplatelet and thrombolytic drugs have no established indications for use in children.

## USE IN OLDER ADULTS

Older adults often develop thromboembolic disorders, especially if mobility is impaired. They are also more likely than younger adults to experience bleeding and other complications of anticoagulant drugs.

With heparin, general principles for safe and effective use apply. With warfarin, dosage should be reduced because impaired liver function and decreased plasma proteins increase the risks of bleeding. Also, many drugs interact with warfarin to increase or decrease its effect, and older adults often take several drugs concurrently. Starting or stopping any drug may require that warfarin dosage be adjusted.

## NURSING ACTIONS: ANTICOAGULANTS

| *Nursing Actions* | *Rationale/Explanation* |
|---|---|
| **1. Administer accurately** | |
| **a.** With *heparin*: | |
| (1) When transcribing a physician's order, write out "units" rather than using the abbreviation "U." | This is a safety precaution to avoid erroneous dosage. For example, 1000 U (1000 units) may be misread as 10,000 units. |
| (2) Check dosage carefully. | Although accurate dosage is important in all drug therapy, it is especially important with anticoagulants because a rather narrow range exists between therapeutic and toxic levels. Therefore, underdosage may cause thromboembolism, and overdosage may cause bleeding. In addition, heparin is available in several concentrations (1000, 2500, 5000, 10,000, 15,000, 20,000, and 40,000 units/ml). |
| (3) For subcutaneous heparin: | |
| (a) Use a 26-gauge, ½-inch needle. | To minimize trauma and risk of bleeding |
| (b) Use a tuberculin syringe and a drug volume of 0.5 ml or less. | To measure accurately and minimize trauma |
| (c) Cleanse injection site gently with an alcohol sponge. | To prevent infection |
| (d) Grasp a fold of tissue between thumb and fingers of the nondominant hand. Do not pinch tightly. | To give the drug in a deep subcutaneous or fat layer |
| (e) Insert the needle at a 90-degree angle into the skin fold, inject without aspirating, and withdraw the needle. | To minimize trauma and risk of bleeding. |
| (f) Apply gentle pressure to the site for 30–60 seconds. Do not rub. | To prevent bleeding |
| (g) Rotate injection sites (abdomen, upper arms, and lateral thighs may be used). Do not inject heparin within 2 inches of the umbilicus. | To minimize tissue irritation and trauma. Avoid the umbilical area to prevent inadvertent injection into umbilical veins. |
| (4) For intermittent IV administration: | |
| (a) Give by direct injection into a heparin lock or tubing injection site. | These methods prevent repeated venipunctures. |
| (b) Dilute the dose in 50 to 100 ml of any IV fluid (usually 5% dextrose in water). | |
| (5) For continuous IV administration: | This is usually the preferred method of administration because it maintains consistent serum drug levels rather than peak levels and trough levels. |

*(continued)*

| Nursing Actions | Rationale/Explanation |
|---|---|
| (a) Use a volume-control device and an infusion-control device. | To regulate dosage and flow rate accurately |
| (b) Add only enough heparin for a few hours. One effective method is to fill the volume-control set (*e.g.*, Volutrol) with 100 ml of 5% dextrose in water and add 5000 units of heparin to yield a concentration of 50 units/ml. Dosage is regulated by varying the flow rate. For example, administration of 1000 units/h requires a flow rate of 20 ml/h.<br><br>Another method is to add 25,000 units of heparin to 500 ml of IV solution. | To avoid inadvertent administration of large amounts. Whatever method is used, it is desirable to standardize concentration of heparin solutions within an institution. Standardization is safer, because it reduces risks of errors in dosage. |
| **b.** After the initial dose of warfarin, check prothrombin time before subsequent dose. *Do not* give the dose if prothrombin time (PT) is more than twice the control value. Notify the physician. | PT is measured daily until a maintenance dose is established, then periodically throughout warfarin therapy. Prolonged PT (*e.g.*, more than 24 seconds with a control value of 12 seconds) indicates high risk of bleeding. |
| **c.** With thrombolytic agents, follow manufacturers' instructions for reconstitution and administration. | |

**2. Observe for therapeutic effects**

**a.** Absence of signs and symptoms when given prophylactically

**b.** Decrease or improvement in signs and symptoms when given therapeutically (*e.g.*, less edema and pain with thrombophlebitis, less chest pain and respiratory difficulty with pulmonary embolism)

**c.** PT (for warfarin) or APPT (for heparin) within therapeutic ranges (1½ to 2 times the control value)

**3. Observe for adverse effects**

| Nursing Actions | Rationale/Explanation |
|---|---|
| **a.** Bleeding: | Bleeding is the major adverse effect of anticoagulant drugs. It may occur anywhere in the body, spontaneously or in response to minor trauma. |
| (1) Record vital signs regularly. | Hypotension and tachycardia may indicate internal bleeding. |
| (2) Check stools for blood (melena). | Gastrointestinal (GI) bleeding is fairly common; risks are increased with intubation. Blood in stools may be bright red, tarry (blood that has been digested by GI secretions), or occult (hidden to the naked eye but present with a guaiac test). Hematemesis also may occur. |
| (3) Check urine for blood (hematuria). | Genitourinary bleeding also is fairly common; risks are increased with catheterization or instrumentation. Urine may be red (indicating fresh bleeding) or brownish or smoky gray (indicating old blood). Or bleeding may be microscopic (red blood cells are visible only on microscopic examination during urinalysis). |
| (4) Inspect the skin and mucous membranes daily. | Bleeding may occur in the skin as petechiae, purpura, or ecchymoses. Surgical wounds, skin lesions, parenteral injection sites, the nose, and gums may be bleeding sites. |
| (5) Assess for excessive menstrual flow. | |
| **b.** Other adverse effects: | |
| (1) With heparin, tissue irritation at injection sites, transient alopecia, reversible thrombocytopenia, paresthesias, hypersensitivity | These effects are uncommon. They are more likely to occur with large doses or prolonged administration. |

## Nursing Actions

## Rationale/Explanation

(2) With warfarin, dermatitis, diarrhea, alopecia

These effects occur only occasionally. Warfarin has been given for prolonged periods without toxicity.

**c.** With thrombolytic drugs, observe for bleeding with all uses and reperfusion arrhythmias when used for acute myocardial infarction.

Bleeding is most likely to occur at sites of venipuncture or other invasive procedures. Reperfusion arrhythmias may occur when blood supply is restored to previously ischemic myocardium.

**4. Observe for drug interactions**
**a.** Drugs that *increase* effects of heparin:

(1) Aspirin, dipyridamole

These drugs inhibit platelet function and therefore increase risks of bleeding.

(2) Warfarin sodium (Coumadin)

Additive anticoagulant effects and increased risks of bleeding

**b.** Drugs that *decrease* effects of heparin:

(1) Antihistamines, digitalis glycosides, tetracyclines

These drugs antagonize the anticoagulant effects of heparin. Mechanisms are not clear.

(2) Protamine sulfate

The antidote for heparin overdose

**c.** Drugs that *increase* effects of warfarin and other coumarins:

(1) Allopurinol, anabolic steroids (*e.g.*, methandrostenolone), cimetidine, tricyclic antidepressants (*e.g.*, amitriptyline), isoniazid (INH), methylphenidate

These drugs potentiate anticoagulant effects (and increase risks of bleeding) by inhibiting hepatic enzymes and slowing the rate of warfarin metabolism. Other mechanisms also may be involved.

(2) Antibiotics

Potentiate anticoagulant effects by decreasing production of vitamin K by intestinal bacteria. In addition, chloramphenicol and tetracyclines act by other mechanisms to increase risks of bleeding. Alternate antibiotics are preferred.

(3) Antidiabetic agents, oral

Displace anticoagulants from plasma protein binding sites

(4) Antilipemics (*e.g.*, clofibrate)

Displace oral anticoagulants from plasma protein binding sites; possibly other mechanisms

(5) Antineoplastics

Additive risks of bleeding because antineoplastic drugs depress bone marrow function and platelet counts

(6) Antiplatelet agents (*e.g.*, aspirin, dipyridamole)

Decrease platelet aggregation

(7) Aspirin, other salicylates and nonsteroidal anti-inflammatory agents (*e.g.*, indomethacin)

These drugs greatly increase risks of bleeding. They displace warfarin from plasma protein binding sites, decrease platelet aggregation, and are ulcerogenic. None of these drugs should be given concurrently with oral anticoagulants.

(8) Heparin

Additive anticoagulant effects

(9) Thyroid preparations (*e.g.*, Synthroid)

Increase metabolism of clotting factors

**d.** Drugs that may *increase* or *decrease* effects of oral anticoagulants:

(1) Alcohol

Alcohol may induce liver enzymes, which *decrease* effects by accelerating the rate of metabolism of the anticoagulant drug. However, with alcohol-induced liver disease (*i.e.*, cirrhosis), effects may be *increased* owing to impaired metabolism of the anticoagulant.

*(continued)*

| Nursing Actions | Rationale/Explanation |
|---|---|
| (2) Corticosteroids | These drugs may *decrease* effects by stimulating synthesis of clotting factors or other mechanisms. They may *increase* risks of bleeding by their ulcerogenic effects. |
| **e.** Drugs that *decrease* effects of warfarin and other coumarins: | |
| (1) Antacids and griseofulvin | May decrease GI absorption of oral anticoagulants |
| (2) Barbiturates and other sedative-hypnotics, carbamazepine, disulfiram, rifampin | These drugs activate liver metabolizing enzymes, which accelerate the rate of metabolism of oral anticoagulant drugs. |
| (3) Cholestyramine | Decreases absorption |
| (4) Diuretics | Increase synthesis and concentration of blood clotting factors |
| (5) Estrogens, including oral contraceptives | Increase synthesis of clotting factors and have thromboembolic effect |
| (6) Vitamin K | Restores prothrombin and other vitamin K–dependent clotting factors in the blood. Antidote for overdose of oral anticoagulants. |
| **5. Teach clients receiving long-term therapy**<br>**a.** Take the drugs as directed. | This is crucial to avoid underdosage (risks of thromboemboli) and overdosage (risks of bleeding). |
| **b.** Do not change from one brand to another. | Different brands may not be equivalent, and either increased or decreased anticoagulant effects may occur. |
| **c.** Do not take any other drugs without the physician's knowledge and consent, especially over-the-counter cold remedies and analgesics. | Oral anticoagulant drugs interact with many other drugs with subsequent increased or decreased anticoagulant effects, either of which may be harmful to the client. Many nonprescription analgesics and cold remedies contain aspirin. Aspirin and any aspirin-containing products are contraindicated with oral anticoagulants because the risks of bleeding are greatly increased. |
| **d.** Do not stop taking any medication without the physician's knowledge and consent. | Dosage of warfarin is carefully regulated or balanced. Stopping a drug may upset the balance and either increase risks of bleeding or increase risks of blood clot formation. |
| **e.** Inform any physician, surgeon, or dentist about anticoagulant drug therapy before any treatment measures are begun. | This is mainly a safety measure to prevent bleeding episodes. |
| **f.** Keep all appointments for laboratory tests. | These tests are required regularly throughout oral anticoagulant therapy for safety (prevention of bleeding) and titration of dosage. |
| **g.** Use safety precautions:<br>(1) Avoid walking barefoot.<br>(2) Avoid contact sports.<br>(3) Use an electric razor.<br>(4) Avoid injections when possible. | To avoid injury and subsequent bleeding |
| **h.** Carry an identification card, necklace, or bracelet (*e.g.*, MedicAlert) stating the name of the drug and the physician's name and telephone number. | |
| **i.** Inspect skin, mucous membranes, urine, and feces for signs of bleeding. Report to the physician if bleeding occurs. | Pinprick hemorrhages, bruising, or frank bleeding may occur in the skin and mucous membranes. Urine may be bright red or smoky gray. Feces may be bright red or black (tarry). |

## Nursing Actions

## Rationale/Explanation

**j.** Apply direct pressure to superficial bleeding sites for 3 to 5 minutes or longer if necessary.

To prevent excessive blood loss

**k.** Do not eat large amounts of green leafy vegetables (*e.g.*, spinach), tomatoes, bananas, or fish.

These foods contain vitamin K, which may decrease anti-coagulant effects.

## Review and Application Exercises

1. What are the major factors in blood clotting?
2. What are the indications for use of heparin and warfarin?
3. How do heparin and warfarin differ in mechanism of action, onset and duration of action, and method of administration?
4. List interventions to protect clients from anti-coagulant-induced bleeding.
5. Why are clients with low levels of serum albumin at high risk of bleeding with warfarin unless dosage is reduced?
6. When is it appropriate to use protamine sulfate as an antidote for heparin?
7. When is it appropriate to use vitamin K as an antidote for warfarin?
8. How do protamine sulfate and vitamin K act to control bleeding?
9. What is the role of platelets in blood coagulation?
10. List commonly used drugs that inhibit platelet aggregation and function.
11. For what conditions are antiplatelet drugs indicated?
12. How do thrombolytic drugs act to dissolve blood clots?
13. When is it appropriate to use a thrombolytic drug?
14. How do aminocaproic acid and tranexamic acid stop bleeding induced by thrombolytics?

## Selected References

Brater, D. C. (1992). Clinical pharmacology of cardiovascular drugs. In W. N. Kelley (Ed.), *Textbook of internal medicine* (2nd ed.) (pp. 315–335). Philadelphia: J.B. Lippincott.

Bullock, B. L. (1992). Normal and altered coagulation. In B. L. Bullock & P. P. Rosendahl (Eds.), *Pathophysiology: Adaptations and alterations in function* (3rd ed.) (pp. 408–423). Philadelphia: J.B. Lippincott.

Bussey, H. I., Force, R. W., Bianco, T. M., & Leonard, A. D. (1992). Reliance on prothrombin time ratios causes significant errors in anticoagulation therapy. *Archives of Internal Medicine, 152,* 278–282.

Byers, J. F. (1993). The use of aspirin in cardiovascular disease. *Journal of Cardiovascular Nursing, 8*(1), 1–18.

(1993). *Drug facts and comparisons*. St. Louis: Facts and Comparisons.

Goodnight, S. H., Coull, B. M., McAnulty, J. H., & Taylor L. M. (1993). Antiplatelet therapy—Part 1. *Western Journal of Medicine, 158,* 385–392.

Gueldner, S. H. (1992). Common problems of the hematologic system. In L. O. Burrell (Ed.), *Adult nursing in hospital and community settings* (pp. 548–573). Norwalk, CT: Appleton & Lange.

Guyton, A. C. (1991). *Textbook of medical physiology* (8th ed.). Philadelphia: W.B. Saunders.

Hoak, J. C. (1992). Disorders associated with thrombosis. In W. N. Kelley (Ed.), *Textbook of internal medicine* (2nd ed.) (pp. 1285–1293). Philadelphia: J.B. Lippincott.

Kayser, S. R. (1992). Thrombosis. In M. A. Koda-Kimble & L. Y. Young (Eds.), *Applied therapeutics: The clinical use of drugs* (5th ed.) (pp. 13-1–13-23). Vancouver, WA: Applied Therapeutics.

Nichols, W. L., & Bowie, E. J. W. (1993). Standardization of the prothrombin time for monitoring orally administered anticoagulant therapy with use of the international normalized ratio system. *Mayo Clinic Proceedings, 68,* 897–898.

Pless, B. S. (1992). Nursing management of adults with disorders of the venous and lymphatic systems. In L. O. Burrell (Ed.), *Adult nursing in hospital and community settings* (pp. 520–534). Norwalk, CT: Appleton & Lange.

Porth, C. M. (1990). *Pathophysiology: Concepts of altered health states* (3rd ed.) (pp. 267–287). Philadelphia: J.B. Lippincott.

Prandoni, P., Lensing, A. W. A., Buller, H. R., Carta, M., Cogo, A., Vigo, M., Casara, D., Ruol, A., & Ten Cate, J. W. (1992). Comparison of subcutaneous low-molecular-weight heparin with intravenous standard heparin in proximal deep-vein thrombosis. *The Lancet, 339,* 441–445.

Shlafer, M. (1993). *The Nurse, pharmacology, and drug therapy: A prototype approach* (2nd ed.). Redwood City, CA, Addison-Wesley.

Stein, F., & Fuster, V. (1990). Role of platelet inhibitor agents in coronary artery disease. In E. J. Topol (Ed.), *Textbook of interventional cardiology* (pp. 3–27). Philadelphia: W.B. Saunders.

### CHAPTER 61

# Antilipemics and Peripheral Vasodilators

## Antilipemic drugs and peripheral vasodilators

**Antilipemic drugs** are used in the treatment of clients with elevated blood lipids, a major risk factor for atherosclerosis. **Peripheral vasodilator drugs** are used in the treatment of clients with arterial insufficiency caused by atherosclerosis or vasospasm.

## Atherosclerosis

Atherosclerosis is the major cause of angina pectoris, myocardial infarction, cerebrovascular accidents (CVAs or strokes), and peripheral vascular disease. Atherosclerosis is characterized by deposition of blood lipids on the lining of the arteries. These fatty plaques (atheromas) interfere with nutrition of the blood vessel lining and lead to necrosis, scarring, and calcification. The normally smooth endothelium becomes roughened and constricted, and the lumen size is reduced. These changes predispose to decreased blood flow, thrombus formation, and eventual occlusion of the vessel. When an artery is gradually occluded by atheromatous plaque, collateral circulation may develop sufficiently to provide oxygen and nutrients at rest. However, tissue ischemia and infarction are likely to develop with strenuous exer-

cise or other conditions that increase tissue demands for oxygen and nutrients.

### DRUGS USED TO TREAT ATHEROSCLEROSIS

Drugs to prevent or treat atherosclerotic cardiovascular disease are needed. Antilipemic drugs are being used increasingly because several effective agents are available and because research studies indicate that lowering blood lipids decreases morbidity and mortality. Peripheral vasodilators are occasionally used despite their questionable efficacy. Although they increase blood flow in normal vessels, they have not been proved to increase flow in atherosclerotic vessels or to decrease ischemia in body tissues. By diverting blood flow to the skin and nonischemic tissues, they may actually decrease flow to ischemic tissues. Also, they may cause hypotension with a resultant decrease in cerebral blood flow. Another type of drug, a hemorrheologic agent, improves blood flow by decreasing blood viscosity and making erythrocytes more flexible. The drug reduces symptoms of intermittent claudication.

### DRUGS USED TO TREAT HYPERLIPIDEMIA

Antilipemic drugs are used to treat hyperlipidemia or hyperlipoproteinemia. Blood lipids are cholesterol, phospholipids, and triglycerides. Lipids are transported in plasma by specific proteins called lipoproteins. Each lipoprotein contains cholesterol, phospholipid, and triglyceride in different and characteristic amounts, which can be measured in the laboratory. The plasma lipoproteins are chylomicrons, very low-density lipoproteins (VLDL), low-density lipoproteins (LDL), and high-density lipoproteins (HDL). When blood lipid levels are elevated, there is an accompanying increase in blood levels of lipoproteins (hyperlipoproteinemia). Hyperlipoproteinemia may be primary (*i.e.*, genetic or familial) or secondary to dietary habits or other diseases (*e.g.*, diabetes mellitus, alcoholism, hypothyroidism, obstructive liver disease). The five major types of hyperlipoproteinemia are as follows:

1. *Type I* is characterized by elevated or normal serum cholesterol, elevated triglycerides, and chylomicronemia. This rare condition may occur in infancy and childhood.
2. *Type IIa* (familial hypercholesterolemia) is characterized by a high level of LDL, a normal level of VLDL, and a normal or slightly increased level of triglycerides. It occurs in children and is a definite risk factor for development of atherosclerosis and coronary artery disease. *Type IIb* (combined familial hyperlipoproteinemia) is characterized by increased levels of LDL, VLDL, cholesterol, and triglycerides and lipid deposits (xanthomas) in the feet, knees, and elbows. It occurs in adults.
3. *Type III* is characterized by elevations of cholesterol and triglycerides plus abnormal levels of LDL and VLDL. This type usually occurs in middle-aged adults (40–60 years) and is associated with accelerated coronary and peripheral vascular disease.
4. *Type IV* is characterized by normal or elevated cholesterol levels, elevated triglycerides, and increased levels of VLDL. This type usually occurs in adults and may be the most common form of hyperlipoproteinemia. Type IV is often secondary to obesity, excessive intake of alcohol, or other diseases. Ischemic heart disease may occur at 40 to 50 years of age.
5. *Type V* is characterized by elevated cholesterol and triglyceride levels with an increased level of VLDL and chylomicronemia. This uncommon type usually occurs in adults. Type V is not associated with ischemic heart disease. Instead, it is associated with fat and carbohydrate intolerance, abdominal pain, and pancreatitis, which are relieved by lowering triglyceride levels.

Antilipemic drugs decrease hyperlipoproteinemias by altering the production, metabolism, or removal of lipoproteins. No drugs currently available are effective in lowering all types of hyperlipoproteinemia. Antilipemic drugs should be used only after dietary therapy for 3 to 6 months has failed to decrease hyperlipoproteinemia to

an acceptable level. Further, the drugs should be given only to clients with signs and symptoms of coronary heart disease, a strong family history of coronary heart disease or hyperlipoproteinemia, or other risk factors for atherosclerotic vascular disease (*e.g.*, hypertension, diabetes mellitus, cigarette smoking). The drugs should generally be discontinued after 2 to 3 months of therapy if blood lipids and lipoproteins are not lowered by at least 10% beyond that occurring with diet alone.

## Individual drugs

Antilipemic drugs are listed in Table 61-1; peripheral vasodilators are listed in Table 61-2.

### HEMORRHEOLOGIC AGENT

**Pentoxifylline** (Trental), a methylxanthine derivative, is a hemorrheologic agent that improves blood flow by decreasing blood viscosity rather than by vasodilation. Specific effects include increased flexibility of red blood cells with subsequent decreases in red blood cell aggregation and local hyperviscosity, decreased platelet aggregation, and decreased fibrinogen concentration.

Pentoxifylline is approved for use in intermittent claudication caused by chronic occlusive arterial insufficiency. It is contraindicated in clients who cannot take methylxanthines, such as theophylline or caffeine. It is generally well tolerated, and adverse reactions (dyspepsia, nausea, vomiting, dizziness, and headache) occur in only 1% to 3% of recipients.

#### Route and dosage range

*Adults:* PO 400 mg three times per day with meals, reduced to 400 mg twice daily if gastrointestinal and central nervous system side effects occur

## *Nursing Process*

### Assessment

Assess the client's status in relation to atherosclerotic vascular disease.
- Identify risk factors:
  - Hypertension
  - Diabetes mellitus
  - High intake of dietary fat and refined sugars
  - Obesity
  - Lack of exercise
  - Cigarette smoking
  - Family history of atherosclerotic disorders
  - Hyperlipidemia
- Signs and symptoms depend on the specific problem:
  - *Hyperlipidemia* is manifested by elevated serum choles-

**TABLE 61-1.   ANTILIPEMIC AGENTS**

| Generic/Trade Name | Clinical Indications (Type of Hyper- lipoproteinemia) | Mechanism of Action | Route and Dosage Ranges | |
|---|---|---|---|---|
| | | | **Adults** | **Children** |
| **Cholestyramine** (Questran) | Type IIa | Binds bile acids in the intestines, resulting in increased oxidation of cholesterol to bile acids and decreased LDL cholesterol in the blood | PO 12–24 g daily, in two to four divided doses, before or during meals and at bedtime | |
| **Clofibrate** (Atromid-S) | Types III, IV, V | Decreases synthesis of triglycerides and re- duces VLDL | PO 2 g daily, in two to four divided doses | |
| **Colestipol** (Colestid) | Type IIa | Same as cholestyr- amine | PO 15–30 g daily, in two to four divided doses, before or during meals and at bedtime | |
| **Dextrothyroxine** (Choloxin) | Type II | Decreases cholesterol by increasing the rate of cholesterol catabo- lism | PO 1 mg daily for 1 mo, increased at monthly intervals until thera- peutic effects of maximal daily doses of 8 mg are achieved | PO 0.05 mg/kg per day initially; maximal daily dose, 4 mg |
| **Gemfibrozil** (Lopid) | Types IV, V | Decreases hepatic pro- duction of triglycer- ides, decreases VLDL, increases HDL | PO 900–1500 mg daily, usually 1200 mg in two divided doses, 30 min before morning and evening meals | |
| **Lovastatin** (Mevacor) | Types IIa and IIb | Decreases hepatic syn- thesis of cholesterol by blocking a neces- sary enzyme, HMG- CoA* reductase | PO 20 mg daily with a meal, ini- tially, increased up to 80 mg daily if necessary. Dosage increments should be at least 4 wk apart. | |
| **Nicotinic acid (niacin)** | Types II, III, IV, V | Decreases synthesis and increases catabo- lism to lower choles- terol, triglycerides, LDL, and VLDL | PO 2–6 g daily, in three or four di- vided doses, with or just after meals | PO 55–87 mg/kg per day, in three or four divided doses, with or just after meals |
| **Pravastatin** (Pravachol) | Types IIa and IIb | Same as lovastatin | PO 10–40 mg once daily at bed- time Elderly, PO 10 mg once daily at bedtime | |
| **Probucol** (Lorelco) | Type II | Decreases cholesterol and LDL | PO 500 mg twice daily, with morn- ing and evening meals | |
| **Simvastatin** (Zocor) | Types IIa and IIb | Same as lovastatin | PO 5–40 mg once daily in the evening Elderly, PO 5–20 mg once daily in the evening | |

* HMG-CoA = hydroxymethylglutarylcoenzyme A. Lovastatin, pravastatin, and simvastatin are called HMG-CoA reductase inhibitors.

terol (above 250 mg/100 ml) or triglycerides (above 150 mg/100 ml) or both.

- *Coronary artery atherosclerosis* is manifested by myocar- dial ischemia (angina pectoris, myocardial infarction).
- *Cerebrovascular insufficiency* may be manifested by syn- cope, memory loss, transient ischemic attacks (TIAs) or CVAs. Impairment of blood flow to the brain is caused primarily by atherosclerosis in the carotid, vertebral, or cerebral arteries.
- *Peripheral arterial insufficiency* is manifested primarily by impaired blood flow in the legs (weak or absent pulses; cool, pale extremities; intermittent claudication; leg pain at rest; and development of gangrene, usually in the toes because they are most distal to blood supply). This condi- tion results from atherosclerosis in the distal abdominal

aorta, the iliac arteries, and the femoral and smaller arte- ries in the legs.

**Nursing diagnoses**

- Altered Tissue Perfusion related to atherosclerotic plaque in coronary, cerebral, or peripheral arteries
- Altered Nutrition: More than Body Requirements of fats and calories
- Anxiety related to risks of atherosclerotic cardiovascular disease
- Body Image Disturbance related to the need for life-style changes
- Pain related to gastrointestinal distress with drug therapy
- Noncompliance related to dietary restrictions and adverse drug reactions

**TABLE 61-2. PERIPHERAL VASODILATORS**

| Generic/ Trade Name | Routes and Dosage Ranges (Adults) |
|---|---|
| Papaverine hydrochloride (Pavabid, others) | PO 100–300 mg three to five times daily. Timed-release capsules, PO 150 mg q12h |
| Cyclandelate (Cyclospasmol) | PO 1.2–1.6 g daily, in four divided doses, before meals and at bedtime. Decreased to 400–800 mg daily, in two to four divided doses, for maintenance |
| Isoxsuprine hydrochloride (Vasodilan) | PO 10–20 mg, three or four times daily IM 5–10 mg, two or three times daily |

- Knowledge Deficit related to drug and diet therapy of hyperlipidemia

**Planning/Goals**

*The client will:*
- Take lipid-lowering drugs as prescribed
- Decrease dietary intake of saturated fats and cholesterol
- Lose weight if obese and maintain the lower weight
- Have periodic measurements of blood lipids
- Avoid preventable adverse drug effects
- Receive positive reinforcement for efforts to lower blood lipid levels
- Feel less anxious and more in control as risks of atherosclerotic cardiovascular disease are decreased

**Interventions**

Use measures to prevent, delay, or minimize atherosclerosis.
- Help clients to control risk factors. Ideally, primary prevention begins in childhood with healthful eating habits (*i.e.*, avoiding excessive fats, meat, and dairy products; obtaining adequate amounts of all nutrients, including dietary fiber; avoiding obesity), exercise, and avoiding cigarette smoking.

    However, changing habits to a more healthful life-style is probably helpful at any time, before or after disease manifestations appear. Weight loss often reduces blood lipids and lipoproteins to a normal range. Changing habits is difficult for most people, even those with severe symptoms.
- Use measures to increase blood flow to tissues:
  - Exercise is helpful in developing collateral circulation in the heart and legs. Collateral circulation involves use of secondary vessels in response to tissue ischemia related to obstruction of the principal vessels. Clients with angina pectoris or previous myocardial infarction require a carefully planned and supervised program of progressive exercise. Those with peripheral arterial insufficiency usually can increase exercise tolerance by walking regularly. Distances should be determined by occurrence of pain and must be individualized.
  - Posture and position may be altered to increase blood flow to the legs in peripheral arterial insufficiency. Elevating the head of the bed and having the legs horizontal or dependent may help. Elevating the feet is usually contraindicated unless edema is present or likely to develop.

- At present, the major treatment of occlusive vascular disease is surgical removal of atherosclerotic plaque or revascularization procedures. Thus, severe angina pectoris may be relieved by a coronary artery bypass procedure that detours around occluded vessels. This procedure also may be done after a myocardial infarction. The goal is to prevent infarction or reinfarction. TIAs may be relieved by carotid endarterectomy; the goal is to prevent a CVA. Peripheral arterial insufficiency may be relieved by aortofemoral, femoral-popliteal, or other bypass grafts that detour around occluded vessels. Although these procedures increase blood flow to ischemic tissues, they do not halt progression of atherosclerosis.

    The nursing role in relation to these procedures is to provide excellent preoperative and postoperative nursing care to promote healing, prevent infection, maintain patency of grafts, and help the client to achieve optimum function.
- The most effective treatment in hyperlipoproteinemia is diet therapy. Specific diets have been developed for each type. Any antilipemic drug therapy must be accompanied by an appropriate diet.

*Teach clients:*
- The most effective measures for preventing hyperlipidemia and atherosclerosis are those related to a healthful life-style (diet low in cholesterol and saturated fats, weight control, exercise, not smoking cigarettes).
- Drug therapy is relatively ineffective without diet therapy. Overeating or gaining weight may decrease or cancel the lipid-lowering effects of the drugs.
- Dietary restrictions and other life-style changes contribute to improved health and decreased risks of heart attack and stroke.

**Evaluation**

- Observe for decreased blood levels of cholesterol and triglycerides.
- Observe and interview regarding compliance with instructions for drug, diet, and other therapeutic measures.
- Observe and interview regarding adverse drug effects.
- Validate the client's ability to identify foods high and low in cholesterol and saturated fats.

# Principles of therapy

## INITIAL TREATMENT

Although several antilipemic drugs are available, none is effective in all types of hyperlipidemia, and all may cause adverse effects. Thus, diet and exercise are the first-line treatment, and drug therapy is used if they are ineffective. In addition, treatment of conditions known to increase blood lipid levels (*e.g.*, diabetes, hypothyroidism, liver disease, corticosteroid drug therapy) may obviate the need for drug therapy.

## DRUG SELECTION

To lower cholesterol, cholestyramine, colestipol, lovastatin, pravastatin, or simvastatin is preferred. Probucol and dextrothyroxine have been used but are not recommended because of adverse effects. To lower both cholesterol and triglycerides, clofibrate, gemfibrozil, lovastatin, pravastatin, simvastatin, and niacin are used. In addition to single-drug therapy, various combinations are being investigated. For example, a bile acid sequestrant (cholestyramine or colestipol) with niacin or lovastatin may be more effective than any one of the drugs used alone.

## DRUG INTERACTIONS

Cholestyramine decreases absorption of many oral medications (*e.g.,* corticosteroids, digitalis glycosides, folic acid, iron preparations, phenobarbital, tetracyclines, thiazide diuretics, thyroid preparations, fat-soluble vitamins, and warfarin). When one of these drugs is ordered concomitantly with cholestyramine, the drug should be given at least 1 hour before or 4 hours after cholestyramine administration. In addition, dosage of the interactive drug may need to be changed when cholestyramine is added or withdrawn.

## USE IN CHILDREN

Hyperlipidemia occurs in children and may lead to atherosclerotic cardiovascular disease, including myocardial infarction, in early adulthood. Thus, early identification and treatment are needed. As with adults, initial treatment consists of diet therapy and treatment of any secondary causes. With primary familial hypercholesterolemia (type IIa), however, these measures are not likely to be effective without drug therapy. Although few studies have been done in children, the bile acid sequestrants are considered the drugs of choice, and niacin also may be used.

The manufacturers of cholestyramine and colestipol do not list pediatric dosages. Jacobson and Lillienfeld (1988) suggest 8 to 20 g daily, with the amount determined by cholesterol level rather than weight. They also recommend starting at low doses and increasing to tolerance. With niacin, they list 100 to 1000 mg to be started at low doses and given with aspirin to decrease flushing.

Although the manufacturer lists pediatric doses for dextrothyroxine, it is not recommended for use in children. The drug has been associated with increased cardiovascular mortality in adults and is also not recommended for them.

## USE IN OLDER ADULTS

Basic principles of using antilipemic drugs in younger adults apply. In addition, older adults often have diabetes, impaired liver function, or other conditions that raise blood lipid levels. They are also likely to have cardiovascular and other disorders that increase the adverse effects of antilipemic drugs. Thus, diet, exercise, weight control, and treatment of secondary causes are especially important. Use of antilipemic drugs should be cautious, with close monitoring for therapeutic and adverse effects.

# NURSING ACTIONS: ANTILIPEMICS AND VASODILATORS

| *Nursing Actions* | *Rationale/Explanation* |
|---|---|
| **1. Administer accurately**<br>**a.** Give cholestyramine before meals; mix with 4 to 6 ounces of water, milk, fruit juice, or other noncarbonated beverage, let stand 1 to 2 minutes, then stir. | The drug is available in a dry form, which should not be swallowed dry because of irritation to mucous membranes and possible obstruction of the esophagus. |
| **b.** Give lovastatin, nicotinic acid, and probucol preparations with meals. | To decrease gastric irritation. This is probably not necessary with timed-release forms. |
| **2. Observe for therapeutic effects**<br>**a.** With antilipemic agents, observe for decreased or normal levels of serum cholesterol (normal range is approximately 150–250 mg/100 ml), serum triglycerides (normal range is approximately 50–150 mg/100 ml), low-density lipoproteins (LDL) and very low-density lipoproteins (VLDL). | With *nicotinic acid*, cholesterol and triglycerides are usually lowered within 1 week and LDL within 3 to 5 weeks.<br>With *clofibrate*, triglycerides and VLDL are usually lowered within 2 to 5 days. Lipid-lowering effects can be canceled by weight gain. |

## Nursing Actions

## Rationale/Explanation

With *cholestyramine*, cholesterol and LDL are usually lowered within 4 to 7 days. When the drug is discontinued, blood lipid levels return to pretreatment values in approximately 3 to 4 weeks.

With *probucol*, maximal decrease in cholesterol and LDL occurs after 1 to 3 months of treatment.

**b.** With vasodilators, observe for increased warmth and improved color of extremities.

**c.** With pentoxifylline, observe for decreased leg pain with exercise.

Improvement in function and symptoms may occur in 2 to 4 weeks.

**3. Observe for adverse effects**

**a.** Gastrointestinal (GI) problems—nausea, vomiting, flatulence, constipation or diarrhea, abdominal discomfort

GI symptoms are the most common adverse effects of antilipemic and vasodilator drugs. Constipation is especially common with cholestyramine and colestipol.

**b.** With clofibrate and gemfibrozil, observe for an influenza-like syndrome (weakness, severe muscle cramps and tenderness); indications of cholelithiasis and cholecystitis; increased angina, thromboembolic disorders, and cardiac arrhythmias.

The mechanism of the influenza-like syndrome is unknown. Increased incidence of gallbladder disease is related to increased lithogenicity of bile. Development or aggravation of cardiovascular symptoms occurs in clients with coronary artery disease. Although all these adverse effects have not been reported with gemfibrozil, they may occur because gemfibrozil is pharmacologically similar to clofibrate.

**c.** With lovastatin, pravastatin, and simvastatin observe for headache, GI upset (see 3a), skin rash, and pruritus.

Adverse effects are usually mild and of short duration. A less common but potentially more serious effect is liver dysfunction. This is usually manifested by increased levels of serum transaminases rather than jaundice or other signs and symptoms. Liver function tests are recommended every 4 to 6 weeks during the first 15 months of drug use and periodically thereafter.

**d.** With vasodilator drugs, tachycardia, hypotension, dizziness, and flushing of the face and neck may occur.

These effects result from vasodilation of nonatherosclerotic blood vessels, including the skin capillaries of the face and neck.

**e.** With nicotinic acid, flushing of the face and neck, pruritus, and skin rash may occur, as well as tachycardia, hypotension, and dizziness.

These symptoms may be prominent when nicotinic acid is used to lower blood lipids because relatively high doses are required. Aspirin 325 mg, given 30 minutes before nicotinic acid, decreases the flushing reaction.

**f.** With pentoxifylline, observe for dyspepsia, nausea, vomiting, dizziness, and headache.

These are the more common adverse effects.

**4. Observe for drug interactions**

**a.** Drugs that *increase* effects of clofibrate:

(1) Acidifying agents (*e.g.*, ascorbic acid)

Decrease urinary excretion of clofibrate

(2) Dextrothyroxine (Choloxin), neomycin

Additive hypolipidemic effects. These drugs are sometimes used alone for treatment of hyperlipoproteinemia.

(3) Probenecid (Benemid)

Impairs renal and metabolic clearance of clofibrate

**b.** Drugs that *decrease* effects of clofibrate:

(1) Estrogens and oral contraceptives that contain estrogens

Estrogens increase blood lipids and thus antagonize effects of clofibrate.

(2) Rifampin

Induces hepatic metabolism of clofibrate

*(continued)*

## Nursing Actions

## Rationale/Explanation

| Nursing Actions | Rationale/Explanation |
|---|---|
| **c.** Drugs that *increase* effects of nicotinic acid and other vasodilating drugs | |
| Alcohol and antihypertensive vasodilating drugs (*e.g.*, hydralazine [Apresoline]) | Additive vasodilation with hypotension and dizziness |
| **5. Teach clients** | |
| **a.** Take cholestyramine and colestipol with ample amounts of fluids, and increase dietary intake of high-fiber foods. | To prevent constipation, a common adverse effect |
| **b.** When taking vasodilator drugs, assume an upright position slowly. | To prevent or decrease vertigo, syncope, and weakness |

## Review and Application Exercises

1. How would you describe hyperlipidemia to a client?
2. What is the goal of treatment for hyperlipidemia?
3. Differentiate lipid-lowering drugs according to their mechanisms of action.
4. Which groups of lipid-lowering drugs are most effective?
5. What are the limitations and adverse effects of peripheral vasodilating drugs?
6. How does pentoxifylline improve circulation?

## Selected References

(1993). *Drug facts and comparisons.* St. Louis: Facts and Comparisons.

Guyton, A. C. (1991). *Textbook of medical physiology* (8th ed.). Philadelphia: W.B. Saunders.

Jacobsen, M. S., & Lillienfeld, D. E. (1988). The pediatrician's role in atherosclerosis prevention. *Journal of Pediatrics, 112*, 836–841.

Kraemer, F. B. (1992). Treatment of endocrine disorders: Lipids. In K. L. Melmon, H. F. Morelli, B. B. Hoffman, & D. W. Nierenberg (Eds.), *Clinical pharmacology: Basic principles in therapeutics* (3rd ed.) (pp. 397–425). New York: McGraw-Hill.

Porth, C. M. (1990). *Pathophysiology: Concepts of altered health states* (3rd ed.) (pp. 267–287). Philadelphia: J.B. Lippincott.

Raasch, R. H. (1992). Hyperlipidemias. In M. A. Koda-Kimble & L. Y. Young (Eds.), *Applied therapeutics: The clinical use of drugs* (5th ed.) (pp. 73-1–73-15). Vancouver, WA: Applied Therapeutics.

Shlafer, M. (1993). *The nurse, pharmacology, and drug therapy: A prototype approach* (2nd ed.). Redwood City, CA: Addison-Wesley.

# Drugs Affecting the Digestive System

### CHAPTER 62

# Physiology of the Digestive System

## The digestive system

The digestive system consists of the alimentary canal (a tube extending from the oral cavity to the anus, about 25–30 ft [7.5–9 meters] long) and the accessory organs (salivary glands, gallbladder, liver, and pancreas). The main function of the system is to provide the body with fluids, nutrients, and electrolytes in a form that can be used at the cellular level. The system also disposes of waste products that result from the digestive process.

The alimentary canal has the same basic structure throughout. The layers of the wall are mucosa, connective tissue, and muscle. Peristalsis propels food through the tract and mixes the food bolus with digestive juices. Stimulation of the parasympathetic nervous system (by vagus nerves) increases motility and secretions. The tract has an abundant blood supply, which increases cell regeneration and healing. Blood flow increases during digestion and absorption. Blood flow decreases with strenuous exercise, sympathetic nervous system stimulation (*i.e.*, "fight or flight"), aging (secondary to decreased cardiac output and atherosclerosis), and conditions that shunt blood away from the digestive tract (*e.g.*, congestive heart failure, atherosclerosis).

## Organs of the digestive system

1. In the *oral cavity*, chewing mechanically breaks food into smaller particles, which can be swallowed more easily and provide a larger surface area for enzyme action. Food is also mixed with saliva, which lubricates the food bolus for swallowing and initiates the digestion of starch.

2. The *esophagus* is a musculofibrous tube about 10 inches (25 cm) long; its main function is to convey food from the pharynx to the stomach. It secretes a small amount of mucus and has some peristaltic movement.

3. The *stomach* is a dilated area that serves as a reservoir. It churns and mixes the food with digestive juices, secretes mucus and enzymes, starts protein breakdown, and secretes intrinsic factor, which is necessary for absorption of vitamin $B_{12}$ from the ileum. Although there is much diffusion of water and electrolytes through the gastric mucosa in both directions, there is very little absorption of these substances. Carbohydrates and amino acids are also poorly absorbed. Only a few highly lipid-soluble substances, such as alcohol and some drugs, are absorbed in moderate quantities from the stomach.

    The inlet of the stomach is the cardiac sphincter at the end of the esophagus, and the outlet is the pyloric sphincter at the beginning of the duodenum. The stomach normally holds about 1000 ml comfortably and empties in about 4 hours. Numerous factors influence the rate of gastric emptying, including the size of the pylorus, gastric motility, type of food, fluidity of chyme (the material produced by gastric digestion of food), and the state of the duodenum. Generally, factors that cause rapid emptying include carbohydrate foods, increased motility, fluid chyme, and an empty duodenum. The stomach empties more

Anne Collins Abrams: CLINICAL DRUG THERAPY, Fourth Edition. © 1995 J.B. Lippincott Company.

slowly with decreased gastric tone and motility, fatty foods, chyme of excessive acidity, and a duodenum that contains fats, proteins, or chyme of excessive acidity. When fats are present, the duodenal mucosa produces a hormone, enterogastrone, that inhibits gastric secretion and motility. This allows a longer time for the digestion of fats in the small intestine.

4. The *small intestine* consists of the duodenum, jejunum, and ileum and is about 20 feet (6 meters) long. The duodenum makes up the first 10 to 12 inches (25–27 cm) of the small intestine. The pancreatic and bile ducts empty into the duodenum at the papilla of Vater. The small intestine contains numerous glands that secrete digestive enzymes, hormones, and mucus. For the most part, digestion and absorption occur in the small intestine, including absorption of most orally administered drugs.

5. The *large intestine* consists of the cecum, colon, rectum, and anus. The ileum opens into the cecum. The colon secretes mucus and absorbs water.

6. The *pancreas* secretes enzymes, which are necessary for the digestion of carbohydrates, proteins, and fats. It also secretes insulin and glucagon, hormones that regulate glucose metabolism and blood sugar levels.

7. The *gallbladder* is a small pouch attached to the underside of the liver that stores and concentrates bile. It has a capacity of about 50 to 60 ml. The gallbladder releases bile when fats are present in the duodenum.

8. The *liver* is a vital organ that performs numerous functions. It receives about 1500 ml of blood per minute, or 25% to 30% of the total cardiac output. About three fourths of the blood flow is venous blood from the stomach, intestines, spleen, and pancreas (portal circulation); the remainder is arterial blood through the hepatic artery. The hepatic artery carries blood to the connective tissue of the liver and bile ducts, then empties into the hepatic sinuses. Arterial blood mixes with blood from the portal circulation. Venous blood from the liver flows into the inferior vena cava for return to the systemic circulation. The ample blood flow facilitates specific hepatic functions, which include the following:

    a. **Blood reservoir**. The liver can eject about 500 to 1000 ml of blood into the general circulation in response to stress, decreased blood volume, and sympathetic nervous system stimulation (*e.g.*, hemorrhagic or hypovolemic shock).

    b. **Blood filter and detoxifier**. Kupffer's cells in the liver phagocytize bacteria carried from the intestines by the portal vein. They also break down worn-out erythrocytes, saving iron for reuse in hemoglobin synthesis, and form bilirubin, a waste product excreted in bile. The liver metabolizes many body secretions and most drugs to prevent accumulation and harmful effects on body tissues.

    Most drugs are active as the parent compound

and are metabolized in the liver to an inactive metabolite that is then excreted by the kidneys. However, some drugs become active only after formation of a metabolite in the liver.

The liver detoxifies or alters substances by oxidation, hydrolysis, or conjugation. Conjugation involves combining a chemical substance with an endogenous substance to produce an inactive or harmless compound. Essentially all steroid hormones, including adrenal corticosteroids and sex hormones, are at least partially conjugated in the liver and secreted into the bile. When the liver is damaged, these hormones may accumulate in body fluids and cause symptoms of hormone excess.

    c. **Metabolism of carbohydrate, fat, and protein**. In carbohydrate metabolism, the liver functions to convert glucose to glycogen for storage and reconvert glycogen to glucose when needed to maintain an adequate blood sugar concentration. Excess glucose that cannot be converted to glycogen is converted to fat. The liver also changes fructose and galactose, which cannot be used by body cells, to glucose, which provides energy for cellular metabolism. Fats are synthesized and catabolized by the liver. Amino acids from protein breakdown may be used to form glycogen, plasma proteins, and enzymes.

    d. **Storage of nutrients**. In addition to glycogen, the liver also stores fat-soluble vitamins (*i.e.*, vitamins A, D, E, K), vitamin $B_{12}$, iron, phospholipids, cholesterol, and small amounts of protein and fat.

    e. **Synthesis** of bile; serum albumin and globulin; prothrombin; fibrinogen; blood coagulation factors V, VII, VIII, IX, XI, and XII; and urea. Formation of urea removes ammonia from body fluids. Large amounts of ammonia are formed by intestinal bacteria and absorbed into the blood. If the ammonia is not converted to urea by the liver, plasma ammonia concentrations rise to toxic levels and cause hepatic coma and death.

    f. **Production of body heat** by continuous cellular metabolism. The liver is the body organ with the highest rate of chemical activity during basal conditions, and it produces about 20% of total body heat.

## Secretions of the digestive system

1. *Mucus* is secreted by mucous glands in every part of the gastrointestinal (GI) tract. The functions of mucus are to protect the lining of the tract from digestive juices, lubricate the food bolus for easier passage, promote adherence of the fecal mass, and neutralize acids and bases.

2. *Saliva* consists of mucus and salivary amylase. It is produced by the salivary glands and totals about 1000 ml daily. Saliva has a slightly acidic to neutral pH (6–7); it lubricates the food bolus and starts starch digestion.
3. *Gastric juice* consists of mucus, digestive enzymes, hydrochloric acid, and electrolytes. The gastric glands secrete about 2000 ml of gastric juice daily. The pH is highly acidic (1–3). Secretion is stimulated by the parasympathetic nervous system (by the vagus nerve), the hormone gastrin, the presence of food in the mouth, and seeing, smelling, or thinking about food.

    The major digestive enzyme in gastric juice is pepsin, a proteolytic enzyme that functions best at a pH of 2 to 3. Hydrochloric acid provides the acid medium to promote pepsin activity. The major function of gastric juice is to begin digestion of proteins. There is also a weak action on fats by gastric lipase and on carbohydrates by gastric amylase. A large amount of mucus is secreted in the stomach to protect the stomach wall from the proteolytic action of pepsin. When mucus is not secreted, gastric ulceration occurs within hours.
4. *Pancreatic juices* are alkaline (pH of 8 or above) secretions that contain amylase for carbohydrate digestion, lipase for fat digestion, and trypsin and chymotrypsin for protein digestion. They also contain large amounts of sodium bicarbonate, a base (alkali) that neutralizes the acid chyme from the stomach by reacting with hydrochloric acid. This protects the mucosa of the small intestine from the digestive properties of gastric juice. The daily amount of pancreatic secretion is about 1200 ml. The hormone cholecystokinin (also called pancreozymin) stimulates secretion of pancreatic juices.
5. *Bile* is an alkaline (pH of about 8) secretion that is formed continuously in the liver, carried to the gallbladder by the bile ducts, and stored there. The hormone cholecystokinin causes the gallbladder to contract and release bile into the small intestine when fats are present in intestinal contents. The liver secretes about 600 ml of bile daily. This amount is concentrated to the 50- to 60-ml capacity of the gallbladder. Bile contains bile salts, cholesterol, bilirubin, fatty acids, and electrolytes. Bile salts are required for digestion and absorption of fats, including fat-soluble vitamins. Most of the bile salts are reabsorbed and reused by the liver (enterohepatic circulation); some are excreted in feces.

# Effects of drugs on the digestive system

The digestive system and drug therapy have a reciprocal relationship. Many common symptoms (*i.e.*, nausea, vomiting, constipation, diarrhea, abdominal pain) relate to GI dysfunction. These symptoms may result from a disorder in the digestive system, disorders in other body systems, or drug therapy. Many GI symptoms and disorders alter the ingestion, dissolution, absorption, and metabolism of drugs. Drugs may be administered to *relieve* these symptoms and disorders, but drugs administered for conditions unrelated to the digestive system may *cause* such symptoms and disorders. GI conditions may alter responses to drug therapy.

Drugs used in digestive disorders primarily alter GI secretion, absorption, or motility. They may act systemically or locally within the GI tract. The drug groups included in this section are drugs used for peptic ulcer disease, laxatives, antidiarrheals, and antiemetics. Other drug groups used in GI disorders include cholinergics (see Chap. 20), anticholinergics (Chap. 21), corticosteroids (Chap. 24), and anti-infective drugs (Section VI).

## Review and Application Exercises

1. What is the main function of the GI system?
2. What is the role of the parasympathetic nervous system in gastrointestinal function?
3. List factors affecting GI motility and secretions.
4. Describe important GI secretions and their functions.
5. What factors stimulate or inhibit GI secretions?

## Selected References

Collins, A., & Bullock, B. L. (1992). Normal function of the gastrointestinal system. In B. L. Bullock & P. P. Rosendahl (Eds.), *Pathophysiology: Adaptations and alterations in function* (3rd ed.) (pp. 770–786). Philadelphia: J.B. Lippincott.

Guyton, A. C. (1991). *Textbook of medical physiology* (8th ed.). Philadelphia: W.B. Saunders.

McDermott, M. M. (1992). Overview of anatomy, physiology, and pathophysiology of the gastrointestinal system. In L. O. Burrell (Ed.), *Adult nursing in hospital and community settings* (pp. 1310–1319). Norwalk, CT: Appleton & Lange.

### CHAPTER 63

# Drugs Used in Peptic Ulcer Disease

## Peptic ulcer disease

Peptic ulcer disease is a common condition characterized by ulcer formation in an area of the gastrointestinal (GI) tract that is exposed to gastric acid. Therefore, peptic ulcers may develop in the esophagus, stomach, or duodenum. Acute ulcers occur more often in the stomach and may be associated with stress (*e.g.*, surgery, shock, head injury, severe burn injuries, major medical illness). These are often called stress ulcers. Acute ulcers also may be caused by certain drugs (*e.g.*, aspirin and other non-steroidal anti-inflammatory drugs [NSAIDs], corticosteroids, antineoplastics, and potassium tablets). Chronic ulcers are more likely to occur in the duodenum.

### CAUSES OF PEPTIC ULCER DISEASE

Peptic ulcer disease is attributed to an imbalance between cell-destructive and cell-protective effects. Cell-destructive effects include those of gastric acid (hydrochloric acid) and pepsin. Gastric acid, a strong acid that can digest the stomach wall, is secreted by the parietal cells in the mucosa of the stomach antrum, near the pylorus. The parietal cells contain receptors for acetylcholine, gastrin, and histamine, substances that stimulate gastric acid production. Acetylcholine is released by vagus nerve endings in response to stimuli, such as thinking about or ingesting food. Gastrin is a hormone released by cells in the stomach and duodenum in response to food ingestion and stretching of the stomach wall. It is secreted into the bloodstream and eventually circulated to the parietal cells. Histamine is released from cells in the gastric mucosa and diffuses into nearby parietal cells.

Once produced, gastric acid is released by activation of an enzyme system (hydrogen, potassium adenosine-triphosphatase, or $H^+,K^+$-ATPase) at the surface of parietal cells. This enzyme system acts as a gastric acid (proton) pump to move gastric acid from parietal cells in the mucosal lining of the stomach into the stomach lumen.

Pepsin is a proteolytic enzyme that also can digest the stomach wall. Pepsin is derived from a precursor called pepsinogen, which is secreted by chief cells in the gastric mucosa. Pepsinogen is converted to pepsin only in a highly acidic environment (*i.e.*, when the pH of gastric juices is about 3 or less).

Autodigestion of stomach and duodenal tissues and ulcer formation are normally prevented by the cell-protective effects of mucus, dilution of gastric acid by food and secretions, prevention of diffusion of hydrochloric acid from the stomach lumen back into the gastric mucosal lining, the presence of certain prostaglandins, alkalinization of gastric secretions by pancreatic juices and bile, and perhaps other mechanisms.

A possible etiologic factor that is receiving increased attention is *Helicobacter pylori*, a bacterium found in the gastric mucosa of most patients with gastric or duodenal ulcers. It is unknown whether *H. pylori* causes initial ulceration, possibly by impairing the usual defense mechanisms of gastric mucosa, or whether it infects damaged mucosa without being a significant factor in ulcer formation. However, eradication of the organism significantly decreases the rate of ulcer recurrence.

Anne Collins Abrams: CLINICAL DRUG THERAPY, Fourth Edition.
© 1995 J.B. Lippincott Company.

# Types of antiulcer drugs

Drugs used in the prevention and treatment of peptic ulcer disease mainly decrease cell-destructive effects, increase cell-protective effects, or both. Thus, a variety of agents may be useful, alone or in combination. *H. pylori* infections are treated with antibiotics and bismuth preparations. Other antiulcer agents are described below.

## GASTRIC ACID INHIBITORS (ANTISECRETORY DRUGS)

### Gastric acid pump inhibitors

These drugs bind with $H^+,K^+$-ATPase to prevent the "pumping" or release of gastric acid into the stomach lumen and therefore block the final step of acid production. Indications for use include treatment of peptic ulcer disease, erosive gastritis, gastroesophageal reflux disease, and Zollinger-Ellison syndrome (a rare condition characterized by excessive secretion of gastric acid).

Omeprazole, the only approved drug in this classification, is generally well tolerated. Nausea, diarrhea, and headache are the most frequently reported adverse effects. However, long-term consequences of profound gastric acid suppression are unknown. Gastric cancer developed in animals given omeprazole for 2 years.

### Histamine-2 receptor blocking agents

Histamine is a substance found in almost every body tissue and released in response to certain stimuli (*e.g.*, allergic reactions, tissue injury). Once released, histamine causes the following reactions: contraction of smooth muscle in the bronchi, GI tract, and uterus; dilation and increased permeability of capillaries; dilation of cerebral blood vessels; and stimulation of sensory nerve endings to produce pain and itching. Another effect of histamine, and the most important effect in relation to peptic ulcer disease, is strong stimulation of gastric acid secretion. Vagal stimulation causes release of histamine from cells in the gastric mucosa. The histamine then acts on receptors located on the parietal cells to increase production of hydrochloric acid. These receptors are called the $H_2$ receptors.

Traditional antihistamines or $H_1$ receptor blocking agents prevent or reduce other effects of histamine but do not block histamine effects on gastric acid production. The $H_2$ receptor blocking drugs were developed to inhibit gastric acid secretion.

Clinical indications for use include prevention and treatment of peptic ulcer disease, Zollinger-Ellison syndrome, acute stress ulcers, and esophagitis resulting from gastroesophageal reflux of gastric acid. There are no known contraindications, but the drugs should be used with caution in children, pregnant women, older adults, and clients with impaired renal or hepatic function.

## Prostaglandins

Naturally occurring prostaglandin E is thought to decrease acid secretion and increase mucus production in gastric mucosa. Thus, it has antisecretory and mucosal protective effects. When prostaglandin synthesis is inhibited, erosion and ulceration of gastric mucosa may occur. This is apparently the mechanism by which aspirin and other NSAIDs cause acute gastric ulcers (see Chap. 6).

Misoprostol (Cytotec) is a synthetic prostaglandin indicated for use with NSAIDs to prevent gastric ulceration, especially in older adults with arthritis who require high doses of NSAIDs and are at high risk of GI bleeding. Misoprostol is the only approved prostaglandin; several others are being investigated.

Prostaglandins are contraindicated in women of childbearing age unless effective contraceptive methods are being used, because the drugs may cause abortion. The most common adverse effects are diarrhea (occurs in 10%–40% of recipients) and abdominal pain.

## GASTRIC ACID NEUTRALIZERS

### Antacids

Antacids are alkaline substances that neutralize acids. Systemic antacids are absorbed into body fluids and may alter acid-base balance. Sodium bicarbonate (see Chap. 32), for example, is used in the treatment of metabolic acidosis. In this chapter, nonsystemic or poorly absorbed antacids are discussed.

Nonsystemic antacids are aluminum, magnesium, and calcium compounds. They react with hydrochloric acid in the stomach to produce neutral, less acidic, or poorly absorbed salts and to raise the pH (alkalinity) of gastric secretions. Raising the pH to about 3.5 neutralizes more than 90% of gastric acid and inhibits conversion of pepsinogen to pepsin.

Gastric antacids differ in the amounts needed to neutralize gastric acid (about 50–80 mEq of acid are produced hourly), in onset of action, and in adverse effects produced. *Aluminum compounds* generally have a low neutralizing capacity (*i.e.*, large doses are required) and a slow onset of action. They can cause constipation. People who ingest large amounts of aluminum-based antacids over a long period may develop hypophosphatemia and osteomalacia because aluminum combines with phosphates in the GI tract and prevents phosphate absorption. Aluminum compounds are rarely used alone. *Magnesium-based antacids* have a relatively high neutralizing capacity and a rapid onset of action. They may cause diarrhea and hypermagnesemia. *Calcium compounds* are effective and have a rapid onset of action but may cause hypersecretion of gastric acid ("acid rebound") and the "milk-alkali syndrome," which includes alkalosis and azotemia. Consequently, calcium compounds are rarely used in peptic ulcer disease. Although gastric antacids are considered nonsystemic drugs, small amounts of aluminum, magnesium, and calcium are absorbed from the GI tract. Normally insignificant, these small amounts may cause serious adverse effects in the presence of renal disease.

The most commonly used antacids are mixtures of aluminum hydroxide and magnesium hydroxide (*e.g.,* Gelusil, Mylanta, Maalox). Some antacid mixtures contain other ingredients, such as simethicone. Simethicone is an antiflatulent drug available alone as Mylicon. When added to antacids, simethicone does not affect gastric acidity. It reportedly decreases gas bubbles, thereby reducing GI distention and abdominal discomfort.

Antacids act primarily in the stomach and are used to prevent or treat peptic ulcer disease, gastroesophageal reflux disease, esophagitis, pyrosis ("heartburn"), gastritis, GI bleeding, and stress ulcers. Aluminum-based antacids also are given to clients with chronic renal failure and hyperphosphatemia to decrease absorption of phosphates in food.

Magnesium-based antacids are contraindicated in clients with renal failure, and sodium-containing antacids should be used cautiously in clients with hypertension or congestive heart failure.

## CYTOPROTECTIVE AGENTS

### Locally active agents

Locally active agents help to heal ulcers and prevent their recurrence by forming a protective barrier between the mucosa and gastric acid, pepsin, and bile salts. They do not alter the secretion of gastric acid. Because the drugs are not absorbed systemically, they are well tolerated and cause few adverse effects. Sucralfate is the only approved drug of this group.

### Prostaglandins

Some prostaglandins inhibit gastric acid secretion (see Prostaglandins, above) and perform protective functions on gastric mucosal cells. Protective functions are attributed to their ability to increase secretion of mucus and bicarbonate, mucosal blood flow, and perhaps mucosal repair.

## Individual drugs

### GASTRIC ACID INHIBITORS

### Gastric acid pump inhibitor

**Omeprazole** (Prilosec) inhibits gastric acid secretion by combining with $H^+,K^+$-ATPase and preventing release of gastric acid into the stomach lumen. It is well absorbed following oral administration, highly bound to plasma proteins (about 95%), metabolized in the liver, and excreted in the urine (about 75%) and bile or feces (about 25%). Acid-inhibiting effects occur within 2 hours and last 72 hours or longer. When the drug is discontinued, effects persist for 3 to 5 days, until the gastric parietal cells can synthesize additional $H^+,K^+$-ATPase.

Omeprazole is formulated as an extended-release capsule containing enteric-coated granules to prevent its destruction by gastric acid. As a result, the capsule should be swallowed whole and not opened or chewed.

#### Route and dosage range

*Adults:* Gastritis, gastroesophageal reflux disease, PO 20 mg/d for 4–8 wk, taken before eating
Zollinger-Ellison syndrome, PO 60 mg once daily initially, increased up to 120 mg three times daily in divided doses if necessary
Peptic ulcer disease (unlabeled use), PO 10–60 mg/d

### Histamine-2 receptor blocking agents

**Cimetidine** (Tagamet) was the first $H_2$ blocker to be developed, and it is still widely used. It decreases the amount and acidity (hydrogen ion concentration) of gastric juices. It is well absorbed following oral administration. After a single dose, peak blood level is reached in 1 to 1.5 hours, and an effective concentration is maintained about 4 hours. The drug is distributed in almost all body tissues. Most of an oral dose is excreted unchanged in the urine within 24 hours; some is excreted in bile and eliminated in feces. For acutely ill clients, cimetidine is given intravenously.

Adverse effects occur infrequently with usual doses and duration of treatment. They are more likely to occur with prolonged use of high doses and in older adults or those with impaired renal or hepatic function. The major clinical indication for the use of cimetidine is peptic ulcer disease. When used therapeutically for gastric or duodenal ulcers, cimetidine promotes healing within 6 to 8 weeks. It is also effective in preventing GI bleeding due to peptic ulcer disease. When used prophylactically, cimetidine can prevent recurrence of chronic ulcers or development of stress ulcers associated with severe burns, trauma, and other serious illnesses. Cimetidine also may be used in the treatment of Zollinger-Ellison syndrome.

There are no known contraindications to the use of cimetidine, but the drug should be used with caution in older adults or people with renal or hepatic impairment, because drug half-life is prolonged and accumulation may occur. It also should be used with caution during pregnancy because it crosses the placenta, and it should not be taken during lactation because it is excreted in breast milk. Experience with cimetidine in children is limited, and the drug is generally not recommended for children younger than 16 years of age.

### Routes and dosage ranges

*Adults:* PO 800 mg once daily at bedtime or 300 mg four times per day with meals and at bedtime
 Prophylaxis of recurrent ulcer, PO 400 mg at bedtime
 IV injection, 300 mg, diluted in 20 ml of 5% dextrose or saline solution and infused over at least 2 min, q6h
 IV intermittent infusion, 300 mg diluted in at least 50 ml of dextrose or saline solution and infused over 15–20 min, q6h
 IM 300 mg q6h (undiluted)
 Impaired renal function, PO, IV 300 mg q8–12h

**Ranitidine** (Zantac) is an $H_2$ receptor blocking agent with the same mechanism of action and clinical indications for use as cimetidine. Its effectiveness in the prevention and treatment of peptic ulcer disease is similar to that of cimetidine. Ranitidine is more potent than cimetidine, so smaller doses can be given less frequently. In addition, ranitidine reportedly causes fewer drug interactions than cimetidine.

Oral ranitidine is 50% to 60% bioavailable, reaches peak blood levels 1 to 3 hours after administration, and is metabolized in the liver; about 30% is excreted unchanged in the urine. Parenteral ranitidine is 90% to 100% bioavailable and reaches peak blood levels in approximately 15 minutes; about 65% to 80% is excreted unchanged in the urine. Because of these pharmacokinetic differences, larger doses are required with oral than with parenteral administration. Ranitidine accumulates in the presence of renal impairment, and dosage should therefore be reduced. Ranitidine can be eliminated from the body by hemodialysis or peritoneal dialysis.

### Routes and dosage ranges

*Adults:* PO 300 mg once daily at bedtime or 150 mg twice daily
 IM 50 mg q6–8h (undiluted)
 IV injection, 50 mg diluted in 20 ml of 5% dextrose or 0.9% sodium chloride solution and injected over at least 5 min q6–8h
 IV intermittent infusion, 50 mg diluted in 100 ml of 5% dextrose or 0.9% sodium chloride solution and infused over 15–20 min

Impaired renal function (creatinine clearance below 50 ml/min), PO 150 mg q24h
 IV, IM 50 mg q18–24h

**Famotidine** (Pepcid) and **nizatidine** (Axid) are chemically different but pharmacologically similar to cimetidine and ranitidine. They are more potent on a weight basis. The drugs cause similar adverse effects but are less likely to cause mental confusion and gynecomastia (antiandrogenic effects) than cimetidine. In addition, they do not affect the cytochrome P450 drug metabolizing system in the liver and therefore do not interfere with the metabolism of other drugs, as does cimetidine. Dosage should be reduced in the presence of renal impairment.

### Famotidine

### Routes and dosage ranges

*Adults:* Acute duodenal ulcer, PO 40 mg once daily at bedtime or 20 mg twice daily for 4–8 wk; maintenance therapy, PO 20 mg once daily at bedtime
 Zollinger-Ellison syndrome, PO 20 mg q6h, increased if necessary
 IV injection, 20 mg q12h, diluted to 5 or 10 ml with 5% dextrose or 0.9% sodium chloride, and injected over at least 2 min
 IV infusion, 20 mg q12h, diluted with 100 ml of 5% dextrose or 0.9% sodium chloride, and infused over 15–30 min
 Impaired renal function (creatinine clearance below 10 ml/min), PO, IV 20 mg q24–48h

### Nizatidine

### Route and dosage range

*Adults:* Acute duodenal ulcer, PO 300 mg once daily at bedtime; maintenance therapy, PO 150 mg once daily at bedtime
 Impaired renal function (creatinine clearance 20–50 ml/min), PO 150 mg daily; (creatinine clearance below 20 ml/min), PO 150 mg q48h

## Prostaglandin

**Misoprostol** is a synthetic form of prostaglandin E. When given concurrently with NSAIDs, the drug protects gastric mucosa from NSAID-induced erosion and ulceration. It is indicated for clients at high risk of GI ulceration and bleeding, such as those taking high doses of NSAIDs for arthritis and older adults. It is contraindicated in women of childbearing potential and during pregnancy because it may induce abortion. Diarrhea is the most common adverse effect.

### Route and dosage range

*Adults:* PO 200 μg four times per day with meals and at bedtime. If diarrhea is bothersome, dosage may be reduced to 100 μg four times per day.

## GASTRIC ACID NEUTRALIZERS

Antacids are listed in Table 63-1.

## CYTOPROTECTIVE AGENTS

### Locally active agent

**Sucralfate** (Carafate) is a preparation of sulfated sucrose and aluminum hydroxide that binds to normal and ulcerated mucosa. It is used to prevent and treat peptic ulcer disease. When an ulcer is present, the drug combines with ulcer exudate, adheres to the ulcer site, and forms a protective coating that decreases further damage by gastric acid, pepsin, and bile salts. Sucralfate is as effective as other antiulcer agents in healing the duodenal ulcer. When an ulcer has healed, sucralfate may be used in small doses as maintenance therapy to prevent ulcer recurrence. Incidence and severity of adverse effects are low; constipation and dry mouth are most often reported.

### Route and dosage range

*Adults:* Treatment of active ulcer, PO 1 g (1000 mg) four times per day on an empty stomach (before meals and at bedtime); maintenance therapy, PO 1 g twice daily

For information about **prostaglandin**, see Misoprostol, above.

## Nursing Process

### Assessment

Assess the client's status in relation to peptic ulcer disease and other conditions in which antiulcer drugs are used.
- Identify risk factors for peptic ulcer disease:
  - Cigarette smoking. Specific effects are thought to include stimulation of gastric acid secretion and decreased blood supply to gastric mucosa. Moreover, patients with peptic ulcers who continue to smoke heal more slowly and have more recurrent ulcers, despite usually adequate treatment, than those who stop smoking.
  - Stress, including physiologic stress (*e.g.*, shock, sepsis, burns, surgery, head injury, severe trauma, or medical illness) and psychological stress. One mechanism may be that stress activates the sympathetic nervous sys-

tem, which in turn causes vasoconstriction in organs not needed for "fight or flight." Thus, stress may lead to ischemia in gastric mucosa, with ulceration if ischemia is severe or prolonged.
  - Genetic influences. Clients with blood type O are more likely to have duodenal ulcers; those with blood type A are more likely to have gastric ulcers. Also, close relatives of clients with peptic ulcer disease have an increased risk of developing ulcers.
  - Male sex. Men have a higher incidence of duodenal (four times) and gastric (two and one half times) ulcers compared with women.
  - Drug therapy with aspirin and other NSAIDs, corticosteroids, and antineoplastics.
- Signs and symptoms depend on the type and location of the ulcer:
  - Periodic epigastric pain, which occurs 1 to 4 hours after eating or during the night and is often described as burning or gnawing, is a characteristic symptom of chronic duodenal ulcer.
  - GI bleeding occurs with acute or chronic ulcers when the ulcer erodes into a blood vessel. Clinical manifestations may range from mild (*e.g.*, occult blood in feces and eventual anemia) to severe (*e.g.*, hematemesis, melena, hypotension, and shock).
- Gastroesophageal reflux disease and esophagitis are often associated with hiatal hernia and are usually characterized by a substernal burning sensation ("heartburn" or indigestion). They also may occur with obesity and overeating as a result of gastric distention. Symptoms are caused by the backward flow of gastric acid onto esophageal mucosa.

### Nursing diagnoses

- Pain related to effects of gastric acid on peptic ulcers
- Ineffective Individual Coping related to acute and chronic manifestations of peptic ulcer disease
- High Risk for Injury: GI bleeding, ulcer perforation, bowel obstruction
- Altered Nutrition: Less than Body Requirements related to anorexia and abdominal discomfort
- Constipation with anticholinergic drugs, aluminum or calcium-containing antacids, or sucralfate
- Diarrhea with magnesium-containing antacids and misoprostol
- High Risk for Injury: Adverse drug effects
- Knowledge Deficit related to the disease process
- Knowledge Deficit related to drug therapy for peptic ulcer disease

### Planning/Goals

*The client will:*
- Take or receive antiulcer drugs accurately
- Experience relief of symptoms
- Avoid situations that cause or exacerbate symptoms, when possible
- Be observed for GI bleeding and other complications of peptic ulcer disease
- Maintain normal patterns of bowel function
- Avoid preventable adverse effects of drug therapy
- Demonstrate use of relaxation techniques

## TABLE 63-1.  REPRESENTATIVE ANTACID PRODUCTS

| Trade Name | Components | | | | | Route and Dosage Ranges (Adults) |
|---|---|---|---|---|---|---|
| | Magnesium Oxide or Hydroxide | Aluminum Hydroxide | Calcium Carbonate | Sodium | Other | |
| Alka-Seltzer effervescent tablets | | | | 296 mg | Sodium bicarbonate 958 mg, citric acid 832 mg, potassium bicarbonate 312 mg | PO 1–2 tablets, dissolved in 2–3 oz of water, q4h as needed; maximal dose: 8 tablets/24 h |
| Aludrox Amphojel | 103 mg/5 ml | 307 mg/5 ml 300 or 600 mg/tab, 320 mg/5 ml | | 1.15 mg/5 ml <7mg/5ml | | PO 10 ml q4h, or as needed PO 10 ml or 600 mg five or six times daily |
| Camalox | 200 mg/5 ml | 225 mg/5 ml | 250 mg/5 ml | 2.5 mg/5 ml | | PO 2–4 tsp four or five times daily or as directed by physician, to maximal dose of 16 tsp/24 h |
| Di-Gel | 87 mg/5 ml | 282 mg/5 ml | | 8.5 mg/5 ml | Simethicone 20 mg/5 ml | PO 2 tsp liquid q2h, after meals or between meals, and at bedtime. Maximal dose, 20 tsp/24 h. Do not use maximal dose longer than 2 wk. |
| Gelusil | 200 mg/5 ml | 200 mg/5ml | | 0.7 mg/5 ml | Simethicone 25 mg/5 ml | PO 10 or more ml or 2 or more tablets after meals and at bedtime or as directed by physician to a maximum of 12 tablets or tsp/24 h |
| Maalox suspension | 200 mg/5 ml | 225 mg/5 ml | | 1.35 mg/5 ml | | PO 30 ml four times daily, after meals and at bedtime or as directed by physician; maximal dose, 16 tsp/24 h |
| Maalox No. 1 tablets | 200 mg/tab | 200 mg/tab | | 0.84 mg/tab | | PO 2–4 tablets, four times daily after meals and at bedtime or as directed by physician; maximal dose, 16 tablets/24 h |
| Maalox No. 2 tablets | 400 mg/tab | 400 mg/tab | | 1.84 mg/tab | | PO 1–2 tablets, four times daily, after meals and at bedtime or as directed by physician; maximal dose, 8 tablets/24 h |
| Maalox Plus | 200 mg/tab, 200 mg/5 ml | 200 mg/tab, 225 mg/5 ml | | 1 mg/tab, 1.3 mg/5 ml | Simethicone 25 mg/tab, 25 mg/5 ml | PO 2–4 tsp or tablets four times daily after meals and at bedtime, or as directed by physician |
| Mylanta | 200 mg/tab, 200 mg/5 ml | 200 mg/tab, 200 mg/5 ml | | 0.77 mg/tab, 0.68 mg/5 ml | Simethicone 20 mg/tab, 20 mg/5 ml | PO 5–10 ml or 1–2 tablets q2–4h, between meals and at bedtime or as directed by physician |
| Mylanta-II | 400 mg/tab, 400 mg/5 ml | 400 mg/tab, 400 mg/5 ml | | 1.3 mg/tab, 1.14 mg/5 ml | Simethicone 30 mg/tab, 30 mg/5 ml | Same as Mylanta |
| Titralac | | | 420 mg/tab, 1 g/5 ml | <0.3 mg/tab, 11 mg/5 ml | Glycine 180 mg/tab, 300 mg/5 ml | PO 1 tsp or 2 tablets, after meals or as directed by physician, to maximal dose of 19 tablets or 8 tsp/24 h |
| WinGel | 160 mg/5 ml | 180 mg/5 ml | | | | PO 1–2 tsp or tablets, up to four times daily, or as directed by physician. Children over age 6 years: same as adults |

## Interventions

Use measures to prevent or minimize peptic ulcer disease and gastric acid-induced esophageal disorders.

- With peptic ulcer disease, helpful interventions may include the following:
  - General health measures such as a well-balanced diet, adequate rest, and regular exercise
  - Avoiding cigarette smoking and gastric irritants (*e.g.*, alcohol, aspirin, caffeine)
  - Reducing psychological stress (*e.g.*, by changing environments) or learning healthful methods of handling it (*e.g.*, relaxation techniques, physical exercise). There is no practical way to avoid psychological stress, because it is part of everyday life.
  - Long-term drug therapy with relatively small doses of $H_2$ receptor antagonists, antacids, or sucralfate. With "active" peptic ulcer disease, helping the client follow the prescribed therapeutic regimen helps to promote healing and prevent serious complications (*i.e.*, hemorrhage, perforation, obstruction).
  - Diet therapy has little role in prevention or treatment of peptic ulcer disease. Because various studies have failed to demonstrate the effectiveness of ulcer diets, some physicians prescribe no dietary restrictions for clients with peptic ulcer disease, while others suggest avoiding highly spiced foods, gas-forming foods, and caffeine-containing beverages.
- With gastric acid-induced esophagitis, helpful measures are those that prevent or decrease gastroesophageal reflux of gastric contents (*e.g.*, elevating the head of the bed, avoiding gastric distention by eating small meals, not lying down for about 1 hour after eating, and avoiding obesity, constipation, or other conditions that increase intra-abdominal pressure).

### Teach clients:

- That conditions for which antiulcer drugs are used are chronic and are usually managed on an outpatient basis. It is important for the client to know about prevention and treatment of the conditions.
- Characteristics of the disease process, nondrug measures to prevent or minimize symptoms, drug therapy, and accurate information related to diet
- To observe for and report signs and symptoms of complications, such as GI bleeding
- Relaxation and stress-management techniques

## Evaluation

- Observe and interview regarding drug usage.
- Observe and interview regarding relief of symptoms.
- Observe for signs and symptoms of complications.
- Observe and interview regarding adverse drug effects.
- Observe and interview regarding relaxation techniques.

# Principles of therapy

## DRUG SELECTION

All of the drugs are effective for indicated uses; thus, the choice of drug may depend on cost, convenience, and acuity of peptic ulcer disease. $H_2$ receptor antagonists are the drugs of first choice in most situations. They are convenient to administer and cause few adverse effects. Of these, cimetidine is the least expensive but the most likely to cause confusion and antiandrogenic effects. Cimetidine also increases the risks of toxicity with several commonly used drugs. Compared with cimetidine, famotidine, nizatidine, and ranitidine are more potent on a weight basis and have a longer duration of action, so they can be given in smaller, less frequent doses. In addition, they do not alter the hepatic metabolism of other drugs.

Antacids are more often used with other agents than alone. The frequent administration of relatively large amounts is inconvenient for many clients. Sucralfate must be taken before meals, and this is inconvenient for some clients. Omeprazole is not recommended for maintenance therapy to prevent ulcer recurrence.

## GUIDELINES FOR THERAPY WITH HISTAMINE-2 RECEPTOR ANTAGONISTS

1. For an acute ulcer, full dosage may be given for up to 8 weeks. When the ulcer heals, the drug may be discontinued or reduced in dosage for maintenance therapy to prevent recurrence. These drugs are effective and convenient in a single daily dose taken at bedtime to suppress nocturnal secretion of gastric acid. Dosage of all these drugs should be reduced in the presence of impaired renal function.
2. Antacids are often given concurrently with $H_2$ receptor blocking agents to relieve pain. They should not be given at the same time because the antacid reduces absorption of the other drug. $H_2$ antagonists relieve pain after about 1 week of administration.

## GUIDELINES FOR THERAPY WITH SUCRALFATE

When sucralfate is used to treat an ulcer, it should be administered for 4 to 8 weeks unless healing is confirmed by radiologic or endoscopic examination. When used long-term to prevent ulcer recurrence, dosage should be reduced.

## GUIDELINES FOR THERAPY WITH ANTACIDS

1. The choice of antacid depends on characteristics of clients and drug preparations and should be individualized. Combination products containing aluminum hydroxide and magnesium oxide or hydroxide are commonly used. Some guidelines include the following:
   a. *Neutralizing capacity*. Use of an agent with high *in vitro* neutralizing capacity is probably better. However, the clinical or *in vivo* capacity may be

different, depending on the amount of gastric acid and rate of gastric emptying. In a fasting state, for example, the antacid leaves the stomach in about 30 minutes and thereafter becomes ineffective. After a meal, acid-neutralizing effects last 3 hours or longer.

b. *Side effects*. Calcium carbonate has a high neutralizing capacity, but doses large and frequent enough to maintain neutralization of gastric acid may cause hypercalcemia and impaired renal function due to systemic absorption. Magnesium hydroxide has a higher buffering capacity than magnesium hydroxide–aluminum hydroxide mixtures, but it may cause diarrhea and hypermagnesemia. Aluminum hydroxide has the least buffering capacity.

c. *Rapid action*. Magnesium hydroxide, magnesium oxide, and calcium carbonate are effective for rapid action. Sodium bicarbonate is rapidly effective but of short duration. It is contraindicated for long-term use because of systemic absorption and possible metabolic alkalosis. Effervescent antacids have a rapid onset but short duration of action, because they leave the stomach quickly.

d. *Dosage form*. Antacid liquid suspensions usually act faster than chewable tablets. However, suspensions have not been proven more effective in neutralizing gastric acid. Chewable tablets may be more convenient in some circumstances.

e. *Antiflatulent*. Simethicone, which is added to several antacid mixtures, has no effect on intragastric pH but may be useful in relieving flatulence or gastroesophageal reflux.

f. *Ingredients*. Antacids with these ingredients or characteristics are contraindicated as follows:
   (1) Magnesium is contraindicated in renal disease because hypermagnesemia may result.
   (2) High sodium content may be contraindicated in edematous states, such as congestive heart failure.
   (3) High sugar content may be contraindicated in diabetes mellitus.

g. *Occasional use*. Although sodium bicarbonate (baking soda) and calcium carbonate are generally contraindicated in the large amounts and long-term usage required for treatment of peptic ulcer disease, occasional use is not likely to be harmful.

h. *Palatability*. Efforts should be made to find an antacid preparation that is acceptable to the client in terms of taste, dosage, and convenience of administration.

2. As a general rule, single drugs are preferable to mixtures. However, antacid combinations have several advantages, including the following:
   a. Combining an antacid with a laxative effect (*e.g.*, magnesium hydroxide) with one that has a con-

stipating effect (*e.g.*, aluminum hydroxide) tends to prevent or reduce the incidence of both symptoms.
   b. Combining fast-acting and slow-acting antacids can prolong gastric acid neutralization.
   c. Mixtures allow smaller dosages of individual ingredients, and adverse effects may be prevented or reduced.
   d. Client compliance with antacid therapy is usually improved.

3. Antacid dosage, including frequency of administration, depends primarily on the purpose for use, buffering capacity of the antacid, and client response. Some guidelines include the following:
   a. To prevent stress ulcers in critically ill clients and to treat acute GI bleeding, nearly continuous neutralization of gastric acid is desirable. Dose and frequency of administration must be sufficient to neutralize about 50 to 80 mEq of gastric acid each hour. This can be accomplished by a continuous intragastric drip through a nasogastric tube or by hourly administration.
   b. When a client has a nasogastric tube in place, antacid dosage may be titrated by aspirating stomach contents, determining pH with Nitrazine paper, and then basing the dose on the pH. (Most gastric acid is neutralized and most pepsin activity is eliminated at a pH above 3.5.)
   c. For most clients, the standard practice of giving an antacid 1 hour before and 3 hours after meals and at bedtime is effective and rational, although gastric acid is buffered intermittently rather than continuously. When an antacid is given on an empty stomach, gastric acid is neutralized for about 30 minutes, depending on gastric emptying time. When an antacid is taken after meals, buffering effects last 3 or more hours.
   d. When antacids are used to relieve pain, they may be taken as needed.
   e. The usual dose of a liquid antacid is 30 ml (2 tbsp or 6 tsp). This amount is higher than doses recommended by most manufacturers (5–20 ml or 1–4 tsp).

## EFFECTS OF ANTIULCER DRUGS ON OTHER DRUGS

**Histamine 2 receptor blocking drugs** may alter the effects of several drugs. Most significant effects occur with cimetidine, which inhibits drug metabolizing enzymes (cytochrome P450 pathway) in the liver and interferes with the metabolism of several commonly used drugs. Consequently, the affected drugs are eliminated more slowly, their serum levels are increased, and they are more likely to cause adverse effects and toxicity unless dosage is reduced.

Interacting drugs include antiarrhythmics (lidocaine,

moricizine, propafenone, quinidine), the anticoagulant warfarin, anticonvulsants (carbamazepine, phenytoin), benzodiazepine antianxiety or hypnotic agents (alprazolam, chlordiazepoxide, diazepam, flurazepam, triazolam), beta-adrenergic blocking agents (labetalol, metoprolol, propranolol), the bronchodilator theophylline, calcium channel-blocking agents (*e.g.*, verapamil), tricyclic antidepressants (*e.g.*, amitriptyline), and sulfonylureas (*e.g.*, oral antidiabetic drugs). In addition, cimetidine may increase serum levels (*e.g.*, fluorouracil, procainamide and its active metabolite) and pharmacologic effects of other drugs (*e.g.*, flecainide, respiratory depression with narcotic analgesics or succinylcholine) by unidentified mechanisms. Cimetidine also may decrease effects of several drugs, including drugs that require an acidic environment for absorption (*e.g.*, iron salts, indomethacin, fluconazole, ketoconazole, tetracyclines) and miscellaneous drugs (*e.g.*, digoxin, tocainide), by unknown mechanisms.

Ranitidine, famotidine, and nizatidine do not inhibit the cytochrome P450 metabolizing enzymes. Ranitidine decreases absorption of diazepam if given at the same time and increases hypoglycemic effects of glipizide. Nizatidine increases serum salicylate levels in people taking high doses of aspirin.

**Antacids** may prevent absorption of most drugs taken at the same time, including benzodiazepine antianxiety drugs, corticosteroids, digoxin, $H_2$ blockers (cimetidine, ranitidine), iron supplements, phenothiazine antipsychotic drugs, phenytoin, quinolone antibacterials, salicylates, and tetracyclines. Antacids increase absorption of a few drugs, including levodopa, quinidine, and valproic acid. These interactions can be avoided or minimized by separating administration times by 1 to 2 hours.

**Omeprazole** increases blood levels of diazepam, phenytoin, and warfarin, probably by inhibiting hepatic metabolism.

**Sucralfate** decreases absorption of cimetidine, ciprofloxacin, digoxin, norfloxacin, phenytoin, ranitidine, tetracycline, and theophylline. Apparently, sucralfate binds to these drugs when both are present in the GI tract. This interaction can be avoided or minimized by giving the interacting drug 2 hours before sucralfate.

## EFFECTS OF ANTIULCER DRUGS ON NUTRIENTS

Dietary folate, iron, and vitamin $B_{12}$ are better absorbed from an acidic environment. When gastric fluids are made less acidic by antisecretory or antacid drugs, deficiencies of these nutrients may occur. In addition, sucralfate interferes with absorption of fat-soluble vitamins, and magnesium-containing antacids interfere with absorption of vitamin A.

## USE IN CHILDREN

Antacids may be given to ambulatory children in doses of 5 to 15 ml every 3 to 6 hours or at 1 and 3 hours after meals and at bedtime, as for adults with acute peptic ulcer disease. For prevention of GI bleeding in critically ill children, 2 to 5 ml may be given to infants and 5 to 15 ml to children every 1 to 2 hours. Safety and effectiveness of other antiulcer drugs have not been established for children.

## USE IN OLDER ADULTS

Older adults often take large doses of NSAIDs for arthritis and therefore are at risk of developing acute gastric ulcers. Thus, they may be candidates for treatment with misoprostol. With $H_2$ receptor antagonists, older adults are more likely to experience adverse effects, especially confusion, agitation, and disorientation with cimetidine. In addition, older adults often have decreased renal function, and doses need to be reduced.

With antacids, older adults usually secrete less gastric acid than younger adults, and smaller doses may be effective. Further, with decreased renal function, older adults are more likely to have adverse effects. These include neuromuscular effects of magnesium-containing antacids and cardiovascular effects (edema, hypertension, congestive heart failure) of sodium-containing antacids, especially if large or frequent doses are taken.

# NURSING ACTIONS: ANTIULCER DRUGS

| *Nursing Actions* | *Rationale/Explanation* |
|---|---|
| **1. Administer accurately** | |
| **a.** Give oral cimetidine with meals or at bedtime. Famotidine, nizatidine, and ranitidine may be given without regard to food intake. | When cimetidine is taken with meals, peak serum drug level coincides with gastric emptying, when gastric acidity is usually highest. When taken at bedtime, cimetidine prevents secretion of gastric acid for several hours. Thus, correct timing of drug administration may promote faster healing of the ulcer. |
| **b.** To give cimetidine or ranitidine intravenously, dilute in 20 ml of 5% dextrose or normal saline solution, and inject over at least 2 minutes. For intermittent infusion, dilute in at least 50 ml of 5% dextrose of 0.9% sodium chloride solution, and infuse over 15 to 20 minutes. | |
| **c.** To give famotidine intravenously, dilute with 5 to 10 ml of 0.9% sodium chloride injection, and inject over at least 2 minutes. For intermittent infusion, dilute in 100 ml of 5% dextrose or 0.9% sodium chloride, and infuse over 15 to 30 minutes. | |
| **d.** Do not give antacids within about 1 hour of oral H$_2$ antagonists or sucralfate. | Antacids decrease absorption and therapeutic effectiveness of the other drugs. |
| **e.** Shake liquid antacids well before measuring the dose. | These preparations are suspensions. Drug particles settle to the bottom of the container on standing and must be mixed thoroughly to give the correct dose. |
| **f.** Instruct clients to chew antacid tablets thoroughly. | To increase the surface area of drug available to neutralize gastric acid |
| **g.** Give sucralfate 1 hour before meals and at bedtime. | To allow the drug to form its protective coating over the ulcer before high levels of gastric acidity. Sucralfate requires an acidic environment. After it has adhered to the ulcer, antacids and food do not affect drug action. |
| **h.** Give omeprazole before food intake. | |
| **i.** Give misoprostol with food. | |
| **2. Observe for therapeutic effects** | Therapeutic effects depend on the reason for use. |
| **a.** Decreased epigastric pain | Antacids should relieve ulcer pain within a few minutes. H$_2$ antagonists relieve pain in about 1 week by healing effects on the ulcer. |
| **b.** Decreased gastrointestinal (GI) bleeding (*e.g.*, absence of visible or occult blood in vomitus, gastric secretions, or feces) | |
| **c.** Higher pH of gastric contents | The minimum acceptable pH with antacid therapy is 3.5. In acute situations the goal may be a pH of 7 (neutral). |
| **d.** Radiologic or endoscopic reports of ulcer healing | |

(*continued*)

| Nursing Actions | Rationale/Explanation |
|---|---|
| **3. Observe for adverse effects**<br>**a.** With H$_2$ antagonists, observe for diarrhea or constipation, headache, dizziness, muscle aches, fatigue, skin rashes, mental confusion, delirium, coma, depression, fever. | Adverse effects are uncommon and usually mild with recommended doses and duration of drug therapy (8 weeks). Central nervous system effects have been associated with high doses in elderly clients or those with impaired renal function. With long-term administration of cimetidine, other adverse effects have been observed. These include decreased sperm count and gynecomastia in men and galactorrhea in women. |
| **b.** With antacids containing magnesium, observe for diarrhea and hypermagnesemia. | Diarrhea may be prevented by combining these antacids with other antacids containing aluminum or calcium. Hypermagnesemia is unlikely in most clients but may occur in those with impaired renal function. These antacids should not be given to clients with renal failure. |
| **c.** With antacids containing aluminum or calcium, observe for constipation. | Constipation may be prevented by combining these antacids with other antacids containing magnesium. A high-fiber diet and adequate fluid intake (2000–3000 ml daily) also help prevent constipation. |
| **d.** With sucralfate, observe for constipation. | Thus far, adverse effects observed with sucralfate have been few and minor. (The drug is not absorbed systemically.) The most common one was constipation (4.7% in 2500 people). |
| **e.** With misoprostol, observe for diarrhea, abdominal pain, nausea, vomiting, headache, uterine cramping, vaginal bleeding. | Diarrhea is the most commonly reported and may be severe enough to indicate dosage reduction or stopping the drug. |
| **f.** With omeprazole, observe for headache, diarrhea, abdominal pain, nausea, and vomiting. | These effects occur infrequently and are usually well tolerated. |
| **4. Observe for drug interactions** | Most significant drug interactions alter the effect of the other drug rather than that of the antiulcer drug. For example, cimetidine may potentiate anticoagulants; antacids alter the absorption of many oral drugs. |
| **a.** Drugs that *decrease* effects of cimetidine and ranitidine:<br><br>Antacids | Antacids decrease absorption of cimetidine and probably ranitidine. The drugs should not be given at the same time. |
| **b.** Drugs that *increase* effects of antacids:<br><br>Anticholinergic drugs (*e.g.*, atropine) | May increase effects by delaying gastric emptying and by decreasing acid secretion themselves |
| **c.** Drugs that *decrease* effects of antacids:<br><br>Cholinergic drugs (*e.g.*, dexpanthenol [Ilopan]) | May decrease effects by increasing GI motility and rate of gastric emptying |
| **d.** Drugs that *decrease* effects of sucralfate:<br><br>Antacids | Antacids should not be given within 1/2 hour before or after administration of sucralfate. |

## Nursing Actions

## Rationale/Explanation

| Nursing Actions | Rationale/Explanation |
|---|---|
| **5. Teach clients**<br>**a.** Take antiulcer drugs as prescribed. | Underuse decreases therapeutic effectiveness; overuse increases adverse effects. For acute peptic ulcer disease, drugs are given in relatively high doses for 4 to 8 weeks to promote healing. For long-term maintenance therapy, dosage is reduced. |
| **b.** Take cimetidine with food; take ranitidine, famotidine, and nizatidine without regard to meals; take sucralfate before meals and at bedtime; take antacids 1 and 3 hours after meals and at bedtime; take misoprostol with food and omeprazole before food intake. | For increased therapeutic effects |
| **c.** Choose antacids carefully. | Because antacids do not require a prescription, many products are readily available. However, these products are not equally safe or effective in all people. |
| (1) Consult with a physician before choosing an antacid for peptic ulcer disease or when heart or kidney disease is present. | Some antacids are safer and more effective than others in the large doses and long-term usage required for peptic ulcer disease. Some antacids should not be taken with heart disease (because of high sodium content with potential fluid retention and edema) or kidney disease (because of drug accumulation and higher risks of toxicity). |
| (2) Do not take baking soda, Alka-Seltzer effervescent antacid tablets, Titralac, or Tums more often than occasionally. | These products may cause serious adverse effects if taken in large amounts or for prolonged periods. Baking soda and Alka-Seltzer effervescent tablets contain large amounts of sodium; the other products contain calcium carbonate. |
| **d.** Take antacids at least 1 hour before or after other drugs. | Antacids decrease absorption of many other drugs, including cimetidine and other H₂ receptor antagonists and sucralfate. |
| **e.** Swallow omeprazole capsules whole. Do not open, chew, or crush the capsules. | To prevent destruction of the drug by stomach acid |

## Review and Application Exercises

1. What are risk factors for peptic ulcer disease?
2. How are ulcers thought to develop? What roles do gastric acid, pepsin, *H. pylori* organisms, prostaglandins, and mucus play in ulcer occurrence?
3. How do the various antiulcer drugs heal ulcers or prevent their recurrence?
4. List advantages and disadvantages of cimetidine in comparison with other H₂ blockers.
5. What is the rationale for taking H₂ blockers at bedtime?
6. What is the rationale for taking sucralfate before meals?
7. What is the rationale for taking antacids after meals?
8. Why are aluminum and magnesium salts often combined in antacid preparations?

9. For a client who smokes cigarettes and is newly diagnosed with peptic ulcer disease, how would you explain that smoking cessation aids ulcer healing?
10. Is diet therapy important in ulcer occurrence, healing, or recurrence? Why or why not?

## Selected References

Collins, A., & Bullock, B. L. (1992). Alterations in gastrointestinal function. In B. L. Bullock & P. P. Rosendahl (Eds.), *Pathophysiology: Adaptations and alterations in function* (3rd ed.) (pp. 787–807). Philadelphia: J.B. Lippincott.

Davis, J., & Sherer, K. (1994). Applied nutrition and diet therapy for nurses (2nd ed.). Philadelphia: W.B. Saunders.

(1994). *Drug facts and comparisons*. St. Louis: Facts and Comparisons

Garcia, G. (1992). Gastrointestinal disorders. In K. L. Melmon, H. F. Morrelli, B. B. Hoffman, & D. W. Nierenberg (Eds.), *Clinical pharmacology: Basic principles in therapeutics* (3rd ed.) (pp. 219–232). New York: McGraw-Hill.

Garnett, W. R., & Dukes, G. E. Jr. (1992). Upper gastrointestinal disorders. In M. A. Koda-Kimble & L. Y. Young (Eds.), *Applied therapeutics: The clinical use of drugs* (5th ed.) (pp. 19-1–19-22). Vancouver, WA: Applied Therapeutics.

Graham, D. Y., Lew, G. M., Klein, P. D., Evans, D. G., Evans, D. J., Saeed, Z. A., & Malaty, H. M. (1992). Effect of treatment of *Helicobacter pylori* infection on the long-term recurrence of gastric or duodenal ulcer: A randomized, controlled study. *Annals of Internal Medicine, 116*(9), 705–708.

Guyton, A. C. (1991). *Textbook of medical physiology* (8th ed.). Philadelphia: W.B. Saunders.

Hentschel, E., Brandstatter, G., Dragosics, B., Hirschl, A. M., Nemec, H., Schutze, K., Taufer, M., & Wurzer, H. (1993). Effect of ranitidine and amoxicillin plus metronidazole on the eradication of *Helicobacter pylori* and the recurrence of duodenal ulcer. *New England Journal of Medicine, 328,* 308–312.

Porth, C. M. (1990). *Pathophysiology: Concepts of altered health states* (3rd ed.) (pp. 697–718). Philadelphia: J.B. Lippincott.

Walsh, J. H. (1992). Acid peptic disorders of the gastrointestinal tract. In W. N. Kelley (Ed.), *Textbook of internal medicine* (2nd ed.) (pp. 457–469). Philadelphia: J.B. Lippincott.

### CHAPTER 64

# Laxatives and Cathartics

## Description

Laxatives and cathartics are drugs used to promote bowel elimination (defecation). The term *laxative* implies mild effects and elimination of soft, formed stool. The term *cathartic* implies strong effects and elimination of liquid or semiliquid stool. Because the different effects depend more on the dose than on the particular drug used, the terms often are used interchangeably.

## Defecation

Defecation is normally stimulated by movements and reflexes in the gastrointestinal (GI) tract. When the stomach and duodenum are distended with food or fluids, gastrocolic and duodenocolic reflexes cause propulsive movements in the colon, which move feces into the rectum and arouse the urge to defecate. When sensory nerve fibers in the rectum are stimulated by the fecal mass, the defecation reflex causes strong peristalsis, deep breathing, closure of the glottis, contraction of abdominal muscles, contraction of the rectum, relaxation of anal sphincters, and expulsion of the fecal mass.

The cerebral cortex normally controls the defecation reflex so that defecation can occur at acceptable times and places. Voluntary control inhibits the external anal sphincter to allow defecation or contracts the sphincter to prevent defecation. When the external sphincter remains contracted, the defecation reflex dissipates, and

the urge to defecate usually does not recur until additional feces enter the rectum or several hours later.

People who often inhibit the defecation reflex or fail to respond to the urge to defecate develop constipation as the reflex weakens. *Constipation* is the infrequent and painful expulsion of hard, dry stools. Although there is no "normal" number of stools because of variations in diet and other factors, most people report more than three bowel movements per week. Normal bowel elimination should produce a soft, formed stool without pain.

## Laxatives and cathartics

Laxatives and cathartics are somewhat arbitrarily classified as bulk-forming laxatives, surfactant laxatives or stool softeners, saline cathartics, irritant or stimulant cathartics, and lubricant or emollient laxatives. Individual drugs are listed in Table 64-1.

### BULK-FORMING LAXATIVES

Bulk-forming laxatives (*e.g.*, methylcellulose, psyllium seed) are substances that are largely unabsorbed from the intestine. When water is added, these substances swell and become gel-like. The added bulk or size of the fecal mass stimulates peristalsis and defecation. The substances also may act by pulling water into the intestinal lumen. Bulk-forming laxatives are the most physiologic laxatives because they act similarly to increased intake of dietary fiber.

Anne Collins Abrams: CLINICAL DRUG THERAPY, Fourth Edition.
© 1995 J.B. Lippincott Company.

**TABLE 64-1. LAXATIVES AND CATHARTICS**

| Generic/Trade Name | Routes and Dosage Ranges | |
|---|---|---|
| | *Adults* | *Children* |
| ***Bulk-Forming Laxatives*** | | |
| **Methylcellulose** (Citrucel) | PO 1 heaping Tbsp one to three times daily with water (8 oz or more) | PO 1 level Tbsp one to three times daily with water (4 oz) |
| **Polycarbophil** (FiberCon, Mitrolan) | PO 1 g four times daily or PRN with 8 oz of fluid; maximum dose, 6 g/24 h | Age 6–12 years, PO 500 mg one to three times daily or PRN; maximum dose, 3 g/24 h<br>Age 2–6 years, PO 500 mg one or two times daily or PRN; maximum dose, 1.5 g/24 h |
| **Psyllium preparations** (Metamucil, Effersyllium, Serutan, Perdiem Plain) | PO 4–10 g (1–2 tsp) one to three times daily, stirred in at least 8 oz of water or other liquid | |
| ***Surfactant Laxatives (Stool Softeners)*** | | |
| **Docusate sodium** (Colace, Doxinate) | PO 50–200 mg daily | Age over 12 years, same dosage as adults<br>Age 3–12 years, 20–120 mg daily<br>Age under 3 years, 10–40 mg daily |
| **Docusate calcium** (Surfak) | PO 50–240 mg daily | Age over 12 years, same dosage as adults<br>Age 2–12 years, 50–150 mg daily<br>Age under 2 years, 25 mg daily |
| **Docusate potassium** (Dialose) | PO 100–300 mg daily | Age 6–12 years, 100 mg at bedtime |
| ***Saline Cathartics*** | | |
| **Magnesium citrate solution** | PO 200 ml at bedtime | |
| **Magnesium hydroxide (milk of magnesia, magnesia magma)** | Regular liquid, PO 15–60 ml at bedtime<br>Concentrated liquid, PO 10–20 ml at bedtime | Regular liquid, PO 2.5–5 ml |
| **Polyethylene glycol-electrolyte solution (PEG 3350, sodium sulfate, sodium bicarbonate, sodium chloride, potassium chloride)** (CoLyte, Colovage, GoLYTELY) | For bowel cleansing before GI examination: PO 240 ml (8 oz) every 10 min until 4 L are consumed | No recommended children's dose |
| **Sodium phosphate and sodium biphosphate** (Fleet Phosphosoda, Fleet Enema) | PO 20–40 ml in 8 oz of water<br>Rectal enema, 60–120 ml | Age 10 years and over, PO 10–20 ml in 8 oz of water<br>Age 5–10 years, PO 5–10 ml in 8 oz of water<br>Rectal enema, 60 ml |
| ***Irritant or Stimulant Cathartics*** | | |
| ***Anthraquinones*** | | |
| **Cascara sagrada** (Cas-Evac) | PO, tablets, 325 mg; fluid extract, 0.5–1.5 ml; aromatic fluid extract, 5 ml | |
| **Senna pod preparations** (Senokot, Black Draught) | Granules, PO 1 level tsp once or twice daily; geriatric, obstetric, gynecologic clients, PO 0.5 level tsp once or twice daily<br>Syrup, PO 2–3 tsp once or twice daily; geriatric, obstetric, gynecologic clients, 1–1½ tsp once or twice daily<br>Tablets, PO 2 tablets once or twice daily; geriatric, obstetric, gynecologic clients, 1 tablet once or twice daily<br>Suppositories, 1 suppository at bedtime | Weight over 27 kg: granules, syrup, tablets, suppositories—½ adult dose |
| ***Diphenylmethane Cathartics*** | | |
| **Bisacodyl** (Dulcolax) | PO 10–15 mg<br>Rectal suppository, 10 mg | Age 6 years and over, PO 5–10 mg<br>Age under 2 years, rectal suppository 5 mg |
| **Phenolphthalein** (Alophen, Feen-a-Mint, Ex-Lax) | PO 30–194 mg daily | |

(continued)

**TABLE 64-1.    LAXATIVES AND CATHARTICS    (Continued)**

| Generic/Trade Name | Routes and Dosage Ranges | |
| --- | --- | --- |
| | **Adults** | **Children** |
| *Other Irritant Cathartics* | | |
| **Castor oil** (Alphamul, Neoloid) | PO 15–60 ml | Age 5–15 years, PO 5–30 ml depending on strength of emulsion Age under 2 years, PO 1.25–7.5 ml depending on strength of emulsion |
| **Glycerin** | Rectal suppository, 3 g | Age under 6 years, rectal suppository 1–1.5 g |
| *Lubricant Laxative* | | |
| **Mineral oil** (Agoral Plain, Milkinol, Fleet Mineral Oil Enema) | PO 15–30 ml at bedtime Rectal enema, 60–120 ml | Age over 6 years, PO 5–15 ml at bedtime Rectal enema, 30–60 ml |
| *Miscellaneous Laxatives* | | |
| **Lactulose** (Chronulac, Cephulac) | PO 15–30 ml daily; maximum dose, 60 ml daily Portal systemic encephalopathy, PO 30–45 ml three or four times daily, adjusted to produce two or three soft stools daily Rectally as retention enema, 300 ml with 700 ml water or normal saline, retained 30–60 minutes, q4–6h | Infants, PO 2.5–10 ml daily in divided doses Older children, PO 40–90 ml daily in divided doses |
| **Sorbitol** | PO 30–50 g daily | |

## SURFACTANT LAXATIVES (STOOL SOFTENERS)

Surfactant laxatives (*e.g.*, docusate sodium) decrease the surface tension of the fecal mass to allow water to penetrate into the stool. They also act as a detergent to facilitate admixing of fat and water in the stool. As a result, stools are softer and easier to expel. These agents have little if any laxative effect. Their main value is to prevent straining while expelling stool.

## SALINE CATHARTICS

Saline cathartics (*e.g.*, magnesium citrate, milk of magnesia, sodium phosphate) are not well absorbed from the intestine. Consequently, they increase osmotic pressure in the intestinal lumen and cause water to be retained. Distention of the bowel leads to increased peristalsis and decreased intestinal transit time for the fecal mass. The resultant stool is semifluid.

## IRRITANT OR STIMULANT CATHARTICS

The irritant or stimulant cathartics are the strongest and most abused laxative products. These drugs act by irritating the GI mucosa and pulling water into the bowel lumen. As a result, feces are moved through the bowel too rapidly to allow colonic absorption of fecal water, so a watery stool is eliminated. These cathartics are subdivided into three groups, which differ in location and time of action but are similar in mechanism of action, pharmacokinetics, and adverse effects. The groups are castor oil, anthraquinones (senna products, cascara sagrada), and diphenylmethanes (bisacodyl, phenolphthalein). Phenolphthalein is the active ingredient in several over-the-counter laxatives (*e.g.*, Ex-Lax, Feen-a-Mint).

In addition to the oral agents, glycerin is administered as a rectal suppository. Glycerin stimulates bowel evacuation by its irritant effects on rectal mucosa and hyperosmotic effects in the colon. Glycerin is not given orally for laxative effects.

## LUBRICANT LAXATIVES

Mineral oil is the only lubricant laxative used clinically. It lubricates the intestine and is thought to soften stool by retarding colonic absorption of fecal water, but the exact mechanism of action is unknown. Mineral oil may cause several adverse effects and is not recommended for long-term use.

## MISCELLANEOUS LAXATIVES

Lactulose is a disaccharide that is not absorbed from the GI tract. It exerts laxative effects by pulling water into the intestinal lumen. It is used to treat constipation and hepatic encephalopathy. The latter condition usually results from alcoholic liver disease in which ammonia accumulates and causes stupor or coma. Ammonia is produced by metabolism of dietary protein and intestinal bacteria. Lactulose decreases production of ammonia in the intestine. The goal of treatment is usually to maintain two to three soft stools daily.

Polyethylene glycol-electrolyte solution (CoLyte, GoLYTELY) is a nonabsorbable, oral solution that induces diarrhea within 30 to 60 minutes and rapidly evacuates the bowel, usually within 4 hours. It is used only for bowel cleansing prior to GI examination (*e.g.*, colonoscopy) and is contraindicated with GI obstruction, gastric retention, colitis, or bowel perforation.

Sorbitol is a monosaccharide that pulls water into the intestinal lumen and has laxative effects. It is often given with sodium polystyrene sulfonate (Kayexalate), a potassium-removing resin used to treat hyperkalemia, to prevent constipation and aid expulsion of the potassium-resin complex.

## INDICATIONS FOR USE

Laxatives and cathartics are widely available on a nonprescription basis. They are among the most frequently used and abused drugs. One reason for overuse is the common misconception that a daily bowel movement is necessary for health and well-being. This notion may lead to a vicious cycle of events in which a person fails to have a bowel movement, takes a strong laxative, again fails to have a bowel movement, and takes another laxative before the fecal column has had time to become reestablished (2–3 days). Thus, a pattern of laxative dependence and abuse is established. Despite widespread abuse of laxatives and cathartics, there are several rational indications for use:

1. To *relieve constipation* in pregnant women, elderly clients whose abdominal and perineal muscles have become weak and atrophied, children with megacolon, and clients receiving drugs that decrease intestinal motility (*e.g.*, narcotic analgesics, anticholinergics, tricyclic antidepressants)
2. To *prevent straining* at stool in clients with coronary artery disease (*e.g.*, postmyocardial infarction), hypertension, cerebrovascular disease, and hemorrhoids and other rectal conditions
3. To *empty the bowel* in preparation for bowel surgery or diagnostic procedures (*e.g.*, proctoscopy, colonoscopy, barium enema)
4. To *accelerate elimination* of potentially toxic substances from the GI tract (*e.g.*, orally ingested drugs or toxic compounds)
5. To *prevent absorption* of intestinal ammonia in clients with hepatic encephalopathy

6. To *obtain a stool specimen* for parasitologic examination
7. To *accelerate excretion of parasites* after anthelmintic drugs have been administered

## CONTRAINDICATIONS FOR USE

Laxatives and cathartics should not be used in the presence of undiagnosed abdominal pain. The danger is that the drugs may cause an inflamed organ (*e.g.*, the appendix) to rupture and spill GI contents into the abdominal cavity with subsequent peritonitis, a life-threatening situation. The drugs also are contraindicated with intestinal obstruction and fecal impaction.

## *Nursing Process*

### Assessment

Assess clients for current or potential constipation.
- Identify risk factors:
  - Diet with minimal fiber (*i.e.*, small amounts of fruits, vegetables, and whole-grain products)
  - Low fluid intake (*e.g.*, less than 2000 ml daily)
  - Immobility or limited activity
  - Drug therapy with central nervous system depressant drugs (*e.g.*, narcotic analgesics), anticholinergics, and others that reduce intestinal motility. Overuse of antidiarrheal agents also may cause constipation.
  - Hemorrhoids, anal fissures, or other conditions characterized by painful bowel elimination
  - Elderly or debilitated clients
- Signs and symptoms include the following:
  - Decreased number and frequency of stools
  - Passage of dry, hard stools
  - Abdominal distention and discomfort
  - Flatulence

### Nursing diagnoses

- Constipation related to decreased activity, inadequate dietary fiber, inadequate fluid intake, drugs, or disease processes
- Pain (abdominal cramping and distention) related to constipation or use of laxatives
- Impaired Tissue Integrity: Loss of normal bowel function related to overuse of laxatives
- Noncompliance with recommendations for nondrug measures to prevent or treat constipation
- Noncompliance with instructions for appropriate use of laxatives
- High Risk for Fluid Volume Deficit related to diarrhea from frequent or large doses of laxatives
- High Risk for Altered Nutrition: Poor absorption of nutrients during laxative-induced diarrhea
- High Risk for Injury: Falls from weakness induced by vigorous bowel cleansing prior to GI surgery or diagnostic tests
- Knowledge Deficit: Nondrug measures to prevent constipation
- Knowledge Deficit: Appropriate use of laxatives

## Planning/Goals

*The client will:*

- Take laxative drugs appropriately
- Use nondrug measures to promote normal bowel function and prevent constipation
- Regain normal patterns of bowel elimination
- Avoid excessive losses of fluids and electrolytes from laxative use
- Be protected from excessive fluid loss, hypotension, and other adverse drug effects, when possible
- Be assisted to avoid constipation when at risk (*i.e.*, has illness or injury that prevents activity, food and fluid intake; has medically prescribed drugs that decrease GI function)
- Be assisted as needed to prevent falls and other injuries when weak from vigorous bowel cleansing prior to surgery or diagnostic tests

## Interventions

When not contraindicated by the client's condition, assist clients with constipation to:

- Increase activity and exercise
- Increase intake of dietary fiber (vegetables, fruits, cereal grains)
- Drink at least 2000 ml of fluid daily
- Establish and maintain a routine for bowel elimination (*e.g.*, going to the bathroom immediately after breakfast)

Monitor client responses:

- Record number, amount, and type of bowel movements.
- For clients who become weak from laxatives and enemas, assist in ambulation or other activities.
- Record vital signs. Hypotension and weak pulse may indicate fluid volume deficit.

*Teach clients:*

- That diet, exercise, and fluid intake influence the frequency and type of bowel movements
- Nondrug measures to promote normal bowel function and prevent constipation:
    - Eat foods high in dietary fiber daily. Fiber is the portion of plant food that is not digested. It is contained in fruits, vegetables, and whole-grain cereals and breads. Bran, the outer coating of cereal grains, such as wheat or oats, is an excellent source of dietary fiber and is available in numerous cereal products.
    - Drink at least 6 to 10 glasses (8 oz each) of fluid daily if not contraindicated.
    - Exercise regularly. Walking and other activities aid movement of feces through the bowel.
    - Establish regular bowel habits. The defecation urge is usually strongest after eating or drinking. This knowledge may help to establish a regular time for defecation. The defecation reflex is weakened or lost if repeatedly ignored. The place chosen for defecation should allow adequate privacy.
- To avoid regular use of self-prescribed laxatives because it may prevent normal bowel function, cause adverse drug reactions, and delay treatment for conditions that cause constipation
- *Never* to take laxatives when acute abdominal pain is present. Doing so may cause a ruptured appendix or other serious complication.

- That 2 to 3 days of normal eating are required to reestablish the fecal column after a strong oral laxative has been taken
- That frequent use of strong oral laxatives promotes laxative dependence
- That bulk-forming laxatives act the same way as increasing fiber in the diet and are usually best for long-term use. When taken daily, these drugs are effective in preventing constipation, but they are not effective in relieving acute constipation.

## Evaluation

- Observe and interview for improved patterns of bowel elimination.
- Observe for use of nondrug measures to promote bowel function.
- Observe for appropriate use of laxatives.
- Observe and interview regarding adverse effects of laxatives.

# Principles of therapy

## DRUG SELECTION

Choice of a laxative or cathartic depends on the reason for use and the client's condition.

1. For long-term use of laxatives or cathartics in clients who are elderly, unable or unwilling to eat an adequate diet, or debilitated, bulk-forming laxatives (*e.g.*, Metamucil, Effersyllium) usually are preferred. However, because obstruction may occur, these agents should not be given to clients with dysphagia, adhesions or strictures in the GI tract, or to those who are unable or unwilling to drink adequate fluids.
2. For clients in whom straining is potentially harmful or painful, stool softeners (*e.g.*, docusate sodium [Colace]) are agents of choice.
3. For occasional use to cleanse the bowel for endoscopic or radiologic examinations, saline or stimulant cathartics are acceptable (*e.g.*, magnesium citrate, polyethylene glycol-electrolyte solution, castor oil, bisacodyl [Dulcolax]). These drugs should not be used more than once per week. Frequent use is likely to produce laxative abuse.
4. Oral use of mineral oil may cause potentially serious adverse effects (decreased absorption of fat-soluble vitamins and some drugs, lipid pneumonia if aspirated into the lungs). Thus, mineral oil is not an oral laxative of choice in any condition, although occasional use in the alert client is unlikely to be harmful. Mineral oil is probably most useful as a retention enema to soften hard, dry feces and aid in their expulsion. Mineral oil should not be used regularly.

5. In fecal impaction, a rectal suppository (*e.g.*, bisacodyl) or an enema (*e.g.*, oil retention or Fleet enema) is preferred. Oral laxatives are contraindicated when fecal impaction is present but may be given after the rectal mass is removed. Once the impaction is relieved, measures should be taken to prevent recurrence. If dietary and other nonpharmacologic measures are ineffective or contraindicated, use of a bulk-forming agent daily or another laxative once or twice weekly may be necessary.

6. Saline cathartics containing magnesium, phosphate, or potassium salts are contraindicated in clients with renal failure because hypermagnesemia, hyperphosphatemia, or hyperkalemia may occur.

7. Saline cathartics containing sodium salts are contraindicated in clients with edema or congestive heart failure because enough sodium may be absorbed to cause further fluid retention and edema. They also should not be used in clients with impaired renal function or those following a sodium-restricted diet for hypertension.

8. Polyethylene glycol-electrolyte solution is formulated for rapid and effective bowel cleansing without significant changes in water or electrolyte balance.

## USE IN CHILDREN

As in adults, increasing fluids, high-fiber foods, and exercise is preferred when possible. For acute constipation, glycerin suppositories are often effective in infants and small children. Stool softeners may be given to older children. Children generally should not use strong, stimulant laxatives. Parents should be advised not to use any laxative more than once a week without consulting a health-care provider.

## USE IN OLDER ADULTS

Constipation is a common problem in older adults, and laxatives are often used or overused. Nondrug measures to prevent constipation (*e.g.*, increasing fluids, high-fiber foods, and exercise) are much preferred to laxatives. If a laxative is required on a regular basis, a psyllium compound (*e.g.*, Metamucil) is best because it is most physiologic in its action. If taken, it should be accompanied by a full glass of fluid. There have been reports of obstruction in the GI tract when taken with insufficient fluid. Strong stimulant laxatives should generally be avoided.

---

## NURSING ACTIONS: LAXATIVES AND CATHARTICS

| *Nursing Actions* | *Rationale/Explanation* |
|---|---|
| **1. Administer accurately** | |
| **a.** Give bulk-forming laxatives with at least 8 oz of water or other fluid. Mix with fluid immediately before administration. | To prevent thickening and expansion in the GI tract with possible obstruction. These substances absorb water rapidly and solidify into a gelatinous mass. |
| **b.** With bisacodyl tablets, instruct the client to swallow the tablets without chewing and not to take them within an hour after ingesting milk or gastric antacids or while receiving cimetidine therapy. | The tablets have an enteric coating to delay dissolution until they reach the alkaline environment of the small intestine. Chewing or giving the tablets close to antacid substances or to cimetidine-treated clients causes premature dissolution and gastric irritation and results in abdominal cramping and vomiting. |
| **c.** Give saline cathartics on an empty stomach with 240 ml of fluid. | To increase effectiveness |
| **d.** Refrigerate magnesium citrate and polyethylene glycol-electrolyte solution before giving. | To increase palatability and retain potency |
| **e.** Castor oil may be chilled and followed by fruit juice or other beverage. | To increase palatability |
| **f.** Insert rectal suppositories to the length of the index finger, next to rectal mucosa. | These drugs are not effective unless they are in contact with intestinal mucosa. |

## Nursing Actions

## Rationale/Explanation

**2. Observe for therapeutic effects**

   **a.** Soft to semiliquid stool

Therapeutic effects occur in approximately 1 to 3 days with bulk-forming laxatives and stool softeners; 6 to 8 hours with bisacodyl tablets, cascara sagrada, phenolphthalein, and senna products; 15 to 60 minutes with bisacodyl and glycerin suppositories.

   **b.** Liquid to semiliquid stool

Effects occur in approximately 1 to 3 hours with saline cathartics and castor oil

   **c.** Decreased abdominal pain when used in irritable bowel syndrome or diverticulosis

   **d.** Decreased rectal pain when used in clients with hemorrhoids or anal fissures

Pain results from straining to expel hard, dry feces.

**3. Observe for adverse effects**

   **a.** Diarrhea—several liquid stools, abdominal cramping. Severe, prolonged diarrhea may cause hyponatremia, hypokalemia, dehydration, and other problems.

Diarrhea is most likely to result from strong, stimulant cathartics (*e.g.*, castor oil, bisacodyl, phenolphthalein, senna preparations) or large doses of saline cathartics (*e.g.*, milk of magnesia).

   **b.** With bulk-forming agents, impaction or obstruction

Impaction or obstruction of the gastrointestinal (GI) tract can be prevented by giving ample fluids with these agents and not giving the drugs to clients with known dysphagia or strictures anywhere in the alimentary canal.

   **c.** With saline cathartics, hypermagnesemia, hyperkalemia, fluid retention, and edema

Hypermagnesemia and hyperkalemia are more likely to occur in clients with renal insufficiency because of impaired ability to excrete magnesium and potassium. Fluid retention and edema are more likely to occur in clients with congestive heart failure or other conditions characterized by edema. Polyethylene glycol-electrolyte solution produces the least change in water and electrolyte balance.

   **d.** With mineral oil, lipid pneumonia and decreased absorption of vitamins A, D, E, and K

Lipid pneumonia can be prevented by not giving mineral oil to clients with dysphagia or impaired consciousness. Decreased absorption of fat-soluble vitamins can be prevented by not giving mineral oil with or shortly after meals or for longer than 2 weeks.

**4. Observe for drug interactions**

   **a.** Drugs that *increase* effects of laxatives and cathartics:

      Cholinergics (*e.g.*, dexpanthenol [Ilopan])

Additive stimulation of intestinal motility. There is probably no reason to use such a combination.

   **b.** Drugs that *decrease* effects of laxatives and cathartics:

      (1) Anticholinergic drugs (*e.g.*, atropine) and other drugs with anticholinergic properties (*e.g.*, phenothiazine antipsychotic drugs, tricyclic antidepressants, some antihistamines, and antiparkinsonism drugs)

These drugs slow intestinal motility. Clients receiving these agents are at risk for developing constipation and requiring laxatives, perhaps on a long-term basis.

      (2) Central nervous system depressants (*e.g.*, narcotic analgesics)

Narcotic analgesics commonly cause constipation.

**5. Teach clients**

   **a.** With bulk-forming laxatives, mix in 8 oz of fluid immediately before taking and follow with additional fluid, if able. *Never* take the drug dry.

Adequate fluid intake is essential with these drugs. GI obstruction has been reported in clients taking the drug dry or with inadequate fluid.

*(continued)*

| *Nursing Actions* | *Rationale/Explanation* |
|---|---|
| **b.** With bisacodyl tablets, swallow whole (do not crush or chew), and do not take with antacids. | The drug is a strong gastric irritant formulated to dissolve in the alkaline fluids of the small intestine. Crushing, chewing, or taking with antacids allows it to dissolve in the stomach. |
| **c.** Do not exceed recommended doses of laxatives. | To avoid adverse effects |
| **d.** Discoloration of the urine may occur with cascara sagrada, phenolphthalein, or senna preparations. | Color of the urine may be pink-red, red-violet, red-brown, or yellow-brown, depending on the acidity or alkalinity of the urine. |

## Review and Application Exercises

1. What are risk factors for developing constipation?
2. Describe nonpharmacologic strategies to prevent constipation.
3. Which type of laxative is generally the most desirable for long-term use? Which is the least desirable?
4. What are the most significant adverse effects of strong laxatives?
5. If an adult client asked you to recommend an over-the-counter laxative, what information about the client's condition would you need, and what would you recommend? Why?

## Selected References

Barnett, J. L. (1992). Approach to the patient with constipation. In W. N. Kelley (Ed.), *Textbook of internal medicine* (2nd ed.) (pp. 629–632). Philadelphia: J.B. Lippincott.

Beare, G., & Myers, J. L. (Eds.) (1990). *Principles and practice of adult health nursing.* St. Louis: C.V. Mosby.

Collins, A., & Bullock, B. L. (1992). Alterations in gastrointestinal function. In B. L. Bullock & P. P. Rosendahl (Eds.), *Pathophysiology: Adaptations and alterations in function* (3rd ed.) (pp. 787–807). Philadelphia: J.B. Lippincott.

(1994). *Drug facts and comparisons.* St. Louis: Facts and Comparisons.

Gerlach, M. J., McDermott, M. M., Burrell, L. O., Lukens, L., McCall, C. Y., Walters, N. G., & Lillis, P. P. (1992). Nursing management of adults with common problems of the gastrointestinal system. In L. O. Burrell (Ed.), *Adult nursing in hospital and community settings* (pp. 1320–1378). Norwalk, CT: Appleton & Lange.

Jinks, M. J., & Fuerst, R. H. (1992). Geriatric therapy. In M. A. Koda-Kimble & L. Y. Young (Eds.), *Applied therapeutics: The clinical use of drugs* (5th ed.) (pp. 79-1–79-19). Vancouver, WA: Applied Therapeutics.

Porth, C. M. (1990). *Pathophysiology: Concepts of altered health states* (3rd ed.) (pp. 697–718). Philadelphia: J.B. Lippincott.

### CHAPTER 65

# Antidiarrheals

## Description

Antidiarrheal drugs are used to treat diarrhea, defined as the frequent expulsion of liquid or semiliquid stools. Diarrhea is a symptom of numerous conditions that increase bowel motility, cause secretion or retention of fluids in the intestinal lumen, and cause inflammation or irritation of the gastrointestinal (GI) tract. As a result, bowel contents are rapidly propelled toward the rectum, and absorption of fluids and electrolytes is limited. Some causes of diarrhea include the following:

1. Excessive use of laxatives
2. Intestinal infections with viruses, bacteria, or protozoa. A common source of infection is ingestion of food or fluid contaminated by *Salmonella, Shigella*, or *Staphylococcus* microorganisms. So-called travelers' diarrhea is usually caused by an enteropathogenic strain of *Escherichia coli*.
3. Undigested, coarse, or highly spiced food in the GI tract. The food acts as an irritant and attracts fluids in a defensive attempt to dilute the irritating agent. This may result from inadequate chewing of food or lack of digestive enzymes.
4. Lack of digestive enzymes. Deficiency of pancreatic enzymes inhibits digestion and absorption of carbohydrates, proteins, and fats. Deficiency of lactase, a sugar-splitting intestinal enzyme, inhibits digestion of milk and milk products.
5. Inflammatory bowel disorders, such as gastroenteritis, diverticulitis, ulcerative colitis, and regional enteritis (Crohn's disease). In these disorders, the inflamed mucous membrane secretes large amounts of fluids into the intestinal lumen. In addition, when the ileum is diseased or a portion is surgically excised, large amounts of bile salts reach the colon, where they act as cathartics and cause diarrhea. Bile salts are normally reabsorbed from the ileum.

6. Drug therapy. Many oral drugs may irritate the GI tract and cause diarrhea. Antibacterial drugs often do so. Antibacterial drugs also may cause diarrhea by altering the normal bacterial flora in the intestine.

Pseudomembranous colitis is a serious condition that results from oral or parenteral antibiotic therapy. By suppressing normal flora, antibiotics allow anaerobic *Clostridium difficile* to proliferate. The organisms produce a toxin that causes fever, abdominal pain, inflammatory lesions of the colon, and severe diarrhea with stools containing mucus, pus, and sometimes blood. Symptoms may develop within a few days or several weeks after the causative antibiotic is discontinued. Pseudomembranous colitis is more often associated with ampicillin, cephalosporins, and clindamycin but may occur with any antibacterial drug that alters intestinal microbial flora.

7. Intestinal neoplasms. Tumors may increase intestinal motility by occupying space and stretching the intestinal wall. Diarrhea sometimes alternates with constipation in colon cancer.
8. Functional disorders. Diarrhea may be a symptom of stress or anxiety in some clients. No organic disease process can be found in such circumstances.
9. Hyperthyroidism. This condition increases bowel motility.
10. Surgical excision or bypass of portions of the intes-

Anne Collins Abrams: CLINICAL DRUG THERAPY, Fourth Edition.
© 1995 J.B. Lippincott Company.

tine, especially the small intestine. Such procedures decrease the absorptive area and increase fluidity of stools.

Diarrhea may be acute or chronic and mild or severe. Most episodes of acute diarrhea are defensive mechanisms by which the body tries to rid itself of irritants, toxins, and infectious agents. These are usually self-limiting and subside within 24 to 48 hours without serious consequences. If severe or prolonged, acute diarrhea may lead to serious fluid and electrolyte depletion, especially in young children and elderly adults. Chronic diarrhea may cause malnutrition and anemia and is often characterized by remissions and exacerbations.

## ANTIDIARRHEAL DRUGS

Antidiarrheal drugs include a variety of agents, most of which are discussed in other chapters. When used for treatment of diarrhea, the drugs may be given to relieve the symptom (nonspecific therapy) or the underlying cause of the symptom (specific therapy). Individual drugs are listed in Table 65-1.

## Nonspecific therapy

For symptomatic treatment of diarrhea, opiates and opiate derivatives (see Chap. 5) are the most effective. These drugs decrease diarrhea by slowing propulsive movements in the small and large intestines. Morphine, codeine, and related drugs are effective in relieving diarrhea but are rarely used for this purpose because of their potentially serious adverse effects. Although paregoric is occasionally useful, other opiates have largely been replaced by the synthetic drugs diphenoxylate, loperamide, and difenoxin, which are used only for treatment of diarrhea and do not cause morphine-like adverse effects in recommended doses.

Other nonspecific agents sometimes used in diarrhea are anticholinergics (see Chap. 21), polycarbophil and psyllium preparations (see Chap. 64), and adsorbent–demulcent products. Anticholinergic drugs, of which atropine is the prototype, are infrequently used because doses large enough to decrease intestinal motility and secretions cause intolerable adverse effects. The drugs are occasionally used to decrease abdominal cramping and pain (antispasmodic effects) associated with acute nonspecific diarrhea and chronic diarrhea associated with inflammatory bowel disease.

Psyllium preparations (*e.g.*, Metamucil) are most often used as bulk-forming laxatives. They are occasionally used in diarrhea to decrease fluidity of stools. The preparations absorb large amounts of water and produce stools of gelatin-like consistency.

Bismuth salts have antibacterial and antiviral activity;

bismuth subsalicylate (Pepto-Bismol, a commonly used over-the-counter drug) also has antisecretory and possibly anti-inflammatory effects attributed to the salicylate component.

Adsorbent–demulcent products include kaolin–pectin preparations. Kaolin is a form of clay that occurs naturally as hydrated aluminum silicate. Pectin is a carbohydrate product obtained from apples and rinds of citrus fruits. Although widely used, there is no reliable evidence that these agents have therapeutic effects in diarrhea. Further, they may adsorb nutrients and other drugs, including antidiarrheal agents if given concurrently.

## Specific therapy

Specific drug therapy for diarrhea depends on the cause of the symptom and may include the use of antibacterial, enzymatic, and bile salt-binding drugs. Antibacterial drugs are recommended for use only in carefully selected cases of bacterial enteritis. Although effective in preventing travelers' diarrhea, antibiotics are generally not recommended because their use may promote the emergence of drug-resistant microorganisms. Although effective in reducing diarrhea due to *Salmonella* and *E. coli* intestinal infections, antibiotics may induce a prolonged carrier state during which the infection can be transmitted to other people.

## INDICATIONS FOR USE

Despite the limitations of drug therapy in prevention and treatment of diarrhea, antidiarrheal drugs are generally indicated in the following circumstances:

1. Severe or prolonged diarrhea (more than 2–3 days), to prevent severe fluid and electrolyte loss
2. Relatively severe diarrhea in young children and elderly adults. These groups are less able to adapt to fluid and electrolyte losses.
3. In chronic inflammatory diseases of the bowel (ulcerative colitis and Crohn's disease), to allow a more nearly normal life-style. Ulcerative colitis also is treated with adrenal corticosteroids and poorly absorbed sulfonamides.
4. In ileostomies or surgical excision of portions of the ileum, to decrease fluidity and volume of stool
5. When specific causes of diarrhea have been determined

## CONTRAINDICATIONS FOR USE

Contraindications for the use of antidiarrheal agents include diarrhea caused by toxic materials, microorganisms that penetrate intestinal mucosa (*e.g.*, pathogenic *E. coli*, *Salmonella*, *Shigella*), or pseudomembranous colitis caused by broad-spectrum antibiotic therapy. In

# TABLE 65-1. ANTIDIARRHEAL DRUGS

| Generic/Trade Name | Characteristics | Clinical Indications | Routes and Dosage Ranges | |
|---|---|---|---|---|
| | | | *Adults* | *Children* |

## Opiates and Related Drugs

| Generic/Trade Name | Characteristics | Clinical Indications | Adults | Children |
|---|---|---|---|---|
| **Camphorated tincture of opium (paregoric)** | 1. Contains 0.04% morphine, alcohol, camphor, anise oil, and benzoic acid<br>2. Antidiarrheal activity is caused by morphine content. Morphine slows propulsive movements in small and large intestines.<br>3. Under Controlled Substances Act, a Schedule III drug when used alone and a Schedule V drug in the small amounts combined with other drugs.<br>4. Recommended doses and short-term duration of administration do not produce euphoria, analgesia, or dependence. | Symptomatic treatment of acute diarrhea | PO 5–10 ml one to four times daily (maximum of four doses) until diarrhea is controlled | PO 0.25–0.5 ml/ kg one to four times daily (maximum of four doses) until diarrhea is controlled |
| **Difenoxin with atropine sulfate (Motofen)** | 1. It is the main active metabolite of diphenoxylate.<br>2. It slows intestinal motility by a local effect on the GI wall.<br>3. Overdose may cause severe respiratory depression and coma.<br>4. Each tablet contains 1 mg of difenoxin and 0.025 mg of atropine. The subtherapeutic dose of atropine is added to discourage overdose and abuse for opiate-like effects<br>5. Contraindicated in children under age 2 years, clients allergic to the ingredients, and clients with hepatic impairment.<br>6. A Schedule IV drug under the Controlled Substances Act | Symptomatic treatment of acute or chronic diarrhea | PO 2 mg initially, then 1 mg after each loose stool or 1 mg q3–4h as needed; maximum dose, 8 mg (8 tablets)/24 h | Safety and effectiveness not established for children under 12 years |
| **Diphenoxylate with atropine sulfate (Lomotil)** | 1. A derivative of meperidine (Demerol) used only for treatment of diarrhea<br>2. Most commonly prescribed antidiarrheal drug. Decreases intestinal motility.<br>3. As effective as paregoric and more convenient to administer<br>4. In recommended doses, does not produce euphoria, analgesia, or dependence. In high doses, produces morphine-like effects, including euphoria, dependence, and respiratory depression. Antidote for overdose is the narcotic antagonist naloxone (Narcan).<br>5. Each tablet or 5 ml of liquid contains 2.5 mg of diphenoxylate and 0.025 mg of atropine. The subtherapeutic dose of atropine is added to discourage drug abuse by producing unpleasant anticholinergic side effects.<br>6. Contraindicated in severe liver disease, glaucoma, and children under 2 years. Safety during pregnancy and lactation has not been established. The drug is excreted in breast milk.<br>7. A Schedule V drug under the Controlled Substances Act | Symptomatic treatment of acute or chronic diarrhea | PO 5 mg (2 tablets or 10 ml of liquid) three or four times daily; maximal daily dose, 20 mg | Liquid preparation recommended<br>Ages 8–12 years, PO 10 mg daily in five divided doses<br>Ages 5–8 years, PO 8 mg daily in four divided doses<br>Ages 2–5 years, PO 6 mg daily in three divided doses<br>Under age 2 years, contraindicated |
| **Loperamide (Imodium)** | 1. A derivative of meperidine (Demerol) used only for treatment of diarrhea<br>2. Decreases intestinal motility<br>3. Compared to diphenoxylate, loperamide is equally effective and may cause fewer adverse reactions in recommended doses. High doses may produce morphine-like effects.<br>4. Safety has not been established for use in pregnancy, lactation, and in children under age 2 years. | Symptomatic treatment of acute or chronic diarrhea | PO 4 mg initially, then 2 mg after each loose stool to a maximal daily dose of 16 mg. For chronic diarrhea, dosage should be reduced to the lowest effective amount (average 4–8 mg daily). | Ages 8–12 years, PO 6 mg daily in three divided doses (as liquid or capsule)<br>Ages 5–8 years, PO 4 mg daily in two divided doses (as liquid or capsule) |

*(continued)*

661

**TABLE 65-1. ANTIDIARRHEAL DRUGS** (*Continued*)

| Generic/ Trade Name | Characteristics | Clinical Indications | Routes and Dosage Ranges | |
|---|---|---|---|---|
| | | | *Adults* | *Children* |
| | 5. Antidote for overdose is the narcotic antagonist naloxone.<br>6. Each capsule or 10 ml of liquid contains 2 mg of loperamide. | | | Ages 2–5 years, PO 3 mg daily in three divided doses (as liquid) Under age 2 years, contrain-dicated |

*Antibacterial Agents*

| Generic/ Trade Name | Characteristics | Clinical Indications | Adults | Children |
|---|---|---|---|---|
| **Ampicillin** (Omnipen, Pen-briten, others) | A broad-spectrum penicillin | 1. Bacillary dysentery caused by sensitive strains of *Shigella*<br>2. Typhoid fever resis-tant to chloram-phenicol<br>3. Typhoid fever to elim-inate the postinfec-tive carrier state | PO, IM, 2–4 g/d, in divided doses, q6h | PO, IM, IV 50–100 mg/kg per day, in di-vided doses, q6h |
| **Chloramphenicol** (Chloromycetin) | | Typhoid fever (gastro-enteritis caused by *Salmonella typhi*) | PO, IV 50 mg/kg per day, in di-vided doses, q6h | PO 50 mg/kg per day, in divided doses, q6h |
| **Colistin sulfate** (Coly-Mycin S) | | Enteritis caused by sus-ceptible strains of *Escherichia coli* and other gram-negative bacilli resistant to less toxic antibiotics | PO 0.5 g/d in di-vided doses, q8h | 10–15 mg/kg per day, in divided doses, q8h |
| **Nalidixic acid** (NegGram) | | Bacillary dysentery caused by strains of *Shigella* that are resis-tant to other antibiotics but sensitive to nalidixic acid | PO 2–3 g/d, in divided doses, q6h | PO 55 mg/kg per day, in divided doses, q6h |
| **Neomycin** | | Same as colistin, above | PO 4 g/d in di-vided doses, q6h | PO 50–100 mg/kg per day in di-vided doses, q6h |
| **Tetracycline** | | 1. Cholera<br>2. Bacillary dysentery caused by sensitive strains of *Shigella* | PO 2 g/d in di-vided doses, q6h | PO 40 mg/kg per day in divided doses, q6h |
| **Trimethoprim-sulfamethoxazole (TMP-SMX)** (Bactrim, Septra) | | 1. Bacillary dysentery caused by suscepti-ble strains of *Shigella*<br>2. Typhoid fever resis-tant to chloram-phenicol and ampicillin<br>3. Enteritis caused by susceptible strains of *E. coli* | PO 160 mg of tri-methoprim and 800 mg of sul-famethoxazole daily, in divided doses, q12h<br>IV 8–10 mg/kg of trimethoprim and 50 mg/kg sul-famethoxazole daily, in two to four divided doses | PO 8 mg/kg of tri-methoprim and 40 mg/kg of sul-famethoxazole daily, in divided doses, q12h<br>IV 8–10 mg/kg of trimethoprim and 50 mg/kg sul-famethoxazole daily, in two to four divided doses |
| **Vancomycin** (Vancocin) | | 1. Pseudomembranous colitis due to sup-pression of normal bacterial flora by antibiotics and overgrowth of *Clostridium* organ-isms<br>2. Staphylococcal colitis due to broad-spec-trum antibiotic ther-apy, combined with parenteral nafcillin (Unipen) | PO 2 g/d in di-vided doses, q6h | PO 44 mg/kg per day in divided doses, q6h |

(*continued*)

## TABLE 65-1.   ANTIDIARRHEAL DRUGS (Continued)

| Generic/ Trade Name | Characteristics | Clinical Indications | Routes and Dosage Ranges | |
|---|---|---|---|---|
| | | | *Adults* | *Children* |
| ***Miscellaneous Drugs*** | | | | |
| **Cholestyramine** (Questran) | Binds and inactivates bile salts in the intestine | Diarrhea due to bile salts reaching the colon and causing a cathartic effect. "Bile salt diarrhea" is associated with Crohn's disease or surgical excision of the ileum. | PO 16–32 g/d in 120–180 ml of water, in two to four divided doses before or during meals and at bedtime | |
| **Colestipol** (Colestid) | Same as cholestyramine, above | Same as colestyramine | PO 15–30 g/d in 120–180 ml of water, in two to four divided doses before or during meals and at bedtime | |
| **Kaolin, pectin, atropine sulfate, hyoscyamine sulfate, hyoscine hydrobromide, alcohol** (Donnagel) | 1. Kaolin and pectin not proven effective in diarrhea; belladonna alkaloids are present in subtherapeutic amounts 2. Not recommended for use | | | |
| **Kaolin and pectin mixture** (Kaopectate) | 1. Ingredients not proven effective and mixture not recommended for use 2. Available over the counter | | | |
| **Kaolin, pectin, and paregoric** (Parepectolin) | 1. Effectiveness, if any, attributed to paregoric (3.7 ml paregoric/30 ml of preparation) 2. Schedule V drug under Controlled Substances Act 3. Not recommended for use | Possibly effective for symptomatic treatment of mild, acute diarrhea | PO 15–30 ml after each loose stool to a maximum of 8 doses/24 h | PO 2.5–10 ml after each loose stool to a maximum of 8 doses/24 h |
| **Lactobacillus** (Bacid, Lactinex) | Not proven effective and not recommended for use | | | |
| **Pancreatin or pancrelipase** (Viokase, Pancrease, Cotazym) | Pancreatic enzymes used only for replacement | Diarrhea and malabsorption due to deficiency of pancreatic enzymes | PO 1–3 tablets or capsules or 1–2 packets of powder with meals and snacks | PO 1–3 tablets or capsules or 1–2 packets of powder with each meal |
| **Psyllium preparations** (Metamucil, Effersyllium) | Absorbs water and decreases fluidity of stools | Possibly effective for symptomatic treatment of diarrhea | PO 6–10 g (1–2 tsp), two or three times daily, in a full glass of water or other fluid, mixed immediately before ingestion | |
| **Sulfasalazine** (Azulfidine) | A poorly absorbed sulfonamide | Ulcerative colitis | PO 2 g/d in four divided doses | Over age 2 months, PO 40–60 mg/kg per day in three to six divided doses initially. Maintenance, PO 30 mg/kg per day in four divided doses |

these circumstances, antidiarrheal agents that slow peristalsis may aggravate and prolong diarrhea. Opiates (morphine, codeine, paregoric) usually are contraindicated in chronic diarrhea because of possible opiate dependence. Difenoxin, diphenoxylate, and loperamide are contraindicated in children under 2 years of age.

## Nursing Process

### Assessment

Assess for acute or chronic diarrhea.
- Try to determine the duration of diarrhea; number of stools per day; amount, consistency, color, odor, and presence of

abnormal components (*e.g.*, undigested food, blood, pus, mucus) in each stool; precipitating factors; accompanying signs and symptoms (*i.e.*, nausea, vomiting, fever, abdominal pain or cramping); and measures used to relieve diarrhea. When possible, observe stool specimens.

- Try to determine the *cause* of the diarrhea. This includes questioning about causes such as chronic inflammatory diseases of the bowel, food intake, possible exposure to contaminated food, living or traveling in areas of poor sanitation, and use of laxatives or other drugs that may cause diarrhea. When available, check laboratory reports on stool specimens (*e.g.*, culture reports).
- With severe or prolonged diarrhea, especially in young children and elderly adults, assess for dehydration, hypokalemia, and other fluid and electrolyte disorders.

### Nursing diagnoses

- Diarrhea related to GI infection or inflammatory disorders, other disease processes, dietary irritants, or overuse of laxatives
- Altered Nutrition: Less than Body Requirements related to impaired absorption of nutrients with diarrhea
- Anxiety related to availability of bathroom facilities
- Body Image Disturbance with chronic diarrhea related to loss of control and possible incontinence of stool
- Social Isolation with chronic diarrhea related to frequent bowel movements
- Fluid Volume Deficit related to excessive losses in liquid stools
- Pain (abdominal cramping) related to intestinal hypermotility and spasm
- Impaired Tissue Integrity: Perianal skin excoriation related to irritants in liquid stools
- High Risk for Self-Care Deficit related to weakness
- High Risk for Constipation related to use of antidiarrheal drugs
- Knowledge Deficit: Factors that cause or aggravate diarrhea
- Knowledge Deficit: Appropriate use of antidiarrheal drugs

### Planning/Goals

*The client will:*
- Take antidiarrheal drugs appropriately
- Obtain relief from acute diarrhea (reduced number of liquid stools, reduced abdominal discomfort)
- Maintain fluid and electrolyte balance
- Maintain adequate nutritional intake
- Be assisted when weak from diarrhea
- Avoid adverse effects of antidiarrheal medications
- Reestablish normal bowel patterns after an episode of acute diarrhea
- Have fewer liquid stools with chronic diarrhea

### Interventions

Use measures to prevent diarrhea:
- Prepare and store food properly and avoid improperly stored foods and those prepared under unsanitary conditions. Dairy products, cream pies, and other foods may cause diarrhea ("food poisoning") if not refrigerated.
- Wash hands before handling any foods, after handling raw poultry or meat, and always before eating.
- Chew food well.
- Do not overuse laxatives (*i.e.*, amount per dose or frequency of use). Many commonly used over-the-counter products contain phenolphthalein, a strong stimulant laxative.

Whether or not antidiarrheal drugs are used, supportive therapy is required for the treatment of diarrhea. Elements of supportive care include the following:

- Replacement of fluids and electrolytes. If diarrhea is not severe, fluids such as weak tea, water, bouillon, clear soup, and gelatin may be sufficient. If diarrhea is severe or prolonged, intravenous fluids may be needed (*i.e.*, solutions containing dextrose, sodium chloride, and potassium chloride). Also, oral intake may be restricted to decrease bowel stimulation.
- Avoid foods and fluids that may further irritate GI mucosa (*e.g.*, highly spiced foods or "laxative" foods, such as raw fruits and vegetables).
- Increase frequency and length of rest periods, and decrease activity. Exercise and activity stimulate peristalsis.
- If perianal irritation occurs because of frequent liquid stools, cleanse the area with mild soap and water after each bowel movement, then apply an emollient, such as white petrolatum (Vaseline).

*Teach clients:*
- To maintain a fluid intake of 2 to 3 quarts daily. This will help prevent dehydration from fluid loss in stools. Clear broths and noncarbonated, caffeine-free beverages are recommended because they are unlikely to cause further diarrhea.
- To avoid highly spiced or "laxative" foods, such as fresh fruits and vegetables, until diarrhea is controlled and peristaltic movements have returned to normal
- Measures to prevent diarrhea (*e.g.*, frequent and thorough handwashing, careful food storage and preparation)
- To consult a health-care provider if diarrhea is accompanied by severe abdominal pain or fever

### Evaluation

- Observe and interview for decreased number of liquid or loose stools.
- Observe for signs of adequate food and fluid intake (*e.g.*, good skin turgor and urine output, stable weight).
- Observe for appropriate use of antidiarrheal drugs.
- Observe and interview for return of prediarrheal patterns of bowel elimination.
- Interview regarding knowledge and use of measures to prevent or minimize diarrhea.

## Principles of therapy

### DRUG SELECTION

Choice of antidiarrheal agent depends largely on the cause, severity, and duration of diarrhea.

1. For symptomatic treatment of diarrhea, difenoxin with atropine (Motofen), diphenoxylate with atropine (Lomotil), or loperamide (Imodium) is probably the drug of choice for most people.
2. In bacterial gastroenteritis or diarrhea, choice of antibacterial drug depends on the causative microorganism and susceptibility tests.

3. In ulcerative colitis, sulfonamides and adrenal corticosteroids are the drugs of choice.

4. In pseudomembranous colitis, stopping the causative drug is the initial treatment. If symptoms do not improve, oral metronidazole or vancomycin is given for 7 to 10 days. Both are effective against *C. difficile*, but metronidazole is much less expensive. Vancomycin may be the first drug of choice for severe disease. For about 6 weeks following recovery, relapse often occurs and requires retreatment. Because relapse is not due to emergence of drug-resistant strains, the same drug used for the initial bout may be used to treat the relapse.

5. In diarrhea caused by enzyme deficiency, pancreatic enzymes are given rather than antidiarrheal drugs.

6. In bile salt diarrhea, cholestyramine (Questran) is the drug of choice. Colestipol (Colestid), a similar drug, is probably effective also.

7. Although morphine and codeine are contraindicated in chronic diarrhea, they may occasionally be used in the treatment of acute, severe diarrhea. Dosages required for antidiarrheal effects are smaller than those required for analgesia. The following oral drugs and dosages are approximately equivalent in antidiarrheal effectiveness: 4 mg morphine, 30 mg codeine, 10 ml paregoric, 5 mg diphenoxylate, and 2 mg loperamide.

## USE IN CHILDREN

Antidiarrheal drugs, including antibiotics, are often used in children to prevent excessive losses of fluids and electrolytes. Small children especially may rapidly develop fluid volume deficit with diarrhea. Drug therapy should be accompanied by appropriate fluid replacement and efforts to decrease further stimuli.

**Difenoxin** and **Diphenoxylate** contain atropine, and signs of atropine overdose may occur with usual doses. Difenoxin, diphenoxylate, and **loperamide** are contraindicated in children younger than 2 years. Loperamide is a nonprescription drug. See Table 65-1 for doses.

## USE IN OLDER ADULTS

Diarrhea is less common than constipation in older adults, but it may occur from laxative abuse and bowel cleansing procedures before GI surgery or diagnostic tests. With diarrhea, older adults may rapidly develop fluid volume deficits. General principles of fluid and electrolyte replacement, measures to decrease GI irritants, and drug therapy apply as for younger adults. Most antidiarrheal drugs may be given to older adults, but cautious use is indicated to avoid inducing constipation.

## NURSING ACTIONS: ANTIDIARRHEALS

| *Nursing Actions* | *Rationale/Explanation* |
|---|---|
| **1. Administer accurately**<br>**a.** With liquid diphenoxylate, use only the calibrated dropper furnished by the manufacturer for measuring dosage. | For accurate measurement |
| **b.** Add at least 30 ml of water to each dose of paregoric. The mixture appears milky. | To add sufficient volume for the drug to reach the stomach |
| **c.** Do not exceed maximal daily doses of diphenoxylate, loperamide, difenoxin, and paregoric. Also, stop the drugs when diarrhea is controlled. | To decrease risks of adverse reactions, including drug dependence |
| **d.** Give cholestyramine and colestipol with at least 120 ml of water. Also, do not give within approximately 4 hours of other drugs. | The drugs may cause obstruction of the gastrointestinal (GI) tract if swallowed in a dry state. They may combine with and inactivate other drugs. |
| **2. Observe for therapeutic effects**<br>**a.** Decreased number, frequency, and fluidity of stools | Therapeutic effects are usually evident within 24 to 48 hours. |
| **b.** Decreased or absent abdominal cramping pains | |
| **c.** Signs of normal fluid and electrolyte balance (adequate hydration, urine output, and skin turgor) | |
| **d.** Resumption of usual activities of daily living | |

*(continued)*

| *Nursing Actions* | *Rationale/Explanation* |
|---|---|
| **3. Observe for adverse effects**<br>  **a.** Constipation | Constipation is the most common adverse effect. It can be prevented by using antidiarrheal drugs only as prescribed and stopping the drugs when diarrhea is controlled. |
|   **b.** Drug dependence | Dependence is unlikely with recommended doses but may occur with long-term use of large doses of paregoric, diphenoxylate, and probably loperamide. |
|   **c.** With diphenoxylate, anorexia, nausea, vomiting, dizziness, abdominal discomfort, paralytic ileus, toxic megacolon, hypersensitivity (pruritus, urticaria, angioneurotic edema), headache, tachycardia | Although numerous adverse reactions have been reported, their incidence and severity are low when diphenoxylate is used appropriately. |
|     With overdoses of a diphenoxylate-atropine or difenoxin-atropine combination, respiratory depression and coma may result from diphenoxylate or difenoxin content and anticholinergic effects (*e.g.*, dry mouth, blurred vision, urinary retention) from atropine content | Deliberate overdose and abuse are unlikely because of unpleasant anticholinergic effects. Overdose can be prevented by using the drug in recommended doses and only when required. Overdose can be treated with naloxone (Narcan) and supportive therapy. |
|   **d.** With loperamide, abdominal cramps, dry mouth, dizziness, nausea and vomiting | Abdominal cramps are the most common adverse effect. No serious adverse effects have been reported with recommended doses of loperamide. Overdose may be treated with naloxone, gastric lavage, and administration of activated charcoal. |
|   **e.** With cholestyramine and colestipol, constipation, nausea, abdominal distention | Adverse effects are usually minor and transient because these drugs are not absorbed from the GI tract. |
| **4. Observe for drug interactions** | Few clinically significant drug interactions have been reported with commonly used antidiarrheal agents. |
|   Drugs that *increase* effects of antidiarrheal agents: | |
|     (1) Central nervous system (CNS) depressants (alcohol, sedative-hypnotics, narcotic analgesics, antianxiety agents, antipsychotic agents) | Additive CNS depression with opiate and related antidiarrheals. Narcotic analgesics have additive constipating effects. |
|     (2) Anticholinergic agents (atropine and synthetic anticholinergic antispasmodics; antihistamines and antidepressants with anticholinergic effects) | Additive anticholinergic adverse effects (dry mouth, blurred vision, urinary retention) with diphenoxylate-atropine (Lomotil) and difenoxin-atropine (Motofen) |
| **5. Teach clients**<br>  **a.** Take antidiarrheal drugs only as prescribed, and stop them when diarrhea is controlled. | To avoid adverse effects |
|   **b.** Report to the physician if diarrhea persists longer than 3 days, if stools contain blood or mucus, and if fever or abdominal pain develops. | These signs and symptoms may indicate more serious disorders for which other treatment measures are needed. |

## Review and Application Exercises

1. What are some common causes of diarrhea?
2. In which patient populations is diarrhea most likely to cause serious problems?
3. Which types of diarrhea do not require antidiarrheal drug therapy and why?
4. How do antidiarrheal drugs decrease frequency or fluidity of stools?
5. What are adverse effects of commonly used antidiarrheal drugs?
6. If a client asked you to recommend an over-the-counter antidiarrheal agent, which would you recommend and why?
7. Would your recommendation differ if the proposed recipient were a child? Why or why not?

## Selected References

Beare, G., & Myers, J. L. (Eds.) (1990). *Principles and practice of adult health nursing*. St. Louis: C.V. Mosby.

Collins, A., & Bullock, B. L. (1992). Alterations in gastrointestinal function. In B. L. Bullock & P. P. Rosendahl (Eds.), *Pathophysiology: Adaptations and alterations in function* (3rd ed.) (pp. 787–807). Philadelphia: J.B. Lippincott.

Danziger, L. H., Itokazu, G. S., & Gross, M. H. (1992). Gastrointestinal infection. In M. A. Koda-Kimble & L. Y. Young (Eds.), *Applied therapeutics: The clinical use of drugs* (5th ed.) (pp. 40-1–40-11). Vancouver, WA: Applied Therapeutics.

(1994). *Drug facts and comparisons*. St. Louis: Facts and Comparisons.

Gerlach, M. J., McDermott, M. M., Burrell, L. O., Lukens, L., McCall, C. Y., Walters, N. G., & Lillis, P. P. (1992). Nursing management of adults with common problems of the gastrointestinal system. In L. O. Burrell (Ed.), *Adult nursing in hospital and community settings* (pp. 1320–1378). Norwalk, CT: Appleton & Lange.

George, W. L., & Finegold, S. M. (1992). Clostridial infections. In W. N. Kelley (Ed.), *Textbook of internal medicine* (2nd ed.) (pp. 1415–1419). Philadelphia: J.B. Lippincott.

Plaut, A. G. (1992). Gastrointestinal infections. In W. N. Kelley (Ed.), *Textbook of internal medicine* (2nd ed.) (pp. 508–514). Philadelphia: J.B. Lippincott.

Porth, C. M. (1990). *Pathophysiology: Concepts of altered health states* (3rd ed.) (pp. 697–718). Philadelphia: J.B. Lippincott.

Powell, D. W. (1992). Approach to the patient with diarrhea. In W. N. Kelley (Ed.). *Textbook of internal medicine* (2nd ed.) (pp. 618–628). Philadelphia: J.B. Lippincott.

### CHAPTER 66

# Antiemetics

## Nausea and vomiting

Antiemetic drugs are used to prevent or treat nausea and vomiting. *Nausea* is an unpleasant sensation of abdominal discomfort accompanied by a desire to vomit. *Vomiting* is the expulsion of stomach contents through the mouth. Nausea may occur without vomiting and vomiting may occur without prior nausea, but the two symptoms most often occur together.

Nausea and vomiting are common symptoms experienced by virtually everyone. These symptoms may accompany almost any illness or stress situation. Causes of nausea and vomiting include the following:

1. Systemic illness or infection
2. Gastrointestinal (GI) infection or inflammation (*e.g.*, any portion of the GI tract, liver, gallbladder, or pancreas)
3. Impaired GI motility and muscle tone (*e.g.*, gastroparesis)
4. Overeating or ingestion of foods or fluids that irritate the GI mucosa
5. Drug therapy. Nausea and vomiting are the most common adverse reactions to drug therapy. Although the symptoms may occur with most drugs, they are especially associated with alcohol, aspirin, anticancer drugs, estrogen preparations, narcotic analgesics, antibiotics, and digitalis preparations.
6. Pain and other noxious stimuli, such as unpleasant sights and odors
7. Emotional disturbances, physical or mental stress
8. Radiation therapy
9. Motion sickness

Vomiting occurs when the vomiting center in the medulla oblongata is stimulated. Stimuli may be relayed to the vomiting center from peripheral (*e.g.*, gastric mucosa, peritoneum, intestines, joints) and central (*e.g.*, cerebral cortex, vestibular apparatus of the ear, and neurons in the fourth ventricle, called the *chemoreceptor trigger zone* or CTZ) sites. The CTZ contains dopamine, opiate, and serotonin receptors, which are thought to be stimulated by emetogenic drugs and toxins circulating in blood and cerebrospinal fluid. Acetylcholine also stimulates the vomiting center. In motion sickness, rapid changes in body motion stimulate receptors in the inner ear (vestibular branch of the auditory nerve, which is concerned with equilibrium), and nerve impulses are transmitted to the CTZ and the vomiting center.

When stimulated, the vomiting center initiates efferent impulses that cause closure of the glottis, contraction of abdominal muscles and the diaphragm, relaxation of the gastroesophageal sphincter, and reverse peristalsis, which moves stomach contents toward the mouth for ejection.

## Antiemetic drugs

Drugs used in nausea and vomiting belong to several different therapeutic classifications, and most have anticholinergic, antidopaminergic, or antihistaminic effects. The drugs are generally more effective in prophylaxis than treatment. Most antiemetics prevent or relieve nausea and vomiting by acting on the vomiting center, CTZ, cerebral cortex, vestibular apparatus, or a combina-

Anne Collins Abrams: CLINICAL DRUG THERAPY, Fourth Edition.
© 1995 J.B. Lippincott Company.

tion of these. Major drugs are described below and in Table 66-1.

## PHENOTHIAZINES

Phenothiazines, of which chlorpromazine (Thorazine) is the prototype, are central nervous system depressants used primarily in the treatment of psychosis and psychotic symptoms in other disorders (see Chap. 9). These drugs have widespread effects on the body. Their therapeutic effects in psychosis and vomiting are attributed to their ability to block dopamine from receptor sites in the brain (antidopaminergic effects). When used as antiemetics, phenothiazines act on the CTZ and the vomiting center. Not all phenothiazines are effective antiemetics.

Phenothiazines are usually effective in preventing or treating nausea and vomiting induced by drugs, radiation therapy, surgery, and most other stimuli but are generally ineffective in motion sickness. Drowsiness usually occurs with these drugs.

## ANTIHISTAMINES

Antihistamines (*e.g.*, hydroxyzine [Vistaril]) are used primarily to prevent histamine from exerting its widespread effects on body tissues (see Chap. 51). Antihistamines used as antiemetic agents are the "classic" antihistamines or H₁ receptor blocking agents (as differentiated from cimetidine [Tagamet] and related drugs, which are H₂ receptor blocking agents). The drugs are thought to relieve nausea and vomiting by blocking the action of acetylcholine in the brain (anticholinergic effects). Antihistamines are especially effective in preventing and treating motion sickness. Not all antihistamines are effective as antiemetic agents.

## CORTICOSTEROIDS

Although corticosteroids are used mainly as antiallergic, anti-inflammatory, and antistress agents (see Chap. 24), dexamethasone (Decadron) and methylprednisolone (Medrol) reportedly have antiemetic effects as well. The mechanism by which the drugs exert antiemetic effects is unknown. Although not Food and Drug Administration-approved for this purpose, they are used in the management of chemotherapy-induced emesis, usually in combination with one or more other antiemetic agents. Regimens vary from a single dose before chemotherapy to doses every 4 to 6 hours for 24 to 48 hours. With this short-term usage, adverse effects are mild (*e.g.*, euphoria, insomnia, mild fluid retention). Dexamethasone is most commonly used, in doses of 10 to 20 mg.

## BENZODIAZEPINE ANTIANXIETY DRUGS

These drugs (see Chap. 8) are not antiemetics, but they are often used in multidrug regimens to prevent nausea and vomiting associated with cancer chemotherapy. They produce sedation and relaxation, especially in clients who experience anticipatory nausea and vomiting prior to administration of anticancer drugs. Lorazepam (Ativan) is commonly used.

## MISCELLANEOUS ANTIEMETICS

Miscellaneous antiemetics include several drugs with varied mechanisms of action, as listed below.

**Benzquinamide** (Emete-Con) apparently acts on the CTZ.

**Cisapride** (Propulsid) is a prokinetic drug structurally related to metoclopramide (Reglan). Prokinetic agents increase gastrointestinal motility and the rate of gastric emptying by increasing the release of acetylcholine from nerve endings in the GI tract (peripheral cholinergic effects). As a result, they can decrease nausea and vomiting associated with gastroparesis and other nonobstructive disorders characterized by gastric retention of food and fluids. Cisapride lacks the antidopaminergic activity of metoclopramide and therefore does not have direct antiemetic effects in the brain and does not cause extrapyramidal effects. Cisapride is well absorbed following oral administration, and the presence of food increases the rate and extent of absorption. Extensive first-pass hepatic metabolism occurs. Peak plasma levels occur in 1 to 2 hours. The drug is 98% protein bound and widely distributed in body tissues. It is eliminated about 50% in urine and 50% in feces. Cisapride reportedly causes fewer adverse effects than metoclopramide but may cause diarrhea.

**Diphenidol** (Vontrol) is thought to act on the vestibular apparatus of the inner ear.

**Dronabinol** (Marinol) is a cannabinoid (derivative of marijuana) used in the management of nausea and vomiting associated with anticancer drugs and unrelieved by other drugs. Dronabinol may cause the same adverse effects as marijuana, including psychiatric symptoms, and has a high potential for abuse. As a result, it is a Schedule II drug under federal narcotic laws.

**Droperidol** (Inapsine) is a butyrophenone related to the antipsychotic drug haloperidol (Haldol). It is often used in combination with fentanyl, a narcotic analgesic, for neuroleptanalgesia. The combination product (Innovar) is usually administered by anesthesiologists, but droperidol may be used alone to prevent nausea and vomiting during surgical or diagnostic procedures. Droperidol may be given preoperatively or during surgery for induction and maintenance of anesthesia.

**Metoclopramide** has central and peripheral anti-

## TABLE 66-1. ANTIEMETIC DRUGS

| Generic/Trade Name | Routes and Dosage Ranges | |
| --- | --- | --- |
| | **Adults** | **Children** |
| **Phenothiazines** | | |
| **Chlorpromazine** (Thorazine) | PO 10–25 mg q4–6h<br>IM 25 mg q3–4h until vomiting stops, followed by oral administration if necessary<br>Rectal suppository 25–100 mg q6–8h | PO 0.5 mg/kg q4–6h<br>IM 0.5 mg/kg q6–8h. Maximal daily dose: up to age 5 years or weight 50 lb, 40 mg; age 5–12 years or weight 50–100 lb, 75 mg<br>Rectal suppository 1 mg/kg q6–8h<br>Not recommended for children under age 6 months |
| **Perphenazine** (Trilafon) | PO 8–16 mg daily in divided doses<br>IM 5 mg as a single dose | |
| **Prochlorperazine** (Compazine) | PO 5–10 mg three or four times daily (sustained-release capsule, 10 mg twice daily)<br>IM 5–10 mg q3–4h to a maximum of 40 mg daily<br>Rectal suppository 25 mg twice daily | Weight over 10 kg: PO 0.4 mg/kg per day, in three or four divided doses<br>IM 0.2 mg/kg as a single dose<br>Rectal suppository 0.4 mg/kg per day, in three or four divided doses |
| **Promethazine** (Phenergan) | PO, IM, rectal suppository 12.5–25 mg q4–6h | Age over 3 months: PO, IM, rectal suppository 0.25–0.5 mg/kg q4–6h |
| **Thiethylperazine** (Torecan) | PO, IM, rectal suppository 10–30 mg/d | |
| **Triflupromazine** (Vesprin) | PO 20–30 mg/d<br>IM 5–15 mg q4–6h; maximal dose, 60 mg/d<br>IV 1–3 mg as a single dose | Age over 2 years: PO, IM 0.2 mg/kg per day in three divided doses; maximal daily dose, 10 mg |
| **Antihistamines** | | |
| **Buclizine** (Bucladin-S) | Motion sickness, PO 50 mg 30 minutes before departure and 4–6 h later, if needed; maintenance dose, 50 mg twice daily | |
| **Cyclizine** (Marezine) | Motion sickness, PO 50 mg 30 minutes before departure, then q4–6h as needed, to a maximal daily dose of 300 mg; IM 50 mg three or four times daily as needed, rectal suppository 100 mg three or four times daily as needed<br>Postoperative vomiting, IM 50 mg preoperatively, 20–30 min before surgery is completed or q4–6h as needed | Age 6–10 years: Motion sickness, PO, IM 3 mg/kg per day in three divided doses; rectal suppository 6 mg/kg per day, in three divided doses<br>Maximal daily dose, 75 mg |
| **Dimenhydrinate** (Dramamine) | PO 50–100 mg q4h<br>IM 50 mg as needed<br>Rectal suppository 100 mg once or twice daily | PO, IM 5 mg/kg/day in four divided doses; maximal daily dose, 150 mg |
| **Diphenhydramine** (Benadryl) | Motion sickness, PO 50 mg 30 minutes before departure and 50 mg before each meal; IM, IV 20–50 mg q2–3h to a maximal daily dose of 400 mg | PO, IM 5 mg/kg per day, in four divided doses; maximal daily dose, 300 mg |
| **Hydroxyzine** (Vistaril, Atarax) | PO, IM 25–100 mg, three or four times daily | Age over 6 years, PO 50–100 mg daily in four divided doses<br>Age under 6 years, PO 50 mg daily in four divided doses |
| **Meclizine** (Antivert, Bonine) | PO 25–100 mg daily | Dosage not established |
| **Miscellaneous Agents** | | |
| **Benzquinamide** (Emete-Con) | IM 0.5–1.0 mg/kg at least 15 min before administering antineoplastic drugs or emergence from anesthesia, then q3–4h as needed<br>IV 0.2–0.4 mg/kg as a single dose, injected over 1–3 min | |
| **Cisapride** (Propulsid) | PO 10–20 mg 15 min before meals and at bedtime (four doses daily) | Dosage not established |
| **Diphenidol** (Vontrol) | PO 25–50 mg four times daily<br>IM 20–40 mg four times daily<br>IV 20 mg, repeated in 1 h if necessary. Subsequent doses should be given PO or IM. | Age over 6 months or weight over 12 kg, PO 5 mg/kg per day in four divided doses; IM 3 mg/kg per day in four divided doses |
| **Dronabinol** (Marinol) | PO 5 mg/m² (square meter of body surface area) 1–3 h before chemotherapy, then q2–4h for a total of four to six doses daily. Dosage can be increased by 2.5 mg/m² increments to a maximal dose of 15 mg/m² if necessary. | |
| **Droperidol** (Inapsine) | Preoperatively, IM 2.5–10 mg 30–60 min before procedure | Age 2–12 years, preoperatively, IM 1–1.5 mg/ 20–25 lb 30–60 min before procedure |

*(continued)*

**TABLE 66-1.  ANTIEMETIC DRUGS** *(Continued)*

| Generic/Trade Name | Routes and Dosage Ranges | |
|---|---|---|
| | **Adults** | **Children** |
| **Metoclopramide** (Reglan) | PO 10 mg 30 min before meals and at bedtime for 2–8 wk<br>IV 2 mg/kg 30 min before injection of cisplatin and 2 h after injection of cisplatin, then 1–2 mg/kg q2–3h if needed, up to four doses | |
| **Ondansetron** (Zofran) | IV 0.15 mg/kg, diluted in 50 ml of 5% dextrose or 0.9% sodium chloride injection, for three doses. First dose, 30 min before emetogenic anticancer drug; second dose 4 h after first dose; third dose 8 h after first dose. | |
| **Trimethobenzamide** (Tigan) | PO 250 mg 3–4 times daily<br>IM, rectal suppository 200 mg three or four times daily | PO, rectal suppository 15 mg/kg per day in three or four divided doses; IM not recommended |
| **Scopolamine** (Transderm Scōp) | Motion sickness, PO, SC 0.6–1 mg as a single dose<br>Transdermal disc (1.5 mg scopolamine) placed behind the ear every 3 days if needed | Motion sickness, PO, SC, 0.006 mg/kg as a single dose |
| **Phosphorated carbohydrate solution** (Emetrol) | PO 15–30 ml repeated at 15-min intervals until vomiting ceases | PO 5–10 ml repeated at 15-min intervals until vomiting ceases |

emetic effects. Centrally, metoclopramide antagonizes the action of dopamine, a catecholamine neurotransmitter. Peripherally, metoclopramide stimulates release of acetylcholine, which in turn stimulates GI motility and increases the rate of gastric emptying. Metoclopramide is given orally in diabetic gastroparesis and esophageal reflux. Large doses of the drug are given intravenously during chemotherapy with cisplatin (Platinol) and other emetogenic antineoplastic drugs.

**Ondansetron** (Zofran) is a unique antiemetic agent that is more effective than most other drugs in preventing nausea and vomiting associated with anticancer drug therapy. Some anticancer drugs apparently cause nausea and vomiting by combining with a subset of serotonin (5-hydroxytryptamine or 5HT) receptors located centrally in the CTZ and peripherally on vagal nerve endings. Ondansetron antagonizes 5-HT₃ receptors and prevents their activation by emetogenic anticancer drugs. It is not yet known whether the drug's antiemetic effects are central, peripheral, or both. The drug is given intravenously, has an elimination half-life of about 4 hours, and is extensively metabolized in the liver. Adverse effects are usually mild to moderate, and the most common ones reported in clinical trials were diarrhea (22%), headache (16%), constipation (11%), and transient elevation of liver enzymes.

**Phosphorated carbohydrate solutions** (Emetrol, Nausetrol) are hyperosmolar carbohydrate solutions with phosphoric acid. They are thought to exert a direct local action on the wall of the GI tract, reducing smooth muscle contraction. These preparations are available over the counter.

**Scopolamine**, an anticholinergic drug (see Chap. 21), is effective in relieving nausea and vomiting associated with motion sickness. A transdermal patch is often used to prevent seasickness.

**Trimethobenzamide** (Tigan) may act on the CTZ but is considered minimally effective.

## INDICATIONS FOR USE

Antiemetic drugs are indicated to prevent and treat nausea and vomiting associated with surgery, pain, motion sickness, cancer chemotherapy, radiation therapy, and other causes. Phenothiazines, because of their relatively high incidence and severity of adverse effects, are indicated only when other antiemetic drugs are ineffective or when only a few doses are expected to be required.

## CONTRAINDICATIONS FOR USE

Antiemetic drugs are generally contraindicated when their use may prevent or delay diagnosis, when signs and symptoms of drug toxicity may be masked (*e.g.*, during digitalis therapy), and for routine use to prevent postoperative vomiting.

## *Nursing Process*

### Assessment

Assess for nausea and vomiting.
- Identify risk factors (*e.g.*, digestive or other disorders in which nausea and vomiting are symptoms; drugs associated with nausea and vomiting).
- Interview regarding frequency, duration, and precipitating causes of nausea and vomiting. Also, question the client about accompanying signs and symptoms, characteristics of vomitus (amount, color, odor, presence of abnormal components, such as blood), and any measures that relieve nausea and vomiting. When possible, observe and measure the vomitus.

**Nursing diagnoses**

- Fluid Volume Deficit related to uncontrolled vomiting
- Altered Nutrition: Less than Body Requirements related to impaired ability to ingest and digest food
- Altered Tissue Perfusion: Hypotension related to fluid volume depletion or antiemetic drug effect
- High Risk for Injury: Trauma related to drug-induced drowsiness and hypotension
- Knowledge Deficit related to nondrug measures to reduce nausea and vomiting
- Knowledge Deficit related to appropriate use of antiemetic drugs

**Planning/Goals**

*The client will:*

- Have antiemetic drugs administered at appropriate times by indicated routes
- Take antiemetic drugs as prescribed for outpatient use
- Obtain relief of nausea and vomiting
- Eat and retain food and fluids
- Have increased comfort
- Maintain body weight
- Maintain normal bowel elimination patterns
- Have fewer vomiting episodes and less discomfort with cancer chemotherapy

**Interventions**

Use measures to prevent or minimize nausea and vomiting:

- Avoid exposure to stimuli when feasible (*e.g.*, unpleasant sights and odors; excessive ingestion of food, alcohol, or aspirin).
- Because pain may cause nausea and vomiting, administration of analgesics before painful diagnostic tests and dressing changes or other therapeutic measures may be helpful.
- Administer antiemetic drugs before radiation therapy, cancer chemotherapy, or travel.
- Many oral drugs cause less gastric irritation, nausea, and vomiting if taken with or just after food. Thus, scheduling and administering drugs may be an important measure in preventing nausea and vomiting. However, food delays or prevents absorption of many drugs and may decrease therapeutic effectiveness. For any drug likely to cause nausea and vomiting, check reference sources to determine whether it can be given with food without altering beneficial effects.
- When nausea and vomiting occur, assess the client's condition and report to the physician. In some instances, a drug (*e.g.*, digitalis, an antibiotic) may need to be discontinued or reduced in dosage. In other instances (*e.g.*, paralytic ileus, GI obstruction), preferred treatment is restriction of oral intake and nasogastric intubation.
- Eating dry crackers before rising in the morning may help prevent nausea and vomiting associated with pregnancy.
- Avoid oral intake of food, fluids, and drugs during acute episodes of nausea and vomiting. Oral intake may increase vomiting and risks of fluid and electrolyte imbalances.
- Avoid activity during acute episodes of nausea and vomiting. Lying down and resting quietly are often helpful.

Give supportive care during vomiting episodes:

- Give replacement fluids and electrolytes. Offer small amounts of food and fluids orally when tolerated and according to client preference.

- Record vital signs, intake and output, and body weight at regular intervals if nausea or vomiting occurs frequently.
- Decrease environmental stimuli when possible (*e.g.*, noise, odors). Allow the client to lie quietly in bed when nauseated. Decreasing motion may decrease stimulation of the vomiting center in the brain.
- Help the client rinse his or her mouth after vomiting. This decreases the bad taste and corrosion of tooth enamel by gastric acid.
- Provide requested home remedies when possible (*e.g.*, a cool wet washcloth to the face and neck).

*Teach clients:*

- To avoid situations that cause or aggravate nausea and vomiting, when possible
- To avoid intake of food, fluids, and medications during acute vomiting episodes
- To avoid or decrease activity during episodes of nausea
- When an antiemetic drug is indicated, take it about 30 to 60 minutes before a nausea-producing event, when possible

**Evaluation**

- Observe and interview for decreased nausea and vomiting.
- Observe and interview regarding ability to maintain adequate intake of food and fluids.
- Compare current weight with baseline weight.
- Observe and interview regarding appropriate use of antiemetic drugs.

# Principles of therapy

## DRUG SELECTION

Choice of an antiemetic drug depends largely on the cause of nausea and vomiting and the client's condition.

1. For ambulatory clients, drugs causing minimal sedation are preferred. However, most antiemetic drugs cause some sedation in usual therapeutic doses.
2. Hydroxyzine and promethazine (Phenergan) are among the most frequently used antiemetic agents. Hydroxyzine is an antihistamine; promethazine is a phenothiazine with potent antihistaminic effects. Promethazine is most often used clinically for its antihistaminic, antiemetic, and sedative effects.
3. Drugs with anticholinergic and antihistaminic properties are preferred for motion sickness.
4. Prokinetic drugs are preferred when nausea and vomiting are associated with nonobstructive gastric retention.
5. Although phenothiazines are effective antiemetic agents, they may cause serious adverse effects (*e.g.*, hypotension, sedation, anticholinergic effects, extrapyramidal reactions that simulate signs and symptoms of Parkinson's disease). Consequently, phenothiazines other than promethazine generally should not be used, especially for pregnant, young, elderly, and postoperative clients, unless vomiting is severe and cannot be controlled by other measures.

## DOSAGE AND ADMINISTRATION FACTORS

Dosage and route of administration depend primarily on the reason for use.

1. Doses of phenothiazines are much smaller for antiemetic effects than for antipsychotic effects.
2. Most antiemetic agents are available in oral, parenteral, and rectal dosage forms. As a general rule, oral dosage forms are preferred for prophylactic use, and rectal or parenteral forms are preferred for therapeutic use.
3. Antiemetic drugs are often ordered PRN (as needed). As for any PRN drug, the client's condition should be assessed before drug administration.

## TIMING OF DRUG ADMINISTRATION

When nausea and vomiting are likely to occur because of travel, administration of emetogenic anticancer drugs, diagnostic tests, or therapeutic procedures, an antiemetic drug should be given prior to the emetogenic event. Pretreatment usually increases patient comfort and allows use of lower drug doses. It also may prevent aspiration and other potentially serious complications of vomiting.

## CHEMOTHERAPY-INDUCED NAUSEA AND VOMITING

Several anticancer drugs may cause severe nausea and vomiting and much discomfort for clients. Cisplatin is one of the most emetogenic drugs. For this reason, new antiemetics are usually compared with older drugs in the treatment of cisplatin-induced nausea and vomiting. Some general guidelines for managing this difficult problem include the following:

1. Chemotherapy may be given during sleeping hours.
2. Some clients may experience less nausea and vomiting if they avoid or decrease food intake for a few hours prior to scheduled chemotherapy.
3. Antiemetic drugs should be given before the emetogenic drug to *prevent* nausea and vomiting when possible. Most often, they are given intravenously for rapid effects.
4. Metoclopramide, given intravenously in high doses, may be used alone or in combination with various other drugs. Diphenhydramine (Benadryl) or another drug with anticholinergic effects may be given at the same time or PRN because high doses of metoclopramide often cause extrapyramidal effects (see Chap. 9).
5. Numerous combinations have been tried, with varying degrees of success. Most of them include two to five antiemetic and sedative-type drugs, usually in moderate to high doses. The client should be closely observed for excessive sedation.

## USE IN CHILDREN

The use of antiemetics in children is not clearly defined. Phenothiazines (*e.g.*, chlorpromazine) are more likely to cause dystonias and other neuromuscular reactions in children than in adults. Promethazine is probably preferred because its action is more like the antihistamines than the phenothiazines. Several other antiemetics are not recommended for use in children younger than age 12 years. These include benzquinamide, buclizine (Bucladin-S), cyclizine (Marezine), and scopolamine. Thus, antiemetic drug therapy should generally be cautious and limited to prolonged vomiting of known etiology.

## USE IN OLDER ADULTS

Most antiemetic drugs cause drowsiness, especially in older adults, and therefore should be used cautiously. Efforts should be made to prevent nausea and vomiting when possible. Older adults are at risk of fluid volume depletion and electrolyte imbalances with vomiting.

## NURSING ACTIONS: ANTIEMETICS

| *Nursing Actions* | *Rationale/Explanation* |
|---|---|
| **1. Administer accurately**<br>**a.** For prevention of motion sickness, give antiemetics about 30 minutes before travel and q3–4h, if necessary. | To allow time for drug dissolution and absorption |
| **b.** For prevention of vomiting with cancer chemotherapy and radiation therapy, give antiemetic drugs 30–60 minutes before treatment. | Drugs are more effective in preventing than in aborting nausea and vomiting. |

*(continued)*

| Nursing Actions | Rationale/Explanation |
|---|---|
| **c.** Inject intramuscular antiemetics deeply into a large muscle mass (*e.g.*, gluteal area). | To decrease tissue irritation. |
| **d.** As a general rule, do not mix parenteral antiemetics in a syringe with other drugs. An exception is promethazine (Phenergan), which is often mixed with meperidine (Demerol) and atropine sulfate for preanesthetic medication. | To avoid physical incompatibilities |
| **e.** Omit antiemetic agents and report to the physician if the client appears excessively drowsy or is hypotensive. | To avoid potentiating adverse effects and central nervous system (CNS) depression |

**2. Observe for therapeutic effects**

**a.** Verbal reports of decreased nausea

**b.** Decreased frequency or absence of vomiting

**3. Observe for adverse effects**

| | |
|---|---|
| **a.** Excessive sedation and drowsiness | Excessive sedation may occur with usual therapeutic doses of antiemetics and is more likely to occur with high doses. This may be minimized by avoiding high doses and assessing the client for responsiveness before each dose. |
| **b.** Anticholinergic effects—dry mouth, urinary retention | These effects are common to many antiemetic agents and are more likely to occur with large doses. |
| **c.** Hypotension, including orthostatic hypotension | May occur with any of the drugs but is most likely with phenothiazines and droperidol |
| **d.** Extrapyramidal reactions—dyskinesia, dystonia, akathisia, parkinsonism | These disorders may occur with phenothiazines and metoclopramide. They are more likely to occur when phenothiazines are used as antipsychotics rather than as antiemetics. |
| **e.** With dronabinol, observe for alterations in mood, cognition, and perception of reality, depersonalization, dysphoria, drowsiness, dizziness, anxiety, tachycardia, and conjunctivitis. | According the the manufacturer, these adverse effects are well tolerated. Tachycardia may be prevented with a beta-adrenergic blocking drug, such as propranolol (Inderal). |

**4. Observe for drug interactions**

Drugs that *increase* effects of antiemetic agents:

| | |
|---|---|
| (1) CNS depressants (alcohol, sedative-hypnotics, antianxiety agents, other antihistamines or antipsychotic agents) | Additive CNS depression |
| (2) Anticholinergics (*e.g.*, atropine) | Additive anticholinergic effects. Some phenothiazines and antiemetic antihistamines have strong anticholinergic properties. |
| (3) Antihypertensive agents | Additive hypotension |

**5. Teach clients**

| | |
|---|---|
| **a.** Take the drugs as prescribed. | To avoid adverse effects |
| **b.** Do not drive an automobile or operate dangerous machinery if drowsy from antiemetic drugs. | To avoid injury |
| **c.** If taking antiemetic drugs regularly, do not take other drugs without the physician's knowledge and consent. | Several drugs interact with antiemetic agents to increase incidence and severity of adverse effects. |
| **d.** Report excessive drowsiness or other adverse reactions. | The drug may need to be discontinued or reduced in dose or frequency of administration. Also, a change in drugs may reduce adverse effects in a particular individual. |
| **e.** With dronabinol, teach clients to take the drug only when they can be supervised by a responsible adult. | To increase safety, owing to the mind-altering effects of the drug. |

## Review and Application Exercises

1. List common causes of nausea and vomiting or circumstances in which nausea and vomiting often occur.
2. How do antiemetic drugs prevent or relieve nausea and vomitng?
3. What are adverse effects of commonly used antiemetics?
4. Are antiemetics more effective if given before, during, or after nausea and vomiting?
5. Which antiemetics are often given to control nausea and vomiting that occurs with certain antineoplastic drugs?

## Selected References

Alpers, D. H. (1992). Approach to the patient with nausea and vomiting. In W. N. Kelley (Ed.), *Textbook of internal medicine* (2nd ed.) (pp. 613–618). Philadelphia: J.B. Lippincott.

Beare, P. G., & Myers, J. L. (Eds.) (1990). *Principles and practice of adult health nursing*. St. Louis: C.V. Mosby.

(1994). *Drug facts and comparisons*. St. Louis: Facts and Comparisons.

Finley, R. S. (1992). Nausea and vomiting. In M. A. Koda-Kimble & L. Y. Young (Eds.), *Applied therapeutics: The clinical use of drugs* (5th ed.) (pp. 6-1–6-13). Vancouver, WA: Applied Therapeutics.

Gerlach, M. J., McDermott, M. M., Burrell, L. O., Lukens, L., McCall, C. Y., Walters, N. G., & Lillis, P. P. (1992). Nursing management of adults with common problems of the gastrointestinal system. In L. O. Burrell (Ed.), *Adult nursing in hospital and community settings* (pp. 1320–1378). Norwalk, CT: Appleton & Lange.

Porth, C. M. (1990). *Pathophysiology: Concepts of altered health states* (3rd ed.) (pp. 697–718). Philadelphia: J.B. Lippincott.

# Drugs Used in Special Conditions

### CHAPTER 67

# Antineoplastic Drugs

Antineoplastic drugs are used in the treatment of cancer. Cancer chemotherapy is a major treatment modality, alone or in conjunction with surgery and radiation therapy. It may cure some malignant tumors and is important in the treatment of many others. To participate effectively in cancer chemotherapy, nurses must know the characteristics of normal and malignant cells and of the drugs used to arrest tumor growth.

## Characteristics of normal cells

Normal cells undergo an orderly process of replication and differentiation into specialized cells that perform specialized functions. Some specific characteristics of normal cells include the following:

1. They reproduce according to a predetermined sequence of events. The normal cell cycle (the interval between the "birth" of a cell and its division into two daughter cells) involves several phases. During the resting phase ($G_0$), cells perform all usual functions except replication. That is, they are not dividing but are capable of doing so when stimulated. Different types of cells spend different lengths of time in this phase, after which they either reenter the cell cycle and differentiate or die. During the first active phase ($G_1$), ribonucleic acid (RNA) and enzymes required for production of deoxyribonucleic acid (DNA) are developed. During the next phase (S), DNA is synthesized for chromosomes. During $G_2$, RNA is synthesized, and the mitotic spindle is formed. Mitosis occurs in the final phase (M). The resulting two daughter cells may

then enter the resting phase ($G_0$) or proceed through the reproductive cycle.
2. Normal cells reproduce in response to a need (*e.g.*, growth or tissue repair) and stop reproduction when the need has been met.
3. They are well differentiated in appearance and function. Thus, they can be examined under a microscope and the tissue of origin determined.

## Characteristics of malignant neoplasms

Malignant neoplasms, malignant tumors, and cancer are terms used to describe a group of more than 200 disease processes. A cancer develops from a single normal cell that is altered or transformed into a malignant cell. The transformation probably begins with a random mutation (abnormal structural changes within the genetic material of a cell). A mutated cell may be destroyed by body defenses (*e.g.*, an immune response), or it may replicate. During succeeding cell divisions, additional changes and mutations may produce cells with progressively fewer normal and more malignant characteristics. Malignant cells differ from normal cells in several ways, including the following:

1. Malignant cells reproduce with the same sequence of events as normal cells, but they tend to grow rapidly in an uncontrolled fashion. They do not differentiate, mature, or function like normal cells, and they can proliferate indefinitely. Generally, it takes years for malignant cells to produce a clinically detectable

mass or tumor. Factors influencing the rate of tumor growth include blood and nutrient supply, the immunocompetence of the host, and hormonal stimulation of some types of cancer.

2. Malignant cells serve no useful purpose in the body. Instead, they occupy space and act as parasites by taking blood and nutrients away from normal tissues.

3. Malignant cells are anaplastic or undifferentiated. This means they have lost the structural and functional characteristics of the cells from which they originated. In comparison to normal cells of the same type, malignant cells are usually larger, more immature or primitive, and differ in appearance from normal cells and other malignant cells. Generally, cells that are more anaplastic or undifferentiated are more malignant. These cells grow into masses that are disorganized and irregular.

4. Malignant cells can invade normal tissues to cause widespread tissue destruction and eventual death unless treatment measures intervene. Owing to a lack of cohesiveness, increased motility, and production of proteolytic enzymes that break down normal tissues, malignant cells are able to break away from the primary tumor and spread to other body parts. Malignant cells invade normal tissues primarily by extending into tissues adjacent to the tumor and by traveling through blood and lymph vessels into tissues distant from the tumor site.

## ETIOLOGIC FACTORS

Despite extensive study, the cause of cancer is not clear. Because "cancer" is actually many diseases, many etiologic factors are probably involved. Most (about 80%) cancers are thought to be environmental in origin. Several carcinogens (cancer-causing agents) and risk factors that predispose people to develop cancer have been identified; Table 67-1 lists some known and probable chemical carcinogens. Other carcinogens include radiation (from radioisotopes, ultraviolet light, and sunlight), physical irritation (*e.g.*, of pigmented moles or of the colon from ulcerative colitis), and viruses. Viruses have been linked to the development of leukemia and cancers of the lymph nodes, liver, pharynx, and cervix and other genitalia.

Risk factors cannot predict whether cancer will occur in a person, but they can help identify people who are more likely to develop cancer. Some risk factors are primarily environmental; others are related to personal characteristics.

### Geographic and racial factors

Breast cancer occurs more often in the United States than in Japan, while the incidence of stomach cancer is higher in Japan. Primary liver cancer is common in some areas of Africa but rare in Europe and North America. These differences have not been fully explained but are probably caused by environmental rather than hereditary or racial factors. Also, people who live in cities are more likely to develop cancer because of greater exposure to air pollutants and other carcinogens. In the United States, African-Americans have higher rates of multiple myeloma and cancers of the lung, prostate, esophagus, and pancreas than white people.

### Age and gender

The incidence of cancer increases with age and reaches a peak as a cause of death in the sixth and seventh decades. A smaller peak in cancer mortality occurs during the first 4 years of life. Lung cancer is the leading cause of cancer death in men and women; colon cancer occurs about equally in both sexes. In addition, men are more likely to have leukemia and cancer of the urinary bladder, stomach, and pancreas. Elderly men have a relatively high risk of prostatic cancer. Women are at risk of developing cancer of the breast, cervix, and endometrium.

### Social customs and life-style

The incidence of lung cancer is greatly increased among people who smoke cigarettes and increased to a lesser extent among nonsmokers who are exposed to other people's smoke. The increased incidence of lung cancer in women is attributed to increased cigarette smoking. Cancers of the mouth, throat, and esophagus are associated with cigarette smoking and alcohol use. There is some evidence that alcohol alone is a carcinogen and, when combined with cigarette smoking, probably acts as a cocarcinogen that increases the cancer-producing effects of cigarette smoking. Oral cancer is associated with smoking a pipe, chewing tobacco, using "smokeless tobacco," smoking cigarettes, and using alcohol. There is also an increased incidence of liver cancer among alcoholics.

Eating habits also influence the occurrence of cancer. Cancers of the colon, breast, prostate gland, ovary, and endometrium are associated with a high intake of carbohydrate, fat, and animal protein and a low intake of fiber. These eating patterns are more prevalent in affluent, industrialized parts of the world.

### Heredity

Hereditary factors are less important than environmental factors in cancer development. Most relatives of people with cancer are generally no more likely to develop cancer than the general population. However, some specific types of cancer are related to heredity. For example, close relatives of premenopausal women with breast cancer are more likely to develop breast cancer; close

**TABLE 67-1.   KNOWN AND PROBABLE CHEMICAL CARCINOGENS**

| Chemical | Source of Exposure | Location of Associated Cancer |
|---|---|---|
| Aflatoxins | Foods contaminated with aspergillus fungus, such as peanuts, soybeans, corn, wheat, and rice. Contamination is most likely with warm, moist storage conditions. | Liver |
| Alcohol | Ingestion of alcoholic beverages, such as whiskey, beer, or wine | Mouth, pharynx, larynx, esophagus, liver |
| Alkylating agents (*e.g.,* melphalan [Alkeran], others) | Cytotoxic, immunosuppressive drugs used in the treatment of several types of cancer | Lymphoid tissue (lymphoma, leukemia), bladder (cyclophosphamide [Cytoxan]) |
| Alpha-naphthyline (1 NA) and beta-naphthylamine (2 NA) | Manufacturing, handling, or storing substances containing this chemical. It is used in a wide variety of products, including herbicides, dyes, food colors, color film, paint, plastics, rubber, and petroleum products. | Bladder |
| Anabolic steroids (androgens) | Large doses used by athletes to gain weight and muscle strength. | Liver |
| Arsenic | Manufacturing sodium arsenate, drinking water contaminated by arsenic | Skin and lung |
| Asbestos | Working in areas where asbestos is used, including shipyards and factories. Several thousand products contain asbestos. These include insulation, floor tiles, and automobile brake linings. Beer, gin, and a number of medicines are filtered through asbestos filters in the manufacturing process. Family members and household contacts of asbestos workers receive considerable exposure from asbestos carried home on clothes. | Bronchi, pleura, peritoneum |
| Benzene | Working with glues and varnishes | Bone marrow (leukemia) |
| Benzidine | Working in chemical plants where benzidine is used in the production of aniline dyes, rubber, plastics, printing inks, fireproofing of textiles, various laboratory chemicals. Living in neighborhoods where such plants are located also may result in significant exposure over the years. | Bladder |
| Bis (chloromethyl) ether (BCME) | Working in chemical plants where BCME is used for water-softening products, to remove impurities such as salt from water or to decolorize or clarify food beverages. BCME is not present in the finished product. | Lung |
| Dichlorbenzidine (DCB) | Working in chemical plants where DCB is used in the production of pigments for printing inks, textile dyes, plastics, and crayons. DCB is destroyed during the manufacturing process and is not contained in the final products. | Liver, bladder, breasts, skin |
| Estrogens | Drugs prescribed for menopausal symptoms and menstrual problems. Estrogen is a component of oral contraceptives. | Uterine endometrium, possibly breasts |
| Hydrocarbons | Cigarette smoke; soot (chimney sweeps may develop cancer of the scrotum); air pollution from industrial wastes, automobile exhausts; coal tar ointments used in treating some skin disorders; gases and particles produced by burning of coal, wood, and oil; foods such as smoked meats, foods burned by charcoal grilling, some vegetables and cereals; food packaging materials; many groups of industrial workers | Lungs, skin |
| Metallic ores (specific agent unknown) | Workers exposed to chromium in production of chromates and nickel refiners | Lungs |
| Polyvinyl chloride (PVC) | Workers in chemical plants that use PVC in the production of floor tiles, shoes, phonograph records, automobile upholstery, blood bags, and many other widely used products | Liver |
| Tobacco | Cigarette smoking, pipe smoking, chewing tobacco | Lungs, mouth, pharynx, larynx, esophagus, bladder |

relatives of people with stomach cancer are more likely to develop this disease; and close relatives of people with bronchogenic carcinoma who also smoke cigarettes are much more likely to develop bronchogenic carcinoma. Finally, familial polyposis strongly increases the incidence of colon cancer.

## Therapeutic drugs

The major drug groups associated with an increased risk of cancer are anticancer drugs (especially the alkylating group), female sex hormones, and immunosuppressants. With alkylating anticancer drugs used to treat Hodgkin's and non-Hodgkin's lymphoma, multiple myeloma, and ovarian, gastric, or colorectal cancer, surviving clients have a relatively high risk of developing acute nonlymphocytic leukemia for about 15 to 20 years. With female sex hormones, risks are increased for breast and endometrial cancers, especially with long-term use of estrogens to treat symptoms of menopause. With immunosuppressants used for solid organ or bone marrow transplant, clients have an increased risk for non-Hodgkin's lymphoma within a few months after transplant and later risks of skin (*e.g.*, squamous cell carcinoma and malignant melanoma) and soft-tissue sarcoma (Kaposi's sarcoma).

## ONCOGENES AND ANTIONCOGENES

Oncogenes (cancer-causing genes) are normal cell structures that have been altered by chromosomal translocations or mutation. They are introduced into the cell by viruses, where they apparently affect cellular growth factors. Tumors of the breast, colon, lung, and bone have been linked to activation of oncogenes. There also may be substances that suppress cancer development (tumor-suppressing genes or antioncogenes). Breast cancer has been associated with the absence of an antioncogene. Other factors are probably also involved, because the incidence of breast and colon cancer varies widely among countries.

## CLASSIFICATION OF MALIGNANT NEOPLASMS

Malignant neoplasms are classified in several different ways according to the type of tissue involved, the rate of growth, and other characteristics. With the exception of the acute leukemias, they are considered chronic diseases. These diseases can be broadly categorized as hematologic or solid neoplasms.

### Hematologic malignancies

Hematologic malignancies involve the bone marrow and lymphoid tissues; they include leukemias, lymphomas, and multiple myeloma.

**Leukemias.** Leukemias are cancers of the bone marrow characterized mainly by overproduction of abnormal white blood cells. These cells range from very primitive and immature to nearly normal in morphology. They cannot function normally as a body defense mechanism against microorganisms and tissue injuries. They also prevent or decrease production of normal red blood cells, white blood cells, and platelets. They eventually infiltrate other organs (liver, spleen, kidneys) and interfere with organ function.

Leukemias are more specifically classified according to the type of abnormal white blood cell. Acute leukemias involve more immature and less functional cells; chronic leukemias involve cells that are more nearly normal and somewhat functional. Granulocytic leukemia indicates abnormal granulocytes, most often neutrophils; myelogenous leukemia indicates that the abnormal cells originate in the bone marrow. Lymphocytic, lymphatic, or lymphogenous leukemia is characterized by abnormal lymphoid tissue.

The four main types of leukemia are acute lymphocytic leukemia, which is more common in children; acute myelogenous leukemia, which occurs in all ages but more often in young adults; chronic lymphocytic leukemia, which is more common in elderly people; and chronic myelogenous leukemia, which is more common in middle age.

**Lymphomas.** Lymphomas are malignant tumors of lymphoid tissue that are characterized by abnormal proliferation of the white blood cells normally found in lymphoid tissue. Lymphomas usually develop within lymph nodes and may occur anywhere in the body, because virtually all body tissues contain lymphoid structures. They develop as a solid tumor mass without involving peripheral blood. They impair immunity and increase susceptibility to infection. As the disease progresses, the liver, spleen, bone marrow, and other organs are involved and functionally impaired. The two main types of malignant lymphomas are known as Hodgkin's disease and non-Hodgkin's lymphoma.

**Multiple myeloma.** Multiple myeloma is a malignant tumor of the bone marrow in which abnormal plasma cells proliferate. Because normal plasma cells produce antibodies or immunoglobulins and abnormal plasma cells cannot fulfill this function, the body's immune system is impaired. As the tumor grows, it crowds out normal cells and interferes with other bone marrow functions. Although multiple myeloma is a slow-growing tumor, the abnormal plasma cells eventually infiltrate bone and cause extensive destruction. Metastasis eventually occurs in tissues outside bone, such as the spleen, liver, and lymph nodes.

### Solid neoplasms

Solid tumors are composed of a mass of malignant cells (parenchyma) and a supporting structure of connective tissue, blood vessels, and lymphatics (stroma). The growing tumor develops its own blood supply as new blood vessels grow from preexisting blood vessels of the host. Apparently, neoplastic cells secrete a substance that acts on capillaries to stimulate their growth into the tumor. The two major classifications of solid malignant neoplasms are carcinomas and sarcomas. Each is then subclassified according to the particular kind of body cell involved.

**Carcinomas.** Carcinomas are derived from epithelial tissues (skin, mucous membrane, linings and coverings of viscera) and are the most common type of malignant tumors. They are further classified by cell type, such as adenocarcinoma or basal cell carcinoma.

**Sarcomas.** Sarcomas are derived from connective tissue (muscle, bone, cartilage, fibrous tissue, fat, blood vessels). They are subclassified by cell type (*e.g.,* osteogenic sarcoma, angiosarcoma).

## EFFECTS OF CANCER ON THE BODY

Effects of cancer on the host vary according to the extent and location of the disease process. There are few effects initially. As the neoplasm grows, effects occur when the tumor becomes large enough to cause pressure, distortion, or deficient blood supply in surrounding tissues; interfere with organ function; obstruct ducts and organs; and cause malnutrition of normal tissues. More specific effects include anemia, malnutrition, pain, infection, hemorrhagic tendencies, thromboembolic problems, hypercalcemia, cachexia, and occurrence of symptoms related to impaired function of affected organs and tissues.

# Characteristics of antineoplastic drugs

1. Many antineoplastic drugs damage body cells (*i.e.,* they are cytotoxic). They kill malignant cells by interfering with cell replication. Nutrients and genetic materials are necessary for cell replication. To be effective, the drugs must interfere with the supply and use of nutrients (amino acids, purines, pyrimidines) or with the genetic materials in the cell nucleus (DNA or RNA).
2. Some antineoplastic drugs act during specific phases of the cell cycle, such as DNA synthesis or formation of the mitotic spindle. These cell cycle-specific (CCS) agents include the antimetabolites, the plant alkaloids, and some miscellaneous agents (*e.g.,* asparaginase, hydroxyurea). These drugs are more effective when administered continuously because this method prolongs exposure of malignant cells to drug action. Other drugs act during any phase of the cell cycle and are called cell cycle-nonspecific (CCNS) agents. This group includes the alkylating agents, the antibiotic antineoplastics, the nitrosureas, and some miscellaneous agents (*e.g.,* cisplatin, dacarbazine). CCNS agents are more effective when administered intermittently.
3. Cytotoxic antineoplastic drugs are most active against rapidly dividing and proliferating cells, although some kill resting and dividing cells. Because the drugs do not act specifically against malignant cells, normal cells are damaged as well. The normal cells especially endangered are the rapidly proliferating cells of the bone marrow, the lining of the gastrointestinal tract, and the hair follicles. The cytotoxic

effects of antineoplastic drugs account for therapeutic and adverse effects.

4. Each dose of antineoplastic drugs kills some but not all malignant cells. The cell kill effect follows "first-order kinetics," meaning that a drug dose kills a specific percentage of cells. If the drug destroys 99% of cells, it reduces 1 million cells to 10,000. Succeeding doses would destroy 99% of remaining cells but not all of them. This is important because all malignant cells must be killed to effect a cure.
5. Antineoplastic drugs are given mainly by oral and intravenous routes of administration. In some circumstances, they may be given topically, intra-arterially, intrathecally, or by instillation into a body cavity.
6. Antineoplastic drugs may induce drug-resistant malignant cells. Mechanisms are unclear but may involve the ability of malignant cells to act on the drug (*e.g.,* by inhibiting drug uptake or activation, increasing the rate of drug inactivation, or pumping the drug out of the cell before it can act) or to act on themselves (*e.g.,* increase cellular repair of DNA damaged by the drugs or alter metabolic pathways and target enzymes of the drugs). Mutant cells also may emerge.
7. Most cytotoxic antineoplastic drugs are potential teratogens.

## CLASSIFICATION OF ANTINEOPLASTIC DRUGS

Antineoplastic drugs are classified in several different ways. Some are described in terms of their mechanisms of action (alkylating agents and antimetabolites), others according to their sources (plant alkaloids, antibiotics, enzymes). Other drugs used in cancer chemotherapy are immunostimulants (see Chap. 47), hormones, antihormones, and miscellaneous agents.

### Alkylating agents

Alkylating agents include nitrogen mustard and its derivatives (busulfan, chlorambucil, cyclophosphamide, and melphalan), nitrosureas (carmustine, lomustine, and streptozocin) and platinum compounds (carboplatin and cisplatin). Nitrogen mustard derivatives interfere with cell division and structure of DNA during dividing and resting stages of the malignant cell cycle. Consequently, their spectrum of activity is relatively broad compared with other antineoplastic drugs. They are most effective in hematologic malignancies but also are used to treat breast, lung, and ovarian tumors. All of these drugs cause significant bone marrow depression. All except nitrogen mustard may be given orally.

Nitrosoureas are classified as alkylating agents, although they also may inhibit essential enzymatic reactions of cancer cells. They have been used in clients with gastrointestinal, lung, and brain tumors. One unique feature of the nitrosureas is their high lipid solubility, which allows them to enter the brain and cerebrospinal fluid more effectively than most antineoplastic drugs. A second unique characteristic is that they cause delayed bone marrow depression, with maximum leukopenia and thrombocytopenia occurring about 5 to 6 weeks after drug administration.

The platinum compounds inhibit DNA synthesis. Cisplatin is widely used to treat cancers of the bladder, cervix, esophagus, head and neck, lung, prostate, and testes. It is also used to treat lymphomas, multiple myeloma, osteosarcoma, and other sarcomas. Adverse effects are mainly renal, neurologic, and otologic damage. Carboplatin is structurally similar to cisplatin but differs in other aspects. For example, it is most often used to treat endometrial and ovarian carcinomas, and it produces bone marrow depression as a major adverse effect.

## Antimetabolites

Antimetabolites include a folic acid antagonist (methotrexate), purine antagonists (mercaptopurine and thioguanine), pyrimidine antagonists (fluorouracil and floxuridine), and an inhibitor of DNA polymerase (cytarabine). The drugs are similar to nutrients needed by the cells for reproduction and are allowed to enter the cells. Once inside the cell, the drugs deprive the cell of necessary substances or cause formation of abnormal DNA. Either action kills the cell.

The antimetabolites have been used to treat the entire spectrum of cancers. Effectiveness of individual drugs varies with different kinds of cancer. Toxic effects mainly involve the bone marrow, epithelial lining of the gastrointestinal tract, and hair follicles.

Some antimetabolites can be given orally and parenterally; others are given only by one route. The effectiveness of these drugs depends greatly on the schedule of administration. They exert their cytotoxic effects during only one phase of the reproductive cycle of the cell (*i.e.*, when DNA is being synthesized). Although there is no way a chemotherapist can determine exactly when a drug is likely to be most effective (*i.e.*, kill the largest number of malignant cells), information has been accumulated empirically through extensive clinical trials. Thus, recommendations regarding dosage schedules should be followed as precisely as possible.

## Plant alkaloids

Plant alkaloids include the podophyllotoxin derivatives (etoposide, teniposide) and the vinca or periwinkle derivatives (vinblastine, vincristine). These drugs exert their cytotoxic effects by inhibiting cell division (antimitotic effects). Etoposide and teniposide are semisynthetic derivatives of the active ingredient in the May apple or mandrake plant. Etoposide is used mainly in a multidrug regimen to treat small-cell lung cancer and to treat testicular cancer that does not respond adequately to surgery, radiation, and other chemotherapy. Teniposide is used mainly in a multidrug regimen to treat childhood acute lymphocytic leukemia.

Common adverse effects are bone marrow depression, nausea and vomiting, and peripheral neuropathy. Vinblastine and vincristine have similar structures but different ranges of antineoplastic activity and adverse effects. Either may be effective in treating Hodgkin's disease and choriocarcinoma. Vinblastine also is useful in testicular carcinoma, and vincristine is used in acute lymphoblastic leukemia, non-Hodgkin's lymphomas, oat-cell carcinoma of the lung, and Wilms' tumor. In terms of adverse effects, vinblastine is more likely to cause bone marrow depression, and vincristine is more likely to cause peripheral nerve toxicity.

## Antineoplastic antibiotics

Antibiotics with antineoplastic activity include bleomycin, dactinomycin, daunorubicin, doxorubicin, idarubicin, mitomycin, mitoxantrone, pentastatin, and plicamycin. These drugs differ in activity and toxicity. They have some anti-infective activity, but they are too toxic for this use. The major toxicity is bone marrow depression. The anthracycline drugs, daunorubicin, doxorubicin, and idarubicin, also cause cardiotoxicity. Bleomycin may cause significant pulmonary toxicity. All of these drugs, except bleomycin, must be given intravenously because they are extremely irritating to tissues and cause tissue necrosis if extravasation occurs.

## Hormones and hormone inhibitors

Hormones used in cancer chemotherapy exert beneficial effects by altering the hormonal environment that promotes cancer growth. The sex hormones (estrogens, progestins, androgens) are useful in cancers of the sex organs, including the breast and prostate gland. The adrenal corticosteroids suppress formation and function of lymphocytes and are therefore most useful in the treatment of acute leukemia in children and of malignant lymphoma. They also may be used in treating complications of cancer, such as intracranial metastases and hypercalcemia. Hormone inhibitors include tamoxifen (Nolvadex), an antiestrogen that competes with estrogen for binding sites in breast tissue; aminoglutethimide (Cytadren), an adrenocorticosteroid-inhibiting agent that produces a ''medical adrenalectomy''; and goserelin

(Zoladex) and leuprolide (Lupron), which inhibit testosterone secretion in advanced prostatic cancer.

## Radioactive iodine

Radioactive iodine ($^{131}I$) is used only for treatment of thyroid cancer.

## Miscellaneous agents

Miscellaneous antineoplastic agents vary greatly in their sources, mechanisms of action, indications for use, and toxic effects.

### INDICATIONS FOR USE

Cytotoxic antineoplastic drugs are used in the treatment of malignant neoplasms. Goals of chemotherapy vary according to the clinical situation. In some cases, chemotherapy is curative; in others, it is palliative. In still others, it induces or maintains remissions (symptom-free periods that last for varying lengths of time).

Chemotherapy is the primary treatment of choice for a few types of cancer, including Burkitt's lymphoma, choriocarcinoma, Hodgkin's disease, acute leukemia, carcinoma of the testes, Wilms' tumor, Ewing's sarcoma, and retinoblastoma. Most of these malignant tumors are relatively rare. Chemotherapy is less effective in cancers of the lung, rectum, pancreas, colon, and prostate gland.

In hematologic neoplasms, drug therapy is the primary treatment of choice because the systemic distribution of the disease precludes use of the other two treatments for cancer (surgery and radiation). In solid tumors, drug therapy is often used to kill malignant cells remaining after surgery or radiation therapy. Chemotherapy is more effective when the tumor mass has been removed or reduced. Chemotherapy used in conjunction with surgery or irradiation is called *adjuvant chemotherapy*. Adjuvant chemotherapy is used to destroy malignant cells in breast and other cancers. Drug therapy also is used in advanced malignant disease for palliation of symptoms. Once metastasized, solid tumors become systemic diseases and are no longer readily accessible to surgical excision or radiation therapy.

Antineoplastic drugs are sometimes used in the treatment of nonmalignant conditions. One of these is polycythemia vera, an uncommon condition characterized by abnormal proliferation of blood cells. Methotrexate may be used, in smaller doses than those used for malignant diseases, to treat rheumatoid arthritis and psoriasis.

## Individual drugs

See Table 67-2.

## Nursing Process

### Assessment

Assess the client's condition before drug therapy is started and frequently throughout the course of treatment. Knowledge about the type of malignancy the client has is necessary for adequate assessment. Useful information includes the main organs affected, whether the tumor grows slowly or rapidly, and usual patterns of metastasis. Specific assessment data include the following:

- Grade of the malignancy. Tumor grading is an attempt to determine the degree of malignancy. It is done by biopsy and histologic examination. Grade 1 and 2 tumors show cellular differentiation and are similar to the normal tissue of origin. Grade 3 and 4 tumors are less differentiated, bear little resemblance to the normal tissue of origin, and are more malignant. Generally, the higher the tumor grade, the poorer the prognosis. Criteria for each grade vary with the type of cancer.
- Stage of the malignancy. Staging is a way to determine the extent of the malignant process (*i.e.*, whether the tumor is localized or has spread). It also determines which organs are involved in the malignant process. One system of staging is the TNM system. $T$ stands for the primary tumor; subcategories ($T_1$, $T_2$, $T_3$) indicate increasing size. $N$ indicates involvement of regional lymph nodes; $N_0$ means no involvement, and $N_1$ and $N_2$ indicate increasing nodal disease. $M$ stands for metastasis; $M_0$ indicates absence of metastasis, and $M_1$ indicates metastatic spread.

   Staging is done by the physician on the basis of a history and physical examination and diagnostic tests, such as x-ray studies, radioisotope scans, tissue biopsies, cytologic examination of various body secretions, endoscopies, liver and other organ function studies, and sometimes exploratory laparotomy or thoracotomy.
- Laboratory test results. Several laboratory tests are useful in cancer chemotherapy. These are usually done before the beginning of drug therapy to establish baseline data for later comparison and during drug therapy to monitor drug effects.
- *Blood tests for "tumor markers."* Alpha-fetoprotein is a fetal antigen normally present during intrauterine and early postnatal life but absent in adulthood. Increased amounts may indicate hepatic or testicular cancer. Carcinoembryonic antigen (CEA) is secreted by several types of malignant cells, especially by cells originating in the gastrointestinal tract. It is not a good screening test because false-positive and false-negative results occur. It can be useful in selected circumstances, however. For example, a rising CEA level may indicate progression of malignant disease and a need for evaluation or treatment. If CEA levels are elevated before surgery and disappear after surgery, this is a good indication of adequate tumor excision. If CEA levels rise later, it probably indicates recurrence of the tumor. In chemotherapy, falling CEA levels indicate drug effectiveness. Other tumor markers are immunoglobulins (elevated levels may indicate multiple myeloma), prostatic acid phosphatase (elevated levels may indicate prostatic cancer), and prostate-

(*Text continues on p. 689*)

## TABLE 67-2. ANTINEOPLASTIC DRUGS

| Generic/Trade Name | Routes and Dosage Ranges* | Clinical Uses | Common or Potentially Severe Adverse Reactions |
|---|---|---|---|
| *Alkylating Drugs* | | | |
| *Nitrogen Mustard Derivatives* | | | |
| **Busulfan** (Myleran) | PO 4–8 mg daily until white blood cell count decreases by half, then maintenance doses up to 4 mg daily | Chronic granulocytic leukemia | Bone marrow depression (leukopenia, thrombocytopenia, anemia), pulmonary toxicity |
| **Chlorambucil** (Leukeran) | PO 0.1–0.2 mg/kg per day for 3–6 wk. If maintenance therapy is required, 0.03–0.1 mg/kg per day | Chronic lymphocytic leukemia, non-Hodgkin's lymphomas, carcinomas of breast and ovary | Bone marrow depression, hyperuricemia |
| **Cyclophosphamide** (Cytoxan) | Induction of therapy, PO 1–5 mg/kg per day; IV 35–40 mg/kg over several days (20–30 mg/kg for clients with prior chemotherapy or radiation) Oral maintenance therapy, 1.5–2 mg/kg daily | Hodgkin's disease, non-Hodgkin's lymphomas, neuroblastoma. Often combined with other drugs for acute lymphoblastic leukemia in children; carcinomas of breast, ovary, and lung; multiple myeloma and other malignancies | Bone marrow depression, anorexia, nausea, vomiting, alopecia, hemorrhagic cystitis |
| **Ifosfamide** (Ifex) | IV 1.2 g/m² per day for 5 consecutive d. Repeat every 3 wk or after WBC and platelet counts return to normal after a dose. | Germ cell testicular cancer | Bone marrow depression, hemorrhagic cystitis, nausea and vomiting |
| **Mechlorethamine (nitrogen mustard)** (Mustargen) | IV 0.4 mg/kg in one or two doses. Repeat in 3–6 wk. Intracavitary 0.4 mg/kg instilled into pleural or peritoneal cavities | Hodgkin's disease and non-Hodgkin's lymphomas, lung cancer, pleural and peritoneal malignant effusions | Bone marrow depression, nausea, vomiting. Extravasation may lead to tissue necrosis. |
| **Melphalan** (Alkeran) | PO 0.25 mg/kg per day for 7 d, followed by 21 drug-free d, then maintenance dose of 2 mg daily | Multiple myeloma | Bone marrow depression, nausea and vomiting |
| **Pipobroman** (Vercyte) | Polycythemia vera, PO 1 mg/kg per day until hematocrit reduced by 50%, then 0.1–0.2 mg/kg per day Chronic granulocytic leukemia, 1.5–2.5 mg/kg per day initially, reduced to maintenance dose of 7–175 mg/d when WBC count approaches 10,000 | Polycythemia vera, chronic granulocytic leukemia | Bone marrow depression |
| *Nitrosoureas* | | | |
| **Carmustine (BCNU)** | IV 200 mg/m² every 6 wk | Hodgkin's disease, malignant melanoma, multiple myeloma, brain tumors | Bone marrow depression, nausea, vomiting, hepatotoxicity |
| **Lomustine (CCNU)** | PO 130 mg/m² every 6 wk | Hodgkin's disease, brain tumors | Bone marrow depression, nausea, vomiting, hepatotoxicity |
| **Streptozocin** (Zanosar) | IV 500 mg/m² for 5 consecutive days every 6 wk | Metastatic islet cell carcinoma of pancreas | Nephrotoxicity, nausea, vomiting |
| *Others* | | | |
| **Carboplatin** (Paraplatin) | IV infusion 360 mg/m² over at least 15 min on day 1 every 4 wk | Palliation of ovarian cancer | Bone marrow depression, nausea and vomiting |
| **Cisplatin** (Platinol) | IV 100 mg/m² once every 4 wk | Carcinomas of testes, bladder, ovary, head and neck, and endometrium | Renal toxicity and ototoxicity |
| *Antimetabolites* | | | |
| **Cytarabine (ARA-C, cytosine arabinoside)** (Cytosar-U) | IV 2 mg/kg per day for 10 d | Leukemias of adults and children | Bone marrow depression, nausea, vomiting, stomatitis, diarrhea |
| **Floxuridine** (FUDR) | Intra-arterial infusion, 0.1–0.6 mg/kg per day until toxicity occurs | Head and neck tumors, carcinomas of the GI tract, liver, pancreas, and biliary tract | Same as cytarabine, above |
| **Fludarabine** (Fludara) | IV 25 mg/m² daily for 5 consecutive d | Chronic lymphocytic leukemia | Bone marrow depression, fever, nausea, vomiting |
| **Fluorouracil (5-FU)** (Adrucil) | IV 12 mg/kg per day for 5 d | Carcinomas of the breast, colon, rectum, stomach, and pancreas | Same as cytarabine, above |

*(continued)*

## TABLE 67-2.  ANTINEOPLASTIC DRUGS  (*Continued*)

| Generic/Trade Name | Routes and Dosage Ranges* | Clinical Uses | Common or Potentially Severe Adverse Reactions |
|---|---|---|---|
| (Efudex, Fluoroplex) | Topical, apply to skin cancer lesion twice daily for several weeks | Solar keratoses, basal cell carcinoma | Pain, pruritus, burning at site of application |
| **Mercaptopurine** (Purinethol) | PO 2.5 mg/kg per day | Acute and chronic leukemias | Bone marrow depression, nausea, hyperuricemia |
| **Methotrexate (MTX, Amethopterin)** (Mexate) | Induction of remission of acute leukemia in children PO, IV 3 mg/m² per day. Maintenance of remission, PO 30 mg/m² two times per week (combined with prednisone for induction and maintenance of remission) Choriocarcinoma, PO, IM 15 mg/m² daily for 5 d | Acute lymphoblastic leukemia in children, lymphocytic lymphoma, choriocarcinoma of the testes, osteogenic carcinoma, others | Bone marrow depression, nausea, diarrhea, stomatitis |
| **Thioguanine** | PO 2 mg/kg per day | Acute and chronic leukemias | Bone marrow depression, nausea |
| ***Antibiotics*** | | | |
| **Bleomycin** (Blenoxane) | IV, IM 0.25–0.5 units/kg once or twice weekly | Squamous cell carcinoma, lymphomas, testicular carcinoma, Hodgkin's disease | Pulmonary toxicity, stomatitis, alopecia, hyperpigmentation and ulceration of skin |
| **Dactinomycin (Actinomycin D)** (Cosmegen) | IV 15 µg/kg per day for 5 d and repeated every 2–4 wk | Rhabdomyosarcoma, Wilms' tumor | Bone marrow depression, anorexia, nausea, vomiting. Extravasation may lead to tissue necrosis. |
| **Daunorubicin** (Cerubidin) | IV 60 mg/m² daily for 3 d every 3–4 wk | Acute granulocytic and acute lymphocytic leukemias, lymphomas | Same as doxorubicin, below |
| **Doxorubicin** (Adriamycin) | Adults, IV 60–75 mg/m² every 21 d Children, IV 30 mg/m² daily for 3 d, repeated every 4 wk | Acute leukemias, lymphomas, carcinomas of breast, lung, and ovary | Bone marrow depression, alopecia, stomatitis, GI upset, cardiomyopathy. Extravasation may lead to tissue necrosis. |
| **Idarubicin** (Idamycin) | IV injection 12 mg/m² daily for 3 d, with concomitant cytarabine | Acute myelogenous leukemia in adults, with other antileukemic drugs | Same as doxorubicin, above |
| **Mitomycin** (Mutamycin) | IV 2 mg/m² per day or 50 µg/kg per day for 5 d, repeated after 2 d. This course of therapy may be repeated after recovery of the bone marrow. | Carcinomas of stomach, colon, rectum, pancreas, bladder, breast, lung, head and neck, and malignant melanoma | Bone marrow depression, nausea, vomiting, diarrhea, stomatitis. Extravasation may lead to tissue necrosis. |
| **Mitoxantrone** (Novantrone) | IV infusion 12 mg/m² on days 1–3, for induction | Acute nonlymphocytic leukemia | Fever, cough, dyspnea, congestive heart failure, cardiac arrhythmias, nausea, vomiting, diarrhea |
| **Pentastatin** (Nipent) | IV 4 mg/m² every other week | Hairy cell leukemia unresponsive to alpha-interferon | Bone marrow depression, hepatotoxicity, nausea, vomiting, fever, skin rash |
| **Plicamycin (formerly known as mithramycin)** (Mithracin) | IV 25–30 µg/kg per day or every other day for eight to ten doses or until toxicity occurs | Testicular tumors, severe hypercalcemia | Toxicity affecting the bone marrow, liver, and kidneys. Extravasation can cause local tissue inflammation. |
| ***Plant Alkaloids*** | | | |
| **Etoposide** (VePesid) | IV 50–100 mg/m² per day on days 1–5, or 100 mg/m² per day on days 1, 3, and 5, every 3–4 wk | Testicular cancer, acute leukemias, lymphomas, small-cell lung cancer | Bone marrow depression, anaphylaxis, nausea, vomiting, alopecia |
| **Teniposide** (Vumon) | IV infusion 165 mg/m² twice weekly (with cytarabine) | Acute lymphocytic leukemia in children | Same as etoposide, above |
| **Vinblastine** (Velban) | IV 0.1 mg/kg weekly, increased gradually by 0.05 mg/kg increments | Metastatic testicular carcinoma, Hodgkin's disease, carcinoma of breast | Bone marrow depression, especially leukopenia, neurotoxicity. Extravasation may lead to tissue necrosis. |
| **Vincristine** (Oncovin) | Adults, IV 0.01–0.03 mg/kg weekly Children, IV 0.4–1.4 mg/m² weekly | Hodgkin's disease and other lymphomas, acute leukemia | Neurotoxicity with possible foot drop from muscle weakness, paresthesias, constipation, and other manifestations. Extravasation may lead to tissue necrosis. |

(continued)

**TABLE 67-2. ANTINEOPLASTIC DRUGS** (*Continued*)

| Generic/Trade Name | Routes and Dosage Ranges* | Clinical Uses | Common or Potentially Severe Adverse Reactions |
|---|---|---|---|
| *Hormones* | | | |
| *Adrenocorticosteroid* | | | |
| **Prednisone** (Meticorten, others) | PO 60–100 mg/m² per day for first few days, then gradual reduction to 20–40 mg/d | Used as adjunct for palliation of symptoms in acute leukemia, Hodgkin's disease, lymphomas, complications of cancer, such as thrombocytopenia, hypercalcemia, intracranial metastases | Potentially toxic to almost all body systems. See Chapter 24. |
| *Estrogens* | | | |
| **Diethylstilbestrol (DES)** (Stilbestrol) | Breast cancer, PO 1–5 mg three times daily<br>Prostate cancer, PO 1–3 mg daily | Carcinoma of prostate gland, carcinoma of breast in post-menopausal women | Feminizing effects in men, anorexia, nausea, vomiting, edema, hypercalcemia, and others. See Chapter 28. |
| **Ethinyl estradiol** (Estinyl, others) | Breast cancer, PO 0.5 mg/d initially, gradually increased to 3 mg/d in three divided doses<br>Prostate cancer, PO 0.15–2 mg daily | Carcinoma of prostate, advanced carcinoma of breast in post-menopausal women | Feminizing effects in men, anorexia, nausea, vomiting, edema, hypercalcemia, and others. See Chapter 28. |
| *Progestins* | | | |
| **Medroxyprogesterone** (Provera, Depo-Provera) | IM 400–800 mg twice weekly<br>PO 200–300 mg/d | Advanced endometrial carcinoma | Usually well tolerated. May cause edema and irritation at injection sites. |
| **Megestrol** (Megace) | PO 40–320 mg/d in divided doses | Advanced endometrial carcinoma, breast carcinoma | Usually produces minimal adverse reactions |
| *Androgen* | | | |
| **Fluoxymesterone** (Halotestin) | PO 10 mg, three times daily (30 mg/d) | Advanced breast carcinoma in premenopausal women | Masculinizing effects, hypercalcemia |
| *Hormone Inhibitors* | | | |
| *Adrenocorticosteroid Inhibitor* | | | |
| **Aminoglutethimide** (Cytadren) | PO 250 mg four times daily | Advanced breast carcinoma | Adrenal insufficiency |
| *Antiandrogen* | | | |
| **Flutamide** (Eulexin) | PO 250 mg every 8 h | Advanced prostatic cancer | Hot flashes, decreased libido, impotence, nausea, vomiting, diarrhea, gynecomastia |
| *Antiestrogen* | | | |
| **Tamoxifen** (Nolvadex) | PO 20–40 mg/d in two divided doses | Advanced breast cancer in post-menopausal women | Hot flashes, nausea and vomiting, ocular toxicity |
| *Gonadotropin-Releasing Hormone Analogues (Antitestosterone Effects)* | | | |
| **Goserelin** (Zoladex) | SC 3.6 mg every 28 d | Advanced prostatic cancer | Worsening of symptoms during first few weeks, especially bone pain |
| **Leuprolide** (Lupron) | SC 1 mg/d | Advanced prostatic cancer | Same as for goserelin, above |
| *Miscellaneous Antineoplastic Agents* | | | |
| **Altretamine** (Hexalen) | PO 260 mg/m² per day for 14 or 21 days in four doses, after meals and at bedtime | Advanced ovarian cancer | Nausea, vomiting, bone marrow depression, peripheral neuropathy |
| **Asparaginase** (Elspar) | IV 1000 IU/kg per day for 10 d | Acute lymphocytic leukemia refractory to other drugs. Usually used in conjunction with other agents. | Abnormal functioning of the liver, kidneys, pancreas, central nervous system, and the blood-clotting mechanism; hypersensitivity reactions |
| **Cladribine** (Leustatin) | IV infusion 0.09 mg/kg per day for 7 consecutive d | Hairy cell leukemia | Bone marrow depression, nausea, vomiting, fever |
| **Dacarbazine** (DTIC-Dome) | IV 3.5 mg/kg per day for 10 d, repeated every 28 d | Malignant melanoma, Hodgkin's disease, sarcoma | Bone marrow depression, nausea and vomiting; increased blood urea nitrogen, aspartate aminotransferase and alanine amino- |

*(continued)*

**TABLE 67-2. ANTINEOPLASTIC DRUGS** (*Continued*)

| Generic/Trade Name | Routes and Dosage Ranges* | Clinical Uses | Common or Potentially Severe Adverse Reactions |
|---|---|---|---|
| | | | transferase. Extravasation may cause severe pain and tissue damage. |
| **Hydroxyurea** (Hydrea) | PO 80 mg/kg as single dose every third day or 20–30 mg/kg as a single dose daily | Chronic granulocytic leukemia, malignant melanoma | Bone marrow depression, GI upset |
| **Levamisole** (Ergamisol) | PO 50 mg every 8 h for 3 d every 2 wk for 1 y | Colon cancer, with fluorouracil | Nausea, vomiting, diarrhea, dermatitis |
| **Mitotane** (Lysodren) | PO 8–10 g daily in three to four divided doses. Maximal daily dose, 19 g. | Inoperable carcinoma of the adrenal cortex | Anorexia, nausea, damage to adrenal cortex |
| **Paclitaxel** (Taxol) | IV 135 mg/m² every 3 wk | Advanced ovarian cancer | Bone marrow depression, allergic reactions, hypotension, bradycardia, peripheral neuropathy, nausea, vomiting, muscle and joint pain, alopecia |
| **Procarbazine** (Matulane) | PO 100–200 mg/d for 1 wk, then 300 mg/d until maximal response or toxicity occurs | Hodgkin's disease | Bone marrow depression, nausea, vomiting |

*Dosages change frequently according to use in different types of cancer and in combination with other antineoplastic drugs.

specific antigen (elevated levels may indicate prostatic cancer).

- *Complete blood count* (*CBC*) to check for anemia and other abnormalities. Of special interest are the leukocyte and platelet counts, because most antineoplastic drugs cause bone marrow depression manifested mainly by leukopenia and thrombocytopenia. A CBC and white blood cell differential are done before each cycle of chemotherapy. The tests are used to determine dosage and frequency of drug administration, to monitor bone marrow function so that fatal bone marrow depression does not occur, and to assist the nurse in planning care. For example, the client is very susceptible to infection when the leukocyte count is low, and bleeding is likely when the platelet count is low. Nursing measures can be taken to prevent or minimize both of these complications of chemotherapy.
- *Other tests*. These include serum calcium, uric acid, and others, depending on the particular organs affected by the malignant disease.
- Clinical manifestations of the malignancy. Common signs and symptoms include anemia, malnutrition, weight loss, pain, and infection; other symptoms depend on the particular organs affected.
- Other disease conditions. Determine whether other diseases are present and, if the client has had previous cancer treatment, the response obtained.
- Emotional and mental status. Anxiety and depression are common features at any point in cancer diagnosis and treatment. Other aspects of nursing assessment include the client's coping mechanisms, family relationships, and financial resources.

**Nursing diagnoses**

- Pain, nausea and vomiting, and weakness related to disease process or drug therapy

- Altered Nutrition: Less than Body Requirements related to disease process or drug therapy
- Activity Intolerance related to anemia and weakness from disease process or drug therapy
- Self-Care Deficit related to debilitation from disease process or drug therapy
- Anxiety related to the disease, its possible progression, and its treatment
- Ineffective Individual Coping related to medical diagnosis of cancer
- Ineffective Family Coping related to illness and treatment of a family member
- Altered Tissue Perfusion related to anemia
- Fluid Volume Deficit related to chemotherapy-induced nausea, vomiting, and diarrhea
- Body Image Disturbance related to drug-induced alopecia
- High Risk for Injury: Infection related to drug-induced neutropenia
- High Risk for Injury: Bleeding related to drug-induced thrombocytopenia
- High Risk for Injury: Stomatitis (mucositis) related to damage of oral mucosal cells
- Sexual Dysfunction related to adverse drug effects
- Knowledge Deficit about cancer
- Knowledge Deficit about cancer chemotherapy

**Planning/Goals**

*The client will:*

- Receive assistance in coping with the diagnosis of cancer
- Experience reduced anxiety and fear
- Receive chemotherapy accurately
- Experience reduction of tumor size, change of laboratory values toward normal, or other therapeutic effects of chemotherapy
- Experience minimal bleeding, infection, nausea and vomiting, and other consequences of adverse drug effects

- Maintain adequate intake of food and fluid
- Maintain body weight
- Receive assistance in activities of daily living when needed
- Be informed about community resources for cancer care (*e.g.,* hospice, Reach to Recovery, other support groups)

**Interventions**

Because all antineoplastic drugs may cause adverse reactions ranging from relatively minor to life threatening, measures are needed to prevent or minimize the incidence and intensity of adverse reactions. If they cannot be prevented, they must be detected as early as possible so that treatment may be started and damaging effects may be decreased.

- *Nausea and vomiting* are common with most antineoplastic drugs. They usually occur within 1 or 2 hours of drug administration and may last for several hours. Various measures to prevent or treat nausea and vomiting have met with varying amounts of success.
  - Giving antineoplastic drugs at bedtime, often with a sedative, may allow the client to sleep through the hours when nausea and vomiting are likely to be most severe.
  - Antiemetic drugs are probably most effective when started before administration of antineoplastic drugs and given on a regular schedule up to 48 hours afterward.
  - Oral intake after drug administration is probably best determined by the client through trial and error. Some clients feel better if they avoid oral intake for a few hours; others tolerate small amounts of liquid and dry carbohydrates, such as crackers. As soon as nausea and vomiting are relieved, a normal diet can be resumed.
- *Anorexia* and altered taste perception are related problems that interfere with nutrition. Well-balanced meals, consisting of foods the client is able and willing to eat, are very important. Also, nutritional supplements can be used to increase intake of protein and calories.
- *Alopecia* occurs with several of the more frequently used antineoplastic drugs, such as cyclophosphamide, doxorubicin, methotrexate, and vincristine. Complete hair loss can be psychologically devastating, especially for women. Measures to help decrease the impact of alopecia include the following:
  - Warn clients before drug therapy is started. Reassure them that alopecia is usually temporary and reversible when drug therapy is stopped. Sometimes hair growth returns even while drug therapy continues. Hair may grow back a different color and texture.
  - Suggest the purchase of wigs, hats, and scarves. This should be done before hair loss is expected to occur.
  - Suggest that clients avoid permanent waves, hair coloring, or other hair treatments that damage the hair and may affect the degree of hair loss.
  - Allow clients to express feelings about altered body image.
- *Stomatitis* occurs often with the antimetabolites, antibiotics, and plant alkaloids used in cancer chemotherapy. It is likely to interfere with nutrition, lead to oral infections and bleeding, and cause considerable discomfort. Some guidelines for minimizing or treating stomatitis follow; most of these can be done by the client after the nurse has explained their purpose, while others must be done by or with the assistance of the nurse:

- Brush the teeth at least twice daily with a soft-bristled toothbrush. Stop brushing the teeth if the platelet count drops below 20,000/mm$^3$ because gingival bleeding is likely. Teeth may then be cleaned with toothettes (soft sponge-tipped devices) or cotton-tipped applicators dipped in a dilute hydrogen peroxide solution.
- Floss teeth daily with unwaxed floss. Stop if the platelet count drops below 20,000/mm$^3$ to prevent gingival bleeding.
- Rinse the mouth several times daily, especially before meals (to decrease unpleasant taste and increase appetite) and after meals (to remove food particles that promote growth of microorganisms). One suggested solution is 1 tsp of table salt and 1 tsp of baking soda in 1 quart of water. Commercial mouthwashes are irritating and drying to oral mucosa and are not recommended for use.
- Encourage the client to drink fluids. Systemic dehydration and local dryness of the oral mucosa contribute to the development and progression of stomatitis. Pain and soreness contribute to dehydration. Fluids usually tolerated by the client with stomatitis include tea, carbonated beverages, and ices, such as popsicles. Gelatin desserts also are usually well tolerated and add to fluid intake. Fruit juices are not usually recommended, especially citrus juices, such as orange and grapefruit, because they may produce pain, burning, and further tissue irritation. They may be tolerated if diluted with water or carbonated beverages, such as Sprite or 7-Up. Drinking fluids through a straw may be more comfortable, because this decreases contact of fluids with painful ulcerations.
- Encourage the client to eat soft, bland, cold, nonacidic foods. Although individual tolerances vary, it is usually better to avoid highly spiced or rough foods.
- Remove dentures entirely or for at least 8 hours daily, because they may irritate oral mucosa.
- Inspect the mouth daily for signs of inflammation and lesions.
- Give medications for pain. Local anesthetic solutions, such as viscous lidocaine, can be used about 15 minutes before meals to make eating more comfortable. Because the mouth and throat are anesthetized, swallowing and detecting the temperature of hot foods may be difficult, and aspiration or burns may occur. Doses should not exceed 15 ml every 3 hours or 120 ml in 24 hours. If systemic analgesics are used, they should be given about 30 to 60 minutes before eating.
- In oral infections resulting from stomatitis, local or systemic anti-infective drugs are used. Fungal infections with *Candida albicans*, which are common, can be treated with antifungal tablets, suspensions, or lozenges. Severe infections may require systemic antibiotics, depending on the causative organism as identified by cultures of mouth lesions.
- *Infection* is common because the disease and its treatment lower host resistance to infection. Measures to prevent infection are aimed toward increasing host resistance and decreasing exposure to pathogenic microorganisms. Measures to minimize infection are aimed toward early detection and treatment.
  - Help the client maintain a well-balanced diet. Oral hygiene before meals and analgesics when appropriate

may increase food intake. High-protein, high-calorie foods and fluids can be given between meals. Several types of nutritional supplements are available commercially and can be taken with or between meals. Provide fluids with high nutritional value (*e.g.*, milkshakes or nutritional supplements) rather than coffee, tea, or carbonated beverages if the client can tolerate them and has an adequate intake of water and other fluids.

- Instruct and assist the client to avoid exposure to infection by avoiding crowds, anyone with a known infection, and contact with fresh flowers, soil, animals, or animal excrement.
- Frequent and thorough handwashing by the client and everyone involved in his or her care is probably the best way to reduce exposure to pathogenic microorganisms.
- The client should take a bath daily and put on clean clothes. In addition, the perineal area should be washed with soap and water after each urination or defecation.
- Avoid indwelling venous and urinary catheters when possible. If they are necessary, take particular care to prevent them from becoming sources of infection. For central venous lines (*e.g.*, Hickman and other catheters), inspect and cleanse around exit sites according to agency policies and procedures. Use strict sterile technique when changing dressings or flushing the catheters. For peripheral venous lines, the same principles of care apply, except that sites should be changed about every 3 days or if signs of phlebitis occur. For urinary catheters, cleansing the perineal area with soap and water at least once daily is recommended.
- Signs and symptoms of infection may not be obvious in the person whose defenses against infection are compromised. Fever is probably the most consistent symptom. If it occurs, assume it is caused by infection, and try to determine the source. Rectal temperature measurements are usually avoided because of the risk of mucosal trauma and subsequent infection.
- When infection is suspected, possible sources are cultured and antibiotics initiated without waiting for culture reports.
- Severe leukopenia can be prevented or its extent and duration minimized by administering colony-stimulating factors (*e.g.*, filgrastim or sargramostim) that stimulate the bone marrow to produce leukocytes (see Chap. 47). If severe leukopenia develops, a protective environment is indicated to decrease exposure to pathogens. Recommendations, resources, and policies vary regarding protective environments, at least partly because most infections are caused by microorganisms from the client's own body rather than exogenous sources. Transfusions of white blood cells may be given in some circumstances.
- *Bleeding* may be caused by thrombocytopenia, and precautions should be instituted if the platelet count drops to 50,000/mm$^3$ or below. Bleeding may occur spontaneously or with seemingly minor trauma. Measures to avoid bleeding include:
  - Avoid trauma, including venipuncture, injections, and rectal temperatures when possible.
  - Use an electric razor for shaving.
  - Check skin, urine, and stool for blood.

- For platelet counts less than 20,000/mm$^3$, stop brushing the teeth. Platelet transfusions may be given.
- *Extravasation* is the leakage of drug into subcutaneous tissues around an intravenous injection site. Many of the cytotoxic antineoplastic drugs cause severe inflammation, pain, and even tissue necrosis if extravasation occurs. Thus, efforts are needed to prevent extravasation if possible or to minimize tissue damage if it occurs.
  - Start an intravenous infusion. Avoid veins that are small, located in an edematous extremity, or located near a joint.
  - With the intravenous infusion running rapidly, inject the drug into the intravenous tubing with a small-gauge needle. This provides for relatively slow administration and rapid dilution of the drug. In addition, if extravasation should occur, it can be detected quickly and stopped when only small amounts of drug have been injected into subcutaneous tissues.
  - After the drug has been injected, continue the rapid flow rate of the intravenous fluid for 2 to 5 minutes to thoroughly flush the vein.
  - If extravasation occurs, various techniques have been suggested to decrease tissue damage. These include aspiration of the drug or injection of hydrocortisone through the intravenous line before it is removed, subcutaneous infiltration of hydrocortisone around the extravasated area, and application of ice bags or cold compresses. Nurses involved in cancer chemotherapy must know the procedure to be followed in their facility if extravasation occurs so that it can be instituted immediately.
- *Hyperuricemia* results from rapid breakdown or destruction of malignant cells, whether it occurs spontaneously or as a result of antineoplastic drugs. Uric acid crystals can cause kidney damage. Uric acid nephropathy is the main danger to the client. The following measures minimize these effects:
  - Maintain a high fluid intake, with intravenous fluids if necessary, and a high urine output.
  - Alkalinize the urine with sodium bicarbonate or other agents.
  - Administer allopurinol (Zyloprim) to inhibit uric acid formation.

Provide supportive care to clients and families.

- Physiologic care includes pain management, comfort measures, and assistance with nutrition, hygiene, ambulation, and other activities of daily living when needed.
- Psychological care includes allowing family members or significant others to be with the client and participate in care when desired and keeping clients and families informed. In addition, mental health professionals may be consulted to assist in coping with the distress that often accompanies cancer and its treatment.

*Teach clients:*

- To practice meticulous personal hygiene, including frequent and thorough handwashing, and to avoid potential sources of infection when possible
- Ways to maintain or improve intake of food and fluids
- To use wigs, scarves, and hats to minimize the impact of alopecia, if expected with chemotherapy. These should be purchased before starting chemotherapy if possible.
- To decrease risks of bleeding by shaving with an electric

razor, avoiding aspirin and other nonsteroidal anti-inflammatory drugs (*e.g.*, ibuprofen), and avoiding injections when possible

- To report fever, mouth soreness or ulcerations, or any sign of bleeding (*e.g.*, bruising, bleeding from gums, nose, seeing blood in urine or feces). If these occur, drug therapy may need to be changed or stopped.
- To inform any other physician, dentist, or health-care provider that chemotherapy is being taken before any diagnostic test or treatment is begun. Some procedures may be contraindicated or require special precautions.
- To keep all appointments for drug therapy and blood tests for maximal benefits and minimal adverse effects

### Evaluation

- Monitor drug administration for accuracy.
- Observe and interview for therapeutic effects of chemotherapy.
- Compare current laboratory reports with baseline values for changes toward normal values.
- Compare weight and nutritional status with baseline values for maintenance or improvement.
- Observe and interview for adverse drug reactions, including interventions to prevent or control them.
- Observe and interview for adequate pain management and other symptom control.
- Observe and interview regarding mental and emotional status of the client and family members.
- Interview for knowledge of resources (*e.g.*, family, health-care providers, hospice, others).

## Principles of therapy

### PLANNING WITH CLIENT AND FAMILY

Once the diagnosis of cancer is made, the tumor is graded and staged, the client's physical and mental status is assessed, and the physician decides that the anticipated benefits of chemotherapy outweigh the disadvantages, additional factors must be discussed with the client and family.

1. *What is the goal of chemotherapy?* It may be to cure the malignant disease, decrease tumor size, relieve symptoms, kill metastatic cells left after surgery or radiation therapy, or prolong life. When the goal is cure or induction of remission, adverse reactions and other disadvantages of chemotherapy may be acceptable. When expected benefit is minimal, even moderate morbidity due to drug therapy may be unacceptable.
2. *What adverse reactions are likely to occur?* Which reactions should be reported to the physician? How will they be managed if they occur? Even if the realities of chemotherapy are quite unpleasant, it is usually better for the client to know what they are than to fear

the unknown. Some specific effects that should be discussed, depending on the drugs to be used, include alopecia, amenorrhea, oligospermia, and possibly permanent sterility. Because most of these drugs are teratogenic, clients in the reproductive years are advised to avoid pregnancy during treatment.

3. *Who will administer the drugs; where and for how long will they be administered?* Cancer chemotherapy is highly specialized. Because the drugs are highly toxic to both normal and malignant body cells and require meticulous techniques of administration, they are preferably given at a cancer treatment center. Some clients undergo chemotherapy at a cancer center far from home; others undergo treatment at a nearby hospital, clinic, physician's office, or even at home. The duration of treatment may be short- or long-term, depending largely on the type of tumor and response to drug therapy. Thus, estimates of weeks, months, or years of drug therapy must be discussed. The time required for one drug treatment should be described as well so that the client can schedule other activities.

   Usual practice requires that blood be drawn for a CBC and perhaps other tests. The results of these tests must be reported before antineoplastic drugs are given. If excessive leukopenia or thrombocytopenia is reported, drug therapy may be discontinued or postponed. Clients should be informed about the frequent venipunctures required for blood tests and drug administration.

4. *How can the client help to maximize therapeutic benefits of chemotherapy and minimize adverse effects?* One self-help measure is to eat a well-balanced diet. This may require great effort in the presence of anorexia, nausea, vomiting, diarrhea, or stomatitis. Another self-help measure is frequent and thorough oral hygiene. A third measure is to keep all appointments for drug administration and blood tests.

### DRUG SELECTION

Choice of drug or combination of drugs depends largely on which drugs have been effective in similar types of cancer. Other factors to be considered include primary tumor sites, presence and extent of metastases, physical status of the client, and other disease conditions that affect chemotherapy, such as liver or kidney disease.

### COMBINATION DRUG THERAPY

Combinations of several drugs are often used in the continuing effort to increase therapeutic effects without increasing toxic effects. The effectiveness of various combinations is determined by clinical testing and is usually expressed as a percentage of the clients who respond favorably. Combinations also may prevent or delay the development of drug resistance. Combinations are based on knowledge of tumor cell kinetics and drug actions. Some general characteristics of effective drug combinations include the following:

1. Each drug should exert antineoplastic activity when used alone.
2. Each drug should act by a different mechanism. Drugs can be combined to produce either sequential inhibition or concurrent inhibition. For example, one drug can be chosen to damage the DNA, RNA, or proteins of the malignant cell, and another drug can be chosen to prevent their repair or synthesis.
3. Drugs should act at different times in the reproductive cycle of the malignant cell. For example, more malignant cells are likely to be destroyed by combining CCS and CCNS drugs. The first group kills only dividing cells; the second group kills cells during any part of the life cycle, including the resting or nondividing phase.
4. Consecutive doses kill a percentage of the tumor cells remaining after earlier doses and further decrease the tumor burden.
5. Toxic reactions of the various drugs should not overlap so that maximal tolerated doses may be given. It is preferable to use drugs that are not toxic to the same organ system (e.g., bone marrow, kidney) and to use drugs that do not exert their toxic effects at the same time. However, adverse reactions to drug combinations may differ considerably from those of each drug when given alone.
6. Combinations may require different dosages and schedules than single-agent drug therapy.
7. Combination chemotherapy undergoes rapid change as new drugs are developed or different combinations and schedules of older drugs are tried. Numerous combinations have been developed for use in specific types of cancer. For information about specific combinations and their clinical uses, see a current reference on cancer chemotherapy.

## DOSAGE AND ADMINISTRATION FACTORS

Antineoplastic drugs are usually given in relatively high doses, on an intermittent or cyclic schedule. This regimen seems to be more effective than low doses given continuously or massive doses given once. It also produces less immunosuppression and provides drug-free periods during which normal tissues can repair themselves from damage inflicted by the drugs. Fortunately, normal cells repair themselves faster than malignant cells. Succeeding doses are given as soon as tissue repair becomes evident, usually when leukocyte and platelet counts return to normal or acceptable levels.

Each antineoplastic drug must be used in the schedule, route, and dose judged to be most effective for a particular type of neoplastic disease. With combinations of drugs, the recommended schedule should be followed precisely because safety and effectiveness may be schedule dependent. When chemotherapy is used as an adjuvant to surgery, it usually should be started as soon as possible after surgery, given in maximal tolerated doses just as if advanced disease were present, and continued for several months (usually 1 year for breast cancer).

Dosage of antineoplastic drugs must be calculated and regulated carefully to avoid unnecessary toxicity. The age, nutritional status, blood count, kidney and liver function, and previous chemotherapy or radiation therapy must all be considered when determining dosage for a client. Additional factors that influence dosage are as follows:

1. Dosage is usually based on the recipient's body weight (mg/kg) or surface area ($mg/m^2$).
2. The usual dosages listed for individual drugs apply only when the drug is used as a single agent. In drug combinations, the amount of each agent must be determined by clinical investigations.
3. Dosage may be reduced on the basis of bone marrow depression (as indicated by leukopenia or thrombocytopenia), liver disease, or kidney disease.
4. Sex hormones used in cancer chemotherapy must be given in larger amounts (pharmacologic doses) than when they are used in hormone replacement therapy (physiologic doses). Consequently, adverse reactions are likely to be increased in incidence and severity.

## GUIDELINES FOR HANDLING ANTINEOPLASTIC DRUGS

Antineoplastic drugs exert adverse effects on nurses and other people who prepare and administer them. These effects include contact dermatitis and mutagenic cells in the urine. The extent and long-term consequences of the mutagenic cells are not yet known. Guidelines for handling the drugs to avoid adverse effects include the following:

1. Avoid contact with solutions for injection by wearing disposable gloves, eye protectors, and protective clothing (e.g., long-sleeved garments).
2. If handling a powder form of a drug, wear a mask to avoid inhaling the powder.
3. Prepare the drugs on disposable trays or towels so that spills can be contained.
4. Dispose of contaminated materials in specific chemo-

therapy waste containers. The containers should be incinerated at temperatures of 1800°F to 2000°F.

## USE IN CHILDREN

Safety and effectiveness of most antineoplastic drugs have not been established, and few controlled studies have been done in children. However, children are at risk for a wide range of malignant diseases, including acute leukemias, lymphomas, brain tumors (neuroblastomas and others), Wilms' tumor (nephroblastoma), and sarcomas of muscle (*e.g.*, rhabdomyosarcoma) and bone (*e.g.*, osteosarcoma, Ewing's sarcoma).

Cancer chemotherapy is often used in conjunction with surgical excision or irradiation. Basic principles of therapy apply to children (*e.g.*, preventing or minimizing adverse effects and others). Long-term effects on growth and development of survivors are not clearly defined. Special efforts are needed to maintain nutrition, organ function, psychological support, and other aspects of growth and development.

## USE IN OLDER ADULTS

Older adults are at risk of developing a wide range of malignant diseases. Although they also are likely to have renal impairment, chronic cardiovascular disorders, and other diseases that increase their risks of serious adverse effects, they should not be denied the potential benefits of chemotherapy on the basis of age alone. Instead, greater vigilance is needed to maximize benefits and minimize hazards of chemotherapy.

With impaired renal function, dosages of cyclophosphamide (Cytoxan) and methotrexate (Mexate) may need to be reduced. Creatinine clearance should be monitored; serum creatinine level is not a reliable indicator of renal function in older adults because of their decreased muscle mass.

With cardiovascular disorders, careful assessment and monitoring of cardiovascular status is required with the use of doxorubicin (Adriamycin) and other cardiotoxic drugs.

Older adults are especially sensitive to the neurotoxic effects of vincristine (Oncovin).

# NURSING ACTIONS: ANTINEOPLASTIC DRUGS

| *Nursing Actions* | *Rationale/Explanation* |
|---|---|
| **1. Administer accurately**<br>**a.** If not accustomed to giving cytotoxic antineoplastic drugs regularly, read package inserts or other recent drug references regarding administration of individual drugs. | Obtaining current information is necessary for several reasons, including the relatively large number and varied characteristics of the drugs, differences in administration according to the type of neoplasm being treated and other client characteristics, continuing development of new dosages, routes, and schedules of administration, and continuing development of combination regimens. |
| **b.** For drugs to be given parenterally:<br><br>(1) Prepare the drug solution immediately before use when possible. | Many of the drugs are available in a powder form, which must be reconstituted before administration. The drugs are usually prepared in the pharmacy under a vertical laminar flow hood. This is the preferred method, because it prevents contamination of the solution and dissemination of drug particles into the environment.<br>Several drugs are unstable in solution and therefore need to be given soon after mixing. Others may be stable for varying lengths of time. |
| (2) If necessary to use a prepared drug solution at a later time, label it with an expiration time, and store it correctly, usually under refrigeration. | Expiration times vary with individual drugs and the method of storage. Most drug solutions last longer when refrigerated. |
| (3) Wear gloves when mixing the drugs (cyclophosphamide, dacarbazine, dactinomycin, doxorubicin, mechlorethamide, vinblastine, and vincristine.) | To avoid chemical burns because a number of the drugs are very irritating to the skin. Safety glasses also are recommended for those who wear contact lenses. If some drug solution gets on the skin despite precautions, wash the area with large amounts of water as with any chemical burn. |

## *Nursing Actions*

## *Rationale/Explanation*

(4) Give IV drugs through a small needle (23–25 gauge) over a period of 2 to 3 minutes or inject into the tubing of a rapidly flowing IV infusion.

To decrease tissue irritation. The second method is recommended for the more irritating drugs, such as doxorubicin, so that extravasation into subcutaneous tissues becomes immediately apparent if it occurs.

c. For drugs to be given orally, the total dose of most drugs can be given at one time. An exception is mitotane, which is given in three or four divided doses.

2. Observe for therapeutic effects
   a. Increased appetite

   b. Increased sense of well-being

   c. Improved mobility

   d. Decreased pain

Therapeutic effects depend to a large extent on the type of malignancy being treated. They may not become evident for several weeks after chemotherapy is begun. Some clients experience anorexia, nausea, and vomiting for 2 to 3 weeks after each cycle of drug therapy.

   e. With busulfan, given for chronic myelogenous leukemia, also observe for decreased white blood cell count and decreased size of the spleen.

Decreased white blood cell count and splenomegaly usually become evident about the second or third week of drug therapy.

   f. With melphalan, given for multiple myeloma, also observe for decreased amounts of abnormal proteins in urine and blood, decreased levels of serum calcium, and increased hemoglobin.

3. Observe for adverse effects

Because they are toxic to both normal and malignant cells, cytotoxic antineoplastic drugs may have adverse effects on almost any body tissue. These adverse effects range from common to rare, from relatively mild to life threatening. Some are expected, such as bone marrow depression, and this is used to guide drug therapy. Most of the adverse effects occur with usual dosage ranges and are likely to be increased in incidence and severity with larger doses.

   a. Hematologic effects:

   (1) Bone marrow depression with leukopenia (decreased white blood cell count), thrombocytopenia (decreased platelets), and anemia (decreased red blood cell count, hemoglobin, and hematocrit)

For most of these drugs, white blood cell count and platelet counts reach their lowest points about 7 to 14 days after drug administration and return toward normal after about 21 days. Normal leukocyte and platelet counts signify recovery of bone marrow function. Anemia may occur later because the red blood cell lives longer than white cells and platelets.

   (2) Decreased antibodies and lymphocytes

Most of these drugs have immunosuppressant effects, which impair body defenses against infection.

   b. Gastrointestinal (GI) effects—anorexia, nausea, vomiting, diarrhea, constipation, stomatitis and other mucosal ulcerations, oral candidiasis

Anorexia, nausea, and vomiting are very common. They usually occur within a few hours of drug administration. Nausea and vomiting often subside within approximately 12 to 24 hours, but anorexia may persist. Constipation is most likely to occur with vincristine. Mucosal ulcerations may occur anywhere in the GI tract and can lead to serious complications (infection, hemorrhage, perforation). Their occurrence is usually an indication to stop drug therapy, at least temporarily. Fungal and bacterial infections may interfere with nutrition. They may be relatively mild or severe.

*(continued)*

## Nursing Actions

## Rationale/Explanation

**c.** Integumentary effects—alopecia, dermatitis, tissue irritation at injection sites

Complete hair loss may take several weeks to occur. Alopecia is most significant in terms of altered body image, possible mental depression, and other psychological effects. Several drugs may cause phlebitis and sclerosis of veins used for injections, as well as pain and tissue necrosis if allowed to leak into subcutaneous tissues around the injection site.

**d.** Renal effects:

(1) Hyperuricemia and uric acid nephropathy

When malignant cells are destroyed by drug therapy, they release uric acid into the bloodstream. Uric acid crystals may precipitate in the kidneys and cause impaired function or even renal failure. Adverse effects on the kidneys are especially associated with methotrexate and cisplatin. Hyperuricemia can be decreased by an ample fluid intake or by administration of allopurinol.

(2) With cyclophosphamide, hemorrhagic cystitis (blood in urine, dysuria, burning on urination)

Hemorrhagic cystitis is thought to occur in about 10% of the clients who receive cyclophosphamide and to result from irritating effects of drug metabolites on the bladder mucosa. The drug is stopped if this occurs. Cystitis can be decreased by an ample fluid intake.

**e.** Pulmonary effects—cough, dyspnea, chest x-ray changes

Adverse reactions affecting the lungs are associated mainly with bleomycin, busulfan, and methotrexate. With bleomycin particularly, pulmonary toxicity may be severe and progress to pulmonary fibrosis.

**f.** Cardiovascular effects—congestive heart failure (dyspnea, edema, fatigue), arrhythmias, ECG changes

Cardiomyopathy is associated primarily with daunorubicin and doxorubicin. This is a life-threatening adverse reaction. The heart failure may be unresponsive to digitalis preparations.

**g.** CNS effects—peripheral neuropathy with vincristine, manifested by muscle weakness, numbness and tingling of extremities, foot drop, and decreased ability to walk

This fairly common effect of vincristine may worsen for several weeks after drug administration. There is usually some recovery of function eventually.

**h.** Endocrine effects—menstrual irregularities, sterility in males and females

**4. Observe for drug interactions**
**a.** Drugs that *increase* effects of cytotoxic antineoplastic drugs:

(1) Allopurinol

Allopurinol is usually given to prevent or treat hyperuricemia, which may occur with cancer chemotherapy. When given with mercaptopurine, allopurinol facilitates the formation of the active metabolite. Consequently, doses of mercaptopurine must be reduced to one-third to one-fourth the usual dose.

(2) Anticoagulants, oral

Increased risk of bleeding

(3) Bone marrow depressants

Increased bone marrow depression

(4) Other antineoplastic drugs

Additive cytotoxic effects, both therapeutic and adverse

**b.** Drugs that *increase* effects of cyclophosphamide:

(1) Anesthetics, inhalation

Lethal combination. Discontinue cyclophosphamide at least 12 hours before general inhalation anesthesia is to be given.

(2) Barbiturates

Potentiate cyclophosphamide by induction of liver enzymes, which accelerate transformation of the drug into its active metabolites

## Nursing Actions                          ## Rationale/Explanation

(3) Other alkylating antineoplastic drugs

Increased bone marrow depression

**c.** Drugs that *increase* effects of methotrexate:

(1) Alcohol

Additive liver toxicity. Avoid concomitant use.

(2) Aspirin; analgesics and antipyretics containing aspirin or other salicylates; barbiturates; phenytoin; sulfonamides

Potentiate methotrexate by displacing it from protein-binding sites in plasma. Salicylates also block renal excretion of methotrexate. This may cause pancytopenia and liver toxicity. Salicylates are present in many prescription and nonprescription drugs, such as headache remedies, pain relievers, and cold remedies.

(3) Other hepatotoxic drugs

Additive liver toxicity

(4) Other antineoplastic drugs

Additive cytotoxic effects, both therapeutic and adverse. Methotrexate is one component of several drug combinations used to treat breast cancer.

**d.** Drugs that *decrease* effects of methotrexate:

Leucovorin (citrovorum factor, folinic acid)

Leucovorin antagonizes the toxic effects of methotrexate and is used as an antidote for high-dose methotrexate regimens or for overdose. It must be given exactly at the specified time, before affected cells become too damaged to respond.

**5. Teach clients**

**a.** With vincristine, eat high-fiber foods, such as raw fruits and vegetables and whole cereal grains, if able. Also try to maintain a high fluid intake. A stool softener or bulk laxative may be prescribed on a daily basis.

To prevent the constipation that may occur during vincristine therapy

**b.** With cyclophosphamide, drink 2 or 3 quarts of fluid daily, if possible, and urinate often, especially at bedtime. If blood is seen in the urine or signs of cystitis occur despite precautions, report this immediately.

Products of cyclophosphamide breakdown are irritating to the bladder lining and may cause bleeding, burning on urination, and other signs of cystitis. High fluid intake and frequent emptying of the bladder help to decrease bladder damage. If blood appears in the urine or if cystitis occurs, the drug should be discontinued.

**c.** With doxorubicin, the urine may turn red for 1 to 2 days after drug administration.

To decrease the anxiety that may occur if the client thinks the red urine is from bleeding. The discoloration is harmless.

**d.** Also with doxorubicin, the client should report edema, shortness of breath, and excessive fatigue.

These are signs of heart failure and require that drug therapy be stopped.

## Review and Application Exercises

1. Compare and contrast normal cells and malignant cells.
2. Which common or major cancers are attributed mainly to environmental factors? Which are attributed to genetic factors?
3. How do cytotoxic antineoplastic drugs destroy malignant cells?
4. Which cytotoxic antineoplastic drugs are associated with bone marrow suppression?
5. Which antineoplastic drugs are cardiotoxic? Which are nephrotoxic? Which are neurotoxic?
6. Which drugs are associated with second malignancies?
7. What is the basis for the anticancer effects of hormones and antihormones?
8. What is the rationale for combination chemotherapy in cancer?
9. Why are antiemetics, drugs for hypercalcemia, and allopurinol often used with clients who are taking antineoplastic drugs?

## Selected References

Bertino, J. R. (1992). Antineoplastic drugs. In K. L. Melmon, H. F. Morrelli, B. B. Hoffman, & D. W. Nierenberg (Eds.), *Clinical pharmacology: Basic principles in therapeutics* (3rd ed.) (pp. 600–641). New York: McGraw-Hill

Blattner, W. A. (1992) Etiology and epidemiology of malignant disease. In W. N. Kelley (Ed.), *Textbook of internal medicine* (2nd ed.) (pp. 1063–1066). Philadelphia: J.B. Lippincott.

Bullock, B. L. (1992). Concepts of altered cellular function. In B. L. Bullock & P. P. Rosendahl (Eds.), *Pathophysiology: Adaptations and alterations in function* (3rd. ed.) (pp. 342–348). Philadelphia: J.B. Lippincott.

Bullock, B. L. (1992). Benign and malignant neoplasia. In B. L. Bullock & P. P. Rosendahl (Eds.), *Pathophysiology: Adaptations and alterations in function* (3rd. ed.) (pp. 349–366). Philadelphia: J.B. Lippincott.

Burrell, N. (1992). Nursing management of adults with cancer. In L. O. Burrell (Ed.), *Adult nursing in hospital and community settings* (pp. 223–259). Norwalk, CT: Appleton & Lange.

Dorr, R. T., & Dalton, W. S. (1993). Cancer chemotherapy. In R. Bressler & M. D. Katz (Eds.), *Geriatric pharmacology* (pp. 535–583). New York: McGraw-Hill.

(1994). *Drug facts and comparisons*. St. Louis: Facts and Comparisons.

Finley, R. S., & LaCivita, C. L. (1992). Neoplastic diseases. In M. A. Koda-Kimble & L. Y. Young (Eds.), *Applied therapeutics: The clinical use of drugs* (5th ed.) (pp. 52-1–52-48). Vancouver, WA: Applied Therapeutics.

Furlong, T. G. (1993). Neurologic complications of immunosuppressive cancer therapy. *Oncology Nursing Forum, 20,* 1337–1354.

Graham, K. M., Pecoraro, D. A., Ventura, M., & Meyer, C. C. (1993). Reducing the incidence of stomatitis using a quality assessment and improvement approach. *Cancer Nursing, 16*(2), 117–122.

Hsing, A. W., Hoover, R. N., McLaughlin, J. K., Co-Chien, H. T., Wacholder, S., Blot, W. J., & Fraumeni, J. F. Jr. (1992). Oral contraceptives and primary liver cancer among young women. *Cancer Causes and Control, 3,* 43–48.

Longo, D. L., & Urba, W. J. (1992). Principles of cancer treatment. In W. N. Kelley (Ed.), *Textbook of internal medicine* (2nd ed.) (pp. 1113–1126). Philadelphia: J.B. Lippincott.

Porth, C. M. (1990). *Pathophysiology: Concepts of altered health states* (3rd ed.) (pp. 57–79). Philadelphia: J.B. Lippincott.

Relling, M. V., & Evans, W. E. (1992). Pediatric neoplastic disorders. In M. A. Koda-Kimble & L. Y. Young (Eds.), *Applied therapeutics: The clinical use of drugs* (5th ed.) (pp. 53-1–53-32). Vancouver, WA: Applied Therapeutics.

Uhlenhopp, M. B. (1992). An overview of the relationship between alkylating agents and therapy-related acute nonlymphocytic leukemia. *Cancer Nursing, 15*(1), 9–17.

# CHAPTER 68

# Drugs Used in Ophthalmic Conditions

## Structures of the eye

The eye is the major sensory organ through which the person receives information about the external environment. An in-depth discussion of vision and ocular anatomy is beyond the scope of this chapter, but some characteristics and functions are described to facilitate understanding of ocular drug therapy. These include the following:

1. The eyelids and lacrimal system function to protect the eye. The *eyelid* is a covering that acts as a barrier to the entry of foreign bodies, strong light, dust, and other potential irritants. The *conjunctiva* is the mucous membrane lining of the eyelids. The *canthi* (singular, canthus) are the angles or corners where upper and lower eyelids meet. The *lacrimal system* produces a fluid that constantly moistens and cleanses the anterior surface of the eyeball. The fluid drains through two small openings in the inner canthus and flows through the nasolacrimal duct into the nasal cavity. When the conjunctiva is irritated or certain emotions are experienced (*e.g.*, sadness), the lacrimal gland produces more fluid than the drainage system can accommodate. The excess fluid overflows the eyelids and becomes *tears*.

2. The eyeball is a spherical structure composed of the sclera, cornea, choroid, and retina, plus special refractory tissues. The *sclera* is a white, opaque fibrous tissue that covers the posterior five sixths of the eyeball. The *cornea* is a transparent, special connective tissue that covers the anterior sixth of the eyeball. The cornea contains no blood vessels. The *choroid*, composed of blood vessels and connective tissue, continues forward to form the iris. The *iris* is composed of pigmented cells, the opening called the *pupil*, and muscles that control the size of the pupil by contracting or dilating in response to stimuli. The *retina* is the innermost layer of the eyeball.

   For vision to occur, light rays must enter the eye through the cornea; travel through the pupil, lens, and vitreous body (see below); and be focused on the retina. Light rays do not travel directly to the retina. Instead, they are deflected in various directions according to the density of the ocular structures through which they pass. This process, called *refraction*, is controlled by the aqueous humor, lens, and vitreous body. The *optic disk* is the area of the retina where ophthalmic blood vessels and the optic nerve enter the eyeball.

3. The structure and function of the eyeball are further influenced by the lens, aqueous humor, and vitreous body. The *lens* is an elastic, transparent structure; its function is to focus light rays to form images on the retina. It is located behind the iris and held in place by suspensory ligaments attached to the ciliary body. The *aqueous humor* is a clear fluid produced by capillaries in the ciliary body. Most of the fluid flows through the pupil into the anterior chamber (between the cornea and the lens and anterior to the iris). A small amount flows into a passage called Schlemm's canal, from which it enters the venous circulation. Under normal circumstances, production and drainage of

Anne Collins Abrams: CLINICAL DRUG THERAPY, Fourth Edition.
© 1995 J.B. Lippincott Company.

aqueous humor are approximately equal, and normal intraocular pressure (about 15–25 mm Hg) is maintained. Impaired drainage of aqueous humor causes increased intraocular pressure. The *vitreous body* is a transparent, jelly-like mass located in the posterior portion of the eyeball. It functions to refract light rays and maintain the normal shape of the eyeball.

## Disorders of the eye

The eye is subject to the development of many disorders that threaten its structure, function, or both. Some disorders in which ophthalmic drugs play a prominent role include the following.

### REFRACTIVE ERRORS

Refractive errors include myopia (nearsightedness), hyperopia (farsightedness), presbyopia, and astigmatism. These conditions impair vision by interfering with the eye's ability to focus light rays on the retina. Ophthalmic drugs are used only in the diagnosis of the conditions; treatment involves prescription of eyeglasses or contact lenses.

### GLAUCOMA

Glaucoma is a common preventable cause of blindness. It occurs when the inflow of aqueous humor into the anterior chamber is greater than the outflow. As a result, intraocular pressure is increased, blood vessels and the optic nerve are compressed, ocular tissues are damaged, and blindness occurs if the condition is not treated effectively.

The most common type of glaucoma is called primary open-angle glaucoma. It is a chronic disorder of unknown cause. A less common but more dramatic type is called narrow-angle glaucoma. Acute glaucoma results from a sudden, severe increase in intraocular pressure and is characterized by progressive ocular damage and loss of vision. Acute glaucoma occurs in people with narrow-angle glaucoma when pupils are dilated, and the outflow of aqueous humor is blocked. Darkness and numerous drugs (*e.g.*, anticholinergics, antihistamines, antipsychotics, and antidepressants) may precipitate acute glaucoma. Secondary glaucoma may follow traumatic or inflammatory conditions of the eye.

### INFLAMMATORY OR
### INFECTIOUS CONDITIONS

Inflammation may be caused by bacteria, viruses, allergic reactions, or irritating chemicals. Infections may result from foreign bodies, contaminated hands, contaminated equipment or solutions used in treatment, or infections in contiguous structures (*e.g.*, nose, face, sinuses). Common inflammatory and infectious disorders include the following:

1. **Conjunctivitis** is often caused by allergic reactions that are characterized by a watery discharge and pruritus. A highly contagious form of conjunctivitis ("pink eye") commonly occurs in children. Chronic conjunctivitis is usually caused by *Staphylococcus aureus, Streptococcus viridans*, or *Diplococcus pneumoniae* and is characterized by mucoid or mucopurulent discharge and red, edematous conjunctiva. Conjunctivitis with a purulent discharge is most often caused by the gonococcus; corneal ulcers and scarring may result.
2. **Blepharitis** is a chronic infection of glands and lash follicles on the margins of the eyelids. A hordeolum (commonly called a sty) is often associated with blepharitis. The most common causes are seborrhea and staphylococcal infections.
3. **Keratitis** (inflammation of the cornea) may be caused by microorganisms, trauma, allergy, ischemia, and drying of the cornea (*e.g.*, from inadequate lacrimation or inability to close the eyelid). The major symptom is pain, which ranges from mild to severe. Vision may not be affected initially. However, if not treated effectively, corneal ulceration, scarring, and impaired vision may result.
4. Bacterial **corneal ulcers** are most often caused by pneumococci and staphylococci. Pseudomonal ulcers are less common but may rapidly progress to perforation. Fungal ulcers may follow topical corticosteroid therapy or injury with vegetable matter, such as a tree branch. Viral ulcers are usually caused by the herpesvirus.

## Ophthalmic drugs

Drugs used to diagnose or treat ophthalmic disorders represent numerous therapeutic classifications, most of which are discussed in other chapters. Some drugs are used primarily by ophthalmologists. Major classes of drugs used in ophthalmology include the following:

1. Anti-infective drugs are used to treat bacterial, viral, and fungal infections (see Chaps. 33–43). They are usually applied topically but may be injected subconjunctivally or intravenously in severe infections.
2. Autonomic drugs are used extensively in ophthalmology for diagnostic and therapeutic purposes (see Chaps. 17–21). Some are used to dilate the pupil before ophthalmologic examinations or surgical procedures; some are used to constrict the pupil and decrease intraocular pressure in glaucoma. Auto-

nomic drugs indicated in one disorder may be contraindicated in another. For example, anticholinergic drugs are usually contraindicated in glaucoma. Adrenergic mydriatics (*e.g.*, epinephrine, phenylephrine) should be used cautiously in clients with hypertension, cardiac arrhythmias, arteriosclerotic heart disease, and hyperthyroidism.

3. Corticosteroids (see Chap. 24) are often used to treat inflammatory conditions of the eye, thereby reducing scarring and preventing loss of vision. Corticosteroids are generally more effective in acute than chronic inflammatory conditions. Because these drugs are potentially toxic, they should not be used to treat minor disorders or disorders that can be effectively treated with safer drugs. When used, corticosteroids should be administered in the lowest effective dose and for the shortest effective time. Long-term use should be avoided when possible. When used in ophthalmologic conditions, corticosteroids may be administered topically, systemically, or both. Corticosteroids are contraindicated in eye infections caused by the herpesvirus because the drugs increase the severity of the infection.

4. Carbonic anhydrase inhibitors and osmotic diuretics are given to decrease intraocular pressure in glaucoma and before certain surgical procedures. Carbonic anhydrase inhibitors were initially used as diuretics, but their effectiveness in lowering intraocular pressure (by decreasing production of aqueous humor) does not depend on diuretic effects.

5. Miscellaneous drugs used by the ophthalmologist include the following:
   a. A chelating agent, edetate disodium (Endrate), is used to remove calcium deposits in the cornea, which cause pain or impair vision. The drug also may be used for emergency treatment of calcium hydroxide burns of the eye. No ophthalmic preparation is available; the intravenous preparation is diluted with sterile normal saline to a concentration of 0.35% to 1.85%. The diluted solution is used to irrigate the eye for about 15 minutes.
   b. Fluorescein (Ful-Glo) is the most commonly used dye. This agent is useful in diagnosing lesions or foreign bodies in the cornea, fitting contact lenses, and studying the lacrimal system and flow of aqueous humor. Rose bengal is another dye that may be used.

Drug therapy of ophthalmic conditions is unique because of the location, structure, and function of the eye. Many systemic drugs are unable to cross the blood-eye barrier and achieve therapeutic concentrations in ocular structures. Some drugs penetrate the eye better than others, however, depending on the serum drug concentration, size of drug molecules, solubility of the drug in fat, extent of drug protein binding, and whether inflammation is present in the eye. Generally, penetration is greater if the drug achieves a high concentration in the blood, has small molecules, is fat soluble, and is poorly bound to serum proteins and if inflammation is present.

## METHODS OF ADMINISTRATION

Because of the difficulties associated with systemic therapy, various methods of administering drugs locally have been developed. The most common method of drug administration in ocular therapeutics is topical application of ophthalmic solutions (eye drops) to the conjunctiva. Drugs are distributed through the tear film covering the eye and may be used for superficial disorders (*e.g.*, conjunctivitis) or for relatively deep ocular disorders (*e.g.*, when epinephrine is given for glaucoma, the drug must penetrate the cornea, anterior chamber, and ciliary processes to exert therapeutic effects). Other topical dosage forms include ophthalmic ointments and a specialized method of administering pilocarpine so that the drug is slowly released over a 1-week period (Ocusert). Ocusert is a small plastic device inserted into the conjunctival area and replaced weekly by the client. It is used for long-term management of glaucoma.

Other methods of local administration of drugs involve special injection techniques used by ophthalmologists. These include injections through the conjunctiva to subconjunctival tissues or under the fibrous capsule beneath the conjunctiva (sub-Tenon's injection). These injections are painful, and topical anesthetic solutions should be applied before the procedure. Antibiotics and corticosteroids are the drugs most likely to be administered by subconjunctival or sub-Tenon's injection. A third type of injection, called retrobulbar injection, involves injecting a drug behind the globe of the eyeball. Corticosteroids and preoperative local anesthetics may be administered this way.

## Individual drugs

See Tables 68-1 and 68-2.

## *Nursing Process*

### Assessment

Assess the client's condition in relation to ophthalmic disorders.
- Determine whether the client has impaired vision and if so, the extent or severity of the impairment. Minimal assessment includes the vision-impaired client's ability to participate in activities of daily living, including safe ambulation. Maximal assessment depends on the nurse's ability and working situation. Some nurses do complete vision testing and ophthalmoscopic examinations.
- Identify risk factors for eye disorders. These include trauma,

(*Text continues on p. 704*)

## TABLE 68-1. DRUGS USED IN OCULAR DISORDERS*

| Ocular Effects | Clinical Indications | Generic/Trade Name | Routes and Dosage Ranges | |
| --- | --- | --- | --- | --- |
| | | | *Adults* | *Children* |
| *Autonomic Drugs* | | | | |
| *Adrenergics* | | | | |
| 1. Decreased production of aqueous humor<br>2. Mydriasis<br>3. Decreased intraocular pressure<br>4. Vasoconstriction<br>5. Photophobia | 1. Glaucoma<br>2. Ophthalmoscopic examination<br>3. Reduction of adhesion formation with uveitis<br>4. Preoperative and postoperative mydriasis<br>5. Local hemostasis | **Dipivefrin (0.1% solution)** (Propine) | Topically, 1 drop in affected eye(s) twice daily q12h | |
| | | **Epinephrine hydrochloride (0.25%, 0.5%, 1%, and 2% solutions)** (Epifrin, Glaucon) | Topically 1 drop in each eye once or twice daily | Same as adults |
| | | **Hydroxyamphetamine (1% solution)** (Paredrine) | Before ophthalmoscopy, topically, 1 drop in each eye | |
| | | **Phenylephrine (2.5% and 10% solutions)** (Neo-Synephrine) | Before ophthalmoscopy or refraction, topically, 1 drop of 2.5% or 10% solution<br>Preoperatively, topically, 1 drop of 2.5% or 10% solution 30–60 min before surgery<br>Postoperatively, topically, 1 drop of 10% solution once or twice daily | Refraction, topically, 1 drop of 2.5% solution |
| *Antiadrenergic (Beta-Blocking) Drugs* | | | | |
| 1. Decreased production of aqueous humor<br>2. Reduced intraocular pressure | Glaucoma | **Betaxolol** (Betoptic) | Topically to each eye, 1 drop q12h | |
| | | **Carteolol** (Ocupress) | Topically to affected eye(s) 1 drop q12h | |
| | | **Levobunolol** (Betagan) | Topically to the affected eye, 1 drop once or twice daily | |
| | | **Metipranolol** (Optipranolol) | Topically to affected eye(s) 1 drop q12h | |
| | | **Timolol maleate** (Timoptic) | Topically, 1 drop of 0.25% or 0.5% solution in each eye twice daily q12h | |
| *Cholinergics* | | | | |
| 1. Increased outflow of aqueous humor<br>2. Miosis | Glaucoma | **Pilocarpine (0.25%–10% solutions)** (Almocarpine, Isopto Carpine, Pilocar, Pilocel, Pilomiotin) | Chronic glaucoma, topically, 1 drop of 1% or 2% solution instilled in each eye q6–8h initially. Then, drug concentration and frequency of administration are adjusted to maintain intraocular pressure in the desired range. Drops are usually instilled four times daily. | |
| | | **Pilocarpine ocular therapeutic system** (Ocusert Pilo-20, Ocusert Pilo-40) | One system placed into conjunctival sac per week, according to package directions. Each system releases 20 or 40 µg pilocarpine per hour for 1 wk. | |
| | | **Carbachol** (Carbacel, Isopto Carbachol) | Topically, 1 drop of 0.75%–3% solution instilled in each eye initially. Then drug concentration and frequency of administration are adjusted to maintain intraocular pressure in the desired range. | |
| *Anticholinesterase Agents* | | | | |
| 1. Increased outflow of aqueous humor<br>2. Miosis | Glaucoma | **Demecarium bromide** (Humorsol) | Topically, 1 drop of 0.125%–0.25% solution in each eye twice a day to twice a week, depending on condition | |
| | | **Echothiophate iodide** (Phospholine Iodide) | Topically, 1 drop of solution (0.03%, 0.06%, 0.125%, or 0.25%) in each eye q12–48h | |
| | | **Isoflurophate** (Floropryl) | Topically, ¼-inch strip of ointment in the lower conjunctival sac of each eye q12–72h | |
| | | **Physostigmine sulfate** (Eserine Sulfate) | Topically, 0.25% ointment three or four times daily | |

(continued)

## TABLE 68-1.   DRUGS USED IN OCULAR DISORDERS* *(Continued)*

| Ocular Effects | Clinical Indications | Generic/Trade Name | Routes and Dosage Ranges | |
|---|---|---|---|---|
| | | | *Adults* | *Children* |
| | | **Physostigmine salicylate** (Isopto Eserine) | Topically, 1–2 drops of 0.25%–0.5% solution in each eye up to four times daily | |
| *Anticholinergics* 1. Mydriasis 2. Cycloplegia 3. Photophobia | 1. Mydriasis for refraction and other diagnostic purposes 2. Pre- and post-operatively in intraocular surgery 3. Treatment of uveitis 4. Treatment of some secondary glaucoma | **Atropine sulfate (0.5%–3% solutions)** | Before intraocular surgery, topically, 1 drop of solution Following intraocular surgery, topically, 1 drop of solution once daily | |
| | | **Cyclopentolate hydrochloride** (Cyclogyl) | For refraction, topically, 1 drop of 0.5% or 2% solution instilled once Before ophthalmoscopy, 1 drop of 0.5% solution | For refraction, topically, 1 drop of 0.5%, 1%, or 2% solution, repeated in 10 min |
| | | **Homatropine hydrobromide (2% and 5% solutions)** (Isopto Homatropine) | Refraction, topically, 1 drop of 5% solution every 5 min for two or three doses or 1–2 drops of 2% solution every 10–15 min for five doses Uveitis, topically, 1 drop of 2% or 5% solution two or three times daily | |
| | | **Scopolamine hydrobromide (0.25% solution)** (Isopto Hyoscine) | Refraction, topically, 1–2 drops in affected eye(s) 1 h before examination | |
| | | **Tropicamide (0.5% and 1% solutions)** (Mydriacyl) | Before refraction or ophthalmoscopy, topically, 1 drop of 0.5% or 1% solution, repeated in 5 min, then every 20–30 min as needed to maintain mydriasis | |
| *Diuretics* | | | | |
| *Carbonic Anhydrase Inhibitors* 1. Decreased production of aqueous humor 2. Decreased intraocular pressure | 1. Glaucoma 2. Preoperatively in intraocular surgery | **Acetazolamide** (Diamox) | PO 250 mg q6h Sustained-release capsules (Diamox Sequels), PO 500 mg q12h IV, IM 500 mg initially, repeated in 2–4 h if necessary | PO 10–15 mg/kg per day in divided doses IV, IM 5–10 mg/kg per day in divided doses, q6h |
| | | **Dichlorphenamide** (Daranide) | PO 50–200 mg q6–8h. Maintenance dosage, 25–50 mg one to three times daily | |
| | | **Methazolamide** (Neptazane) | PO 50–100 mg q8h | |
| *Osmotic Agents* 1. Reduced volume of vitreous humor 2. Decreased intraocular pressure | 1. Preoperatively in intraocular surgery 2. Treatment of acute glaucoma | **Glycerin** (Osmoglyn) | PO 1–1.5 g/kg, usually given as a 50% or 75% solution 1–1½ h before surgery | Same as adults |
| | | **Isosorbide** (Ismotic) | Emergency reduction of intraocular pressure (*e.g.,* acute angle-closure glaucoma), PO 1.5 g/kg up to four times daily if necessary | |
| | | **Mannitol** (Osmitrol) | IV 1.5–2 g/kg given as a 20% solution over 30–60 min | Same as adults |
| *Miscellaneous Agents* | | | | |
| *Anesthetics, Local* Surface anesthesia of conjunctiva and cornea | 1. Tonometry 2. Subconjunctival injections | **Proparacaine hydrochloride** (Alcaine, Ophthaine) | Minor procedures, topically, 1–2 drops of 0.5% solution; instillation may be repeated for deeper anesthesia | |

*(continued)*

**TABLE 68-1. DRUGS USED IN OCULAR DISORDERS\*** *(Continued)*

| Ocular Effects | Clinical Indications | Generic/Trade Name | Routes and Dosage Ranges | |
|---|---|---|---|---|
| | | | *Adults* | *Children* |
| | 3. Removal of foreign bodies<br>4. Removal of sutures | **Tetracaine hydrochloride** (Pontocaine) | Minor procedures, topically, 1–2 drops of 0.5% solution; 2–4 instillations are required for deeper anesthesia | |
| *Antiallergic Agent* | Allergic keratitis or conjunctivitis | **Cromolyn sodium** (Opticrom) | 1–2 drops in each eye four to six times daily at regular intervals | Same as adults |
| *Antiseptic* | Prophylaxis of gonorrheal ophthalmia neonatorum | **Silver nitrate ophthalmic** | | Newborns, topically, 2 drops of 1% solution in each eye |
| *Lubricants*<br>Serve as "artificial tears" | 1. Prevent damage to the cornea in clients with keratitis<br>2. Protect the cornea during gonioscopy and other procedures<br>3. Moisten contact lenses<br>4. Lubricate artificial eyes | **Methylcellulose** (Methulose, Visculose, others)<br><br>**Polyvinyl alcohol** (Liquifilm, others) | Topically, 1–2 drops as needed<br><br><br><br>Topically, 1–2 drops as needed | |

\* Anti-infective and anti-inflammatory agents are listed in Table 68-2.

allergies, infection in one eye (a risk factor for infection in the other eye), use of contact lenses, infections of facial structures or skin, and occupational exposure to chemical irritants or foreign bodies.

- Signs and symptoms vary with particular disorders:
  - Pain is usually associated with corneal abrasions or inflammation. Sudden, severe pain may indicate acute angle-closure glaucoma. Acute glaucoma requires immediate treatment to lower intraocular pressure and minimize damage to the eye.
  - Signs of inflammation (redness, edema, heat, tenderness) are especially evident with infection or inflammation of external ocular structures, such as the eyelids and conjunctiva. A mucoid or purulent discharge also often occurs.
  - Pruritus is most often associated with allergic conjunctivitis.
  - Photosensitivity commonly occurs with keratitis.

### Nursing diagnoses

- Sensory-Perceptual Alteration: Impaired vision
- Pain in eyes related to infection, inflammation, or increased intraocular pressure (glaucoma)
- High Risk for Injury: Blindness related to inadequately treated glaucoma or ophthalmic infections
- High Risk for Injury: Trauma related to blurred vision from disease process or drug therapy
- Impaired Physical Mobility related to impaired vision

- Body Image Disturbance related to impaired vision and chronic illness
- Anxiety related to acute and chronic disturbances in vision
- Knowledge Deficit related to prevention and treatment of ocular disorders

### Planning/Goals

*The client will:*

- Take ophthalmic medications as prescribed
- Follow safety precautions to protect eyes from trauma and disease
- Experience improvement in signs and symptoms (*e.g.,* decreased drainage with infections, decreased eye pain with glaucoma)
- Avoid injury from impaired vision (*e.g.,* falls)
- Avoid systemic effects of ophthalmic drugs
- Have intraocular pressure measured regularly to monitor effects of antiglaucoma drugs

### Interventions

Use measures to minimize ocular disorders.

- Treat eye injuries appropriately:
  - For chemical burns, irrigate the eyes with copious amounts of water as soon as possible (*i.e.,* near the area where the injury occurred). Do not wait for transport to a first-aid station, hospital, or other health-care facility. Damage continues as long as the chemical is in contact with the eye.

**TABLE 68-2. OPHTHALMIC ANTI-INFECTIVE AND ANTI-INFLAMMATORY AGENTS**

| Generic/Trade Name | Routes and Dosage Ranges | |
| --- | --- | --- |
| | *Adults* | *Children* |
| ***Antibacterial Agents*** | | |
| **Bacitracin** (Baciguent) | Ophthalmic ointment, topically, instill in infected eye one to three times daily | |
| **Chloramphenicol** (Chloromycetin) (Chloroptic [0.5% solution, 1% ointment]) | Mild conjunctivitis: topically, 1 drop of 0.5% ophthalmic solution q1–2h or ointment instilled three or four times daily Severe conjunctivitis, corneal ulcers: topically, 1 drop of 0.5% solution every 30 min | Topically, same as adults |
| **Ciprofloxacin ophthalmic solution** (Ciloxan) | Corneal ulcers, topically to affected eye. Day 1, 2 drops q15min for 6 h, then q30min for rest of day; day 2, 2 drops q1h; days 3–14, 2 drops q4h. Conjunctivitis, 1–2 drops q2h while awake for 2 d, then 1–2 drops q4h while awake for 5 d | Safety and effectiveness not established for children younger than 12 years |
| **Erythromycin** (Ilotycin ophthalmic [0.5% ointment]) | | Prevention of neonatal gonococcal or chlamydial conjunctivitis, topically, 0.5–1 cm in each eye |
| **Gentamicin sulfate** (Garamycin) | Topically, ophthalmic solution (0.3%) 1 drop q1–4h; ophthalmic ointment (0.3%), instill two or three times daily | Topically, same as adults |
| **Norfloxacin ophthalmic solution** (Chibroxin) | Topically to affected eye(s), 1–2 drops four times daily, up to 7 d | Same as adults for children 1 year and older; safety not established for children younger than 1 year |
| **Polymyxin B sulfate** | Corneal ulcers due to *Pseudomonas aeruginosa*: topically, 1 drop of a freshly prepared solution (20,000 units/ml), instilled two to ten times hourly | |
| **Sulfacetamide sodium** (Bleph-10 Liquifilm [10% solution or ointment] Isopto Cetamide [15% solution]) (Cetamide [10% ointment] Sodium Sulamyd [10% and 30% solution, 10% ointment]) (Also available generically as 10% and 30% solutions) | Acute catarrhal conjunctivitis caused by *Staphylococcus aureus, Diplococcus pneumoniae, Haemophilus influenzae, Neisseria catarrhalis*: topically, 1 drop of 10% or 15% solution every 10–30min Chronic conjunctivitis due to *Proteus* organisms: topically, 10% ointment instilled three or four times daily Chronic blepharoconjunctivitis due to *S. aureus*: topically, 1 drop of 30% solution three or four times daily Corneal ulcers due to *Escherichia coli* or *Klebsiella pneumoniae*: 1 drop of 10% solution every 30 min or 10% ointment instilled three or four times daily | |
| **Sulfisoxazole diolamine** (Gantrisin [4% solution]) | Topically, 2–3 drops in affected eye three or more times daily | |
| **Tetracycline** (Achromycin) | Inclusion conjunctivitis: topically, 1% solution or ointment instilled three or four times daily for 30 d | Conjunctivitis, same as adults Prevention of neonatal gonococcal or chlamydial conjunctivitis, 0.5–1 cm of ointment into each eye |
| **Tobramycin** (Tobrex [0.3% solution and ointment]) | Topically, 1–2 drops two to six times daily or ointment two or three times daily | |
| ***Antiviral Agents*** | | |
| **Idoxuridine** (Herplex) | Herpes simplex infection of eyelids, conjunctiva, and cornea: topically, 1 drop of 0.1% solution q1h during daytime hours and q2h at night, or 0.5% ointment instilled four or five times daily. Treatment should be continued for at least 2 wk. | |
| **Trifluridine** (Viroptic) | Keratoconjunctivitis or corneal ulcers caused by herpes simplex virus: topically, 1 drop of 1% solution q2h while awake (maximal daily dose, 9 drops) until corneal ulcer heals, then 1 drop q4h (minimal dose, 5 drops daily for 7 d) | |
| **Vidarabine** (Vira-A) | Keratoconjunctivitis caused by herpes simplex virus: topically, 3% ointment instilled q3h | |
| ***Antifungal Agent*** | | |
| **Natamycin** (Natacyn) | Topically, 1 drop of 5% suspension q1–2h | |

*(continued)*

**TABLE 68-2. OPHTHALMIC ANTI-INFECTIVE AND ANTI-INFLAMMATORY AGENTS** (*Continued*)

| Generic/Trade Name | Routes and Dosage Ranges | |
| | *Adults* | *Children* |
| --- | --- | --- |
| ***Corticosteroids*** | | |
| **Dexamethasone**<br>(Decadron Phosphate Ophthalmic [0.1% solution, 0.05% ointment] Maxidex [0.1% solution, 0.05% ointment]) | Topically, 1 drop of solution q1–2h until response is obtained, then less frequently; ointment, apply three or four times daily | |
| **Fluorometholone**<br>(FML Liquifilm [0.1% suspension]) | Topically, 1 drop q1–2h until response is obtained, then less frequently | |
| **Medrysone**<br>(HMS Liquifilm [1% suspension]) | Topically, 1 drop q1–2h until response is obtained, then less frequently | |
| **Prednisolone acetate**<br>(Econopred [0.125% or 1% suspension]) | Topically, 1 drop q1–2h until response is obtained, then less frequently | |
| **Prednisolone sodium phosphate**<br>(Inflamase [0.125% and 1% solution])<br>(Metreton [0.5% solution]) | Topically, 1 drop q1–2h until response is obtained, then less frequently; ointment, apply three or four times daily | |

- For thermal burns, apply cold compresses to the area.
- Superficial foreign bodies may be removed by irrigation with water. Foreign bodies embedded in ocular structures must be removed by a physician.
- Warm wet compresses are often useful in ophthalmic inflammation or infections. They relieve pain and promote healing by increasing the blood supply to the affected area.

*Teach clients:*
- Wear safety goggles when working in high-risk areas. These are often provided by employers.
- Avoid overwearing contact lenses. This is a common cause of corneal abrasion and may cause corneal ulceration. The lens wearer should consult a physician when eye pain occurs. Antibiotics are often prescribed for corneal abrasions to prevent development of ulcers.
- Avoid regular use of nonprescription eye drops (*e.g.*, Murine, Visine). Persistent eye irritation and redness should be reported to a physician.
- Avoid eyestrain by using appropriate lighting for reading and handwork. Also, limit periods of reading, watching television, and other visual activities.
- Minimize exposure to dust, smog, cigarette smoke, and other eye irritants when possible.
- Have regular eye examinations and testing for glaucoma after 40 years of age.
- Avoid straining at stool (use laxatives or stool softeners if necessary), heavy lifting, bending over, coughing, and vomiting when possible. These activities increase intraocular pressure, which may cause ocular damage in glaucoma and after intraocular surgery.

**Evaluation**
- Observe and interview for compliance with instructions regarding drug therapy and follow-up care.

- Observe and interview for relief of symptoms.
- Observe for systemic adverse effects of ophthalmic drugs (*e.g.*, tachycardia and arrhythmias with adrenergics; bradycardia and congestive heart failure with beta-blockers).

# Principles of therapy

## OCULAR INFECTIONS

For drug therapy for ocular infections, guidelines regarding choice of drug, dosage, and route of administration include the following:

1. Drug therapy is usually initiated as soon as culture material (eye secretions) has been obtained, often with a broad-spectrum antibacterial agent or a combination of two or more antibiotics.
2. Topical administration is used most often, and recommended drugs include bacitracin, colistimethate, chloramphenicol, polymyxin B, and sulfacetamide. These agents are rarely given systemically. They do not cause sensitization to commonly used systemic antibiotics and do not promote growth of drug-resistant microorganisms.
3. In severe infections, antibacterial drugs may be given both topically and systemically. Because systemic antibiotics penetrate the eye poorly, large doses are required to attain therapeutic drug concentrations in ocular structures. Drugs that reach therapeutic levels in the eye when given in proper dosage include amp-

icillin and dicloxacillin. Gentamicin and other antibiotics penetrate the eye when inflammation is present.

4. Combination products containing two or more antibacterials are available for topical treatment of external ocular infections. These products are most useful when therapy must be initiated before the infecting microorganism is identified. Mixtures provide a broader spectrum of antibacterial activity than a single drug. Most of the available combination products contain various amounts of polymyxin B, neomycin, and bacitracin (*e.g.*, Neosporin).

5. Fixed-dose combinations of an antibacterial agent and corticosteroid are available for topical use in selected conditions (*e.g.*, staphylococcal keratitis, blepharoconjunctivitis, allergic conjunctivitis, and some postoperative inflammatory reactions). Chloramphenicol and corticosteroid mixtures include Chloromycetin-Hydrocortisone and Chloroptic. A combination of chloramphenicol, polymyxin B, and corticosteroid is available as Ophthocort. Neomycin and corticosteroid mixtures include Neo-Cortef and NeoDecadron. Neomycin, polymyxin B, and corticosteroid mixtures include Poly-Pred and Maxitrol. Neomycin, polymyxin B, bacitracin, and corticosteroid mixtures include Cortisporin and Coracin. Sulfacetamide and corticosteroid mixtures include Blephamide, Cetapred, Metimyd, Optimyd, and Vasocidin.

6. Trifluridine (Viroptic) is the drug of choice in eye infections caused by the herpes simplex virus.

7. In fungal infections, natamycin (Natacyn) may be preferred because it has a broad spectrum of antifungal activity and is nonirritating and nontoxic.

## GLAUCOMA

For drug therapy of chronic, primary open-angle glaucoma, pilocarpine was commonly used, but more recently beta-adrenergic blocking agents have become preferred drugs. They are effective in lowering intraocular pressure and do not cause miosis as pilocarpine does. Several beta-blockers are now available for ophthalmic use. Most adverse effects occurring with systemic beta-blockers also have been reported with ophthalmic preparations.

## USE OF OPHTHALMIC OINTMENTS

Many ophthalmic drugs are available as eye drops (solutions or suspensions) and ointments. Ointments do not need to be administered as frequently and often produce higher concentrations of drug in target tissues. However, ointments also cause blurred vision, which limits their daytime use, at least for ambulatory clients. In some situations, drops may be used during waking hours and ointments at bedtime. However, the two formulations are *not* interchangeable.

## USE IN CHILDREN

Topical ophthalmic drug therapy in children differs little from that in adults. Few studies of ophthalmic drug therapy in children have been reported, and many conditions for which adults need therapy (*e.g.*, cataract, glaucoma) rarely occur in children. A major use of topical ophthalmic drugs in children is to dilate the pupil and paralyze accommodation for ophthalmoscopic examination. As a general rule, the short-acting mydriatics and cycloplegics (*e.g.*, cyclopentolate, tropicamide) are preferred because they cause fewer systemic adverse effects than atropine and scopolamine. In addition, lower drug concentrations are usually given empirically because of the smaller size of children and the potential risk of systemic adverse effects.

## USE IN OLDER ADULTS

Older adults are at risk for developing ocular disorders, especially glaucoma and cataracts. General principles of ophthalmic drug therapy are the same as for younger adults. In addition, older adults are likely to have cardiovascular disorders, which may be aggravated by systemic absorption of topical eye medication. Thus, accurate dosage and occlusion of the nasolacrimal duct in the inner canthus of the eye are needed to prevent adverse drug effects (*e.g.*, hypertension, tachycardia, or arrhythmias with adrenergic drugs and bradycardia or congestive heart failure with beta-blockers).

## NURSING ACTIONS: OPHTHALMIC DRUGS

| *Nursing Actions* | *Rationale/Explanation* |
|---|---|
| **1. Administer accurately** | |
| **a.** Read labels of ophthalmic medications carefully. | To avoid error. For example, many drugs are available in several concentrations. The correct concentration and the correct drug must be given. |
| **b.** Read medication orders carefully and accurately. | To avoid error. Abbreviations (*e.g.*, O.S., O.D., O.U.) are often used in physicians' orders and must be interpreted accurately. |
| **c.** For hospitalized clients, keep eye medications at the bedside when possible. | Eye medications should be ordered for and used by one person only. They are dispensed in small amounts for this purpose. This minimizes cross-contamination and risk of infection. |
| **d.** Wash hands before approaching the client for instillation of eye medications. | To reduce risks of infection |
| **e.** To administer eye drops, have the client lie down or tilt the head backward and look upward. Then, pull down the lower lid to expose the conjunctival sac, and drop the medication into the sac.<br><br>Alternate method: gently grasp the lower lid and pull it outward to form a pouch into which medication is instilled.<br><br>After instillation, have the client close the eyes gently, and apply pressure to the inner canthus briefly (nurse or client). | Absorption of the drug and its concentration in ocular tissues depend partly on the length of time the medication is in contact with ocular tissues. Contact time is increased by the "pouch" method of administration, closing the eyes (delays outflow into the nasolacrimal) duct), and pressure on the inner canthus (delays outflow and decreases side effects resulting from systemic absorption). |
| **f.** When instilling ophthalmic ointments, position the client as above, and apply a one-quarter-inch to one-half-inch strip of ointment to the conjunctiva. | |
| **g.** Do not touch the dropper tip or ointment top to the eye or anything else. | To avoid contamination of the medication and infection |
| **h.** When crusts or secretions are present, cleanse the eye prior to administering medication. | If the eye is not cleansed, the drug may not be absorbed. |
| **i.** When two or more eye drops are scheduled for the same time, they should be instilled about 5 minutes apart. | To avoid drug loss by dilution and outflow into the nasolacrimal duct |
| **2. Observe for therapeutic effects** | Therapeutic effects depend on the reason for use. |
| **a.** With mydriatics, observe for dilation of the pupil. | Mydriasis begins within 5 to 15 minutes after instillation. |
| **b.** With miotics, observe for constriction of the pupil. | |
| **c.** With anti-infective drugs, observe for decreased redness, edema, and drainage. | |
| **d.** With osmotic agents, observe for decreased intraocular pressure. | With oral glycerin, maximal decrease in intraocular pressure occurs approximately 1 hour after administration, and effects persist for about 5 hours. With IV mannitol, maximal decrease in intraocular pressure occurs within 30 to 60 minutes, and effects last 6 to 8 hours. |

| *Nursing Actions* | *Rationale/Explanation* |
|---|---|

**3. Observe for adverse effects**

**a.** Local effects:

(1) Irritation and discomfort, lacrimation, contact dermatitis of eyelids, allergic conjunctivitis

These effects may occur with any topical ophthalmic agents, from the drug itself, or from the preservatives in the formulation.

(2) With antibacterial agents—superinfection or sensitization

Superinfection caused by drug-resistant organisms may occur. Sensitization means that topical application induces antibody formation. Therefore, if the same or a related drug is subsequently administered systemically, an allergic reaction may occur. The allergic reaction most often involves dermatitis; occasionally urticaria or anaphylaxis occurs. Penicillin is the most frequently involved drug. Other drugs include streptomycin, neomycin, gentamicin, and sulfonamides (with the exception of sulfacetamide sodium). Sensitization can be prevented or minimized by avoiding topical administration of antibacterial agents that are commonly given systemically.

(3) With anticholinergics, adrenergics, topical corticosteroids—glaucoma

Mydriatic drugs (anticholinergics and adrenergics) may cause an acute attack of angle-closure glaucoma in clients with narrow angles by blocking outflow of aqueous humor. Topical corticosteroids raise intraocular pressure in some clients. The "glaucomatous" response occurs most often in clients with chronic, primary open-angle glaucoma and their relatives. It also may occur in clients with myopia or diabetes mellitus. The magnitude of increased intraocular pressure depends on the concentration, frequency of administration, duration of therapy, and anti-inflammatory potency of the corticosteroid. Increased intraocular pressure has been reported most often with 0.1% dexamethasone (Decadron). This adverse effect can be minimized by checking intraocular pressure every 2 months in clients receiving long-term therapy with topical corticosteroids.

(4) Cataract formation

This is most likely to occur with long-term use of anticholinesterase agents.

(5) With miotic drugs—decreased vision in dim light

These agents prevent pupil dilation, which normally occurs in dim light or darkness.

**b.** Systemic effects:

Systemic absorption and adverse effects of eye drops can be prevented or minimized by applying pressure to the inner canthus during and after instillation of the medications. Pressure may be applied by the nurse or the client.

(1) With miotics—sweating, nausea, vomiting, diarrhea, abdominal pain, bradycardia, hypotension, bronchoconstriction. Toxic doses produce ataxia, confusion, convulsions, coma, respiratory failure, and death.

These cholinergic or parasympathomimetic effects occur rarely with pilocarpine or carbachol. They are more likely to occur with the long-acting anticholinesterase agents, especially echothiophate (Phospholine Iodide). Acute toxicity may be reversed by an anticholinergic agent, atropine, given IV.

(2) With anticholinergic mydriatics—dryness of the mouth and skin, fever, rash, tachycardia, confusion, hallucinations, delirium

These effects are most likely to occur with atropine and in children and older adults. Tropicamide (Mydriacyl) rarely causes systemic reactions.

(3) With adrenergic mydriatics—tachycardia, hypertension, premature ventricular contractions, tremors, headache

Systemic effects are uncommon. They are more likely to occur with repeated instillations of high drug concentrations (*e.g.* epinephrine 2%, phenylephrine [Neo-Synephrine] 10%).

(4) With carbonic anhydrase inhibitors—anorexia, nausea, vomiting, diarrhea, paresthesias, weakness, lethargy

Nausea, malaise, and paresthesias (numbness and tingling of extremities) commonly occur.

*(continued)*

| *Nursing Actions* | *Rationale/Explanation* |
|---|---|
| (5) With osmotic diuretics—dehydration, nausea, vomiting, headache; hyperglycemia and glycosuria with glycerin (Osmoglyn) | These agents may produce profound diuresis and dehydration. Oral agents (*e.g.*, glycerin) are less likely to cause severe systemic effects than IV agents (*e.g.*, mannitol). These agents are usually given in a single dose, which decreases the risks of serious adverse reactions unless large doses are given. |
| (6) With corticosteroids, see Chapter 24. | Serious adverse effects may occur with long-term use of corticosteroids. |
| (7) With antibacterial agents, see Chapter 33 and the chapter on the individual drug group. | Adverse effects may occur with all antibacterial agents. |
| **4. Observe for drug interactions**<br>**a.** Drugs that *increase* effects of adrenergic (sympathomimetic) ophthalmic drugs: | |
| (1) Anticholinergic ophthalmic drugs | The combination (*e.g.*, atropine and phenylephrine) produces additive mydriasis. |
| (2) Systemic adrenergic drugs | Additive risks of adverse effects (*e.g.*, tachycardia, cardiac arrhythmias, hypertension) |
| **b.** Drugs that *decrease* effects of adrenergic ophthalmic preparations: | |
| Cholinergic and anticholinesterase ophthalmic drugs | Antagonize mydriatic effects of adrenergic drugs |
| **c.** Drugs that *increase* effects of antiadrenergic ophthalmic preparations: | |
| Systemic antiadrenergics (*e.g.*, propranolol, atenolol, metoprolol, nadolol, timolol) | When the client is receiving a topical beta-blocker in ocular disorders, administration of systemic beta-blocking agents in cardiovascular disorders may cause additive systemic toxicity. |
| **d.** Drugs that *increase* effects of anticholinergic ophthalmic drugs: | |
| (1) Adrenergic ophthalmic agents | Additive mydriasis |
| (2) Systemic anticholinergic drugs (*e.g.*, atropine) and other drugs with anticholinergic effects (*e.g.*, some antihistamines, antipsychotic agents, and tricyclic antidepressants) | Additive anticholinergic effects (mydriasis, blurred vision, tachycardia). These drugs are hazardous in glaucoma. |
| **e.** Drugs that *decrease* effects of cholinergic and anticholinesterase ophthalmic drugs: | |
| (1) Anticholinergics and drugs with anticholinergic effects (*e.g.*, atropine, antipsychotic agents, tricyclic antidepressants, some antihistamines) | Antagonize antiglaucoma (miotic) effects of cholinergic and anticholinesterase drugs |
| (2) Corticosteroids | Long-term use of corticosteroids, topically or systemically, raises intraocular pressure and may cause glaucoma. Therefore, corticosteroids decrease effects of all drugs used for glaucoma. |
| (3) Sympathomimetic drugs | Antagonize miotic (antiglaucoma) effects |
| **5. Teach clients**<br>**a.** The correct procedure for administering eye medications (including maintenance of sterility) | If the client cannot administer the drugs, a family member may be taught the procedure. Written instructions are preferred to verbal ones. |
| **b.** To discard cloudy or discolored solutions | These changes indicate deterioration. Phenylephrine (Neo-Synephrine) solutions become cloudy, epinephrine solutions turn brown, and physostigmine becomes pink or red. |

| *Nursing Actions* | *Rationale/Explanation* |
|---|---|
| **c.** With glaucoma: | |
| (1) Do not take any drugs without the physician's knowledge and consent. | Many drugs given for purposes other than eye disorders may cause or aggravate glaucoma. |
| (2) Wear a MedicAlert bracelet or carry identification that states that the person has glaucoma. | To avoid administration of drugs that aggravate glaucoma or to maintain treatment of glaucoma, in emergencies |
| **d.** With eye infections: | |
| (1) Avoid touching the unaffected eye. | These measures are indicated to avoid spreading the infection to the unaffected eye or to other people. |
| (2) Wash hands before and after contact with the infected eye. | |
| (3) Use a separate towel. | |

## Review and Application Exercises

1. What is the main function of the eye?
2. List common disorders of the eye for which drug therapy is indicated.
3. Do ophthalmic medications need to be sterile? Why or why not?
4. What are important principles and techniques related to the nurse's administration of ophthalmic drugs?
5. For a client with newly-prescribed eye drops, how would you teach self-administration principles and techniques?

## Selected References

Abel, S. R. (1992). Eye disorders. In M. A. Koda-Kimble & L. Y. Young (Eds.), *Applied therapeutics: The clinical use of drugs* (5th ed.) (pp. 66-1–66-23). Vancouver, WA: Applied Therapeutics.

Curtis, S. M., & Carroll, E. M. (1994). Alterations in vision. In C. M. Porth (Ed.), *Pathophysiology: Concepts of altered health states* (4th ed.) (pp. 1113–1153). Philadelphia: J.B. Lippincott.

(1994) *Drug facts and comparisons.* St. Louis: Facts and Comparisons.

Sneed, S. R., & Lichter, P. R. (1992). Medical ophthalmology. In W. N. Kelley (Ed.), *Textbook of internal medicine* (2nd ed.) (pp. 51–53). Philadelphia: J.B. Lippincott.

# CHAPTER 69

# Drugs Used in Dermatologic Conditions

## Functions of the skin

The skin, the largest organ of the body, is the interface between the body's internal and external environments. The skin is composed of the epidermis and dermis. Epidermal or epithelial cells begin in the basal layer of the epidermis and migrate outward, undergoing degenerative changes in each layer. The outer layer, called the *stratum corneum*, is composed of dead cells and keratin. The dead cells are constantly being shedded (desquamated) and replaced by newer cells. Normally, about 1 month is required for cell formation, migration, and desquamation. When dead cells are discarded, keratin remains on the skin. Keratin is a tough protein substance that is insoluble in water, weak acids, and weak bases. Hair and nails, which are composed of keratin, are referred to as appendages of the skin.

*Melanocytes* are pigment-producing cells located at the junction of the epidermis and the dermis. These cells produce yellow, brown, or black skin coloring in response to genetic influences, melanocyte-stimulating hormone released from the anterior pituitary gland, and exposure to ultraviolet light (*e.g.*, sunlight).

The dermis is composed of elastic and fibrous connective tissue. Dermal structures include blood vessels, lymphatic channels, nerves and nerve endings, sweat glands, sebaceous glands, and hair follicles. The dermis is supported underneath by subcutaneous tissue, which is composed primarily of fat cells.

The skin has numerous functions, most of which are protective. Functions include the following:

1. Serves as a physical barrier against loss of fluids and electrolytes and against entry of potentially harmful substances (*e.g.*, microorganisms and other foreign bodies)
2. Detects sensations of pain, pressure, touch, and temperature through sensory nerve endings
3. Assists in regulating body temperature through production and elimination of sweat
4. Serves as a source of vitamin D when exposed to sunlight or other sources of ultraviolet light. Skin contains a precursor for vitamin D.
5. Serves as an excretory organ. Water, sodium, chloride, lactate, and urea are excreted in sweat.
6. Inhibits growth of many microorganisms by its acidic pH (about 4.5–6.5)

Mucous membrane is composed of a surface layer of epithelial cells, a basement membrane, and a layer of connective tissue. Mucous membranes line body cavities that communicate with the external environment (*i.e.*, mouth, vagina, anus). They receive an abundant blood supply. Capillaries lie just beneath the epithelial cells.

Dermatologic disorders may be primary (*i.e.*, originate in the skin or mucous membranes) or secondary (*i.e.*, result from a systemic condition, such as measles, lupus erythematosus, or adverse drug reactions). This chapter focuses on primary skin disorders and the topical medications used to prevent or treat them.

Anne Collins Abrams: CLINICAL DRUG THERAPY, Fourth Edition.
© 1995 J.B. Lippincott Company.

# Disorders of the skin

Because the skin is constantly exposed to the external environment, it is susceptible to numerous disorders. Dermatologic disorders include the following.

## INFLAMMATORY DISORDERS

### Dermatitis

*Dermatitis* is a general term denoting an inflammatory response of the skin to various injuries from irritants, allergens, or trauma. *Eczema* is often used as a synonym for dermatitis. Whatever the cause, dermatitis is usually characterized by erythema, pruritus, and skin lesions. Dermatitis may be acute or chronic.

1. **Atopic dermatitis** is a chronic disorder characterized primarily by pruritus. Its cause is uncertain but may involve allergic, hereditary, or psychological elements.
2. **Contact dermatitis** results from irritants (*e.g.*, strong soaps, detergents, acids, alkalis) or allergens (*e.g.*, clothing materials or dyes, jewelry, cosmetics, hair dyes). Irritants cause dermatitis in anyone with sufficient contact or exposure. Allergens cause dermatitis only in sensitized or hypersensitive people. The location of the dermatitis may indicate the cause (*e.g.*, facial dermatitis may indicate an allergy to cosmetics).
3. **Seborrheic dermatitis** is a disease of the sebaceous glands characterized by excessive production of sebum. A simple form of seborrheic dermatitis involving the scalp is dandruff, which is characterized by flaking and itching of the skin. More severe forms of seborrheic dermatitis are characterized by greasy, yellow scales or crusts with variable amounts of erythema and itching. Seborrheic dermatitis may occur on the scalp, face, or trunk.
4. **Urticaria** ("hives") is an allergic reaction to external agents (*e.g.*, insect bites) or to internal allergens that reach the skin through the bloodstream (*e.g.*, from foods or drugs). The characteristic skin lesion of urticaria is the wheal, a raised edematous area with a pallid center and erythematous border, which itches severely. Topical medications may be applied to relieve itching, but systemic drug therapy with antihistamines and perhaps epinephrine is the major element of drug therapy.

### Psoriasis

*Psoriasis* is a chronic skin disorder characterized by erythematous, dry, scaling lesions. The lesions may occur anywhere on the body but commonly involve the skin covering bony prominences, such as the elbows and knees. The disease is characterized by remissions and exacerbations. It is not contagious.

The cause of psoriasis is unknown. The pathophysiology involves excessively rapid turnover of epidermal cells. Instead of approximately 30 days from formation to elimination of normal epidermal cells, epidermal cells involved in psoriasis are abnormal in structure and have a life span of about 4 days.

Skin lesions may be tender, but they do not usually cause severe pain or itching. However, the lesions are unsightly and usually cause embarrassment and mental distress.

## DERMATOLOGIC INFECTIONS

### Bacterial infections

Bacterial infections of the skin are common; they are most often caused by streptococci or staphylococci.

1. **Cellulitis** is characterized by erythema, tenderness, and edema, which may spread to subcutaneous tissue. Erysipelas is a form of cellulitis. Generalized malaise, chills, and fever may occur.
2. **Folliculitis** is an infection of the hair follicles that most often occurs on the scalp or bearded areas of the face.
3. **Furuncles** and **carbuncles** are infections usually caused by staphylococci. Furuncles (boils) may result from folliculitis. They usually occur in the neck, face, axillae, buttocks, thighs, and perineum. Furuncles tend to recur. Carbuncles involve many hair follicles and include multiple pustules. Carbuncles may cause fever, malaise, leukocytosis, and bacteremia. Healing of carbuncles often produces scar tissue.
4. **Impetigo** is a superficial skin infection caused by streptococci or staphylococci. An especially contagious form is caused by group A beta-hemolytic streptococci. This form occurs most often in children.

### Fungal infections

Fungal infections of the skin and mucous membranes are most often caused by *Candida albicans*.

1. **Oral candidiasis** (thrush) involves mucous membranes of the mouth. It often occurs as a superinfection following the use of broad-spectrum systemic antibiotics.
2. **Candidiasis of the vagina and vulva** occurs with systemic antibiotic therapy and in women with diabetes mellitus.
3. **Intertrigo** involves skin folds or areas where two skin surfaces are in contact (*e.g.*, groin, pendulous breasts).

4. **Tinea** infections (ringworm) are caused by fungi (dermatophytes). These infections may involve the scalp (tinea capitis), the body (tinea corporis), the foot (tinea pedis), and other areas of the body. Tinea pedis, commonly called "athlete's foot," is the most common type of ringworm infection.

## Viral infections

Viral infections of the skin include veruccal (warts) and herpes infections. There are two types of herpes simplex infections. Type 1 infections usually involve the face or neck (*e.g.*, fever blisters or cold sores on the lips), and type 2 infections involve the genital organs. Other herpes infections include herpes zoster (shingles) and varicella (chickenpox).

## TRAUMA

Trauma refers to a physical injury that disrupts the skin. When the skin is broken, it may not be able to function properly. The major problem associated with skin wounds is infection. Common wounds include lacerations (cuts or tears), abrasions (shearing or scraping of the skin), and puncture wounds; surgical incisions; and burn wounds.

## ULCERATIONS

Cutaneous ulcerations are usually caused by trauma and impaired circulation. They may become inflamed or infected.

1. **Pressure ulcers** may occur anywhere on the body where external pressure decreases blood flow. Common sites include the sacrum, trochanters, ankles, and heels. Cutaneous ulcers also may result from improper moving and lifting techniques. For example, when a person is pulled across bed linens rather than lifted, friction and shearing force may cause skin abrasions. Abraded skin is susceptible to infection and ulcer formation.

   Pressure ulcers are most likely to develop in clients who are immobilized, incontinent, malnourished, and debilitated.
2. **Venous stasis ulcers** are commonly located on the lower extremities.

## ACNE

Acne is a common disorder characterized by excessive production of sebum and obstruction of hair follicles, which normally carry sebum to the skin surface. As a result, hair follicles expand and form comedones (black-heads and whiteheads). The most severe form of acne is acne vulgaris, in which follicles become infected, and irritating secretions leak into surrounding tissues to form pustules, cysts, and abscesses.

Acne occurs most often on the face, upper back, and chest because large numbers of sebaceous glands are located in these areas. Etiologic factors include increased secretion of male hormones (which occurs at puberty in males and females); bacteria, which cause sebum to break down into irritating fatty acids; oil-based cosmetics, which plug hair follicles; and certain medications (*e.g.*, phenytoin [Dilantin], corticosteroids, and iodides). There is no evidence that certain foods and emotional stress cause acne.

## EXTERNAL OTITIS

External otitis is a general term for inflammatory processes involving the external ear. The external ear, including the meatus, canal, and tympanic membrane (eardrum), is lined with epidermal tissue. The epidermal tissue is susceptible to the same skin disorders that affect other parts of the body. External otitis may be acute or chronic, and it may be treated with topical medications.

## ANORECTAL DISORDERS

Hemorrhoids and anal fissures are common anorectal disorders characterized by pruritus, bleeding, and pain. Inflammation and infection may occur.

# Types of Dermatologic Drugs

Many different agents are used to prevent or treat dermatologic disorders. Most agents fit into one or more of the following categories:

1. **Antiseptics** kill or inhibit the growth of bacteria, viruses, or fungi. They are used primarily to prevent infection. They are occasionally used to treat dermatologic infections. Soaps and detergents are not antiseptics because they do not kill or inhibit growth of microorganisms. However, soaps and detergents facilitate mechanical cleansing of the skin, especially when applied with friction. Skin surfaces should generally be clean before application of antiseptics. Antiseptics are sometimes called "skin disinfectants," but generally the term *disinfectant* refers to agents used for sterilizing inanimate objects (*e.g.*, instruments). Disinfectants are usually too strong for application to the skin and mucous membranes.
2. **Anti-infective agents** are used to treat infections caused by bacteria, fungi, and viruses. (These drugs

are extensively discussed in Chaps. 33–43). When used in dermatologic infections, anti-infective drugs may be administered locally (topically) or systemically (orally or parenterally). In many bacterial infections (*e.g.*, furuncles), systemic antibiotics are preferred. Generally, topical antibiotics have limited clinical use in bacterial infections. However, topical therapy of fungal infections is effective. Topical antiviral therapy is available for treatment of ophthalmic viral infections (see Chap. 68); herpes genitalis, an infectious viral disease transmitted primarily by sexual contact; and herpes labialis ("fever blisters") in immunosuppressed clients (see Chap. 42).

3. **Anti-inflammatory agents** are used to treat the inflammation present in many dermatologic conditions. The major anti-inflammatory agents are the adrenal corticosteroids (see Chap. 24). When used in dermatologic conditions, corticosteroids are most often applied topically. However, they also may be administered orally and parenterally in severe dermatologic disorders.

4. **Astringents** (*e.g.*, dilute solutions of aluminum salts) are used for their drying effects on exudative lesions.

5. **Emollients** or lubricants (*e.g.*, mineral oil, lanolin, petrolatum) are used to relieve pruritus and dryness of the skin.

6. **Enzymes** are used to débride burn wounds, decubitus ulcers, and venous stasis ulcers. They promote healing by removing necrotic tissue.

7. **Keratolytic agents** (*e.g.*, salicylic acid) are used to remove warts, corns, calluses, and other keratin-containing skin lesions.

8. **Sunscreens** are used to protect the skin from excessive exposure to sunlight, thereby preventing sunburn and decreasing skin cancer and wrinkles. Sunscreen preparations are labeled in terms of "sun protection factor" (SPF); an SPF of 15 or above is the most protective. Agents with high SPF values are recommended for people with fair skin who sunburn easily, people allergic to sunlight, and people who are using topical or systemic medications with photosensitizing or phototoxic characteristics (*e.g.*, tetracycline). Agents with low SPF values may be used by people who wish to tan the skin without experiencing sunburn.

9. Agents affecting skin pigmentation may be used with variable degrees of effectiveness to increase or decrease pigmentation. **Melanizing agents** (*e.g.*, trioxsalen, methoxsalen) may be used to increase skin pigmentation in vitiligo, a disorder characterized by white patches of skin surrounded by normally pigmented skin. **Demelanizing agents** (*e.g.*, hydroquinone, monobenzone) are occasionally used for hyperpigmented areas of the skin, such as freckles or chronic inflammatory lesions.

## APPLICATION OF DERMATOLOGIC DRUGS

Most dermatologic medications are applied topically. To be effective, topical agents must be in contact with the underlying skin or mucous membrane. Numerous dosage forms have been developed for topical application of drugs to various parts of the body and for various therapeutic purposes. Basic components of topical agents are one or more active ingredients and a usually inactive vehicle. The vehicle is a major determinant of the drug's ability to reach affected skin and mucous membranes. Many topical preparations contain other additives (*e.g.*, preservatives, emulsifiers, emollients, dispersing agents) that further facilitate application to skin and mucous membranes. Commonly used vehicles and dosage forms include ointments, creams, lotions, powders, sprays, aerosols, gels, otic solutions, and vaginal and rectal suppositories. Many topical drug preparations are available in several dosage forms.

Topical medications are used primarily for local effects when systemic absorption is undesirable. Factors that influence percutaneous absorption of topical agents include the following:

1. *Degree of skin hydration*. Drug penetration and percutaneous absorption are increased when keratin in the outermost layer of the epidermis is well hydrated.

2. *Drug concentration*. Because percutaneous absorption occurs by passive diffusion, higher concentrations increase the amount of drug absorbed.

3. *Skin condition*. Absorption from abraded or damaged skin is much greater than from intact skin.

4. *Length of contact time*. Absorption is increased when drugs are left in place for prolonged periods.

5. *Size of area*. Absorption is increased when topical medications are applied to large areas of the body.

6. *Location of area*. Absorption from mucous membranes and facial skin is comparatively rapid. Absorption from thick-skinned areas (*e.g.*, palms of hands and soles of feet) is comparatively slow.

## Individual drugs

See Tables 69-1 to 69-3.

## *Nursing Process*

### Assessment

Assess the client's skin for any characteristics or lesions that may indicate current or potential dermatologic disorders.

● When a skin rash is present, interview the client and inspect the area to determine the following:

(*Text continues on p. 718*)

## TABLE 69-1. ANTISEPTICS

| Generic/Trade Name | Characteristics | Clinical Indications |
| --- | --- | --- |
| *Alcohols* | | |
| **Ethanol (ethyl alcohol) Isopropyl alcohol** (Rubbing Alcohol U.S.P. [70% ethanol]) (Isopropyl Alcohol [99% solution], Isopropyl Rubbing Alcohol [70% solution]) | 1. Bactericidal to common bacteria. When applied to skin, kills approximately 90% of bacteria within 2 min if the area is kept moist for that period. When applied in a single wipe and left to evaporate (*e.g.*, before injections), approximately 75% of bacteria are killed. 2. Erratic against viruses and fungi; ineffective against spores 3. Irritating to intact skin with prolonged contact. Irritating to denuded skin areas or open wounds; causes burning type of pain, increases tissue injury, and coagulates protein to form a mass under which bacteria may proliferate 4. Isopropyl alcohol is slightly more antiseptic than ethyl alcohol. It has the same indications for use. | Cleansing of intact skin before injections or surgical incisions |
| *Biguanide* | | |
| **Chlorhexidine gluconate** (Hibiclens [4% Aqueous Emulsion]) | 1. Effective against gram-positive and gram-negative bacteria 2. Some studies indicate chlorhexidine (4%) is more effective than 3% hexachlorophene (pHisoHex) or povidone-iodine (Betadine) for handwashing and surgical scrubs. 3. Little, if any, absorption occurs through the skin of adults. Absorption from the skin of neonates is unknown but probably slight. 4. Some gram-negative organisms are resistant to the drug, and infection may occur. | 1. Handwashing 2. Preoperative skin cleansing for client and health-care personnel (surgical scrub) 3. Treatment of superficial cutaneous infections 4. Wound cleansing 5. Neonatal skin cleansing to reduce incidence of staphylococcal and streptococcal infections 6. Treatment of oral ulcers (as an ingredient in mouthwashes) 7. Prevention of dental caries |
| *Iodine Preparations* | | |
| **Iodine tincture, U.S.P. (2% iodine and 2.4% sodium iodide diluted in 50% ethanol) Iodine topical solution U.S.P. (2% iodine and 2.4% sodium iodide in water) Povidone-iodine (a 10% solution contains 1% available iodine)** (Betadine, Isodine, others) | 1. Iodine preparations kill most microorganisms (bacteria, fungi, viruses). When applied to the skin, a 1% solution kills approximately 90% of bacteria within 90 seconds. 2. Antiseptic activity depends on the concentration of iodine. Sodium iodide increases solubility; polyvinyl-pyrrolidone (povidone) is a carrier substance that increases solubility of iodine and releases iodine slowly for a sustained action. 3. Betadine, a commonly used iodine preparation, is available in numerous concentrations and dosage forms. These include the following (concentrations expressed in terms of available iodine): aerosol spray 0.5%; ointment 1%; shampoo 0.75%; skin cleanser 0.75%; solution 1%; surgical scrub 0.75%; vaginal douche solution and vaginal gel 1%. 4. Iodine topical solution should not be confused with strong iodine solution (Lugol's solution) used for the treatment of hyperthyroidism. | 1. Prevention or treatment of infections of the skin, scalp, and mucous membranes of the mouth and vagina 2. Preoperative cleansing of the skin 3. Treatment of wounds and abrasions |
| *Chlorine Preparations* | | |
| **Sodium hypochlorite solution, diluted** (Modified Dakin's solution) | 1. Exerts bactericidal action by releasing hypochlorous acid 2. Irritating to tissues 3. Dissolves necrotic materials 4. Dissolves blood clots and delays clotting 5. Undiluted solutions are too strong for use as antiseptics. | Infected wounds when other methods or agents are not available |
| **Sodium oxychlorosene** (Clorpactin sodium) | A mixture of sodium hypochlorite solution and alkylbenzene sulfonates. The alkylbenzene sulfonates have surfactant properties that increase penetration and antibacterial effects. | Treatment of infected wounds |
| *Metallic Antiseptics* | | |
| **Silver nitrate** | Silver nitrate is available in solid form (Toughened silver nitrate U.S.P.) for use as a caustic in removing warts and cauterizing wounds; an ophthalmic solution for use in newborn infants; and a solution (0.5%) for use in treating burn wounds. It is infrequently used in burn treatment because it stains the skin black and causes hypochloremia. | 1. Cauterizing warts or wounds 2. Prophylaxis of ophthalmia neonatorum in newborns 3. Treatment of burn wounds |

(continued)

**TABLE 69-1. ANTISEPTICS** (*Continued*)

| Generic/Trade Name | Characteristics | Clinical Indications |
| --- | --- | --- |
| **Silver sulfadiazine** (Silvadene) | 1. Silver sulfadiazine is widely used in treatment of burn wounds. <br> 2. Exerts antibacterial action against *Pseudomonas* and many other organisms that infect burn wounds. The drug penetrates eschar. <br> 3. Does not stain the skin or cause pain at application sites. | Prevention of infection in burn wounds |
| **Zinc oxide** (Zinc Oxide Ointment [20% zinc oxide]) (Calamine Lotion U.S.P. [8% calamine and 8% zinc oxide]) | 1. Available in many preparations and dosage forms (powders, ointments, pastes, lotions) <br> 2. Also has astringent properties | 1. Eczema <br> 2. Impetigo <br> 3. Tinea infections (ringworm) <br> 4. Venous stasis ulcers <br> 5. Pruritus <br> 6. Psoriasis |
| **Zinc pyrithione** (Zincon, others) | 1. Used in concentrations of 0.1%–2% <br> 2. A common ingredient in over-the-counter dandruff shampoos | 1. Seborrhea <br> 2. Dandruff |

*Oxidizing Agents*

| Generic/Trade Name | Characteristics | Clinical Indications |
| --- | --- | --- |
| **Hydrogen peroxide topical solution U.S.P. (3% hydrogen peroxide in water)** | 1. Hydrogen peroxide is more effective as a débriding and cleansing agent than as an antiseptic. It is of doubtful value on intact skin. However, when it comes in contact with wounds or blood, it rapidly decomposes into oxygen and water. The liberated oxygen exerts a brief antibacterial effect and loosens infected material. <br> 2. Prolonged use of hydrogen peroxide as a mouthwash, even at half strength, may cause hypertrophy of filiform papillae of the tongue ("hairy tongue"). This condition is reversible when hydrogen peroxide is discontinued. | 1. Wound cleansing <br> 2. Mouthwash (diluted in equal parts with water or normal saline and a commercial mouthwash such as Cepacol) <br> 3. To remove cerumen from the external ear <br> 4. Cleansing of tracheostomy tubes (inner cannulae) |
| **Benzoyl peroxide** (Benzoyl peroxide lotion U.S.P. [5% or 10% hydrous benzoyl peroxide]) | 1. Benzoyl peroxide slowly releases oxygen and is bactericidal for anaerobic bacteria (*e.g. Corynebacterium*). <br> 2. This agent also has irritant, keratolytic, and antiseborrheic properties | Acne |

*Phenol Derivatives*

| Generic/Trade Name | Characteristics | Clinical Indications |
| --- | --- | --- |
| **Hexachlorophene and entsufon sodium emulsion** (pHisoHex) | 1. pHisoHex is a commonly used preparation of hexachlorophene. It contains 3% hexachlorophene and entsufon sodium, a detergent. <br> 2. Bacteriostatic against gram-positive bacteria, including staphylococci. Relatively ineffective against gram-negative organisms and fungi. Gram-negative bacterial and fungal infections may increase in incidence during chronic use of hexachlorophene preparations. <br> 3. A single washing with a hexachlorophene substance is no more effective than soap in reducing the number of microorganisms on the skin. Repeated washings leave a residual film on the skin that produces a steady reduction in bacterial flora. Cleansing with alcohol or washing with soap removes the antibacterial residual film. <br> 4. Hexachlorophene is absorbed systemically from intact skin, especially after repeated applications. Systemic absorption is increased if the skin is broken; thus, hexachlorophene should *not* be applied to open wounds. <br> 5. Use should be followed by thorough rinsing. | 1. Handwashing, especially for healthcare personnel and food handlers <br> 2. Preoperative skin cleansing |
| **Resorcinol** | 1. Bactericidal and fungicidal <br> 2. Also has mild irritant and keratolytic characteristics <br> 3. Usually applied as a 10% ointment or lotion | 1. Acne <br> 2. Ringworm (tinea) infections <br> 3. Dermatitis <br> 4. Psoriasis <br> 5. Other cutaneous lesions |

*Miscellaneous Antiseptics*

| Generic/Trade Name | Characteristics | Clinical Indications |
| --- | --- | --- |
| **Acetic acid** | 1. Bactericidal to many microorganisms, including *Pseudomonas aeruginosa*, in a 5% concentration <br> 2. Bacteriostatic in concentrations lower than 5% | 1. Irrigations and dressings of surgical wounds (1% solution), bladder irrigations (0.25% solution) <br> 2. Vaginal infections due to *Trichomonas, Candida,* or *Haemophilus* organisms. Administered as a vaginal douche. <br> 3. External otitis (2% solution, instilled in the auditory canal) |

(*continued*)

**TABLE 69-1.  ANTISEPTICS** *(Continued)*

| Generic/Trade Name | Characteristics | Clinical Indications |
|---|---|---|
| **Gentian violet U.S.P.** (Gentian Violet Topical Solution U.S.P. [1% gentian violet in 10% ethanol]) (Gentian Violet Cream [1.35% gentian violet in an absorbable base]) (Genapax tampons) (Hyva vaginal tablets) | 1. Effective against gram-positive bacteria (bacteriostatic and bactericidal) and many fungi; ineffective against gram-negative and acid-fast (*e.g.*, tuberculosis) bacteria<br>2. Stains granulation tissue; should not be applied to ulcerative facial lesions | 1. Oral and vaginal fungal infections<br>2. Infected wounds and mucous membranes |
| **Sulfur** | 1. Has fungicidal and keratolytic properties<br>2. May be used alone or in combination with other keratolytic agents (*e.g.*, coal tar, resorcinol, 2% salicylic acid<br>3. Widely used in dermatology | 1. Psoriasis<br>2. Seborrhea<br>3. Dermatitis |

- *Appearance of individual lesions*. Lesions should be described as specifically as possible so that changes can be identified. Terms commonly used in dermatology include *macule* (flat spot), *papule* (raised spot), *nodule* (small solid swelling), *vesicle* (blister), *pustule* (pus-containing lesion), *petechia* (flat, round, purplish-red spot the size of a pinpoint, caused by intradermal or submucosal bleeding), and *erythema* (redness). Lesions also may be described as weeping or dry and scaly or crusty.
- *Location or distribution*. Some skin rashes occur exclusively or primarily on certain parts of the body (*e.g.*, face, extremities, trunk), and distribution may indicate the cause.
- *Accompanying symptoms*. Pruritus occurs with most dermatologic conditions. Fever, malaise, and other symptoms may occur as well.
- *Historic development*. Appropriate questions include:
  - When and where did the skin rash appear?
  - How long has it been present?
  - Has it changed in appearance or location?
  - Has it occurred previously?
- *Etiologic factors*. In many instances, appropriate treatment is determined by the cause. Some etiologic factors include the following:
  - *Drug therapy*. Many commonly used drugs may cause skin lesions, including antibiotics (*e.g.*, penicillins, sulfonamides, tetracyclines), barbiturates, narcotic analgesics, phenothiazine antipsychotic agents (*e.g.*, chlorpromazine [Thorazine]), and thiazide diuretics. Skin rashes due to drug therapy are usually generalized and appear abruptly.
  - *Irritants or allergens* may cause contact dermatitis. For example, dermatitis involving the hands may be caused by soaps, detergents, or various other cleansing agents. Dermatitis involving the trunk may result from allergic reactions to clothing.
  - *Communicable diseases* (*i.e.*, measles, scarlatina, chickenpox) cause characteristic skin rashes and systemic signs and symptoms.
- When skin lesions other than rashes are present, assess appearance, size or extent, amount and character of any drainage, and whether the lesion appears infected or contains necrotic material. Bleeding into the skin is usually described as *petechiae* (pinpoint hemorrhages) or *ecchymoses* (bruises). Burn wounds are usually described in terms of depth (partial or full thickness of skin) and percentage of body surface area. Burn wounds with extensive skin damage are rapidly colonized with potentially pathogenic microorganisms. Venous stasis, pressure, and other cutaneous ulcers are usually described in terms of diameter and depth.
- When assessing the skin, consider the age of the client. Infants are likely to have "diaper" dermatitis, miliaria (heat rash), and tinea capitis (ringworm infection of the scalp). School-age children have a relatively high incidence of measles, chickenpox, and tinea infections. Adolescents often have acne. Older adults are more likely to have dry skin, actinic keratoses, and skin neoplasms.
- Assess for skin neoplasms. *Basal cell carcinoma* is the most common type of skin cancer. It may initially appear as a pale nodule, most often on the head and neck. *Squamous cell carcinomas* may appear as ulcerated areas. These lesions may occur anywhere on the body but are more common on sun-exposed parts, such as the face and hands. *Malignant melanoma* is the most serious skin cancer. It involves melanocytes, the pigment-producing cells of the skin. Malignant melanoma may occur in pigmented nevi (moles) or previously normal skin. In nevi, malignant melanoma may be manifested by enlargement and ulceration. In previously normal skin, lesions appear as irregularly shaped pigmented areas. Although it can occur in almost any area, malignant melanoma is most likely to be located on the back in white people and in toe webs and soles of the feet in African-American or Asian people.
- When assessing dark-skinned clients, color changes and skin rashes are more difficult to detect. Some guidelines include the following:
  - Adequate lighting is required. Nonglare daylight is best. The illumination provided by overbed lights or flashlights is inadequate for most purposes.
  - Some skin rashes may be visible on oral mucous membranes.

## TABLE 69-2. DERMATOLOGIC ANTI-INFECTIVE AND ANTI-INFLAMMATORY AGENTS

| Generic/Trade Name | Routes and Dosage Ranges (Adults and Children) | Generic/Trade Name | Routes and Dosage Ranges (Adults and Children) |
|---|---|---|---|
| **Antibacterial Agents** | | **Antiviral Agent** | |
| **Bacitracin** (Baciguent ointment) | Topically to skin lesions once or twice daily | **Acyclovir** (Zovirax) | Herpes genitalis (initial lesions) and herpes labialis in immunosuppressed clients: topically to lesions q3h or at least six times daily for 7 d |
| **Neomycin sulfate** (Myciguent ointment) | Topically to skin once or twice daily | | |
| **Nitrofurazone** (Furacin) | Topically to burn wounds once daily or every few days when dressings are changed | | |
| **Combination Agents** | | **Corticosteroids** | |
| **Bacitracin and poly- myxin B** (Polysporin ointment) | Topically to skin two to five times daily | **Alclometasone** (Aclovate) | Topically to skin two to four times daily |
| **Polymyxin B sulfate, neomycin sulfate, and bacitracin** (Neosporin ointment) | Topically to skin two to five times daily | **Amcinonide** (Cyclocort) | Topically to skin two to three times daily |
| | | **Betamethasone** (Benisone, Valisone) | Topically to skin one to four times daily |
| **Antifungal Agents** | | **Clobetasol** (Temovate) | Topically to skin two to four times daily |
| **Acrisorcin** (Akrinol) | Tinea versicolor: topically to skin, morning and night | **Clocortolone** (Cloderm) | Topically to skin one to three times daily |
| **Amphotericin B** (Fungizone) | Cutaneous candidiasis: topically to skin two to four times daily | **Desonide** (Tridesilon) | Topically to skin two or three times daily |
| **Clotrimazole** (Lotrimin, Mycelex) | Cutaneous dermatophytosis, cutaneous and vaginal candidiasis: topically to skin or vaginal mucosa once daily | **Desoximetasone** (Topicort) | Topically to skin one or two daily |
| **Ciclopirox** (Loprox) | Same as econazole | **Dexamethasone** (Decaderm, Decadron) | Topically to skin two to three times daily |
| **Econazole** (Spectazole) | Tinea infections, cutaneous candidiasis: topically to skin twice daily for 2–4 wk | **Diflorasone** (Florone, Maxiflor) | Topically to skin two to three times daily |
| **Haloprogin** (Halotex) | Tinea pedis (athlete's foot), cutaneous candidiasis: topically to skin twice daily for 2–4 wk | **Fluocinonide** (Lidex, Synalar) | Topically to skin three or four times daily |
| **Iodochlorhydroxyquin** (Vioform) | Localized dermatophytosis: topically to skin several times daily | **Flurandrenolide** (Cordran) | Topically to skin two or three times daily |
| **Miconazole** (Micatin) | Dermatophytosis, cutaneous candidiasis: topically to skin once or twice daily for 4 wk | **Halcinonide** (Halog) | Topically to skin two or three times daily |
| **Nystatin** (Mycostatin) | Candidiasis of skin and oral mucous membranes: topically to lesions two or three times daily. Vaginal candidiasis: topically to vaginal mucosa once or twice daily for 14 d | **Hydrocortisone** (Cortril, Hydrocortone) | Topically to skin three or four times daily |
| | | **Methylprednisolone acetate** (Medrol acetate) | Topically to skin one to four times daily, then reduced when disease process is controlled |
| **Oxiconazole** (Oxistat) | Tinea infections: topically to skin twice daily for 2 to 4 wk | **Triamcinolone acetonide** (Aristocort, Kenalog, others) | Topically to skin three or four times daily |
| **Tolnaftate** (Tinactin) | Dermatophytosis: topically to skin twice daily | | |
| **Undecylenic acid** (Desenex, others) | Dermatophytosis, especially tinea pedis (athlete's foot): topically to skin or mucous membranes. Dosage recommendations vary among manufacturers. | | |

- Petechiae are not visible on dark-brown or black skin, but they may be visible on oral mucous membranes or the conjunctiva.
- When skin disorders are present, assess the client's psychological response to the condition. Many clients, especially those with chronic disorders, feel self-conscious and depressed.

**Nursing diagnoses**

- Body Image Disturbance related to visible skin lesions
- Anxiety related to potential for permanent scarring or disfigurement
- Pain related to skin lesions and pruritus
- High Risk for Injury: Infection related to entry of microbes through damaged skin

**TABLE 69-3. MISCELLANEOUS DERMATOLOGIC AGENTS**

| Generic/Trade Name | Dermatologic Effects | Clinical Indications | Method of Administration |
|---|---|---|---|
| **Demelanizing Agents** | | | |
| **Hydroquinone** (Eldoquin) | Decreases skin pigmentation | 1. Freckles<br>2. Melasma | Topically to hyperpigmented areas of the skin one or two times daily |
| **Monobenzone** (Benoquin) | Decreases skin pigmentation | Vitiligo—for permanent depigmentation of areas containing normal pigmentation (*i.e.*, to relieve "spotted" appearance) | Topically, to pigmented areas only, two or three times daily |
| **Melanizing Agents** | | | |
| **Methoxsalen** (Oxsoralen-ultra) | Increases skin pigmentation | 1. Vitiligo<br>2. Psoriasis | Topically to small lesions, followed by sunlight or ultraviolet light<br>Psoriasis, PO 10–40 mg daily, followed in 2 h by sunlight or ultraviolet light |
| **Trioxsalen** (Trisoralen) | Increases skin pigmentation | 1. Vitiligo<br>2. Increase tolerance to sunlight | Vitiligo: PO 10 mg daily, followed in 2 h by exposure to sunlight<br>To increase tolerance to sunlight: PO 10 mg daily for no longer than 14 d |
| **Enzymes** | | | |
| **Collagenase** (Santyl) | Débriding effects | Enzymatic débridement of infected wounds (*e.g.* burn wounds, decubitus ulcers) | Topically once daily until the wound is cleansed of necrotic material |
| **Fibrinolysin-deoxyribonuclease** (Elase) | See collagenase, above | See collagenase, above | See collagenase, above |
| **Papain** (Panafil) | Débriding effects | Débridement of surface lesions | Topically one or two times daily |
| **Sutilains** (Travase) | Débriding effects | Débridement of wounds | Topically to wound three or four times daily |
| **Trypsin** (Granulex) | Débriding effects | Débridement of infected wounds (*e.g.*, decubitus and varicose ulcers) | Topically by spray twice daily |
| **Other Agents** | | | |
| **Aluminum acetate solution (Burow's solution)** | Astringent, antipruritic, anti-inflammatory | 1. Weeping or "wet" skin lesions due to infection or inflammation<br>2. External otitis | Topically to skin, as wet dressings<br>Topically to external ear, as irrigating solution to remove debris |
| **Coal tar** (Balnetar, Zetar, others) | Irritant | 1. Psoriasis<br>2. Dermatitis | Topically to skin, in various concentrations and preparations (*e.g.*, creams, lotions, shampoos, bath emulsion). Also available in combination with hydrocortisone and other substances |
| **Colloidal oatmeal** (Aveeno) | Antipruritic | Pruritus | Topically as a bath solution (1 cup in bathtub of water) |
| **Fluorouracil** (Efudex) | Antineoplastic | 1. Actinic keratoses<br>2. Superficial basal cell carcinomas | Topically to skin lesions twice daily for 2–6 wk |
| **Isotretinoin** (Accutane) | Inhibits sebum production and keratinization | 1. Severe cystic acne<br>2. Disorders characterized by excessive keratinization (*e.g.*, pityriasis, ichthyosis)<br>3. *Mycosis fungoides* | PO 1–2 mg/kg per day, in two divided doses, for 15–20 wk |
| **Salicylic acid** | Keratolytic, antifungal | 1. Removal of warts, corns, calluses<br>2. Superficial fungal infections<br>3. Seborrheic dermatitis<br>4. Acne<br>5. Psoriasis | Topically to lesions |
| **Selenium sulfide** (Selsun) | Antifungal, antidandruff | 1. Dandruff<br>2. Tinea versicolor | Topically to scalp as shampoo once or twice weekly |
| **Tretinoin** (Retin-A) | Irritant | Acne vulgaris | Topically to skin lesions once daily |

- Knowledge Deficit related to prevention and treatment of skin disorders

### Planning/Goals

*The client will:*
- Apply topical drugs correctly
- Experience relief of symptoms
- Use techniques to prevent or minimize skin damage and disorders
- Avoid scarring and disfigurement when possible
- Be encouraged to express concerns about acute and chronic body image changes

### Interventions

Use measures to prevent or minimize skin disorders.
- Use general measures to promote health and increase resistance to disease (*i.e.*, maintain nutrition, rest, and exercise).
- Practice good personal hygiene, with at least once daily cleansing of skin areas with high bacterial counts, such as underarms and perineum.
- Practice safety measures to avoid injury to the skin. Any injury, especially one that disrupts the integrity of the skin (*e.g.*, lacerations, puncture wounds, scratching of skin lesions), increases the likelihood of skin infections.
- Avoid known irritants or allergens. Have the client substitute nonirritating soaps or cleaning supplies for irritating ones; use hypoallergenic jewelry and cosmetics if indicated; wear cotton clothing if indicated.
- Use measures to relieve dry skin and pruritus. Dry skin causes itching, and itching promotes scratching. Scratching relieves itching only if it is strong enough to damage the skin and serve as a counterirritant. Skin damaged or disrupted by scratching is susceptible to invasion by pathogenic microorganisms. Thus, dry skin may lead to serious skin disorders. Older adults are especially likely to have dry, flaky skin. Measures to decrease skin dryness include the following:
  - Alternating complete and partial baths. For example, the client may alternate a complete shower or tub bath with a sponge bath (of face, hands, underarms, and perineal areas). Warm water, mild soaps, and patting dry are recommended because hot water, harsh soaps, and rubbing with a towel have drying effects on the skin.
  - Liberal use of lubricating creams, lotions, and oils. Bath oils, which usually contain mineral oil or lanolin oil and a perfume, are widely available. If bath oils are used, precautions against falls are necessary, because the oils make bathtubs and shower floors slippery. Creams and lotions may be applied several times daily.
- Prevent pressure ulcers by avoiding trauma to the skin and prolonged pressure on any part of the body. In clients at high risk for developing pressure ulcers, major preventive measures include frequent changes of position and correct lifting techniques. Various pressure-relieving devices also are useful. These include water beds, air or foam rubber mattresses, and chair pads. Daily inspection of the skin is needed for early detection and treatment of beginning pressure ulcers.
- Avoid excessive exposure to sunlight and other sources of ultraviolet light. Although controlled amounts of ultraviolet light are beneficial in some dermatologic disorders (*i.e.*, acne, psoriasis), excessive amounts cause wrinkling, dryness, and malignancies. If prolonged exposure is necessary, protective clothing and sunscreening lotions decrease skin damage.
- When skin rashes are present, cool, wet compresses or baths are often effective in relieving pruritus. Water or normal saline may be used alone or with additives, such as aluminum acetate solution (Burow's solution), colloidal oatmeal (Aveeno), or baking soda. A cool environment also tends to decrease pruritus. The client's fingernails should be cut short and kept clean to avoid skin damage and infection from scratching.

### Teach clients:

- To promote healthy skin by a balanced diet, personal hygiene measures, avoiding excessive exposure to sunlight, avoiding skin injuries, and lubricating dry skin. Healthy skin is less susceptible to inflammation, infections, and other disorders. It also heals more rapidly when disorders or injuries occur.
- To avoid scratching, squeezing, or rubbing skin lesions. These behaviors cause additional skin damage.
- Ways to mask unavoidable lesions or scars (*e.g.*, with makeup or clothing)

### Evaluation

- Observe and interview regarding use of dermatologic drugs.
- Observe for improvement in skin lesions and symptoms.
- Interview regarding use of measures to promote healthy skin and prevent skin disorders.

## Principles of therapy

### DRUG SELECTION IN VARIOUS SKIN CONDITIONS

The choice of dermatologic agents depends primarily on the reason for use and client response. Some guidelines include the following:

1. For routine handwashing of health-care personnel and preoperative skin cleansing of surgical staff and clients, chlorhexidine (Hibiclens) and povidone-iodine (Betadine) are the antiseptics of first choice. Alcohol is effective but too drying for routine use. pHisoHex is not effective against gram-negative bacteria and is absorbed systemically from intact skin.
2. Topical medications for inflammatory and noninflammatory skin disorders vary greatly. Generally, though, astringents and lotions are used as drying agents for "wet," oozing lesions, and ointments and creams are used as "wetting" agents for dry, scaling lesions. Topical corticosteroids are available in several dosage forms for use in acute and chronic inflamma-

tory disorders. Hydrocortisone is the topical corticosteroid of choice for use on the face or other cosmetically important areas. It is available over the counter in a 0.5% concentration. The fluorinated corticosteroids may cause skin eruptions, dermatitis, and acne; therefore, these compounds are generally used on areas other than the face.

3. For topical antibiotic therapy, bacitracin, neomycin, and polymyxin are usually preferred. These drugs are often used in combination, and various preparations are available (*e.g.*, Neosporin). Although other antibiotics are available in dosage forms for topical use (*e.g.*, gentamicin, chloramphenicol, tetracyclines), these drugs generally should not be used. These drugs may cause sensitization when used topically. If a sensitized client receives the drug systemically at a later time, serious allergic reactions may occur.

4. In acne, benzoyl peroxide, 5% or 10%, is one of the most effective topical agents. Systemic tetracycline in low doses may be used for long-term treatment of acne. Because of potentially severe adverse effects, isotretinoin is recommended for use only in severe cystic acne that is resistant to other treatments. Because of teratogenic effects, it is contraindicated during pregnancy. Women of childbearing potential should use an effective method of contraception during and for at least 1 month after isotretinoin therapy.

5. In external otitis, otic preparations of various dermatologic medications are used. Polymyxin B (Cortisporin Otic Solution) and neomycin (Otobiotic Otic Solution) are the most commonly used antibiotics, although others (*e.g.*, tetracyclines, sulfonamides, gentamicin) are available. Acetic acid solution 2% also may be administered as an otic anti-infective agent. Acetic acid is effective against *Pseudomonas* and many other organisms that cause external ear disease. It establishes an acidic environment, which prevents growth of the organisms, and does not produce resistant organisms. Hydrocortisone is the corticosteroid most often included in topical otic preparations. It relieves pruritus and inflammation in chronic external otitis. Local anesthetics, usually benzocaine, are included in some otic formulations. However, local anesthetics are not well absorbed from the ear and are generally ineffective in relieving the severe pain associated with acute external otitis or otitis media. Systemic analgesics are usually required.

6. In pressure ulcers, the only clear-cut guideline for treatment is avoiding further pressure on the affected area. Many topical agents are used, most often with specific procedures for dressing changes, skin cleansing, and so on. No one agent or procedure is clearly superior. Consistent implementation of a protocol (*i.e.*, position changes, inspection of current or potential pressure areas, dressing changes, use of an air mattress) may be more effective than drug therapy.

7. In anorectal disorders, most preparations contain a local anesthetic, emollients, and perhaps a corticosteroid. These preparations relieve pruritus and pain but do not cure the underlying condition. Some preparations contain ingredients of questionable value, such as vasoconstrictors, astringents, and weak antiseptics. No particular mixture is clearly superior.

## DOSAGE FORMS

The choice of dosage form for topical drug therapy depends largely on the reason for use. Guidelines include the following:

1. *Ointments* are oil-based substances that usually contain a medication in an emollient vehicle, such as petrolatum or lanolin. Ointments occlude the skin and promote retention of moisture. Thus, they are especially useful in chronic skin disorders characterized by dry lesions. Ointments should generally be avoided in hairy, moist, and intertriginous areas of the body because of potential maceration, irritation, and secondary infection.

2. *Creams* (emulsions of oil in water, which may be greasy or nongreasy) and *gels* (transparent colloids, which dry and leave a film over the area) retain moisture in the skin but are less occlusive than ointments. These preparations are cosmetically acceptable for use on the face and other visible areas of the body. They also may be used in hairy, moist, intertriginous areas. Creams and gels are especially useful in subacute dermatologic disorders.

3. *Lotions* are suspensions of insoluble substances in water. They cool, dry, and protect the skin. They are most useful in subacute dermatologic disorders. *Sprays* and *aerosols* are similar to lotions.

4. *Powders* have absorbent, cooling, and protective effects. Generally, powders should not be applied in acute, exudative disorders or on denuded areas because they tend to cake, occlude the lesions, and retard healing. Also, some powders (*e.g.*, cornstarch) may lead to secondary infections by promoting growth of bacteria and fungi.

5. *Pastes* are semisolid preparations composed primarily of powder. Pastes adhere strongly to the area of application and are difficult to remove. They are generally less macerating, penetrating, and occlusive than ointments. Pastes should not be used on hairy areas of the body.

6. Topical otic medications are usually delivered in a liquid vehicle. However, creams or ointments may be used for dry, crusted lesions, and powders may be used for drying effects.

7. Topical vaginal medications may be applied as douche solutions, vaginal tablets, or vaginal creams used with an applicator.

8. Dosage of corticosteroids applied topically to skin depends on the potency of the preparation (percentage of drug contained in the ointment, lotion, or other vehicle), the area of application, and the method of application. The skin covering the face, scalp, scrotum, and axillae is more permeable to corticosteroids than other skin surfaces, and these areas can usually be treated with less potent formulations, smaller amounts, or less frequent applications. In addition, drug absorption is increased by applying an occlusive dressing over the affected area. Systemic toxicity may occur. For this reason, drug application is usually done less frequently when occlusive dressings are used.

9. Anorectal medications may be applied as ointments, creams, foams, and rectal suppositories.

## USE IN CHILDREN

Children are at risk of developing a wide range of dermatologic disorders, including dermatitis and skin rashes in younger children and acne in adolescents. Few guidelines have been developed for drug therapy of these disorders. Infants, and perhaps older children, have more permeable skin and are more likely to absorb topical drugs than adults. In addition, absorption is increased in the presence of broken or damaged skin. Therefore, cautious use of topical agents is advised.

With topical corticosteroids, suppression of the hypothalamic-pituitary-adrenal axis (see Chap. 24), Cushing's disease, and intracranial hypertension have been reported. Signs of impaired adrenal function may include delayed growth in height and weight and low plasma cortisol levels. Signs of intracranial hypertension may include headaches, bulging fontanelles, and swelling of the optic nerve (papilledema) on ophthalmoscopic examination. The latter may lead to blindness if pressure on the optic nerve is not relieved. These drugs should be used only if clearly indicated, in the least effective dose, and for the shortest effective time.

## USE IN OLDER ADULTS

Older adults often have dry skin and are at risk of pressure ulcers if mobility, nutrition, or elimination is impaired. Principles of topical drug therapy are the same as for younger adults.

## NURSING ACTIONS: DERMATOLOGIC DRUGS

| *Nursing Actions* | *Rationale/Explanation* |
|---|---|
| **1. Administer accurately**<br>**a.** Use the correct preparation for the intended use (*i.e.*, dermatologic, otic, vaginal, anorectal) | Preparations may differ in drug contents and concentrations. |
| **b.** For topical application to skin lesions: | |
| (1) Wash the skin, and pat it dry. | To cleanse the skin and remove previously applied medication. This facilitates drug contact with the affected area of the skin. |
| (2) Apply a small amount of the drug preparation, and rub it in well. | A thin layer of medication is effective and decreases the incidence and severity of adverse effects. |
| (3) For burn wounds, broken skin, or open lesions, apply the drug with sterile gloves or sterile cotton-tipped applicators. | To prevent infection |
| (4) Use the drug only for the individual client (*i.e.*, do not use the same tube for more than one client). | To avoid bacterial cross-contamination between clients |
| (5) Wash hands before and after application. | Wash hands before to avoid exposing the client to infection; wash hands afterward to avoid transferring the drug to your own face or eyes and causing adverse reactions. |
| **2. Observe for therapeutic effects**<br>**a.** With dermatologic conditions, observe for healing of skin lesions. | Therapeutic effects depend on the medication being used and the disorder being treated. |

*(continued)*

*Nursing Actions*                                    *Rationale/Explanation*

**b.** With external otitis, observe for decreased pain and pruritus.

**c.** With vaginal disorders, observe for decreased vaginal discharge and pruritus.

**d.** With anorectal disorders, observe for decreased pain and pruritus.

**3. Observe for adverse effects**                    Incidence of adverse effects is low with topical agents.

    **a.** Local irritation or inflammation—erythema, skin rash, pruritus

Local adverse effects may occur with antiseptics (*e.g.,* iodine preparations), local anesthetics (*e.g.,* in anorectal preparations), and antibiotics. When topical antibiotics are applied to the external ear, the drugs may cause a cutaneous reaction that resembles the disorder being treated.

    **b.** With topical corticosteroids, observe for acneiform facial lesions and other skin changes (atrophy, thinning, development of striae).

Facial lesions occur with chronic use of fluorinated corticosteroids. They can be avoided by using hydrocortisone on facial lesions. Other skin changes occur with prolonged use of topical corticosteroids.

    **c.** With topical antibiotics, superinfection and sensitization may occur.

Superinfection with drug-resistant organisms may occur with any antibacterial agent. It is less likely to occur with mixtures that have a broad spectrum of antibacterial activity. Sensitization may cause serious allergic reactions if the same drug is given systemically at a later time.

    **d.** With isotretinoin, observe for hypervitaminosis A (nausea, vomiting, headache, blurred vision, eye irritation, conjunctivitis, skin disorders, abnormal liver function, musculoskeletal pain, increased plasma triglycerides, others).

Adverse effects commonly occur with usual doses but are more severe with higher doses.

**4. Observe for drug interactions**                   Clinically significant drug interactions rarely occur with topical agents.

**5. Teach clients**

    **a.** Use topical medications only as prescribed or according to the manufacturer's instructions (for over-the-counter products).

Most topical agents are safe if used properly but may cause adverse effects if used improperly.

    **b.** For minor wounds and abrasions, cleansing with soap and water is usually adequate. If an antiseptic is used, an iodine preparation (*e.g.,* aqueous iodine solution 1%) is preferred.

Iodine preparations are effective in preventing infection. Alcohol should not be applied to open wounds. Hydrogen peroxide may facilitate mechanical cleansing, but it is a weak antiseptic. Common household agents, for instance, merbromin (Mercurochrome) and thimerosal (Merthiolate), are weak antiseptics. These mercury compounds are generally not recommended for use.

    **c.** With isotretinoin, avoid vitamin supplements containing vitamin A and excessive exposure to sunlight

To decrease risks of excessive vitamin A intake and photosensitivity

## Review and Application Exercises

1. What are the main functions of the skin?
2. Describe interventions to promote skin health and integrity.

3. During initial assessment of a client, what signs and symptoms may indicate common skin disorders?
4. Which client groups are at risk of developing common skin disorders (*e.g.,* skin infections, pressure ulcers)?

5. Compare topical and systemic corticosteroids in terms of adverse effects.
6. Given an adolescent client with acne who asks your advice about over-the-counter topical drugs, which would you recommend and why?
7. List general principles of using topical agents for common skin disorders.

## Selected References

Allman, R. M. (1992). Pressure ulcers in the elderly. In W. N. Kelley (Ed.), *Textbook of internal medicine* (2nd ed.) (pp. 2425–2428). Philadelphia: J.B. Lippincott.

Bond, C. A. (1992). Skin disorders I. In M. A. Koda-Kimble & L. Y. Young (Eds.), *Applied therapeutics: The clinical use of drugs* (5th ed.) (pp. 64-1–64-16). Vancouver, WA: Applied Therapeutics.

(1994). *Drug facts and comparisons.* St. Louis: Facts and Comparisons.

Goslen, J. B., Tabas, M., & Bauer, E. A. (1992). Management of acute and chronic diseases of the skin. In W. N. Kelley (Ed.), *Textbook of internal medicine* (2nd ed.) (pp. 1041–1045). Philadelphia: J.B. Lippincott.

Porth, C. M. (1990). *Pathophysiology: Concepts of altered health states* (3rd ed.) (pp. 697–718). Philadelphia: J.B. Lippincott.

Ricketts, J. L., & Williamson, N. B. (1992). Nursing management of adults with disorders of the skin. In L. O. Burrell (Ed.), *Adult nursing in hospital and community settings* (pp. 2015–2041). Norwalk, CT: Appleton & Lange.

Ricketts, J. L., & Williamson, N. B. (1992). Nursing management of adults with common problems of the skin. In L. O. Burrell (Ed.), *Adult nursing in hospital and community settings* (pp. 1986–2014). Norwalk, CT: Appleton & Lange.

West, D. P., & Rumsfield, J. A. (1992). Skin disorders II: Acne, psoriasis, photosensitivity, photoallergic, fungal. In M. A. Koda-Kimble & L. Y. Young (Eds.), *Applied therapeutics: The clinical use of drugs* (5th ed.) (pp. 65-1–65-14). Vancouver, WA: Applied Therapeutics.

### CHAPTER 70

# Drug Use During Pregnancy and Lactation

Drug use during pregnancy and lactation requires special consideration because the fetus or infant, as well as the mother, is affected. Few drugs are considered safe, and drug use is generally contraindicated. Ideally, drugs should be avoided during these periods, but realistically many pregnant or lactating women take drugs for one reason or another. Common reasons include acute disorders that may or may not be associated with pregnancy, chronic disorders that require continued treatment during pregnancy or lactation and habitual use of nontherapeutic drugs (*e.g.*, alcohol, tobacco, others).

## Pregnancy and lactation

Pregnancy is a dynamic state: mother and fetus undergo physiologic changes that influence drug effects. In the pregnant woman, physiologic changes alter drug pharmacokinetics (Table 70-1), and drug effects are less predictable than in the nonpregnant state. The major purpose of this chapter is to describe potential drug effects on the fetus and maternal drug therapy to protect the fetus while providing therapeutic effects to the pregnant woman. Most of the drugs mentioned in this chapter are described more fully elsewhere; they are discussed here in relation to pregnancy and lactation. Other drugs are used mainly to influence some aspect of pregnancy and lactation. These drugs are discussed in greater detail and

include those used to induce abortion (abortifacients), drugs used to stop preterm labor (tocolytics), and drugs used during labor and delivery.

## Maternal-placental-fetal circulation

Drugs ingested by the pregnant woman reach the fetus through the maternal-placental-fetal circulation, which is completed about the third week after conception. On the maternal side, arterial blood pressure carries blood and drugs to the placenta. In the placenta, maternal and fetal blood are separated by a few thin layers of tissue over a large surface area. Drugs readily cross the placenta, mainly by passive diffusion. This process, called placental transfer, begins about the fifth week after conception. When drugs are given on a regular schedule, serum levels reach equilibrium, with fetal blood containing 50% to 100% of the amount in maternal blood.

After drugs enter the fetal circulation, relatively large amounts are pharmacologically active because the fetus has low levels of serum albumin and thus low levels of drug binding. Drug molecules are distributed in two ways. Most are transported to the liver, where they are metabolized. Metabolism occurs slowly because the fetal liver is immature in quantity and quality of drug-metabolizing enzymes. Drugs metabolized by the fetal liver are

Anne Collins Abrams: CLINICAL DRUG THERAPY, Fourth Edition.
© 1995 J.B. Lippincott Company.

**TABLE 70-1. PREGNANCY: PHYSIOLOGIC AND PHARMACOKINETIC CHANGES**

| Physiologic Change | Pharmacokinetic Change |
|---|---|
| Increased plasma volume and body water, approximately 50% in a normal pregnancy | Once absorbed into the bloodstream, a drug (especially if water soluble) is distributed and "diluted" more than in the nonpregnant state. Drug dosage requirements may increase. However, this effect may be offset by other pharmacokinetic changes of pregnancy. |
| Increased weight (average 25 lb) and body fat | Drugs (especially fat-soluble ones) are distributed more widely. Drugs that are distributed to fatty tissues tend to linger in the body because they are slowly released from storage sites into the bloodstream. |
| Decreased serum albumin. The rate of albumin production is increased. However, serum levels fall because of plasma volume expansion. Also, many plasma protein-binding sites are occupied by hormones and other endogenous substances that increase during pregnancy. | The decreased capacity for drug binding leaves more free or unbound drug available for therapeutic or adverse effects on the mother and for placental transfer to the fetus. Thus, a given dose of a drug is likely to produce greater effects than it would in the nonpregnant state. Some commonly used drugs with higher unbound amounts during pregnancy include dexamethasone (Decadron), diazepam (Valium), lidocaine (Xylocaine), meperidine (Demerol), phenobarbital, phenytoin (Dilantin), propranolol (Inderal), and sulfisoxazole (Gantrisin). |
| Increased renal blood flow and glomerular filtration rate secondary to increased cardiac output | Increased excretion of drugs by the kidneys, especially those excreted primarily unchanged in the urine. These include penicillins, digoxin (Lanoxin), and lithium. In late pregnancy, the increased size and weight of the uterus may decrease renal blood flow when the woman assumes a supine position. This may result in decreased excretion and prolonged effects of renally excreted drugs. |

excreted by fetal kidneys into amniotic fluid. Excretion also is slow and inefficient owing to immature development of fetal kidneys. In addition, the fetus swallows some amniotic fluid, and some drug molecules are recirculated.

Other drug molecules are transported directly to the heart, which then distributes them to the brain and coronary arteries. Drugs enter the brain easily because the blood-brain barrier is poorly developed in the fetus. About half of the drug-containing blood is then transported through the umbilical arteries to the placenta where it reenters the maternal circulation. Thus, the mother can metabolize and excrete some drug molecules for the fetus.

# Drug effects on the fetus

The multiple factors of exposure to any drugs circulating in maternal blood, small size of the developing fetus, low levels of protein binding, and weak capacity for metabolizing and excreting drugs combine to make the fetus sensitive to drug effects. Once drug molecules reach the fetus, they may cause teratogenicity (anatomic malformations) or other adverse effects.

Drug teratogenicity is most likely to occur when drugs are taken during the first trimester of pregnancy, when fetal organs are formed (Table 70-2). For drugs taken during the second and third trimesters, adverse effects are usually manifested in the neonate (birth–1 month) or infant (1 month–1 year) as growth retardation, respiratory problems, infection, or bleeding. Specific effects depend primarily on the amount of drug and the level of fetal growth and development when exposed to the drug(s).

Therapeutic and nontherapeutic drugs may affect the fetus. Effects of commonly used therapeutic drugs are listed in Table 70-3. Nontherapeutic drugs include alcohol, caffeine, cigarettes, cocaine, marijuana, and heroin.

Alcohol is contraindicated during pregnancy; no amount is considered safe. Heavy intake may cause fetal alcohol syndrome, a condition characterized by multiple congenital defects and mental retardation. Caffeine intake above 300 mg daily is thought to be associated with an increased incidence of spontaneous abortion, stillbirth, and premature birth. One cup of coffee contains about 150 mg of caffeine. Caffeine also is present in tea and cola drinks, over-the-counter analgesics, and antisleep preparations.

Cigarette smoking (nicotine and carbon monoxide ingestion) also is contraindicated. It decreases infant birth weight and increases the incidence of premature delivery, abortion, and neonatal death. Nicotine causes vasoconstriction and decreases blood flow to the fetus; carbon monoxide decreases the oxygen available to the fetus. Chronic fetal hypoxia from heavy smoking has been associated with mental retardation.

Cocaine, marijuana, and heroin are illegal drugs of abuse. Use of these drugs during pregnancy is particularly serious. Cocaine may cause maternal vasoconstriction, tachycardia, hypertension, cardiac arrhythmias, and seizures. These effects increase the risk of spontaneous abortion during the first and second trimesters. During the third trimester, cocaine causes increased uterine contractility, vasoconstriction and decreased blood flow in the placenta, fetal tachycardia, and increased risk of fetal distress and abruptio placentae. These life-threatening effects on mother and fetus are even more likely to occur with "crack" cocaine, a highly purified and potent form.

**TABLE 70-2. FDA DRUG CATEGORIES REGARDING PREGNANCY**

| Category | Drugs |
|---|---|
| A. Adequate studies in pregnant women demonstrate no risk to the fetus | Digitalis preparation: digoxin |
| B. Animal studies indicate no risk to the fetus, but there are no adequate studies in pregnant women; or animal studies show adverse effects, but adequate studies in pregnant women have not demonstrated a risk. | Thyroid hormones: levothyroxine, others |
|  | Antiarrhythmics: lidocaine |
|  | Antibiotics: penicillins, cephalosporins, erythromycin, cinoxacin, aztreonam |
|  | Antihypertensives: guanadrel, guanfacine |
|  | Antidepressant: maprotiline |
|  | Beta adrenergic blocking agents: acebutolol, metoprolol, pindolol |
|  | Histamine-1 antagonists: azatadine, brompheniramine, chlorpheniramine, clemastine, cyproheptadine, dexchlorpheniramine, diphenhydramine, triprolidine |
|  | Histamine-2 antagonists: famotidine, ranitidine |
|  | Thiazide diuretics: hydrochlorothiazide, others |
|  | Miscellaneous drugs: cromolyn, ketoprofen, naproxen, terbutaline |
| C. A potential risk, usually because animal studies have either not been performed or indicated adverse effects, and there are no data from human studies. These drugs may be used when potential benefits outweigh the potential risks. | Adrenergics: albuterol, epinephrine, ephedrine, bitolterol, isoetharine, metaproterenol |
|  | Antianxiety drugs: diazepam, others |
|  | Antiarrhythmics: flecainide, mexilitene, procainamide, quinidine, tocainide |
|  | Antibiotics: aminoglycosides, imipenem/cilastatin, norfloxacin, vancomycin |
|  | Anticholinergics: atropine, scopolamine |
|  | Antidepressants: amitriptyline and other tricyclics, trazodone |
|  | Antihypertensives: captopril, guanabenz, minoxidil, nitroprusside |
|  | Beta adrenergic blocking agents: atenolol, labetalol, nadolol, propranolol, timolol |
|  | Calcium channel blocking agents: diltiazem, nifedipine, verapamil |
|  | Histamine-1 antagonists: carbinoxamine, terfenadine |
|  | Narcotic analgesics |
|  | Nitrate antianginals: nitroglycerin |
|  | Miscellaneous: digitoxin, diphenoxylate/atropine, heparin |
| D. There is evidence of human fetal risk, but the potential benefits to the mother may be acceptable despite the potential risk. | Antimanic agent: lithium |
|  | Salicylate: aspirin |
| X. Studies in animals or humans or adverse reaction reports or both have demonstrated fetal abnormalities; the risk of use in a pregnant woman clearly outweighs any possible benefit. | Antiacne drug: isotretinoin |
|  | Anticonvulsant: trimethadione |
|  | Antiviral: ribavirin |

Marijuana impairs formation of deoxyribonucleic acid and ribonucleic acid, the basic genetic material of body cells. It also may decrease the oxygen supply of mother and fetus. Heroin ingestion increases the risks of pregnancy-induced hypertension, malpresentation, third-trimester bleeding, complications of labor and delivery, and postpartum morbidity.

## Fetal therapeutics

Although the major concern about drugs ingested during pregnancy is adverse effects on the fetus, a few drugs are given to the mother specifically for their therapeutic effects on the fetus. These include digoxin (Lanoxin) for fetal tachycardia or congestive heart failure, levothyroxine (Synthroid) for hypothyroidism, penicillin for exposure to maternal syphilis, and corticosteroids to promote lung function and decrease respiratory distress syndrome in preterm infants.

## Maternal therapeutics

Thus far, the main emphasis on drug use during pregnancy has related to actual or potential adverse effects on the fetus. Despite the general principle that drug use should be avoided when possible, pregnant women may require drug therapy for increased nutritional needs, pregnancy-induced problems, chronic disease processes, treatment of preterm labor, induction of labor, and pain management during labor.

### PREGNANCY-INDUCED SYMPTOMS AND THEIR MANAGEMENT

#### Anemias

Three types of anemia are common during pregnancy. One is physiologic anemia, which results from expanded blood volume. A second is iron-deficiency anemia,

*(Text continues on p. 732)*

## TABLE 70-3. DRUG EFFECTS IN PREGNANCY

| | |
|---|---|
| *Adrenergics* | These drugs stimulate the heart to increase rate and force of contractions. They also may increase blood pressure. Several are teratogenic and embryocidal in animal studies, but no adequate studies have been done in pregnant women. These drugs are common ingredients in over-the-counter decongestants, cold remedies, and appetite suppressants.<br><br>Oral and parenteral adrenergics may inhibit uterine contractions during labor; cause hypokalemia, hypoglycemia, and pulmonary edema in the mother; and cause hypoglycemia in the neonate. These effects are unlikely with inhaled adrenergics. Oral albuterol (Proventil, Ventolin) and oral or intravenous terbutaline (Brethine) relax uterine muscle and inhibit preterm labor. Terbutaline is used therapeutically for this purpose. |
| *Analgesics, Narcotic* | Safety is not established. The drugs rapidly cross the placenta and reach the fetus. Maternal addiction and neonatal withdrawal symptoms result from regular use. Use of *codeine* during the first trimester has been associated with congenital defects. *Alfentanil* (Alfenta) and *sufentanil* (Sufenta) had embryocidal effects in animal studies.<br><br>When given to women in labor, narcotic analgesics may decrease uterine contractility and slow progress toward delivery. They also may cause respiratory depression in the neonate. *Meperidine* (Demerol) reportedly causes less neonatal respiratory depression than other narcotics and is usually preferred for obstetric analgesia. If respiratory depression occurs, it can be reversed by administration of *naloxone* (Narcan), a narcotic antagonist. |
| *Angiotensin-Converting Enzyme (ACE) Inhibitors* | In animal studies, captopril (Capoten) was embryocidal, and enalapril (Vasotec) produced conflicting data. There are no adequate studies in pregnant women. |
| *Antianginal Agents (Nitrates)* | Animal studies have not been conducted, and safety for use has not been established. Because the drugs lower blood pressure, a potential effect is decreased blood supply to the fetus. |
| *Antianxiety and Sedative-Hypnotic Agents (Benzodiazepines)* | These drugs should generally be avoided. The benzodiazepines and their metabolites cross the placenta freely and accumulate in fetal blood. If taken during the first trimester, they may cause physical malformations. If taken during labor, they may cause sedation, respiratory depression, hypotonia, lethargy, and sucking difficulties in the neonate. Neonatal tremors and irritability also have been attributed to maternal use of the drugs. |
| *Antiarrhythmics* | *Quinidine* (Quinaglute) crosses the placenta and reaches fetal serum levels similar to maternal levels. However, there are no reports of congenital defects. Neonatal thrombocytopenia has been reported. *Procainamide* (Pronestyl, Procan) crosses the placenta. Although adverse effects on the fetus have not been identified, quinidine is preferred because of more clinical experience in its use. *Disopyramide* (Norpace) has been found in human fetal blood, and it may stimulate contraction of the pregnant uterus. Adequate studies have not been done, and experience in its use is limited. *Lidocaine* (Xylocaine) has not been established as safe. In animal studies with large doses, *tocainide* (Tonocard) was not teratogenic but apparently increased the incidence of abortions and stillbirths. *Mexilitene* (Mexitil) has not been studied adequately. *Flecainide* (Tambocor) had teratogenic and embryotoxic effects in animal studies. |
| *Antibiotics* | |
| *Beta Lactams* | *Penicillins* cross the placenta but apparently produce no adverse effects on the fetus. They are considered safer than other antibiotics. *Cephalosporins* cross the placenta and seem to be safe, although they have not been studied extensively in pregnancy. They apparently have shorter half-lives, lower serum concentrations, and a faster rate of elimination during pregnancy. *Aztreonam* (Azactam) crosses the placenta and enters fetal blood, but fetal effects are unknown. *Imipenem/cilastatin* (Primaxin) showed no teratogenicity in animal studies but has not been studied in pregnant women. |
| *Aminoglycosides* | *Aminoglycosides* cross the placenta, and fetal serum levels may reach 15% to 50% of maternal levels. Deafness has been reported in children whose mothers received streptomycin during pregnancy. Serious adverse effects on the fetus or neonate have not been reported with other aminoglycosides, but there is potential for harm because the drugs are nephrotoxic and ototoxic. |
| *Tetracyclines* | *Tetracyclines* are contraindicated during pregnancy. They cross the placenta, and fetal serum levels reach 60% to 70% of maternal levels. They interfere with development of teeth and bone in the fetus. Animal studies indicate embryotoxicity. |
| *Sulfonamides* | *Sulfonamides* should not be used during the last 2 wk of pregnancy because they displace bilirubin from binding sites on serum albumin and may cause kernicterus in the neonate. |
| *Erythromycin* | *Erythromycin* (E-Mycin, others) crosses the placenta to reach fetal serum levels up to 20% of maternal level, but no fetal abnormalities have been reported. |
| *Nitrofurantoin* | *Nitrofurantoin* (Macrodantin) should not be used during late pregnancy because of possible hemolytic anemia in the neonate. |
| *Clindamycin* | *Clindamycin* (Cleocin) should be used only when infection with *Bacteroides fragilis* is suspected. |
| *Antitubercular Drugs* | *Isoniazid* (INH) was embryocidal in some animal studies and should be used only if necessary. *Ethambutol* (Myambutol) was teratogenic in animal studies, but administration to pregnant women produced no detectable effects on the fetus. The effects of combination with other antitubercular drugs are unknown. *Rifampin* (Rifadin) was teratogenic in animal studies. |

*(continued)*

## TABLE 70-3.  DRUG EFFECTS IN PREGNANCY  *(Continued)*

| | |
|---|---|
| *Antiviral Agents* | *Acyclovir* (Zovirax), *amantadine* (Symmetrel), *vidarabine* (Vira-A), and *zidovudine* (Retrovir) were teratogenic in animal studies. None of these drugs should be given unless clearly necessary, and *ribavarin* (Virazole) is contraindicated. |
| *Miscellaneous* | *Trimethoprim* (Proloprim), often given in combination with *sulfamethoxazole* (Bactrim, Septra), was teratogenic in small animals. It crosses the placenta to reach levels in fetal serum and amniotic fluid that are similar to those in maternal serum. It may interfere with folic acid metabolism in the fetus. A few studies in pregnant women have not indicated teratogenic effects. |
| **Anticholinergics** | *Atropine* crosses the placenta rapidly with IV injection; effects on the fetus depend on the maturity of its parasympathetic nervous system. *Scopolamine* may cause respiratory depression in the neonate and may contribute to neonatal hemorrhage by reducing vitamin K-dependent clotting factors in the neonate. |
| **Anticoagulants** | *Heparin* does not cross the placenta and has not been associated with congenital defects. However, its use during pregnancy has been associated with 13% to 22% unfavorable outcomes, including stillbirths and prematurity. *Warfarin* (Coumadin) crosses the placenta and fetal hemorrhage, spontaneous abortion, prematurity, stillbirth, and congenital anomalies may occur. About 31% of fetuses exposed to warfarin may experience a problem related to the anticoagulant. If a woman becomes pregnant during warfarin therapy, inform her of the potential risks to the fetus, and discuss the possibility of terminating the pregnancy. |
| **Anticonvulsants** | Although a large majority of women receiving anticonvulsant drugs deliver normal infants, reports suggest an increased incidence of birth defects. Data are more extensive with *phenytoin* (Dilantin) and *phenobarbital*. The drugs may be discontinued before and during pregnancy when the type, frequency, and severity of seizures do not seriously threaten the client's well-being. They should not be discontinued when given for major seizures because of the risk of precipitating status epilepticus with resultant hypoxia and risk to mother and fetus. It is not known whether minor seizures cause fetal risk. Maternal ingestion of these drugs, especially barbiturates, may cause neonatal bleeding during the first 24 h after birth. This neonatal coagulation defect is characterized by decreased levels of vitamin K-dependent clotting factors and prolongation of either the prothrombin time or partial thromboplastin time or both. This may be prevented by giving vitamin K to the mother 1 mo prior to delivery and during delivery and to the infant immediately after birth. |
| **Antidepressants** | Tricyclic antidepressants such as *amitriptyline* (Elavil) have been associated with teratogenicity and embryotoxicity when given in large doses, and there have been reports of congenital malformations and neonatal withdrawal syndrome. *Trazodone* (Desyrel), in animal studies with large doses, caused increased fetal resorption and congenital anomalies. Monoamine oxidase inhibitors, such as *phenelzine* (Nardil), were associated with fewer viable offspring and growth retardation in animal studies with large doses. Overall, clinical experience with these drugs in pregnant women is limited. |
| **Antidiabetic Drugs** | *Insulin* is the only acceptable hypoglycemic drug during pregnancy. Dosage requirements usually change, generally increasing during the second and third trimesters. Blood sugar must be monitored closely. Oral antidiabetic drugs are contraindicated. They cross the placenta and may cause hypoglycemia and death in the fetus. They also may be teratogenic. |
| **Antidiarrheals** | *Diphenoxylate* (Lomotil) has been used without reported teratogenic or other adverse effects. *Loperamide* (Imodium) has not been studied in relation to pregnancy. |
| **Antiemetics** | None of the available antiemetic drugs has been proven safe for use. Nondrug measures are preferred for controlling nausea and vomiting because of possible drug effects on the fetus. |
| **Antihistamines** | Histamine-1 receptor blocking agents, such as *diphenhydramine* (Benadryl), have been associated with teratogenic effects, but the extent and significance are unknown. Safety has not been established. The drugs should not be used during the third trimester because of possible convulsions and other adverse effects in the neonate. Histamine-2 receptor blocking agents, such as *cimetidine* (Tagamet), have not been established as safe. Animal studies indicated no harmful effects on the fetus, but studies in pregnant women have not been done. |
| **Antihypertensives** | Beta-blocking agents, such as *propranolol* (Inderal) and others, apparently improve fetal survival. *Methyldopa* (Aldomet) crosses the placenta and reaches fetal concentrations similar to those of maternal serum. However, no teratogenic effects have been reported despite widespread use during pregnancy. Neonates of mothers receiving methyldopa may have decreased blood pressure for about 48 h. *Hydralazine* (Apresoline) is often used and is generally considered safe. *Captopril* (Capoten), *clonidine* (Catapres), *guanabenz* (Wytensin), and *guanfacine* (Tenex) are not recommended because effects in pregnant women are unknown. |
| **Antimanic Agent** | *Lithium* crosses the placenta. About 11% of infants exposed to lithium during the first trimester had major congenital defects, 72% of which were cardiovascular. In the neonate, lithium has a prolonged half-life due to slow elimination and has caused bradycardia, cyanosis, diabetes insipidus, hypotonia, hypothyroidism, and ECG abnormalities. Most of these effects resolve within 1 to 2 wk. |

*(continued)*

**TABLE 70-3.  DRUG EFFECTS IN PREGNANCY** *(Continued)*

| | |
|---|---|
| *Antipsychotic Drugs* | Phenothiazines, such as *chlorpromazine* (Thorazine) and related drugs, readily cross the placenta. Several studies indicate that the drugs are not teratogenic, but animal studies indicate potential embryotoxicity, increased neonatal mortality, and decreased performance. The possibility of permanent neurologic damage cannot be excluded. Use near term may cause abnormal movements, abnormal reflexes, and jaundice in the neonate and hypotension in the mother. |
| *Antithyroid Drugs* | The drugs readily cross the placenta and can cause fetal goiter and cretinism. If given, dosage must be carefully regulated so that sufficient but not excessive amounts are given. In some women, thyroid function decreases as pregnancy progresses, and dosage must be reduced. Propylthiouracil is the preferred antithyroid drug. Neonatal goiter occurs in about 10% of cases. |
| *Aspirin* | *Aspirin* is generally contraindicated because of potential adverse effects on the mother and fetus. Maternal effects include prolonged gestation, prolonged labor, and antepartal and postpartal hemorrhage. Fetal effects include constriction of the ductus arteriosus, low birth weight, and increased incidence of stillbirth and neonatal death. However, for the pregnant client with rheumatoid arthritis, aspirin is considered the nonsteroidal anti-inflammatory of choice. The lowest possible doses should be given. For analgesic and antipyretic effects during pregnancy, acetaminophen (Tylenol) is preferred. |
| *Beta-Adrenergic Blocking Agents* | Safety for use of propranolol (Inderal) and related drugs has not been established. Animal studies with large doses indicated embryotoxicity. Teratogenicity has not been reported in humans. However, problems have been reported during delivery. These include maternal bradycardia and neonatal bradycardia, hypoglycemia, apnea, low Apgar scores, and low birth weight. Neonatal effects may last up to 72 hours. |
| *Bronchodilators (Xanthine)* | *Theophylline* (Theo-Dur, Aminophylline) has not been associated with teratogenic effects, but adequate studies have not been done in animals or humans. Thus, drug effects during pregnancy are unknown. Theophylline crosses the placenta and therapeutic serum levels have been found in neonates. There have been reports of tachycardia and irritability in neonates whose mothers took the drug until labor and delivery. |
| *Calcium Channel-Blocking Agents* | Teratogenic and embryotoxic effects occurred in small animals given large doses. Diltiazem (Cardizem) caused fetal death, skeletal abnormalities, and increased incidence of stillbirths. Verapamil (Calan) crosses the placenta, but effects are unknown. Adequate studies have not been done in pregnant women. Because the drugs decrease blood pressure, there is a potential risk of inadequate blood flow to the placenta and the fetus. |
| *Corticosteroids* | These drugs cross the placenta. Animal studies indicate that large doses of cortisol early in pregnancy may produce cleft palate, stillborn fetuses, and decreased fetal size. Chronic maternal ingestion during the first trimester has shown a 1% incidence of cleft palate in humans. Adequate human reproduction studies have not been done. Infants of mothers who received substantial amounts of corticosteroids during pregnancy should be closely observed for signs of adrenal insufficiency. |
| *Digitalis Preparations* | *Digoxin* (Lanoxin) is apparently safe for use during pregnancy. It crosses the placenta to reach fetal serum levels that are 50% to 80% those of maternal serum. Fetal toxicity and neonatal death have occurred with maternal overdose. Dosage requirements may be less predictable during pregnancy, and serum drug levels and other assessment parameters must be closely monitored. Digoxin also has been administered to the mother for treatment of fetal tachycardia and congestive heart failure. *Digitoxin* (Crystodigin) also crosses the placenta and reaches fetal serum levels similar to those of digoxin. |
| *Diuretics* | Thiazide diuretics such as *hydrochlorothiazide* (HydroDiuril) cross the placenta. They are not associated with teratogenesis, but they may cause other adverse effects. Because the drugs decrease plasma volume, decreased blood flow to the uterus and placenta may occur with resultant impairment of fetal nutrition and growth. Other adverse effects may include fetal or neonatal jaundice, thrombocytopenia, hyperbilirubinemia, hemolytic jaundice, fluid and electrolyte imbalances, and impaired carbohydrate metabolism. These drugs are not indicated for treatment of dependent edema caused by uterine enlargement and restriction of venous blood flow. They also are not effective in prevention or treatment of pregnancy-induced hypertension (preeclampsia). They may be used for treatment of pathologic edema from cardiovascular and other conditions.<br>Loop diuretics such as *furosemide* (Lasix) have not been studied adequately in pregnant women. Teratogenesis has not been reported, but animal studies indicated fetal toxicity and death. Like the thiazides, loop diuretics may decrease plasma volume and blood flow to the placenta and fetus.<br>Potassium-conserving diuretics, such as *triamterene* (an ingredient in Dyazide and Maxide), cross the placenta in animal studies, but effects on the human fetus are unknown. |
| *Laxatives* | If a laxative is required, a bulk-forming agent, such as Metamucil, is preferred. It is more physiologic than other laxatives and is not absorbed systemically. It is unlikely to harm the fetus.<br>Mineral oil should be avoided because it interferes with absorption of fat-soluble vitamins. Strong laxatives such as castor oil or bisacodyl (Dulcolax) or excessive use of any laxative may cause fluid and electrolyte imbalances or initiate labor. |

*(continued)*

**TABLE 70-3. DRUG EFFECTS IN PREGNANCY** *(Continued)*

| | |
|---|---|
| *Nonsteroidal Anti-Inflammatory Drugs (NSAIDs)* | Use of *ibuprofen* (Motrin, Advil, others) and other NSAIDs has not been established as safe during pregnancy and should be avoided. There are no adequate studies in pregnant women. In animal studies, delayed delivery occurred. <br><br> Because the drugs inhibit prostaglandin synthesis, they may cause premature closure of the ductus arteriosus and other adverse effects on the fetus. If taken during the third trimester, they may delay onset of labor and delivery. If taken within 1 week of labor and delivery, they increase risks of excessive bleeding. |
| *Thyroid Hormones* | These drugs do not readily cross the placenta. No adverse effects have been reported in human fetuses, and the drugs are apparently safe to use in appropriate dosages. When given as replacement therapy in hypothyroid women, the drugs should be continued through pregnancy. *Levothyroxine* (Synthroid) also has been given to the mother to treat hypothyroidism in the fetus. |

which is often related to long-term nutritional deficiencies. Iron supplements are usually given for prophylaxis (*e.g.*, ferrous sulfate 300 mg three times daily or ferrous gluconate 600 mg three times daily). Iron preparations should be given with food to decrease gastric irritation. A third type is megaloblastic anemia, caused by folic acid deficiency. A folic acid supplement (0.8 mg daily) is often prescribed for prophylaxis.

## Constipation

Constipation often occurs during pregnancy, probably from decreased peristalsis. Preferred treatment, if effective, is to increase intake of fluids and high-fiber foods. If a laxative is required, a bulk-producing agent (*e.g.*, Metamucil) is the most physiologic for the mother and safest for the fetus because it is not absorbed systemically. A stool softener, such as docusate (Colace), may be used occasionally. Mineral oil should be avoided because it interferes with absorption of fat-soluble vitamins. Strong laxatives or any laxative used in excess may initiate uterine contractions and labor.

## Heartburn

Heartburn (pyrosis) often occurs in the later months of pregnancy, when increased abdominal pressure and a relaxed cardiac sphincter allow gastric acid to regurgitate into the esophagus and cause irritation and discomfort. Interventions to decrease abdominal pressure (*e.g.*, eating small meals, sitting in an upright position, avoiding gas-producing foods and constipation) may be helpful. Antacids may be used if necessary. Because little systemic absorption occurs, the drugs are unlikely to harm the fetus if used in recommended doses.

## Nausea and vomiting

Nausea and vomiting often occur, especially during early pregnancy. Dietary management (*e.g.*, eating a few crackers when awakening and waiting a few minutes

before arising) and maintaining fluid and electrolyte balance are recommended. Antiemetic drugs should be given only if nausea and vomiting are severe enough to threaten the mother's nutritional or metabolic status. Meclizine (Antivert), 25–50 mg daily, and dimenhydrinate (Dramamine), 50 mg q3–4h, are thought to have low teratogenic risks. However, possible teratogenesis cannot be ruled out.

## Pregnancy-induced hypertension

Pregnancy-induced hypertension includes preeclampsia and eclampsia. These serious complications endanger the lives of mother and fetus. Preeclampsia is most likely to occur during the last 10 weeks of pregnancy or during labor. It is characterized by edema, hypertension, and proteinuria. Nonpharmacologic management includes bed rest, in a left lateral position, and a high-protein, high-carbohydrate, low-salt, low-fat diet. The left lateral position increases blood flow to the kidneys and placenta, promotes diuresis, and lowers blood pressure. Drug therapy includes intravenous hydralazine (Apresoline), which does not cause adverse fetal effects.

Eclampsia, characterized by severe symptoms and convulsions, occurs if preeclampsia is not treated effectively. Intravenous magnesium sulfate is the drug of choice to prevent or treat convulsive seizures. Delivery of the fetus is the only known cure for preeclampsia or eclampsia.

## MANAGEMENT OF CHRONIC DISEASES DURING PREGNANCY

### Asthma

Pharmacologic treatment of pregnant women with asthma is similar to treatment of nonpregnant women. For mild symptoms or infrequent attacks, inhaled adrenergic bronchodilators, such as albuterol (Proventil, Ventolin) or metaproterenol (Alupent), are the drugs of choice. For more severe or more frequent attacks, oral theophylline, oral terbutaline, or an inhaled corticosteroid, such as beclomethasone (Vanceril), may be required. Severe episodes or status asthmaticus are managed as in nonpregnant women. Although large doses of corticosteroids in early pregnancy are teratogenic, cautious use of smaller amounts may benefit the mother sufficiently to risk adverse effects on the fetus. Cromolyn and nedocromil, which are prophylactic agents, are not recommended during pregnancy because their safety and fetal effects are unknown.

## Diabetes mellitus

For diabetic women who become pregnant, maintaining normal or near-normal blood sugar levels is required for successful outcomes because poor glycemic control increases the risks of birth defects. Pregnancy causes significant metabolic changes, and insulin is the only hypoglycemic drug acceptable for use during pregnancy. Because insulin requirements vary according to the stage of pregnancy, the diabetic client's condition must be monitored very closely and insulin therapy individualized. At the same time, careful dietary control and other treatment measures are necessary. Some guidelines for insulin therapy during antepartal, intrapartal, and postpartal periods are as follows.

Antepartal period. Pregnancy has a diabetogenic effect because of several hormonal changes. First, human placental lactogen (HPL) exerts an increasing diabetogenic effect throughout pregnancy. This hormone increases mobilization of free fatty acids and decreases effects of maternal insulin. Second, estrogen levels increase as pregnancy advances; estrogen is thought to be an insulin antagonist. Third, progesterone may decrease insulin effectiveness. Fourth, cortisol from the adrenal cortex is thought to increase gluconeogenesis and thus cause maternal hyperglycemia.

Some women first show signs of diabetes during pregnancy. This is called *gestational diabetes*. These women may revert to a nondiabetic state when pregnancy ends, but they are at increased risk of developing diabetes at a later time. Other women, who were previously able to control diabetes with diet alone, may become insulin dependent during pregnancy. Still other women, already insulin dependent, are likely to need larger doses as pregnancy advances.

More specifically, insulin requirements usually decrease during the first trimester and increase during the second and third trimesters. During the first trimester, decreased need for insulin is attributed to fetal use of maternal glucose for growth and development. This lowers maternal blood glucose levels and may cause hypoglycemia. During the second trimester, insulin requirements increase along with increasing blood levels of HPL, estrogen, progesterone, and cortisol. It is recommended that women be screened for diabetes between 24 and 28 weeks (by measuring blood sugar after an oral glucose dose of 50 or 100 g). During the third trimester, insulin requirements increase still further, and the largest amounts are likely to be needed near term.

It is especially important that sufficient insulin is given to prevent maternal acidosis. Uncontrolled acidosis is likely to interfere with neurologic development of the fetus.

Intrapartal period. Women with diabetes usually deliver at 37 to 38 weeks of gestation because of increased incidence of fetal death closer to full term. Early delivery is usually induced by oxytocin (Pitocin) or accomplished by cesarean section. Either method precipitates a high-risk situation. During labor, for example, strenuous muscular contractions increase cellular use of glucose and deplete glycogen stores. Thus, less insulin is needed, and hypoglycemia may occur. If a cesarean section is done, the stress of surgery may increase insulin requirements. Regular, short-acting insulin and frequent blood sugar tests are used to control diabetes during labor and delivery as during other acute situations.

Postpartal period. Insulin requirements continue to fluctuate during the immediate postpartal period because stress, trauma, infection, surgery, or other factors associated with delivery tend to increase blood glucose levels and insulin requirements. At the same time, termination of the pregnancy reverses the diabetogenic hormonal changes and decreases insulin requirements. Usually, women are at higher risk of hypoglycemia during the first 24 to 48 hours after delivery, and some may require no insulin during this time. As during the intrapartal period, regular, short-acting insulin is given, and dosage is based on frequent measurements of blood sugar. Once the insulin requirement is stabilized, the client can return to the prepregnancy treatment regimen unless she is breast-feeding. Insulin does not enter breast milk; however, breast-feeding may decrease insulin requirements. Gestational diabetes usually subsides within 6 weeks after delivery.

Oral antidiabetic drugs are contraindicated in pregnancy and lactation. In pregnancy, they cross the placenta, stimulate the fetal pancreas, and may cause fetal hypoglycemia or death. They also increase the risk of congenital anomalies and may cause overt diabetes in women with gestational diabetes because they stimulate an already overstimulated pancreas. If these drugs are taken by a woman of childbearing potential, they should be discontinued before conception if possible or as soon as pregnancy is suspected. In lactation, chlorpropamide (Diabinese) and tolbutamide (Orinase) are excreted in breast milk. The status of other oral agents is unknown. Because there is a risk of hypoglycemia in the nursing infant, it is recommended that the mother stop the drug or stop breast-feeding.

## Seizure disorders

Women with seizure disorders, whether receiving anticonvulsant drugs or not, are more likely to have children with congenital defects and mental retardation than women who do not have epilepsy. Thus, the disease and anticonvulsant drugs have potential teratogenic effects, and none of the drugs has been proven safe for use. Despite this, however, women on medication have a 90% chance of having a normal child. Because seizures adversely affect the fetus, the goal of drug therapy is to prevent seizures with the fewest possible effects on the fetus.

If a client has been seizure free for several years, it may be possible to discontinue drug therapy prior to pregnancy. If drug therapy is required, phenytoin (Dilantin) or carbamazepine (Tegretol) is probably preferred. Because dosage requirements may be altered during pregnancy, serum drug levels should be measured monthly and the dosage adjusted accordingly.

Valproic acid (Depakene) is considered the most teratogenic and should not be given to women of childbearing potential.

## Hypertension

Chronic hypertension (hypertension beginning prior to conception or up to 20 weeks of pregnancy) is associated with increased maternal and fetal risks. Thus, appropriate management is mandatory. Nonpharmacologic interventions (avoiding excessive weight gain, sodium restriction, increased rest) should be emphasized. If drug therapy is required, methyldopa (Aldomet) is probably the most commonly used drug. For acute episodes of hypertension, intravenous hydralazine (Apresoline) is commonly used.

Although diuretics are widely used in the treatment of hypertension at other times and in other groups of people, they should not be given during pregnancy. They decrease blood volume, cardiac output, and blood pressure and may cause fluid and electrolyte imbalances, all of which may have adverse effects on the fetus.

## Abortifacients

Abortion is the termination of pregnancy prior to 20 weeks. It may occur spontaneously or be intentionally induced. Prostaglandins are commonly used to terminate pregnancy during the second trimester (Table 70-4 lists individual drugs). In the female reproductive sys-

tem, prostaglandins E and F are found in the ovaries, myometrium, and menstrual fluid. They stimulate uterine contraction and are probably important in initiating and maintaining the normal birth process. Drug preparations of prostaglandins are capable of inducing labor at any time during pregnancy.

## Tocolytics

Drugs given to inhibit labor and maintain the pregnancy are called tocolytics. Uterine contractions between about 20 and 37 weeks of gestation are considered premature labor. Nonpharmacologic treatment includes bed rest, hydration, and sedation. Drug therapy is most effective when the cervix is dilated less than 4 cm, and membranes are intact.

Ritodrine (Yutopar), terbutaline (Brethine), and magnesium sulfate are used as tocolytics (see Table 70-4). Ritodrine and terbutaline are beta-adrenergic agents that relax uterine smooth muscle and thereby slow or stop uterine contractions. Magnesium sulfate is most often used as an anticonvulsant in the treatment of pregnancy-induced hypertension (preeclampsia), but it also inhibits preterm labor. Hypermagnesemia may occur because tocolytic serum levels (about 4–7 mEq/L) are higher than normal levels (1.5–2.5 mEq/L). Close monitoring of serum levels and signs of hypermagnesemia is required.

## Drugs used during labor and delivery at term

At the end of gestation, labor usually begins spontaneously and proceeds through delivery of the neonate. Drugs often used during labor, delivery, and the immediate postpartal period include oxytocics, analgesics, anesthetics, and lactation suppressors.

### OXYTOCICS

Oxytocic drugs include oxytocin and ergot alkaloids (see Table 70-4). Oxytocin is a hormone produced in the hypothalamus and released by the posterior pituitary gland (see Chap. 23). Oxytocin functions in childbirth by stimulating uterine contractions and in lactation by promoting milk "letdown" (movement of breast milk from the glands to the nipples). Pitocin is a synthetic form used to induce labor at or near full-term gestation and to stimulate labor when uterine contractions are weak and ineffective. It also is used to prevent or control uterine bleeding after delivery, to complete an incom-

## TABLE 70-4. ABORTIFACIENTS, TOCOLYTICS, OXYTOCICS, AND LACTATION SUPPRESSOR

| Generic/Trade Name | Routes and Dosage Ranges |
| --- | --- |
| **Abortifacients (Prostaglandins)** | |
| **Carboprost tromethamine** (Hemabate) | IM 250 μg q1.5–3.5h, depending on uterine response, increased to 500 μg per dose if uterine contractility is inadequate after several 250-μg doses |
| **Dinoprostone** (Prostin E₂) | Intravaginally 20 mg, repeated q3–5h until abortion occurs |
| **Tocolytics** | |
| **Ritodrine** (Yutopar) | IV infusion 0.1 mg/min initially, increased by 50 μg/min every 10 min to a maximal dose of 350 μg/min if necessary to stop labor. The infusion should be continued for 12 h after uterine contractions cease. PO 10 mg 30 min before discontinuing the IV infusion, then 10 mg q2h for 24 hr, then 10–20 mg q4–6h as long as necessary to maintain the pregnancy. Maximal oral dose, 120 mg daily. |
| **Terbutaline** (Brethine) | IV infusion 10 μg/min, titrated up to a maximum dose of 80 μg/min until contractions cease PO 2.5 mg q4–6h as maintenance therapy until term |
| **Magnesium sulfate** | IV infusion, loading dose 3–4 g mixed in 5% dextrose injection and administered over 15–20 min. Maintenance dose 1–2 g/h, according to serum magnesium levels and deep tendon reflexes. PO 250–450 mg q3h, to maintain a serum level of 2.0–2.5 mEq/L. |
| **Oxytocics** | |
| **Oxytocin** (Pitocin) | During labor and delivery, IV 2 milliunits/min, gradually increased to 20 milliunits/min, if necessary, to produce three or four contractions within 10-min periods. Prepare solution by adding 10 units (1 ml) of oxytocin to 1000 ml of 0.9% sodium chloride or 5% dextrose in 0.45% sodium chloride. To control postpartal hemorrhage, IV 10–40 units added to 1000 ml of 0.9% sodium chloride, infused at a rate to control bleeding To prevent postpartal bleeding, IM 3–10 units (0.3–1 ml) as a single dose To promote milk ejection, topically, 1 spray of nasal solution to one or both nostrils 2–3 min before nursing |
| **Ergonovine maleate** (Ergotrate) | After delivery of the placenta, IM 0.2 mg, repeated in 2–4 h if bleeding is severe Severe uterine bleeding, IV 0.2 mg To prevent excessive postpartal bleeding, PO 0.2 mg two to four times daily for 2–7 d if necessary |
| **Methylergonovine maleate** (Methergine) | Same as ergonovine maleate, above |
| **Lactation Suppressor** | |
| **Bromocriptine** (Parlodel) | PO 2.5 mg twice daily for 14 d |

plete abortion, and to promote milk ejection during lactation. It is contraindicated for antepartal use in the presence of fetal distress, cephalopelvic disproportion, preterm labor, placenta previa, previous uterine surgery, and severe preeclampsia. Ergot alkaloids markedly increase the force and frequency of uterine contractions. They are used after delivery of the infant and placenta to prevent postpartum uterine atony and hemorrhage.

## ANALGESICS

Parenteral narcotic analgesics are used to control discomfort and pain during labor and delivery. They may prolong labor and cause sedation and respiratory depression in the mother and neonate. Meperidine (Demerol) is usually the drug of choice because it may cause less neonatal depression than other narcotic analgesics. If neonatal respiratory depression does occur, it can be reversed by the narcotic antagonist naloxone (Narcan).

## ANESTHETICS

Local anesthetics also are used to control discomfort and pain. They are injected by physicians for regional anesthesia in the pelvic area. Paracervical blocks involve injection of the anesthetic agent around the cervix; epidural blocks involve injection into the epidural space of the spinal cord. With regional anesthesia, the mother is usually conscious and comfortable, and the neonate is rarely depressed.

## LACTATION SUPPRESANTS

Bromocriptine (Parlodel) is the drug of choice for suppression of lactation in mothers who do not plan to breast-feed. It suppresses lactation by inhibiting secretion of prolactin, a pituitary hormone. Route and dosage are listed in Table 70-4.

# Neonatal therapeutics

In the neonate, any drug must be used cautiously. Drugs are usually given less often because they are metabolized and excreted slowly. Immature liver and kidney function prolong drug action and increase risks of toxicity. Also, drug therapy should be initiated with low doses, especially with drugs that are highly bound to plasma proteins. Neonates have few binding proteins, which leads to increased amounts of free, active drug and increased risk of toxicity even at lower doses. When assessing the neonate, drugs received by the mother during pregnancy, labor and delivery, and lactation must be considered.

At birth, some drugs are routinely administered to prevent hemorrhagic disease of the newborn and ophthalmia neonatorum. Hemorrhagic disease of the newborn occurs because the intestinal tract lacks the bacteria that normally synthesize vitamin K. Vitamin K is required for liver production of several clotting factors, including prothrombin. Thus, the neonate is at increased risk of bleeding during approximately the first week of life. One dose of phytonadione (AquaMephyton) 0.5 to 0.1 mg is given intramuscularly in the thigh at delivery or on admission to the nursery.

Ophthalmia neonatorum, an eye infection that may cause ulceration and blindness, is usually caused by exposure to *Neisseria gonorrhoeae* during passage through the birth canal. It is a sexually transmitted disease for which prophylaxis is legally required. Another serious eye infection is caused by *Chlamydia trachomatis*, also a sexually transmitted microorganism. Erythromycin 0.5% or tetracycline 1% is applied to each eye at delivery. The drugs are effective against gonorrheal and chlamydial infections. Silver nitrate 1% is used less often than formerly because it is effective only against the gonococcus.

## *Nursing Process*

### Assessment

Assess each female client of reproductive age for possible pregnancy. If the client is known to be pregnant, assess status in relation to pregnancy, as follows:
- Length of gestation
- Use of prescription, over-the-counter, nontherapeutic, and illegal drugs
- Acute or chronic health problems that may influence the pregnancy and drug therapy
- With premature labor, length of gestation, the frequency and quality of uterine contractions, the amount of vaginal bleeding or discharge, and the length of labor. Also determine whether any tissue has been expelled from the vagina. When abortion is inevitable, oxytocics may be given. When stopping labor is possible or desired, a tocolytic may be given.
- When spontaneous labor occurs in normal, full-term pregnancy, frequency and quality of uterine contractions, amount of cervical dilatation, fetal heart rate and quality, and maternal blood pressure

Assess antepartal women for intention to breast-feed.

### Nursing diagnoses
- High Risk for Injury: Damage to fetus or neonate from maternal ingestion of drugs
- High Risk for Injury: Damage to the pregnant client from acute and chronic health problems
- High Risk for Altered Nutrition: Less than Body Requirements related to pregnancy-induced anemia and nausea and vomiting
- High Risk for Altered Nutrition: More than Body Requirements related to excessive weight gain with pregnancy
- Anxiety about outcome of pregnancy
- Noncompliance related to drug ingestion during actual or potential pregnancy
- Pain related to uterine contractions
- High Risk for Injury related to possible damage to mother or infant during the birth process
- Knowledge Deficit: Drug effects during pregnancy and lactation

### Planning/Goals

*The client will:*
- Avoid unnecessary drug ingestion when pregnant or likely to become pregnant
- Use nondrug measures to relieve symptoms associated with pregnancy or other health problems when possible
- Maintain nutritional status and appropriate weight gain to support maternal health and fetal growth and development
- Obtain optimal care during pregnancy, labor and delivery, and the postpartal period
- Avoid complications of pregnancy and labor and delivery
- Breast-feed safely and successfully if desired

### Interventions
- Use nondrug measures to prevent the need for drug therapy during actual or potential pregnancy.
- Provide optimal prenatal care and counseling to promote a healthy pregnancy (*e.g.,* regular monitoring of blood pressure, weight, blood sugar, urine protein, and counseling about nutrition and other health-promotion activities).
- Help clients and families cope with complications of pregnancy, including therapeutic abortion.
- Counsel candidates for therapeutic abortion about methods and expected outcomes; counsel postabortion clients about contraceptive techniques.

*Teach clients:*
- That any drug taken by a pregnant woman reaches the fetus and may interfere with fetal growth and development. For most drugs, safety during pregnancy has not been established, and all drugs are relatively contraindicated. Therefore, any drug usage (including prescription drugs) must be cautious and minimal to avoid potential damage to the fetus.
- To avoid drugs when possible and use them very cautiously when necessary. If women who are sexually active and not

## TABLE 70-5.  DRUG EFFECTS IN LACTATION

| | |
|---|---|
| *Adrenergics* | Parenteral *epinephrine* (Adrenalin) is excreted in breast milk; the status of other adrenergic bronchodilators is not known. *Albuterol* (Proventil, Ventolin) had tumorigenic effects in animals; if considered necessary, breast-feeding should be discontinued. Oral drugs used as nasal decongestants (*e.g., pseudoephedrine* [Sudafed], others) are contraindicated in nursing mothers because of higher than usual risks to infants from sympathomimetic drugs. |
| *Analgesics* | *Acetaminophen* (Tylenol) is excreted in breast milk in low concentrations. No adverse effects have been reported, and it is probably the analgesic-antipyretic drug of choice for nursing mothers. Salicylates (*e.g., aspirin*) are excreted in breast milk in small amounts. Adverse effects on nursing infants have not been reported but are a potential risk. Narcotic analgesics such as *meperidine* (Demerol) are excreted in breast milk, but amounts may not be enough to cause adverse effects in the nursing infant. Some authorities recommend waiting 4 to 6 h after a dose before nursing. *Alfentanil* (Alfenta) should probably not be given. Significant amounts were found in breast milk 4 h after a dose. |
| *Angiotensin-Converting Enzyme (ACE) Inhibitors* | *Captopril* (Capoten) is excreted in breast milk, but effects on the infant are unknown. It is not known whether *enalapril* (Vasotec) or *lisinopril* (Prinivil, Zestril) is excreted in breast milk. In general, nursing is not recommended while taking these drugs. |
| *Antianginal Agents (Nitrates)* | Safety for use in the nursing mother has not been established. |
| *Antianxiety and Sedative-Hypnotic Agents (Benzodiazepines)* | *Diazepam* (Valium) and other benzodiazepines should generally be avoided. They are excreted in breast milk and may cause lethargy and weight loss in the infant. The drugs and their metabolites may accumulate to toxic levels in neonates because of slow drug metabolism. |
| *Antiarrhythmics* | When these agents are required for a nursing mother, breast-feeding should generally be discontinued. *Quinidine* (Quinaglute), *disopyramide* (Norpace), and *mexiletine* (Mexitil) are excreted in breast milk; it is unknown whether *procainamide* (Pronestyl, Procan), *lidocaine* (Xylocaine), and *flecainide* (Tambocor) are excreted. There is a potential for serious adverse effects on infants. |
| *Antibiotics* | *Penicillins* are excreted in breast milk in low concentrations and may cause diarrhea, candidiasis, or allergic responses in nursing infants. *Cephalosporins* are excreted in small amounts and may alter bowel flora, cause pharmacologic effects, and interfere with interpretation of culture reports with fever or infection. *Aztreonam* (Azactam) is excreted in small amounts; discontinuing breast-feeding temporarily is probably indicated. It is unknown whether *imipenem/cilastatin* (Primaxin) is excreted. The aminoglycosides *netilmicin* (Netromycin) and *streptomycin* are excreted in small amounts. Because these drugs are nephrotoxic and ototoxic, the immature kidney function of neonates and infants should be considered. *Tetracyclines* are excreted in breast milk and should be avoided. *Sulfonamides* are excreted and generally contraindicated. They may cause kernicterus in the neonate and diarrhea and skin rash in the nursing infant. *Erythromycin* is excreted and may become concentrated in breast milk. No adverse effects on nursing infants have been reported. However, the potential exists for alteration in bowel flora, pharmacologic effects, and interference with fever workup. *Nitrofurantoin* (Macrodantin) is excreted in very small amounts. However, safety for use in nursing mothers has not been established, and infants with glucose-6-phosphate dehydrogenase (G-6-PD) deficiency may be adversely affected. *Clindamycin* (Cleocin) is excreted. Breast-feeding is probably best discontinued if the drug is necessary, to avoid potential problems in the infant. *Cinoxacin* (Cinobac) and *norfloxacin* (Noroxin) are probably excreted, and there is a potential for severe adverse effects in nursing infants. Depending on the mother's need for the drug, either the drug or breast-feeding should be discontinued. *Isoniazid* (INH) and *rifampin* (Rifadin) are excreted in breast milk, and nursing infants should be observed for adverse drug effects. *Trimethoprim* (Proloprim, Bactrim) is excreted and may interfere with folic acid metabolism in the infant. |
| *Anticholinergics* | *Atropine* and others are excreted and may cause infant toxicity or decreased breast milk production. Safety for use is not established. |
| *Anticoagulants* | *Heparin* is not excreted in breast milk; *warfarin* (Coumadin) is excreted, but some evidence suggests no harm to the nursing infant. More data are needed, and heparin is preferred if anticoagulant therapy is required. |
| *Anticonvulsants* | *Phenytoin* (Dilantin) and other hydantoins are excreted and may cause serious adverse effects in nursing infants. The drug or breast-feeding should be discontinued. *Phenobarbital* is excreted in small amounts and may cause drowsiness in the infant. |
| *Antidepressants* | Tricyclic antidepressants such as *amitriptyline* (Elavil) and others are excreted in small amounts; effects on nursing infants are not known. Other antidepressants have not been established as safe for use. |

*(continued)*

**TABLE 70-5. DRUG EFFECTS IN LACTATION** *(Continued)*

| | |
|---|---|
| *Antidiabetic Drugs* | *Insulin* does not enter breast milk and is not known to affect the nursing infant. However, insulin requirements of the mother may be decreased while breast-feeding. Oral agents *chlorpropamide* (Diabinese) and *tolbutamide* (Orinase) are excreted in breast milk; the status of other sulfonylureas is unknown. There is a potential for hypoglycemia in nursing infants. |
| *Antidiarrheals* | *Diphenoxylate* (Lomotil) and *loperamide* (Imodium) should be used cautiously during lactation; effects on the nursing infant are unknown. |
| *Antiemetics* | Although information is limited, most of the drugs (*e.g.*, phenothiazines such as *promethazine* [Phenergan] and antihistamines such as *dimenhydrinate* [Dramamine]) are apparently excreted in breast milk and may cause drowsiness and possibly other effects in nursing infants. Antihistamines used for antiemetic effects also may inhibit lactation. *Metoclopramide* (Reglan) is excreted and concentrated in breast milk; it should be used cautiously, if at all. |
| *Antihistamines* | Histamine-1 receptor antagonists such as *diphenhydramine* (Benadryl) may inhibit lactation by their drying effects and may cause drowsiness in nursing infants. For most of the commonly used drugs, including over-the-counter allergy and cold remedies, little information is available about excretion in breast milk or effects on nursing infants. Histamine-2 receptor antagonists such as *cimetidine* (Tagamet) and *ranitidine* (Zantac) are excreted in breast milk. *Famotidine* (Pepcid) was excreted in animals, but it is not known whether it is excreted in human breast milk. It is generally recommended that either the drug or nursing be discontinued. |
| *Antihypertensives* | Beta-adrenergic blocking agents should generally be avoided by nursing mothers. *Propranolol* (Inderal) and *metoprolol* (Lopressor) are excreted in low concentrations; *acebutolol* (Sectral) and its major metabolite are excreted; it is unknown whether *nadolol* (Corgard) and *timolol* (Blocadren) are excreted. *Methyldopa* (Aldomet) is excreted; effects on nursing infants are unknown. It is unknown whether *hydralazine* (Apresoline) is excreted; safety for use is not established. *Captopril* (Capoten), *clonidine* (Catapres), *guanabenz* (Wytensin), and *guanfacine* (Tenex) are not generally recommended because information about effects on nursing infants is limited. Calcium channel-blocking drugs should not be given to nursing mothers. *Verapamil* (Calan) and *diltiazem* (Cardizem) are excreted in breast milk. |
| *Antimanic Agent* | *Lithium* is excreted in breast milk and reaches about 40% of the mother's serum level. Infant serum and milk levels are about equal. If the drug is required, nursing should be discontinued. |
| *Antipsychotic Drugs* | Little information is available considering the extensive use of these drugs. *Chlorpromazine* (Thorazine) and *haloperidol* (Haldol) have been detected in breast milk in small amounts. Safety has not been established. |
| *Antithyroid Drugs* | Nursing is contraindicated for clients on the antithyroid drugs *propylthiouracil* and *methimazole* (Tapazole). |
| **Beta-Adrenergic Blocking Agents** | See **Antihypertensives**. |
| **Bronchodilators (Xanthine)** | *Theophylline* (Theo-Dur) enters breast milk readily; use with caution. |
| **Calcium Channel-Blocking Agents** | See **Antihypertensives**. |
| *Corticosteroids* | *Prednisone* (Deltasone), *dexamethasone* (Decadron), and others appear in breast milk and could suppress growth, interfere with endogenous corticosteroid production, or cause other adverse effects in nursing infants. Advise mothers taking pharmacologic doses not to breast-feed. |
| *Digitalis* | *Digoxin* (Lanoxin) is excreted. However, infants receive very small amounts, and no adverse effects have been reported. |
| *Diuretics* | If diuretic drug therapy is required, nursing mothers should discontinue breast-feeding. Thiazide diuretics such as *hydrochlorothiazide* (HydroDiuril) and the loop diuretic *furosemide* (Lasix) are excreted in breast milk. It is unknown whether *bumetanide* (Bumex) and *ethacrynic acid* (Edecrin) are excreted. Little information is available about potassium-sparing diuretics, such as *amiloride* (Midamor), *triamterene* (Dyrenium, Dyazide, Maxide), and *spironolactone* (Aldactone). They are not recommended for use. |
| *Laxatives* | *Cascara sagrada* is excreted in breast milk and may cause diarrhea in the nursing infant. It is not known whether *docusate* (Colace) is excreted. |
| *Nonsteroidal Anti-Inflammatory Drugs* | Most of the drugs, such as *ibuprofen* (Motrin, Advil), are excreted in breast milk, and nursing is not recommended. However, occasional use of therapeutic doses is probably acceptable. |
| *Thyroid Hormones* | Small amounts are excreted in breast milk. The drugs are not associated with adverse effects on nursing infants but should be used with caution in nursing mothers. |

using contraception take *any* drugs, there is a high risk that potentially harmful agents may be ingested before pregnancy is suspected or confirmed.

- Measures to prevent the need for drug therapy, such as a healthful life-style (adequate nutrition, exercise, rest and sleep; avoiding alcohol and cigarette smoking) and avoiding infection (personal hygiene, avoiding contact with people known to have infections, maintaining indicated immunizations)
- Nondrug measures to relieve common health problems (positioning, adequate food and fluid intake, deep breathing)
- To see a health-care provider as soon as pregnancy is suspected
- To inform any health-care provider from whom treatment is sought if there is a possibility of pregnancy
- That many drugs are excreted in breast milk to some extent and reach the nursing infant

### Evaluation

- Interview regarding actions taken to promote reproductive and general health.
- Observe and interview regarding compliance with instructions for promoting and maintaining a healthy pregnancy.
- Interview regarding ingestion of therapeutic and nontherapeutic drugs during prepregnant, pregnant, and lactating states.
- Observe and interview regarding the health status of the mother and neonate.

## Principles of therapy

### GENERAL GUIDELINES: PREGNANCY

1. Give medications only when clearly indicated, weighing anticipated benefits to the mother against the risk of harm to the fetus.
2. When drug therapy is required, the choice of drug should be based on the stage of pregnancy and available drug information (see Tables 70-2 and 70-3). During the first trimester, for example, an older drug that has not been associated with teratogenic effects is usually preferred over a newer drug of unknown teratogenicity.
3. Any drugs used during pregnancy should be given in the lowest effective doses and for the shortest effective time.

### GENERAL GUIDELINES: LACTATION

1. Many drugs given to the mother reach the infant in breast milk. For some, the amount of drug is too small to cause significant effects; for others, effects on the nursing infant are unknown or potentially adverse. For the latter drugs, it is usually recommended that the mother stop the drug or stop breast-feeding. Effects of commonly used therapeutic drugs are listed in Table 70-5.
2. Give medications only when clearly indicated, weighing potential benefit to the mother against possible harm to the nursing infant.
3. Any drugs used during lactation should be given in the lowest effective dose for the shortest effective time.

### USE OF OXYTOCIN

Oxytocin is the drug of choice for induction or augmentation of labor because physiologic doses produce a rhythmic uterine contraction-relaxation pattern that approximates the normal labor process. It is also the drug of choice for prevention or control of postpartal uterine bleeding because it is less likely to cause hypertension than the ergot alkaloids.

## NURSING ACTIONS: ABORTIFACIENTS, TOCOLYTICS, OXYTOCICS, AND LACTATION SUPPRESSOR

| *Nursing Actions* | *Rationale/Explanation* |
|---|---|
| **1. Administer accurately** | |
| **a.** Give abortifacients IM or intravaginally. | Physicians administer intra-amniotic agents. |
| **b.** Give tocolytics IV initially, then PO. With IV ritodrine, have the client lie in the left lateral position. | The side-lying position decreases risks of hypotension. |
| **c.** For IV oxytocin, dilute the drug in an IV sodium chloride solution, and piggyback the solution into a primary IV line. Use an infusion pump to administer. | Oxytocin has an antidiuretic effect and may cause water intoxication. This is less likely to occur if the drug is given in a saline solution rather than a water solution, such as 5% dextrose in water. Piggybacking allows regulation of the |

*(continued)*

| Nursing Actions | Rationale/Explanation |
|---|---|
| | oxytocin drip without interrupting the main IV line. Infusion pumps deliver more accurate doses and minimize the possibility of overdosage. |
| **d.** Give IM oxytocin immediately after delivery of the placenta. | To prevent excessive postpartal bleeding |
| **e.** Give bromocriptine with food. | To decrease nausea and vomiting |
| **2. Observe for therapeutic effects** | |
| **a.** When prostaglandins are given to induce abortion, observe for the onset of labor and the expulsion of the fetus and placenta. | Abortion usually occurs within 24 hours. Uterine contractions may be perceived by the client as abdominal cramping or low back pain. |
| **b.** When a tocolytic drug is given in threatened abortion or premature labor, observe for absent or decreased uterine contractions. | The goal of drug therapy is to stop the labor process. |
| **c.** When oxytocin is given to induce or augment labor, observe for firm uterine contractions at a rate of three to four per 10 minutes. Each contraction should be followed by a palpable relaxation period. Examine periodically for cervical dilatation and effacement. | Oxytocin is given to stimulate the normal labor process. Contractions should become regular and increase in duration and intensity. |
| **d.** When oxytocin or an ergot alkaloid is given to prevent or control postpartal bleeding, observe for a small, firm uterus and minimal vaginal bleeding. | These agents control bleeding by causing strong uterine contractions. The uterus can be palpated in the lower abdomen. |
| **e.** When bromocriptine is given to suppress lactation, observe for absent or decreased breast engorgement and secretion. | |
| **3. Observe for adverse effects** | |
| **a.** With prostaglandins, observe for: | |
| (1) Nausea, vomiting, diarrhea | These are the most common adverse effects. They occur with all routes of prostaglandin administration and result from drug-induced stimulation of gastrointestinal smooth muscle. |
| (2) Fever, cardiac arrhythmias, bronchospasm, convulsive seizures, chest pain, muscle aches | These effects occur less frequently and are not clearly related to prostaglandin administration. Bronchospasm is more likely to occur in clients with asthma; seizures are more likely in clients with known epilepsy. |
| **b.** With ritodrine, observe for: | |
| (1) Change in fetal heart rate | This is a common adverse effect and may be significant if changes are extreme or prolonged. |
| (2) Maternal effects, such as changes in heart rate, arrhythmias, palpitations, nausea and vomiting, tremors, hypokalemia, hyperglycemia, dyspnea, chest pain, and anaphylactic shock | |
| **c.** With oxytocin, observe for: | |
| (1) Excessive stimulation of uterine contractility (hypertonicity, tetany, rupture, cervical and perineal lacerations, fetal hypoxia, arrhythmias, death or damage from rapid, forceful propulsion through the birth canal) | Most likely to occur when excessive doses are given to initiate or augment labor |
| (2) Hypotension or hypertension | Usual obstetric doses do not cause significant change in blood pressure. Large doses may cause an initial drop in blood pressure, followed by a sustained elevation. |

| *Nursing Actions* | *Rationale/Explanation* |
|---|---|
| (3) Water intoxication (convulsions, coma) | Unlikely with usual doses but may occur with prolonged administration of large doses (more than 20 milliunits/min) |
| (4) Allergic reactions, including anaphylactic shock | |
| (5) Nausea and vomiting | |
| **d.** With ergot preparations, observe for: | |
| (1) Nausea, vomiting, diarrhea | These drugs have a direct effect on the vomiting center of the brain and stimulate contraction of gastrointestinal smooth muscle. |
| (2) Symptoms of ergot poisoning—coolness, numbness and tingling of extremities, headache, vomiting, dizziness, thirst, convulsions, weak pulse, confusion, chest pain, tachycardia or bradycardia, muscle weakness and pain, cyanosis, gangrene of the extremities | The ergot alkaloids are highly toxic; poisoning may be acute or chronic. Acute poisoning is rare; chronic poisoning usually results from overdosage. Circulatory impairments may result from vasoconstriction and vascular insufficiency. Large doses also damage capillary endothelium and may cause thrombosis and occlusion. Gangrene of extremities rarely occurs with usual doses unless peripheral vascular disease or other contraindications also are present. |
| (3) Hypertension | Blood pressure may rise as a result of generalized vasoconstriction induced by the ergot preparation. Hypertension is most likely to occur when ergonovine or methylergonovine is given to postpartal women with previous hypertension or to those who have had regional anesthesia with vasoconstrictive agents (*e.g.*, epinephrine). |
| (4) Allergic reactions—local edema, pruritus, anaphylactic shock | Allergic reactions are relatively uncommon. |
| **e.** With bromocriptine, observe for hypotension, headache, nausea and vomiting, and dizziness. | These are the most common adverse effects. These effects are usually mild when the drug is used for inhibition of physiologic lactation. |
| **4. Observe for drug interactions** | |
| **a.** Drugs that alter effects of prostaglandins: | |
| Aspirin and other nonsteroidal anti-inflammatory agents, such as ibuprofen (Motrin) | These drugs inhibit effects of prostaglandins. When given concurrently with abortifacient prostaglandins, the abortive process is prolonged. |
| **b.** Drugs that alter effects of ritodrine: | |
| (1) Beta-adrenergic blocking agents, such as propranolol (Inderal) | Decreased effectiveness of ritodrine, which is a beta-adrenergic stimulating (agonist) agent |
| (2) Corticosteroids | Increased risk of pulmonary edema |
| **c.** Drugs that alter effects of oxytocin: | |
| Vasoconstrictors, such as epinephrine (Adrenalin) and other adrenergic drugs | Additive vasoconstriction with risks of severe, persistent hypertension and intracranial hemorrhage |
| **d.** Drugs that alter effects of ergot alkaloids: | |
| (1) Propranolol (Inderal) | Additive vasoconstriction |
| (2) Vasoconstrictors | See oxytocin, above. |
| **e.** Drugs that alter effects of bromocriptine: | |
| Antihypertensives | Additive hypotension and risk of fainting. |
| **5. Teach clients**<br>Purpose and expected effects of drugs | The drugs are indicated for short-term use, with close supervision by a health-care provider. |

## Review and Application Exercises

1. Why should drugs be avoided during pregnancy and lactation when possible?
2. How does insulin therapy for diabetes mellitus differ during pregnancy?
3. What is the rationale for using methyldopa and hydralazine to treat hypertension during pregnancy?
4. Which anticonvulsant agents are generally preferred during pregnancy? Which should not be given during pregnancy?
5. In a client receiving ritodrine or terbutaline to inhibit uterine contractions, how and when would you assess the client for adverse drug effects?
6. In a client receiving an oxytocin infusion to induce or augment labor, what interventions are needed to increase safety and decrease adverse drug effects?
7. Which drugs may be used to increase uterine muscle tone and decrease postpartum hemorrhage?

## Selected References

Briggs, G. G. (1992). Drugs in pregnancy and lactation. In M. A. Koda-Kimble & L. Y. Young (Eds.), *Applied therapeutics: The clinical use of drugs* (5th ed.) (pp. 69-1–69-33). Vancouver, WA: Applied Therapeutics.

(1994). *Drug facts and comparisons.* St. Louis: Facts and Comparisons.

May, K. A., & Mahlmeister, L. R. (1990). *Comprehensive maternity nursing: Nursing process and the childbearing family* (2nd ed.). Philadelphia: J.B. Lippincott.

Porth, C. M. (1990). *Pathophysiology: Concepts of altered health states* (3rd ed.). Philadelphia: J.B. Lippincott.

Rubin, P. C. (1992). Drugs in special patient groups: Pregnancy and nursing. In K. L. Melmon, H. F. Morrelli, B. B. Hoffman, & D. W. Nierenberg (Eds.), *Clinical pharmacology: Basic principles in therapeutics* (3rd ed.) (pp. 805–825). New York: McGraw-Hill.

Sagraves, R., & Letassy, N. A. (1992). Obstetrics. In M. A. Koda-Kimble & L. Y. Young (Eds.), *Applied therapeutics: The clinical use of drugs* (5th ed.) (pp. 68-1–68-31). Vancouver, WA: Applied Therapeutics.

# APPENDIX A.
# Miscellaneous Drugs

| Generic/Trade Name | Clinical Use | Characteristics | Routes and Dosage Ranges |
|---|---|---|---|
| **Beractant** (Survanta) | To prevent or treat neonatal respiratory distress syndrome | • Natural lung surfactant from bovine lungs<br>• Stabilizes alveoli against collapse | Intratracheal instillation, dosage individualized according to birth weight, four doses during first 48 h of life, at least 6 h apart |
| **Chenodiol** (Chenix) | To dissolve gallstones in clients who are not candidates for surgical removal | • Contraindicated in liver disease<br>• Adverse effects include diarrhea, abdominal pain, and hepatotoxicity | PO 13–16 mg/kg per day in two divided doses, morning and evening |
| **Colfosceril** (Exosurf) | To prevent or treat respiratory distress syndrome in premature newborn infants | • Synthetic lung surfactant<br>• Stabilizes alveoli against collapse | Intratracheal instillation, 5 mg/kg of birth weight, first dose immediately after birth, second dose 12 h after first, third dose 24 h after first dose if infant on mechanical ventilation |
| **Dornase alfa** (Pulmozyme) | To decrease risks of respiratory infection and improve lung function in patients with cystic fibrosis | • A mucolytic enzyme<br>• Main adverse effects, hoarseness and sore throat | Inhalation, 2.5–10 mg q12h |
| **Epoetin alfa** (Epogen, Procrit) | Treatment of anemia associated with end-stage renal disease, human immunodeficiency virus (HIV) infection, zidovudine therapy, or chemotherapy of non-myeloid malignancies | • A recombinant DNA form of erythropoietin<br>• Stimulates production of red blood cells<br>• Contraindicated in uncontrolled hypertension<br>• Generally well tolerated and adverse effects consistent with underlying disease process (*e.g.*, hypertension with chronic renal failure, fever with HIV infection and cancer chemotherapy) | Patients with chronic renal failure, Epogen IV or SC 50–100 U/kg three times weekly, adjusted according to hematocrit<br>Patients receiving zidovudine, Epogen IV or SC 100 U/kg three times weekly for 8 wk, then adjusted according to hematocrit<br>Patients receiving cancer chemotherapy, Procrit SC 150 U/kg three times weekly |
| **Etretinate** (Tegison) | Treatment of severe psoriasis | • Contraindicated in pregnancy<br>• Adverse effects commonly occur and resemble those of excessive vitamin A | PO 0.75–1 mg/kg per day in divided doses |
| **Finasteride** (Proscar) | Treatment of symptomatic benign prostatic hyperplasia (BPH) | • Inhibits an intracellular enzyme that produces dihydrotestosterone (DHT) in prostate gland. Reduced serum DHT leads to regression of the enlarged prostate gland.<br>• Improves ability to empty the urinary bladder | PO 5 mg once daily for at least 6 mo |
| **Monoctanoin** (Moctanin) | Dissolution of cholesterol gallstones remaining in the biliary tract after cholecystectomy | • Dissolves or reduces size of approximately 30%–65% of stones<br>• Adverse effects are common, especially nausea, vomiting, diarrhea, and abdominal discomfort | Perfusion into biliary tract through catheter, 3–5 ml/h for 2–10 d |
| **Masoprocol** (Actinex) | Treatment of actinic keratoses | • Mechanism of action is unknown<br>• Adverse effects include burning, erythema, itching, bleeding, crusting, soreness. These local | Topically to skin lesions after washing and drying affected areas, morning and evening for 28 d. Apply evenly, avoiding eyes and mucous membranes of the |

(continued)

| Generic/Trade Name | Clinical Use | Characteristics | Routes and Dosage Ranges |
|---|---|---|---|
| | | skin reactions are common, but usually subside within 2 wk of stopping the drug. | mouth and nose. Do *not* cover with occlusive dressings, and do *not* use other skin care products or makeup on medicated areas. |
| **Mesna** (Mesnex) | Prevention of ifosfamide-induced hemorrhagic cystitis | • Combines with the ifosfamide metabolite that causes hemorrhagic cystitis<br>• Adverse effects include nausea, vomiting, diarrhea, and allergic reactions. | Adults, IV injection, 20% of ifosfamide dose for three doses; first dose at time of ifosfamide administration; repeat at 4 h and 8 h after ifosfamide dose. (Total dose, 60% of ifosfamide dose) |
| **Minoxidil** (Rogaine) | Treatment of male pattern baldness | • Initial hair growth usually requires at least 4 mo of regular use.<br>• When treatment is stopped, new hair growth is usually shed within a few months.<br>• Adverse effects include dermatitis, redness and itching at site of application | Topically to dry hair and scalp, 1 ml morning and evening |
| **Mupirocin** (Bactroban) | Impetigo | • Adverse effects include burning, itching, pain, or stinging at site of application | Topically to skin, adults and children, three times daily |
| **Nicotine** (Habitrol, Nicoderm, Nicorette, ProStep) | Smoking deterrent in a smoking cessation program | • Contraindicated in people with significant cardiovascular disease (angina pectoris, arrhythmias, or recent myocardial infarction) and during pregnancy<br>• Adverse effects include soreness of mouth, throat, and jaw (with gum); nausea; vomiting; dizziness; hypertension; arrhythmias; confusion; and skin rash or irritation at site of transdermal patch application.<br>• Should not be used while continuing to smoke because of high risk of serious adverse effects | Habitrol or Nicoderm transdermal patch, 21 mg/d for 6 wk, then 14 mg/d for 2 wk, then 7 mg/d for 2 wk<br>ProStep transdermal patch, 22 mg/d for 4–8 wk, then 11 mg/d for 2–4 wk<br>Nicorette gum, 10–12 pieces daily (maximum dose, 30 pieces daily) |
| **Rifabutin** (Mycobutin) | Prophylaxis of *Mycobacterium avium* complex disease in patients with advanced HIV infection | • An antimycobacterial drug chemically related to rifampin<br>• Should not be given to patients with active tuberculosis but may be given concurrently with isoniazid (INH) to patients who need prophylaxis against both *Mycobacterium tuberculosis* and *M. avium* complex<br>• Adverse effects include skin rash, nausea, vomiting, diarrhea, and neutropenia | PO 300 mg once daily |
| **Tacrine** (Cognex) | Treatment of memory deficit in patients with Alzheimer's disease | • Centrally acting indirect cholinergic agent<br>• Increases acetylcholine in the brain by blocking pseudocholinesterase, the enzyme that normally inactivates acetylcholine<br>• Does not cure or delay progression of Alzheimer's disease<br>• Adverse effects include abdominal discomfort, diarrhea, nausea, increased urination, and sweating. | PO 40–160 mg daily |
| **Ursodiol** (Actigall) | To dissolve gallstones in clients who are not candidates for surgical excision | • Decreases hepatic synthesis and secretion of cholesterol<br>• Decreases intestinal absorption of cholesterol<br>• Contraindicated with calcified or radiopaque gallstones and with chronic liver disease | PO 8–10 mg/kg per day, in two or three divided doses, usually for several months |

# APPENDIX B.

# The International System of Units

The International System of Units (Systeme International d'Unites or SI units), which is based on the metric system, has been adopted by many countries in an attempt to standardize reports of clinical laboratory data among nations and disciplines. A major reason for using SI units is that biologic substances react in the human body on a molar basis.

The international system, like the conventional system, uses the kilogram for measurement of mass or weight and the meter for measurement of length. The major difference is that the international system uses the mole for measurement of amounts per volume of a substance. A mole is the amount of a chemical compound of which its weight in grams equals its molecular weight. Thus, the concentration of solutions is expressed in moles, millimoles, or micromoles per liter (mol/L, mmol/L, $\mu$mol/L) rather than the conventional measure-ment of mass per volume, such as grams or milligrams per 100 ml or dl. A few laboratory values are the same in conventional and SI units, but many differ dramatically. Moreover, "normal values" in both systems often vary, depending on laboratory methodologies and reference sources. Thus, laboratory data should be interpreted in light of the client's clinical status and with knowledge of the "normal values" of the laboratory performing the test.

In addition to other laboratory tests, measuring the amount of a drug in blood plasma or serum is often useful in the clinical management of various disorders. For example, serum drug levels may be used to guide drug dosage (*e.g.*, aminoglycoside antibiotics such as gentamicin), to evaluate an inadequate therapeutic response, and to diagnose drug toxicity.

# APPENDIX C.
# Therapeutic Serum Drug Concentrations for Selected Drugs

Listed below are generally accepted therapeutic serum drug concentrations, in conventional and SI units, for several commonly used drugs. In addition, toxic concentrations are listed for selected drugs. SI units have not been established for some drugs.

| Drug | Conventional Units | SI units |
|------|--------------------|----------|
| Acetaminophen | 0.2–0.6 mg/dL | 13–40 μmol/L |
| | Toxic >5 mg/dL | > 300 μmol/L |
| Amikacin | (peak) 16–32 μg/mL | 20–30 mg/L |
| | (trough) 8 μg/mL or less | |
| Amitriptyline | 110–250 ng/mL | 375–900 nmol/L |
| Carbamazepine | 4–12 μg/mL | 17–50 μmol/L |
| Desipramine | 125–300 ng/mL | 470–825 nmol/L |
| Digoxin | 0.5–2.2 ng/mL | 1–2.6 nmol/L |
| Disopyramide | 2–8 μg/mL | 6–18 μmol/L |
| Ethosuximide | 40–110 μg/mL | 280–780 μmol/L |
| Gentamicin | (peak) 4–8 μg/mL | 5–10 mg/L |
| | (trough) 2 μg/mL or less | |
| Imipramine | 200–350 ng/mL | 530–950 nmol/L |
| Lidocaine | 1.5–6 μg/mL | 6–21 μmol/L |
| Lithium | 0.5–1.5 mEq/L | 0.5–1.5 mmol/L |
| Maprotiline | 50–200 ng/mL | 180–270 nmol/L |
| Netilmicin | (peak) 6–10 μg/mL | 5–10 mg/L |
| | (trough) 2 μg/mL or less | |
| Nortriptyline | 50–150 ng/mL | 190–570 nmol/L |
| Phenobarbital | 15–50 μg/mL | 65–170 μmol/L |
| Phenytoin | 10–20 μg/mL | 40–80 μmol/L |
| Primidone | 5–12 μg/mL | 25–45 μmol/L |
| Procainamide | 4–8 μg/mL | 17–40 μmol/L |
| Propranolol | 50–200 ng/mL | 190–770 nmol/L |
| Protriptyline | 100–300 ng/mL | 380–1140 nmol/L |
| Quinidine | 2–6 μg/mL | 4.6–9.2 μmol/L |
| Salicylate | 100–200 mg/L | 724–1448 μmol/L |
| | Toxic >200 mg/L | >1450 μmol/L |
| Theophylline | 10–20 μg/mL | 55–110 μmol/L |
| Tobramycin | (peak) 4–8 μg/mL | 5–10 mg/L |
| | (trough) 2 μg/mL or less | |
| Valproic acid | 50–100 μg/mL | 350–700 μmol/L |
| Vancomycin | (peak) 30–40 μg/mL | (peak) 20–40 mg/L |
| | (trough) 5–10 μg/mL | (trough) 5–10 mg/L |

μg = microgram; ng = nanogram; μmol = micromole.

## References

(1993). *Compendium of pharmaceuticals and specialties* (28th ed.) (pp. B82–B85). Ottawa, Ontario, Canada: Canadian Pharmaceutical Association.

(1994). *Drug facts and comparisons* (p. 3062). St. Louis: Facts and Comparisons.

Spencer, R. T., Nichols, L. W., Lipkin, G. B., Henderson, H. S., & West, F. M. (1993). *Clinical pharmacology and nursing management* (4th ed.) (pp. 1360–1361). Philadelphia: J.B. Lippincott.

Young, L. Y., & Smith, G. H. (1992). Interpretation of clinical laboratory tests. In M. A. Koda-Kimble & L. Y. Young (Eds.), *Applied therapeutics: The clinical use of drugs* (5th ed.) (pp. 3-1–3-17). Vancouver, WA: Applied Therapeutics.

# APPENDIX D.
# Canadian Drug Laws and Standards

Two national laws, with their amendments, regulate drug-related standards and practices. The Health Protection Branch of the Department of National Health and Welfare is responsible for administering and enforcing the laws, which are described below.

The Food and Drugs Act, initially passed in 1953 and amended periodically since then, regulates the manufacture, distribution, advertising, labeling, and use of drugs. Specific provisions:

- Empower the government to control the marketing of drugs according to proof of safety and effectiveness
- Require that drugs comply with the standards under which the drugs are approved for sale or the standards listed in "specific pharmacopeiae"
- Direct the government to supervise the manufacturing processes of some drugs
- Classify drugs (*e.g.*, antihypertensives, antimicrobials, hormones) that require a prescription and specify that refills must be designated on the original prescription and obtained within 6 months (Schedule F)
- Specify symbols to be placed on containers of the different classifications of drugs
- Require proof of appropriate drug release from oral dosage formulations
- Prohibit advertising of prescription and controlled drugs to the public
- Prohibit the sale of contaminated, adulterated, or unsafe drugs
- Establish requirements for labeling
- Prohibit false, misleading, or deceptive labeling of drug products

The Narcotic Control Act, originally passed in 1961 and amended periodically since then, restricts the sale, possession, and use of opiates, cocaine, marijuana, and methadone. Additional provisions:

- Restrict possession of the above drugs to authorized people
- Require people possessing the drugs to keep them in a secure place, maintain strict dispensing records, and promptly report any thefts or other losses
- Require prescriptions for dispensing narcotics
- Require that containers with prescribed narcotics be labeled with the symbol N
- Specify four levels of controlled drugs. The first level, narcotics, includes single drugs and preparations containing camphorated tincture of opium (paregoric), cocaine, codeine, heroin, hydrocodone, hydromorphone, methadone, morphine, oxycodone, and pentazocine. The second level, controlled drugs or Schedule G, includes nonnarcotic prescription drugs, the use of which is restricted to treatment of certain disorders (*e.g.*, amphetamines, methylphenidate, pentobarbital, and secobarbital). The third level restricts anabolic steroids, amobarbital, phenobarbital, diethylpropion, and nalbuphine. The fourth level (Schedule H), includes substances with no recognized medicinal uses (*e.g.*, hallucinogens such as LSD).

Nurses in Canada are governed by these national laws; there also may be local and provincial laws. Legal possession of a narcotic by a nurse is restricted to the following circumstances:

- When administering to a client according to a physician's order
- When performing custodial care of narcotics as an agent of a health-care facility
- When receiving a prescribed narcotic for medical treatment.

## References

(1993). *Compendium of pharmaceuticals and specialties* (28th ed.) (p. B111). Ottawa, Ontario, Canada: Canadian Pharmaceutical Association.

Spencer, R. T., Nichols, L. W., Lipkin, G. B., Henderson, H. S., & West, F. M. (1993). *Clinical pharmacology and nursing management* (4th ed.) (p. 13). Philadelphia: J.B. Lippincott.

# APPENDIX E.
# Canadian Drug Names

Many drugs are distributed by international pharmaceutical companies, and most names (generic and trade) are the same in the United States and Canada. To assist the Canadian reader in identifying the drugs discussed in this book, generic names and Canadian trade names are listed below. Generic names used in Canada but not in the United States are designated by an asterisk. The chapter number is listed in parentheses. Canadian trade names that include Apo, Novo, or Nu are drugs manufactured by Apotex, Novo-Pharm and Nu-Pharm companies, respectively.

## Generic/Canadian Trade Names

**Acebutolol (19)**
Monitan, Rhotral, Sectral

**Acetaminophen (6)**
**Paracetamol***
APAP, Abenol, Atasol, Panadol, Tantaphen, Tempra, Tylenol

**Acetazolamide (68)**
Diamox

**Acetohexamide (27)**
Dimelor

**Acetylcysteine (49)**
Mucomyst

**Acyclovir (42, 69)**
Zovirax

**Albuterol**
**Salbutamol***
Novo-Salmol, Ventodisc, Ventolin, Volmax

**Alfentanil (5)**
Alfenta

**Allopurinol (6)**
Purinol, Zyloprim

**Alprazolam (8)**
Apo-Alpraz, Novo-Alprazol, Nu-Alpraz, Xanax

**Alteplase (60)**
Activase rt-PA

**Aluminum hydroxide (63)**
Amphojel

**Aluminum hydroxide gel/magnesium hydroxide (63)**
Diovol Ex, Maalox, Mylanta, Neutralca-S

**Amantadine (12, 42)**
Symmetrel

**Amcinonide (69)**
Cyclocort

**Amikacin (36)**
Amikin

**Amiloride (59)**
Apo-Amilzide, Moduret, Novamilor, Nu-Amilzide

**Aminocaproic acid (60)**
Amicar

## Generic/Canadian Trade Names

**Aminoglutethimide (67)**
Cytadren

**Aminophylline (16, 50)**
Phyllocontin

**Amiodarone (55)**
Cordarone

**Amitriptyline (10)**
Elavil

**Amlodipine (56)**
Norvasc

**Amobarbital (7)**
**Amylobarbitone***
Amytal, Novamobarb

**Amoxapine (10)**
Asendin

**Amoxicillin (34)**
Amoxil, Apo-Amoxi, Novamoxin, Nu-Amoxi

**Amoxicillin/potassium clavulanate (34)**
Clavulin

**Amphotericin B (43)**
Fungizone

**Ampicillin (34)**
Ampicin, Apo-Ampi, Nu-Ampi, Penbriten

**Amrinone (54)**
Inocor

**Antithymocyte globulin (48)**
Atgam

**Ascorbic acid (31)**
Apo-C, Ce-Vi-Sol

**Asparaginase (67)**
**Colaspase***
Kidrolase

**Aspirin (6)**
Entrophen, Novasen

**Astemizole (51)**
Hismanal

**Atenolol (19, 56, 58)**
Apo-Atenol, Novo-Atenol, Nu-Atenol, Tenormin

**Atracurium (14)**
Tracium

## Generic/Canadian Trade Names

**Atopine sulfate (21, 68)**
Atropisol, Isopto Atropine, R.O.-Atropine

**Azatadine (51)**
Optimine

**Azathioprine (48)**
Imuran

**Bacampicillin (34)**
Penglobe

**Bacitracin (68, 69)**
Baciguent, Bacitin

**Baclofen (13)**
Lioresal

**Beclomethasone (24, 50)**
Beclodisk, Becloforte, Beclovent, Beconase, Propaderm, Vancenase, Vanceril

**Bendroflumethiazide (59)**
**Bendrofluazide***
Naturetin

**Benzocaine (14)**
Topicaine

**Benzoyl peroxide (69)**
Acetoxyl, Acnomel, Benoxyl, Benzac, Benzagel, Dermoxyl, Desquam-X, Loroxide, Panoxyl, Solugel

**Benztropine (12, 21)**
Cogentin

**Betamethasone (24, 69)**
Beben, Betacort, Betaderm, Betnesol, Betnovate, Celestoderm, Celestone, Diprosone, Occlucort, Rhoprosone, Tara-Sone, Valisone

**Betaxolol (58, 68)**
Betoptic

**Bethanechol (20)**
Duvoid, Myotonachol, Urecholine

**Biperiden (12, 21)**
Akineton

**Bisacodyl (64)**
Dulcolax

**Bleomycin (67)**
Blenoxane

| Generic/Canadian Trade Names | Generic/Canadian Trade Names | Generic/Canadian Trade Names |
| --- | --- | --- |

**Bretylium (55)**
Bretylate

**Bromocriptine (12)**
Parlodel

**Brompheniramine (51)**
**Parabromdylamine***
Dimetane

**Bupivacaine (14)**
Marcaine

**Busulfan (67)**
Myleran

**Calcitonin-salmon (26)**
Calcimar

**Calcitriol (26)**
Calcijex, Rocaltrol

**Calcium carbonate (26)**
Apo-Cal, Calsan, Caltrate, Nu-Cal, Os-Cal, Tums

**Captopril (58)**
Apo-Capto, Capoten, Novo-Captoril, Nu-Capto

**Carbachol (68)**
Isopto Carbachol, Miostat

**Carbamazepine (11)**
Novo-Carbamaz, Tegretol

**Carbenicillin (34)**
Geopen, Pyopen

**Carboplatin (67)**
Paraplatin

**Carisoprodol (13)**
**Isomeprobamate***
Soma

**Carmustine (67)**
BiCNU

**Cefaclor (35)**
Ceclor

**Cefadroxil (35)**
Duricef

**Cefamandole (35)**
Mandol

**Cefazolin (35)**
Ancef, Kefzol

**Cefoperazone (35)**
Cefobid

**Cefotaxime (35)**
Claforan

**Cefotetan (35)**
Cefotan

**Cefoxitin (35)**
Mefoxin

**Ceftazidime (35)**
Ceptaz, Tazidime

**Ceftizoxime (35)**
Cefizox

**Ceftriaxone (35)**
Rocephin

**Cefuroxime (35)**
Ceftin, Kefurox, Zinacef

**Cephalexin (35)**
Apo-Cephalex, Keflex, Novo-Lexin, Nu-Cephalex

**Cephalothin (35)**
Keflin

**Cephradine (35)**
Velosef

**Chlorambucil (67)**
Leukeran

**Chloramphenicol (39, 68)**
Chloromycetin, Diochloram, Ophtho-Chloram, Sopamycetin

**Chlordiazepoxide (8)**
Librium, Solium

**Chlorhexidine (69)**
Hexifoam, Hibidil, Hibitane

**Chlorpheniramine (51)**
**Chlorphenamine***
Chlor-Tripolon

**Chloroprocaine (14)**
Nesacaine

**Chloroquine (44)**
Aralen

**Chlorpromazine (9, 66)**
Largactil

**Chlorpropamide (27)**
Diabinese

**Chlorthalidone (59)**
Hygroton

**Cholestyramine resin (61)**
Questran

**Ciclopirox (69)**
Loprox

**Cimetidine (63)**
Novo-Cimetine, Nu-Cimet, Peptol, Tagamet

**Ciprofloxacin (39, 68)**
Ciloxin, Cipro

**Cisapride (66)**
Prepulsid

**Cisplatin, *cis*-platinum (67)**
Platinol AQ

**Clarithromycin (38)**
Biaxin

**Clemastine (51)**
Tavist

**Clindamycin (39)**
Dalacin

**Clofibrate (61)**
Atromid-S

**Clomipramine (8)**
Anafranil

**Clonazepam (8)**
Rivotril

**Clonidine (58)**
Catapres, Dixarit

**Clorazepate (8)**
Novo-Clopate, Tranxene

**Clotrimazole (43)**
Canesten, Clotrimaderm, Myclo

**Cloxacillin (34)**
Apo-Cloxi, Novo-Cloxin, Nu-Cloxi, Orbenin, Tegopen

**Clozapine (9)**
Clozaril

**Coal tar (69)**
Balnetar, Estar, Ionil T Plus, Tersa-Tar, Zetar

**Colestipol (61)**
Colestid

**Cortisone (24)**
Cortone

**Cromolyn (50)**
**Sodium cromoglycate***
Intal, Opticrom, Rynacrom

**Crotamiton (44)**
Eurax

**Cyanocobalamin (31)**
Rubion, Rubramin

**Cyclandelate (61)**
Cyclospasmol

**Cyclizine (51)**
Marezine

**Cyclobenzaprine (13)**
Flexeril

**Cyclopentolate (68)**
Cyclogyl, Diopentolate

**Cyclophosphamide (67)**
Cytoxan, Procytox

**Cyclosporine (48)**
Sandimmune

**Cyproheptadine (51)**
Periactin

**Cytarabine, cytosine arabinoside (67)**
Cytosar

**Dacarbazine (67)**
DTIC

**Dactinomycin (Actinomycin D) (67)**
Cosmegen

**Danazol (29)**

**Dantrolene (13)**
Dantrium

**Daunorubicin (daunomycin) (67)**
Cerubidine

**Deferoxamine (32)**
Desferal

**Demeclocycline (37)**
Declomycin

**Desipramine (10)**
Norpramin, Pertofrane

**Desonide (69)**
Tridesilon

**Desoximetasone (69)**
Topicort

**Dexamethasone (24, 68, 69)**
Decadron, Dexasone, Diodex, Hexadrol, Maxidex, Oradexon, Spersadex

**Dexchlorpheniramine (51)**
Polaramine

**Dextroamphetamine (16)**
**Dexamphetamine***
Dexedrine

**Dextromethorphan (52)**
Balminil DM, Benylin DM, Formula 44, Koffex DM, Robidex

**Diazepam (8)**
Diazemuls, Valium, Vivol

**Diazoxide (58)**
Hyperstat, Proglycem

**Dibucaine (14)**
Nupercainal

## Generic/Canadian Trade Names

**Diclofenac (6)**
Apo-Diclo, Novo-Difenac, Nu-Diclo, Voltaren

**Dicyclomine (21)**
Bentylol

**Didanosine (42)**
Videx

**Dienestrol (28)**
**Dienoestrol***
Ortho Dienestrol Creme

**Diethylpropion (30)**
Tenuate

**Diflorasone (69)**
Florone

**Diflunisal (6)**
Dolobid

**Digitoxin (54)**
Digitaline

**Digoxin (54)**
Lanoxin

**Digoxin immune Fab (54)**
**Digoxin-specific antibody fragments***
Digibind

**Dihydrotachysterol (26)**
Hytakerol

**Diltiazem (55, 56, 58)**
Apo-Diltiaz, Cardizem, Novo-Diltazem, Nu-Diltiaz

**Dimenhydrinate (51, 66)**
Gravol, Nauseatol, Travel Aid, Travel-Eze

**Dinoprostone (prostaglandin E$_2$) (70)**
Prepidil, Prostin E$_2$

**Diphenhydramine (12, 51, 66)**
Allerdryl, Benadryl, Nytol, Sleep-Eze

**Diphenoxylate (65)**
Lomotil

**Dipivefrin (68)**
Propine

**Dipyridamole (60)**
Novo-Dipiradol, Persantine

**Disopyramide (55)**
Norpace, Rythmodan

**Dobutamine (18, 57)**
Dobutrex

**Docusate calcium (64)**
Calax, Colax-C, Doxate-C, Surfak

**Docusate sodium (64)**
Colace, Colax-S, Doxate-S, Selax, Silace

**Dopamine (18, 57)**
Intropin, Revimine

**Doxacurium (14)**
Nuromax

**Doxazosin (58)**
Cardura

**Doxepin (9)**
Sinequan, Triadapin

**Doxorubicin (67)**
Adriamycin

**Doxycycline (37)**
Apo-Doxy, Doryx, Doxycin, Novo-Doxylin, Vibramycin, Vibra-Tabs

**Droperidol (14, 66)**
Inapsine

**Echothiophate (68)**
Phospholine

## Generic/Canadian Trade Names

**Econazole (43)**
Ecostatin

**Edrophonium (20)**
Enlon, Tensilon

**Enalapril (58)**
Vasotec

**Enflurane (14)**
Ethrane

**Epinephrine (18, 50, 57)**
Adrenalin, Bronkaid Mistometer, EpiPen, Vaponefrin

**Ergocalciferol (26)**
Calciferol, Drisdol, Ostoforte, Radiostol

**Ergonovine (70)**
**Ergometrine***
Ergotrate

**Ergotamine (6)**
Ergomar, Gynergen

**Ergotamine/caffeine**
Cafergot

**Erythromycin (38, 68)**
Apo-Erythro, Diomycin, EES, E-Mycin, Erybid, Eryc, Eryped, Erythrocin, Erythromid, Ilosone, Ilotycin, Novo-Rythro

**Esmolol (55)**
Brevibloc

**Estradiol (28)**
Delestrogen, Estraderm, Estrase

**Estrogens, conjugated (28)**
Congest, Premarin

**Estrogens, esterified (28)**
Neo-Estrone

**Estrone (28)**
Neo-Estrone, Oestrilin

**Estropipate (28)**
**Piperazine estrone sulfate***
Ogen

**Ethacrynic acid (59)**
Edecrin

**Ethambutol (41)**
Myambutol

**Ethinyl estradiol (28)**
Estinyl

**Ethinyl estradiol/ethynodiol (28)**
Demulen

**Ethinyl estradiol/levonorgestrel (28)**
Min-Ovral, Triphasil, Triquilar

**Ethinyl estradiol/norethindrone (28)**
Brevicon, Loestrin, Minestrin, Norlestrin, Ortho 0.5/35, Ortho 1/35, Ortho 7/7/7, Ortho 10/11, Synphasic

**Ethinyl estradiol/norgestrel (28)**
Ovral

**Ethopropazine (12)**
Parsitan

**Ethosuximide (11)**
Zarontin

**Etidronate (26)**
Didronel

**Etoposide (67)**
VePesid

**Famotidine (63)**
Pepcid

## Generic/Canadian Trade Names

**Felodipine (56)**
Plendil

**Fenfluramine (30)**
Ponderal, Pondimin

**Fenoprofen (6)**
Nalfon

**Fentanyl (5)**
Duragesic, Sublimaze

**Ferrous sulfate (32)**
Fer-In-Sol, Fero-Grad, Slow-Fe

**Fibrinolysin/desoxyribonuclease (69)**
Elase

**Filgrastim (47)**
Neupogen

**Flavoxate (21)**
Urispas

**Flecainide (55)**
Tambocor

**Fluconazole (43)**
Diflucan

**Flucytosine (43)**
Ancotil

**Fludarabine (67)**
Fludara

**Fludrocortisone (24)**
Florinef

**Flumazenil (8)**
Anexate

**Flunisolide (24, 50)**
Bronalide, Rhinalar

**Fluocinolone (69)**
Lidemol, Lidex, Lyderm, Topsyn Gel

**Fluocinolone acetonide (69)**
Dermalar, Fluoderm, Fluonide, Synalar, Synamol

**Fluorometholone (68)**
Flarex

**Fluorouracil, 5-FU (67)**
Adrucil, Efudex, Fluoroplex

**Fluoxetine (10)**
Prozac

**Fluoxymesterone (29)**
Halotestin

**Fluphenazine (9)**
Moditen

**Flurazepam (7)**
Dalmane, Somnol

**Flurbiprofen (6)**
Froben, Ocufen

**Flutamide (67)**
Euflex

**Folic acid (31)**
Folvite

**Fosinopril (58)**
Monopril

**Furosemide (26, 59)**
**Frusemide***
Lasix, Uritol

**Gallamine (14)**
Flaxedil

**Ganciclovir (42)**
Cytovene

**Gemfibrozil (61)**
Lopid

## Generic/Canadian Trade Names

**Gentamicin (36, 68)**
Alcomicin, Cidomycin, Diogent, Garamycin, Gentacidin, R.O.-Gentycin

**Glyburide (27)**
**Glibenclamide***
DiaBeta, Euglucon, Gen-Glybe

**Glycopyrrolate (21)**
**Glycopyrronium***
Robinul

**Goserelin (67)**
Zoladex

**Guaifenesin (52)**
**Glyceryl guaiacolate***
Balminil Expectorant, Benylin-D, Resyl, Robitussin

**Griseofulvin (43)**
Fulvicin, Grisovin

**Haemophilus B conjugate vaccine (46)**
HibTITER, Pedvax HIB

**Halcinonide (69)**
Halog

**Haloperidol (9)**
Haldol

**Halothane (14)**
Fluothane

**Heparin sodium (60)**
Hepalean

**Hepatitis B immune globulin, human (46)**
Hyperhep

**Hepatitis B vaccine, recombinant (46)**
Engerix-B, Recombivax-HB

**Hexachlorophene (69)**
pHisoHex

**Hydralazine (58)**
Apresoline, Novo-Hylazin, Nu-Hydral

**Hydrochlorothiazide (59)**
Apo-Hydro, HydroDiuril

**Hydrocodone (5, 52)**
Hycodan, Robidone

**Hydrocortisone (24, 50, 69)**
A-Hydrocort, Cortacet, Cortate, Cortef, Cortenema, Corticreme, Cortiment, Cortifoam, Cortoderm, Hyderm, Solu-Cortef

**Hydromorphone (5, 52)**
Dilaudid

**Hydroquinone (69)**
Eldopaque, Eldoquin, NeoStrata HQ, Solaquin

**Hydroxychloroquine (44)**
Plaquenil

**Hydroxyurea (67)**
Hydrea

**Hydroxyzine (8, 51, 66)**
Multipax

**Ibuprofen (6)**
Actiprofen, Advil, Medipren, Motrin, Novo-Profen

**Idarubicin (67)**
Idamycin

**Ifosfamide (67)**
Ifex

**Imipramine (10)**
Tofranil

**Imipenem/cilastatin (39)**
Primaxin

**Immune serum globulin (human) (ISG-IM) (46)**
Gammabulin

**Immune serum globulin (IV) (46)**
Gamimune N, Iveegam

**Indapamide (59)**
Lozide

**Indomethacin (6)**
Indocid, Novo-methacin, Nu-Indo

**Influenza vaccines (46)**
Fluviral, Fluzone

**Insulins, animal (27)**
**Regular**
Iletin Regular, Insulin-Toronto, Velosulin
**Isophane (NPH)**
Iletin NPH, Insulatard, NPH Insulin
**Zinc suspension**
Iletin Semilente, Iletin Lente, Iletin Ultralente, Insulin Semilente, Insulin Lente, Insulin Ultralente
**Mixtures**
Mixtard 30/70 (30% regular, 70% isophane), Initard 50/50 (50% regular, 50% isophane)

**Insulins, human (27)**
**Regular**
Humulin-R, Novolin-Toronto, Velosulin Human (Regular)
**Isophane (NPH)**
Humulin-N, Insulatard Human NPH, Novolin-NPH
**Zinc suspension**
Humulin-L, Humulin-U, Novolin-Lente, Novolin-Ultralente
**Mixtures**
Humulin 30/70 (30% regular, 70% isophane), Mixtard 15/85 human, Novolin 30/70

**Interferon alfa-2a (47)**
Roferon A

**Interferon alfa-2b (47)**
Intron A

**Iodochlorhydroxyquin (69)**
**Clioquinol***
Vioform

**Ipratropium (50)**
Atrovent

**Isoflurane (14)**
Forane

**Isoproterenol (18, 50)**
**Isoprenaline***
Isuprel

**Isosorbide dinitrate (56)**
**Sorbide nitrate***
Apo-ISDN, Cedocard-SR, Coradur, Coronex, Isordil

**Isotretinoin (69)**
Accutane, Isotrex

**Ketamine (14)**
Ketalar

**Ketoconazole (43)**
Nizoral

**Ketoprofen (6)**
Apo-Keto, Novo-Keto, Orudis, Oruvail, Rhodis

**Ketorolac (6)**
Acular, Toradol

**Labetalol (58)**
Trandate

**Lactulose (64)**
Cephulac, Chronulac, Comalose-R, Gel-Ose, Lactulax, Rhodialax, Rhodialose

**Leuprolide (67)**
Lupron

**Levobunolol (19, 68)**
Betagan

**Levodopa (12)**
Larodopa

**Levorphanol (5)**
Levo-Dromoran

**Levothyroxine (25)**
Eltroxin, Synthroid

**Lidocaine (14, 55)**
**Lignocaine***
Xylocaine, Xylocard

**Liothyronine (25)**
Cytomel

**Lisinopril (58)**
Prinivil, Zestril

**Lithium (10)**
Carbolith, Duralith, Lithane

**Lomustine (67)**
CCNU, CeeNu

**Loperamide (65)**
Imodium

**Loratadine (51)**
Claritin

**Lorazepam (8)**
Ativan, Novo-Lorazem, Nu-Loraz

**Lovastatin (61)**
Mevacor

**Loxapine (9)**
**Oxilapine***
Loxapac

**Magnesium citrate (64)**
Citro-Mag

**Mannitol (59, 68)**
Osmitrol

**Maprotiline (10)**
Ludiomil

**Mazindol (30)**
Sanorex

**Measles, mumps, and rubella vaccine (46)**
M-M-R II

**Mebendazole (44)**
Vermox

**Meclizine (51, 66)**
**Histamethizine***
Bonamine

**Mechlorethamine (nitrogen mustard), chlormethine (67)**
Mustargen

**Medroxyprogesterone (28)**
Depo-Provera, Provera

**Megestrol (28)**
Megace

**Melphalan (67)**
Alkeran

## Generic/Canadian Trade Names

**Meperidine (5)**
  **Pethidine***
  Demerol
**Mepivacaine (14)**
  Carbocaine, Polocaine
**Mercaptopurine (67)**
  Purinethol
**Mesoridazine (9)**
  Serentil
**Mestranol/norethindrone (28)**
  Norinyl, Ortho 1/50
**Methoxsalen (69)**
  Oxsoralen, UltraMOP
**Metoclopramide (66)**
  Apo-Metoclop, Maxeran, Reglan
**Metolazone (59)**
  Zaroxolyn
**Metaproterenol (18, 50)**
  **Orciprenaline***
  Alupent
**Methazolamide (68)**
  Neptazane
**Methenamine (40)**
  Dehydral, Hip-Rex, Mandelamine
**Methimazole (25)**
  **Thiamazole***
  Tapazole
**Methocarbamol (13)**
  Robaxin
**Methohexital (14)**
  Brietal
**Methotrexate (48)**
  **Amethopterin***
  Rheumatrex
**Methyclothiazide (59)**
  Duretic
**Methylcellulose (64)**
  Citrucel, Murocel
**Methyldopa (58)**
  Aldomet, Novo-Medopa, Nu-Medopa
**Methylphenidate (16)**
  Ritalin
**Methylprednisolone (24, 50, 69)**
  Depo-Medrol, Medrol, Solu-Medrol
**Methyltestosterone (29)**
  Metandren
**Methysergide (6)**
  Sansert
**Metocurine (14)**
  Metubine
**Metoprolol (19, 58)**
  Betaloc, Lopressor, Novo-Metoprol,
  Nu-Metop
**Metronidazole (39, 44)**
  Flagyl, Metrogel, Novo-Nidazol, Trikacide
**Mexiletine (55)**
  Mexitil
**Miconazole (43, 69)**
  Micatin, Monistat
**Midazolam (8)**
  Versed
**Minocycline (37)**
  Minocin
**Minoxidil (58)**
  Apo-gain, Loniten, Rogaine

## Generic/Canadian Trade Names

**Misoprostol (6, 61)**
  Cytotec
**Mitomycin (67)**
  Mutamycin
**Mitotane (67)**
  Lysodren
**Mitoxantrone (67)**
  Novantrone
**Morphine (5, 52)**
  MOS, MS Contin, MSIR, Oramorph,
  Statex
**Mumps vaccine (46)**
  Mumpsvax
**Muromonab-CD3 (48)**
  Orthoclone OKT 3
**Nadolol (19, 56, 58)**
  Apo-Nadol, Corgard
**Nafcillin (34)**
  Unipen
**Nalbuphine (5)**
  Nubain
**Nalidixic acid (40)**
  NegGram
**Naloxone (5)**
  Narcan
**Nandrolone (29)**
  Deca-Durabolin, Durabolin
**Naphazoline (18, 52)**
  Diopticon, Privine, Naphcon, R.O.-Naphz,
  Vasocon
**Naproxen (6)**
  Anaprox, Naprosyn, Naxen, Novo-Naprox,
  Nu-Naprox, Synflex
**Nedocromil (50)**
  Tilade
**Neomycin (36)**
  Mycifradin, Myciguent
**Neostigmine (20)**
  Prostigmin
**Netilmicin (36)**
  Netromycin
**Nicardipine (56)**
  Cardene
**Nifedipine (56)**
  Adalat, Apo-Nifed, Novo-Nifedin, Nu-Nifed
**Nimodipine (56)**
  Nimotop
**Nitrofurantoin (40)**
  Macrodantin
**Nitroprusside (58)**
  Nipride
**Nitroglycerin (56)**
  **Glyceryl trinitrate***
  Nitro-Bid, Nitro-Dur, Nitrogard-SR, Nitrol,
  Nitrolingual, Nitrong, Nitrostat, Trans-
  derm-Nitro, Tridil
**Nizatidine (63)**
  Axid
**Norepinephrine (18, 57)**
  **Levarterenol**
  **Noradrenaline***
  Levophed
**Norethindrone (28)**
  Norlutate

## Generic/Canadian Trade Names

**Norfloxacin (39, 68)**
  Noroxin
**Nortriptyline (10)**
  Aventyl
**Nystatin (43, 69)**
  Mycostatin, Nadostine, Nilstat, Nyaderm
**Ofloxacin (39)**
  Floxin
**Omeprazole (63)**
  Prilosec
**Ondansetron (66)**
  Zofran
**Orphenadrine (12, 13)**
  Disipal, Norflex
**Oxazepam (8)**
  Serax
**Oxycodone (5)**
  Supeudol
**Oxymetazoline (18, 52)**
  Ocuclear
**Oxymetholone (29)**
  Anapolon
**Oxymorphone (5)**
  Numorphan
**Oxytocin (23, 70)**
  Syntocinon, Toesen
**Pamidronate (26)**
  Aredia
**Pancreatin (30)**
  Entozyme
**Pancrelipase (30)**
  Cotazym, Creon, Pancrease, Viokase
**Pancuronium (14)**
  Pavulon
**Penicillamine (32)**
  Cuprimine, Depen
**Penicillin G benzathine (34)**
  Bicillin, Megacillin
**Penicillin G potassium (34)**
  **Benzylpenicillin potassium***
  Megacillin
**Penicillin G procaine (34)**
  Ayercillin, Wycillin
**Penicillin V (34)**
  **Phenoxymethyl penicillin***
  Apo-Pen VK, Ledercillin VK, Nadopen-V,
  Novo-Pen-VK, Nu-Pen-VK, Pen-Vee, V-Cil-
  lin K
**Pentaerythritol (56)**
  Peritrate
**Pentamidine (44)**
  Pentacarinat, Pneumopent
**Pentazocine (5)**
  Talwin
**Pentobarbital (7)**
  Nembutal
**Pentoxifylline (61)**
  Trental
**Pergolide (12)**
  Permax
**Perphenazine (9)**
  Trilafon
**Phenazopyridine (40)**
  Pyridium

## Generic/Canadian Trade Names

**Phenelzine (10)**
Nardil

**Phenobarbital (7, 11)**
**Phenobarbitone***
Fastin, Ionamin

**Phentermine (30)**
Fastin, Ionamin

**Phenylephrine (18, 52)**
Dionephrine, Mydfrin, Neo-Synephrine, Novahistine decongestant

**Phenytoin (11)**
Dilantin

**Phytonadione (vitamin K) (60)**
**Phytomenadione***
Konakion

**Pilocarpine (68)**
Diocarpine, Isopto Carpine, Miocarpine, Pilopine, R.O.-Carpine, Spersacarpine

**Pindolol (19, 58)**
Apo-Pindol, Novo-Pindol, Nu-Pindol, Visken

**Piperacillin (34)**
Pipracil

**Piperazine (44)**
Entacyl

**Piroxicam (6)**
Feldene, Novo-Pirocam, Nu-Pirox

**Pneumococcal vaccine (46)**
Pneumovax 23

**Polycarbophil (64)**
Mitrolan

**Polymyxin B (39, 68)**
Aerosporin

**Polyvinyl alcohol (68)**
Hypotears, PMS-Artificial Tears, R.O.-Dry Eyes

**Potassium chloride (32)**
Apo-K, Kalium, Kaochlor, D-Dur, K-Long, K-Lor, K-Med, K-10, Micro-K, Roychlor, Slow-K

**Povidone-iodine (44, 69)**
Betadine, Proviodine

**Pramoxine (14)**
**Pramocaine***
Tronothane

**Pravastatin (61)**
Pravachol

**Prazosin (58)**
Apo-Prazo, Minipress, Novo-Prazin, Nu-Prazo

**Prednisolone (24)**
**Delta hydrocortisone***
**Metacortandrolone***
Diopred, Inflamase, Ophtho-Tate, R.O. Predphate

**Prednisone (24)**
**Delta cortisone***
**Metacortandracin***
Deltasone, Winpred

**Prilocaine (14)**
Citanest

**Primidone (11)**
Mysoline

**Probenecid (6)**
Benemid

**Probucol (61)**
Lorelco

## Generic/Canadian Trade Names

**Procainamide (55)**
Procan-SR, Pronestyl

**Procaine (14)**
Novocain

**Procarbazine (67)**
Natulan

**Prochlorperazine (9)**
Stemetil

**Procyclidine (12)**
Kemadrin, Procyclid

**Promethazine (9, 51, 66)**
Histanil, Phenergan

**Propafenone (55)**
Rythmol

**Propantheline (21)**
Banlin, Pro-Banthine

**Proparacaine (14)**
**Proxymetacaine***
Alcaine, Diocaine

**Propofol (14)**
Diprivan

**Propranolol (19, 55, 56)**
Inderal

**Propylthiouracil (25)**
Propyl-Thyracil

**Protriptyline (10)**
Triptil

**Pseudoephedrine (52)**
Eltor, Maxenal, Pseudofrin, Robidrine, Sudafed

**Psyllium hydrophilic muciloid (64)**
Fibrepur, Metamucil, Novo-Mucilax, Prodiem Plain

**Pyrantel pamoate (44)**
Combantrin

**Pyrazinamide (41)**
Tebrazid

**Pyridostigmine (20)**
Mestinon, Regonol

**Pyridoxine (31)**
Hexa-Betalin

**Pyrimethamine (44)**
Daraprim

**Quinapril (58)**
Accupril

**Quinidine (55)**
Biquin, Cardioquin, Quinidex, Quinaglute

**Rabies immune globulin (human) (46)**
Hyperab, Imogam Rabies

**Ranitidine (63)**
Novo-Ranidine, Nu-Ranit, Zantac

**Rho (D) immune globulin (human) (46)**
HypRho-D, Win Rho

**Ribavirin (42)**
Virazole

**Rifampin (41)**
Rifadin, Rimactane, Rofact

**Ritodrine (70)**
Yutopar

**Scopolamine (21, 66)**
Transderm-V

**Secobarbital (7)**
Novo-Secobarb, Seconal

**Selegiline (12)**
Eldepryl

## Generic/Canadian Trade Names

**Selenium sulfide (69)**
Selsun, Versel

**Sertraline (10)**
Zoloft

**Silver sulfadiazine (40)**
Flamazine

**Simvastatin (61)**
Zocor

**Sodium hypochlorite (69)**
Hygeol Solution

**Sodium polystyrene sulfonate (32)**
Kayexelate

**Sotalol (19, 55)**
Sotacor

**Spectinomycin (39)**
Trobicin

**Spironolactone (59)**
Aldactone, Novo-Spiroton

**Streptokinase (60)**
Streptase

**Streptozocin (67)**
Zanosar

**Succinylcholine (14)**
**Suxamethonium***
Anectine, Quelicin

**Sucralfate (63)**
Sulcrate

**Sufentanil (5)**
Sufenta

**Sulfacetamide (68)**
Cetamide, Diosulf, Ophtho-Sulf, Sodium Sulamyd, Sulfex

**Sulfamethoxazole/trimethoprim (40)**
**Co-trimoxazole***
Apo-Sulfatrim, Bactrim, Novo-Trimel, Nu-Cotrimix, Roubac, Septra

**Sulfasalazine (40)**
Salazopyrin

**Sulfinpyrazone (5)**
Anturane, Novo-Pyrazone

**Sulfisoxazole/phenazopyridine (40)**
Azo Gantrisin

**Sulindac (6)**
Apo-Sulin, Clinoril, Novo-Sudac

**Sumatriptan (6)**
Imitrex

**Sutilains (69)**
Travase

**Tamoxifen (67)**
Apo-Tamox, Nolvadex, Tamofen, Tamone, Tamoplex

**Temazepam (7)**
Restoril

**Teniposide (67)**
Vumon

**Terazosin (58)**
Hytrin

**Terbutaline (18, 50)**
Bricanyl

**Terconazole (43)**
Terazol

**Terfenadine (51)**
Seldane

**Testosterone (29)**
Andriol, Delatestryl

| Generic/Canadian Trade Names | Generic/Canadian Trade Names | Generic/Canadian Trade Names |
|---|---|---|
| **Tetracaine (14)**<br>Pontocaine, Supracaine | **Tranexamic acid (60)**<br>Cyklokapron | **Vecuronium (14)**<br>Norcuron |
| **Tetracycline (37, 68)**<br>Achromycin, Apo-Tetra, Novo-Tetra, Nu-Tetra, Tetracyn | **Tranylcypromine (10)**<br>Parnate | **Verapamil (55, 56, 58)**<br>Apo-Verap, Isoptin, Novo-Veramil, Nu-Verap |
| **Tetrahydrozoline (18)**<br>R.O.-Eye Drops | **Trazodone (10)**<br>Desyrel | **Vidarabine (42, 68)**<br>Vira-A |
| **Theophylline (16, 50)**<br>Pulmophylline, Slo-Bid, Somophyllinn, Theochron, Theo-Dur, Theolair, Theo-SR, Uniphyl | **Tretinoin (retinoic acid) (69)**<br>Retin-A, StieVAA, Vitamin A Acid | **Vinblastine (67)**<br>Velbe |
| **Thiamine (31)**<br>Betaxin, Bewon | **Triamterene (59)**<br>Dyrenium | **Vincristine (67)**<br>Oncovin |
| **Thiabendazole (44)**<br>Mintezol | **Triazolam (7)**<br>Apo-Triazo, Halcion, Novo-Triolam, Nu-Triazo | **Vitamin A (31)**<br>**Retinol***<br>Aquasol A |
| **Thiethylperazine (66)**<br>Torecan | **Triamcinolone (24, 50, 69)**<br>Aristocort, Aristospan, Azmacort, Kenalog, Nasacort, Oracort, Triaderm, Trimacort | **Vitamin B$_1$ (31)**<br>Betaxin, Bewon |
| **Thioguanine (67)**<br>Lanvis | **Trifluoperazine (9)**<br>Stelazine | **Vitamin B$_6$ (31)**<br>Hexa-Betalin |
| **Thiopental (14)**<br>Pentothal | **Trifluridine (42, 68)**<br>Viroptic | **Vitamin B$_{12}$ (31)**<br>Rubion, Rubramin |
| **Thioridazine (9)**<br>Mellaril | **Trihexyphenidyl (12)**<br>**Benzhexol***<br>Apo-Trihex, Artane | **Vitamin C (31)**<br>Apo-C, Ce-Vi-Sol |
| **Thiothixene (9)**<br>Navane | **Trimeprazine (51)**<br>**Alimemazine***<br>Panectyl | **Vitamin D (26)**<br>Calcijex, Rocaltrol |
| **Ticarcillin (34)**<br>Ticar | **Trimethoprim (40)**<br>Proloprim | **Vitamin E (31)**<br>**Tocofersolan, alpha-tocopheryl***<br>Aquasol E |
| **Ticarcillin/potassium clavulanate (34)**<br>Timentin | **Trimipramine (10)**<br>Apo-Trimip, Novo-Tripramine, Rhotrimine, Surmontil | **Vitamin K (31, 60)**<br>**Phytomenadione***<br>Konakion |
| **Ticlopidine (60)**<br>Ticlid | **Trioxsalen (69)**<br>Trisoralen | **Warfarin (60)**<br>Coumadin, Warfilone |
| **Timolol (19, 58, 68)**<br>Apo-Timol, Apo-Timop, Blocadren, Novo-Timol, Timoptic | **Tripelennamine (51)**<br>Pyribenzamine | **Xylometazoline (18, 52)**<br>Otrivin |
| **Tioconazole (43)**<br>Gyno-Trosyd, Trosyd | **Tropicamide (68)**<br>Diotrope, Mydriacyl, R.O.-Tropamide | **Zalcitabine (42)**<br>Hivid |
| **Tobramycin (36, 68)**<br>Nebcin, Tobrex | **Tubocurarine (14)**<br>Tubarine | **Zidovudine (42)**<br>**Azidothymidine, AZT**<br>Novo-AZT, Retrovir |
| **Tocainide (55)**<br>Tonocard | **Urokinase (60)**<br>Abbokinase | **Zinc oxide (69)**<br>Prevex, Zincofax |
| **Tolbutamide (27)**<br>Orinase | **Valproic acid (11)**<br>Depakene | **Zinc sulfate (69)**<br>Anusol, PMS-Egozinc |
| **Tolmetin (6)**<br>Tolectin | **Vancomycin (39)**<br>Vancocin | |
| **Tolnaftate (43, 69)**<br>Pitrex, Tinactin | | |

## Reference

(1993). *Compendium of pharmaceuticals and specialties* (28th ed.)
Ottawa, Ontario, Canada: Canadian Pharmaceutical Association.

# INDEX

Page numbers followed by *t* indicate tabular material.
Drug names beginning with a lower case letter indicate generic drugs, and those with a capital indicate trade names.

## A

Abbokinase (urokinase), 615, 617–618
    as Canadian trade name, 754
Abenol (acetaminophen), as Canadian
        trade name, 748
abortifacients
    nursing actions for, 739–741
    pregnancy and, 734, 735t
abortion, abortifacients for, 734, 735t
absorption
    defined, 10
    geriatric patient and, 15, 40t
    intramuscular drug administration and,
        25
    in pediatric patient, 38t
    subcutaneous drug administration and, 24
abuse. *See* drug abuse
Accupril (quinapril), 591t
    as Canadian trade name, 753
Accutane (isotretinoin), 720t
    as Canadian trade name, 751
acebutolol (Sectral), 198, 199t, 200, 565,
        591t
    Canadian trade name for, 748
    lactation and, 738t
Acel-Imune (DTaP) (diphtheria and tetanus
        toxoids and acellular pertussis
        vaccine), 477t
acellular pertussis vaccine and diphtheria
        and tetanus toxoids (DTaP) (Acel-
        Imune, Tripedia), 477t
acetaminophen (Tylenol), 66, 68
    Canadian trade name for, 748
    in geriatrics, 76
    indications for, 68, 68t
    lactation and, 737t
    in pediatrics, 76
    pregnancy and, 731t
    therapeutic serum drug concentrations
        for, 746
    therapy guidelines for, 74–75
    toxic concentrations of, 746
acetazolamide (Diamox)
    Canadian trade name for, 748
    in glaucoma, 218
    in ocular disorders, 703t
acetic acid, 717t
acetohexamide (Dymelor), 284t, 284–285
    Canadian trade name for, 748
acetophenazine (Tindal), 101t
Acetoxyl (benzoyl peroxide), as Canadian
        trade name, 748
acetylcholine, 49
    cholinergic drugs and, 207
acetylcysteine (Mucomyst), 535t
    Canadian trade name for, 748
acetylsalicylic acid (aspirin), 68–69, 615
    adverse effects of, 67–68
    Canadian trade name for, 748
    in geriatrics, 76
    indications for, 68, 68t
    mechanism of action in, 67
    in pediatrics, 76
    perioperative use of, 75–76
    pregnancy and, 731t

rheumatoid arthritis and, 75
    routes and dosage ranges for, 69
    therapy guidelines for, 74
Achromycin (tetracycline), 403t, 451
    as Canadian trade name, 754
    in ocular disorders, 705t
acid-base disorders. *See also* acidosis; alkalosis
    agents used in, 348–350
    neurotransmission and, 48
    nursing process for, 356–357
    principles of therapy for, 360
acidifying agent, 348
acidosis, metabolic, 349–350, 360. *See also*
        acid-base disorders
Aclovate (alclometasone), 719t
acne
    dermatologic drugs for, 722
    description of, 714
Acnomel (benzoyl peroxide), as Canadian
        trade name, 748
acrisorcin (Akrinol), 719t
Acthar (corticotropin), 230
ACTH (corticotropin), 230
Actidil (triprolidine hydrochloride), 527t
Actifed, 536t
Actigall (ursodiol), 744t
Actimmune (interferon-gamma-1b), 489t
Actinex (masoprocol), 743t–744t
actinomycin D (dactinomycin) (Cos-
        megen), 687
Actiprofen (ibuprofen), as Canadian trade
        name, 751
Activase (alteplase), 615, 617
Activase rt-PA (alteplase), as Canadian
        trade name, 748
Actrapid (insulin injection), 283t
Acular (ketorolac), as Canadian trade
        name, 751
Acutrim (phenylpropanolamine), 322
acyclovir (Zovirax), 435, 436t, 719t
    Canadian trade name for, 748
    pregnancy and, 730t
Adalat (nifedipine), 574t, 592t
    as Canadian trade name, 752
Adapin (doxepin), 117t
Addison's disease, 238
additive effects, pharmacologic, 14
Adenocard (adenosine), 566
adenosine (Adenocard), 566
adrenal cortex
    disorders of, 238–239
    hormones produced by, 228–229. *See also*
        *specific hormones*; cortisone
adrenal hyperplasia, 239
Adrenalin (epinephrine), 187t, 187–188,
        515–516
    as Canadian trade name, 750
    in hypotension and shock, 582
    lactation and, 737t
adrenal insufficiency, thyroid drugs and,
        259–260
adrenergic drugs, 186–194, 187t
    administration of, 190, 191–192
    adverse effects of, 193
    in anaphylaxis, 190

in bronchoconstrictive disorders,
        515–517
    in cardiopulmonary resuscitation, 190
    client teaching with, 189–190, 194
    contraindications to, 186
    description of, 186
    drug interactions with, 193–194
    in geriatrics, 191
    in hypotension, 190
    indications for, 186, 187t
    individual, 187t, 187–189
    lactation and, 737t
    mechanism of action with, 186
    nursing actions for, 191–194
    nursing process for, 189–190
    in ocular disorders, 702t
    in pediatrics, 190–191
    in pregnancy, 733–734
    pregnancy and, 729t
    principles of therapy with, 190
    selection of, 190
    in shock, 190
    therapeutic effects of, 192
adrenergic receptors, 184, 184t
    mechanisms of action in, 184
adrenocortical insufficiency, 238–239
adrenocorticotropic hormone (ACTH), 229
adrenogenital syndromes, 239
Adriamycin (doxorubicin), 687t
    as Canadian trade name, 750
Adrucil (fluorouracil), 686t–687t
    as Canadian trade name, 750
adult development, testosterone in, 310
adverse effects of drugs, 17–18
    nursing process and, 43
Advil (ibuprofen)
    as Canadian trade name, 751
    in pregnancy, 732t
    lactation and, 738t
Aerobid (flunisolide), 241t, 517–518
Aerosporin (polymyxin B), 412–413
    as Canadian trade name, 753
aflatoxins, 681t
African-Americans, beta-adrenergic drugs
        in, 202
Afrin (oxymetazoline hydrochloride), 187t,
        535t
age
    cancer and, 680
    drug action and, 15–16
agonists, defined, 13
Agoral Plain (mineral oil), 653t
A-Hydrocort (hydrocortisone), as Canadian
        trade name, 751
Akineton (biperiden), 137t, 216
    as Canadian trade name, 748
Akrinol (acrisorcin), 719t
albuterol (Proventil, Ventolin), 187t, 516
    Canadian trade name for, 748
    lactation and, 737t
    in pediatrics, 191
    pregnancy and, 729t
Alcaine (proparacaine), 156t
    as Canadian trade name, 753
    in ocular disorders, 703t–704t

alclometasone (Aclovate), 719t
alcohol
 absorption of, 166
 abuse of, 163–164, 166–169. *See also* drug
   abuse
   acute, 173
   cardiovascular effects of, 167
   central and peripheral nervous system
     effects of, 166–167
   chronic, 172–173
   description of, 164
   drug interactions with, 168–169
   endocrinologic effects of, 168
   gastrointestinal effects of, 167
   hematologic effects of, 167–168
   hepatic effects of, 167
   muscular effects of, 168
   nursing process for, 170–171
   prevention of, 171–172
   skeletal effects of, 168
   treatment of, 172–173
   withdrawal from, 173
 as carcinogen, 681t
 metabolism of, 166
 pregnancy and, 172, 727
alcohol, hyoscine hydrobromide, hyoscyamine sulfate, atropine sulfate,
   pectin, kaolin (Donnagel), 663t
alcohols, dermatologic, 716t
Alcomicin (gentamicin), as Canadian trade
   name, 751
Aldactazide (hydrochlorothiazide and
   spironolactone), 603t
Aldactone (spironolactone), 602t
 as Canadian trade name, 753
aldesleukin (Proleukin), 487, 489t
Aldomet (methyldopa), 591t
 as Canadian trade name, 752
 lactation and, 738t
 pregnancy and, 730t
Aldoril (methyldopa and hydrochlorothiazide), 593t
Alfenta (alfentanil), 55, 153t
 as Canadian trade name, 748
 pregnancy and, 729t
alfentanil (Alfenta), 55, 153t
 Canadian trade name for, 748
 pregnancy and, 729t
Alferon N (interferon-alfa-n3), 489t
alkalinizing agents, 349–350
alkaloids. *See also* antineoplastic drugs
 belladonna, 215–216
 plant, 684, 687t
alkalosis, metabolic, 360. *See also* acid-base
   disorders
 hyperchloremic, 350t
Alka-Seltzer, 643t
Alkeran (melphalan), 686t
 as Canadian trade name, 751
alkylamines, 525, 527t. *See also* antihistamines
alkylating agents, 683–684, 686t. *See also*
   antineoplastic drugs
Allerdryl (diphenhydramine), as Canadian
   trade name, 750
Allerest, 536t
allergic reactions. *See* hypersensitivity
   reactions
allergic rhinitis, antihistamines for, 526
allopurinol (Zyloprim), 71
 Canadian trade name for, 748
 in hyperuricemia, 76
Almocarpine (pilocarpine), in ocular
   disorders, 702t
alopecia, antineoplastic drugs and, 690
Alophen (phenolphthalein), 652t
alpha-adrenergic blocking drugs, 197, 198, 201
 administration of, 203
 adverse effects of, 203–204
 client teaching with, 201, 205

contraindications to, 197–198
 description of, 196
 drug interactions with, 204
 indications for, 197
 individual, 198
 mechanism of action with, 196
 nursing actions for, 203–205
 principles of therapy with, 201
 therapeutic effects of, 203
Alphamul (castor oil), 653t
alpha-tocopheryl, (vitamin E)
 Canadian trade name for, 754
alprazolam (Xanax), 91t
 Canadian trade name for, 748
Altace (ramipril), 591t
alteplase (Activase), 615, 617
 Canadian trade name for, 748
altretamine (Hexalen), 688t
Aludrox, 643t
aluminum acetate solution (Burow's solution), 720t
aluminum hydroxide, Canadian trade name
   for, 748
aluminum hydroxide gel and magnesium
   hydroxide, Canadian trade name for,
   748
Alupent (metaproterenol), 187t, 516–517
 as Canadian trade name, 752
 in pediatrics, 191
Alurate (aprobarbital), 82t, 83
amantadine (Symmetrel), 435, 436t
 Canadian trade name for, 748
 pregnancy and, 730t
ambenonium (Mytelase), 208
Ambien (zolpidem), 82t, 83
amcinonide (Cyclocort), Canadian trade
   name for, 748
amebiasis, 448
 nursing process for, 455
amebicides, 450–451. *See also* antiparasitics
Americaine (benzocaine), 156t
*American Hospital Formulary Service*, 4
amethopterin. *See* methotrexate (MTX)
Amicar (aminocaproic acid), 618
 as Canadian trade name, 748
Amidate (etomidate), 153t
amikacin (Amikin), 397
 Canadian trade name for, 748
 therapeutic serum drug concentrations
   for, 746
Amikin (amikacin), 397
 as Canadian trade name, 748
amiloride and hydrochlorothiazide (Moduretic), 603t
amiloride (Midamor), 602t
 Canadian trade name for, 748
 lactation and, 738t
Amin-Aid, 324
aminocaproic acid (Amicar), 618
 Canadian trade name for, 748
aminoglutethimide (Cytadren), 688t
 Canadian trade name for, 748
aminoglycosides, 396–401
 administration of, 400
 adverse effects of, 400
 client teaching with, 401
 contraindications to, 397
 dosage of, 399
 drug interactions with, 400–401
 in geriatrics, 399
 indications for, 396–397
   limitations on, 399
 individual, 397–398
 mechanism of action with, 396
 nursing actions for, 400–401
 nursing process for, 398
 in pediatrics, 399
 penicillins with, 384
 pharmacokinetics of, 396

pregnancy and, 729t
 in renal impairment, 399
 selection of, 399
 therapeutic effects of, 400
 toxicity and, 399
 in urinary tract infections, 399
aminophylline, Canadian trade name for,
   748
Aminophylline (theophylline), 518t
 pregnancy and, 731t
Aminosyn (crystalline amino acid solutions), 324
amiodarone (Cordarone), 565, 568
 Canadian trade name for, 748
amitriptyline (Elavil, Endep), 117t
 Canadian trade name for, 748
 lactation and, 737t
 pregnancy and, 730t
 therapeutic serum drug concentrations
   for, 746
amlodipine (Norvasc), 574t, 592t
 Canadian trade name for, 748
ammonium chloride (NH4Cl), 348
amobarbital, Canadian trade name for, 748
amobarbital sodium (Amytal), 82t, 83
amoxapine (Asendin), 117t
 Canadian trade name for, 748
amoxicillin (Amoxil, Larotid), 381, 382t
 Canadian trade name for, 748
amoxicillin and potassium clavulanate
   (Augmentin), 383t
 Canadian trade name for, 748
Amoxil (amoxicillin), 382t
 as Canadian trade name, 748
amphetamines. *See also* central nervous system stimulants
 abuse of, 164
   treatment of, 174
 description of, 176
 individual, 177
Amphojel (aluminum hydroxide), 643t
 as Canadian trade name, 748
amphotericin, Canadian trade name for,
   748
amphotericin B (Fungizone), 444t, 719t
 in geriatrics, 445
 in pediatrics, 445
ampicillin and sulbactam (Unasyn), 383t
ampicillin (Omnipen, Penbriten), 381, 382t,
   662t
 Canadian trade name for, 748
ampicillins, 381, 382t
Ampicin (ampicillin), as Canadian trade
   name, 748
ampules, 24
amrinone (Inocor), 551
 administration of, 556
 adverse effects of, 557–558
 Canadian trade name for, 748
amyl nitrite (Vaporole), 575
amylobarbitone, Canadian trade name for,
   748
Amytal (amobarbital), 82t, 83
 as Canadian trade name, 748
anabolic steroids, 309, 310–315. *See also*
   testosterone
 abuse of, 310
 administration of, 314
 adverse effects of, 310, 314–315
 in breast cancer, 311, 312t, 314
 characteristics of, 311
 client teaching with, 315
 contraindications to, 311
 description of, 309
 drug interactions with, 315
 in geriatrics, 314
 indications for, 311
 individual, 312t
 mechanism of action with, 311

nursing actions for, 314–315
nursing process for, 311, 313
in pediatrics, 313–314
preparations of, 312t
principles of therapy with, 313–314
therapeutic effects of, 314
Anadrol-50 (oxymetholone), 312t
Anafranil (clomipramine), 90, 92
as Canadian trade name, 749
analeptics. *See also* central nervous system
stimulants
description of, 176
individual, 177
analgesic-antipyretic-anti-inflammatory
drugs, 66–79
adverse effects of, 77–78
in ankylosing spondylitis, 68t
client teaching with, 79
contraindications to, 68
description of, 66
drug interactions with, 78–79
in fever, 67
in geriatrics, 76
in gout and hyperuricemia, 71–72
indications for, 68, 68t
individual, 68–73
in inflammation, 67
mechanism of action with, 67–68
in migraine, 72–73
nursing actions for, 76–79
nursing process for, 73–74
in osteoarthritis, 68t
in pain, 67, 68t
in pediatrics, 76
perioperative use of, 75–76
principles of therapy for, 74–76
in rheumatoid arthritis, 68t, 75
in tendinitis, 68t
analgesics
in cold, cough, and allergy remedies,
536t–537t
lactation and, 737t
narcotic. *see* narcotic analgesics
pregnancy and, 735
urinary tract, 422
anaphylactic shock, 581, 584
adrenergic drugs for, 190
from penicillins, 384, 385
Anapolon (oxymetholone), as Canadian
trade name, 752
Anaprox (naproxen), 68, 69
as Canadian trade name, 752
Anaspaz (hyoscyamine), 215–216
Ancef (cefazolin), 390, 391t, 393
as Canadian trade name, 749
Ancobon (flucytosine), 444t
Ancotil (flucytosine), as Canadian trade
name, 750
Andriol (testosterone), as Canadian trade
name, 753
androgens. *See also* testosterone
abuse of, 310
administration of, 314
adverse effects of, 310
adverse reactions to, 314–315
characteristics of, 311
client teaching with
contraindications to, 311
description of, 309
drug interactions with, 315
endogenous, 309
in geriatrics, 314
indications for, 311
mechanism of action with, 311
as antineoplastic drugs, 684
nursing actions for, 314–315
nursing process for, 311, 313
in pediatrics, 313
preparations of, 312t

principles of therapy with, 313–314
therapeutic effects of, 314
tumor production of, 239
Android-T (testosterone), 312t
Anectine (succinylcholine), 155t
as Canadian trade name, 753
chlolinergic drugs and, 208
anemia
iron-deficiency, treatment of, 359–360
pregnancy and, 728, 732
anesthesia. *See also* anesthetics
defined, 150
anesthetics, 150–162
adjuncts to
antianxiety agents and sedative-
hypnotics, 151
anticholinergics, 152
narcotic analgesics, 152
neuromuscular blocking agents, 152,
155t
administration of, 157–158
adverse effects of, 159
client teaching with, 161–162
in delivery, 735
drug interactions with, 160–161
general, 150, 152t–154t
individual, 153t–154t, 156t
during labor and delivery, 735
local, 156t
administration of, 157
client teaching with, 162
nursing process for, 152, 153–155
ophthalmic, 703t–704t
principles of therapy for, 155–157
regional, 150–151
therapeutic effects of, 158–159
topical, 151
Anexate (flumazenil), as Canadian trade
name, 750
angina pectoris
antianginal drugs for, 572–580. *See also*
antianginal drugs
description of, 572
nonpharmacologic treatment of, 572
angiotensin-converting enzyme (ACE) inhibitors
in congestive heart failure, 549
hypertension and, 589–590, 591t, 595
lactation and, 737t
pregnancy and, 729t
anisotropine methylbromide (Valpin), 214t
anistreplase (Eminase), 615, 617
ankylosing spondylitis, drugs used in, 68t
anorectal disorders, 714
dermatologic drugs for, 722, 723
anorexiants, 319, 322, 323t
administration of, 330
adverse effects of, 331
client teaching with, 326, 331
drug interactions with, 331
nursing actions for, 330–331
in obesity, 328
principles of therapy with, 328
therapeutic effects of, 330
Ansaid (flurbiprofen), 68, 69
indications for, 68, 68t
Anspor (cephradine), 390t, 391t
antacids
administration of, 647
adverse effects of, 648
client teaching for, 649
description of, 639–640
drug interactions with, 645–646, 648
effect on nutrients, 646
in geriatrics, 646
guidelines for therapy with, 644–645
mechanism of action with, 13
nursing actions for, 647–649
in pediatrics, 646

pregnancy and, 732
representative products, 643t
therapeutic effects of, 647
antagonism, pharmacologic, 13
Antepar (piperazine citrate), 454
anthelmintics, 453–455. *See also* antiparasitics
antiadrenergic drugs, 196–205
administration of, 203
adverse effects of, 203–204
alpha-adrenergic blocking drugs as, 197,
198, 201
beta-adrenergic blocking drugs as, 197,
198, 199t, 201–202
client teaching with, 201, 205
contraindications to, 197–198
description of, 196
drug interactions with, 204–205
genetic or ethnic considerations with,
202
in geriatrics, 202–203
hypertension and, 590, 591t, 595
indications for, 197
individual, 198, 199t, 200
mechanism of action with, 196–197
nursing actions for, 203–205
nursing process for, 200–201
in ocular disorders, 702t
in pediatrics, 202
principles of therapy with, 201–202
therapeutic effects of, 203
antianginal drugs, 571–580
administration of, 578
adverse effects of, 579
beta-adrenergic blocking agents as, 573,
575
calcium channel-blocking agents as, 573,
574t
client teaching with, 579–580
drug interactions with, 579
in geriatrics, 577
individual, 574–575
lactation and, 737t
nursing actions for, 578–580
nursing process for, 575–577
organic nitrates as, 572–573, 574–575
in pediatrics, 577
pregnancy and, 729t
principles of therapy with, 577
selection of, 577
therapeutic effects of, 578
titration of, 577
antianxiety drugs, 89–98
administration of, 95–96
adverse effects of, 97
anesthesia and, 151
anxiety and, 89
benzodiazepines as, 89–90, 91t
client teaching with, 98
contraindications to, 90
dosage of, 94
drug interactions with, 97–98
in geriatrics, 95
in hypoalbuminemia, 95
indications for, 90
individual, 90–92
lactation and, 737t
in liver disease, 95
mechanism of action with, 90
with narcotic analgesics, 94
nonbenzodiazepine, 90, 92
nursing actions for, 95–98
nursing process for, 92–93
in pediatrics, 95
pregnancy and, 729t
principles of therapy for, 93–95
rational use of, guidelines for, 93–94
scheduling of, 94
therapeutic effects of, 96–97

antiarrhythmic drugs, 560–570
  administration of, 569–569
  adverse effects of, 569–570
  classification of, 562–566
  client teaching for, 570
  drug interactions with, 570
  in geriatrics, 568
  indications for, 562
  individual, 562–566
  lactation and, 737t
  mechanisms of action with, 562
  nursing actions for, 568–570
  nursing process for, 566–567
  in pediatrics, 568
  pregnancy and, 729t
  principles of therapy with, 567–568
  selection of, 567–568
  therapeutic effects of, 569
  unclassified, 566–567
antiasthmatic drugs, 515–523.
        *See also* bronchodilating drugs
  administration of, 522
  adverse effects of, 522–523
  client teaching with, 523
  contraindications to, 515
  dosage factors with, 521
  drug interactions with, 523
  in geriatrics, 521
  indications for, 515
  individual, 515–519, 518t
  mechanism of action in, 515
  nursing actions for, 522–523
  nursing process for, 519–520
  in pediatrics, 521
  principles of therapy with, 520–521
  selection of, 520
  therapeutic effects of, 522
antibacterial drugs. *See also* anti-infective
        drugs
  as antidiarrheals, 662
  dermatologic, 719t
  ophthalmic, 705t
antibiotics. *See also* anti-infective drugs
  as antineoplastic drugs, 684, 687t
  lactation and, 737t
  pregnancy and, 729t
anticholinergic drugs, 213–221
  adjunctive to anesthesia, 152
  administration of, 219
  adverse effects of, 219–220
  anesthesia and, 152
  antiparkinson drugs as, 136, 137t
  as antispasmodics, 213, 214
  belladonna alkaloids and derivatives as,
        213, 215–216
  in biliary colic, 217
  in bronchoconstrictive disorders, 515, 517
  client teaching for, 217, 220–221
  contraindications to, 215
  description of, 213
  drug interactions with, 220
  effects of, 213
  in extrapyramidal reactions, 218
  in gastrointestinal disorders, 213, 214,
        214t, 218
  in genitourinary disorders, 214, 216–217
  in geriatrics, 218
  in glaucoma, 217–218
  indications for, 214
  individual, 215–217
  lactation and, 737t
  mechanism of action with, 213–214
  nursing actions for, 219–221
  nursing process for, 217
  in ophthalmology, 213, 214, 703t
  overdosage in, 218
  in Parkinson's disease, 215, 216, 218
  in pediatrics, 218
  pregnancy and, 730t

preoperative, 215, 217–218
  principles of therapy with, 217–218
  in renal colic, 217
  in respiratory disorders, 213, 214–215
  synthetic, 214, 214t, 216
  therapeutic effects of, 219
anticholinesterases, 207
  in ocular disorders, 702t
anticoagulants, 613–625
  administration of, 621–622
  adverse effects of, 622–623
  antidotes to, 616, 617
  client teaching with, 624–625
  description of, 613, 614–615
  dosage of, 619–620
  drug interactions with, 623–624
  in geriatrics, 621
  individual, 615–617
  lactation and, 737t
  nursing actions for, 621–625
  nursing process for, 618–619
  in pediatrics, 620
  pregnancy and, 730t
  principles of therapy with, 619–620
  selection of, 619
  therapeutic effects of, 622
anticonvulsant drugs, 125–135
  administration of, 132
  adverse effects of, 133
  barbiturates as, 127
  benzodiazepines as, 127–128
  client teaching with, 130, 134–135
  contraindications to, 126
  dosage of, 130–131
  drug interactions with, 133–134
  duration of therapy with, 131
  epilepsy and, 125–126
  in geriatrics, 131–132
  indications for, 126
  individual, 126–129
  lactation and, 737t
  mechanism of action with, 126
  monitoring of, 131
  nursing actions for, 132–135
  nursing process for, 129–130
  in pediatrics, 131
        parent teaching for, 134–135
  pregnancy and, 730t, 734
  principles of therapy with, 130–131
  seizure disorders and, 125
  selection of, 130
  status epilepticus and, 125–126, 131
  therapeutic effects of, 132–133
antidepressants, 113–123
  administration of, 117t, 119, 121
  adverse effects of, 121–122
  client teaching with, 123
  contraindications to, 116
  depression and, 113–114
  dosage of, 117t, 119
  drug interactions with, 122–123
  duration of therapy with, 119
  in geriatrics, 117t, 120–121
  indications for, 116
  individual, 117t
  lactation and, 737t
  mechanism of action of, 116
  monoamine oxidase inhibitors, 114–115,
        115t
  mood stabilizing, 115–116, 117t. *See also*
        lithium
  nursing actions for, 121–123
  nursing process for, 116, 118–119
  overdosage of, 120
  in pediatrics, 117t, 120
  perioperative, 120
  pregnancy and, 730t
  principles of therapy with, 118–121
  selection of, 118–119

serotonin reuptake inhibitors, 115, 117t,
        118
  therapeutic effects of, 121
  toxicity of, 120
  tricyclic, 114, 117t
antidiabetic drugs, 278–295. *See also* hypo-
        glycemic drugs, oral; insulin
  administration of, 291–292
  adverse reactions to, 293
  client teaching with, 294–295
  description of, 278–279
  drug interactions with, 293–294
  nursing actions for, 291–295
  nursing process for, 285–287
  principles of therapy with, 287–291
  therapeutic effects of, 292
antidiarrheals, 660–666
  administration of, 665
  adverse effects of, 666
  antibacterial agents as, 662t
  client teaching with, 666
  contraindications to, 660, 662
  description of, 659–660
  drug interactions with, 666
  in geriatrics, 665
  indications for, 660
  individual, 661t–663t
  lactation and, 738t
  nonspecific, 660
  nursing actions for, 665–666
  nursing process for, 663–664
  opiates as, 661t–662t
  in pediatrics, 665
  pregnancy and, 730t
  principles of therapy with, 664–665
  selection of, 664
  specific, 660
  therapeutic effects of, 665
antidiuretic hormone (ADH), 50, 229,
        232–233
antidotes
  in heparin overdosage, 616
  in thrombolytic overdosage, 618
  in warfarin overdosage, 617
antiemetics, 668–674, 670t–671t
  administration of, 673–674
        timing of, 673
  adverse effects of, 674
  antihistamines as, 669, 670t
  chemotherapy and, 673
  client teaching with, 674
  contraindications to, 671
  corticosteroids as, 669
  dosage of, 673
  drug interactions with, 674
  in geriatrics, 673
  indications for, 671
  lactation and, 738t
  mechanism of action in, 668–669
  nursing actions for, 673–674
  nursing process for, 671–672
  in pediatrics, 673
  phenothiazines as, 669, 670t
  pregnancy and, 730t, 732
  principles of therapy with, 672–673
  selection of, 672
  therapeutic effects of, 674
antiepileptic drugs. *See* anticonvulsants
antifungal drugs, 442–446, 444t
  administration of, 445
  adverse effects of, 446
  client teaching for, 446
  dermatologic, 719t
  diagnostic and therapeutic factors and, 443
  drug interactions with, 446
  in geriatrics, 445
  individual, 444t
  mechanism of action in, 443
  nursing actions for, 445–446

nursing process for, 443
ophthalmic, 705t
in pediatrics, 444t, 445
principles of therapy with, 443, 445
therapeutic effects of, 445
antihistamines, 525–531
administration of, 530
adverse effects of, 531
as antiemetics, 669, 670t
client teaching with, 531
in cold, cough, and allergy remedies,
536t–537t
contraindications to, 526
description of, 525–526
drug interactions with, 531
in geriatrics, 530
indications for, 526
individual, 527t–529t
lactation and, 738t
mechanism of action with, 526
nonsedating, 526, 528t
nursing actions for, 530–531
nursing process for, 529
in pediatrics, 530
pregnancy and, 730t
principles of therapy with, 529–530
as sedative-hypnotics, 83–84
therapeutic effects of, 530
antihypertensive drugs, 589–599, 591t–593t
administration of, 598
adverse effects of, 598–599
angiotensin-converting enzyme inhibitors as, 589–590, 591t, 595
antiadrenergic drugs as, 590, 591t, 595
calcium channel-blocking agents as, 590,
592t, 595
client teaching for, 599
combination products, 593t, 595
diuretics as, 590
dosage of, 596
drug interactions with, 598–599
duration of therapy with, 596
genetic/ethnic considerations and, 596
in geriatrics, 597
lactation and, 738t
nursing actions for, 598–599
nursing process for, 593–595
in pediatrics, 596–597
pregnancy and, 730t
principles of therapy with, 595–597
regimens of, 595
renal impairment and, 596
selection of, 595
sodium restriction and, 596
surgery and, 596
therapeutic effects of, 598
vasodilators as, 590, 592t–593t, 595
anti-infective drugs, 369–378, 411–417. *See
also named class*
administration of, 376–377, 414–415
route of, 375
adverse effects of, 377–378, 415–416
beta lactams as, 411
characteristics of, 371–372
client teaching with, 373, 378, 417
combination therapy with, 374
dermatologic, 714–715, 722
dosage of, 374–375
drug interactions with, 416–417
duration of therapy with, 375
in geriatrics, 376
host defense mechanisms and, 369
indications for, 372
in liver disease, 375
macrolides as, 407
mechanism of action with, 371
microorganisms and, 369–371, 371t
nursing actions for, 376–378, 414–415
nursing process for, 371–373

ophthalmic, 700, 705t
in pediatrics, 375–376
polymyxins as, 412–414
principles of therapy with, 374–376, 414
quinolones as, 411–412
rational use of, 374
in renal insufficiency, 375
selection of, 374
specimen collection and, 374
therapeutic effects of, 377, 415
anti-inflammatory drugs. *See also* analgesic-
antipyretic-anti-inflammatory drugs;
corticosteroids
dermatologic, 715, 721–722
ophthalmic, 705t
antilipemic drugs, 626–632, 628t
administration of, 630
adverse effects of, 631
client teaching with, 632
drug interactions with, 630, 631–632
in geriatrics, 630
individual, 628t
mechanism of action with, 627
nursing actions for, 629–632
nursing process for, 627–629
in pediatrics, 630
principles of therapy with, 629–630
selection of, 630
therapeutic effects of, 630–631
antilymphocyte antibody preparations.
*See also* immunosuppressants
for immunosuppression, 499–500
antimalarial drugs, 451–453. *See also* antiparasitics
antimanic drug, 115–116, 117t
lactation and, 738t
pregnancy and, 730t
antimetabolites, 684, 686t–687t. *See also*
antineoplastic drugs
antimicrobial drugs. *See* anti-infective drugs
Antiminth (pyrantel pamoate), 454
antineoplastic drugs, 679–697, 686t–689t
administration of, 693, 694–695
adverse effects of, 695–696
characteristics of, 683
client and family planning in, 692
client teaching with, 697
combinations of, 692–693
dosage of, 693
drug interactions with, 696–697
in geriatrics, 694
handling of, 693–694
indications for, 685
individual, 685t–689t
nursing actions for, 694–696
nursing process for, 685, 689–692
in pediatrics, 694
principles of therapy with, 692–694
selection of, 692
therapeutic effects of, 695
antioncogenes, 682
antiparasitics, 448–459
administration of, 457
adverse effects of, 458
amebicides as, 450–451
anthelmintics as, 453–454
antimalarials as, 451–453
antitrichomonal agents as, 453
client teaching for, 459
drug interactions with, 459
nursing actions for, 457–459
nursing process for, 455–456
pediculocides as, 455
principles of therapy with, 456
scabicides as, 455
therapeutic effects of, 457–458
antiparkinson drugs, 136–143
administration of, 141
adverse effects of, 141–142

anticholinergic drugs as, 136, 137t
client teaching with, 143
contraindications to, 137
dopaminergic drugs as, 136
dosage of, 140
drug interactions with, 142–143
in geriatrics, 140
indications for, 137
individual, 136, 137t–139
mechanism of action with, 136–137
nursing actions for, 141–143
nursing process for, 139
Parkinson's disease and, 136
in pediatrics, 140
principles of therapy with, 140
selection of, 140
therapeutic effects of, 141
antiplatelet drugs, 615
aspirin as, 619
individual, 617
nursing process for, 618–619
principles of therapy with, 619
selection of, 619
anti-*Pneumocystis carinii* agent, 453. *See also*
antiparasitics
antipseudomonal penicillins, 381,
382t–385t
antipsychotic drugs, 99–111
administration of, 106, 107–108
adverse effects of, 108–110
client teaching with, 105, 111
contraindications to, 100
dosage of, 106
drug interactions with, 110–111
duration of therapy, 106
ethnic or genetic considerations in, 106
extrapyramidal effects of, 106
in geriatrics, 107
goals of treatment with, 105
indications for, 100
limitations on, 105
individual, 101t–102t, 103–104
lactation and, 738t
mechanism of action with, 100
nonphenothiazines, 103–104
nursing actions for, 107–111
nursing process for, 104–105
in pediatrics, 107
perioperative, 106–107
phenothiazines, 100, 101t–102t
pregnancy and, 731t
principles of therapy with, 105–107
psychosis and, 99–100
selection of, 105–106
therapeutic effects of, 108
antirabies serum, equine, 480t
antisecretory drugs. *See* gastric acid inhibitors
antiseptics
dermatologic, 714, 716t–718t, 721
metallic, 716t–717t
ophthalmic, 704t
urinary, 418, 421–425
antispasmodics, urinary, 216–217
antithymocyte globulin, Canadian trade
name for, 748
antithymocyte globulin (ATG)
for immunosuppression, 499–500
selection of, 502
antithyroid drugs
administration of, 261
adverse effects of, 262
client teaching with, 263
dose of, 260
drug interactions with, 263
duration of therapy with, 260
in geriatrics, 260
individual, 257–258
nursing actions for, 261–263

antithyroid drugs (*continued*)
  in pediatrics, 260
  pregnancy and, 260, 731t
  therapeutic effects of, 261–262
  thyroid disorders and, 254t, 254–256
antitoxins, 478, 479t–480t
antitrichomonal drugs, 453. *See also* antiparasitics
antitubercular drugs, 427–433
  administration of, 431
  adverse effects of, 431–432
  characteristics of, 428
  client teaching with, 432–433
  contraindications to, 428
  drug interactions with, 432
  in geriatrics, 431
  indications for, 428
  lactation and, 737t
  mechanisms of action with, 428
  nursing actions for, 431–433
  nursing process for, 430
  in pediatrics, 431
  pregnancy and, 729t
  primary, 428–429
  principles of therapy with, 430–431
  regimens for, 427, 430–431
  secondary, 429–430
  therapeutic effects of, 431
antitussives, 534, 535t, 536t
  administration of, 540
  adverse effects of, 540
  description of, 534
  drug interactions with, 540–541
  in geriatrics, 539
  indications for, 534
  narcotic, 535t, 536t–537t
  nonnarcotic, 535t
  nursing actions for, 539–541
  nursing process for, 534, 537–538
  principles of therapy with, 538
  selection of, 539
  therapeutic effects of, 540
antiulcer drugs, 639–649. *See also* peptic
  ulcer disease, drugs used in
Antivert (meclizine), 528t, 670t
antiviral drugs, 434–440, 436t
  administration of, 438
  adverse effects of, 439
  client teaching with, 437, 440
  dermatologic, 719t
  description of, 435
  drug interactions with, 439–440
  in geriatrics, 438
  individual, 435, 436t, 437
  mechanism of action with, 435
  nursing actions for, 438–440
  nursing process for, 437
  ophthalmic, 705t
  in pediatrics, 438
  pregnancy and, 730t
  principles of therapy with, 438
  therapeutic effects of, 439
Anturane (sulfinpyrazone), 72
  as Canadian trade name, 753
Anusol (zinc sulfate), as Canadian trade
  name, 754
anxiety, defined, 89. *See also* antianxiety drugs
APAP (acetaminophen), as Canadian trade
  name, 748
Apo-Alpraz (alprazolam), as Canadian trade
  name, 748
Apo-Amoxi (amoxicillin), as Canadian
  trade name, 748
Apo-Ampi (ampicillin), as Canadian trade
  name, 748
Apo-Atenol (atenolol), as Canadian trade
  name, 748
Apo-Cal (calcium carbonate), as Canadian
  trade name, 749

Apo-Capto (captopril), as Canadian trade
  name, 749
Apo-C (ascorbic acid, vitamin C), as Canadian trade name, 748, 754
Apo-Cephalex (cephalexin), as Canadian
  trade name, 749
Apo-Cloxi (cloxacillin), as Canadian trade
  name, 749
Apo-Diclo (diclofenac), as Canadian trade
  name, 750
Apo-Ditiaz (diltiazem), as Canadian trade
  name, 750
Apo-Doxy (doxycycline), as Canadian trade
  name, 750
Apo-Erythro (erythromycin), as Canadian
  trade name, 750
Apo-gain (minoxidil), as Canadian trade
  name, 752
Apo-Hydro (hydrochlorothiazide), as Cana-
  dian trade name, 751
Apo-ISDN (isosorbide dinitrate), as Cana-
  dian trade name, 751
Apo-Keto (ketoprofen), as Canadian trade
  name, 751
Apo-K (potassium chloride), as Canadian
  trade name, 753
Apo-Metoclop (metoclopramide), as Canadian trade name, 752
Apo-Nadol (nadolol), as Canadian trade
  name, 752
Apo-Nifed (nifedipine), as Canadian trade
  name, 752
Apo-Pen VK (penicillin V), as Canadian
  trade name, 752
Apo-Pindol (pindolol), as Canadian trade
  name, 753
Apo-Prazo (prazosin), as Canadian trade
  name, 753
Apo-Sulfatrim (sulfamethoxazole and
  trimethoprim), as Canadian trade
  name, 753
Apo-Sulin (sulindac), as Canadian trade
  name, 753
Apo-Tamox (tamoxifen), as Canadian trade
  name, 753
Apo-Tetra (tetracycline), as Canadian trade
  name, 754
Apo-Timol (timolol), as Canadian trade
  name, 754
Apo-Timop (timolol), as Canadian trade
  name, 754
Apo-Triazo (triazolam), as Canadian trade
  name, 754
Apo-Trihex (trihexyphenidyl), as Canadian
  trade name, 754
Apo-Trimip (trimipramine), as Canadian
  trade name, 754
Apo-Verap (verapamil), as Canadian trade
  name, 754
Apresoline (hydralazine), 592t
  as Canadian trade name, 751
  lactation and, 738t
  in pediatrics, 597
  pregnancy and, 730t
aprobarbital (Alurate), 82t, 83
Aqua-Mephyton (phytonadione), routes
  and dosage ranges for, 340t
Aquasol A (vitamin A)
  as Canadian trade name, 754
  routes and dosage ranges for, 340t
Aquasol E (vitamin E)
  as Canadian trade name, 754
  routes and dosage ranges for, 340t
ARA-C (cytarabine, cytosine arabinoside)
  (Cytosar-U), 686t
  Canadian trade name for, 749
Aralen (chloroquine), 451–452
  as amebicide, 450
  as Canadian trade name, 749

Aramine (metaraminol), 187t, 582–583
Arduan (pipecuronium), 155t
Aredia (pamidronate), 271
  as Canadian trade name, 752
Arfonad (trimethaphan camsylate), 591t
Aristocort diacetate (triamcinolone diacetate), 242t
Aristocort (triamcinolone), 719t
  as Canadian trade name, 754
Aristospan (triamcinolone), 242t
  as Canadian trade name, 754
arrhythmias
  cardiac, 561–562
  drug therapy for, 562–570. *See also* antiar-
    rhythmic drugs
  nonpharmacologic treatment of, 562
Artane (trihexyphenidyl), 137t, 216
  as Canadian trade name, 754
arterial dilators, in congestive heart failure,
  549
arthritis, rheumatoid, 68t, 75
artificial tears, 704t
asbestos, 681t
ascariasis (roundworm infections), 449
ascorbic acid (vitamin C), 336t
  Canadian trade name for, 748
  imbalance of, 339t
  preparations of, 340t
Asendin (amoxapine), 117t
  as Canadian trade name, 748
Asian heritage
  antipsychotic drugs and, 106
  beta-adrenergic drugs in, 202
asparaginase (Elspar), 688t
  Canadian trade name for, 748
aspartic acid, 49
aspartic acid, endogenous, 49
aspirin (acetylsalicylic acid), 68–69, 615,616
  adverse effects of, 67–68
  Canadian trade name for, 748
  in geriatrics, 76
  indications for, 68, 68t
  mechanism of action in, 67
  in pediatrics, 76
  perioperative use of, 75–76
  pregnancy and, 731t
  rheumatoid arthritis and, 75
  routes and dosage ranges for, 69
  therapy guidelines for, 74
astemizole (Hismanal), 528t
  Canadian trade name for, 748
asthma. *See also* antiasthmatic drugs;
    bronchodilating drugs
  characteristics of, 514
  in pregnancy, 732–733
astringents, dermatologic, 715
Atarax (hydroxyzine), 525–526, 529t, 670t
Atasol (acetaminophen), as Canadian trade
  name, 748
atenolol and chlorthalidone (Tenoretic),
  593t
atenolol (Tenormin), 198, 199t, 575, 591t
  Canadian trade name for, 748
Atgam (antithymocyte globulin), as Canadian trade name, 748
atherosclerosis
  description of, 626
  drug therapy for, 626–632
    hemorrheologic agents in, 627
    nursing actions for, 629–632
    nursing process for, 627–629
    principles of, 629–630
    vasodilators in, peripheral, 629t
Ativan (lorazepam), 90, 91t
  as Canadian trade name, 751
atopic dermatitis, 713
atovaquone (Mepron), 453
atracurium (Tracrium), 155t
  Canadian trade name for, 748

atrial arrhythmias. *See also* antiarrhythmic drugs
   fibrillation, 561–562, 568
   flutter, 561–562, 568
Atromid-S (clofibrate), 628t, 630
Atromid-S (clofibrate), as Canadian trade name, 749
atropine, 213, 215
   as antidote to cholinergic drugs, 210
   colic and, 61, 217
   lactation and, 737t
   in pediatrics, 218
   pregnancy and, 730t
atropine sulfate, Canadian trade name for, 748
atropine sulfate, in ocular disorders, 703t
atropine sulfate, pectin, kaolin, hyoscyamine sulfate, hyoscine hydrobromide, alcohol (Donnagel), 663t
atropine sulfate and difenoxin (Motofen), 661t
atropine sulfate and diphenoxylate (Lomotil), 661t
Atropisol (atopine sulfate), as Canadian trade name, 748
Atrovent (ipratropium), 517
   as Canadian trade name, 751
attention-deficit-hyperactivity disorder (ADHD), central nervous system stimulants for, 176, 178
Attenuvax (measles vaccine), 474t
Augmentin (amoxicillin and potassium clavulanate), 383, 383t
autoimmune disorders, 470, 496–497. *See also* immunosuppressants
automaticity, cardiac, 560
autonomic drugs, in ocular disorders, 700–701, 702t
autonomic nervous system
   drugs affecting, 185
   physiology of, 183–185, 184t
Aveeno (colloidal oatmeal), 720t
Aventyl (nortriptyline), 117t
   as Canadian trade name, 752
Axid (nizatidine), 641
   as Canadian trade name, 752
Ayercillin (penicillin G procaine), as Canadian trade name, 752
Azactam (aztreonam), 411
   lactation and, 737t
   pregnancy and, 729t
azatadine, Canadian trade name for, 748
azatadine maleate (Optimine), 529t
azathioprine (Imuran), 497t, 499
   Canadian trade name for, 748
   dosage of, 502–503
   selection of, 502
azidothymidine, Canadian trade name for, 754
azithromycin (Zithromax), 407, 408
Azmacort (triamcinolone), 242t, 517, 518
   as Canadian trade name, 754
Azo Gantanol (sulfamethoxazole phenazopyridine), 420t
Azo Gantrisin (sulfisoxazole phenazopyridine), 420t
   as Canadian trade name, 753
AZT (azidothymidine), Canadian trade name for, 754
aztreonam (Azactam), 411
   lactation and, 737t
   pregnancy and, 729t
Azulfidine (sulfasalazine), 419t, 663t

**B**

Bacid (lactobacillus), 663t
Baciguent (bacitracin), 719t
   as Canadian trade name, 748
   in ocular disorders, 705t

Bacillus Calmette-Guérin (BCG) vaccine
   as immunostimulant, 476t–477t, 488
   for neoplastic disease, 491–492
Bacillus Calmette-Guérin (TheraCys, TICE BCG), 476t–477t, 488, 489t
Bacitin (bacitracin), as Canadian trade name, 748
bacitracin, neomycin sulfate, and polymyxin B sulfate (Neosporin ointment), 719t
bacitracin and polymyxin B (Polysporin ointment), 719t
bacitracin (Baciguent, Bacitin), 719t
   Canadian trade name for, 748
   in ocular disorders, 705t
baclofen (Lioresal), 146t
   Canadian trade name for, 748
bacteria. *See also* anti-infective drugs; microorganisms
   classification of, 370
   gram-positive and gram-negative, common, 371t
Bactrim (TMP-SMX) (trimethoprim-sulfamethoxazole), 419t–420t, 662t
   as Canadian trade name, 753
   lactation and, 737t
   pregnancy and, 730t
Bactroban (mupirocin), 744t
Balminil DM (dextromethorphan), as Canadian trade name, 749
Balminil Expectorant (guaifenesin), as Canadian trade name, 751
Balnetar (coal tar), 720t
   as Canadian trade name, 749
Banlin (propantheline), as Canadian trade name, 753
Banthine (methantheline bromide), 214t
barbiturates, 82t
   abuse of, 164
      treatment of, 173–174
   as anticonvulsants, 127
   long-acting, 82t
   overdose of, 173–174
   as sedative-hypnotics, 81, 82t, 83
   short-acting, 82t
basal ganglia, structure and function of, 51
BCG vaccine. *See* Bacillus Calmette-Guérin
BCME. *See* bis (chloromethyl) ether
BCNU. *See* carmustine
B-complex vitamins
   disorders of, 342
   imbalances of, 338t–339t
   as nutrients, 335t–336t
   preparations of, 340t
Beben (betamethasone), as Canadian trade name, 748
becampicillin (Spectrobid), 381, 382t
   Canadian trade name for, 748
Beclodisk (beclomethasone), as Canadian trade name, 748
Becloforte (beclomethasone), as Canadian trade name, 748
beclomethasone (Beclovent, Beconase, Vancenase, Vanceril), 241t, 517
   Canadian trade name for, 748
Beclovent (beclomethasone), 241t, 517
   as Canadian trade name, 748
Beconase (beclomethasone), 241t
   as Canadian trade name, 748
belladonna alkaloids and derivatives, 215–216. *See also* anticholinergic drugs
belladonna tincture, 215
Benadryl (diphenhydramine), 84, 137t, 525, 527t, 670t
   as Canadian trade name, 750
   lactation and, 738t
   pregnancy and, 730t

benazepril (Lotensin), 591t
bendrofluazide, Canadian trade name for, 748
bendroflumethiazide and nadolol (Corzide), 593t
bendroflumethiazide (Naturetin), 602t
   Canadian trade name for, 748
Benemid (probenecid), 72
   as Canadian trade name, 753
Benisone (betamethasone), 719t
Benoquin (monobenzone), 720t
Benoxyl (benzoyl peroxide), as Canadian trade name, 748
Bentyl (dicyclomine hydrochloride), 214t
Bentylol (dicyclomine), as Canadian trade name, 750
Benylin-D (guaifenesin), as Canadian trade name, 751
Benylin DM (dextromethorphan), 535t
   as Canadian trade name, 749
Benzac (benzoyl peroxide), as Canadian trade name, 748
Benzagel (benzoyl peroxide), as Canadian trade name, 748
Benzedrex (propylhexedrine), 187t, 535t
benzene, 681t
benzhexol, Canadian trade name for, 754
benzidine, 681t
benzocaine (Americaine), 156t
   Canadian trade name for, 748
benzodiazepines
   abuse of, 164
      treatment of, 173–174
   as anticonvulsants, 127–128
   as antiemetics, 669
   contraindications to, 90
   in geriatrics, 85, 95
   in hypoalbuminemia, 95
   indications for, 90
   individual, 91t
   in liver disease, 95
   mechanism of action with, 90
   overdose of, 173–174
   in pediatrics, 85, 87, 95
   pharmacologic properties of, 90
   pregnancy and, 731t
   scheduling of, 94
   as sedative-hypnotics, 82t, 83
   toxicity of, 94–95
      antidote to, 85
   withdrawal from, 94, 95
benzonatate (Tessalon), 535t
benzoyl peroxide (Benzoyl peroxide lotion U.S.P.), 717t
   Canadian trade name for, 748
Benzoyl peroxide lotion U.S.P. (benzoyl peroxide), 717t
benzphetamine (Didrex), 323t
benzquinamide (Emete-Con), 670t, 699
benzthiazide (Exna), 602t
benztropine (Cogentin), 137t, 216
   Canadian trade name for, 748
benzylpenicillin potassium, Canadian trade name for, 752
bepridil (Vascor), 574t
beractant (Survanta), 743t
beta-adrenergic blocking drugs, 197, 198, 199t, 201–202. *See also* antiadrenergic drugs
   activity of, 200
   administration of, 200, 203
   adverse effects of, 204
   for angina pectoris, 573
   client teaching with, 201, 205
   drug interactions with, 204–205
   duration of action of, 200
   effects of, 196–197
   elimination of, 200
   in geriatrics, 202–203

beta-adrenergic blocking drugs (*continued*)
    indications for, 197, 198
    individual agents, 199t
    lactation and, 738t
    mechanism of action with, 196, 197f
    in pediatrics, 202
    pregnancy and, 731t
    principles of therapy with, 201–202
    receptor selectivity of, 198, 200
    therapeutic effects of, 203
Betacort (betamethasone), as Canadian
        trade name, 748
Betaderm (betamethasone), as Canadian
        trade name, 748
Betadine (povidone-iodine), 453, 716t
    as Canadian trade name, 753
Betagan (levobunolol), 198, 199t, 200
    as Canadian trade name, 751
    in ocular disorders, 702t
beta lactams, 411
    pregnancy and, 729t
Betaloc (metoprolol), as Canadian trade
        name, 752
betamethasone acetate and sodium phos-
        phate (Celestone Soluspan), 241t
betamethasone (Benisone, Celestone,
        Valisone), 241t, 719t
    Canadian trade name for, 748
Betapace (sotalol), 198, 199t, 200, 565, 566,
        568
Betaxin (thiamine, vitamin B₁), as Cana-
        dian trade name, 754
betaxolol (Betoptic, Kerlone), 198, 199t,
        200, 592t
    Canadian trade name for, 748
    in ocular disorders, 702t
bethanechol (Urecholine), 207–208
    Canadian trade name for, 748
    in pediatrics, 210
Betnesol (betamethasone), as Canadian
        trade name, 748
Betnovate (betamethasone), as Canadian
        trade name, 748
Betoptic (betaxolol), 198, 199t, 200
    as Canadian trade name, 748
    in ocular disorders, 702t
Bewon (thiamine, vitamin B₁), as Canadian
        trade name, 754
Biavax-II (rubella and mumps vaccine),
        476t
Biaxin (clarithromycin), 407, 408
    as Canadian trade name, 749
Bicillin (penicillin G benzathine), 382t
    as Canadian trade name, 752
BiCNU (carmustine), as Canadian trade
        name, 749
biguanide, dermatologic, 716t
biliary colic, anticholinergics in, 217
biotransformation
    children and, 38t
    defined, 10
    older adults and, 40t
biperiden (Akineton), 137t, 216
    Canadian trade name for, 748
Biquin (quinidine), as Canadian trade
        name, 753
bisacodyl (Dulcolax), 652t
    Canadian trade name for, 748
    pregnancy and, 731t
bis (chloromethyl) ether (BCME)
    as carcinogen, 681t
bisoprolol (Zebeta), 198, 199t, 200
bitolterol (Tornalate), 187t, 516
    in pediatrics, 191
Black Draught (senna pod preparations), 652t
blastomycosis, 442–443
bleeding
    antineoplastic drugs and, 691
    uterine, estrogens and, 301t

Blenoxane (bleomycin), 687t
    as Canadian trade name, 748
bleomycin (Blenoxane), 687t
    Canadian trade name for, 748
blepharitis, 700. *See also* ophthalmic drugs
Bleph-10 Liquifilm (sulfacetamide sodium),
        in ocular disorders, 705t
Blocadren (timolol), 198, 199t, 200, 592t
    as Canadian trade name, 754
    lactation and, 738t
blood
    coagulation of
        coagulation phase in, 614
        estrogens and, 298
        factors in, 614t
        liver and, 636
        platelet phase in, 613–614
    disorders of
        from alcohol abuse, 167–168
        corticosteroids in, 240
        drug-induced, 17
    physiology of, 546–547
blood pressure. *See also* hypertension; hypo-
        tension; shock
    hypothalamus and, 50
    regulation of, 728. *See also* antihyperten-
        sive drugs
blood vessels, physiology of, 546
B lymphocytes, in immune response, 467
body heat, liver and, 636
body-surface nomograms, 39
body temperature, hypothalamus and, 50
body weight, drug action and, 16
Bonamine (meclizine), as Canadian trade
        name, 751
bone, testosterone effect on, 310
bone marrow transplants. *See also* immuno-
        suppressants
    graft-versus-host disease with, 498
Bonine (meclizine), 670t
botulism antitoxin, 480t
bradykinin, in inflammation and immunity,
        7
brain metabolism, 51
brain stem, structure of, 50
breasts
    cancer of
        drug therapy for, 301t, 311, 312t,
                314
        estrogen and, 297
    postpartum enlargement of, 301t, 302t
breathing, defined, 512
Brethine (terbutaline), 187t
    pregnancy and, 729t, 735t
Bretylate (bretylium), as Canadian trade
        name, 749
bretylium (Bretylol), 565–568
    Canadian trade name for, 749
Bretylol (bretylium), 565–568
Brevibloc (esmolol), 198, 199t, 200, 565
    as Canadian trade name, 750
Brevicon (ethinyl estradiol and norethin-
        drone), 304t
    as Canadian trade name, 750
Brevital (methohexital sodium), 154t
Bricanyl (terbutaline), as Canadian trade
        name, 754
Brietal (methohexital), as Canadian trade
        name, 752
bromocriptine (Parlodel), 136, 138–139
    Canadian trade name for, 749
    lactation and, 735
    pregnancy and, 735t
brompheniramine, Canadian trade name
        for, 749
brompheniramine maleate (Dimetane),
        527t
Bronalide (flunisolide), as Canadian trade
        name, 750

bronchitis, chronic. *See* chronic obstructive
        pulmonary disease (COPD)
bronchodilating drugs, 515–523
    administration of, 520, 522
    adrenergics as, 515–517
    adverse effects of, 522–523
    anticholinergic, 517
    client teaching with, 523
    contraindications to, 515
    dosage factors with, 521
    drug interactions with, 523
    in geriatrics, 521
    indications for, 515
    individual, 515–517, 518t
    lactation and, 738t
    mechanisms of action in, 515
    nursing actions for, 522–523
    nursing process for, 519–520
    in pediatrics, 521
    in pregnancy, 733–734
    pregnancy and, 731t
    principles of therapy with, 520
    selection of, 520
    theophylline preparations, 518t
    therapeutic effects of, 522
    xanthines, 515, 517
Bronkaid (epinephrine), 515–517
Bronkaid Mistometer (epinephrine), as
        Canadian trade name, 750
Bronkometer (isoetharine), 516
Bronkosol (isoetharine), 187t, 516
Bucladin-S (buclizine), 670t
buclizine (Bucladin-S), 670t
bulk-forming laxatives, 651, 652t
bumetanide (Bumex), 602t
    lactation and, 738t
Bumex (bumetanide), 602t
    lactation and, 738t
bupivacaine (Marcaine), 156t
    Canadian trade name for, 749
buprenex (Buprenorphine), 57
Buprenorphine (buprenex), 57
bupropion (Wellbutrin), 115, 117t
burns, sulfonamides in, 418, 424
Burow's solution (aluminum acetate solu-
        tion), 720t
bursitis, drugs used in, 68t
busulfan (Myleran), 686t
    Canadian trade name for, 749
butabarbital sodium (Butisol), 82t, 83
butamben (Butesin), 156t
Butesin (butamben), 156t
Butisol (butabarbital sodium), 82t, 83
butoconazole (Femstat), 444t

**C**

Cafergot (ergotamine and caffeine), 72
    as Canadian trade name, 750
caffeine, 177, 178
    pregnancy and, 731t
caffeine and ergotamine (Cafergot), 72
Calamine Lotion U.S.P. (zinc oxide), 717t
Calan SR (verapamil) (sustained-release),
        592t
Calan (verapamil), 566, 568, 574t, 592t
    lactation and, 738t
    in pediatrics, 597
    pregnancy and, 731t
Calax (docusate calcium), as Canadian trade
        name, 750
calcifediol (Calderol), 268t
calciferol (ergocalciferol, vitamin D), 266
    as Canadian trade name, 750
Calcijex (calcitriol, vitamin D), as Canadian
        trade name, 749, 754
Calcimar (calcitonin-salmon), 270
    as Canadian trade name, 749
calcitonin, calcium metabolism and, 266

calcitonin-human (Cibacalcin), 271
calcitonin-salmon (Calcimar), 270
  Canadian trade name for, 749
calcitriol (Rocaltrol), 268t
  Canadian trade name for, 749
calcium, 266–267
  daily requirement for, 267
  functions of, 266–267
  metabolism of
    calcitonin and, 266
    disorders in. See hypercalcemia;
      hypocalcemia
    hormones in, 265–266
    parathyroid hormone and, 265–266
    vitamin D and, 266
  preparations of, 268t, 268t, 268–270
calcium carbonate (Os-Cal 500), 268t
  Canadian trade name for, 749
calcium channel-blocking agents
  for angina pectoris, 573, 574t
  hypertension and, 590, 592t, 595
  lactation and, 738t
  pregnancy and, 731t
calcium chloride, 268t
calcium glubionate (Neo-Calglucon), 268t
calcium gluceptate, 268t
calcium gluconate (Kalcinate), 268t
calcium lactate, 268t
calcium pantothenate (B₅), routes and
  dosage ranges for, 340t
calcium phosphate dibasic (Dical-D), 268t
calcium-vitamin D combinations, 270
Calderol (calcifediol), 268t
calorie, defined, 319
Calsan (calcium carbonate), as Canadian
  trade name, 749
Caltrate (calcium carbonate), as Canadian
  trade name, 749
Camalox, 643t
camphorated tincture of opium (paregoric),
  661t
Canadian trade names, 748–754
cancer. See also antineoplastic drugs; neoplasms, malignant
  breast, drug therapy for, 301t, 311, 312t,
    314
  carcinogens and, 681t
  drug-induced, 681–682
  effects on body, 683
  endometrial, drug therapy for, 301t–302t
  estrogens in, 301t–302t, 305
  immune dysfunction and, 470
  immunostimulants in, 491–492
  progestins in, 303t, 305
  prostate, drug therapy for, 301t–302t, 305
  uterine, drug therapy for, 301t–302t
candidiasis, 442, 443
  oral, 713
  principles of therapy in, 443, 445
  vulvovaginal, 713
Canesten (clotrimazole), as Canadian trade
  name, 749
cannabis preparations, abuse of, 164–165,
  169–170
Cantil (mepenzolate bromide), 214t
Capastat (capreomycin), 429, 430
Capoten (captopril), 549
  as Canadian trade name, 749
  lactation and, 737t, 738t
  in pediatrics, 597
  pregnancy and, 730t
Capozide (captopril and hydrochlorothiazide), 593t
capreomycin (Capastat), 429, 430
captopril and hydrochlorothiazide
  (Capozide), 593t
captopril (Capoten), 549, 591t
  Canadian trade name for, 749
  lactation and, 737t, 738t

in pediatrics, 597
pregnancy and, 730t
Carbacel (carbachol), in ocular disorders,
  702t
carbachol (Carbacel, Isopto Carbachol)
  Canadian trade name for, 749
  in ocular disorders, 702t
carbamazepine (Tegretol), 128
  Canadian trade name for, 749
  therapeutic serum drug concentrations
    for, 746
carbapenem, 411
carbenicillin, 381
  Canadian trade name for, 749
carbenicillin indanyl sodium (Geocillin),
  382t
carbidopa (Lodosyn), 136, 138
carbinoxamine maleate (Clistin), 527t
Carbocaine (mepivacaine), 156t
  as Canadian trade name, 752
carbohydrates
  imbalances of, 322t. See also nutritional
    products
  metabolism of
    glucocorticoids and, 229
    insulin effect on, 278–279
    liver and, 636
Carbolith (lithium), as Canadian trade
  name, 751
carbonic anhydrase inhibitors, ophthalmic,
  701, 703t
carboplatin (Paraplatin), 686t
  Canadian trade name for, 749
carboprost tromethamine (Hemabate),
  pregnancy and, 735t
carbuncles, 713
carcinogenicity, defined, 18
carcinogens, 681t
Cardene (nicardipine), 574t, 592t
  as Canadian trade name, 752
Cardene SR (nicardipine), 592t
cardiac arrhythmias. See arrhythmias
Cardilate (erythrityl tetranitrate), 575
cardiogenic shock, 581, 584
cardiopulmonary resuscitation, adrenergic
  drugs in, 190
Cardioquin (quinidine), 563
  as Canadian trade name, 753
cardioselective beta-blocking agents,
  199t
cardiotonic-inotropic drugs, 548–558. See
  also adrenergic drugs
  administration of, 556–557
  adverse effects of, 557–558
  amrinone, 551
  client teaching with, 558
  in congestive heart failure, 548, 549
  contraindications to, 550
  digitalis preparations, 549, 550–551,
    553–554. See also digitalis
  drug interactions with, 558
  in geriatrics, 555
  indications for, 550
  individual agents, 550–553
  mechanism of action with, 549–550
  milrinone, 551
  nursing actions for, 556–558
  nursing process for, 551–553
  in pediatrics, 555
  principles of therapy with, 553–555
cardiovascular system
  alcohol abuse and, 167
  disorders of
    diabetes and, 281
    drug therapy in, 547
  physiology of, 545–547

Cardizem SR (diltiazem) (sustained-
  release), 592t
Cardizem (diltiazem), 566, 574
  as Canadian trade name, 750
  pregnancy and, 731t
Cardura (doxazosin), 591t
  as Canadian trade name, 750
carisoprodol (Rela, Soma), 146t
  Canadian trade name for, 749
carmustine (BCNU), 686t
  Canadian trade name for, 749
carteolol (Cartrol, Ocupress), 198, 199t,
  200, 592t
  in ocular disorders, 702t
Cartrol (carteolol), 198, 199t, 200, 592t
cascara sagrada (Cas-Evac), 652t
Casec, 324
Cas-Evac (cascara sagrada), 652t
castor oil (Alphamul, Neoloid), 653t
  pregnancy and, 731t
Catapres (clonidine), 591t
  as Canadian trade name, 749
  lactation and, 738t
  pregnancy and, 730t
cathartics, 651–658. See also laxatives
  administration of, 656
  adverse effects of, 657
  client teaching for, 657–658
  contraindications to, 654
  definition of, 651
  drug interactions with, 657
  in geriatrics, 656
  indications for, 654
  irritant or stimulant, 652t–653t, 653,
    654
  nursing actions for, 656–658
  nursing process for, 654–655
  in pediatrics, 656
  principles of therapy with, 655–656
  saline, 653, 656
  selection of, 655, 656
  therapeutic effects of, 657
cation exchange resin (Kayexalate), 350,
  353
caudal anesthesia, 151
CCNU (lomustine), as Canadian trade
  name, 751
Ceclor (cefaclor), 390t
  as Canadian trade name, 749
Cedilanid-D (deslanoside), 551, 554
Cedocard-SR (isosorbide dinitrate), as
  Canadian trade name, 751
CeeNu (lomustine), as Canadian trade
  name, 751
cefaclor (Ceclor), 390t
  Canadian trade name for, 749
cefadroxil (Duricef, Ultracef), 390t
  Canadian trade name for, 749
Cefadyl (cephapirin), 390, 391t
cefamandole (Mandol), 391t
  Canadian trade name for, 749
cefazolin (Ancef, Kefzol), 390, 391t, 393
  Canadian trade name for, 749
cefixime (Suprax), 390t
Cefizox (ceftizoxime), 392t, 393
  as Canadian trade name, 749
cefmetazole (Zefazone), 391t
Cefobid (cefoperazone), 392t, 393
  as Canadian trade name, 749
cefonocid (Monocid), 391t
cefoperazone (Cefobid), 392t, 393
  Canadian trade name for, 749
ceforanide (Precef), 391t
Cefotan (cefotetan), 391t
  as Canadian trade name, 749
cefotaxime (Claforan), 392t
  Canadian trade name for, 749
cefotetan (Cefotan), 391t
  Canadian trade name for, 749

cefoxitin (Mefoxin), 391t
  Canadian trade name for, 749
cefpodoxime (Vantin), 390t
cefprozil (Cefzil), 390t
ceftazidime (Fortaz), 392t
  Canadian trade name for, 749
Ceftin (cefuroxime), 392t
  as Canadian trade name, 749
ceftizoxime (Cefizox), 392t, 393
  Canadian trade name for, 749
ceftriaxone (Rocephin), 392t
  Canadian trade name for, 749
cefuroxime (Ceftin, Kefurox, Zinacef), 390t,
    392t
  Canadian trade name for, 749
Cefzil (cefprozil), 390t
Celestoderm (betamethasone), as Canadian
    trade name, 748
Celestone (betamethasone), 241t
Celestone (betamethasone), as Canadian
    trade name, 748
Celestone Soluspan (betamethasone acetate
    and sodium phosphate), 241t
cells
  immune, 465–469
  injury to, 8
    inflammatory and immune responses
      of, 8–10
  malignant, 679–680
  normal, 6, 8
    characteristics of, 679
cellulitis, 713
central nervous system
  abnormalities of
    psychiatric symptoms and, 48, 49
  alcohol effect on, 166–167
  drug distribution in, 10–11
  drugs affecting, classification of, 51–52
  drug therapy for
    classification of, 51–52
  narcotic antagonist effect on, 54
  pain and, 53
  physiology of, 47–52
central nervous system stimulants, 52,
    176–180
  administration of, 179
  adverse effects of, 179
  amphetamines, 176, 177
  analeptic agent, 176, 177, 179
  in attention-deficit-hyperactivity disorder,
    176
  client teaching with, 180
  contraindications to, 177
  drug interactions with, 179–180
  in geriatrics, 179
  indications for, 177
  individual, 177–178
  in narcolepsy, 176
  nursing actions for, 178–179
  nursing process for, 178
  in pediatrics, 179
  principles of therapy and, 178–179
  therapeutic effects of, 179
  types of, 176–177
  xanthines, 176, 178
Centrax (prazepam), 91t
cephalexin (Keflex), 390t
  Canadian trade name for, 749
cephalosporins, 388–394, 390t, 391t. See
    also anti-infective drugs
  administration of, 393
  adverse effects of, 394
  client teaching with, 394
  contraindications to, 389
  description of, 388–389
  dosage of, 393
  drug interactions with, 394
  first-generation, 388, 389–390, 390t, 391t
  in geriatrics, 393

indications for, 389
lactation and, 737t
mechanism of action with, 389
nursing actions for, 393–394
nursing process for, 389
oral, 390t
parenteral, 391t
in pediatrics, 393
perioperative use of, 393
principles of therapy with, 389–390, 393
in renal failure or impairment, 393
second-generation, 388, 390, 390t,
    391t–392t
selection of, 389–390
therapeutic effects of, 394
third-generation, 388, 390, 390t, 392t
cephalothin (Keflin), 391t
  Canadian trade name for, 749
cephapirin (Cefadyl), 390, 391t
cephradine (Anspor, Velosef), 390t, 391t
  Canadian trade name for, 749
Cephulac (lactulose), 653t
  as Canadian trade name, 751
Ceptaz (ceftazidime), as Canadian trade
    name, 749
cerebellum, structure and function of, 51
cerebral cortex, structure and function of,
    50
Cerubidine (daunomycin, daunorubicin),
    687t
  as Canadian trade name, 749
Cetamide (sulfacetamide), as Canadian
    trade name, 753
Ce-Vi-Sol (ascorbic acid, vitamin C), as
    Canadian trade name, 748, 754
chelating agents, 354
  in ocular disorders, 701. See also oph-
    thalmic drugs
Chemet (succimer), 354
chemotherapy. See antineoplastic drugs
Chenix (chenodiol), 743t
chenodiol (Chenix), 743t
Cheracol D Cough Liquid, 536t
Cheracol Syrup, 536t
Chibroxin (Norfloxacin ophthalmic solu-
    tion), in ocular disorders, 705t
children. See also infant; neonate; pediatrics
  absorption in, 38t
  biotransformation in, 38t
  distribution in, 38t
  drug action in, 15
  drug therapy in, 38t, 38–40
  excretion in, 38t
  immune function and, 469
  metabolism and, 38t
  protein binding and, 38t
  shock and, 584
chloral hydrate, 82t, 83
chlorambucil (Leukeran), 686t
  Canadian trade name for, 749
chloramphenicol (Chloromycetin, Chlor-
    optic), 412, 662t
  Canadian trade name for, 749
  in ocular disorders, 705t
chlordiazepoxide (Librium), 91t
  in anxiety, 89–90
  Canadian trade name for, 749
  in pediatrics, 85, 95
chlorhexidine, Canadian trade name for,
    749
chlorhexidine gluconate (Hibiclens), 716t
chloride
  imbalances of, 350t
  preparations of, 347t
chlorine preparations, dermatologic, 716t
Chloromycetin (chloramphenicol), 412,
    662t
  as Canadian trade name, 749
  in ocular disorders, 705t

chloroprocaine (Nesacaine), 156t
  Canadian trade name for, 749
Chloroptic (chloramphenicol), in ocular dis-
    orders, 705t
chloroquine (Aralen), 451–452
  as amebicide, 450
  Canadian trade name for, 749
chloroquine phosphate (Aralen), 452
chlorothiazide (Diuril), 602t
chlorotrianisene (Tace), 301t
chlorphenamine, Canadian trade name for,
    749
chlorphenesin (Maolate), 146t
chlorpheniramine, Canadian trade name
    for, 749
chlorpheniramine maleate (Chlor-
    Trimeton), 525, 527t
chlorpromazine (Thorazine), 101t, 669t,
    670t
  Canadian trade name for, 749
  lactation and, 738t
  pregnancy and, 731t
chlorpropamide (Diabinese), 284t, 284–285
  Canadian trade name for, 749
  lactation and, 738t
chlorprothixene (Taractan), 103
chlorthalidone and atenolol (Tenoretic),
    593t
chlorthalidone (Hygroton), 602t
  Canadian trade name for, 749
Chlor-Trimeton (chlorpheniramine
    maleate), 525, 527t
Chlor-Tripolon (chlorpheniramine), as
    Canadian trade name, 749
chlorzoxazone (Paraflex), 146t
cholecalciferol (Delta-D), 268t
Choledyl (oxtriphylline), 518t
cholera vaccine, 473t
cholestyramine (Questran), 628t, 630,
    663t
cholestyramine resin, Canadian trade name
    for, 749
cholinergic blocking drugs. See anticholiner-
    gic drugs
cholinergic crisis, treatment of, 210
cholinergic drugs, 207–212
  administration of, 211
  adverse effects of, 211
  antidote to, 210
  client teaching with, 209, 212
  contraindications to, 209
  description of, 207
  direct-acting, 207, 208
  drug interactions with, 211
  in geriatrics, 210
  indications for, 207–208
  indirect-acting, 207, 208–209
  individual, 208–209
  mechanism of action with, 207
  in myasthenia gravis, 209–210
  nursing actions for, 211–212
  nursing process for, 209
  in ocular disorders, 702t. See also oph-
    thalmic drugs
  in pediatrics, 210
  principles of therapy with, 209–210
  therapeutic effects of, 211
Choloxin (dextrothyroxine), 628t, 630
chromium, 351t
chronic obstructive pulmonary disease
    (COPD). See also bronchodilating drugs
  drug therapy in, 515–516
Chronulac (lactulose), 653t
  as Canadian trade name, 751
Cibacalcin (calcitonin-human), 271
ciclopirox (Loprox), 444t, 719t
  Canadian trade name for, 749
Cidomycin (gentamicin), as Canadian trade
    name, 751

cigarette smoking
  as carcinogen, 681t
  estrogen and, 300
  oral contraceptives and, 300
  pregnancy and, 727
cilastatin and imipenem (Primaxin), 411
  Canadian trade name for, 751
  lactation and, 737t
  pregnancy and, 729t
Ciloxan (ciprofloxacin ophthalmic solution), 705t
Ciloxin (ciprofloxacin), as Canadian trade name, 749
cimetidine (Tagamet), 640–641, 644, 645
  Canadian trade name for, 749
  lactation and, 738t
  pregnancy and, 730t
Cinobac (cinoxacin), 412, 421
  lactation and, 737t
cinoxacin (Cinobac), 412, 421
  lactation and, 737t
Cipro (ciprofloxacin), 412
  as Canadian trade name, 749
ciprofloxacin (Cipro), 412
  Canadian trade name for, 749
ciprofloxacin ophthalmic solution (Ciloxan), 705t
circulation, maternal-placental-fetal, 726–727
circulatory system, in respiration, 512
cisapride (Propulsid), 670t, 699
  Canadian trade name for, 749
cisplatin (Platinol), 686t
  Canadian trade name for, 749
cis-platinum, Canadian trade name for, 749
Citanest (prilocaine), 156t
  as Canadian trade name, 753
citrate and potassium bicarbonate (K-Lyte), 355
Citro-Mag (magnesium citrate), as Canadian trade name, 751
Citrotein, 324
Citrucel (methylcellulose), 652t
  as Canadian trade name, 752
cladribine (Leustatin), 688t
Claforan (cefotaxime), 392t
  as Canadian trade name, 749
clarithromycin (Biaxin), 407, 408
  Canadian trade name for, 749
Claritin (loratadine), 525, 528t
  as Canadian trade name, 751
clavulanate-ticarcillin (Timentin), 383t
Clavulin (amoxicillin and potassium clavulanate), as Canadian trade name, 748
clemastine, Canadian trade name for, 749
clemastine fumarate (Tavist), 527t
Cleocin (clindamycin), 413
Cleocin Pediatric (clindamycin palmitate hydrochloride), 413
clidinium bromide (Quarzan), 214t
clindamycin (Cleocin), 413
  Canadian trade name for, 749
  pregnancy and, 729t
clindamycin palmitate hydrochloride (Cleocin Pediatric), 413
clinical trials, 5
Clinoril (sulindac), 70, 71
  as Canadian trade name, 753
  indications for, 68, 68t
clioquinol, Canadian trade name for, 751
Clistin (carbinoxamine maleate), 527t
clobetasol (Temovate), 719t
clocortolone (Cloderm), 719t
Cloderm (clocortolone), 719t
clofibrate (Atromid-S), 628t, 630
  Canadian trade name for, 749
clomipramine (Anafranil), 90, 92
  Canadian trade name for, 749

clonazepam (Klonopin), 91t, 127–128
  Canadian trade name for, 749
clonidine and chlorthalidone (Combipres), 593t
clonidine (Catapres), 591t
  Canadian trade name for, 749
  lactation and, 738t
  pregnancy and, 730t
clorazepate (Tranxene), 91t, 128
  Canadian trade name for, 749
Clorpactin sodium (sodium oxychlorosene), 716t
Clotrimaderm (clotrimazole), as Canadian trade name, 749
clotrimazole (Gyne-Lotrimin, Lotrimin, Mycelex), 444t, 719t
  Canadian trade name for, 749
cloxacillin (Tegopen), 381, 382t
  Canadian trade name for, 749
clozapine (Clozaril), 103–104
  Canadian trade name for, 749
Clozaril (clozapine), 103–104
  as Canadian trade name, 749
coagulation
  estrogens and, 298
  factors in, 614t
  liver and, 608
  phases of, 613–613
coal tar (Balnetar, Zetar), 720t
  Canadian trade name for, 749
cobalt, 351t
cocaine, 156t. See also drug abuse
  abuse of, 165
    treatment of, 174–175
  effects of, 169
  pregnancy and, 727
coccidioidomycosis, 442, 443
codeine, 55–56
  as antitussive, 535t, 536t–537t
  in geriatrics, 539
Codone (hydrocodone), 56
Cogentin (benztropine), 137t, 216
  as Canadian trade name, 748
Cognex (tacrine), 744t
Colace (docusate), 652t
  as Canadian trade name, 750
  lactation and, 738t
colaspase, Canadian trade name for, 748
Colax-C (docusate calcium), as Canadian trade name, 750
Colax-S (docusate sodium), as Canadian trade name, 750
colchicine, 71–72
  in hyperuricemia, 76
cold remedies, 534, 536t–537t
  administration of, 538, 539
  adverse effects of, 540
  client teaching with, 541
  combination, 536t–537t
  description of, 534
  drug interactions with, 540–541
  in geriatrics, 539
  nursing actions for, 539–541
  nursing process for, 537–538
  in pediatrics, 539
  selection of, 538
  therapeutic effects of, 539–540
Colestid (colestipol), 628t, 630, 663t
  as Canadian trade name, 749
colestipol (Colestid), 628t, 630, 663t
  Canadian trade name for, 749
colfosceril (Exosurf), 743t
colistin sulfate (Coly-Mycin S), 662t
collagenase (Santyl), 720t
colloidal oatmeal (Aveeno), 720t
colony-stimulating factors (CSF), 468t, 468–469, 486–487
  preparations of, 489t
Colovage (polyethylene glycol-electrolyte solution), 652t

Coly-Mycin S (colistin sulfate), 662t
CoLyte (polyethylene glycol-electrolyte solution), 652t
Comalose-R (lactulose), as Canadian trade name, 751
Combantrin (pyrantel pamoate), as Canadian trade name, 753
Combipres (clonidine and chlorthalidone), 593t
Compazine (prochlorperazine), 102t, 670t
Compleat, 322
complement, in inflammation and immunity, 7
compliance, pulmonary, 512
Comprehensive Drug Abuse Prevention and Control Act of 1970, 4
Comtrex, 536t
conductivity, cardiac, 560–561
Congest (Estrogens), as Canadian trade name, 750
congestive heart failure
  antacids in, 640
  description of, 548
  diet and, 553
  principles of therapy for, 553
  treatment of, 549–558. See also cardiotonic-inotropic drugs
conjugated estrogens (Premarin), 301t
conjunctivitis, 700. See also ophthalmic drugs
constipation
  description of, 651
  in pregnancy, 732
Contac, 536t
contact dermatitis, 713
contraceptives, oral, 304t. See also oral contraceptives
controlled substances
  anorexiants as, 322
  benzodiazepines as, 90
  categories of, 5b
  storage and dispensing of, 21
Controlled Substances Act, 4, 5
copper, 351t
Coradur (isosorbide dinitrate), as Canadian trade name, 751
Cordarone (amiodarone), 565, 568
  as Canadian trade name, 748
Cordran (flurandrenolide), 719t
Corgard (nadolol), 198, 199t, 200, 575, 592t
  as Canadian trade name, 752
  lactation and, 738t
Coricidin, 536t
Coricidin D, 536t
corneal ulcers, 700. See also ophthalmic drugs
Coronex (isosorbide dinitrate), as Canadian trade name, 751
Cortacet (hydrocortisone), as Canadian trade name, 751
Cortate (hydrocortisone), as Canadian trade name, 751
Cortef (hydrocortisone), 241t
  as Canadian trade name, 751
Cortenema (hydrocortisone), as Canadian trade name, 751
corticosteroids, 236–251, 241t–242t
  administration of, 247–248
    routes for, 246
  adrenal sex hormones as, 238
  adverse effects of, 248–249
  as antiemetics, 669
  in bronchoconstrictive disorders, 515, 517–519
  client teaching with, 244–245, 250–251
  contraindications to, 243
  dermatologic, 719t
    topical, 722

corticosteroids (*continued*)
　dosage for, 245–246
　drug interactions with, 249–250
　endogenous, 236–238
　in geriatrics, 247
　glucocorticoids as, 237–238
　for immunosuppression, 498
　　dosage of, 503
　　selection of, 502
　indications for, 240, 243
　individual, 241t–242t
　lactation and, 738t
　mechanisms of action with, 239–240
　mineralocorticoids as, 238
　nursing actions for, 247–251
　nursing process for, 243–245
　in ocular disorders, 701, 706t
　in pediatrics, 247
　in pregnancy, 734
　pregnancy and, 731t
　principles of therapy with, 245–247
　risk-benefit factors in, 245
　scheduling of, 246–247
　secretion of, 236–237
　selection of, 245
　therapeutic effects of, 248
corticotropin (ACTH, Acthar), 230
corticotropin-releasing hormone, 228
Corticreme (hydrocortisone), as Canadian
　　trade name, 751
Cortifoam (hydrocortisone), as Canadian
　　trade name, 751
Cortiment (hydrocortisone), as Canadian
　　trade name, 751
cortisol, endogenous, 237
cortisone, endogenous, 237
cortisone (Cortone), 241t
　Canadian trade name for, 749
Cortoderm (hydrocortisone), as Canadian
　　trade name, 751
Cortone (cortisone), 241t
　as Canadian trade name, 749
Cortril (hydrocortisone), 719t
Cortrosyn (cosyntropin), 230
Corzide (nadolol and bendroflumethiazide),
　　593t
Cosmegen (actinomycin D, dactinomycin),
　　687
　as Canadian trade name, 749
cosyntropin (Cortrosyn), 230
Cotazym (pancreatin or pancrelipase),
　　663t
Cotazym (pancrelipase), as Canadian trade
　　name, 752
co-trimoxazole, Canadian trade name for,
　　753
CoTylenol cold formula, 536t
CoTylenol liquid, 536t
cough. *See also* antitussives
　defined, 533
　remedies for, 534, 536t–537t
Coumadin (warfarin)
　as Canadian trade name, 754
　lactation and, 737t
　pregnancy and, 730t
crack. *See* cocaine
creams, dermatologic, 722
Creon (pancrelipase), as Canadian trade
　　name, 752
cromolyn (Intal, Nasalcrom, Opticrom),
　　519, 704t
　Canadian trade name for, 749
cross-tolerance, drug, 18
crotamiton (Eurax), 455
　Canadian trade name for, 749
crystalline amino acid solutions (Aminosyn,
　　Freamine), 324
Crystodigin (digitoxin), 549, 551, 554
CSF. *See* colony-stimulating factors

Cuprimine (penicillamine), 354
　as Canadian trade name, 752
Cushing's disease, 239
cyanocobalamin (vitamin B$_{12}$) (Rubramin),
　　334t
　Canadian trade name for, 749
　imbalance of, 338t
　routes and dosage ranges for, 340t
cyclandelate (Cyclospasmol), 629t
　Canadian trade name for, 749
cyclizine hydrochloride (Marezine hydro-
　　chloride), 528t
cyclizine (Marezine), 670t
　Canadian trade name for, 749
cyclobenzaprine (Flexeril), 146t
　Canadian trade name for, 749
Cyclocort (amcinonide), 719t
　as Canadian trade name, 748
Cyclogyl (cyclopentolate)
　as Canadian trade name, 749
　in ocular disorders, 703t
　in pediatrics, 218
cyclooxygenase, 67
cyclopentolate (Cyclogyl)
　Canadian trade name for, 749
　in ocular disorders, 703t
　in pediatrics, 218
cyclophosphamide (Cytoxan), 686t
　Canadian trade name for, 749
cyclopropane, 153t
cycloserine (Seromycin), 429, 430
Cyclospasmol (cyclandelate), 629t
　as Canadian trade name, 749
cyclosporine, 499. *See also* immuno-
　　suppressants
　dosage of, 503
　selection of, 502
cyclosporine (Sandimmune), 497t
　Canadian trade name for, 749
Cyklokapron (tranexamic acid), 618
　as Canadian trade name, 754
Cylert (pemoline), 177
cyproheptadine (Periactin), 529t
　Canadian trade name for, 749
Cytadren (aminoglutethimide), 688t
　as Canadian trade name, 748
cytarabine (ARA-C, cytosine arabinoside)
　　(Cytosar-U), 686t
　Canadian trade name for, 749
CytoGam (cytomegalovirus immune globu-
　　lin, IV, human (GMV-IGIV)), 479t
cytokines
　in immune response, 460, 467, 468t
　in inflammation and immunity, 7
cytomegalovirus immune globulin, IV,
　　human (GMV-IGIV) (CytoGam), 479t
Cytomel (liothyronine), as Canadian trade
　　name, 751
cytoprotective agents, 640
Cytosar (cytarabine, cytosine arabinoside),
　　as Canadian trade name, 749
Cytosar-U (ARA-C, cytarabine, cytosine
　　arabinoside), 686t
cytosine arabinoside (ARA-C, cytarabine)
　　(Cytosar-U), 686t
　Canadian trade name for, 749
Cytotec (misoprostol), 639, 641–642
　as Canadian trade name, 752
　in geriatrics, 646
cytotoxic drugs. *See also* immuno-
　　suppressants
　for immunosuppression, 498–499
Cytovene (ganciclovir), 435, 436t, 437
　as Canadian trade name, 750
Cytoxan (cyclophosphamide), 686t
　as Canadian trade name, 749

**D**

dacarbazine (DTIC-Dome), 688t–689t
　Canadian trade name for, 749

dactinomycin (actinomycin D) (Cosmegen),
　　687t
　Canadian trade name for, 749
Dakin's solution modified (sodium
　　hypochlorite solution, diluted), 716t
Dalacin (clindamycin), as Canadian trade
　　name, 749
Dalgan (dezocine), 57
Dalmane (flurazepam), 82t, 83
　as Canadian trade name, 750
danazol (Danocrine), 312t
　as Canadian trade name, 749
Danocrine (danazol), 312t
Dantrium (dantrolene), 145, 146t
　as Canadian trade name, 749
dantrolene (Dantrium), 145, 146t
　Canadian trade name for, 749
Daranide (dichlorphenamide), in ocular dis-
　　orders, 703t
Daraprim (pyrimethamine), 453
　as Canadian trade name, 753
Darbid (isopropamide chloride), 214t
Daricon (oxyphencyclimine bromide), 214t
Darvon (propoxyphene), 57
daunorubicin (daunomycin) (Cerubidin),
　　687t
　Canadian trade name for, 749
DCB. *See* dichlorbenzidine
DDAVP (desmopressin acetate), 231
ddC. *See* dideoxycytidine
ddI. *See* Videx
D-Dur (potassium chloride), as Canadian
　　trade name, 753
debridement, enzymes in, 715
Decaderm (dexamethasone), 719t
Decadron (dexamethasone), 241t, 719t
　as antiemetic, 669
　as Canadian trade name, 749
　lactation and, 738t
Decadron Phosphate (dexamethasone),
　　706t
Decadron Respihaler (dexamethasone
　　sodium phosphate), 241t
Decadron Turbinaire (dexamethasone
　　sodium phosphate), 241t
Decadron with Xylocaine (dexamethasone
　　and lidocaine), 241t
Deca-Durabolin (nandrolone), 312t
　as Canadian trade name, 752
Declomycin (demeclocycline), 403t
　as Canadian trade name, 749
defecation, 651
deferoxamine, Canadian trade name for,
　　749
deferoxamine mesylate (Desferal), 354
Dehydral (methenamine), as Canadian
　　trade name, 752
Delalutin (hydroxyprogesterone caproate),
　　303t
Delatestryl (testosterone), 312t
　as Canadian trade name, 753
Delestrogen (estradiol), 302t
　as Canadian trade name, 750
delivery
　anesthetics for, 735
　ergot alkaloids following, 735, 735t
Delta-Cortef (prednisolone), 242t
delta cortisone, Canadian trade name for, 753
Delta-D (cholecalciferol), 268t
delta hydrocortisone, Canadian trade name
　　for, 753
Deltasone (prednisone), 242t
　as Canadian trade name, 753
　hypercalcemia and, 271
　lactation and, 738t
demecarium bromide (Humorsol), in ocular
　　disorders, 702t
demeclocycline (Declomycin), 403t
　Canadian trade name for, 749

demelanizing drugs, 715, 719t
Demerol (meperidine), 56
  as Canadian trade name, 752
  lactation and, 737t
  pregnancy and, 729t
Demulen (ethinyl estradiol and ethyno-
    diol), 304t
  as Canadian trade name, 750
Depakene (valproic acid), 129
  as Canadian trade name, 754
Depen (penicillamine), as Canadian trade
    name, 752
Depo-Estradiol (estradiol cypionate), 301t
Depo-Medrol (methylprednisolone), as
    Canadian trade name, 752
Depo-Provera (medroxyprogesterone),
    303t, 688t
  as Canadian trade name, 751
Depo-Testosterone (testosterone cypio-
    nate), 312t
depression. *See also* antidepressants
  description of, 113
  dysthymic, 113–114
  etiology of, 114
  major, 113
  pharmacologic management of, 114–115,
    116
Dermalar (fluocinolone acetonide), as
    Canadian trade name, 750
dermatitis, types of, 713
dermatologic disorders
  antihistamines for, 526
  corticosteroids in, 240
dermatologic drugs, 712–724
  absorption of, 10
  administration of, 26, 723
    nursing action in, 31
  adverse effects of, 724
  anti-infective drugs as, 714–715
  anti-inflammatory agents as, 715, 719t
  antiseptics as, 714, 716t–718t
  application of, 715
  client teaching with, 724
  demelanizing agents as, 715, 720t
  dosage forms of, 722–723
  emollients as, 715
  enzymes as, 715, 720t
  in geriatrics, 723
  individual, 716t–718t, 719t, 720t
  keratolytic agents as, 715
  melanizing agents as, 715, 720t
  nursing actions for, 723–724
  nursing process for, 715, 718–719, 721
  in pediatrics, 723
  principles of therapy with, 721–723
  selection guidelines for, 721–722
  sunscreens as, 715
  therapeutic effects of, 723–724
  types of, 714–715
dermatophytes, 442
Dermoxyl (benzoyl peroxide), as Canadian
    trade name, 748
DES. *See* diethylstilbestrol
Desenex (undecylenic acid, zinc unde-
    cylenate), 444t, 719t
Desferal (deferoxamine), 354
  as Canadian trade name, 749
desflurane (Suprane), 153t
desipramine
  Canadian trade name for, 749
  therapeutic serum drug concentrations
    for, 746
deslanoside (Cedilanid-D), 551, 554
desmopressin acetate (DDAVP, Stimate),
    231
desonide (Tridesilon), 719t
  Canadian trade name for, 749
desoximetasone (Topicort), 719t
  Canadian trade name for, 749

Desoxyn (methamphetamine), 177
Desquam-X (benzoyl peroxide), as Cana-
    dian trade name, 748
Desyrel (trazodone), 115, 117t
  as Canadian trade name, 754
  pregnancy and, 730t
dexamethasone acetate, 241t
dexamethasone and lidocaine (Decadron
    with Xylocaine), 241t
dexamethasone (Decaderm, Decadron,
    Maxidex), 241t, 706t, 719t
  as antiemetic, 669
  Canadian trade name for, 749
  lactation and, 738t
dexamethasone sodium phosphate
    (Decadron Respihaler, Decadron
    Turbinaire), 241t
dexamphetamine, Canadian trade name
    for, 749
Dexasone (dexamethasone), as Canadian
    trade name, 749
Dexatrim (phenylpropanolamine), 187t,
    322
dexchlorpheniramine, Canadian trade
    name for, 749
dexchlorpheniramine maleate (Po-
    laramine), 527t
Dexedrine (dextroamphetamine), 177
  as Canadian trade name, 749
dextroamphetamine (Dexedrine), 177
  Canadian trade name for, 749
dextromethorphan (Benylin DM), 535t
  Canadian trade name for, 749
dextrose and sodium chloride injection,
    324
dextrose injection, 324
dextrothyroxine (Choloxin), 628t, 630
  in pediatrics, 630
dezocine (Dalgan), 57
DHE (dihydroergotamine mesylate), 72
DiaBeta (glyburide), 284t, 284–285
  as Canadian trade name, 751
diabetes, gestational, 280, 733
diabetes mellitus. *See also* hypoglycemic
    drugs, oral; insulin
  characteristics of, 279
  complications of, 280–282
  drug therapy for, 282, 283t–284t, 284t,
    284–285
  etiology of, 280
  insulin-dependent, 279–280
  non-insulin-dependent, 280
  nursing process for, 285–286
  in pregnancy, 733–734
  principles of therapy for, 287–291
  signs and symptoms of, 280
diabetic ketoacidosis
  insulin therapy for, 289
  principles of therapy for, 289
diabetic nephropathy, 281
diabetogenic hormones, 280
Diabinese (chlorpropamide), 284t, 284–285
Diabinese (chlorpropamide)
  as Canadian trade name, 749
  lactation and, 738t
*Diagnostic and Statistical Manual*
  anxiety in, 89
  depression in, 113
  psychosis in, 99
Dialose (docusate potassium), 652t
Diamox (acetazolamide)
  as Canadian trade name, 748
  glaucoma and, 218
  in ocular disorders, 218, 703t
diarrhea. *See also* antidiarrheals
  antidiarrheal therapy for, 660–666,
    661t–663t
  causes of, 659–660
  types of, 660

Diazemuls (diazepam), as Canadian trade
    name, 749
diazepam (Valium), 90, 91t, 146t
  acute or chronic disorders and, 145
  anesthesia and, 151
  Canadian trade name for, 749
  lactation and, 737t
  in pediatrics, 85, 95
  seizure disorders and, 128
diazoxide (Hyperstat), 592t
  Canadian trade name for, 749
Dibenzyline (phenoxybenzamine), 198
dibucaine (Nupercainal, Nupercaine), 156t
  Canadian trade name for, 749
Dical-D (calcium phosphate dibasic), 268t
dichlorbenzidine (DCB), as carcinogen,
    681t
dichlorphenamide (Daranide), in ocular
    disorders, 703t
diclofenac (Voltaren), 71
  Canadian trade name for, 750
  indications for, 68, 68t
dicloxacillin (Dynapen), 381, 382t
dicyclomine, Canadian trade name for, 750
dicyclomine hydrochloride (Bentyl), 214t
didanosine (Videx), 436t, 437
  Canadian trade name for, 750
dideoxycytidine (ddC) (Zalcitabine), 436t,
    437
Didrex (benzphetamine), 323t
Didronel (etidronate), 271
  as Canadian trade name, 750
dienestrol (DV), 301t
  Canadian trade name for, 750
diet. *See also specific component*; nutritional
    products
  in congestive heart therapy, 553
  constipation and, 656
  drug interactions with, 14
    monoamine oxidase inhibitors, 14,
    115t
  hypokalemia and, 358
diethylpropion (Tenuate), 323t
  Canadian trade name for, 750
diethylstilbestrol (DES) (Stilbestrol), 301t,
    688t
diethylstilbestrol diphosphate
    (Stilphostrol), 301t
difenoxin and atropine sulfate (Motofen),
    661t
diffusion
  defined, 10
  in geriatric patient, 40t
  in pediatric patient, 38t
diflorasone (Florone, Maxiflor), 719t
  Canadian trade name for, 750
Diflucan (fluconazole), 444t
  as Canadian trade name, 750
diflunisal (Dolobid), 69
  Canadian trade name for, 750
  indications for, 68, 68t
Di-Gel, 643t
digestants, 319
digestive system
  drug effects on, 637
  physiology of, 635–637
  secretions of, 636–637
Digibind (digoxin immune fab), as Cana-
    dian trade name, 750
Digitaline (digitoxin), as Canadian trade
    name, 750
digitalis
  atrial flutter and fibrillation and, 567
  congestive heart failure and, 548–559
    contraindications for, 550
    dosage of, 554
    electrolyte balance and, 554
    in geriatrics, 555
    guidelines for, 553–555

digitalis, congestive heart failure and
(*continued*)
indications for, 550
maintenance therapy with, 554
mechanism of action in, 549–550
nursing actions for, 556–558
nursing process for, 551–553
in pediatrics, 555
preparations of, 550–551
toxicity with, 554–555
diuretics and, 607
lactation and, 738t
pregnancy and, 731t
digitoxin (Crystodigin), 549, 551, 554
Canadian trade name for, 750
digoxin immune fab, Canadian trade name
for, 750
digoxin (Lanoxin), 549, 550–551, 553–554
Canadian trade name for, 750
lactation and, 738t
pregnancy and, 731t
therapeutic serum drug concentrations
for, 746
digoxin-specific antibody fragments, Canadian trade name for, 750
dihydroergotamine mesylate (DHE 45), 72
dihydrotachysterol (Hytakerol), 268t
Canadian trade name for, 750
diiodohydroxyquin (Yodoxin), 451
Dilantin (phenytoin), 127
as Canadian trade name, 753
digitalis intoxication and, 564
lactation and, 737t
pregnancy and, 730t
Dilaudid (hydromorphone), 56, 535t
as Canadian trade name, 751
diltiazem (Cardizem, Cardizem SR), 566,
574t, 592t
Canadian trade name for, 750
lactation and, 738t
pregnancy and, 731t
Dimelor (acetohexamide), as Canadian
trade name, 748
dimenhydrinate (Dramamine), 527t, 670t
Canadian trade name for, 750
lactation and, 738t
Dimetane (brompheniramine), 527t
as Canadian trade name, 749
Dimetapp Elixir, 536t
Dimetapp Extentabs, 536t
Dimetapp Tablets, 536t
dinoprostone (prostaglandin E$_2$) (Prostin E$_2$)
Canadian trade name for, 750
pregnancy and, 735t
Diocaine (proparacaine), as Canadian trade
name, 753
Diocarpine (pilocarpine), as Canadian trade
name, 753
Diochloram (chloramphenicol), as Canadian trade name, 749
Diodex (dexamethasone), as Canadian
trade name, 749
Diogent (gentamicin), as Canadian trade
name, 751
Diomycin (erythromycin), as Canadian
trade name, 750
Dionephrine (phenylephrine), as Canadian
trade name, 753
Diopentolate (cyclopentolate), as Canadian
trade name, 749
Diopred (prednisolone), as Canadian trade
name, 753
Diopticon (naphazoline), as Canadian trade
name, 752
Diosulf (sulfacetamide), as Canadian trade
name, 753
Diotrope (tropicamide), as Canadian trade
name, 754

Diovol Ex (aluminum hydroxide gel and
magnesium hydroxide), as Canadian
trade name, 748
diphenhydramine (Benadryl), 84, 137t,
525, 527t, 670t
Canadian trade name for, 750
lactation and, 738t
pregnancy and, 730t
diphenidol (Vontrol), 670t, 699
diphenoxylate and atropine sulfate
(Lomotil), 661t
diphenoxylate (Lomotil)
Canadian trade name for, 750
lactation and, 738t
pregnancy and, 730t
diphtheria and tetanus toxoids, adsorbed
(pediatric type), 477t
diphtheria and tetanus toxoids, adsorbed
(adult type), 478t
diphtheria and tetanus toxoids and acellular
pertussis vaccine (DTaP) (Acel-
Imune, Tripedia), 477t
diphtheria and tetanus toxoids and whole-
cell pertussis and *Haemophilus influenzae* type B conjugate vaccines (DTwP-
HibTITER) (Tetramune), 477t
diphtheria and tetanus toxoids and whole-
cell pertussis vaccine (DTwP) (Tri-Immunol), 477t
diphtheria antitoxin, 480t
dipivefrin (Propine)
Canadian trade name for, 750
in ocular disorders, 702t
Diprivan (propofol), 154t
as Canadian trade name, 753
Diprosone (betamethasone), as Canadian
trade name, 748
dipyridamole (Persantine), 615, 616
Canadian trade name for, 750
Disipal (orphenadrine), 137t
as Canadian trade name, 752
disopyramide (Norpace), 563, 568
Canadian trade name for, 750
lactation and, 737t
pregnancy and, 729t
therapeutic serum drug concentrations
for, 746
displacement, pharmacologic, 15
distribution
defined, 10–11
in geriatric patient, 40t
in pediatric patient, 38t
Ditropan (oxybutynin), in pediatrics, 218
diuretics, 601–612
administration of, 609
adverse effects of, 610–611
client teaching for, 611
in congestive heart failure, 549
description of, 601, 604–605
digitalis with, 607
dosage of, 607
drug interactions with, 611
in edema, 607
in geriatrics, 609
hypertension and, 590, 593t, 595
lactation and, 738t
loop, 602t, 605
nursing actions for, 609–611
nursing process for, 606–607
in ocular disorders, 703t. *See also* ophthalmic drugs
osmotic, 606
in pediatrics, 609
potassium imbalances and, 607–608
potassium-sparing, 602t–603t, 605–606
in pregnancy, 734
pregnancy and, 731t
principles of therapy with, 607
renal physiology and, 601, 603–604

selection of, 607
therapeutic effects of, 609
thiazide, 602t, 605
Diuril (chlorothiazide), 602t
Dixarit (clonidine), as Canadian trade
name, 749
dobutamine (Dobutrex), 187t, 582
Canadian trade name for, 750
Dobutrex (dobutamine), 187t, 582
as Canadian trade name, 750
docusate calcium (Surfak), 652t
Canadian trade name for, 750
docusate potassium (Dialose), 652t
docusate sodium (Colace, Doxinate), 652t
Canadian trade name for, 750
lactation and, 738t
Dolobid (diflunisal), 69
as Canadian trade name, 750
indications for, 68, 68t
Dolophine (methadone), 56
Donnagel (kaolin, pectin, atropine sulfate,
hyoscyamine sulfate, hyoscine hydrobromide, alcohol), 663t
dopamine, endogenous, 48, 49
dopamine (Intropin), 187t, 582
Canadian trade name for, 750
dopaminergic drugs, in Parkinson's disease,
136, 137–139
Dopram (doxapram), 177
Doral (quazepam), 82t, 83
dornase alfa (Pulmozyme), 743t
Doryx (doxycycline), as Canadian trade
name, 750
dosage
abbreviations for, 21t
International System of Units, 745
calculation of
equivalents in, 22t
mathematical, 22–23
in pediatrics, 38–39
systems of measurement in, 22, 22t
defined, 14
forms of, 22
general considerations and, 20
International System of Units in, 745
lethal, 14
toxic, 14
doxacurium (Nuromax), 155t
Canadian trade name for, 750
doxapram (Dopram), 177
Doxate-C (docusate calcium), as Canadian
trade name, 750
Doxate-S (docusate sodium), as Canadian
trade name, 750
doxazosin (Cardura), 591t
Canadian trade name for, 750
doxepin (Adapin, Sinequan), 117t
Canadian trade name for, 750
Doxinate (docusate sodium), 652t
doxorubicin (Adriamycin), 687t
Canadian trade name for, 750
Doxycin (doxycycline), as Canadian trade
name, 750
doxycycline (Vibramycin), 403t
Canadian trade name for, 750
Dramamine (dimenhydrinate), 527t, 670t
lactation and, 738t
Drisdol (ergocalciferol), 268t
as Canadian trade name, 750
Dristan, 536t
Drixoral, 537t
dronabinol (Marinol), 670t, 699
droperidol and fentanyl (Innovar), 154t
droperidol (Inapsine), 670t, 699
Canadian trade name for, 750
drug abuse, 163–175

alcohol and. *See* alcohol, abuse of
amphetamines and, 164
anabolic steroids and, 310
androgenic steroids and, 310
anorexiants and, 319
barbiturates and, 164
benzodiazepines and, 164
cocaine and, 165
defined, 163
dependence versus, 163
hallucinogens and, 165
marijuana and, 164–165
nursing process for, 170–171
opiates and, 165
prevention of, 171–172
principles of therapy for, 171–175
treatment of, 172–175
types of, 164–166
volatile solvents and, 165–166
drug administration, 20–31
cautions for, 20
drug preparation form and, 22
general considerations for, 20
nursing actions for
general, 27–32
intramuscular injections and, 30
intravenous injections and, 30–31
nasal medications and, 32
nasogastric tube and, 29
ophthalmic medications and, 31
oral medications and, 28–29
otic medications and, 32
rectal suppositories and, 32
subcutaneous injections and, 29–30
topical medications and, 31
vaginal medications, 32
times of, abbreviations in, 21t
unit-dose system for, 21
drug dependence. *See also* drug abuse
alcohol-type, 164
amphetamine-type, 164
barbiturate-type, 164
benzodiazepine-type, 164
cocaine-type, 165
defined, 18, 163
hallucinogen-type, 165
marijuana-type, 164–165
opiate-type, 165
physical, 163
psychological, 163
types of, 164–166
volatile solvent-type, 165–166
*Drug Facts and Comparisons*, 4
drugs
absorption of, 10
pathologic conditions and, 17
action of
cellular physiology in, 6, 8
nonreceptor, 13
receptor theory of, 12–13
variables affecting, 13–17
administration of
routes for, 14, 24–26
times for, abbreviations for, 21t
adverse effects of, 17–18
age and, 15–16
approval processes for, 4–5
body weight and, 16
in children, 38–39
Canadian trade names for, 748–754
controlled
dispensing of, 21
laws and standards for, 4, 5
diffusion of, 10
distribution of, 10–11, 17
dosage. *See* dosage
dosage forms of, 22
in etiology of psychiatric symptoms, 49
excretion of, 11–12

gender and, 17
genetic and ethnic characteristics and, 16
information sources for, 4
interactions with
diet in, 14
drug, 14–15
laws regulating, 4, 5
Canadian, 747
metabolism of, 11
nomenclature for, 3–4
orders for, 21
pharmacodynamics and, 12–13
pharmacokinetics and, 10–12
preparations and dosage forms of, 22
prototypes for, 33–34
psychological considerations, 17
routes of administration for, 14, 24–26
serum half-life of, 12
sources of, 3
standards for, 4
therapeutic serum concentrations of, selected, 746
tolerance to, 18
transport of, 10
drug therapy
administration in, 41
adverse reactions in, 41–42
client teaching with, 42
dosage considerations in, 41–43
drug selection and, 37–38
general guidelines in, 37
geriatric, 15–16, 40t, 40–41
nursing actions for, 41–43
nursing process in, 33–43
pediatric, 15, 38t, 38–40
psychological considerations in, 17
DTaP. *See* diphtheria and tetanus toxoids and acellular pertussis vaccine
DTIC (dacarbazine), as Canadian trade name, 749
DTIC-Dome (dacarbazine), 688t–689t
DTwP. *See* diphtheria and tetanus toxoids and whole-cell pertussis vaccine
DTwP-HibTITER. *See* diphtheria and tetanus toxoids and whole-cell pertussis and *Haemophilus influenzae* type B conjugate vaccines
Dulcolax (bisacodyl), 652t
as Canadian trade name, 748
pregnancy and, 731t
Durabolin (nandrolone), 312t
as Canadian trade name, 752
Duragesic (fentanyl), as Canadian trade name, 750
Duralith (lithium), as Canadian trade name, 751
Duranest (etidocaine), 156t
Duretic (methyclothiazide), as Canadian trade name, 752
Duricef (cefadroxil), 390t
as Canadian trade name, 749
Duvoid (bethanechol), as Canadian trade name, 748
DV (dienestrol), 301t
Dyazide (hydrochlorothiazide and triamterene), 603t
Dyazide (triamterene)
lactation and, 738t
pregnancy and, 731t
Dyclone (dyclonine), 156t
dyclonine (Dyclone), 156t
Dymelor (acetohexamide), 284t, 284–285
DynaCirc (isradipine), 574t, 592t
Dynapen (dicloxacillin), 382t
Dyrenium (triamterene), 603t
as Canadian trade name, 754
lactation and, 738t
dysmenorrhea, drugs used in, 68t
dysthymia, 113–114

**E**
ear medications, instillation of, 32
echothiophate, Canadian trade name for, 750
echothiophate iodide (Phospholine Iodide), in ocular disorders, 702t
eclampsia, in pregnancy, 732
econazole (Spectazole), 444t, 719t
Canadian trade name for, 750
Econopred (prednisolone acetate), 706t
Ecostatin (econazole), as Canadian trade name, 750
Edecrin (ethacrynic acid), 602t
as Canadian trade name, 750
lactation and, 738t
edema
description of, 604
diuretics for, 607
edrophonium (Tensilon), 208
Canadian trade name for, 750
E.E.S. (erythromycin ethylsuccinate), 408t
EES (erythromycin), as Canadian trade name, 750
Effersyllium (psyllium preparations), 652t, 663t
Efudex (fluorouracil), 686t–687t, 720t
as Canadian trade name, 750
Elase (fibrinolysin-desoxyribonuclease), 720t
as Canadian trade name, 750
Elavil (amitriptyline), 117t
as Canadian trade name, 748
lactation and, 737t
pregnancy and, 730t
Eldepryl (selegiline), 136, 139
as Canadian trade name, 753
Eldopaque (hydroquinone), as Canadian trade name, 751
Eldoquin (hydroquinone), 720t
as Canadian trade name, 751
electrolytes, 346–365. *See also specific electrolyte*
description of, 346, 348
in geriatrics, 361
imbalances of, 348t, 348–350, 349t, 353t
individual, 347t
multiple preparations of, 356
in pediatrics, 361
elemental diets, for oral or tube feeding, 322–324
elimination half-time, 12
Elixophyllin (theophylline anhydrous), 518t
Elspar (asparaginase), 688t
Eltor (pseudoephedrine), as Canadian trade name, 753
Eltroxin (levothyroxine), as Canadian trade name, 751
Emete-Con (benzquinamide), 670t, 699
emetine hydrochloride, 450–451
Emetrol (phosphorated carbohydrate solutions), 671, 671t
Eminase (anistreplase), 615, 617
emollients, dermatologic, 715
emphysema. *See* chronic obstructive pulmonary disease (COPD)
E-Mycin (erythromycin), 408t
as Canadian trade name, 750
pregnancy and, 729t
enalapril and hydrochlorothiazide (Vaseretic), 593t
enalapril (Vasotec), 591t
Canadian trade name for, 750
lactation and, 737t
enanthate and fluphenazine decanoate (Prolixin decanoate; Prolixin enanthate), 101t
Endep (amitriptyline), 117t

endocrine system
  alcohol abuse and, 168
  disorders of
    corticosteroids in, 240
  interaction with nervous system, 225–226
  physiology of, 225–227
endometrial cancer, drug therapy for, 301t–302t, 305
endometriosis, drug therapy for, 303t, 305
endorphins, 54
Enduron (methyclothiazide), 602t
Enfamil, 324
enflurane (Ethrane), 153t
  Canadian trade name for, 750
Engerix-B (hepatitis B vaccine), 473t–474t
  as Canadian trade name, 751
enkephalins, 54
Enlon (edrophonium), as Canadian trade name, 750
enoxacin (Penetrex), 412
enoxaparin (Lovenox), 616
Ensure, 322
Entacyl (piperazine), as Canadian trade name, 753
enteral feedings
  administration of, 331–332
  elemental diets for, 322–324
  nursing actions for, 329
  in pediatrics, 328
  therapeutic effects of, 330
  for undernutrition, 326
    guidelines for, 326–327
enteric-coated tablets or capsules, 22
enterobiasis (pinworm infections), 449
Entozyme (pancreatin), as Canadian trade name, 752
Entrophen (aspirin), as Canadian trade name, 748
entsufon sodium emulsion and hexa-
    chlorophene (pHisoHex), 717t
enzymes
  dermatologic, 715, 719t
  hepatic, 11
  pancreatic, 325, 330, 331
ephedrine, 187t, 188, 516
ephedrine hydrochloride, theophylline, and
    phenobarbital (Tedral), 518t
ephedrine sulfate, 535t
ephedrine sulfate, theophylline, and hy-
    droxyzine hydrochloride (Marax), 518t
epidural anesthesia, 151
  administration of, 157
Epifrin (epinephrine hydrochloride),
  in ocular disorders, 702t
epilepsy, 125–126. See also anticonvulsants
epinephrine (Adrenalin, Bronkaid), 49,
    187t, 187–188, 515–516
  anaphylaxis and, 190
  in bronchoconstrictive disorders, 515–516
  Canadian trade name for, 750
  cardiopulmonary resuscitation and, 190
  hypotension and shock and, 582
  lactation and, 737t
  in pediatrics, 191
epinephrine hydrochloride (Epifrin, Glau-
    con), in ocular disorders, 702t
EpiPen (epinephrine), as Canadian trade name, 750
epoetin alfa (Epogen, Procrit), 486, 743t
Epogen (epoetin alfa), 486, 743t
Equanil (meprobamate), 92
Ergamisol (levamisole), 689t
ergocalciferol (Drisdol), 268t
  Canadian trade name for, 750
Ergomar (ergotamine), 72
  as Canadian trade name, 750
ergometrine, Canadian trade name for, 750

ergonovine (Ergotrate)
  Canadian trade name for, 750
  pregnancy and, 735t
ergotamine and caffeine (Cafergot), 72
  Canadian trade name for, 750
ergotamine (Ergomar), 72
  Canadian trade name for, 750
Ergotrate (ergonovine)
  as Canadian trade name, 750
  pregnancy and, 735t
Erthrocin (erythromycin), as Canadian trade name, 750
Erybid (erythromycin), as Canadian trade name, 750
Eryc (erythromycin), as Canadian trade name, 750
Eryped (erythromycin), as Canadian trade name, 750
erythrityl tetranitrate (Cardilate), 575
Erythrocin stearate (erythromycin stearate), 408t
Erythromid (erythromycin), as Canadian trade name, 750
erythromycin, 407–410
  administration of, 409
  adverse effects of, 409–410
  client teaching with, 410
  contraindications to, 408
  drug interactions with, 409, 410
  in geriatrics, 409
  indications for, 407
  individual, 408
  lactation and, 737t
  nursing actions for, 409–410
  in pediatrics, 409
  pregnancy and, 729t
  preparations of, 408t
  principles of therapy with, 408–409
  therapeutic effects of, 409
erythromycin (E-Mycin), Canadian trade name for, 750
erythromycin estolate (Ilosone), 408t
erythromycin ethylsuccinate (E.E.S.), 408t
erythromycin (Ilotycin ophthalmic), in ocu-
    lar disorders, 705t
erythromycin lactobionate, 408t
erythromycin stearate (Erythrocin stearate), 408t
Eserine Sulfate (physostigmine sulfate),
    in ocular disorders, 702t–703t
Esidrix (hydrochlorothiazide), 602t
esmolol (Brevibloc), 198, 199t, 200, 565
  Canadian trade name for, 750
esophagus, 635
Estar (coal tar), as Canadian trade name, 749
estazolam (ProSom), 82t, 83
esterified estrogens (Estratab), 301t
Estinyl (ethinyl estradiol), 302t, 688t
  as Canadian trade name, 750
Estrace (estradiol), 301t
Estraderm (estradiol), 302t
  as Canadian trade name, 750
estradiol cypionate (Depo-Estradiol), 301t
estradiol (Estrace, Estraderm), 301t, 302t
  Canadian trade name for, 750
estradiol valerate (Delestrogen), 302t
Estradurin (polyestradiol phosphate), 302t
Estrase (estradiol), as Canadian trade name, 750
Estratab (esterfied estrogens), 301t
estrogens
  administration of, 306
  adverse reactions to, 306–307
  in cancer, 305
  as carcinogenic, 681t, 684
  client teaching with, 307
  conjugated, Canadian trade name for, 750
  contraindications for, 299–300

drug interactions with, 307
  esterified, Canadian trade name for, 750
  in geriatrics, 305
  indications for, 299
  mechanism of action with, 299
  in menopause, 299, 303, 305
  nursing actions for, 306–307
  nursing process for, 300
  in oral contraceptives, 305
  in pediatrics, 305
  preparations of, 298–299, 301t–302t
  principles of therapy with, 302–303, 305
  production and function of, 297–298
estrone (Theelin), 302t
  Canadian trade name for, 750
estropipate (Ogen), 302t
  Canadian trade name for, 750
Estrovis (quinestrol), 302t
ethacrynic acid (Edecrin), 602t
  Canadian trade name for, 750
  lactation and, 738t
ethambutol (Myambutol), 429
  Canadian trade name for, 750
ethanolamines, 525, 527t–528t. See also
    antihistamines
ethanol (ethyl alcohol), 716t
ethchlorvynol (Placidyl), 82t, 83
ethinyl estradiol and ethynodiol, Canadian
    trade name for, 750
ethinyl estradiol and levonorgestrel, Cana-
    dian trade name, for, 750
ethinyl estradiol and norgestrel, Canadian
    trade name for, 750
ethinyl estradiol (Estinyl, Feminone)
  Canadian trade name for, 750
  in malignancy, 688t
  in oral contraceptives, 304t
  routes and dosage ranges for, 302t
ethionamide (Trecator SC), 429, 430
Ethmozine (moricizine), 564–565
ethopropazine (Parsidol), 137t
  Canadian trade name for, 750
ethosuximide, Canadian trade name for, 750
ethosuximide (Zarontin), 128
  therapeutic serum drug concentrations
    for, 746
Ethrane (enflurane), 153t
  as Canadian trade name, 750
ethyl alcohol (ethanol), 716t
ethynodiol and ethinyl estradiol, Canadian
    trade name for, 750
etidocaine (Duranest), 156t
etidronate (Didronel), 271
  Canadian trade name for, 750
etodolac (Lodine), 70
  indications for, 68, 68t
etomidate (Amidate), 153t
etoposide (VePesid), 687t
  Canadian trade name for, 750
etretinate (Tegison), 743t
Euflex (flutamide), as Canadian trade name, 750
Euglucon (glyburide), as Canadian trade name, 751
Eulexin (flutamide), 688t
Eurax (crotamiton), 455
  as Canadian trade name, 749
Euthroid (liotrix), 256–257
excretion, defined, 11–12
Exelderm (sulconazole), 444t
Ex-Lax (phenolphthalein), 652t
Exna (benzthiazide), 602t
Exosurf (colfosceril), 743t
expectorants, 534, 535t
extrapyramidal system
  anticholinergics in, 218
  structure and function of, 51

eye
  disorders of, 700. *See also* ophthalmic drugs
  structures of, 699–700

**F**

Factrel (gonadorelin hydrochloride), 230
famotidine (Pepcid), 641
  Canadian trade name for, 750
  lactation and, 738t
Fastin (phentermine), 323t
  as Canadian trade name, 753
fat emulsions (Intralipid, Liposyn), 317,
    324, 327
fats, 321t. *See also* lipids
  metabolism of
    insulin effect on, 279
    liver and, 636
fat-soluble vitamins, 334t, 341–342
  client teaching with, 341
  imbalances of, 337t, 341
    preparations of, 340t
    nursing actions with, 343–344
fecal impaction, treatment of, 656
Federal Drug Administration, drug cate-
    gories and pregnancy, 728t
Federal Food, Drug and Cosmetics Act of
    1938, 4
Feen-a-Mint (phenolphthalein), 652t
Felbatol (felbamate), 126–127
Feldene (piroxicam), 71
  as Canadian trade name, 753
  indications for, 68, 68t
felodipine (Plendil), 574t, 592t
  Canadian trade name for, 750
Feminone (ethinyl estradiol), 302t
Femotrone (progesterone), 303t
Femstat (butoconazole), 444t
fenfluramine (Pondimin), 323t
  Canadian trade name for, 750
fenoprofen (Nalfon), 68–69
  Canadian trade name for, 750
  indications for, 68, 68t
fentanyl and droperidol (Innovar), 154t
fentanyl (Sublimaze), 55
  Canadian trade name for, 750
Feosol (ferrous sulfate), 354–355
Fer-In-Sol (ferrous sulfate), as Canadian
    trade name, 750
Fernisolone (prednisolone acetate), 242t
Fero-Grad (ferrous sulfate), as Canadian
    trade name, 750
ferrous gluconate (Fergon), 354
ferrous sulfate (Feosol), 354–355
  Canadian trade name for, 750
fetus
  drug effects on, 727–728, 728t
  immune function in, 469
  testosterone in development of, 309
  therapeutics in, 728
fever
  analgesic-antipyretic-antiinflammatory
    drugs in, 67, 68t
  definition of, 67
FiberCon (polycarbophil), 652t
Fibrepur (psyllium hydrophilic muciloid),
    as Canadian trade name, 753
fibrillation. *See also* antiarrhythmic drugs
  atrial, 561
  ventricular, 562
fibrinolysin-desoxyribonuclease (Elase),
    720t
fibrinolysin-desoxyribonuclease (Elase),
    Canadian trade name, for, 750
field block, 151
filgrastim (Neupogen), 486–487, 489t
  Canadian trade name for, 750
finasteride (Proscar), 743t
first-pass effect, defined, 11

Flagyl (metronidazole), 413, 451, 453
  as Canadian trade name, 752
Flamazine (silver sulfadiazine), as Canadian
    trade name, 753
Flarex (fluorometholone), as Canadian
    trade name, 750
flavoxate (Urispas)
  Canadian trade name for, 750
  in pediatrics, 218
Flaxedil (gallamine), 155t
  as Canadian trade name, 750
flecainide (Tambocor), 564, 568
  Canadian trade name for, 750
  lactation and, 737t
  pregnancy and, 729t
Fleet Enema (sodium phosphate and
    sodium biphosphate), 652t
Fleet Mineral Oil Enema (mineral oil),
    653t
Fleet Phosphosoda (sodium phosphate and
    sodium biphosphate), 652t
Fleet Theophylline (theophylline
    monothanolamine), 518t
Flexeril (cyclobenzaprine), 146t
  as Canadian trade name, 749
Florinef (fludrocortisone), 242t
  as Canadian trade name, 750
Florone (diflorasone), 719t
  as Canadian trade name, 750
Floropryl (isoflurophate), in ocular dis-
    orders, 702t
Floxin (ofloxacin), 412
  as Canadian trade name, 752
floxuridine (FUDR), 686t
fluconazole (Diflucan), 444t
  Canadian trade name for, 750
flucytosine (Ancobon), 444t
  Canadian trade name for, 750
fludarabine (Fludara), 686t
  Canadian trade name for, 750
Fludara (fludarabine), 686t
  as Canadian trade name, 750
fludrocortisone (Florinef), 242t
  Canadian trade name for, 750
fluid deficiency, treatment of, 326
fluid excess, treatment of, 326
fluids
  adverse effects of, 330
  intravenous, 324
flumazenil (Romazicon)
  in benzodiazepine toxicity, 85, 94–95
  Canadian trade name for, 750
flunisolide (Aerobid, Nasalide), 241t,
    517–518
  Canadian trade name for, 750
fluocinolone acetonide, Canadian trade
    name for, 750
fluocinonide (Lidex, Synalar), 719t
Fluoderm (fluocinolone acetonide),
    as Canadian trade name, 750
Fluogen (influenza vaccine), 474t
Fluonide (fluocinolone acetonide),
    as Canadian trade name, 750
fluoride, 351t
fluorometholone (FML Liquifilm), 706t
  Canadian trade name for, 750
Fluoroplex (fluorouracil), 686t–687t
  as Canadian trade name, 750
fluorouracil (5-FU) (Adrucil, Efudex, Fluo-
    roplex), 686t–687t, 720t
  as Canadian trade name, 750
  Canadian trade name for, 750
Fluothane (halothane), 153t
  as Canadian trade name, 751
fluoxetine (Prozac), 117t
  Canadian trade name for, 750
fluoxymesterone (Halotestin), 312t, 688t
  Canadian trade name for, 750
fluphenazine, Canadian trade name for,
    750

fluphenazine decanoate and enanthate
    (Prolixin decanoate; Prolixin enan-
    thate), 101t
fluphenazine hydrochloride (Permitil, Pro-
    lixin), 101t
flurandrenolide (Cordran), 719t
flurazepam (Dalmane), 82t, 83
  Canadian trade name for, 750
flurbiprofen (Ansaid), 68, 69
  Canadian trade name for, 750
  indications for, 68, 68t
flutamide (Eulexin), 688t
  Canadian trade name for, 750
Fluviral (influenza vaccines), as Canadian
    trade name, 751
Fluzone (influenza vaccines), as Canadian
    trade name, 751
FML Liquifilm (fluorometholone), 706t
folate (folic acid), 335t
  imbalance of, 338t
folic acid (folate) (Folvite), 335t
  Canadian trade name for, 750
  imbalance of, 338t
  routes and dosage ranges for, 340t
follicle-stimulating hormone, 229
folliculitis, 713
Follutein (human chorionic gonadotropin),
    231
Folvite (folic acid)
  as Canadian trade name, 750
  routes and dosage ranges for, 340t
food, drug interaction with, 14, 115t
Food and Drug Administration, 4, 5–6
Forane (isoflurane), 153t
  as Canadian trade name, 751
Formula 44 (dextromethorphan), as Cana-
    dian trade name, 749
Fortaz (ceftazidime), 392t
foscarnet (Foscavir), 435, 436t, 437
Foscavir (foscarnet), 435, 436t, 437
fosinopril (Monopril), 591t
  Canadian trade name for, 750
Freamine (crystalline amino acid solu-
    tions), 324
Frofen (flurbiprofen), as Canadian trade
    name, 750
frusemide, Canadian trade name for,
    750
5-FU. *See* fluorouracil
FUDR (floxuridine), 686t
Fulvicin (griseofulvin), 444t
  as Canadian trade name, 751
fungal infection, 442–443. *See also* anti-
    fungal drugs; candidiasis
  client teaching in, 443
  cutaneous, 713–714
fungi, definition of, 370
Fungizone (amphotericin), 444t, 719t
  as Canadian trade name, 748
  in geriatrics, 445
  in pediatrics, 445
Fungoid (triacetin), 444t
Furacin (nitrofurazone), 719t
Furadantin (nitrofurantoin), 421
furosemide (Lasix), 602t
  Canadian trade name for, 750
  in congestive heart failure, 549
  in hypercalcemia, 271
  lactation and, 738t
  pregnancy and, 731t
furuncles, 713

**G**

GABA. *See* gamma-aminobutyric acid
gallamine (Flaxedil), 155t
  Canadian trade name for, 750
gallbladder, 636
gallium (Ganite), 271

Gamene (gamma benzene hexachloride, lindane), 455
Gamimune (immune serum globulin, IV [IGIV]), 479t
Gamimune N (immune serum globulin (IV)), as Canadian trade name, 751
gamma-amino-butyric acid (GABA), 48, 49
gamma benzene hexachloride (Gamene, Kwell), 455
Gammabulin (immune serum globulin (human) (ISG-IM)), as Canadian trade name, 751
Gammar (immune serum globulin, human (ISG)), 479t
Gamulin Rh (rh₀(D) immune globulin, human), 479t
ganciclovir (Cytovene), 435, 436t, 437
   Canadian trade name for, 750
ganglionic-blocking agents, 590, 591t
Ganite (gallium), 271
Gantanol (sulfamethoxazole), 419t
Gantrisin (sulfisoxazole), 419t
   in ocular disorders, 705t
Garamycin (gentamicin), 397
   as Canadian trade name, 751
   in ocular disorders, 705t
gastric acid inhibitors, in peptic ulcer disease, 639, 640
gastric acid neutralizers, in peptic ulcer disease, 639–640
gastric pump inhibitors, in peptic ulcer disease, 639
gastrointestinal system
   adverse drug effects on, 17
   alcohol abuse and, 167
   disorders of
      anticholinergics in, 214, 214t, 218
      corticosteroids in, 240
      peptic ulcer disease, 638
gastrostomy tubes, in medication administration, 24, 29
Gel-Ose (lactulose), as Canadian trade name, 751
Gelusil, 643t
gemfibrozil (Lopid), 628t, 630
   Canadian trade name for, 750
Genapax tampons (gentian violet U.S.P.), 718t
gender
   cancer and, 680
   pharmacokinetics and, 17
generic, defined, 4
genetic considerations, antipsychotic drugs and, 106
Gen-Glybe (glyburide), as Canadian trade name, 751
genitourinary disorders, anticholinergics in, 214, 216–217
Genora (ethinyl estradiol and norethindrone) (mestranol and levonorgestrel), 304t
Gentacidin (gentamicin), as Canadian trade name, 751
gentamicin (Garamycin), 397
   Canadian trade name for, 751
   in ocular disorders, 705t
   therapeutic serum drug concentrations for, 746
Gentian Violet Cream (gentian violet U.S.P.), 718t
Gentian Violet Topical Solution U.S.P. (gentian violet U.S.P.), 718t
gentian violet U.S.P. (Genapax tampons, Gentian Violet Cream, Gentian Violet Topical Solution U.S.P., Hyva vaginal tablets), 718t
Geocillin (carbenicillin indanyl sodium), 382t
geographic factors, cancer and, 680

geriatrics
   absorption in, 40t
   acetaminophen in, 76
   adrenergic drugs in, 191
   aminoglycosides in, 399
   anabolic steroids in, 314
   analgesic-antipyretic-anti-inflammatory drugs in, 76
   androgens in, 314
   antacids in, 646
   antiadrenergic drugs in, 202–203
   antianginal drugs in, 577
   antiarrhythmic drugs in, 568
   antiasthmatic drugs in, 521
   anticholinergics in, 218
   anticoagulants in, 621
   anticonvulsants in, 131–132
   antidepressants in, 120–121
   antidiabetic drugs in, 291
   antidiarrheals in, 665
   antiemetics in, 673
   antifungal drugs in, 445
   antihistamines in, 530
   antihypertensive drugs in, 597
   anti-infective drugs in, 376
   antilipemic drugs in, 630
   antineoplastic drugs in, 694
   antiparkinson drugs in, 140
   antitubercular drugs in, 431
   antiviral drugs in, 438
   benzodiazepines in, 96
   beta-adrenergic drugs in, 202–203
   bronchodilators in, 521
   cardiotonic-inotropic drugs in, 555
   cathartics in, 656
   central nervous system stimulants in, 179
   cephalosporins in, 393
   cholinergic drugs in, 210
   codeine in, 539
   cold remedies in, 539
   corticosteroids in, 247
   dermatologic drugs in, 723
   distribution in, 40t
   diuretics in, 609
   drug action in, 15–16
   drug therapy in, 40t, 40–41
   erythromycin in, 409
   estrogens in, exogenous, 305
   hypercalcemia drugs in, 273
   hypoglycemia in, 270
   hypotension in, 584
   hypothyroidism in, 260
   immune function in, 469–470
   immunization in, 482
   immunostimulants in, 492
   immunosuppressants in, 503
   laxatives in, 656
   metabolism in, 15, 40t
   minerals in, 361
   mucolytics in, 539
   narcotic analgesics in, 61
   nasal decongestants in, 539
   nutritional support in, 328
   ophthalmic drugs in, 707
   penicillins in, 385
   pharmacodynamics in, 15–16
   protein binding in, 40t
   sedative-hypnotics in, 85
   shock and, 584
   skeletal muscle relaxants in, 147
   tetracyclines in, 404
   theophylline in, 521
   vitamins in, 342
gestational diabetes, 280, 733
Gevral Protein, 324
giardiasis, 449
gilbenclamide, Canadian trade name for, 751
glaucoma, 700
   drug therapy for, 707
      anticholinergics in, 217–218

Glaucon (epinephrine hydrochloride), in ocular disorders, 702t
glipizide (Glucotrol), 284t, 284–285
glomerular filtration, in renal physiology, 601, 603
glucocorticoids
   effects of, 237–238
   secretion of, 237
glucose, in brain metabolism, 51
glucose-6-phosphate dehydrogenase (G-6-PD), lactation and, 737t
glucosuria, in diabetes, 280
Glucotrol (glipizide), 284t, 284–285
glutamate, endogenous, 48, 49
glutamic acid (glutamate), 49
glyburide (DiaBeta, Micronase), 284t, 284–285
   Canadian trade name for, 751
glycerin (Osmoglyn), 603t, 653t
   in ocular disorders, 703t
glyceryl guaiacolate, Canadian trade name for, 751
glyceryl guaiacolate (guaifenesin) (Robitussin), 535t
glyceryl trinitrate, Canadian trade name for, 752
glycine, endogenous, 49
glycopyrrolate (Robinul), 214t
   Canadian trade name for, 751
   in pediatrics, 218
glycopyrronium, Canadian trade name for, 751
goiter, 254
GoLYTELY (polyethylene glycol-electrolyte solution), 652t
gonadorelin acetate (Lutrepulse), 230
gonadorelin hydrochloride (Factrel), 230
gonadotropin-releasing hormone (GnRH), 228
goserelin (Zoladex), 688t
   Canadian trade name for, 751
gout
   drugs used in, 68t, 71
      therapy guidelines for, 76
G-6-PD. See glucose-6-phosphate dehydrogenase
graft-versus-host disease, 498. See also immunosuppressants
Granulex (trypsin), 720t
Gravol (dimenhydrinate), as Canadian trade name, 750
griseofulvin (Fulvicin), 444t
   Canadian trade name for, 751
Grisovin (griseofulvin), as Canadian trade name, 751
growth hormone, 229, 230–231
growth hormone release-inhibiting hormone, 229
growth hormone-release-inhibiting hormone, 228
growth hormone-releasing factor, 228
guaifenesin (glyceryl guaiacolate) (Robitussin), 535t
   Canadian trade name for, 751
guanabenz (Wytensin), 591t
   lactation and, 738t
   pregnancy and, 730t
guanadrel (Hylorel), 591t
guanethidine sulfate (Ismelin), 591t
guanfacine (Tenex), 591t
   lactation and, 738t
   pregnancy and, 730t
Gyne-Lotrimin (clotrimazole), 444t
Gynergen (ergotamine), as Canadian trade name, 750
Gyno-Trosyd (tioconazole), as Canadian trade name, 754

## H

Habitrol (nicotine), 744t
*Haemophilus* B conjugate vaccine (Hib-TITER, Pedvax HIB, ProHibit), 473t
   Canadian trade name for, 751
*Haemophilus influenzae* type B and diphtheria and tetanus toxoids and whole-cell pertussis conjugate vaccines (DTwP-HibTITER) (Tetramune), 477t
hair, testosterone effect on, 310
halazepam (Paxipam), 91t
halcinonide (Halog), 719t
   Canadian trade name for, 751
Halcion (triazolam), 82t, 83
   as Canadian trade name, 754
Haldol (haloperidol), 103
   as Canadian trade name, 751
   lactation and, 738t
Halfan (halofantrine), 452
half-life, serum, defined, 12
hallucinogens, abuse of, 165, 170. *See also* drug abuse
halofantrine (Halfan), 452
Halog (halcinonide), 719t
   as Canadian trade name, 751
haloperidol (Haldol), 103
   Canadian trade name for, 751
   lactation and, 738t
haloprogin (Halotex), 444t, 719t
Halotestin (fluoxymesterone), 312t, 688t
   as Canadian trade name, 750
Halotex (haloprogin), 444t, 719t
halothane (Fluothane), 153t
   Canadian trade name for, 751
H-BIG (hepatitis B immune globulin, human), 479t
hCG. *See* human chorionic gonadotropin
HDCV. *See* human diploid cell rabies vaccine
heart
   electrophysiology of, 560–562
   physiology of, 545–546
heartburn, in pregnancy, 732
helminthiasis, 449–450, 453–455, 455. *See also* antiparasitics
Hemabate (carboprost tromethamine), pregnancy and, 735t
hematopoiesis, immune cell formation and, 465
hemorrheologic drug, in atherosclerosis, 627
Hepalean (heparin sodium), as Canadian trade name, 751
heparin
   antidote for, 616
   dosage for, 619
   lactation and, 737t
   pregnancy and, 730t
heparin sodium (Lipo-Hepin, Liquaemin), 615–616
   Canadian trade name for, 751
hepatitis B immune globulin, human (H-BIG, Hep-B-Gammagee, Hyper-Hep), 479t
   Canadian trade name for, 751
hepatitis B vaccine (Engerix B, Recombivax HB), 473t–474t
   recombinant, Canadian trade name for, 751
hepatotoxicity
   with acetaminophen, 74–75
   with aminoglycosides, 399, 400
   with antitubercular drugs, 432
   drug-induced, 17–18
   with erythromycin, 410
   of isoniazid, 431
   with tetracyclines, 405
Hep-B-Gammagee (hepatitis B immune globulin, human), 479t

heredity
   cancer and, 680
   drug responsivity and, 16
heroin, 169. *See also* drug abuse
Herplex (idoxuridine), 436t, 437
   in ocular disorders, 705t
Hexa-Betalin (pyridostigmine, vitamin B$_6$), as Canadian trade name, 753, 754
hexachlorophene, Canadian trade name for, 751
hexachlorophene and entsufon sodium emulsion (pHisoHex), 717t
Hexadrol (dexamethasone), as Canadian trade name, 749
Hexalen (altretamine), 688t
Hexifoam (chlorhexidine), as Canadian trade name, 749
Hibiclens (chlorhexidine gluconate), 716t
Hibidil (chlorhexidine), as Canadian trade name, 749
Hibitane (chlorhexidine), as Canadian trade name, 749
HibTITER (*Haemophilus* B conjugate vaccine), 473t
   as Canadian trade name, 751
Hip-Rex (methenamine), as Canadian trade name, 752
Hiprex (methenamine hippurate), 421
Hismanal (astemizole), 528t
   as Canadian trade name, 748
histamethizine, Canadian trade name for, 751
histamine
   action of, 525
   in inflammation and immunity, 7
histamine antagonists. *See* antihistamines
histamine-1 receptor blocking drugs
   lactation and, 738t
   pregnancy and, 730t
histamine-2 receptor blocking drugs
   description of, 639
   drug interactions with, 645–646
   individual, 640–641
   pregnancy and, 730t
   therapy guidelines for, 644
Histanil (promethazine), as Canadian trade name, 753
histoplasmosis, 442, 443
history, medication, 36
hives. *See* urticaria
Hivid (zalcitabine), as Canadian trade name, 754
HMS Liquifilm (medrysone), 706t
Homapin (homatropine methylbromide), 215
homatropine hydrobromide (Isopto Homatropine), in ocular disorders, 703t
homatropine methylbromide (Homapin), 215
hookworm infections, 449. *See also* antiparasitics
hormone inhibitors, as antineoplastic drugs, 684–685, 688t
hormones, 226–227. *See also* named hormone
   action at cellular level, 226
   adrenal cortex, 226–227
   as antineoplastic drugs, 684, 688t
   calcium metabolism and, 265–277
   diabetogenic, 280
   as drugs, 227
   functions of, 226–227
   general characteristics of, 226
   hypothalamic, 228, 230
   nursing process for, 232
   parathyroid, 227, 265–266
   phosphorus metabolism and, 265–277
   pituitary, 226, 227, 228–229, 230–232
   therapeutic, 227
   thyroid, 253–254

host defense mechanisms
   anti-infective drugs and, 369
   in immunity, 463
human chorionic gonadotropin (hCG) (Follutein), 231
human diploid cell rabies vaccine (HDCV) (Imovax), 476t
Humatin (paromomycin sulfate), 397, 398
Humatrope (somatropin), 230, 231
Humorsol (demecarium bromide), in ocular disorders, 702t
Humulin 70/30 (insulin mixtures), 283t
Humulin-L (zinc suspension), as Canadian trade name, 751
Humulin-N (isophane, NPH), as Canadian trade name, 751
Humulin N (isophane insulin suspension), 283t
Humulin R (insulin injection), 283t
Humulin-U (zinc suspension), as Canadian trade name, 751
Hycodan (hydrocodone), as Canadian trade name, 751
Hydeltrasol (prednisolone sodium phosphate), 242t
Hydeltra-TBA (prednisolone tebutate), 242t
Hyderm (hydrocortisone), as Canadian trade name, 751
hydralazine (Apresoline), 592t
   Canadian trade name for, 751
   lactation and, 738t
   in pediatrics, 597
   pregnancy and, 730t
Hydrea (hydroxyurea), 689t
   as Canadian trade name, 751
hydrocarbons, 681
hydrochlorothiazide and amiloride (Moduretic), 603t
hydrochlorothiazide and captopril (Capozide), 593t
hydrochlorothiazide and enalapril (Vaseretic), 593t
hydrochlorothiazide and methyldopa (Aldoril), 593t
hydrochlorothiazide and spironolactone (Aldactazide), 603t
hydrochlorothiazide and timolol (Timolide), 593t
hydrochlorothiazide and triamterene (Dyazide, Maxzide), 603t
hydrochlorothiazide (Esidrix, HydroDiuril, Oretic), 602t
   Canadian trade name for, 751
   lactation and, 738t
   pregnancy and, 731t
hydrocodone bitartrate, 535t
hydrocodone (Codone), 56
   Canadian trade name for, 751
hydrocortisone (Cortef, Cortril, Hydrocortone, Solu-Cortef), 241t, 518, 719t
   Canadian trade name for, 751
   in hypercalcemia, 271
Hydrocortone (hydrocortisone), 241t, 719t
HydroDiuril (hydrochlorothiazide), 602t
   as Canadian trade name, 751
   lactation and, 738t
   pregnancy and, 731t
hydroflumethiazide (Saluron), 602t
hydrogen peroxide topical solution U.S.P., 717t
hydromorphone (Dilaudid), 56, 535t
   Canadian trade name for, 751
Hydromox (quinethazone), 602t
hydroquinone (Eldoquin), 720t
   Canadian trade name for, 751
hydroxyamphetamine (Paredrine), in ocular disorders, 702t

hydroxychloroquine (Plaquenil), 452
  Canadian trade name for, 751
hydroxyprogesterone caproate (Delalutin),
  303t
hydroxyurea (Hydrea), 689t
  Canadian trade name for, 751
hydroxyzine (Atarax, Vistaril), 92, 670t
  anesthesia and, 151
  Canadian trade name for, 751
hydroxyzine hydrochloride, ephedrine sulfate and theophylline (Marax), 518t
hydroxyzine hydrochloride and hydroxyzine pamoate (Atarax, Vistaril),
  525–526, 529t
hydroxyzine pamoate and hydroxyzine hydrochloride (Atarax, Vistaril),
  525–526, 529t
Hygeol Solution (sodium hypochlorite), as
  Canadian trade name, 753
Hygroton (chlorthalidone), 602t
  as Canadian trade name, 749
Hylorel (guanadrel), 591t
hyoscine hydrobromide, hyoscyamine sulfate, atropine sulfate, pectin, kaolin,
  alcohol (Donnagel), 663t
hyoscyamine (Anaspaz), 215–216
hyoscyamine sulfate, atropine sulfate,
  pectin, kaolin, hyoscine hydrobromide, alcohol (Donnagel), 663t
Hyperab (rabies immune globulin, human),
  479t, 753
hyperaldosteronism, 239
hypercalcemia
  description of, 268
  drugs used in
    administration of, 275
    adverse effects of, 276
    client teaching with, 272, 277
    drug interactions with, 276
    in geriatrics, 273
    individual, 270
    nursing actions in, 275–277
    nursing process for, 272
    in pediatrics, 273
    principles of therapy in, 273
    therapeutic effects of, 275–276
hyperchloremic metabolic acidosis, chloride
  imbalances in, 350t
hyperglycemia, diabetogenic hormones in,
  280
hyperglycemic hyperosmolar nonketotic
  coma, 281
Hyper-Hep (hepatitis B immune globulin,
  human), 479t
  as Canadian trade name, 751
hyperkalemia
  description of, 349t
  treatment of, 359
hyperkinetic syndrome. See attention-
  deficit-hyperactivity disorder (ADHD)
hyperlipidemia. See also antilipemic drugs
  antilipemic drugs for, 626–627, 628t
  initial treatment of, 629
  types of, 627
hypermagnesemia
  description of, 350t
  treatment of, 359
hypernatremia, description of, 348t
hyperosmolar nonketotic diabetic coma, insulin therapy for, 289
hyperplasia, adrenal, 239
hypersensitivity reaction
  to aminoglycosides, 400
  antihistamines for, 526
  to antitubercular drugs, 432
  corticosteroids in, 240
  drug-induced, 18
  immune dysfunction and, 470
  to penicillins, 384, 385

Hyperstat (diazoxide), 592t
  as Canadian trade name, 749
hypertension. See also antihypertensive
    drugs
  antacids in, 640
  description of, 589
  in pregnancy, 732, 734
Hyper-Tet (tetanus immune globulin,
  human), 479t
hyperthyroidism, 254t, 255–256. See also
    antithyroid drugs
  antithyroid drugs for, 257–258
  drug metabolism and, 259, 260
  in geriatric patient, 260
  and iodine, 260
  nursing process for, 258–259
  in pediatric patient, 260
hyperuricemia
  analgesic-antipyretic-anti-inflammatory
    drugs for, therapy guidelines for, 76
  antineoplastic drugs and, 691
  drugs used in, 71–72
hypoalbuminemia, benzodiazepines in, 96
hypocalcemia
  description of, 268
  drugs used in, 268t, 268–270
    administration of, 273
    adverse effects of, 274
    calcium-vitamin D combinations, 270
    client teaching with, 269, 275
    drug interactions with, 270, 274
    in geriatrics, 270
    nursing actions for, 273–275
    nursing process in, 268–269
    in pediatrics, 270
    principles of therapy with, 269–270
    therapeutic effects of, 273–274
hypochloremic metabolic alkalosis, 348,
  350t, 360
  therapy for, 349–350
hypoglycemia, 51. See also hypoglycemic
    drugs, oral
  treatment of, 290
hypoglycemic drugs, oral, 282, 284–285. See
    also insulin
  in geriatrics, 291
  individual, 284t
  lactation and, 733–734, 738t
  in pediatrics, 291
  pregnancy and, 733–734
  therapy guidelines for, 290
hypogonadism, female, drug therapy for,
  301t–302t
hypokalemia
  description of, 349t
  treatment of, 358
hypomagnesemia
  description of, 350t
  treatment of, 359
hyponatremia, description of, 348t
Hypotears (polyvinyl alcohol), as Canadian
  trade name, 753
hypotension. See also shock
  adrenergic drugs in, 190
  description of, 581
  drugs used in, 581–586
    administration of, 585
    adverse effects of, 585–586
    client teaching with, 586
    drug interactions with, 586
    individual, 582–583
    nursing actions for, 585–586
    nursing process for, 583
    principles of therapy with, 584
    therapeutic effects of, 585
hypothalamic hormones, 229–235
  administration of, 233
  adverse effects of, 233–234
  client teaching with, 235

  description of, 228
  drug interactions with, 234
  individual, 230–232
  nursing actions for, 233–235
  nursing process with, 232
  principles of therapy with, 232
  therapeutic effects of, 233
  therapeutic limitations of, 229–230
hypothalamus, structure and function of,
  50
hypothyroidism, 254t, 254–255. See also
    thyroid drugs
  drug metabolism in, 259
  in geriatric patient, 260
  nursing process for, 258–259
  in pediatric patient, 260
  thyroid agents for, 256–257
hypovolemic shock, 581, 584
hypoxia, neurotransmission and, 48
HypRho-D (rh₀(D) immune globulin,
  human), 479t
HypRho-D (rho D immune globulin
  [human]), as Canadian trade name,
  753
Hytakerol (dihydrotachysterol), 268t
  as Canadian trade name, 750
Hytrin (terazosin), 591t
  as Canadian trade name, 753
Hyva vaginal tablets (gentian violet U.S.P.),
  718t


**I**

ibuprofen (Advil, Motrin), 68, 69, 732t
  Canadian trade name for, 751
  lactation and, 738t
  rheumatoid arthritis and, 75
Idamycin (idarubicin), 687t
  as Canadian trade name, 751
idarubicin (Idamycin), 687t
  Canadian trade name for, 751
idiosyncratic reaction, defined, 18
idoxuridine (Herplex), 436t, 437
  in ocular disorders, 705t
Ifex (ifosfamide), 686t
  as Canadian trade name, 751
IFN. See interferons
ifosfamide (Ifex), 686t
  Canadian trade name for, 751
Iletin II (isophane insulin suspension), 283t
Iletin Lente (zinc suspension), as Canadian
  trade name, 751
Iletin NPH (isophane NPH), as Canadian
  trade name, 751
Iletin Regular (insulin), as Canadian trade
  name, 751
Iletin Semilente (zinc suspension), as Canadian trade name, 751
Iletin Ultralente (zinc suspension), as Canadian trade name, 751
Ilosone (erythromycin), 408t
  as Canadian trade name, 750
Ilotycin (erythromycin)
  as Canadian trade name, 750
  in ocular disorders, 705t
imipenem and cilastatin (Primaxin), 411
  Canadian trade name for, 751
  lactation and, 737t
  pregnancy and, 729t
imipramine (Tofranil), 117t
  Canadian trade name for, 751
  therapeutic serum drug concentrations
    for, 746
Imitrex (sumatriptan), 72–73
  as Canadian trade name, 753
immune serum globulin (ISG) (Gammar,
  Gamimune, Sandoglobulin), 479t
  Canadian trade name for, 751
immune serums, 478, 479t–480t

immune system
  disorders of, 470–471
  physiology of, 463–471
    age and, 469–470
    antigens in, 464–465
    B lymphocytes in, 467
    cytokines in, 467, 468t, 469
    in fetal and neonatal periods, 469
    in geriatric patient, 469–470
    host defense mechanisms in, 463
    immune cells in, 465–469
    immunity in, 463–465
    monocytes in, 466
    neutrophils in, 466
    nutritional status and, 470
    stress and, 470
    T lymphocytes in, 466–467
immunity, types of, 464
immunization, 472. See also vaccines
  client teaching for, 481
  recommendations for, 481–482
immunizing agents
  for active immunity, 472, 473t–478t
    administration of, 483–484
    adverse effects of, 484
    client teaching with, 485
    contraindications to, 478
    drug interactions with, 484
    in geriatrics, 482
    in healthy young adults, 482
    in immunosuppression, 482
    indications for, 472
    information sources for, 481
    nursing actions for, 483–485
    nursing process for, 478, 480–481
    for passive immunity, 478, 479t–480t
    in pediatrics, 481–482
    principles of therapy with, 481–482
    selection of, 481
    storage of, 481
immunodeficiency disorders, immune dys-
    function and, 470
immunostimulants, 486–494, 489t
  administration of, 492
    inpatient versus outpatient, 490
  adverse effects of, 493
  in cancer, 491–492
  client teaching for, 490, 494
  contraindications to, 488
  description of, 486–488
  dosage of, 491
  drug interactions with, 493–494
  in geriatrics, 492
  indications for, 488
  mechanisms of action with, 488
  monitoring of, 491
  nursing actions for, 492–494
  nursing process for, 488–490
  in pediatrics, 492
  principles of therapy with, 490–492
  therapeutic effects of, 493
immunosuppressants, 496–506, 497t. See
    also named class
  administration of, 504
    schedules for, 503
  adverse effects of, 504–505
  antilymphocyte antibody preparations,
    499–500
  in autoimmune disease, 496–497, 497t
  client teaching for, 506
  combinations of, 502
  corticosteroids as, 498
  cyclosporine, 499
  cytotoxic agents as, 498–499
  description of, 496
  dosage factors with, 502–503
  drug interactions with, 506
  in geriatrics, 503
  individual, 497t

  monitoring of, 503
  monoclonal antibodies as, 499–500
  nursing actions for, 504–506
  nursing process for, 500–501
  in pediatrics, 503
  principles of therapy with, 501–503
  in rejection reactions, 497–498
  risk-benefit factors with, 501–502
  selection of, 502
  therapeutic effects of, 504
  in transplantation, 497
immunosuppression
  corticosteroids in, 240
  immunizing agent in, 482
immunotherapy, 471. See also immuno-
    stimulants; immunosuppressants
Imodium (loperamide), 661t–662t
  as Canadian trade name, 751
  lactation and, 738t
  pregnancy and, 730t
Imogam (rabies immune globulin, human),
    479t
  as Canadian trade name, 753
Imovax (rabies vaccine), 476t
impetigo, 713
Imuran (azathioprine), 497t
  as Canadian trade name, 748
Inapsine (droperidol), 670t, 699
  as Canadian trade name, 750
indapamide (Lozol), 602t
  Canadian trade name for, 751
Inderal (propranolol), 198, 199t, 200,
    257–258, 565, 568, 575, 592t
  as Canadian trade name, 753
  lactation and, 738t
  in pediatrics, 202
  pregnancy and, 730t, 731t
Inderide (propranolol and hydrochloro-
    thiazide), 593t
Indocid (indomethacin), as Canadian trade
    name, 751
Indocin (indomethacin), 70
  indications for, 68, 68t
indomethacin (Indocin), 70
  Canadian trade name for, 751
  indications for, 68, 68t
infant
  drug action in, 15
  drug metabolism in, 11, 15
  drug therapy for, 38, 39
infant formulas, 324
infection
  antineoplastic drugs and, 690–691
  dermatologic, 713–714
    bacterial, 713
    fungal, 713–714
    viral, 714
  diabetes and, 282
  ocular, 700
    anti-infectives for, 700, 705t. See also
      ophthalmic drugs
    drug therapy for, 705t, 706–707
InFeD (iron dextran injection), 355
infiltration anesthesia, 151
Inflamase (prednisolone), 706t
  as Canadian trade name, 753
inflammation
  analgesic-antipyretic-antiinflammatory
    drugs in, 67, 68t
  cutaneous, 713
  defining, 67
  description of, 67
  glucocorticoids and, 237
  ocular, 700. See also ophthalmic drugs
    corticosteroids for, 701
inflammatory response, 8–10, 67
  chemical mediators of, 7–8
influenza vaccine (Fluogen), 474t
  Canadian trade name for, 751

INH (isoniazid) (Laniazid, Nydrazid),
    428–429
  lactation and, 737t
  pregnancy and, 729t
injection
  drugs for, 24
  equipment for, 24
  intramuscular, 27, 39
  intravenous, 30–31
  nursing actions in, 27–32
  routes for, 24–26
  subcutaneous, 29–30
Innovar (fentanyl and droperidol), 154t
Inocor (amrinone), 551
  as Canadian trade name, 748
insomnia, 81
  chronic, 85
Insulatard Human NPH (isophane),
    as Canadian trade name, 751
Insulatard (isophane), as Canadian trade
    name, 751
Insulatard NPH (isophane insulin suspen-
    sion), 283t
insulin
  administration of, 291–292
    needle for, 24
  adverse reactions to, 293
  Canadian trade name for, 751
  choice of, 287–288
  client teaching with, 294–295
  contraindications to, 285
  in diabetic ketoacidosis, 289
  dosage for, 288
  drug interactions with, 293–294
  endogenous, 278
    effects of, 278–279
  food intake and, 288–289
  guidelines for therapy, 287–290
  in hyperosmolar nonketoacidotic diabetic
    coma, 289
  indications for, 285
  intermediate-acting, 282t
  lactation and, 738t, 738t
  long-acting, 282t
  mechanism of action with, 285
  nursing actions for, 291–295
  in pediatrics, 291
  perioperative use, 289–290
  in pregnancy, 733
  pregnancy and, 730t
  preparations of, 282, 283t–284t
  selection of, 287
  short-acting, 282t
  therapeutic effects of, 292
  in unconscious patient, 289
insulin injection (Actrapid, Humulin R,
    Novolin R, Regular Iletin I, Regular
    Iletin II, Velosulin), 283t
Insulin Lente (zinc suspension), as Cana-
    dian trade name, 751
insulin mixtures (Humulin 70/30, Mixtard
    70/30, Novolin 70/30), 283t
Insulin Semilente (zinc suspension), as
    Canadian trade name, 751
Insulin-Toronto (insulin), as Canadian
    trade name, 751
Insulin Ultralente (zinc suspension), as
    Canadian trade name, 751
insulin zinc suspension, extended (Ultra-
    lente, Ultratard), 283t
insulin zinc suspension, prompt (Semilente
    Iletin I, Semilente Insulin, Semi-
    tard), 283t
insulin zinc suspension (Lente Iletin I,
    Lente Iletin II, Lente Insulin, Lente
    purified pork, Novolin L), 283t
Intal (cromolyn), 519
  as Canadian trade name, 749

interactions
   drug-diet, 14
   drug-drug, 14–15
      with narcotic analgesics, 63–64
      nursing process and, 42
interference, pharmacologic, 15
interferon-alfa-2a (Roferon-A), 489t
   Canadian trade name for, 751
interferon-alfa-2b (Intron-A), 489t
   Canadian trade name for, 751
interferon-alfa-n3 (Alferon N), 489t
interferon-gamma-1b (Actimmune), 489t
interferons (IFN), 468t, 469, 487. *See also*
      immunostimulants
   in neoplastic disease, 491
interleukin-2, preparation of, 489t
interleukins (IL), 468t, 469, 487. *See also*
      immunostimulants
   in neoplastic disease, 491
International System of Units, 745
interstitial cell-stimulating hormone. *See*
      luteinizing hormone
intertrigo, 713
intestines, 636
Intopin (dopamine), as Canadian trade
      name, 750
intoxication
   alcohol, 173
   salicylate, 74
Intralipid (fat emulsions), 324
intramuscular drugs
   absorption of, 10
   administration of, 25
      in deltoid muscle, 25
      in dorsogluteal site, 26
      nursing actions for, 27, 30
      in vastus lateralis, 27
      in ventrogluteal area, 26
intravenous drugs, administration of, 30–31
intravenous fluids, preparations of, 324
Intron-A (interferon-alfa-2b), 489t
   as Canadian trade name, 751
Intropin (dopamine), 187t, 582
iodine, 352t
   in hyperthyroidism, 260
   preparations of
      topical, 716t
iodine solutions, 257
iodine tincture, U.S.P., 716t
iodine topical solution U.S.P., 716t
iodochlorhydroxyquin (Vioform), 719t
   Canadian trade name for, 751
iodoquinol (Yodoxin), 451
Iodotope (sodium iodide ¹³¹I), 257
Ionamin (phentermine resin), 323t
Ionil T Plus (coal tar), as Canadian trade
      name, 749
IPOL (poliomyelitis vaccine, inactivated),
      475t
ipratropium (Atrovent), 517
   Canadian trade name for, 751
iron, 352t
   excess of, treatment of, 354
   imbalances of, 353t
   ingestion of, hyperthyroidism and, 260
   overdosage of, treatment of, 360
   preparations of, 354–355
iron deficiency anemia, treatment of,
      359–360
iron dextran injection (InFeD), 355
irritant cathartics, 652t–653t, 654
ISG. *See* immune serum globulin, human
Ismelin (guanethidine sulfate), 591t
Ismo (isosorbide mononitrate), 575
Ismotic (isosorbide), 603t
   in ocular disorders, 703t
Isocal, 322
isocarboxazid (Marplan), 117t
Isodine (povidone-iodine), 716t

isoetharine (Bronkometer, Bronkosol),
      187t, 516
isoflurane (Forane), 153t
   Canadian trade name for, 751
isoflurophate (Floropryl), in ocular disor-
      ders, 702t
isomeprobamate, Canadian trade name for,
      749
Isomil, 323
isoniazid (INH) (Laniazid, Nydrazid)
   lactation and, 737t
   pregnancy and, 729t
isophane insulin suspension (Humulin N,
      Iletin II, Insulatard NPH, Novolin N,
      NPH Iletin I, NPH Insulin, NPH puri-
      fied pork), 283t
isophane (NPH), Canadian trade name for,
      751
isoprenaline, Canadian trade name for, 751
isopropamide chloride (Darbid), 214t
Isopropyl Alcohol (isopropyl alcohol), 716t
isopropyl alcohol (Isopropyl Alcohol, Iso-
      propyl Rubbing Alcohol, Rubbing Al-
      cohol U.S.P.), 716t
Isopropyl Rubbing Alcohol (isopropyl alco-
      hol), 716t
isoproterenol (Isuprel), 187t, 188, 516, 567
   Canadian trade name for, 751
   hypotension and shock and, 582
   in pediatrics, 191
Isoptin SR (verapamil) (sustained-release),
      592t
Isoptin (verapamil), 566, 568, 574t, 592t
   as Canadian trade name, 754
   in pediatrics, 597
Isopto Atropine (atropine sulfate), as Cana-
      dian trade name, 748
Isopto Carbachol (carbachol)
   as Canadian trade name, 749
   in ocular disorders, 702t
Isopto Carpine (pilocarpine)
   as Canadian trade name, 753
   in ocular disorders, 702t
Isopto Cetamide (sulfacetamide sodium), in
      ocular disorders, 705t
Isopto Eserine (physostigmine salicylate), in
      ocular disorders, 703t
Isopto Homatropine (homatropine hydro-
      bromide), in ocular disorders, 703t
Isopto Hyoscine (scopolamine hydrobro-
      mide), in ocular disorders, 703t
Isordil (isosorbide dinitrate), 575
   as Canadian trade name, 751
isosorbide dinitrate (Isordil, Sorbitrate), 575
   Canadian trade name for, 751
isosorbide (Ismotic), 603t
   in ocular disorders, 703t
isosorbide mononitrate (Ismo), 575
isotonic diet, 323
isotretinoin (Accutane), 720t
   Canadian trade name for, 751
Isotrex (isotretinoin), as Canadian trade
      name, 751
isoxsuprine hydrochloride (Vasodilan), 629t
isradipine (DynaCirc), 574t, 592t
Isuprel (isoproterenol), 187t, 188, 516, 567
   as Canadian trade name, 751
   in hypotension and shock, 582
itraconazole (Sporanox), 444t
Iveegam (immune serum globulin (IV)), as
      Canadian trade name, 751


**K**

Kalcinate (calcium gluconate), 268t
Kalium (potassium chloride), as Canadian
      trade name, 753
kanamycin (Kantrex), 397
Kantrex (kanamycin), 397

Kaochlor (potassium chloride), as Canadian
      trade name, 753
kaolin, pectin, and paregoric (Parepectolin),
      663t
kaolin, pectin, atropine sulfate,
      hyoscyamine sulfate, hyoscine hy-
      drobromide, alcohol (Donnagel), 663t
kaolin and pectin mixture (Kaopectate),
      663t
Kaon (potassium gluconate), 355
Kaopectate (kaolin and pectin mixture),
      663t
Kayexalate (sodium polystyrene sulfonate),
      as Canadian trade name, 753
Keflex (cephalexin), 390t
   as Canadian trade name, 749
Keflin (cephalothin), 391t
   as Canadian trade name, 749
Kefurox (cefuroxime), 392t
   as Canadian trade name, 749
Kefzol (cefazolin), 390, 391t, 393
   as Canadian trade name, 749
Kemadrin (procyclidine), 137t, 216
   as Canadian trade name, 753
Kenacort diacetate (triamcinolone diac-
      etate), 242t
Kenalog (triamcinolone), 719t
   as Canadian trade name, 754
Kenalog-40 (triamcinolone acetonide), 242t
keratitis, 700. *See also* ophthalmic drugs
keratolytic drugs, 715
Kerlone (betaxolol), 198, 199t, 200, 592t
Ketalar (ketamine), 154t
   as Canadian trade name, 751
ketamine (Ketalar), 154t
   Canadian trade name for, 751
ketoacidosis, diabetic, 281
ketoconazole (Nizoral), 444t
   Canadian trade name for, 751
ketoprofen (Orudis), 68, 69
   Canadian trade name for, 751
   indications for, 68, 68t
ketorolac (Toradol), 70, 71
   Canadian trade name for, 751
   indications for, 68, 68t
kidney. *See also entries beginning with renal*
   physiology of, 601, 603–604
Kidrolase (asparaginase), as Canadian trade
      name, 748
K-Long (potassium chloride), as Canadian
      trade name, 753
Klonopin (clonazepam), 91t, 127–128
K-Lor (potassium chloride), as Canadian
      trade name, 753
K-Lyte (potassium bicarbonate and citrate),
      355
K-Med (potassium chloride), as Canadian
      trade name, 753
Koffex DM (dextromethorphan), as Cana-
      dian trade name, 749
Konakion (phytonadione, vitamin K), as
      Canadian trade name, 753, 754
K-10 (potassium chloride), as Canadian
      trade name, 753
Kwell (gamma benzene hexachloride, lin-
      dane), 455


**L**

labetalol (Normodyne, Trandate), 198, 199t,
      200, 592t
   Canadian trade name for, 751
labor
   anesthetics in, 735
   inhibition of, tocolytics in, 734, 735t
   initiation of, oxytocics in, 734–735, 735t
lactation
   description of, 726
   drug effects on, 737t–738t

drug use in
    effects of, 737t–738t
    guidelines for, 739
    hypoglycemic drugs in, oral, 733–734
    oxytocics for, 734, 735t
    principles of therapy during, 739
    suppression of. *See* lactation suppressor
lactation suppressor, 735, 735t
    nursing actions for, 739–741
Lactinex (lactobacillus), 663t
lactobacillus (Bacid, Lactinex), 663t
Lactulax (lactulose), as Canadian trade
    name, 751
lactulose, as laxative, 653–654
lactulose (Cephulac, Chronulac), 653t
    Canadian trade name for, 751
Laniazid (isoniazid) (INH), 428–429
Lanoxin (digoxin), 549, 550–551, 553–554
    as Canadian trade name, 750
    lactation and, 738t
    pregnancy and, 731t
Lanvis (thioguanine), as Canadian trade
    name, 754
Largactil (chlorpromazine), as Canadian
    trade name, 749
large intestine, 636
Lariam (mefloquine), 452
Larodopa (levodopa), 136, 137–138
    as Canadian trade name, 751
Larotid (amoxicillin), 382t
larynx, defined, 511
Lasix (furosemide), 602t
    as Canadian trade name, 750
    congestive heart failure and, 549
    hypercalcemia and, 271
    lactation and, 738t
    pregnancy and, 731t
laxatives, 651–658. *See also* cathartics
    administration of, 656
    adverse effects of, 657
    bulk-forming, 651, 652t
    client teaching for, 657–658
    contraindications to, 654
    definition of, 651
    drug interactions with, 657
    in geriatrics, 656
    indications for, 654
    lactation and, 738t
    lactulose as, 653–654
    lubricant, 653, 653t
    nursing actions for, 656–658
    nursing process for, 654–655
    in pediatrics, 656
    polyethylene glycol-electrolyte as, 654
    pregnancy and, 731t
    principles of therapy with, 655–656
    selection of, 655–656
    sorbitol as, 654
    surfactant, 652t, 653
    therapeutic effects of, 657
Ledercillin VK (penicillin V), as Canadian
    trade name, 752
legal responsibilities, in nursing process,
    34
Lente Iletin II (insulin zinc suspension),
    283t
Lente Iletin I (insulin zinc suspension),
    283t
Lente Insulin (insulin zinc suspension),
    283t
Lente purified pork (insulin zinc suspen-
    sion), 283t
lethal dose, 14
leukemia, 682
Leukeran (chlorambucil), 686t
    as Canadian trade name, 749
Leukine (sargramostim), 489t
leukotrienes, in inflammation and immu-
    nity, 7

leuprolide (Lupron), 688t
    Canadian trade name for, 751
Leustatin (cladribine), 688t
levamisole (Ergamisol), 689t
levarterenol (Levophed), 187t, 198, 583
    Canadian trade name for, 752
Levatol (penbutolol), 198, 199t, 200,
    592t
Levlen (ethinyl estradiol and norethin-
    drone acetate), 304t
levobunolol (Betagan), 198, 199t, 200
    Canadian trade name for, 751
    in ocular disorders, 702t
levodopa (Larodopa), 136, 137–138
    Canadian trade name for, 751
Levo-Dromoran (levorphanol), 56
    as Canadian trade name, 751
levonorgestrel, in oral contraceptives, 304t
levonorgestrel and ethinyl estradiol, Cana-
    dian trade name for, 750
Levophed (levarterenol), 187t, 198, 583
    as Canadian trade name, 752
levorphanol (Levo-Dromoran), 56
    Canadian trade name for, 751
Levothroid (levothyroxine), 256, 258
levothyroxine (Levothroid, Synthroid),
    256, 258, 732t
    Canadian trade name for, 751
Librium (chlordiazepoxide), 91t
    anxiety and, 89–90
    as Canadian trade name, 749
    in pediatrics, 85, 95
Lidemol (fluocinolone), as Canadian trade
    name, 750
Lidex (fluocinolone, fluocinonide), 719t
    as Canadian trade name, 750
lidocaine and dexamethasone (Decadron
    with Xylocaine), 241t
lidocaine (Xylocaine), 156t, 563–564, 568
    Canadian trade name for, 751
    lactation and, 737t
    pregnancy and, 729t
    therapeutic serum drug concentrations
        for, 746
life-style, cancer and, 680
limbic system, structure and function of, 51
lindane (Gamene, Kwell), 455
Lioresal (baclofen), 146t
    as Canadian trade name, 748
liothyronine (Cytomel, Triostat), 256
    Canadian trade name for, 751
liotrix (Euthroid, Thyrolar), 256–257
lipids. *See also* fats; hyperlipidemia
    defined, 626–627
Lipo-Hepin (heparin sodium), 615–616
Lipomul, 324
Liposyn (fat emulsions), 324
Liquaemin (heparin sodium), 615–616
Liquifilm (polyvinyl alcohol), in ocular dis-
    orders, 704t
lisinopril (Prinivil, Zestril), 591t
    Canadian trade name for, 751
    lactation and, 737t
Lithane (lithium), as Canadian trade name,
    751
lithium, 115–116, 117t
    Canadian trade name for, 751
    lactation and, 738t
    pregnancy and, 730t
    therapeutic serum drug concentrations
        for, 746
lithium carbonate (Eskalith), 115–116, 117t
liver
    alcohol abuse and, 167
    disorders of
        antianxiety drugs in, 95
        anti-infective drugs in, 397
        benzodiazepines in, 95
        corticosteroids in, 240

drug metabolism in, 11
    structure and function of, 636
local anesthesia, 150–151
    administration of, 151, 157
    agents for, 156t
Lodine (etodolac), 70
    indications for, 68, 68t
Lodosyn (carbidopa), 136, 138
Loestrin (ethinyl estradiol and norethin-
    drone), 304t
    as Canadian trade name, 750
Loestrin Fe (ethinyl estradiol and
    norgestrel), 304t
Lofenalac, 322
lomefloxacin (Maxaquin), 412
Lomotil (diphenoxylate), 661t
    as Canadian trade name, 750
    lactation and, 738t
    pregnancy and, 730t
lomustine (CCNU), 686t
    Canadian trade name for, 751
Lonalac, 324
Lonamin (phentermine), as Canadian trade
    name, 753
Loniten (minoxidil), 593t
    as Canadian trade name, 752
loop diuretics, 605
Lo/Ovral (ethinyl estradiol and norethin-
    drone), 304t
loperamide (Imodium), 661t–662t
    Canadian trade name for, 751
    lactation and, 738t
    pregnancy and, 730t
Lopid (gemfibrozil), 628t, 630
    as Canadian trade name, 750
Lopressor (metoprolol), 198, 199t, 200,
    592t, 593t
    as Canadian trade name, 752
    lactation and, 738t
Loprox (ciclopirox), 444t, 719t
    as Canadian trade name, 749
Lorabid (loracarbef), 390t
loracarbef (Lorabid), 390t
loratadine (Claritin), 525, 528t
    Canadian trade name for, 751
lorazepam (Ativan), 90, 91t
    Canadian trade name for, 751
    in seizure disorders, 128
Lorelco (probucol), 628t, 630
    as Canadian trade name, 753
Loroxide (benzoyl peroxide), as Canadian
    trade name, 748
Lotensin (benazepril), 591t
lotions, dermatologic, 722
Lotrimin (clotrimazole), 444t, 719t
lovastatin (Mevacor), 628t, 630
    Canadian trade name for, 751
Lovenox (enoxaparin), 616
Loxapac (loxapine), as Canadian trade
    name, 751
loxapine (Loxitane), 103–104
    Canadian trade name for, 751
Loxitane (loxapine), 103–104
Lozide (indapamide), as Canadian trade
    name, 751
Lozol (indapamide), 602t
lubricant laxatives, 653, 653t
lubricants, ophthalmic, 704t
Ludiomil (maprotiline), 115, 117t
    as Canadian trade name, 751
Lugol's solution (strong iodine solution),
    257
Luminal (phenobarbital), 82t, 83
lungs, defined, 512
Lupron (leuprolide), 688t
    as Canadian trade name, 751
luteinizing hormone, 229
Lutrepulse (gonadorelin acetate), 230
Lyderm (fluocinolone), as Canadian trade
    name, 750

lymphocyte immune globulin, antithymocyte globulin (Equine), 497t
lymphocyte immune globulin antilymphocyte globulin, 499–500
lymphocytes, immune system and, 466–467
lymphomas, 682
lypressin, 231–232
lysergic acid diethylamide (LSD), 165, 170
Lysodren (mitotane), 689t
as Canadian trade name, 752

**M**
Maalox (aluminum hydroxide gel and magnesium hydroxide), as Canadian
trade name, 748
Maalox Plus, 643t
Maalox suspension, 643t
Maalox tablets, 643t
Macrodantin (nitrofurantoin), 421
lactation and, 737t
pregnancy and, 729t
macrolides, 407–410. *See also* anti-infective
drugs; erythromycin
administration of, 409
adverse effects of, 409–410
client teaching with, 410
contraindications to, 408
drug interactions with, 410
indications for, 407
individual, 408
mechanism of action with, 407
nursing actions for, 409–410
principles of therapy with, 408–409
specimen collection and, 408
therapeutic effects of, 409
mafenide (Sulfamylon), 420t
magnesia magma (magnesium hydroxide),
652t
magnesium
description of, 347t
imbalances of, 350t
treatment of, 359
preparation of, 355
magnesium citrate, 652t
Canadian trade name for, 751
magnesium hydroxide and aluminum hydroxide gel, Canadian trade name
for, 748
magnesium hydroxide (magnesia magma,
milk of magnesia), 652t
magnesium sulfate, 355
pregnancy and, 735t
malaria, 448–449, 451–453, 455. *See also*
antimalarial drugs
malathion (Ovide), 455
malignancies. *See* neoplasms, malignant
Mandelamine (methenamine), 421
as Canadian trade name, 752
Mandol (cefamandole), 391t
as Canadian trade name, 749
mannitol (Osmitrol), 603t
Canadian trade name for, 751
in ocular disorders, 703t
Maolate (chlorphenesin), 146t
maprotiline (Ludiomil), 115, 117t
Canadian trade name for, 751
therapeutic serum drug concentrations
for, 746
Marax (theophylline, ephedrine sulfate and
hydroxyzine hydrochloride), 518t
Marcaine (bupivacaine), 156t
as Canadian trade name, 749
Marezine (cyclizine), 670t
as Canadian trade name, 749
marijuana. *See also* drug abuse
abuse of, 164–165
treatment of, 169–170
pregnancy and, 727–728

Marinol (dronabinol), 670t, 699
Marplan (isocarboxazid), 117t
masoprocol (Actinex), 743t–744t
mast cell stabilizers, in bronchoconstrictive
disorders, 515, 519
maternal therapeutics, 728
Matulane (procarbazine), 689t
Maxair (pirbuterol), 187t, 516
Maxaquin (lomefloxacin), 412
Maxenal (pseudoephedrine), as Canadian
trade name, 753
Maxeran (metoclopramide), as Canadian
trade name, 752
Maxide (triamterene)
lactation and, 738t
pregnancy and, 731t
Maxidex (dexamethasone), 706t
as Canadian trade name, 749
Maxiflor (diflorasone), 719t
Maxzide (hydrochlorothiazide and triamterene), 603t
mazindol, Canadian trade name for, 751
mazindol (Sanorex), 323t
MBF, 323
MCT Oil, 324
measles, mumps, and rubella vaccine
(M-M-R II), 474t
Canadian trade name for, 751
measles and rubella vaccine (M-R-Vax II),
474t
measles vaccine (Attenuvax), 474t
Mebaral (mephobarbital), 82t, 83
mebendazole (Vermox), 453–454
Canadian trade name for, 751
mechlorethamine (nitrogen mustard) (Mustargen), 686t
Canadian trade name for, 751
meclizine (Antivert, Bonine), 528t, 670t
Canadian trade name for, 751
meclofenamate (Meclomen), 71
Meclomen (meclofenamate), 71
medication. *See* drug; drug therapy
medication history, 36
medication orders, 21
medication system, 21
Medipren (ibuprofen), as Canadian trade
name, 751
Medrol acetate (methylprednisolone acetate), 719t
Medrol (methylprednisolone), 242t
as antiemetic, 669
as Canadian trade name, 752
medroxyprogesterone (Depo-Provera),
303t, 688t
Canadian trade name for, 751
medrysone (HMS Liquifilm), 706t
medulla oblongata, structure and function
of, 50
mefenamic acid (Ponstel), 71
mefloquine (Lariam), 452
Mefoxin (cefoxitin), as Canadian trade
name, 749
Megace (megestrol), 303t
as Canadian trade name, 751
Megacillin (penicillin G benzathine), as
Canadian trade name, 752
Megacillin (penicillin G potassium), as
Canadian trade name, 752
megestrol (Megace), 303t, 688t
Canadian trade name for, 751
melanizing drugs, 715, 719t
melanocyte-stimulating hormone, 228
melanocyte-stimulating hormone-inhibiting
factor, 228
melanocyte-stimulating hormone-releasing
factor, 228
Mellaril (thioridazine), 102t
as Canadian trade name, 754
melphalan (Alkeran), 686t
Canadian trade name for, 751

menadione sodium diphosphate
(Synkayvite), routes and dosage
ranges for, 340t
meningitis vaccine (Menomune A/C,
Menomune A/C/Y/W-135), 474t
Menomune A/C (meningitis vaccine), 474t
Menomune A/C/Y/W-135 (meningitis vaccine), 474t
menopause, estrogen replacement in, 299,
301t–302t, 303, 305
menotropins (Pergonal), 231
menstrual cycle, estrogens during, 298
mepenzolate bromide (Cantil), 214t
meperidine (Demerol), 56
Canadian trade name for, 752
lactation and, 737t
pregnancy and, 729t
mephobarbital (Mebaral), 82t, 83, 127
Mephyton (phytonadione), 617
routes and dosage ranges for, 340t
mepivacaine (Carbocaine), 156t
Canadian trade name for, 752
meprobamate (Equanil, Miltown), 92
Mepron (atovaquone), 453
mercaptopurine (Purinethol), 687t
Canadian trade name for, 752
Meritene, 322
Meruvax II (rubella vaccine), 476t
mescaline, 165, 170. *See also* drug abuse
mesna (Mesnex), 744t
Mesnex (mesna), 744t
mesoridazine (Serentil), 101t
Canadian trade name for, 752
Mestinon (pyridostigmine), 209
as Canadian trade name, 753
mestranol 50
in oral contraceptives, 304t
mestranol and norethindrone, Canadian
trade name for, 752
metabolic acidosis, 349–350, 350t
metabolic alkalosis, 350t, 360
metabolism
brain, 51
defined, 11
estrogens and, 298
in geriatric patient, 40t
glucocorticoids and, 229
in hypothyroidism, 259
in pediatric patient, 15, 38t
metacortandracin, Canadian trade name
for, 753
metacortandrolone, Canadian trade name
for, 753
Metahydin (trichlormethiazide), 602t
metal chelating agents, mechanism of action in, 13
metallic antiseptics
dermatologic, 716t–717t
metallic ores, 681t
Metamucil (psyllium preparations), 652t,
663t
as Canadian trade name, 753
pregnancy and, 731t
Metandren (methyltestosterone), as Canadian trade name, 752
metaproterenol (Alupent), 187t, 516–517
Canadian trade name for, 752
in pediatrics, 191
metaraminol (Aramine), 187t, 582–583
metaxalone (Skelaxin), 146t
methadone (Dolophine), 56
methamphetamine (Desoxyn), 177
methantheline bromide (Banthine), 214t
methazolamide (Neptazane)
Canadian trade name for, 752
in ocular disorders, 703t
methdilazine and methdilazine hydrochloride (Tacaryl, Tacaryl hydrochloride),
528t

methenamine, Canadian trade name for, 752
methenamine hippurate (Hiprex), 421
methenamine mandelate (Mandelamine), 421
Methergine (methylergonovine maleate), pregnancy and, 735t
methicillin (Staphcillin), 381, 382t
methimazole (Tapazole), 257
  Canadian trade name for, 752
  lactation and, 738t
methocarbamol (Robaxin), 146t
  acute or chronic disorders and, 145
  Canadian trade name for, 752
methohexital, Canadian trade name for, 752
methohexital sodium (Brevital), 154t
methotrexate (amethopterin, MTX) (Mexate, Rheumatrex), 497t, 499, 687t
  Canadian trade name for, 752
  dosage of, 503
  selection of, 502
methoxamine (Vasoxyl), 187t, 583
methoxsalen (Oxsoralen-ultra), 720t
  Canadian trade name for, 752
methoxyflurane (Penthrane), 153t
methscopolamine (Pamine), 216
Methulose (methylcellulose), in ocular disorders, 704t
methyclothiazide (Enduron), 602t
  Canadian trade name for, 752
methylcellulose (Citrucel, Methulose, Visculose), 652t
  Canadian trade name for, 752
  in ocular disorders, 704t
methyldopa (Aldomet), 591t
  Canadian trade name for, 752
  lactation and, 738t
  pregnancy and, 730t
methyldopa and hydrochlorothiazide (Aldoril), 593t
methylergonovine maleate (Methergine), pregnancy and, 735t
methylphenidate (Ritalin), 177
  Canadian trade name for, 752
methylprednisolone acetate (Medrol acetate), 719t
methylprednisolone (Medrol, Solu-Medrol), 242t, 519
  as antiemetic, 669
  Canadian trade name for, 752
methyltestosterone (Oreton methyl), 312t
  Canadian trade name for, 752
methysergide, Canadian trade name for, 752
Meticortelone soluble (prednisolone sodium succinate), 242t
Meticorten (prednisone), 688t
metipranolol (OptiPranolol), 198, 199t, 200, 702t
metoclopramide (Reglan), 669, 671, 671t
  Canadian trade name for, 752
metocurine (Metubine), 155t
  Canadian trade name for, 752
metolazone (Mykrox, Zaroxolyn), 602t
  Canadian trade name for, 752
metoprolol (Lopressor), 198, 199t, 200, 592t, 593t
  Canadian trade name for, 752
  lactation and, 738t
Metreton (prednisolone sodium phosphate), 706t
metric system, 22, 22t
Metrogel (metronidazole), as Canadian trade name, 752
metronidazole (Flagyl), 413, 451, 453
  Canadian trade name for, 752
Metubine (metocurine), 155t
  as Canadian trade name, 752

Mevacor (lovastatin), 628t, 630
  as Canadian trade name, 751
Mexate (amethopterin, methotrexate), 687t
mexiletine (Mexitil), 564
  Canadian trade name for, 752
  lactation and, 737t
  pregnancy and, 729t
Mexitil (mexiletine), 564
  as Canadian trade name, 752
  lactation and, 737t
  pregnancy and, 729t
Mezlin (mezlocillin), 383t
mezlocillin (Mezlin), 381, 383t
Micatin (miconazole), 719t
  as Canadian trade name, 752
miconazole (Micatin, Monistat), 444t, 719t
  Canadian trade name for, 752
Micro-K (potassium chloride), as Canadian trade name, 753
Micronase (glyburide), 284t, 284–285
Micronor (norethindrone), 304t
microorganisms, classification of, 369–370
Microsulfon (sulfadiazine), 419t
Midamor (amiloride), 602t
  lactation and, 738t
midazolam (Versed), 90, 91t, 154t
  Canadian trade name for, 752
migraine
  caffeine in, 178
  drugs used in, 72–73, 76
Mikinol (mineral oil), 653t
milk of magnesia (magnesium hydroxide), 652t
milrinone IV (Primacor), 551
  adverse effects of, 558
Miltown (meprobamate), 92
mineral-electrolyte preparations, 356
mineralocorticoids, 238
mineral oil (Agoral Plain, Fleet Mineral Oil Enema, Mikinol), 653t
  pregnancy and, 731t
minerals, 346–365. See also specific minerals
  administration of, 361–363
  adverse effects of, 364
  client teaching with, 357, 365
  description of, 346, 348
  disorders of, 358–361
  drug interactions with, 364–365
  excess of
    chelation therapy for, 354
    prevention of, 357
  in geriatrics, 361
  imbalances of, 349t, 350t
    acidifying agents in, 348
    alkalinizing agents in, 349–350
    chelating agents in, 354
    preparations for, 354–356
  as macronutrients, 346, 347t, 348
  as micronutrients (trace elements), 348
    selected, 351t–353t
  multiple, preparations of, 356
  nursing actions for, 361–365
  nursing process for, 356–357
  in pediatrics, 361
  principles of therapy with, 357, 358–360
  selection of, 357–358
  supplemental, 357
  therapeutic effects of, 363
  uses for, 346, 348
Minestrin (ethinyl estradiol and norethindrone), as Canadian trade name, 750
Minipress (prazosin), 549, 591t
  as Canadian trade name, 753
Minizide (prazosin and polythiazide), 593t
Minocin (minocycline), 403t
  as Canadian trade name, 752

minocycline (Minocin), 403t
  Canadian trade name for, 752
Min-Ovral (ethinyl estradiol and levonorgestrel), as Canadian trade name, 750
minoxidil (Loniten, Rogaine), 593t, 744t
  Canadian trade name for, 752
Mintezol (thiabendazole), 454–455
  as Canadian trade name, 754
Miocarpine (pilocarpine), as Canadian trade name, 753
Miostat (carbachol), as Canadian trade name, 749
misoprostol (Cytotec), 639, 641–642
  Canadian trade name for, 752
  in geriatrics, 646
Mithracin (plicamycin), 272, 687t
mithramycin. See plicamycin
mitomycin (Mutamycin), 687t
  Canadian trade name for, 752
mitotane (Lysodren), 689t
  Canadian trade name for, 752
mitoxantrone (Novantrone), 687t
  Canadian trade name for, 752
Mitrolan (polycarbophil), 652t
  as Canadian trade name, 753
Mivacron (mivacurium), 155t
mivacurium (Mivacron), 155t
Mixtard 70/30 (insulin mixtures), 283t
M-M-R II (measles, mumps, and rubella vaccine)
  as Canadian trade name, 751
Moban (molindone), 104
Moctanin (monoctanoin), 743t
Modicon (ethinyl estradiol and norethindrone), 304t
Moditen (fluphenazine), as Canadian trade name, 750
Moduret (amiloride), as Canadian trade name, 748
Moduretic (hydrochlorothiazide and amiloride), 603t
molindone (Moban), 104
Monistat (miconazole), 444t
  as Canadian trade name, 752
Monitan (acebutolol), as Canadian trade name, 748
monoamine oxidase inhibitors, 114–115, 117t
  interactions with, food and drug, 14, 115t
  overdosage of, 120
  selection of, 118–119
monobactams, 411
monobenzone (Benoquin), 720t
Monocid (cefonocid), 391t
monoclonal antibodies, 499. See also immunosuppressants
monoctanoin (Moctanin), 743t
Monopril (fosinopril), 591t
  as Canadian trade name, 750
moricizine (Ethmozine), 564–565
morphine, 54–55, 535t. See also narcotic analgesics
  administration of, 54–55
  Canadian trade name for, 752
  classification of, 5
  dosage for, 55
  in geriatrics, 62
  naloxone and, 58
  in pediatrics, 61–62
  as prototype, 54
  route and dosage ranges for, 55
  in severe pain, 60
MOS (morphine), as Canadian trade name, 752
Motofen (difenoxin with atropine sulfate), 661t

Motrin (ibuprofen), 68, 69, 732t
  as Canadian trade name, 751
  indications for, 68, 68t
  lactation and, 738t
moxalactam (Moxam), 390, 392t
Moxam (moxalactam), 390, 392t
M-R-Vax II (measles and rubella vaccine), 474t
MS Contin (morphine), as Canadian trade name, 752
MSOR (morphine), as Canadian trade name, 752
MTX. *See* methotrexate
mucolytics, 534, 535t
  administration of, 538, 539
  in geriatrics, 539
  nursing process for, 534, 537–538
  in pediatrics, 539
  principles of therapy with, 538–539
  selection of, 538
Mucomyst (acetylcysteine), 535t
  as Canadian trade name, 748
mucous membranes, local anesthesia administration in, 157
Multipax (hydroxyzine), as Canadian trade name, 751
multiple myeloma, 682
mumps vaccine (Mumpsvax), 475t
  Canadian trade name for, 752
Mumpsvax (mumps vaccine), 475t
  as Canadian trade name, 752
mupirocin (Bactroban), 744t
Murocel (methylcellulose), as Canadian trade name, 752
muromonab-CD3 (Orthoclone OKT3), 497t, 500, 502, 503
  Canadian trade name for, 752
muscle spasm, defined, 145
musculoskeletal system
  alcohol abuse and, 168
  in respiration, 512
Mustargen (mechlorethamine, nitrogen mustard), 686t
  as Canadian trade name, 751
Mutamycin (mitomycin), 687t
  as Canadian trade name, 752
Myambutol (ethambutol), 429
  as Canadian trade name, 750
myasthenia gravis, cholinergic drugs in, 209–210
Mycelex (clotrimazole), 444t, 719t
Mycifradin (neomycin), 397–398
  as Canadian trade name, 752
  in pediatrics, 399
Myciguent (neomycin), as Canadian trade name, 752
Myciguent ointment (neomycin sulfate), 719t
Myclo (clotrimazole), as Canadian trade name, 749
*Mycobacterium tuberculosis*, 427. *See also* antitubercular drugs
Mycobutin (rifabutin), 744t
Mycostatin (nystatin), 444t, 719t
  as Canadian trade name, 752
Mydfrin (phenylephrine), as Canadian trade name, 753
Mydriacyl (tropicamide)
  as Canadian trade name, 754
  ocular disorders and, 703t
  in pediatrics, 218
Mykrox (metolazone), 602t
Mylanta (aluminum hydroxide gel and magnesium hydroxide), 643t
  as Canadian trade name, 748
Mylanta-II, 643t
Myleran (busulfan), 686t
  as Canadian trade name, 749
Myotonachol (bethanechol), as Canadian trade name, 748

Mysoline (primidone), 128
  as Canadian trade name, 753
Mytelase (ambenonium), 208


**N**

nabumetone (Relafen), 70, 71
  indications for, 68, 68t
nadolol and bendroflumethiazide (Corzide), 593t
nadolol (Corgard), 198, 199t, 200, 575, 592t
  Canadian trade name for, 752
  lactation and, 738t
Nadopen-V (penicillin V), as Canadian trade name, 752
Nadostine (nystatin), as Canadian trade name, 752
nafarelin (Synarel), 230
nafcillin (Unipen), 381, 382t
  Canadian trade name for, 752
naftifine (Naftin), 444t
Naftin (naftifine), 444t
nalbuphine (Nubain), 57
  Canadian trade name for, 752
Nalfon (fenoprofen), 68–69
  as Canadian trade name, 750
  indications for, 68, 68t
nalidixic acid (NegGram), 421, 662t
  Canadian trade name for, 752
naloxone (Narcan), 58
  Canadian trade name for, 752
  pregnancy and, 729t
naltrexone (Trexan), 58
nandrolone, Canadian trade name for, 752
nandrolone decanoate (Deca-Durabolin), 312t
nandrolone phenpropionate (Durabolin), 312t
naphazoline, Canadian trade name for, 752
naphazoline hydrochloride (Privine), 187t, 535t
Naphcon (naphazoline), as Canadian trade name, 752
Naprosyn (naproxen), 68, 69
  as Canadian trade name, 752
  indications for, 68, 68t
naproxen (Anaprox, Naprosyn), 68, 69
  Canadian trade name for, 752
  indications for, 68, 68t
Naqua (trichlormethiazide), 602t
Narcan (naloxone), 58
  as Canadian trade name, 752
  pregnancy and, 729t
narcolepsy, central nervous system stimulants for, 176, 178
narcotic analgesics, 53–64. *See also* narcotic antagonists
  administration route for, 60
  adverse effects of, 63
  agonist, 54–57
  agonists-antagonists, 57–58
  anesthesia and, 152
  in burns, 61
  in colic, 61
  contraindications to, 55
  dosage of, 60–61
  drug interactions with, 63–64
  in effective pain management, 59–60
  in geriatrics, 61
  indications for, 54, 61
  mechanism of action of, 54
  in neoplastic disease, 61
  nursing actions for, 62–65
  nursing process for, 58–59
  overdose of, management of, 61
  in pediatrics, 61–62
  postoperative, 61
  pregnancy and, 729t
  principles of therapy for, 59–62

scheduling of, 60
selection of, 60
narcotic antagonists, 58
  central nervous system effects of, 54
narcotic antitussives, 535t, 536t
Nardil (phenelzine), 117t
  as Canadian trade name, 753
  pregnancy and, 730t
Nasacort (triamcinolone), 242t
  as Canadian trade name, 754
nasal congestion, 533. *See also* nasal decongestants
Nasalcrom (cromolyn), 519
nasal decongestants, 533–541
  administration of, 538
  adverse effects of, 540
  client teaching with, 541
  description of, 534, 535t
  drug interactions with, 540–541
  in geriatrics, 539
  nursing actions for, 539–541
  nursing process for, 534, 537–538
  in pediatrics, 539
  principles of therapy with, 538–539
  selection of, 538
Nasalide (flunisolide), 241t, 518
nasal sprays, administration of, 32
nasogastric tube, drug administration and, 24, 29
Natacyn (natamycin), 444t
  in ocular disorders, 705t
natamycin (Natacyn), 444t
  in ocular disorders, 705t
Natulan (procarbazine), as Canadian trade name, 753
Naturetin (bendroflumethiazide), 602t
  as Canadian trade name, 748
nausea. *See also* antiemetics
  antiemetic therapy for, 668–674
  antineoplastic drugs and, 690
  causes of, 668
  in pregnancy, 732
Nauseatol (dimenhydrinate), as Canadian trade name, 750
Nausetrol (phosphorated carbohydrate solutions), 671, 671t
Navane (thiothixene), 103
  as Canadian trade name, 754
Naxen (naproxen), as Canadian trade name, 752
Nebcin (tobramycin), as Canadian trade name, 754
NebuPent (pentamidine isethionate), 453
nedocromil (Tilade), 519
  Canadian trade name for, 752
N.E.E. (ethinyl estradiol and norethindrone), 304t
needles, 24
NegGram (nalidixic acid), 421, 662t
  as Canadian trade name, 752
Nelova (ethinyl estradiol and norethindrone), 304t
Nelova (mestranol and norethindrone), 304t
Nembutal (pentobarbital), 82t, 83
  as Canadian trade name, 752
Neo-Calglucon (calcium glubionate), 268t
Neo-Estrone (estrone), as Canadian trade name, 750
Neoloid (castor oil), 653t
neomycin (Mycifradin, Otobiotic), 397–398, 662t
  Canadian trade name for, 752
  in pediatrics, 399
neomycin sulfate, polymyxin B sulfate, and bacitracin (Neosporin ointment), 719t
neomycin sulfate (Myciguent ointment), 719t

neonate
cephalosporins in, 375
digoxin in, 555
drug action in, 15
drug metabolism in, 11, 15
drugs used for, 736
drug therapy in, 38, 39
immune system in, 469
penicillins in, 375
pharmacodynamics in, 11, 15
neoplasms, malignant. *See also* antineoplastic drugs; cancer
characteristics of, 679–680
classification of, 682
etiology of, 680–682, 681t
hematologic, 682
solid, 682–683
Neosporin ointment (polymyxin, neomycin sulfate, and bacitracin), 719t
neostigmine (Prostigmine), 208
Canadian trade name for, 752
in pediatrics, 210
NeoStrata HQ (hydroquinone), as Canadian trade name, 751
Neo-Synephrine (phenylephrine), 187t, 188–189, 535t, 583
as Canadian trade name, 753
in ocular disorders, 702t
nephron, in renal physiology, 601
nephropathy, diabetic, 281
nephrotoxicity
with aminoglycosides, 399, 400
with antitubercular drugs, 432
drug-induced, 18
Neptazane (methazolamide)
as Canadian trade name, 752
in ocular disorders, 703t
nerve block, 151
Nesacaine (chloroprocaine), 156t
as Canadian trade name, 749
netilmicin (Netromycin), 398
Canadian trade name for, 752
lactation and, 737t
therapeutic serum drug concentrations for, 746
Netromycin (netilmicin), 398
lactation and, 737t
Neupogen (filgrastim), 489t
as Canadian trade name, 750
neurologic disorders
corticosteroids in, 240
diabetes mellitus and, 281
neuromuscular blocking drugs
anesthesia and, 152, 155t
individual, 155t
neurons, structure and function of, 47
neuropathy, diabetic, 281–282
neurotoxicity, of antitubercular drugs, 431–432
neurotransmission
autonomic nervous system in, 183, 184, 184t
impairment of, depression from, 114
neurotransmitters, 47–48
abnormalities in, 114
excitatory and inhibitory, 49
factors affecting, 48
small-molecule, 496
Neutralca-S (aluminum hydroxide gel-magnesium hydroxide), as Canadian trade name, 748
Neutra-Phos (phosphate salts), 272
neutrophils, 466
niacinamide (nicotinamide), routes and dosage ranges for, 340t
niacin (nicotinic acid, vitamin B₃), 628t, 630
routes and dosage ranges for, 340t

nicardipine (Cardene, Cardene SR), 574t, 592t
Canadian trade name for, 752
Niclocide (niclosamide), 454
niclosamide (Niclocide), 454
Nicoderm (nicotine), 744t
Nicorette (nicotine), 744t
nicotinamide (niacinamide), routes and dosage ranges for, 340t
nicotine (Habitrol, Nicoderm, Nicorette, ProStep), 744t
nicotinic acid (niacin), 628t, 630
routes and dosage ranges for, 340t
nifedipine (Adalat, Procardia), 574t, 592t
Canadian trade name for, 752
nifedipine (sustained-release) (Procardia XL), 592t
Nilstat (nystatin), as Canadian trade name, 752
nimodipine (Nimotop), 574t
Nimotop (nimodipine), 574t
as Canadian trade name, 752
Nipent (pentastatin), 687t
Nipride (sodium nitroprusside), 593t
nitrates
lactation and, 737t
long-acting, tolerance to, 577
organic, for angina pectoris, 572–573, 574–575
Nitro-Bid (nitroglycerin), 574
as Canadian trade name, 752
Nitro-Dur (nitroglycerin), as Canadian trade name, 752
nitrofurantoin (Furadantin, Macrodantin), 421
Canadian trade name for, 752
lactation and, 737t
pregnancy and, 729t
nitrofurazone (Furacin), 719t
Nitrogard-SR (nitroglycerin), as Canadian trade name, 752
nitrogen diet, 323
nitroglycerin (Nitro-Bid), 574
Canadian trade name for, 752
Nitrolingual (nitroglycerin), as Canadian trade name, 752
Nitrol (nitroglycerin), as Canadian trade name, 752
Nitrong (nitroglycerin), as Canadian trade name, 752
nitroprusside, Canadian trade name for, 752
Nitrostat (nitroglycerin), as Canadian trade name, 752
nitrous oxide, 153t
nizatidine (Axid), 641
Canadian trade name for, 752
Nizoral (ketoconazole), 444t
as Canadian trade name, 751
nodal arrhythmias, 562
Nolvadex (tamoxifen), 688t
as Canadian trade name, 753
nomogram, in drug calculation, 39
nonsteroidal anti-inflammatory drugs (NSAIDS). *see also* analgesic-antipyretic-anti-inflammatory drugs
lactation and, 738t
perioperative use of, 75–76
pregnancy and, 732t
therapy guidelines for, 75
noradrenaline, Canadian trade name for, 752
Norcept-E (ethinyl estradiol and levonorgestrel), 304t
Norcuron (vecuronium), as Canadian trade name, 754
Nordette (ethinyl estradiol and norethindrone), 304t

norepinephrine, 49
Canadian trade name for, 752
in hypotension and shock, 583
norethindrone acetate (Norlutate), 303t
norethindrone and mestranol, Canadian trade name for, 752
norethindrone (Norlutin)
Canadian trade name for, 752
in oral contraceptives, 304t
routes and dosage ranges for, 303t
Norethin (ethinyl estradiol and norethindrone), 304t
Norethin (mestranol and norethindrone), 304t
Norflex (orphenadrine), as Canadian trade name, 752
norfloxacin (Noroxin), 412
Canadian trade name for, 752
lactation and, 737t
norfloxacin ophthalmic solution (Chibroxin), 705t
norgestrel and ethinyl estradiol, Canadian trade name for, 750
norgestrel (Ovrette), 303t
in oral contraceptives, 304t
Norinyl (ethinyl estradiol and norethindrone), 304t
Norinyl (mestranol and norethindrone), as Canadian trade name, 752
Norinyl (mestranol and norethindrone acetate), 304t
Norlestrin (ethinyl estradiol and norethindrone), 304t
as Canadian trade name, 750
Norlutate (norethindrone), 303t
as Canadian trade name, 752
Norlutin (norethindrone), 303t
normal saline (sodium chloride injection), 272
Normodyne (labetalol), 198, 199t, 200, 592t
Noroxin (norfloxacin), 412
as Canadian trade name, 752
lactation and, 737t
Norpace (disopyramide), 563, 568
as Canadian trade name, 750
lactation and, 737t
pregnancy and, 729t
Norpramin (desipramine), as Canadian trade name, 749
Nor-Q.D. (norethindrone), 304t
nortriptyline (Aventyl, Pamelor), 117t
Canadian trade name for, 752
therapeutic serum drug concentrations for, 746
Norvasc (amlodipine), 574t, 592t
as Canadian trade name, 748
nose drops
administration of, 32
Novahistine decongestant (phenylephrine), as Canadian trade name, 753
Novahistine DH, 537t
Novahistine DMX, 537t
Novahistine Elixir, 537t
Novahistine Expectorant, 537t
Novamilor (amiloride), as Canadian trade name, 748
Novamobarb (amobarbital), as Canadian trade name, 748
Novamoxin (amoxicillin), as Canadian trade name, 748
Novantrone (mitoxantrone), 687t
as Canadian trade name, 752
Novasen (aspirin), as Canadian trade name, 748
Novo-Alprazol (alprazolam), as Canadian trade name, 748
Novo-Atenol (atenolol), as Canadian trade name, 748

Novo-AZT (zidovudine), as Canadian trade name, 754
Novocaine (procaine), 156t
Novocain (procaine), as Canadian trade name, 753
Novo-Captoril (captopril), as Canadian trade name, 749
Novo-Carbamaz (carbamazepine), as Canadian trade name, 749
Novo-Cimetine (cimetidine), as Canadian trade name, 749
Novo-Clopate (clorazepate), as Canadian trade name, 749
Novo-Cloxin (cloxacillin), as Canadian trade name, 749
Novo-Difenac (diclofenac), as Canadian trade name, 750
Novo-Diltazem (diltiazem), as Canadian trade name, 750
Novo-Dipiradol (dipyridamole), as Canadian trade name, 750
Novo-Doxylin (doxycycline), as Canadian trade name, 750
Novo-Hylazin (hydralazine), as Canadian trade name, 751
Novo-Keto (ketoprofen), as Canadian trade name, 751
Novo-Lexin (cephalexin), as Canadian trade name, 749
Novolin 70/30 (insulin mixtures), 283t
Novolin (isophane insulin suspension), 283t
Novolin-Lente (zinc suspension), as Canadian trade name, 751
Novolin L (insulin zinc suspension), 283t
Novolin-NPH (isophane, NPH), as Canadian trade name, 751
Novolin R (insulin injection), 283t
Novolin-Toronto (insulin), as Canadian trade name, 751
Novo-Lorazem (lorazepam), as Canadian trade name, 751
Novo-Medopa (methyldopa), as Canadian trade name, 752
Novo-methacin (indomethacin), as Canadian trade name, 751
Novo-Metoprol (metoprolol), as Canadian trade name, 752
Novo-Mucilax (psyllium hydrophilic muciloid), as Canadian trade name, 753
Novo-Naprox (naproxen), as Canadian trade name, 752
Novo-Nidazol (metronidazole), as Canadian trade name, 752
Novo-Nifedin (nifedipine), as Canadian trade name, 752
Novo-Pen-VK (penicillin V), as Canadian trade name, 752
Novo-Pindol (pindolol), as Canadian trade name, 753
Novo-Pirocam (piroxicam), as Canadian trade name, 753
Novo-Prazin (prazosin), as Canadian trade name, 753
Novo-Profen (ibuprofen), as Canadian trade name, 751
Novo-Pyrazone (sulfinpyrazone), as Canadian trade name, 753
Novo-Ranidine (ranitidine), as Canadian trade name, 753
Novo-Salmol (albuterol), as Canadian trade name, 748
Novo-Secobarb (secobarbital), as Canadian trade name, 753
Novo-Spiroton (spironolactone), as Canadian trade name, 753
Novo-Sudac (sulindac), as Canadian trade name, 753
Novo-Tetra (tetracycline), as Canadian trade name, 754

Novo-Timol (timolol), as Canadian trade name, 754
Novo-trimel (sulfamethoxazole and trimethoprim), as Canadian trade name, 753
Novo-Triolam (triazolam), as Canadian trade name, 754
Novo-Tripramine (trimipramine), as Canadian trade name, 754
Novo-Tythro (erythromycin), as Canadian trade name, 750
Novo-Veramil (verapamil), as Canadian trade name, 754
NPH Iletin I (isophane insulin suspension), 283t
NPH Insulin (isophane insulin suspension), 283t
NPH Insulin (isophane NPH), as Canadian trade name, 751
NPH purified pork (isophane insulin suspension), 283t
Nu-Alpraz (alprazolam), as Canadian trade name, 748
Nu-Amilzide (amiloride), as Canadian trade name, 748
Nu-Amoxi (amoxicillin), as Canadian trade name, 748
Nu-Ampi (ampicillin), as Canadian trade name, 748
Nu-Atenol (atenolol), as Canadian trade name, 748
Nubain (nalbuphine), 57
  as Canadian trade name, 752
Nu-Cal (calcium carbonate), as Canadian trade name, 749
Nu-Capto (captopril), as Canadian trade name, 749
Nu-Cephalex (cephalexin), as Canadian trade name, 749
Nu-Cimet (cimetidine), as Canadian trade name, 749
Nu-Cloxi (cloxacillin), as Canadian trade name, 749
Nu-Cotrimix (sulfamethoxazole and trimethoprim), as Canadian trade name, 753
Nu-Diclo (diclofenac), as Canadian trade name, 750
Nu-Diltiaz (diltiazem), as Canadian trade name, 750
Nu-Hydral (hydralazine), as Canadian trade name, 751
Nu-Indo (indomethacin), as Canadian trade name, 751
Nu-Loraz (lorazepam), as Canadian trade name, 751
Nu-Medopa (methyldopa), as Canadian trade name, 752
Nu-Metop (metoprolol), as Canadian trade name, 752
Numorphan (oxymorphone), 56–57
  as Canadian trade name, 752
Nu-Naprox (naproxen), as Canadian trade name, 752
Nu-Nifedin (nifedipine), as Canadian trade name, 752
Nu-Pen-VK (penicillin V), as Canadian trade name, 752
Nuperainal (dibucaine), as Canadian trade name, 749
Nupercainal (dibucaine), 156t
Nu-Pindol (pindolol), as Canadian trade name, 753
Nu-Pirox (piroxicam), as Canadian trade name, 753
Nu-Prazo (prazosin), as Canadian trade name, 753
Nu-Ranit (ranitidine), as Canadian trade name, 753

Nuromax (doxacurium), 155t
  as Canadian trade name, 750
nursing diagnoses, 35, 36
nursing process
  assessment in, 35, 36
  in drug therapy, 33–34
  evaluation in, 36
  general considerations in, 33–34
  interventions in, 35, 36
  legal responsibilities in, 34
  monitoring drug therapy in, 41–43
  nursing diagnoses in, 35, 36
  planning and goals in, 35, 36
Nursoy, 323
Nu-Tetra (tetracycline), as Canadian trade name, 754
Nutramigen, 323
Nu-Triazo (triazolam), as Canadian trade name, 754
nutrients, antacid effect on, 646
nutrition, parenteral, 227–228
nutritional products, 319. See also diet; vitamins
  administration of, 329–330
  adverse effects of, 330–331
  client teaching with, 331
  for general use, 322
  infant formulas, 324
  intravenous, 227–228, 324
  nursing actions for, 329–331
  nursing process for, 325–327
  for oral or tube feeding, 322–324
  pancreatic enzymes as, 330–331
  for specific use, 322–324
  supplemental, 324
  therapeutic effects of, 330
nutritional status, immune function and, 470
Nu-Verap (verapamil), as Canadian trade name, 754
Nyaderm (nystatin), as Canadian trade name, 752
Nydrazid (isoniazid) (INH), 428–429
nystatin (Mycostatin), 444t, 719t
  Canadian trade name for, 752
Nytol (diphenhydramine), as Canadian trade name, 750

**O**
obesity
  in diabetes mellitus, 280
  management of, 328
Occlucort (betamethasone), as Canadian trade name, 748
Ocuclear (oxymetazoline), as Canadian trade name, 752
Ocufen (flurbiprofen), as Canadian trade name, 750
ocular disorders, 700, 706–707
Ocupress (carteolol), 198, 199t, 200
  in ocular disorders, 702t
Ocusert (pilocarpine ocular therapeutic system), in ocular disorders, 702t
Oestrilin (estrone), as Canadian trade name, 750
ofloxacin (Floxin), 412
  Canadian trade name for, 752
Ogen (estropipate), 302t
  as Canadian trade name, 750
ointments
  dermatologic, 722
  ophthalmic, 707
omeprazole (Prilosec), 639, 640, 646
  Canadian trade name for, 752
Omnipen (ampicillin), 382t, 662t
oncogenes, 682
Oncovin (vincristine), 687t
  as Canadian trade name, 754

ondansetron (Zofran), 671, 671t
Canadian trade name for, 752
Ophthaine (proparacaine hydrochloride),
703t–704t
ophthalmia neonatorum, 736
ophthalmic drugs, 701–711
administration of, 708
methods of, 701
adverse effects of, 709–710
antiallergic, 704t
anticholinergics as, 214
antifungal drugs as, 705t
anti-infective drugs as, 700, 705t
antiseptic as, 704t
antiviral drugs as, 705t
autonomic drugs as, 700–701, 702t
carbonic anhydrase inhibitors as, 701
chelating agent as, 701
client teaching in, 710–711
corticosteroids as, 240
diuretics as, 703t
drug interactions with, 710
edetate disodium (Endrate) as, 701
fluorescein as, 701
in geriatrics, 707
in glaucoma, 707
individual, 702t–704t
instillation of, 26, 31
local anesthetics as, 703t–704t
lubricants as, 704t
nursing actions for, 708–711
nursing process for, 701, 706
in ocular infections, 706–707
ointments, 707
in pediatrics, 707
principles of therapy with, 706–707
therapeutic effects of, 708
Ophtho-Chloram (chloramphenicol), as
Canadian trade name, 749
Ophtho-Sulf (sulfacetamide), as Canadian
trade name, 753
Ophtho-Tate (prednisolone), as Canadian
trade name, 753
opiates. *See also* narcotic analgesics
abuse of, 165
treatment of, 174
as antidiarrheals, 662f
receptors for, 54t
opium, camphorated tincture of (paregoric), 661t
Opticrom (cromolyn), 519
as Canadian trade name, 749
in ocular disorders, 704t
Optimine (azatadine), 529t
as Canadian trade name, 748
OptiPranolol (metipranolol), 198, 199t, 200
in ocular disorders, 702t
Oracort (triamcinolone), as Canadian trade
name, 754
Oradexon (dexamethasone), as Canadian
trade name, 749
oral cavity, 635
oral contraceptives, 304t
administration of, 306
adverse reactions to, 306–307
client teaching with, 307
contraindications for, 299–300
description of, 299
drug interactions with, 307
estrogen in, 305
indications for, 299
mechanism of action with, 299
nursing actions for, 306
nursing process for, 300
postcoital, 303
preparations of, 304t
principles of therapy with, 302, 305
progestin in, 305
therapeutic effects of, 306

oral feedings
administration of, 331
nutritional products for, 322
for undernutrition, 326
oral medications
absorption of, 10
administration of, 24
nursing actions for, 28–29
routes for, 24–26
Oramorph (morphine), as Canadian trade
name, 752
Orap (pimozide), 104
Orbenin (cloxacillin), as Canadian trade
name, 749
orciprenaline, Canadian trade name for,
752
Oretic (hydrochlorothiazide), 602t
Oreton methyl (methyltestosterone),
312t
Oreton (testosterone), 312t
organ transplants, rejection of, 496–497.
*See also* immunosuppressants
Orimune (poliovirus vaccine), 475t
Orinase (tolbutamide), 284t, 284–285
as Canadian trade name, 754
lactation and, 738t
orphenadrine, 146t
Canadian trade name for, 752
orphenadrine hydrochloride (Disipal),
137t
Orthoclone OKT3 (muromonab-CD3), 497t
as Canadian trade name, 752
Ortho Dienestrol Creme (dienestrol), as
Canadian trade name, 750
Ortho 0.5/35 (ethinyl estradiol and
norethindrone), as Canadian trade
name, 750
Ortho 1/35 (ethinyl estradiol and norethindrone), as Canadian trade name,
750
Ortho 7/7/7 (ethinyl estradiol and
norethindrone), as Canadian trade
name, 750
Ortho 10/11 (ethinyl estradiol and
norethindrone), as Canadian trade
name, 750
Ortho 1/50 (mestranol and norethindrone),
as Canadian trade name, 752
Ortho-Novum (ethinyl estradiol and
norethindrone), 304t
Ortho-Novum (mestranol and norethindrone), 304t
Orudis (ketoprofen), 68, 69
as Canadian trade name, 751
indications for, 68, 68t
Oruvail (ketoprofen), as Canadian trade
name, 751
Os-Cal 500 (calcium carbonate), 268t
Os-Cal (calcium carbonate), as Canadian
trade name, 749
Osmitrol (mannitol), 603t
as Canadian trade name, 751
in ocular disorders, 703t
Osmoglyn (glycerin), 603t
in ocular disorders, 703t
Osmolite, 322
osmotic diuretics, 606
mechanism of action with, 13
ophthalmic, 701, 703t. *See also*
ophthalmic drugs
osteoarthritis, drugs used in, 68t
osteoporosis, estrogens and, 305
Ostoforte (ergocalciferol), as Canadian
trade name, 750
otic drugs, instillation of, 31
otitis, external, 714
dermatologic drugs for, 722
Otobiotic (neomycin), 397–398
in pediatrics, 399

ototoxicity
with aminoglycosides, 400
with neomycin, 399
Otrivin (xylometazoline), 187t, 535t
as Canadian trade name, 754
ovarian hormones, 227
Ovcon (ethinyl estradiol and norethindrone), 304t
Ovcon (ethinyl estradiol and norgestrel),
304t
overdosage
of alcohol and drugs of abuse, 172
of antidepressants, 120
of atropine, 218
of barbiturates, 173–174
of opiates, 174
overweight, management of, 328
Ovide (malathion), 455
Ovral (ethinyl estradiol), 304t
Ovral (ethinyl estradiol and norgestrel), as
Canadian trade name, 750
Ovrette (norethindrone), 304t
Ovrette (norgestrel), 303t
oxacillin (Prostaphlin), 381, 382t
Oxandrin (oxandrolone), 312t
oxandrolone (Oxandrin), 312t
oxazepam (Serax), 91t
Canadian trade name for, 752
oxiconazole (Oxistat), 444t, 719t
oxidizing drugs, antiseptic, 717t
oxilapine, Canadian trade name for, 751
Oxistat (oxiconazole), 444t, 719t
Oxsoralen (methoxsalen), as Canadian
trade name, 752
Oxsoralen-ultra (methoxsalen), 720t
oxtriphylline (Choledyl), 518t
oxybutynin (Ditropan), in pediatrics, 218
oxycodone, Canadian trade name for, 752
oxygen, in brain metabolism, 51
oxymetazoline, Canadian trade name for,
752
oxymetazoline hydrochloride (Afrin), 187t,
535t
oxymetholone (Anadrol-50), 312t
Canadian trade name for, 752
oxymorphone (Numorphan), 56–57
Canadian trade name for, 752
oxyphencyclimine bromide (Daricon),
214t
oxytetracycline (Terramycin), 403t, 451
oxytocics
nursing actions for, 739–741
pregnancy and, 734–735, 735t
oxytocin, endogenous, 50, 229
oxytocin (Pitocin), 50, 232
Canadian trade name for, 752
pregnancy and, 735t

**P**

paclitaxel (Taxol), 689t
pain
acute, 53, 60
analgesic-antipyretic-anti-inflammatory
drugs in, 67, 68t
antianxiety drugs in, 94
chronic, 53, 60
deep, 53
management of, effective, 59
narcotic analgesics for, 53–54
nursing process for, 58–59
receptors for, 53
response to, 53
in children, 62
superficial, 53
Pamelor (nortriptyline), 117t
pamidronate (Aredia), 271
Canadian trade name for, 752
Pamine (methscopolamine), 216

Panadol (acetaminophen), as Canadian trade name, 748
Panafil (papain), 720t
Pancrease (pancreatin or pancrelipase), 663t
  as Canadian trade name, 752
pancreatic enzymes, 325
  administration of, 330
  client teaching with, 331
pancreatic hormones, 227
pancreatin (pancrelipase) (Cotazym, Pancrease, Viokase), 325, 663t
  Canadian trade name for, 752
pancrelipase (pancreatin) (Cotazym, Pancrease, Viokase), 663t
  Canadian trade name for, 752
pancuronium (Pavulon), 155t
  Canadian trade name for, 752
Panectyl (trimeprazine), as Canadian trade name, 754
Panoxyl (benzoyl peroxide), as Canadian trade name, 748
pantothenic acid (vitamin B₅), 335t
  imbalance of, 338t
Panwarfin (warfarin), 615, 616
  antidote for, 617
  dosage for, 619–620
papain (Panafil), 720t
papaverine hydrochloride (Pavabid), 629t
para-aminosalicylic acid (PAS), 429
parabromdylamine, Canadian trade name for, 749
paracetamol, Canadian trade name for, 748
Paraflex (chlorzoxazone), 146t
Paraplatin (carboplatin), 686t
  as Canadian trade name, 749
parasitic diseases, 448–450. See also antiparasitics
parasympathetic nervous system, 185
parasympatholytic drugs. See anticholinergic drugs
parasympathomimetics. See cholinergic drugs
parathyroid hormone, 227
  calcium metabolism and, 265–266
Paredrine (hydroxyamphetamine), in ocular disorders, 702t
paregoric, pectin, and kaolin (Parepectolin), 663t
paregoric (camphorated tincture of opium), 661t
parenteral feedings
  administration of, 327–328, 331
  adverse effects of, 330
  client teaching with, 331
  in pediatrics, 328
  therapeutic effects of, 330
  for undernutrition, 327
    guidelines for, 327–328
parenteral medications, administration of, 24–30
Parepectolin (kaolin, pectin, and paregoric), 663t
Parkinson's disease, 136. See also antiparkinson drugs
  anticholinergics in, 215, 216
  substantia nigra and, 51
Parlodel (bromocriptine), 136, 138–139
  as Canadian trade name, 749
  lactation and, 735
  pregnancy and, 735t
Parnate (tranylcypromine), 117t
  as Canadian trade name, 754
paromomycin sulfate (Humatin), 397, 398
paroxetine (Paxil), 117t
Parsidol (ethopropazine hydrochloride), 137t
Parsitan (ethopropazine), as Canadian trade name, 750
PAS (para-aminosalicylic acid), 429

pastes, dermatologic, 722
Pathilon (tridihexethyl), 214t
Pavabid (papaverine hydrochloride), 629t
Pavulon (pancuronium), 155t
  as Canadian trade name, 752
Paxil (paroxetine), 117t
Paxipam (halazepam), 91t
PBZ (tripelennamine hydrochloride), 528t
pectin, kaolin, and paregoric (Parepectolin), 663t
pectin, kaolin, atropine sulfate, hyoscyamine sulfate, hyoscine hydrobromide, alcohol (Donnagel), 663t
pectin and kaolin mixture (Kaopectate), 663t
pediatrics. See also children; infant; neonate
  acetaminophen in, 76
  adrenergic drugs in, 190–191
  aminoglycosides in, 399
  anabolic steroids in, 314
  analgesic-antipyretic-anti-inflammatory drugs in, 76
  androgens in, 314
  antacids in, 646
  antiadrenergic drugs in, 202
  antianginal drugs in, 577
  antianxiety drugs in, 96
  antiarrhythmic drugs in, 568
  antiasthmatic drugs in, 521
  anticholinergics in, 218
  anticoagulants in, 620
  anticonvulsants in, 131, 134
  antidepressants in, 120
  antidiabetic drugs in, 291
  antidiarrheals in, 665
  antiemetics in, 673
  antifungal drugs in, 444t, 445
  antihistamines in, 530
  antihypertensive drugs in, 596–597
  anti-infective drugs in, 375–376
  antilipemic drugs in, 630
  antineoplastic drugs in, 694
  antiparkinson drugs in, 140
  antithyroid drugs in, 260
  antitubercular drugs in, 431
  antiviral drugs in, 438
  benzodiazepines in, 96
  beta-adrenergic drugs in, 202
  bronchodilators in, 521
  cardiotonic-inotropic drugs in, 555
  cathartics in, 656
  central nervous system stimulants in, 179
  cephalosporins in, 393
  cholinergic drugs in, 210
  cold remedies in, 539
  corticosteroids in, 247
  dermatologic drugs in, 723
  diuretics in, 609
  dosage calculation in, 38–39
  drug therapy in, 15
  electrolytes in, 346–365
  erythromycin in, 409
  estrogens in, exogenous, 305
  hypercalcemia drugs in, 273
  hypocalcemia in, 270
  hypotension in, 584
  immunization in, 481–482, 482t
  immunostimulants in, 492
  immunosuppressants in, 503
  laxatives in, 656
  macrolides in, 409
  minerals in, 361
  mucolytics in, 539
  narcotic analgesics in, 61–62
  nasal decongestants in, 539
  nutritional support in, 328
  ophthalmic drugs in, 707
  penicillins in, 385
  pharmacodynamics in, 15

  sedative-hypnotics in, 85
  skeletal muscle relaxants in, 147
  theophylline in, 521
  tube feedings in, 328
  vitamins in, 342
pediculocides, 455. See also antiparasitics
pediculosis, 450, 455. See also antiparasitics
Pedvax HIB (Haemophilus b conjugate vaccine), 473t
  as Canadian trade name, 751
PEG 3350 (polyethylene glycol-electrolyte solution), 652t
pemoline (Cylert), 177
Penbriten (ampicillin), 382t, 662t
  as Canadian trade name, 748
penbutolol (Levatol), 198, 199t, 200, 592t
Penetrex (enoxacin), 412
Penglobe (bacampicillin), as Canadian trade name, 748
penicillamine (Cuprimine), 354
  Canadian trade name for, 752
penicillin G, 381, 382t
penicillin G benzathine (Bicillin), 382t
  Canadian trade name for, 752
penicillin G potassium (Pentids, Pfizerpen), 382t
  Canadian trade name for, 752
penicillin G procaine (Wycillin), 382t
  Canadian trade name for, 752
penicillin G sodium, 382t
penicillins, 380–386, 382t–383t
  administration of, 385
    route of, 384
  adverse effects of, 385–386
  with aminoglycoside, 384
  ampicillins, 381
  antipseudomonal, 381, 382t–383t
  client teaching for, 386
  contraindications to, 381
  description of, 380
  dosing of, 384
  drug interactions with, 386
  electrolyte disturbances and, 384–385
  extended-spectrum, 381
  in geriatrics, 375, 385
  hypersensitivity to, 384
  indications for, 380
  individual, 382t–383t
  lactation and, 737t
  mechanism of action with, 380
  nursing actions for, 385–386
  nursing process for, 383–384
  in pediatrics, 375–376, 385
  penicillinase-resistant, 381
  penicillin-beta-lactamase combination, 383
  penicillin G, 381
  penicillin V, 381
  principles of therapy with, 383–385
  with probenecid, 384
  selection of, 384
  in sexually transmitted diseases, 384
  in streptococcal infections, 384
  therapeutic effects of, 385
penicillin V (PenVee K, V-Cillin K), 381, 382t
  Canadian trade name for, 752
Pentacarinat (pentamidine), as Canadian trade name, 752
pentaerythritol, Canadian trade name for, 752
pentaerythritol tetranitrate (Peritrate), 575
pentamidine, Canadian trade name for, 752
pentamidine isethionate (NebuPent, Pentam 300), 453
Pentam 300 (pentamidine isethionate), 453
pentastatin (Nipent), 687t
pentazocine (Talwin), 57–58
  Canadian trade name for, 752

Penthrane (methoxyflurane), 153t
Pentids (penicillin G potassium), 382t
pentobarbital, Canadian trade name for, 752
pentobarbital sodium (Nembutal), 82t, 83
Pentothal (thiopental), 154t
  as Canadian trade name, 754
pentoxifylline (Trental), 627
  Canadian trade name for, 752
PenVee K (penicillin V), 382t
Pen-Vee (penicillin V), as Canadian trade
    name, 752
Pepcid (famotidine), 641
  as Canadian trade name, 750
  lactation and, 738t
peptic ulcer disease, 638
  causes of, 638
  drugs used in, 639–649. *See also named
      class*
    administration of, 647
    adverse effects of, 648
    antacid products, 639–640, 643t, 646
    classes of, 641–642
    client teaching for, 649
    cytoprotective drugs, 640
    drug interactions with, 645–646, 648
    gastric acid inhibitors, 639, 640–642
    gastric acid neutralizers, 639–640, 642,
        643t, 646
    in geriatrics, 646
    histamine-2 receptor blocking agents,
        639
    nursing actions for, 647–649
    nursing process for, 642, 644
    nutrients and, 646
    in pediatrics, 646
    principles of therapy with, 644–646
    prostaglandins, 639
    therapeutic effects of, 647
Peptol (cimetidine), as Canadian trade
    name, 749
Perdiem Plain (psyllium preparations), 652t
pergolide, Canadian trade name for, 752
Pergonal (menotropins), 231
Periactin (cyproheptadine), 529t
  as Canadian trade name, 749
Peritrate (pentaerythritol), 575
  as Canadian trade name, 752
Permax (pergolide), as Canadian trade
    name, 752
Permitil (fluphenazine hydrochloride), 101t
perphenazine (Trilafon), 102t, 670t
  Canadian trade name for, 752
Persantine (dipyridamole), 615, 616
  as Canadian trade name, 750
Pertofrane (desipramine), as Canadian
    trade name, 749
pertussis vaccine, 477t
pethidine, Canadian trade name for, 752
Pfizerpen (penicillin G potassium), 382t
pharmacoanthropology
  pharmacokinetics and, 16
pharmacodynamics, 12–13
pharmacogenetics
  pharmacokinetics and, 16
pharmacokinetics, 10–12
  in pregnancy, 727t
pharmacology, prototype approach to,
    33–34
pharynx, defined, 511
phenazopyridine (Pyridium), 422
  Canadian trade name for, 752
phendimetrazine (Plegine), 323t
phenelzine (Nardil), 117t
  Canadian trade name for, 753
  pregnancy and, 730t
Phenergan (promethazine), 100, 528t, 670t
  anesthesia and, 151
  as Canadian trade name, 753
  lactation and, 738t

Phenergan VC, 537t
phenobarbital, ephedrine hydrochloride,
    and theophylline (Tedral), 518t
phenobarbital (Luminal), 82t, 83, 753
  pregnancy and, 730t
  seizure disorders and, 127
  therapeutic serum drug concentrations
      for, 746
phenobarbitone, 753
phenolphthalein (Alophen, Ex-Lax, Feen-
    a-Mint), 652t
phenothiazines, 525, 528t. *See also* antihist-
    amines
  as antiemetics, 669, 670t, 673
phenoxybenzamine (Dibenzyline), 198
phenoxymethyl penicillin, Canadian trade
    name for, 752
phentermine, Canadian trade name for, 753
phentermine hydrochloride (Fastin), 323t
phentermine resin (Ionamin), 323t
phentolamine (Regitine), 198
phenylephrine (Neo-Synephrine), 187t,
    188–189, 535t, 583
  Canadian trade name for, 753
  in geriatrics, 191
  in ocular disorders, 702t
  in pediatrics, 191
phenylpropanolamine (Acutrim, Dexatrim,
    Propagest), 187t, 322, 535t
  in pediatrics, 191–191
phenytoin (Dilantin), 127
  Canadian trade name for, 753
  digitalis intoxication and, 564
  lactation and, 737t
  pregnancy and, 730t
  therapeutic serum drug concentrations
      for, 746
pHisoHex (hexachlorophene and entsufon
    sodium emulsion), 717t
  as Canadian trade name, 751
phosphate salts (Neutra-Phos), 272
Pholphine (echothiophate), as Canadian
    trade name, 750
Pholphine Iodide (echothiophate iodide),
    in ocular disorders, 702t
phosphorated carbohydrate solutions
    (Emetrol, Nausetrol), 671, 671t
phosphorus, 266, 267
  in calcium metabolism, 267
  daily requirement for, 267
  metabolic functions of, 267
Phyllocontin (aminophylline), as Canadian
    trade name, 748
*Physicians' Desk Reference*, 4
physostigmine salicylate (Antilirium, Isopto
    Eserine), 208–209
  in ocular disorders, 702t–703t
physostigmine sulfate (Eserine Sulfate), in
    ocular disorders, 702t–703t
phytomenadione, Canadian trade name for,
    753
phytonadione (vitamin K) (Aqua-Mephy-
    ton, Mephyton), 617
  Canadian trade name for, 753
  routes and dosage ranges for, 340t
Pilocar (pilocarpine), in ocular disorders,
    702t
pilocarpine (Almocarpine, Isopto Carpine,
    Pilocar, Pilocel, Pilomiotin)
  Canadian trade name for, 753
  in glaucoma, 218
  in ocular disorders, 702t
pilocarpine ocular therapeutic system
    (Ocusert Pilo-20, Ocusert pilo-40),
    702t
Pilocel (pilocarpine), in ocular disorders,
    702t
Pilomiotin (pilocarpine), in ocular disor-
    ders, 702t

Pilopine (pilocarpine), as Canadian trade
    name, 753
pimozide (Orap), 104
pindolol (Visken), 198, 199t, 200, 592t
  Canadian trade name for, 753
pinworm infections (enterobiasis), 449. *See
    also* antiparasitics
pipecuronium (Arduan), 155t
piperacillin and tazobactam (Zosyn), 383t
piperacillin (Pipracil), 383t
  Canadian trade name for, 753
piperazine, Canadian trade name for, 753
piperazine citrate (Antepar), 454
piperazine estrone sulfate, Canadian trade
    name for, 750
piperazines, 454, 525, 528t, 528t, 750, 753.
    *See* also antihistamines
pipobroman (Vercyte), 686t
Pipracil (piperacillin), 383t
  as Canadian trade name, 753
pirbuterol (Maxair), 187t, 516
piroxicam (Feldene), 71
  Canadian trade name for, 753
  indications for, 68, 68t
Pitocin (oxytocin), 232
  pregnancy and, 735t
Pitrex (tolnaftate), as Canadian trade name,
    754
pituitary gland, anterior
  estrogens and, 298
  testosterone effect on, 310
pituitary hormones
  administration of, 233
  adverse effects of, 233–234
  anterior, individual, 230–231
  client teaching with, 235
  description of, 228–229
  drug interactions with, 234–235
  nursing actions for, 233–235
  nursing process for, 232
  posterior, individual, 231–232
  principles of therapy with, 232–233
  therapeutic limitations of, 229–230
placental hormones, 227
Placidyl (ethchlorvynol), 82t, 83
plague vaccine, 475t
plant alkaloids, 684, 687t
Plaquenil (hydroxychloroquine), 452
  as Canadian trade name, 751
platelets, defined, 615
Platinol AQ (*cis*-platin), as Canadian trade
    name, 749
Platinol (cisplatin), 686t
Plegine (phendimetrazine), 323t
Plendil (felodipine), 574, 592t
  as Canadian trade name, 750
pleura, defined, 512
plicamycin (Mithracin), 272, 687t
PMS-Artificial Tears (polyvinyl alcohol), as
    Canadian trade name, 753
PMS-Egozinc (zinc sulfate), as Canadian
    trade name, 754
pneumococcal vaccine (Pneumovax 23,
    Pnu-Imune 23), 475t
  Canadian trade name for, 753
*Pneumocystis carinii* pneumonia (PCP), 449,
    453
Pneumopent (pentamidine), as Canadian
    trade name, 752
Pneumovax 23 (pneumococcal vaccine),
    475t
  as Canadian trade name, 753
Pnu-Imune 23 (pneumococcal vaccine),
    475t
Polaramine (dexchlorpheniramine), 527t
  as Canadian trade name, 749
poliomyelitis vaccine, inactivated (IPOL),
    475t
poliovirus vaccine (Orimune), 475t

Polocaine (mepivacaine), as Canadian trade name, 752
polycarbophil (FiberCon, Mitrolan), 652t
  Canadian trade name for, 753
Polycose, 324
polyestradiol phosphate (Estradurin), 302t
polymyxin B sulfate, in ocular disorders, 705t
polymyxin B (Aerosporin), 412–413
  Canadian trade name for, 753
polymyxin B and bacitracin (Polysporin ointment), 719t
polymyxin B sulfate, neomycin sulfate, and bacitracin (Neosporin ointment), 719t
polymyxins, 412–414
  administration of, 415
  adverse effects of, 416
  drug interactions with, 417
  principles of therapy with, 414
polyphagia, in diabetes, 280
Polysporin ointment (bacitracin and polymyxin B), 719t
polythiazide and prazosin (Minizide), 593t
polythiazide (Renese), 602t
polyvinyl alcohol (Liquifilm)
  Canadian trade name for, 753
  in ocular disorders, 704t
polyvinyl chloride (PVC), as carcinogen, 681t
Ponderal (fenfluramine), as Canadian trade name, 750
Pondimin (fenfluramine), 323t
  as Canadian trade name, 750
Ponstel (mefenamic acid), 71
pons varolii, 50
Pontocaine (tetracaine), 156t
  as Canadian trade name, 754
  in ocular disorders, 704t
Portagen, 323
postganglionic-active drugs, 590, 591t
potassium
  description of, 347t
  imbalances of, 349t
    diuretics and, 607–608
    treatment of, 358–359
  preparations of, 355
potassium bicarbonate and citrate (K-Lyte), 355
potassium clavulanate and amoxicillin (Augmentin), 383t
potassium clavulanate and ticarcillin, Canadian trade name for, 754
potassium gluconate (Kaon), 355
potassium iodine solution, 257
potassium-sparing diuretics, 605–606
potentiation, pharmacologic, 14–15
Povan (pyrvinium pamoate), 454
povidone-iodine (Betadine, Isodine), 453, 716t
  Canadian trade name for, 753
powders, dermatologic, 722
pramocaine, Canadian trade name for, 753
pramoxine (Tronothane), 156t
  Canadian trade name for, 753
Pravachol (pravastatin), 628t, 630
  as Canadian trade name, 753
pravastatin (Pravachol), 628t, 630
  Canadian trade name for, 753
prazepam (Centrax), 91t
prazosin and polythiazide (Minizide), 593t
prazosin (Minipress), 549, 591t
  Canadian trade name for, 753
Precef (ceforanide), 391t
prednisolone acetate (Econopred, Fernisolone), 242t, 706t
prednisolone (Delta-Cortef, Sterane), 242t
  Canadian trade name for, 753
prednisolone sodium phosphate (Hydeltrasol, Inflamase, Metreton), 242t, 706t

prednisolone sodium succinate (Meticortelone soluble), 242t
prednisolone tebutate (Hydeltra-TBA), 242t
prednisone (Deltasone, Meticorten), 242t, 519, 688t
  Canadian trade name for, 753
  in hypercalcemia, 271
  lactation and, 738t
Pregestimil, 323
pregnancy. See also delivery; labor
  antithyroid drugs and, 260
  circulation in, maternal-placental-fetal, 726–727
  description of, 726
  drug use during, 726–741
    abortifacients, 734, 735t
    administration of, 739–740
    adverse effects of, 740–741
    analgesics and, 735
    anemia and, 728, 730
    anesthetics and, 735
    asthma and, 732–733
    chronic disease and, 733–734
    client teaching with, 741
    constipation and, 732
    diabetes mellitus and, 733–734
    drug interactions with, 741
    effects of, 729t–731t
    epilepsy and, 734
    FDA categories for, 728t
    guidelines for, 739
    heartburn and, 732
    hypertension and, 734
    hypoglycemics, oral, 733–734
    for labor and delivery, 734–735, 735t
    maternal-placental-fetal circulation and, 726–727
    nausea and vomiting and, 732
    nursing actions for, 739–741
    nursing process for, 736, 738
    oxytocics, 734–735, 735t, 739
    physiology and, 727, 727t
    pregnancy-induced hypertension and, 732
    principles of therapy for, 739
    seizures disorders, 734
    teratogenic drugs and, 727
    therapeutic effects of, 740
    tocolytics in, 734, 735t
  estrogens during, 298
  hypertension in, 732, 734
  physiologic and pharmacokinetic changes in, 727t
  symptoms in, 728, 732
pregnancy-induced hypertension, 732
Premarin (conjugated estrogens), 301t
  as Canadian trade name, 750
Prepidil (dinoprostone, prostaglandin E₂), as Canadian trade name, 750
Prepulsid (cisapride), as Canadian trade name, 749
pressure ulcer, dermatologic drugs for, 722
Prevex (zinc oxide), as Canadian trade name, 754
prilocaine (Citanest), 156t
  Canadian trade name for, 753
Prilosec (omeprazole), 639, 640, 646
  as Canadian trade name, 752
Primacor (milrinone IV), 551
primaquine phosphate, 452–453
Primaxin (imipenem and cilastatin)
  as Canadian trade name, 751
  lactation and, 737t
  pregnancy and, 729t
primidone (Mysoline), 128
  Canadian trade name for, 753
  therapeutic serum drug concentrations for, 746

Prinivil (lisinopril), 591t
  as Canadian trade name, 751
  lactation and, 737t
Privine (naphazoline), 187t, 535t
  as Canadian trade name, 752
Pro-Banthine (propantheline), 214t
  as Canadian trade name, 753
probenecid, penicillins with, 384
probenecid (Benemid), 72
  Canadian trade name for, 753
  in hyperuricemia, 76
probucol (Lorelco), 628t, 630
  Canadian trade name for, 753
procainamide (Procan, Pronestyl), 563, 568
  Canadian trade name for, 753
  lactation and, 737t
  pregnancy and, 729t
  therapeutic serum drug concentrations for, 746
procaine (Novocaine), 156t
  Canadian trade name for, 753
Procan (procainamide), 563, 568
  lactation and, 737t
  pregnancy and, 729t
Procan-SR (procainamide), as Canadian trade name, 753
procarbazine (Matulane), 689t
  Canadian trade name for, 753
Procardia (nifedipine), 574t, 592t
Procardia XL (nifedipine) (sustained-release), 592t
prochlorperazine (Compazine), 102t, 670t
  Canadian trade name for, 753
Procrit (epoetin alfa), 486, 743t
procyclidine (Kemadrin), 137t, 216
  Canadian trade name for, 753
Procyclid (procyclidine), as Canadian trade name, 753
Procytox (cyclophosphamide), as Canadian trade name, 749
Prodiem Plain (psyllium hydrophilic muciloid), as Canadian trade name, 753
Progagest (phenylpropanolamine hydrochloride), 187t
Progelan (progesterone), 303t
progesterone, 298. See also progestins
  indications for, 299
  lipid metabolism and, 298
  in pregnancy, 298
progesterone (Femotrone, Progelan), 298, 303t
progestin, as oral contraceptive, 304t
progestins
  administration of, 306
  adverse reactions to, 306–307
  cancer and, 303t, 305, 684
  client teaching with, 307
  in contraception, 304t, 305
  contraindications for, 299–300
  drug interactions with, 307
  indications for, 299
  mechanism of action with, 299
  nursing actions for, 306–307
  nursing process for, 300
  preparations of, 298–299, 303t
  principles of therapy with, 302, 305
  supervision of, 302
  therapeutic effects of, 306
Proglycem (diazoxide), as Canadian trade name, 749
ProHibit (*Haemophilus* B conjugate vaccine), 473t
Prokine (sargramostim), 489t
prolactin, 50, 229
prolactin-inhibitory factor (PIF), 228
prolactin-releasing factor, 228
Proleukin (aldesleukin), 489t
Prolixin decanoate (fluphenazine decanoate and enanthate), 101t

Prolixin enanthate (fluphenazine decanoate and enanthate), 101t
Prolixin (fluphenazine hydrochloride), 101t
Proloprim (trimethoprim), 422
  as Canadian trade name, 754
  lactation and, 737t
  pregnancy and, 730t
promazine (Sparine), 102t
promethazine (Phenergan), 100, 528t, 670t
  anesthesia and, 151
  Canadian trade name for, 753
  lactation and, 738t
Pronestyl (procainamide), 563, 568
  as Canadian trade name, 753
  lactation and, 737t
  pregnancy and, 729t
Propaderm (beclomethasone), as Canadian trade name, 748
propafenone (Rythmol), 564, 568
  Canadian trade name for, 753
Propagest (phenylpropanolamine hydrochloride), 535t
propantheline, Canadian trade name for, 753
propantheline bromide (Pro-Banthine), 214t
proparacaine (Alcaine, Ophthaine), 156t
  Canadian trade name for, 753
  in ocular disorders, 703t–704t
Propine (dipivefrin)
  as Canadian trade name, 750
  in ocular disorders, 702t
propofol (Diprivan), 154t
  Canadian trade name for, 753
propoxyphene (Darvon), 57
propranolol and hydrochlorothiazide (Inderide), 593t
propranolol (Inderal), 198, 199t, 200, 257–258, 565, 568, 575, 592t
  Canadian trade name for, 753
  lactation and, 738t
  pregnancy and, 730t, 731t
  therapeutic serum drug concentrations for, 746
propranolol (Inderal), in pediatrics, 202
Propulsid (cisapride), 670t, 699
propylhexedrine (Benzedrex), 187t, 535t
propylthiouracil, 257
  Canadian trade name for, 753
  lactation and, 738t
  pregnancy and, 731t
Propyl-Thyracil (propylthiouracil), as Canadian trade name, 753
Proscar (finasteride), 743t
ProSobee, 323
ProSom (estazolam), 82t, 83
prostaglandin E₂ (dinoprostone) (Prostin E₂)
  Canadian trade name for, 750
  pregnancy and, 750
prostaglandins
  as abortifacients, 735t
  in inflammation and immunity, 7, 66–67, 67t
  in peptic ulcer disease, 639, 641–642
prostaglandin synthetase, analgesic-antipyretic-anti-inflammatory drugs and, 67
Prostaphlin (oxacillin), 382t
prostate cancer, drug therapy for, 301t–302t, 305
ProStep (nicotine), 744t
Prostigmine (neostigmine), 208
  in pediatrics, 210
Prostin E₂ (dinoprostone, prostaglandin E₂)
  as Canadian trade name, 750
  pregnancy and, 735t
protamine sulfate, 616

protein binding
  in drug distribution, 11
  in geriatric patient, 40t
  in pediatric patient, 11, 38t
proteins
  description of, 320t–321t
  imbalances of, 322t
  metabolism of
    glucocorticoids and, 229
    insulin and, 279
    liver and, 636
protirelin (Relefact, Thypinone), 230
protozoal infections, 448–450. *See also* antiparasitics
protriptyline (Vivactil), 117t
  Canadian trade name for, 753
  therapeutic serum drug concentrations for, 746
Protropin (somatrem), 230–231
Proventil (albuterol), 187t, 516
  lactation and, 737t
  in pediatrics, 191
  pregnancy and, 729t
Provera (medroxyprogesterone), 688t
  as Canadian trade name, 751
Proviodine (povidone-iodine), as Canadian trade name, 753
proxymetacaine, Canadian trade name for, 753
Prozac (fluoxetine), 117t
  as Canadian trade name, 750
pseudoephedrine (Sudafed), 188, 535t
  Canadian trade name for, 753
  in pediatrics, 190–191
Pseudofrin (pseudoephedrine), as Canadian trade name, 753
psoriasis, 713
psychosis
  description of, 99
  drug therapy in. *See* antipsychotic drugs
  etiology of, 99–100
  types of, 99
psyllium hydrophillic mucioid Canadian trade name for, 753
psyllium preparations (Effersyllium, Metamucil, Perdiem Plain, Serutan), 652t, 663t
puberty
  delayed, drug therapy for, 301t–302t
  testosterone and, 297
Pulmocare, 323
Pulmophylline (theophylline), as Canadian trade name, 754
Pulmozyme (dornase alfa), 743t
pump delivery systems, 22
Purinethol (mercaptopurine), 687t
  as Canadian trade name, 752
Purinol (allopurinol), as Canadian trade name, 748
PVC. *See* polyvinyl chloride
Pyopen (carbenicillin), as Canadian trade name, 749
pyramidal system, structure and function of, 51
pyrantel pamoate (Antiminth), 454
  Canadian trade name for, 753
pyrazinamide, 429
  Canadian trade name for, 753
Pyribenzamine (tripelennamine)
  as Canadian trade name, 754
Pyridium (phenazopyridine), 422
  as Canadian trade name, 752
pyridostigmine (Mestinon), 209
  Canadian trade name for, 753
pyridoxine (vitamin B₆), 335t
  Canadian trade name for, 753
  imbalance of, 338t
  routes and dosage ranges for, 340t
pyrilamine maleate, 525, 527t

pyrimethamine (Daraprim), 453
  Canadian trade name for, 753
pyrvinium pamoate (Povan), 454


**Q**

Quarzan (clidinium bromide), 214t
quazepam (Doral), 82t, 83
Quelicin (succinylcholine), as Canadian trade name, 753
Questran (cholestyramine), 628t, 630, 663t
  as Canadian trade name, 749
Quibron (theophylline and guaifenesin), 518t
Quinaglute (quinidine), 563
  as Canadian trade name, 753
  lactation and, 737t
  pregnancy and, 729t
quinapril (Accupril), 591t
  Canadian trade name for, 753
quinestrol (Estrovis), 302t
quinethazone (Hydromox), 602t
Quinidex (quinidine), as Canadian trade name, 753
quinidine polygalacturonate (Cardioquin), 563
quinidine (Quinaglute), 562–563, 568
  Canadian trade name for, 753
  lactation and, 737t
  pregnancy and, 729t
  therapeutic serum drug concentrations for, 746
quinidine sulfate (Quinora), 563
quinine sulfate (Quinamm), 453
quinolones
  administration of, 415
  adverse effects of, 416
  client teaching with, 417
  description of, 411–412
  drug interactions with, 416
  principles of therapy with, 414
Quinora (quinidine sulfate), 563


**R**

rabies immune globulin, human (Hyperab, Imogam), 479t
  Canadian trade name for, 753
rabies vaccine (Imovax), 476t
racial factors, cancer and, 680
Radiostol (ergocalciferol), as Canadian trade name, 750
ramipril (Altace), 591t
ranitidine (Zantac), 641, 646
  Canadian trade name for, 753
  lactation and, 738t
reabsorption, 603
receptors
  adrenergic, 184, 184t
  neurotransmitter, 114
  opiate, 54t
receptor theory of drug action, 12–13
Recombivax HB (hepatitis B vaccine), 473t–474t
  as Canadian trade name, 751
rectal suppositories, insertion of, 32
Regitine (phentolamine), 198
Reglan (metoclopramide), 669, 671, 671t
  as Canadian trade name, 752
Regonal (pyridostigmine), as Canadian trade name, 753
Regular Iletin II (insulin injection), 283t
Regular Iletin I (insulin injection), 283t
Rela (carisoprodol), 146t
Relafen (nabumetone), 70, 71
  indications for, 68, 68t
Relefact (protirelin), 230
renal colic, anticholinergics in, 217

renal disorders
  antihypertensives in, 596
  corticosteroids in, 240, 596
renal failure
  antacids in, 640
  cephalosporins in, 393
  diabetes mellitus and, 281–282
renal insufficiency, anti-infective drugs in, 375
renal physiology, 601, 603–604
Renese (polythiazide), 602t
Renoquid (sulfacytine), 419t
reserpine (Serpasil), 591t
resorcinol, 717t
respiration
  defined, 511–512
  requirements for, 512
respiratory system
  disorders of, 512–513, 514
    anticholinergics for, 214
    corticosteroids for, 240, 243
    drug therapy for, 513, 514–515
    signs and symptoms of, 533–534
  physiology of, 511–513
Restoril (temazepam), 82t, 83
  as Canadian trade name, 753
Resyl (guaifenesin), as Canadian trade name, 751
reticular activating system, structure and function of, 50–51
Retin-A (retinoic acid, tretinoin), 720t
  as Canadian trade name, 754
retinol (vitamin A), 334t
  Canadian trade name for, 754
  imbalance of, 337t
retinopathy, diabetic, 281
Retrovir (zidovudine), 436t, 437
  as Canadian trade name, 754
  pregnancy and, 730t
Revimine (dopamine), as Canadian trade name, 750
rheumatic disorders, corticosteroids for, 243
rheumatoid arthritis, analgesic-antipyretic-anti-inflammatory drugs in, 68t, 75
Rheumatrex (methotrexate, MTX), 497t
  as Canadian trade name, 752
Rhinalar (flunisolide), as Canadian trade name, 750
Rhodialax (lactulose), as Canadian trade name, 751
Rhodialose (lactulose), as Canadian trade name, 751
rho₀(D) immune globulin, human (Gamulin Rh, HypRho-D, RhoGAM), 479t
  Canadian trade name for, 753
Rhodis (ketoprofen), as Canadian trade name, 751
RhoGAM (rho₀(D) immune globulin, human), 479t
rho immune globulin, human (HypRho-D), as Canadian trade name, 753
Rhoprosone (betamethasone), as Canadian trade name, 748
Rhotral (acebutolol), as Canadian trade name, 748
Rhotrimine (trimipramine), as Canadian trade name, 754
ribavirin (Virazole), 436t, 437
  Canadian trade name for, 753
  pregnancy and, 730t
riboflavin (vitamin B₂), 335t
  imbalance of, 339t
  routes and dosage ranges for, 340t
rifabutin (Mycobutin), 744t
Rifadin (rifampin)
  as Canadian trade name, 753
  lactation and, 737t
  pregnancy and, 729t

rifampin (Rifadin), 429
  Canadian trade name for, 753
  lactation and, 737t
  pregnancy and, 729t
Rimactane (rifampin), as Canadian trade name, 753
Ritalin (methylphenidate), 177
  as Canadian trade name, 752
ritodrine (Yutopar)
  Canadian trade name for, 753
  pregnancy and, 735t
Rivotril (clonazepam), as Canadian trade name, 749
R.O.-Atropine (atropine sulfate), as Canadian trade name, 748
R.O.-Carpine (pilocarpine), as Canadian trade name, 753
R.O.-Dry Eyes (polyvinyl alcohol), as Canadian trade name, 753
R.O.-Eye Drops (tetrahydrozoline), as Canadian trade name, 754
R.O.-Gentycin (gentamicin), as Canadian trade name, 751
R.O.-Naphz (naphazoline), as Canadian trade name, 752
R.O.-Predphate (prednisolone), as Canadian trade name, 753
R.O.-Tropamide (tropicamide), as Canadian trade name, 754
Robaxin (methocarbamol), 146t
  in acute or chronic disorders, 145
  as Canadian trade name, 752
Robidex (dextromethorphan), as Canadian trade name, 749
Robidone (hydrocodone), as Canadian trade name, 751
Robidrine (pseudoephedrine), as Canadian trade name, 753
Robinul (glycopyrrolate), 214t
  as Canadian trade name, 751
  in pediatrics, 218
Robitussin A-C, 537t
Robitussin-CF, 537t
Robitussin-DAC, 537t
Robitussin-DM, 537t
Robitussin (glyceryl guaiacolate, guaifenesin), 535t
  as Canadian trade name, 751
Robitussin-PE, 537t
Rocaltrol (calcitriol, vitamin D), 268t
  as Canadian trade name, 749, 754
Rocephin (ceftriaxone), 392t
  as Canadian trade name, 749
Rofact (rifampin), as Canadian trade name, 753
Roferon A (interferon-alfa-2a), as Canadian trade name, 751
Roferon (interferon-alfa-2a), 489t
Rogaine (minoxidil), 744t
  as Canadian trade name, 752
Romazicon (flumazenil), in benzodiazepine toxicity, 85, 94–95
Roubac (sulfamethoxazole and trimethoprim), as Canadian trade name, 753
roundworm infections (ascariasis), 449. See also antiparasitics
route, drug administration
  abbreviations for, 21t
  drug action and, 14
  intramuscular, 25, 26, 27
  intravenous, 25
  nasogastric, 29
  nursing process for, 43
  oral, 24
  parenteral, 24
  subcutaneous, 15–24, 25
  topical, 26
    nursing actions for, 31–32
Roychlor (potassium chloride), as Canadian trade name, 753

Rubbing Alcohol U.S.P. (isopropyl alcohol), 716t
rubella and mumps vaccine (Biavax-II), 476t
rubella vaccine (Meruvax II), 476t
Rubion (cyanocobalamin, vitamin B₁₂), as Canadian trade name, 749, 754
Rubramin (cyanocobalamin, vitamin B₁₂)
  as Canadian trade name, 749
  routes and dosage ranges for, 340t
Rynacrom (Cromolyn), as Canadian trade name, 749
Rythmodan (disopyramide), as Canadian trade name, 750
Rythmol (propafenone), 564, 568
  as Canadian trade name, 753

**S**

Sabin vaccine (Orimune), 475t
Salazopyrin (sulfasalazine), as Canadian trade name, 753
salbutamol, Canadian trade name for, 748
salicylic acid, 720t
salicylism, 74
saline cathartics, 653, 656
Saluron (hydroflumethiazide), 602t
Sandimmune (cyclosporine), 497t
  as Canadian trade name, 749
Sandoglobulin (immune serum globulin, IV (IGIV)), 479t
Sanorex (mazindol), 323t
  as Canadian trade name, 751
Sansert (methysergide), as Canadian trade name, 752
Santyl (collagenase), 720t
sargramostim (Leukine, Prokine), 486, 487, 489t
saturated solution of potassium iodide (SSKI), 257
scabicides, 455. See also antiparasitics
scabies, 450, 455. See also antiparasitics
scopolamine hydrobromide (Isopto Hyoscine), in ocular disorders, 703t
scopolamine (Scop-Transderm), 216, 671, 671t
  Canadian trade name for, 753
  in pediatrics, 218
  pregnancy and, 730t
seasonal affective disorder, 114
seborrheic dermatitis, 713
secobarbital (Seconal), 82t, 83
  Canadian trade name for, 753
Seconal (secobarbital), 82t, 83
  as Canadian trade name, 753
secretion
  digestive system, 636–637
  in renal physiology, 603–604
  respiratory, 533
Sectral (acebutolol), 198, 199t, 200, 565, 591t
  as Canadian trade name, 748
  lactation and, 738t
sedative-hypnotics, 81–88
  abuse of, 83
  administration of, 86
  adverse effects of, 86–87
  anesthesia and, 151
    client teaching with, 161–162
  antihistamines as, 83–84
  barbiturates as, 81, 82t, 83
  benzodiazepines as, 82t, 83
  client teaching with, 87–88
  contraindications to, 84
  description of, 81
  drug interactions with, 87
  enzyme induction and, 83
  in geriatrics, 85
  indications for, 84

lactation and, 737t
mechanism of action with, 84
nursing actions for, 86–88
nursing process for, 84–85
in pediatrics, 85
pregnancy and, 729t
principles of therapy for, 85
REM sleep suppression and, 81, 83
scheduling of, 85
selection of, 85
therapeutic effects of, 86
seizure disorders, 125. See anticonvulsants
in pregnancy, 734
Selax (docusate sodium), as Canadian trade name, 750
Seldane (terfenadine), 525, 528t
as Canadian trade name, 753
selegiline (Eldepryl), 136, 139
Canadian trade name for, 753
selenium, description of, 352t
selenium sulfide (Selsun), 720t
Canadian trade name for, 753
Selsun (selenium sulfide), 720t
as Canadian trade name, 753
Semilente Iletin I (insulin zinc suspension, prompt), 283t
Semilente Insulin (insulin zinc suspension, prompt), 283t
Semitard (insulin zinc suspension, prompt), 283t
senna pod preparations (Black Draught, Senokot), 652t
Senokot (senna pod preparation), 652t
septic shock, 581, 584
Septra (sulfamethoxazole-trimethoprim), 419t–420t, 662t
as Canadian trade name, 753
pregnancy and, 730t
Serax (oxazepam), 91t
as Canadian trade name, 752
Serentil (mesoridazine), 101t
as Canadian trade name, 752
Seromycin (cycloserine), 429, 430
serotonin
endogenous, 48, 49
in inflammation and immunity, 7
serotonin reuptake inhibitors, 115, 117t. See also antidepressants
dosage and administration of, 119
overdosage of, 120
selection of, 118
sertraline (Zoloft), 117t
Canadian trade name for, 753
Serutan (psyllium preparation), 652t
sex hormones
female. See estrogens; progestins
male. See anabolic steroids; androgens; testosterone
sexually transmitted disease, penicillins in, 384
shock
description of, 581
drugs used in, 581–586
administration of, 585
adrenergic drugs, 190
adverse effects of, 585–586
client teaching for, 586
corticosteroids, 243
in geriatrics, 584
individual, 582–583
nursing actions for, 585–586
nursing process for, 583, 585–586
in pediatrics, 584
principles of therapy with, 584
therapeutic effects of, 585
types of, 581
Silace (docusate sodium), as Canadian trade name, 750
Silvadene (silver sulfadiazine), 420t, 717t

silver nitrate, 704t, 716t
silver sulfadiazine (Silvadene), 420t, 717t
Canadian trade name for, 753
Similac, 324
simvastatin (Zocor), 628t, 630
Canadian trade name for, 753
Sine-Off, 537t
Sinequan (doxepin), 117t
as Canadian trade name, 750
sinus arrhythmias, 561
Sinutab, 537t
Sinutab II, 537t
Skelaxin (metaxalone), 146t
skeletal muscle relaxants, 145–149, 146t.
See also neuromuscular blocking agents
administration of, 147–148
adverse effects of, 148–149
client teaching with, 149
contraindications to, 146
drug interactions with, 149
in geriatrics, 147
indications for, 145
individual, 146t
mechanism of action with, 145
nursing actions for, 147–148
nursing process for, 146–147
in pediatrics, 147
selection of, 147
therapeutic effects of, 148
skeletal muscles, testosterone effect on, 310
skeleton
alcohol abuse and, 168
estrogens and, 297
skin
disorders of, 713–715
estrogen and, 298
functions of, 712
testosterone and, 310
sleep, defined, 81
sleep aids, nonprescription, 84
Sleep-Eze (diphenhydramine), as Canadian trade name, 750
Slo-Bid (theophylline), as Canadian trade name, 754
Slow-Fe (ferrous sulfate), as Canadian trade name, 750
Slow-K (potassium chloride), as Canadian trade name, 753
SMA, 324
small intestine, 636
smallpox vaccine, 476t
smoking. See cigarette smoking
social customs, cancer and, 680
sodium
description of, 347t
imbalances of, 348t
treatment of, 358
preparations of, 355–356
restriction of
with antihypertensive drugs, 596
sodium benzoate and caffeine, 178
sodium chloride injection, 272, 355–356
sodium cromoglycate, Canadian trade name for, 749
sodium hypochlorite, Canadian trade name for, 753
sodium hypochlorite solution, diluted (Dakin's solution modified), 716t
sodium iodide $^{131}$I (Iodotope), 257
sodium nitroprusside (Nipride), 593t
sodium oxychlorosene (Clorpactin sodium), 716t
sodium phosphate and betamethasone acetate (Celestone Soluspan), 241t
sodium phosphate and sodium biphosphate (Fleet Enema, Fleet Phosphosoda), 652t

sodium polystyrene sulfonate (Kayexalate), 350, 353
Sodium Sulamyd (sulfacetamide)
as Canadian trade name, 753
in ocular disorders, 705t
Solaquin (hydroquinone), as Canadian trade name, 751
Solium (chlordiazepoxide), as Canadian trade name, 749
Solu-Cortef (hydrocortisone)
as Canadian trade name, 751
in hypercalcemia, 271
Solugel (benzoyl peroxide), as Canadian trade name, 748
Solu-Medrol (methylprednisolone), 242t, 519
as Canadian trade name, 752
Soma (carisoprodol), 146t
as Canadian trade name, 749
somatostatin. See growth hormone release-inhibiting hormone
somatotropin. See growth hormone
somatrem (Protropin), 230–231
somatropin (Humatrope), 230, 231
Somnol (flurazepam), as Canadian trade name, 750
Somophyllinn (theophylline), as Canadian trade name, 754
Sopamycetin (chloramphenicol), as Canadian trade name, 749
sorbide nitrate, Canadian trade name for, 751
sorbitol, 653t, 654
Sorbitrate (isosorbide dinitrate), 575
Sotacor (sotalol), as Canadian trade name, 753
sotalol (Betapace), 198, 199t, 200, 565, 566, 568
Canadian trade name for, 753
Soyalac, 323
Sparine (promazine), 102t
spasticity, defined, 145
Spectazole (econazole), 444t, 719t
spectinomycin (Trobicin), 413
Canadian trade name for, 753
Spectrobid (bacampicillin), 382t
Spersacarpine (pilocarpine), as Canadian trade name, 753
Spersadex (dexamethasone), as Canadian trade name, 749
spinal anesthesia, 151
administration of, 157
spinal cord, structure and function of, 51
spironolactone (Aldactone), 602t
Canadian trade name for, 753
spironolactone and hydrochlorothiazide (Aldactazide), 603t
Sporanox (itraconazole), 444t
sprays, dermatologic, 722
SSKI (saturated solution of potassium iodide), 257
stanazolol (Winstrol), 312t
Staphcillin (methicillin), 382t
Statex (morphine), as Canadian trade name, 752
status epilepticus, 125–126
in anticonvulsant drug withdrawal, 131
Stelazine (trifluoperazine), 102t
as Canadian trade name, 754
Stemetil (prochlorperazine), as Canadian trade name, 753
Sterane (prednisolone), 242t
StieVAA (tretinoin (retinoic acid)), as Canadian trade name, 754
Stilbestrol (diethylstilbestrol), 301t, 688t
Stilphostrol (diethylstilbestrol diphosphate), 301t
Stimate (desmopressin acetate), 231
stimulant cathartics, 652t–653t, 653, 654

stomach, 635–636
stomatitis, antineoplastic drugs and, 690
stool softeners, pregnancy and, 732
Streptase (streptokinase), as Canadian trade
    name, 753
Streptase (streptokinase), 615, 617
streptokinase (Streptase), 615, 617
    Canadian trade name for, 753
streptomycin, 429
    lactation and, 737t
streptozocin (Zanosar), 686t
    Canadian trade name for, 753
stress, immune function and, 470
strong iodine solution (Lugol's solution), 257
strongyloidiasis (threadworm infections),
    450. See also antiparasitics
subcutaneous drug administration, 24–25
    injection sites for, 25
    nursing actions for, 29–30
Sublimaze (fentanyl), 55
Sublimaze (fentanyl), as Canadian trade
    name, 750
substance abuse. See alcohol, abuse of; drug
    abuse
substantia nigra, 51
succimer (Chemet), 354
succinylcholine (Anectine), 155t
    Canadian trade name for, 753
    chlolinergic drugs and, 208
sucralfate (Carafate), 642, 644, 646
    Canadian trade name for, 753
Sudafed (pseudoephedrine), 535t
    as Canadian trade name, 753
sufentanil (Sufenta), 55, 154t
    Canadian trade name for, 753
    pregnancy and, 729t
Sufenta (sufentanil), 55, 154t
    as Canadian trade name, 753
    pregnancy and, 729t
sulbactam and ampicillin (Unasyn), 383t
sulconazole (Exelderm), 444t
Sulcrate (sucralfate), as Canadian trade
    name, 753
sulfacetamide, Canadian trade name for,
    753
sulfacetamide sodium (Bleph-10 Liquifilm,
    Isopto Cetamide, Sodium Sulamyd),
    in ocular disorders, 705t
sulfacytine (Renoquid), 419t
sulfadiazine (Microsulfon), 419t
sulfamethizole (Thiosulfil), 419t
sulfamethoxazole (Gantanol), 419t
    pregnancy and, 730t
sulfamethoxazole-trimethoprim (TMP-
    SMX) (Bactrim, Septra), 419t–420t,
    662t
    in Canada, 737t
    Canadian trade name for, 753
    lactation and, 737t
    pregnancy and, 730t
Sulfamylon (mafenide), 420t
sulfasalazine (Azulfidine), 419t, 663t
    Canadian trade name for, 753
Sulfex (sulfacetamide), as Canadian trade
    name, 753
sulfinpyrazone (Anturane), 72
    Canadian trade name for, 753
    in hyperuricemia, 76
sulfisoxazole (Gantrisin), 419t
    in ocular disorders, 705t
sulfisoxazole-phenazopyridine (Azo
    Gantrisin), 420t
    Canadian trade name for, 753
sulfonamides, 418–425
    administration of, 423–424
    adverse effects of, 424
    client teaching with, 425
    combination agents, 419t–420t
    contraindications to, 421

description of, 418
drug interactions with, 424–425
in geriatrics, 423
indications for, 418
individual, 419t
lactation and, 737t
nursing actions for, 423–425
nursing process for, 422
in pediatrics, 423
pregnancy and, 729t
preparations of, 419t–420t
principles of therapy with, 422–423
therapeutic effects of, 424
topical, 420t
sulfonylureas, 282, 284t, 284–285. See also
    hypoglycemic drugs, oral
sulfur, 718t
sulindac (Clinoril), 70, 71
    Canadian trade name for, 753
    indications for, 68, 68t
sumatriptan (Imitrex), 72–73
    Canadian trade name for, 753
sunscreens, 715
Supeudol (oxycodone), as Canadian trade
    name, 752
suppositories
    narcotic, 62
    placement of, 32
Supracaine (tetracaine), as Canadian trade
    name, 754
Suprane (desflurane), 153t
Suprax (cefixime), 390t
surfactant laxatives, 652t, 653
Surfak (docusate calcium), 652t
    as Canadian trade name, 750
Surital (thiamylal sodium, thiopental
    sodium), 154t
Surmontil (trimipramine), 117t
    as Canadian trade name, 754
Survanta (beractant), 743t
Sustacal, 322
Sustagen, 322
sutilains (Travase), 720t
    Canadian trade name for, 753
suxamethonium, Canadian trade name for,
    753
Symmetrel (amantadine), 435, 436t
    as Canadian trade name, 748
    pregnancy and, 730t
sympathetic nervous system, 183–184,
    184t. See also autonomic nervous sys-
    tem
Synalar (fluocinolone), as Canadian trade
    name, 750
Synalar (fluocinonide), 719t
Synamol (fluocinolone acetonide), as Cana-
    dian trade name, 750
synapse, 47, 48
Synarel (nafarelin), 230
synergism, pharmacologic, 14–15
Synflex (naproxen), as Canadian trade
    name, 752
Synkayvite (menadione sodium diphos-
    phate), routes and dosage ranges for,
    340t
Synphasic (ethinyl estradiol and norethin-
    drone), as Canadian trade name, 750
synthetic drugs, defined, 3
Synthroid (levothyroxine), 256, 258, 732t
    as Canadian trade name, 751
Syntocinon (oxytocin), as Canadian trade
    name, 752
syringes, 24


T

Tacaryl (methdilazine, methdilazine
    hydrochloride), 528t
Tace (chlorotrianisene), 301t

tachyphylaxis, 18
tacrine (Cognex), 744t
Tagamet (cimetidine), 640–641, 644, 645
    as Canadian trade name, 749
    lactation and, 738t
    pregnancy and, 730t
Talwin (pentazocine), 57–58
    as Canadian trade name, 752
Tambocor (flecainide), 564, 568
    as Canadian trade name, 750
    lactation and, 737t
    pregnancy and, 729t
Tamofen (tamoxifen), as Canadian trade
    name, 753
Tamone (tamoxifen), as Canadian trade
    name, 753
Tamoplex (tamoxifen), as Canadian trade
    name, 753
tamoxifen (Nolvadex), 688t
    Canadian trade name for, 753
Tantaphen (acetaminophen), as Canadian
    trade name, 748
Tapazole (methimazole)
    as Canadian trade name, 752
    lactation and, 738t
tapeworms, 449–450. See also antiparasitics
Taractan (chlorprothixene), 103
Tara-Sone (betamethasone), as Canadian
    trade name, 748
Tavist (clemastine), 527t
    as Canadian trade name, 749
Taxol (paclitaxel), 689t
Tazidime (ceftazidime), as Canadian trade
    name, 749
tazobactam and piperacillin (Zosyn), 383t
Tebrazid (pyrazinamide), as Canadian trade
    name, 753
Tedral (theophylline, ephedrine hydrochlo-
    ride and phenobarbital), 518t
Tegison (etretinate), 743t
Tegopen (cloxacillin), 382t
    as Canadian trade name, 749
Tegretol (carbamazepine), 128
    as Canadian trade name, 749
Temaril (trimeprazine tartrate), 528t
temazepam (Restoril), 82t, 83
    Canadian trade name for, 753
Temovate (clobetasol), 719t
Tempra (acetaminophen), as Canadian
    trade name, 748
tendinitis, drugs used in, 68t
Tenex (guanfacine), 591t
    lactation and, 738t
    pregnancy and, 730t
teniposide (Vumon), 687t
    Canadian trade name for, 753
Tenoretic (atenolol and chlorthalidone), 593t
Tenormin (atenolol), 198, 199t, 575, 591t
    as Canadian trade name, 748
Tensilon (edrophonium), 208
    as Canadian trade name, 750
Tenuate (diethylpropion), 323t
    as Canadian trade name, 750
teratogenicity, defined, 18
Terazol (terconazole), 444t
    as Canadian trade name, 753
terazosin (Hytrin), 591t
    Canadian trade name for, 753
terbutaline (Brethine), 187t
    Canadian trade name for, 753
    in pediatrics, 191, 729
    pregnancy and, 735t
terconazole (Terazol), 444t
    Canadian trade name for, 753
terfenadine (Seldane), 525, 528t
    Canadian trade name for, 753
Terramycin (oxytetracycline), 451
Tersa-Tar (coal tar), as Canadian trade
    name, 749

Teslac (testolactone), 312t
Tessalon (benzonatate), 535t
Testaqua (testosterone), 312t
testicular hormones, 227
Testoject (testosterone), 312t
testolactone (Teslac), 312t
testosterone, effects of, 309–310
testosterone (Android-T, Testaqua, Testo-
    ject, Oreton), 312t
    Canadian trade name for, 753
testosterone cypionate (Depo-Testos-
    terone), 312t
testosterone enanthate (Delatestryl), 312t
testosterone propionate (Various), 312t
tetanus and diphtheria toxoids, adsorbed
    (adult type), 478t
tetanus immune globulin, human (Hyper-
    Tet), 479t
tetanus toxoid, adsorbed, 477t–478t
tetanus toxoid, adsorbed, and diphtheria
    (pediatric type), 477t
tetanus toxoid and diphtheria and acellular
    pertussis vaccine (DTaP) (Acel-
    Imune, Tripedia), 477t
tetanus toxoid and diphtheria and whole-
    cell pertussis and *Haemophilus in-
    fluenzae* type B conjugate vaccines
    (DTwP-HibTITER) (Tetramune), 477t
tetracaine (Pontocaine), 156t
    Canadian trade name for, 754
    in ocular disorders, 704t
tetracycline (Achromycin), 403t, 451, 662t
    Canadian trade name for, 754
    lactation and, 737t
    in ocular disorders, 705t
    pregnancy and, 729t
tetracyclines, 402–406, 403t
    administration of, 404
    adverse effects of, 404–405
    client teaching with, 405–406
    contraindications to, 402–403
    description of, 402
    drug interactions with, 405
    in geriatrics, 404
    indications for, 402
    lactation and, 737t
    mechanism of action in, 402
    nursing actions for, 404–406
    in pediatrics, 404
    pregnancy and, 729t
    principles of therapy with, 404
    therapeutic effects of, 404
Tetracyn (tetracycline), as Canadian trade
    name, 754
tetrahydrozoline hydrochloride (Tyzine,
    Visine), 187t, 535t
tetrahydrozoline, Canadian trade name for,
    754
Tetramune (diphtheria and tetanus tox-
    oids and whole-cell pertussis and
    *Haemophilus influenzae* type conju-
    gate vaccines (DTwP-HibTITER)),
    477t
TGF. *See* T lymphocyte growth factor
thalamus, structure and function of, 50
Theelin (estrone), 302t
Theobid (theophylline anhydrous), 518t
Theochron (theophylline), as Canadian
    trade name, 754
Theoclear LA (theophylline anhydrous),
    518t
Theo-Dur (theophylline), 518t
    as Canadian trade name, 754
    lactation and, 738t
    pregnancy and, 731t
Theolair-SR (theophylline anhydrous),
    518t
Theolair (theophylline), 518t
    as Canadian trade name, 754

theophylline, ephedrine hydrochloride and
    phenobarbital (Tedral), 518t
theophylline, ephedrine sulfate and hy-
    droxyzine hydrochloride (Marax),
    518t
theophylline (Aminophylline, Theo-Dur),
    178, 515, 517, 521
    Canadian trade name for, 754
    lactation and, 738t
    pregnancy and, 731t
    preparations of, 518t
    therapeutic serum drug concentrations
        for, 746
theophylline anhydrous (Elixophyllin,
    Theobid, Theoclear LA, Theo-Dur,
    Theolair, Theolair-SR), 518t
theophylline ethylenediamine (Amino-
    phylline), 518t
theophylline and guaifenesin (Quibron),
    518t
theophylline monothanolamine (Fleet
    Theophylline), 518t
theophylline salts, 178
Theo-SR (theophylline), as Canadian trade
    name, 754
TheraCys (Bacillus Calmette-Guérin), 489t
thiabendazole (Mintezol), 454–455
    Canadian trade name for, 754
thiamazole, Canadian trade name for, 752
thiamine deficiency, 51
thiamine (vitamin B$_1$), 51, 336t
    Canadian trade name for, 754
    imbalance of, 339t
    routes and dosage ranges for, 340t
thiamylal sodium (Surital), 154t
thiazide diuretics, 602t, 605
thiethylperazine (Torecan), 670t
    Canadian trade name for, 754
thioguanine, 687t
    Canadian trade name for, 754
thiopental, Canadian trade name for, 754
thiopental sodium (Pentothal, Surital), 154t
thioridazine (Mellaril), 102t
    Canadian trade name for, 754
Thiosulfil (sulfamethizole), 419t
thiothixene (Navane), 103
    Canadian trade name for, 754
Thorazine (chlorpromazine), 101t, 669t,
    670t
    lactation and, 738t
    pregnancy and, 731t
threadworm infections (strongyloidiasis),
    450. *See also* antiparasitics
thromboembolic disorders, 613
    drug therapy for, 613–615
        individual agents in, 615–618
        nursing actions for, 621–625
        nursing process for, 618–619
        principles of therapy for, 619–621
thrombolytic drugs, 615, 617
    administration of, 620
    antidotes to, 618
    individual, 618
    nursing process for, 618–619
    preparations of, 615, 617–618, 753
    principles of therapy with, 620
thrombotic disorders, 613
    drug therapy for, 613–625
        individual agents in, 615–619
        nursing actions for, 621–625
        nursing process for, 618–619
        principles of therapy for, 619–621
    nursing actions for, 621–625
thrush, 713
Thypinone (protirelin), 230
thyroid drugs. *See also* antithyroid drugs
    administration of, 261
    adrenal insufficiency and, 259–260
    adverse effects of, 262

client teaching with, 263
dosage for, 259
drug interactions with, 263
duration of therapy with, 259
in geriatrics, 260
in hypothyroidism, 256–257
in infants, 259
nursing actions for, 261–263
nursing process for, 258–259
in pediatrics, 260
principles of therapy for, 259–260
selection of, 259
therapeutic effects of, 261–262
thyroid gland
    disorders of, 254t
        hyperthyroidism, 255–256. *See also*
            antithyroid drugs
        hypothyroidism, 254–255. *See also*
            thyroid drugs
thyroid hormones, 227, 253–254
    lactation and, 738t
    pregnancy and, 732t
thyroid-stimulating hormone (TSH), 229
thyroid tablets, desiccated, 256
Thyrolar (liotrix), 256–257
thyrotropin. *See* thyroid-stimulating
    hormone
thyrotropin-releasing hormone (TRH), 228
thyrotropin (Thytropar), 231
Thytropar (thyrotropin), 231
ticarcillin-clavulanate (Timentin), 383t
ticarcillin-potassium clavulanate, Canadian
    trade name for, 754
ticarcillin (Ticar), 381, 382t
    Canadian trade name for, 754
Ticar (ticarcillin), 382t
    as Canadian trade name, 754
TICE BCG (Bacillus Calmette-Guérin),
    489t
Ticlid (ticlopidine), 615, 616
    as Canadian trade name, 754
ticlopidine (Ticlid), 615, 616
    Canadian trade name for, 754
Tigan (trimethobenzamide), 671, 671t
Tilade (nedocromil), 519
    as Canadian trade name, 752
Timentin (ticarcillin-clavulanate), 383, 383t
Timentin (ticarcillin-potassium clavu-
    lanate), as Canadian trade name,
    754
Timolide (timolol and hydrochloro-
    thiazide), 593t
timolol and hydrochlorothiazide (Timo-
    lide), 593t
timolol (Blocadren, Timoptic), 198, 199t,
    200, 592t
    Canadian trade name for, 754
    lactation and, 738t
timolol maleate (Timoptic), in ocular disor-
    ders, 702t
Timoptic (timolol), 198, 199t, 200
    as Canadian trade name, 754
    in ocular disorders, 702t
Tinactin (tolnaftate), 444t, 719t
    as Canadian trade name, 754
Tindal (acetophenazine), 101t
tinea, 714
tioconazole (Vagistat), 444t
    Canadian trade name for, 754
tissue transplants, rejection of, 496. *See also*
    immunosuppressants
Titralac, 643t
T lymphocyte growth factor (TGF), 467,
    468t
T lymphocytes, in immune response,
    466–467
TMP-SMX. *See* trimethoprim-sulfamethox-
    azole
TNF. *See* tumor necrosis factor

tobacco, as carcinogen, 681t. *See also* cigarette smoking
tobramycin (Tobrex)
Canadian trade name for, 754
in ocular disorders, 705t
therapeutic serum drug concentrations
for, 746
Tobrex (tobramycin)
as Canadian trade name, 754
in ocular disorders, 705t
tocainide (Tonocard), 564
Canadian trade name for, 754
pregnancy and, 729t
tocofersolan, Canadian trade name for,
754
tocolytics
nursing actions for, 739–741
pregnancy and, 734, 735t
Toesen (oxytocin), as Canadian trade name,
752
Tofranil (imipramine), 117t
as Canadian trade name, 751
tolazamide (Tolinase), 284t, 284–285
tolbutamide (Orinase), 284t, 284–285
Canadian trade name for, 754
lactation and, 738t
Tolectin (tolmetin), 70, 71
as Canadian trade name, 754
indications for, 68, 68t
tolerance
drug, 18
to nitrates, long-acting, 577
Tolinase (tolazamide), 284t, 284–285
tolmetin (Tolectin), 70, 71
Canadian trade name for, 754
indications for, 68, 68t
tolnaftate (Tinactin), 444t, 719t
Canadian trade name for, 754
Tonocard (tocainide), 564
as Canadian trade name, 754
pregnancy and, 729t
Topicaine (benzocaine), as Canadian trade
name, 748
topical anesthesia, 151
Topicort (desoximetasone), 719t
as Canadian trade name, 749
Topsyn Gel (fluocinolone), as Canadian
trade name, 750
Toradol (ketorolac), 70, 71
as Canadian trade name, 751
indications for, 68, 68t
Torecan (thiethylperazine), 670t
as Canadian trade name, 754
Tornalate (bitolterol), 187t, 516
in pediatrics, 191
total parenteral nutrition (TPN). *See* parenteral feedings
toxic dose, 14
toxoids. *See also* immunizing agents
clinical indications for, 472
contraindications to, 478
trace elements. *See* minerals, micronutrients
(trace elements)
trachea, defined, 512
Tracrium (atracurium), 155t
as Canadian trade name, 748
trade name, defined, 4
Trandate (labetalol), 198, 199t, 200, 592t
as Canadian trade name, 751
tranexamic acid (Cyklokapron), 618
Canadian trade name for, 754
Transderm-Nitro (nitroglycerin), as Canadian trade name, 752
Transderm (scopolamine), 671, 671t
Transderm-V (scopolamine), as Canadian
trade name, 753
transport, defined, 4, 10
Tranxene (clorazepate), 91t, 128
as Canadian trade name, 749

tranylcypromine (Parnate), 117t
Canadian trade name for, 754
trauma, dermatologic, 714
TraumaCal, 323
Travase (sutilains), 720t
as Canadian trade name, 753
Travel Aid (dimenhydrinate), as Canadian
trade name, 750
Travel-Eze (dimenhydrinate), as Canadian
trade name, 750
trazodone (Desyrel), 115, 117t
Canadian trade name for, 754
pregnancy and, 730t
Trental (pentoxifylline), 627
as Canadian trade name, 752
tretinoin (Retin-A) (retinoic acid), 720t
Canadian trade name for, 754
Trexan (naltrexone), 58
triacetin (Fungoid), 444t
Triadapin (doxepin), as Canadian trade
name, 750
Triaderm (triamcinolone), as Canadian
trade name, 754
triamcinolone acetonide (Aristocort,
Kenalog, Nasacort), 242t, 719t
triamcinolone (Azmacort), 517, 518
Canadian trade name for, 754
triamcinolone diacetate (Aristocort diacetate, Kenacort diacetate), 242t
triamcinolone hexacetonide (Aristospan),
242t
triamterene (Dyazide, Dyrenium, Maxide),
603t
Canadian trade name for, 754
lactation and, 738t
pregnancy and, 731t
triazolam (Halcion), 82t, 83
Canadian trade name for, 754
trichinosis, 450. *See also* antiparasitics
trichlormethiazide (Metahydrin, Naqua),
602t
trichomoniasis, 449, 453, 455. *See also*
antiparasitics
trichuriasis (whipworm infection), 450. *See
also* antiparasitics
tricyclic antidepressants, 114, 117t. *See also*
antidepressants
administration of, 119
dosage of, 117t, 119
duration of therapy with, 119
overdosage of, 120
selection of, 118
Tridesilon (desonide), 719t
as Canadian trade name, 749
tridihexethyl (Pathilon), 214t
Tridil (nitroglycerin), as Canadian trade
name, 752
trifluoperazine (Stelazine), 102t
Canadian trade name for, 754
triflupromazine (Vesprin), 670t
trifluridine (Viroptic), 436t, 437
Canadian trade name for, 754
in ocular disorders, 705t
trihexyphenidyl (Artane), 137t, 216
Canadian trade name for, 754
Tri-Immunol (diphtheria and tetanus toxoids and whole-cell pertussis vaccine
(DTwP)), 477t
Trikacide (metronidazole), as Canadian
trade name, 752
Trilafon (perphenazine), 102t, 670t
as Canadian trade name, 752
Tri-Levlen (ethinyl estradiol and levonorgestrel), 304t
Trimacort (triamcinolone), as Canadian
trade name, 754
trimeprazine, Canadian trade name for,
754
trimeprazine tartrate (Temaril), 528t

trimethaphan camsylate (Arfonad), 591t
trimethobenzamide (Tigan), 671, 671t
trimethoprim (Bactrim, Proloprim,
Trimpex), 422
Canadian trade name for, 754
lactation and, 737t
pregnancy and, 730t
trimethoprim-sulfamethoxazole (TMP-
SMX) (Bactrim, Septra), 419t–420t,
662t
lactation and, 737t
pregnancy and, 730t
trimipramine, Canadian trade name for,
754
trimipramine maleate (Surmontil), 117t
Trimpex (trimethoprim), 422
Tri-Norinyl (ethinyl estradiol and norethindrone), 304t
trioxsalen (Trisoralen), 720t
Canadian trade name for, 754
Tripedia (diphtheria and tetanus toxoids
and acellular pertussis vaccine
(DTaP)), 477t
tripelennamine, Canadian trade name for,
754
tripelennamine hydrochloride (PBZ), 528t
Triphasil (ethinyl estradiol and levonorgestrel), 304t
as Canadian trade name, 750
triprolidine hydrochloride (Actidil), 527t
Triptil (protriptyline), as Canadian trade
name, 753
Triquilar (ethinyl estradiol and levonorgestrel), as Canadian trade
name, 750
Trisoralen (trioxsalen), 720t
as Canadian trade name, 754
Trobicin (spectinomycin), 413
as Canadian trade name, 753
Tronothane (pramoxine), 156t
as Canadian trade name, 753
tropicamide (Mydriacyl)
Canadian trade name for, 754
in ocular disorders, 703t
in pediatrics, 218
Trosyd (tioconazole), as Canadian trade
name, 754
trypsin (Granulex), 720t
Tuamine (tuaminoheptane), 187t
tuaminoheptane (Tuamine), 187t
Tubarine (tubocurarine), as Canadian trade
name, 754
tube feedings. *See also* enteral feedings
nutritional products for, 322
tuberculosis, 427. *See also* antitubercular
drugs
multidrug resistant, 427
treatment regimens for, 427–428
tuberculosis vaccine (TICE BCG), 476t–477t
tubocurarine, 155t
Canadian trade name for, 754
tubular reabsorption, in renal physiology,
603
tubular secretion, in renal physiology,
603–604
tumor necrosis factor (TNF), 468t, 469
Tums (calcium carbonate), as Canadian
trade name, 749
Tylenol (acetaminophen)
as Canadian trade name, 748
indications for, 68, 68t
lactation and, 737t
pregnancy and, 731t
typhoid vaccine (Vivotif Berna), 477t
tyramine-containing foods, monoamine
oxidase inhibitors and, 14, 115t
Tyzine (tetrahydrozoline hydrochloride),
187t, 535t

## U

ulcers. *See also* peptic ulcer disease
  corneal, 700. *See also* ophthalmic drugs
    cutaneous, 714
    decubitus, 714
    pressure, 714
    venous stasis, 714
Ultracef (cefadroxil), 390t
Ultralente (insulin zinc suspension, extended), 283t
UltraMOP (methoxsalen), as Canadian trade name, 752
Ultratard (insulin zinc suspension, extended), 283t
Unasyn (ampicillin-sulbactam), 383, 383t
undecylenic acid (Desenex), 719t
undernutrition. *See also* nutritional products
  enteral feedings for, 326–327
  oral feedings for, 326
  parenteral feedings for, 327
  parenteral nutrition for
    home administration of, 327–328
  principles of therapy for, 326–328
Unipen (nafcillin), 382t
  as Canadian trade name, 752
Uniphyl (theophylline), as Canadian trade name, 754
*United States Pharmacopeia*, 4
Urecholine (bethanechol)
  as Canadian trade name, 748
  in pediatrics, 210
urinary antiseptics, 418, 421–425
  administration of, 424
  adverse effects of, 424
  client teaching for, 425
  drug interactions with, 425
  indications for, 418
  individual, 421
  nursing actions for, 424–425
  nursing process for, 411
  principles of therapy with, 423
  therapeutic effects of, 424
  urine cultures and sensitivity tests for, 423
  urine pH and, 423
urinary antispasmodics, 217–218
urinary tract infections, drug therapy for, 418, 421–425
Urispas (flavoxate)
  as Canadian trade name, 750
  in pediatrics, 218
Uritol (furosemide), as Canadian trade name, 750
urokinase (Abbokinase), 615, 617–618
  Canadian trade name for, 754
ursodiol (Actigall), 744t
urticaria, 713

## V

vaccine. *See also* names of specific vaccines
  measles, 474t
  measles, mumps, and rubella, 474t
    Canadian trade name for, 751
  measles and rubella, 474t
  mumps, 475t
    Canadian trade name for, 752
  mumps, measles, and rubella
    Canadian trade name for, 751
  mumps and rubella, 476t
  rabies, 476t
  rubella, 476t
  rubella and measles, 474t
  rubella and mumps, 476t
  smallpox, 476t
  tetanus toxoid, diphtheria, and acellular pertussis, 477t
  tetanus toxoid, diphtheria, whole-cell pertussis, and *Haemophilus influenzae* type B conjugate, 477t

tuberculosis, 476t–477t
  typhoid, 477t
  yellow fever, 477t
vaccines, 473t–478t. *See also* immunizing agents
  clinical indications for, 472
  contraindications to, 478
  storage of, 481
vagina, fungal infection of, 713
vaginal medications, 44t, 442t, 722
  administration of, 32
vaginitis, 444t
Vagistat (tioconazole), 444t
Valisone (betamethasone), 719t
  as Canadian trade name, 748
Valium (diazepam), 90, 91t, 146t
  acute or chronic disorders and, 145
  anesthesia and, 151
  as Canadian trade name, 749
  lactation and, 737t
  in pediatrics, 85, 95
Valpin (anisotropine methylbromide), 214t
valproic acid (Depakene), 129
  Canadian trade name for, 754
  therapeutic serum drug concentrations for, 746
Vancenase (beclomethasone), 241t
  as Canadian trade name, 748
Vanceril (beclomethasone), 241t, 517
  as Canadian trade name, 748
Vancocin (vancomycin), 413–414, 662t
  as Canadian trade name, 754
vancomycin (Vancocin), 413–414, 662t
  Canadian trade name for, 754
  therapeutic serum drug concentrations for, 746
Vantin (cefpodoxime), 390t
Vaponefrin (epinephrine), as Canadian trade name, 750
Vaporole (amyl nitrite), 575
varicella-zoster immune globulin, human (VZIG) (Varicella-zoster immune globulin), 480t
Various (testosterone propionate), 312t
Vascor (bepridil), 574t
vascular disorders, antihistamines for, 526
Vaseretic (enalapril and hydrochlorothiazide), 593t
Vasocon (naphazoline), as Canadian trade name, 752
Vasodilan (isoxsuprine hydrochloride), 629t
vasodilators
  atherosclerosis and, 629t
  in congestive heart failure, 549
  hypertension and, 590, 592t–593t, 595
  peripheral, 626–632, 629t
    adverse effects of, 631
    client teaching for, 632
    drug interactions with, 632
    individual, 629t
    nursing actions for, 630–632
    nursing process for, 627–629
    selection of, 630
    therapeutic effects of, 630–631
vasomotor tone, 50
Vasopressin (Pitressin), 232
Vasotec (enalapril), 591t
  as Canadian trade name, 750
  lactation and, 737t
Vasoxyl (methoxamine), 187t, 583
V-Cillin K (penicillin V), 382t
  as Canadian trade name, 752
vecuronium (Norcuron), 155t
  Canadian trade name for, 754
Velban (vinblastine), 687t
Velbe (vinblastine), as Canadian trade name, 754
Velosef (cephradine), 390t, 391t
  as Canadian trade name, 749

Velosulin (insulin), 283t
  as Canadian trade name, 751
venous stasis ulcers, 714
Ventodisc (albuterol), as Canadian trade name, 748
Ventolin (albuterol)
  as Canadian trade name, 748
  lactation and, 737t
  pregnancy and, 729t
ventricular arrhythmias, 562
VePesid (etoposide), 687t
  as Canadian trade name, 750
verapamil (Calan, Isoptin), 566, 568, 574t, 592t
  Canadian trade name for, 754
  lactation and, 738t
  in pediatrics, 597
  pregnancy and, 731t
Vercyte (pipobroman), 686t
Vermox (mebendazole), 453–454
  as Canadian trade name, 751
Versed (midazolam), 90, 91t, 154t
  as Canadian trade name, 752
Versel (selenium sulfide), as Canadian trade name, 753
Vesprin (triflupromazine), 670t
vials, 24
Vibramycin (doxycycline), 403t
  as Canadian trade name, 750
Vibra-Tabs (doxycycline), as Canadian trade name, 750
vidarabine (Vira-A)
  Canadian trade name for, 754
  in ocular disorders, 705t
  pregnancy and, 730t
Videx (ddI) (didanosine), 436t, 437
  as Canadian trade name, 750
vinblastine (Velban), 687t
  Canadian trade name for, 754
vincristine (Oncovin), 687t
  Canadian trade name for, 754
Vioform (iodochlorhydroxyquin), 719t
  as Canadian trade name, 751
Viokase (pancreatin or pancrelipase), 663t
  as Canadian trade name, 752
Vira-A (vidarabine)
  as Canadian trade name, 754
  in ocular disorders, 705t
  pregnancy and, 730t
viral infection. *See also* antiviral drugs
  cutaneous, 714
  general characteristics of, 434–435
Virazole (ribavirin), 436t, 437
  as Canadian trade name, 753
  pregnancy and, 730t
Viroptic (trifluridine), 436t, 437
  as Canadian trade name, 754
  in ocular disorders, 705t
viruses. *See also* antiviral drugs
  definition of, 370
  general characteristics of, 434–435
Visculose (methylcellulose), in ocular disorders, 704t
Visine (tetrahydrozoline hydrochloride), 187t
Visken (pindolol), 198, 199t, 200, 592t
  as Canadian trade name, 753
Vistaril (hydroxyzine), 92, 525–526, 529t, 670t
  anesthesia and, 151
vitamin A, disorders of, 341
Vitamin A Acid (tretinoin [retinoic acid])
  as Canadian trade name, 754
vitamin A (retinol) (Aquasol A), 334t
  Canadian trade name for, 754
  imbalance of, 337t
  preparations of, 340t
vitamin B, preparations of, 340t

vitamin B₁₂ (cyanocobalamin), 334t
  Canadian trade name for, 754
  imbalance of, 338t
vitamin B₃ (niacin), 335t
  imbalance of, 338t
vitamin B₅ (pantothenic acid), 335t
  imbalance of, 338t
vitamin B₆ (pyridoxine), 335t
  Canadian trade name for, 754
  imbalance of, 338t
vitamin B₂ (riboflavin), 335t
  imbalance of, 339t
vitamin B₁ (thiamine), 336t
  Canadian trade name for, 754
  imbalance of, 339t
vitamin C, disorders of, 342
vitamin C (ascorbic acid), 336t
  Canadian trade name for, 754
  imbalance of, 339t
  preparations of, 340t
vitamin D (calciferol), 266, 268t, 334t
  Canadian trade name for, 754
  imbalance of, 337t
vitamin D (Calciferol), calcium metabolism
    and, 266
vitamin D-calcium combinations, 270
vitamin E (Aquasol E), 334t
  Canadian trade name for, 754
  imbalance of, 337t
  preparations of, 340t
vitamin K, disorders of, 341–342
vitamin K (phytonadione), 334t, 617
  Canadian trade name for, 754
  imbalance of, 337t
  preparations of, 340t
vitamins, 333–344, 334t–337t. *See also*
    *B-complex vitamins; names of specific*
    *vitamins*
  administration of, 343
  adverse reactions to, 344
  client teaching with, 341, 344
  description of, 333
  disorders of, 341–342
  drug interactions with, 344
  fat-soluble, 334t, 341–342, 343, 344
    client teaching with, 341
    imbalances of, 337t, 341
    preparations of, 340t
  in geriatrics, 342
  imbalances of, 337t–339t
  nonprescription, 333, 336
  nursing actions for, 343–344
  nursing process for, 336, 339–341
  as nutrients, 334t–336t
  in pediatrics, 342
  preparations of, 340t
  prescription, 333
  principles of therapy with, 341–342
  therapeutic effects of, 343–344
  water-soluble, 334t–336t, 343
    imbalances of, 338t–339t, 341
    preparations of, 340t
Vivactil (protriptyline), 117t
Vivol (diazepam), as Canadian trade name,
    749
Vivonex, 324
Vivotif Berna (typhoid vaccine), 477t
voice, testosterone effect on, 310
volatile solvents, abuse of, 165–166
Volmax (albuterol), as Canadian trade
    name, 748
Voltaren (diclofenac), 71
  as Canadian trade name, 750
  indications for, 68, 68t

vomiting. *See also* antiemetics
  antineoplastic drugs and, 690
  causes of, 668
  in pregnancy, 732
Vontrol (diphenidol), 670t, 699
vulva, fungal infection of, 713
Vumon (teniposide), 687t
  as Canadian trade name, 753
VZIG. *See* varicella-zoster immune globulin,
    human

**W**

warfarin (Coumadin, Panwarfin), 615, 616
  antidote for, 617
  Canadian trade name for, 754
  dosage for, 619–620
  lactation and, 737t
  pregnancy and, 730t
Warfilone (warfarin), as Canadian trade
    name, 754
water
  description of, 320t
  imbalances of, 322t
water-soluble vitamins, 334t–336t
  client teaching with, 341
  imbalances of, 338t–339t
  preparations of, 340t
weight, body, drug dosage and, 38–39
Wellbutrin (bupropion), 115, 117t
Wernicke-Korsakoff syndrome, 51
whipworm infections (trichuriasis), 450. *See
    also* antiparasitics
whole-cell pertussis and *Haemophilus in-
    fluenzae* type B and tetanus toxoid
    and diphtheria (DTwP-HibTITER)
    (Tetramune), 477t
WinGel, 643t
Winpred (prednisone), as Canadian trade
    name, 753
Win Rho (rho immune globulin, human),
    as Canadian trade name, 753
Winstrol (stanazolol), 312t
withdrawal
  from alcohol, 164
  from alcohol and drug abuse
    treatment of, 174
  from anticonvulsant drugs
    status epilepticus in, 126
  from barbiturates, 164
    treatment of, 174
  from benzodiazepines, 94, 164, 174
  from opiates, 165
  from sedative-hypnotics, in geriatrics, 85
Wycillin (penicillin G procaine), 382t
  as Canadian trade name, 752
Wytensin (guanabenz), 591t
  lactation and, 738t
  pregnancy and, 730t

**X**

Xanax (alprazolam), 91t
  as Canadian trade name, 748
xanthines
  caffeine as, 177, 178
  as central nervous system stimulants,
    176, 178, 518t
  lactation and, 738t
  in pregnancy, 731t
Xylocaine (lidocaine), 156t, 563–564, 568
  as Canadian trade name, 751
  lactation and, 737t
  pregnancy and, 729t

Xylocard (lidocaine), as Canadian trade
    name, 751
xylometazoline, Canadian trade name for,
    754
xylometazoline hydrochloride (Otrivin),
    187t, 535t

**Y**

yellow fever vaccine (YF-Vax), 477t
YF-Vax (yellow fever vaccine), 477t
Yodoxin (diiodohydroxyquin, iodoquinol),
    451
Yutopar (ritodrine)
  as Canadian trade name, 753
  pregnancy and, 735t

**Z**

Zalcitabine, Canadian trade name for, 754
Zalcitabine (dideoxycytidine), 436t, 437
Zanosar (streptozocin), 686t
  as Canadian trade name, 753
Zantac (ranitidine), 641, 646
  as Canadian trade name, 753
  lactation and, 738t
Zarontin (ethosuximide), 128
  as Canadian trade name, 750
Zaroxolyn (metolazone), 602t
  as Canadian trade name, 752
Zebeta (bisoprolol), 198, 199t, 200
Zefazone (cefmetazole), 391t
Zestril (lisinopril), 591t
  as Canadian trade name, 751
  lactation and, 737t
Zetar (coal tar), 720t
  as Canadian trade name, 749
zidovudine (Retrovir), 436t, 437
  Canadian trade name for, 754
  pregnancy and, 730t
Zinacef (cefuroxime), 392t
  as Canadian trade name, 749
zinc, description of, 352t
Zincofax (zinc oxide), as Canadian trade
    name, 754
Zincon (zinc pyrithione), 717t
zinc oxide (Calamine Lotion U.S.P., Zinc
    Oxide Ointment), 717t
  Canadian trade name for, 754
Zinc Oxide Ointment (zinc oxide), 717t
zinc pyrithione (Zincon), 717t
zinc sulfate, 356
  Canadian trade name for, 754
zinc suspension, Canadian trade name for,
    751
zinc undecylenate (Desenex), 444t
Zithromax (azithromycin), 407, 408
Zocor (simvastatin), 628t, 630
  as Canadian trade name, 753
Zofran (ondansetron), 671, 671t
  as Canadian trade name, 752
Zoladex (goserelin), 688t
  as Canadian trade name, 751
Zoloft (sertraline), 117t
  as Canadian trade name, 753
zolpidem (Ambien), 82t, 83
Zosyn (piperacillin-tazobactam), 383,
    383t
Zovirax (acyclovir), 435, 436t, 719t
  as Canadian trade name, 748
  pregnancy and, 730t
Zyloprim (allopurinol), 71
  as Canadian trade name, 748

# LIPPINCOTT...the only study partner you'll need!